Essentials of General Surgery

Third Edition

Medical Student Editors
Rod McKinlay, M.D.
Ric Rasmussen, M.D.
Jennifer Tittensor, M.D.

Illustrated by Lydia Kibiuk and Holly R. Fischer

About the Cover

"Portrait of Professor Gross," also called "The Gross Clinic," was painted by Thomas Eakins in 1875. Eakins had attended lectures at Jefferson Medical College during Samuel David Gross' tenure as Chairman of Surgery. Eakins' students and friends posed as spectators of the operation, and a self-portrait of Eakins himself sketching the procedure (removal of a piece of bone diseased by osteomyelitis) can be found at the center of the painting. The law at that time required the presence of a relative for surgery on a charity patient *(note woman at lower left)*, a situation permitted by doctors who even then wished to avoid malpractice suits. This nearly life-size painting has hung at Jefferson Medical College since 1879.

(Courtesy of Jefferson Medical College, Thomas Jefferson University, Philadelphia, Pennsylvania)

Essentials of General Surgery

Third Edition

Senior Editor
Peter F. Lawrence, M.D.

Professor of Surgery
Vice President of UCI Healthsystem
Associate Dean
University of California, Irvine
Irvine, California

Editors

Richard M. Bell, M.D.

Professor and Chairman
Department of Surgery
University of South Carolina School of Medicine
Columbia, South Carolina

Merril T. Dayton, M.D.

Professor of Surgery
Chief, Gastrointestinal Surgery
Department of Surgery
The University of Utah School of Medicine
Salt Lake City, Utah

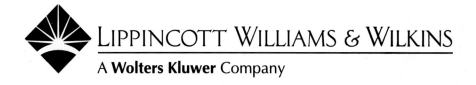

LIPPINCOTT WILLIAMS & WILKINS
A **Wolters Kluwer** Company

BS

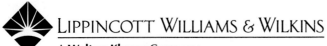

LIPPINCOTT WILLIAMS & WILKINS

A **Wolters Kluwer** Company

Philadelphia • Baltimore • New York • London
Buenos Aires • Hong Kong • Sydney • Tokyo

Acquisitions Editor: Elizabeth A. Nieginski

Editorial Director of Development: Julie P. Scardiglia

Development Editors: Catherine C. Council and Karla M. Schroeder

Senior Managing Editor: Amy G. Dinkel

Marketing Manager: Jennifer Conrad

3rd edition

9 8 7 6 5 4 3 2

Library of Congres Cataloging-in-Publication Data

Essentials of general surgery / series editor, Peter F. Lawrence ;
  editors, Richard M. Bell, Merril T. Dayton. — 3rd ed.
     p.   cm.
  Includes bibliographical references and index.
  ISBN 0–683–30133–0 (pbk.)
  1. Surgery. I. Lawrence, Peter F. II. Bell, Richard M.
III. Dayton, Merril T.
  [DNLM: 1. Surgical Procedures, Operative. WO 500 E782 1999]
RD31.E737 1999
617—dc21
DNLM/DLC
for Library of Congress   99–37812
                                    CIP

10/29/03

Preface

The primary responsibility of medical schools is to educate medical students to become competent clinicians. Because most physicians practice medicine in a nonacademic setting, clinical training is paramount. The third year of medical school, which focuses on basic clinical training, is the foundation for most physicians' clinical training. These realities do not diminish the other critical functions of medical school, including basic science education for M.D. and Ph.D. candidates, basic and clinical research, and the education of residents and practicing physicians. However, the central role of providing clinical education for medical students cannot be overemphasized.

The education of students, residents, and practicing surgeons is often seen as a continuum, although it may be fragmented at times. Because of the length of time needed to completely train surgeons, surgical residents remain "students" for three to nine years beyond medical school. As a result of this extensive training period, most medical schools have large numbers of surgical residents, and resident training makes up the bulk of their educational efforts. Student education is part of the continuum of surgical education that starts in the first or second year of medical school, continues through residency, and never ends, because continuing education is essential for surgeons. Although the goal of continuity in surgical education is admirable for students who plan a career in surgery, attempts to meet this goal led to a loss of focus on the primary role of the surgical education of students who do not plan a surgical career.

To address concerns that medical students, especially those entering a nonsurgical field, were becoming less and less the focus of most clinical departments in medical schools, several medical education organizations, including the Association of American Medical Colleges, collaborated to produce the General Professional Education of Physicians report. This report on the general education of medical students found that students were often being educated in each clinical discipline as though they planned a career in that field. The report concluded that all students need a general education, and that educators in the clinical disciplines, including surgery, must assume responsibility for medical students who are not planning a surgical career as well as for those who are.

This series of textbooks and educational materials was produced with the goal of developing an educational program in surgery for medical students who are not necessarily planning a surgical career. The planning process began by asking the question, "What do all medical students need to know about surgery to be effective clinicians in their chosen field?" Rather than using traditional textbook writing techniques to address this question, members of the Association for Surgical Education (ASE), an organization of surgeons dedicated to undergraduate education, conducted extensive research. The ASE asked residents and practicing physicians in every medical field, faculty educators, and surgery department chairs to help define the content and skills needed for an optimal medical education program in surgery. Somewhat surprisingly, there was consensus among these disparate groups (including practicing surgeons, internists, and even psychiatrists) about the knowledge and skills needed by all physicians. The information from this research became the basis for this textbook. The research process also identified some technical skills, such as suturing skin, that should be mastered by all physicians and are best learned by such methods as viewing a videotape or working in a suturing laboratory. Additionally, the ASE and several other educational organizations developed methods other than a textbook approach, such as videotapes and clinical simulations, for teaching and practicing some of these skills. Alternative teaching methods were devised as part of this educational package. Finally, in recognition of the need to allow students and faculty to measure students' progress, this text contains multiple-choice questions, oral examination questions, and clinical skills training and testing. The answers and explanations that are provided allow students to review incorrect answers and study further any areas of the text that are incompletely understood.

A separate set of multiple-choice and oral examination questions is available to faculty and educators. These questions were written by the same authors who wrote the chapters and practice questions. The additional questions can help students gauge their progress and predict the likelihood of success on the final examinations. Students can prepare for the final examinations by reading the textbook and taking the practice examinations. These questions are a good predictor of performance. This approach is different from that of many other multiple-choice examinations that are not based on a defined curriculum and may include questions on unfamiliar material. It is virtually impossible to prepare for this type of examination.

A companion textbook on the surgical specialties, *Essentials of Surgical Specialties,* is based on a similar approach to the specialty and subspecialty fields of surgery. This text is separate from *Essentials of General Surgery* because some medical schools teach the specialties in the third year and others teach them in the fourth year. Students who complete both the general surgery and specialty programs and answer the practice oral and multiple-choice questions will acquire the essential surgical knowledge and problem-solving skills that all physicians need.

You are entering the most exciting and dynamic phase of your academic life. This educational package is designed to help you achieve your goal of becoming an adept clinician. Best wishes for success in your endeavor.

Acknowledgments

This project was nurtured by many members of the Association for Surgical Education (ASE), whose advice and expertise I would like to acknowledge. At its annual meetings, the ASE provided an excellent forum to discuss and test ideas about the content of the surgical curriculum and methods to teach and evaluate what has been learned.

My thanks go as well to Cathy Council, my editor in Salt Lake City, who has spent two years editing, revising, and coordinating all components of this project. I also thank my two teams of editors at Lippincott Williams & Wilkins: Crystal Taylor, Nancy Evans, and Jane Velker, followed by Amy Dinkel, Julie Scardiglia, and Elizabeth Nieginski. Overseeing them all was Tim Satterfield, who has been guiding these textbooks for more than ten years.

Finally, I owe thanks to three medical students—Rod McKinlay, Ric Rasmussen, and Jennifer Tittensor—for their detailed reviews of the text and questions. Their high level of commitment to the project and their perspective produced suggestions that clarified much of the information found in this book.

Contributors

Kimberly D. Anderson, Ph.D.
Assistant Professor
Department of Surgery
Michigan State University
East Lansing, Michigan

Dorothy A. Andriole, M.D.
Assistant Professor of Surgery
Washington University School of Medicine
St. Louis, Missouri

Peter Angelos, M.D., Ph.D.
Assistant Professor of Surgery
Assistant Professor of Medical Ethics and Humanities
Northwestern University
Chicago, Illinois

David Antonenko, M.D., Ph.D.
Professor of Surgery
University of North Dakota
Grand Forks, North Dakota

Todd R. Arcomano, M.D.
Assistant Professor of Surgery
University of Nevada School of Medicine
Reno, Nevada

Richard M. Bell, M.D.
Professor of Surgery
University of South Carolina School of Medicine
Columbia, South Carolina

Kirby I. Bland, M.D.
J. Murray Beardsley Professor and Chairman
Department of Surgery
Brown University School of Medicine
Providence, Rhode Island

Richard A. Bomberger, M.D.
Associate Professor of Surgery
University of Nevada School of Medicine
Reno, Nevada

Anthony P. Borzotta, M.D.
Medical Director, Trauma ICU
Legacy Emanuel Hospital
Clinical Assistant Professor of Surgery
Oregon Health Sciences University
Portland, Oregon

Kenneth W. Burchard
Associate Professor of Surgery
Dartmouth-Hitchcock Medical Center
Lebanon, New Hampshire

William C. Chapman, M.D.
Associate Professor of Surgery
Vanderbilt University Medical School
Nashville, Tennessee

Kevin C. Chung, M.D., M.S.
Assistant Professor of Surgery
Plastic and Reconstructive Surgery
University of Michigan
Ann Arbor, Michigan

Nicholas P. W. Coe, M.D.
Professor of Surgery
Tufts University
Baystate Medical Center
Springfield, Massachusetts

Debra A. DaRosa, Ph.D.
Professor of Surgery
Northwestern University Medical School
Chicago, Illinois

Rudy G. Danzinger, M.D.
Professor of Surgery
University of Manitoba
Winnipeg, Manitoba, Canada

Merril T. Dayton, M.D.
Professor of Surgery
Chief of Gastrointestinal Surgery
University of Utah School of Medicine
Salt Lake City, Utah

Gary L. Dunnington, M.D.
Professor of Surgery
Southern Illinois University
School of Medicine
Springfield, Illinois

Pablo R. Duran, M.D.
Surgical Oncology Fellow
University of Pittsburgh
Pittsburgh, Pennsylvania

Virginia A. Eddy, M.D.
Associate Professor of Surgery
Vanderbilt University School of Medicine
Nashville, Tennessee

Donald E. Fry, M.D.
Professor and Chairman of Surgery
Department of Surgery
University of New Mexico
Albuquerque, New Mexico

Richard N. Garrison, M.D.
Professor of Surgery
University of Louisville School of Medicine
Louisville, Kentucky

Stephen M. Gemmett, M.D.
Vascular Surgical Fellow
Department of Surgery
University of Arkansas for Medical Sciences
Little Rock, Arkansas

Bruce L. Gewertz, M.D.
Professor of Surgery and Phemister Chair
The University of Chicago School of Medicine
Chicago, Illinois

Mitchell H. Goldman, M.D.
Professor and Chief
Division of Vascular/Transplant Surgery
Department of Surgery
University of Tennessee Medical Center at Knoxville
Knoxville, Tennessee

Alan Graham, M.D.
Associate Professor of Surgery
Chief of Vascular Surgery
Robert Wood Johnson School of Medicine
New Brunswick, New Jersey

Charles D. Hanf, M.D.
Assistant Professor of Surgery
Albert Einstein College of Medicine
Bronx, New York

James C. Hebert, M.D.
Professor of Surgery
University of Vermont
Burlington, Vermont

Anthony L. Imbembo, M.D.
Professor of Surgery
Department of Surgery
University of Maryland

Chris Jamieson, M.B., B.S.
Professor of Surgery
Dalhousie University
Halifax, Nova Scotia

Daniel J. Jurusz, M.D.
Assistant Professor of Surgery
Louisiana State University School of Medicine
New Orleans, Louisiana

Susan Kaiser, M.D., Ph.D.
Associate Professor of Surgery
The Mount Sinai Medical Center
Mount Sinai School of Medicine
New York, New York

Nicholas P. Lang, M.D.
Professor of Surgery
University of Arkansas for Medical Sciences
Little Rock, Arkansas

Steven B. Leapman, M.D.
Professor of Surgery
Indiana University Medical Center
Indianapolis, Indiana

Glenn H. Lytle, M.D.
Professor of Surgery
University of Oklahoma College of Medicine–Tulsa
Tulsa, Oklahoma

Bruce V. MacFadyen, Jr., M.D.
Professor of Surgery
The University of Texas–Houston Medical School
Houston, Texas

Mary C. Mancini, M.D.
Associate Professor of Surgery
Louisiana State University Medical Center, Shreveport
Shreveport, Louisiana

Anne T. Mancino, M.D.
Assistant Professor of Surgery
University of Mississippi Medical Center
Jackson, Mississippi

Alan B. Marr, M.D.
Medical Director Surgical ICU
Director of Nutritional Support Services
Overton Brooks VA Medical Center
Assistant Professor of Surgery
Louisiana State University Medical Center
New Orleans, Louisiana

James A. McCoy, M.D.
Assistant Professor of Surgery/Psychiatry
Morehouse School of Medicine
Atlanta, Georgia

D. Byron McGregor, M.D.
Professor of Surgery
University of Nevada School of Medicine
Reno, Nevada

James F. McKinsey, M.D.
Assistant Professor of Surgery
The University of Chicago School of Medicine
Chicago, Illinois

Michael K. McLeod, M.D.
Associate Professor of Surgery
Michigan State University
College of Human Medicine
Kalamazoo, Michigan

David W. Mercer, M.D.
Associate Professor of Surgery
The University of Texas–Houston Medical School
Houston, Texas

Hollis W. Merrick, III, M.D.
Professor of Surgery
Director, Surgery Clerkship Program
Medical College of Ohio
Toledo, Ohio

Leigh Neumayer, M.D., M.S.
Associate Professor of Surgery
University of Utah School of Medicine
Salt Lake City, Utah

Jeffrey A. Norton, M.D.
Professor of Surgery
University of California, San Francisco
San Francisco Veterans Affairs
   Medical Center
San Francisco, California

J. Patrick O'Leary, M.D
The Isidore Cohn, Jr., Professor and Chairman of Surgery
Louisiana State University School of Medicine
New Orleans, Louisiana

L. Beaty Pemberton, M.D.
Professor and Chairman
Department of Surgery
University of Missouri–Kansas City School of Medicine
Kansas City, Missouri

Walter E. Pofahl, M.D.
Assistant Professor of Surgery
University of South Alabama
Mobile, Alabama

Hiram C. Polk, Jr., M.D.
Ben A. Reid, Sr., Professor and Chairman of Surgery
University of Louisville School of Medicine
Louisville, Kentucky

John R. Potts, III, M.D.
Professor of Surgery
The University of Texas–Houston Medical School
Houston, Texas

Martin C. Robson, M.D.
Chief of Dept. of Veterans Affairs Medical Center
Bay Pines, Florida

Ajit K. Sachdeva
Professor of Surgery
Vice Chairman for Educational Affairs,
Department of Surgery
MCP Hahnemann School of Medicine
Philadelphia, Pennsylvania

Jeffrey R. Saffle, M.D.
Professor of Surgery
Director, Intermountain Burn Center
The University of Utah School of Medicine
Salt Lake City, Utah

Kennith H. Sartorelli, M.D.
Assistant Professor of Surgery
University of Vermont
Burlington, Vermont

Kenneth W. Sharp, M.D.
Associate Professor of Surgery
Vanderbilt University Medical Center
Nashville, Tennessee

Harvey H. Sigman, M.D., M.Sc.
Professor of Surgery
McGill University
Montreal, Quebec, Canada

David J. Smith, Jr., M.D.
Professor of Surgery
Plastic and Reconstructive Surgery
University of Michigan
Ann Arbor, Michigan

Mary R. Smith, M.D.
Professor of Clinical Medicine and Pathology
Associate Dean for Undergraduate and Graduate
   Medical Education
Medical College of Ohio
Toledo, Ohio

Glen Steeb, M.D.
Assistant Professor of Surgery
Louisiana State University School of Medicine
New Orleans, Louisiana

Judith L. Trudel, M.D.
Assistant Professor of Surgery
McGill University
Montreal, Quebec

Delford G. Williams, III, M.D.
Associate Professor of Surgery
Chief of General Surgery
Chief of Vascular Surgery
Charles R. Drew University of Medicine and Science
Los Angeles, California

Table of Contents

1

How to Survive and Excel in a Surgery Clerkship

Debra A. DaRosa, Ph.D.
Kimberly D. Anderson, Ph.D.
Gary L. Dunnington, M.D.

Typically, third-year medical students either thoroughly enjoy or profoundly dislike their surgery clerkship. Different factors contribute to this perception, but several problems and concerns arise consistently. This chapter provides suggestions for dealing with six common problem areas: (1) unclear expectations; (2) overwhelming reading requirements; (3) lack of feedback; (4) stress; (5) preparing for examinations; and (6) not knowing what is required to become an honors student. Reading this chapter before, or at the start of, your clerkship will maximize your enjoyment and minimize your difficulties.

Problem One: What Exactly Is My Role? What Are the Expectations?

Principles for Meeting Clerkship Expectations

- Be first and foremost a student rather than an "extra house officer." Read first to prepare for formal teaching sessions (e.g., teaching rounds, lectures, conferences), second for patient care, and third for test preparation.
- Strive to know more about your patients and their diseases than anyone else on the service does.
- Prepare before you go into the operating room. Review the anatomy and the planned procedure; prepare questions about the procedure or disease process; and consider the postoperative orders.
- Focus on critical thinking skills (e.g., Why is the patient presenting this way? What is the underlying problem? Why are we doing this procedure?) when developing patient assessments.
- Be enthusiastic, punctual, aggressive in assuming responsibility, and respectful of the medical hierarchy. Recognize that what is taught and learned in a surgery clerkship is important to the discipline that you ultimately choose.

Perhaps the most startling difference between the first 2 years of medical school and the clinical clerkship year is the loss of a defined daily structure and the consequent difficulty in determining what is expected of you as a student. During the surgical clerkship, the content to be learned is less well defined than in the basic sciences. In addition, patient care responsibilities may be poorly defined or defined differently, depending on whether you ask a house officer or a faculty member (or sometimes even different faculty members). Ideally, your surgery clerkship will have learning objectives to guide your reading and study as well as a list of clinical responsibilities. Whether these guidelines exist or are poorly defined, the following recommendations may be helpful.

Remember That Your Goal Is to Learn

During the surgical clerkship, the student is expected to be a student, not an extra house officer or an extra pair of hands to complete the work of the ward. Although these roles may often conflict, if you maintain your perspective as a learner, acquiring a sound knowledge base should always take precedence over learning intern survival skills. Keep in mind that ward work (e.g., changing dressings, obtaining arterial blood gases) is not scut work when it is associated with your patients.

Your reading should focus on three areas:

- Managing the clinical problems that you encounter
- Preparing for teaching rounds, student presentations, didactic sessions, or any planned teaching sessions that your institution holds
- Preparing for the final examination

If your institution uses a National Board subtest, you can expect approximately 60% of the test to cover general surgery (including vascular surgery and trauma) and 40% to cover surgical specialties.

Know Your Ward Responsibilities

During the day, the setting for your patient care activities may be the ward, the operating room, the clinic or office, or the ambulatory setting (outpatient operating room). Give yourself plenty of time to evaluate the patients assigned to you before morning rounds, including a chart review (i.e., nursing notes from the previous night, bedside chart, and a focused history and examination). You should be sensitive to patient needs in planning these early morning preround activities. Your morning presentation should include data from the previous 24 hours. In contrast, afternoon presentations traditionally cover only the previous 8 hours.

For typical ward patients who are recovering from surgery, your presentation format should be flexible enough to meet the demands of the service. However, you should generally include subjective and objective data as well as your assessment (supported by the data and examination findings) and a plan for care. Request feedback when your assessments are considered inappropriate or when the treatment plans selected are different from the ones that you proposed.

For patients who have complicated cases and are being treated in the intensive care unit, and for patients with multiple ongoing problems, your presentation is best delivered with an organ system approach. In this approach, subjective and objective data, assessments, and plans are presented for each area for which there are ongoing problems (e.g., neurologic, cardiovascular, pulmonary, gastrointestinal, genitourinary, infection, nutrition). In the beginning, if surgery is your first rotation, practice a presentation with an intern or a classmate.

Because most of the team must be in the operating room at an early hour, remember to keep your presentations succinct. You will receive the most praise for this quality in your presentation skills. To allow time for a thorough assessment and care plan after discussion with the ward team, plan to write your daily progress notes before or after morning rounds. These notes should be finished before you or your team goes to the operating room. Your evening presentations should focus on significant events of the day and should provide the results of diagnostic studies that were performed. Your credibility will increase if you have discussed the studies with the appropriate persons (e.g., radiology faculty member or resident for radiographic studies). Be careful to ensure that your data are accurate. For example, if you do not remember the exact numbers, it is better to say so than to estimate.

In addition to work rounds on the wards, you will probably participate in attending rounds or teaching rounds. When you are asked to present a patient, be sure to know every detail of the patient's history, initial presentation, and hospital course to date. Rehearse your presentation so that you can deliver it in a polished, succinct manner, with only minimal references to notes. Although you can use notes to refresh your memory, do not read your presentation. Most attending physicians and chief residents emphasize **presentation skills** in their overall student evaluations.

Know Your Operating Room Responsibilities

The key to deriving the most benefit from your operating room experience is **advance preparation.** In addition to familiarizing yourself with all aspects of your patient's presentation and hospital course to date, review an anatomy textbook to prepare for the operative dissection. Also, review the planned procedure in Chapter 26 of this textbook so that you have a preliminary understanding of the technical approach. You may need to check the surgical schedule 1 to 2 days in advance to allow time to prepare adequately. Ask questions at appropriate times in the operating room if they are not answered by your observation. Some common operating room questions (e.g., pertaining to anatomy or pathology) can be answered in this textbook or a text such as Abernathy and Harken's *Surgical Secrets.* During the operation, do not restrain your impulse to be a helpful assistant. As the patient's assigned student, you should be one of the first to arrive in the operating room. After surgery, accompany your patient to the recovery room. Think about the postoperative orders you will write in the recovery room (e.g., type of dressing change, type of drain).

Know Your Clinic or Office Responsibilities

Most clerkships provide students with the opportunity to participate in outpatient offices. This participation is becoming a vital aspect of surgical education. Many of the surgical problems you will face are managed in the ambulatory setting, especially if you ultimately practice primary care. If clinic participation is optional, make every effort to participate, focusing on the problems that you will not see on the inpatient service (e.g., breast lumps and mammographic abnormalities, benign perianal disease, intermittent claudication, venous insufficiency).

Know Your Call Schedule Responsibilities

The call schedule is typically prepared by the first day of the rotation. It is important to be flexible and to do your share; however, it is also important to ensure that you can meet your personal and family obligations. If you have an important personal event on your calendar, be certain to notify whoever creates the schedule well in advance of the date. People who create call schedules are usually willing to accommodate special or significant events, but they must consider the needs of many other people. If you are scheduled to be on call when you have a conflict, do not complain to the person who created the call schedule; take care of the problem yourself. First, find out if you can switch call; if switching is permitted, trade with one of your classmates. Remember to reciprocate when classmates get into a similar bind. Complaints about the number of calls you are taking or the number of weekends you are covering are usually not well received by those who create the schedule; again, work with your peers to resolve issues, and inform those in charge of the changes. As far as possible, try to be on call with your assigned preceptor (if attending preceptors are assigned) or with a member of your resident team. Being on call with team members enhances both your team relationships and the continuity of patient care.

Know to Whom You Are Responsible

If you will work with a variety of faculty and residents while on call, find out to whom you are accountable. Talk with this faculty member or resident before call begins to identify his or her expectations. If you have a beeper, be sure that you have given out the correct beeper number. If your institution uses an overhead paging system, make certain that the operator is informed that you are on call. You must be easily accessible to the faculty member or resident; become his or her shadow. Faculty members or residents typically make an effort to call you and inform you of ongoing developments, but if you do not respond to pages or are difficult to reach, they will not search for you. Call is often exhausting, but it can also be exhilarating and can provide you with unique learning opportunities.

At no time should you be alone in the decision-making process. However, you should formulate an assessment and a plan and then discuss them with the faculty member or resident. These steps are important for practicing clinical reasoning and self-assessment of what you know and what else you need to know to make a sound plan or decision.

Plan for the Worst, but Expect the Best

When you are scheduled to be on call, plan on being on call. Period. Do not try to find time for your scheduled reading. When you create your reading schedule (see Problem Two), allot your assignments to days when you are not on call. If your night on call affords some downtime, read to get ahead in your schedule, or use the time for review. Most important, do not try to schedule family time or promise to try to attend events when you are on call. Trying to "fit" other responsibilities into a call night sets up false expectations and often results in disappointment, frustration, and resentment among those you care about most. Plan quality time with family and friends when you have control over your time.

Plan Ahead

You probably will not have the opportunity to go home between a night on call and the next working day. This limitation is not an excuse to practice your "post-call look." Keep a prepacked on-call bag that includes:

- Nutritious snacks (so you don't eat junk food on the run)
- Toiletries
- Alarm clock (to ensure that you are on time)
- Change of shoes (paper booties can only do so much)
- Change of socks or hosiery and clothing
- Required reading for the clerkship

Maintain a Positive Attitude

In addition to the expectations outlined previously, there are six general expectations of all students on surgical clerkships.

1. Be enthusiastic, regardless of the number of patients you are assigned, your degree of sleep deprivation, or your feelings about a particular clinical encounter. Although this attitude may appear artifi-

cial, an enthusiastic approach sets a frame of mind that is conducive to optimal learning.
2. Be punctual for all assigned responsibilities. A stellar performance in any clinical setting is seldom appreciated if that performance begins late.
3. Accept additional responsibilities without referring to the inequality of caseloads among fellow students or the hour of the day. This attitude shows that you understand that the surgical clerks who have the most clinical experiences learn the most.
4. Show that you understand the hierarchy that exists in all of medical education. Discuss concerns about patient care (e.g., an early "scoop" about a diagnostic study) with the surgical intern, not with a more senior resident or surgical faculty member. Although it is easy to criticize this hierarchy when you first encounter it, the concept promotes a team effort and provides clear lines of responsibility.
5. Admit when you do not know something. Although it is nearly impossible to anticipate every question that you will be asked, it is never acceptable to generalize data or "shoot from the hip." Admitting that you "don't know" is uncomfortable, but it is a vital element of professional growth. Following up "I'm sorry, I don't know" with "but I will find out" shows the attending physician or resident that you are concerned about the patient and about improving your knowledge base.
6. Finally, during your surgical rotation, immerse yourself in the experience without concentrating on your future career choice.

Problem Two: There Is Not Enough Time to Read

Principles for Managing Overload

- Develop a reading plan that includes determining what core material you must read and when and where you read best. Take advantage of time windows, which are short, unscheduled blocks of free time (e.g., waiting for an operating room case to begin, waiting for an attending physician to begin teaching rounds).
- Read actively.
- Evaluate how well you retain what you read.

The primary source of frustration for students, residents, and academic and private practice physicians is probably lack of time. For this reason, the ability to set priorities and manage time effectively and efficiently is critical. The following tips will help you to use your reading time wisely.

Develop a Reading Plan

Adhering to a reading plan requires both persistence and good time management skills. You can accomplish your reading goal by realistically determining at the start of the clerkship what you want to have read by the end of the clerkship and establishing a schedule that includes benchmarks or deadlines for maintaining a consistent pace and volume. You can identify what you must read by the end of your clerkship by reviewing old examinations (if they are available), reviewing the learning objectives for the clerkship, talking with students who completed the clerkship and did well, and speaking with the clerkship director or with faculty members. The Association for Surgical Education established learning objectives for third-year students. These objectives are used in this text. To avoid becoming frustrated, devise a plan that is realistic. Keep in mind that content that is read but not learned is a waste of time. Plan a reading schedule that allows time to process the information. When you read text, your brain should sort, select, and link new information to related areas of knowledge. Simply running your eyes across the words does not count.

Differentiating important from nice-to-know content when reading the text is a critical skill that keeps students from becoming overwhelmed. There is an enormous volume of information, and the successful student uses the cues provided by textbook authors and publishers to help readers to identify key concepts and organize information for optimal understanding and learning. Schwenker and colleagues[1] described the following cues:

1. Numeric and categorical cues: Authors often enumerate or classify major concepts and key points.
2. Print format cues: Many textbooks highlight important information with boldface or italicized type. Headings, subheadings, and bulleted summaries are used to show hierarchical relations. Summaries at the end of chapters emphasize main points.
3. Graphic cues: Tables, charts, diagrams, and different colors are typically used to display key information and show relations between information. Some students copy tables, charts, and diagrams and glue them to index cards to use for review.
4. Semantic cues: If the author took the time to provide an example to clarify a point or concept, the point is probably important. Also, certain terms are often used to define relations (e.g., superior and inferior, major and minor, most common and least common).
5. Frequency and scope cues: If a principle or concept is explained fully in the text, illustrated in a figure, and elaborated in a table, it must be important. Also, if the author provides more detail about one disease or principle than about others, the author must consider it important.
6. Word structure cues: Unfamiliar terms can be remembered more easily by analyzing their prefix, root, and suffix. For example, the word hemigastrectomy can be broken down into the prefix *hemi-*, which means half; the root *gastr-*, which refers to the stomach; and the suffix *-ectomy*, which means removal of. Therefore, hemigastrectomy is a surgical procedure in which half of the stomach is removed.

Much of your reading will center around your patients' problems. Concentrate on learning about the involved anatomy, physiology, and pathology. Then read about the clinical signs and symptoms, diagnostic options, differential diagnosis, and alternative methods of therapy. As a surgery clerk, you do not need to know the detailed operative technique and principles. However, you should go to the operating room with an understanding of the treatment or modification of the pathologic process intended by the operation, the prognosis, and the postoperative care of the patient. You should also be aware of possible complications and how to address them.

Your patient-related reading should be done as soon as possible. Rather than waiting until evening to begin reading, try to find a fairly quiet place where you can do some abbreviated reading during the day. Because using information organizes and reinforces it, you are more likely to retain what you read if you use the information shortly afterward.

Our biological clocks are not all the same. Some students have greater powers of concentration in the morning; others are more alert later in the day, or even at night. You may not always have a choice, but try to schedule your core reading for the time when you are most alert. Some students find it helpful to copy the "core reading" chapters that they are scheduled to read that day and carry them in their pockets. Students spend a significant amount of time waiting for lectures, rounds, or conferences to begin. Using these 10 or 20 minutes here and there to read is an effective use of time. Cumulatively over the clerkship period, there are significant waiting periods in the operating room lounge before surgery. If you carry a book or copied pages, you can make good use of this time by catching up on your reading.

Read Actively

While reading, active readers think about how the material might be tested. They also stop occasionally to think about what they are studying. They create outlines or draw diagrams, concept maps, charts, or tables to summarize important information and to show relations between parts and the whole. These study aids can be used as flash cards or review materials to prepare for examinations. Good readers remember what they read, not because they have photographic memories, but because they read to understand. They picture how they can apply the information to future experiences, and they tie what they are learning to what they know. Fitting new information into a logical framework aids recall.

Taking the time to summarize information after reading a section or chapter, either mentally, verbally, on audiotape, or in writing, helps readers to reflect on what they learned. An audiotape can be played back (e.g., while driving) or listened to through headphones (e.g., while exercising). Rereading written summaries is a more welcome review tool than rereading an entire text to prepare for an examination. Summarizing is also a study process that can provide a sense of satisfaction and mastery.

In summary, read deliberately, asking yourself questions as you proceed (e.g., Does this information relate to what I already know or have experienced? What are the key points? Now that I have read this chapter, do I know how to detect and treat a patient who has this problem? What details are critical for me to remember?). After you read the chapter, go back and determine whether you can meet the chapter objectives proficiently (e.g., Can you list the four signs and symptoms of a malignant nevus?). Finally, answer the study questions.

Evaluate Your Reading Retention

To evaluate how well you retained what you read, use the self-testing questions at the end of each chapter, find a good review book that contains test questions, or ask interns or residents to quiz you. Your answers to these questions can help you to determine whether you can recall important facts and concepts and use them in a clinical problem-solving situation or a multiple-choice format. Multiple-choice questions are often used in surgery clerkship examinations, licensure examinations, and certification assessments. The questions that are included in this book can help you to determine whether you can apply the information to common clinical problems. Additionally, many clerkships now use standardized case studies and oral examinations to evaluate students' grasp of material. Preparation for these examinations should emphasize understanding and synthesis of clinical problems, rather than factual recall.

It is also useful for students to quiz each other. As a student, a surgeon colleague carried 3- × 5-inch index cards to jot down acronyms, mnemonics, or important information that she acquired from reading, rounds, or wherever such "pearls" surfaced. She reviewed the cards during free minutes, day or night. Fellow students did the same, and they exchanged cards and quizzed each other. Repetition and reinforcement aid in learning key facts and concepts.

Problem Three: I Am Getting Little or No Feedback

Principles of Feedback

- Recognize the importance of feedback for learning.
- Make constructive use of positive and negative feedback.
- To get effective feedback, be assertive and ask for it.

Good feedback is descriptive (not judgmental), timely, and specific. It is a crucial aspect of learning. Identify areas in which you need feedback, and ask for it. Most faculty and residents are pleased to see that students care enough about what they are learning to ask

for feedback, and they are happy to oblige. Student performance evaluation forms can be an excellent source of feedback. If feedback is not a formal part of your clerkship experience, "midterm" in the clerkship is an ideal time to ask for it. Schedule a time to speak with your supervising faculty member, resident, or clerkship coordinator in a one-on-one setting. Stopping this person in the hall is unlikely to lead to thoughtful commentary about your performance. Explain why you scheduled the meeting and what you hope to accomplish. Provide a self-evaluation of your performance, including specific areas (i.e., skills, knowledge, interpersonal qualities) in which you think you have met or exceeded expectations; areas of skill, knowledge, or behavior that you are working to improve; and your plan for improvement. Ask for specific feedback about your performance and your plan for improvement.

Many medical students report that they receive little or no feedback. Typically, students assume that they are doing fine unless they hear otherwise. This assumption can be misleading. Some students who receive poor ratings do not recognize that they are performing poorly. This type of surprise can be avoided by asking for feedback.

Feedback is a critical part of education because it reinforces what is known and points out errors of omission or commission before they become habitual. To be helpful, feedback must be specific. A comment that something was "poorly done" may let you know that you made a mistake, but it does not tell you exactly what was wrong. If you receive this type of comment, speak up and ask, "Could you please be more specific so that I have a clearer understanding of where I need to improve?" Asking for details should provide you with the detailed feedback that you need. It also shows interest and indicates that you want to learn from your mistakes.

Faculty and residents are busy and have differing personalities, so you should be practical in recognizing how much feedback to expect and how frequently you can expect to receive it. Obviously, you cannot expect to receive explicit feedback on everything you say or do, so ask for feedback only in those areas in which you lack confidence or need reinforcement. If you sense that it is not a good time to ask for feedback (e.g., the resident or faculty member seems preoccupied), request an appointment for this purpose. Fortunately, most residents and faculty members are more than willing to offer feedback to the mature student who seeks it. If they are not, view their reluctance as a reflection on them, not on you.

Several skills that are learned and practiced in a surgery clerkship should be evaluated and commented on by a faculty member, associated health professional, or designated resident. If you do not receive feedback routinely, be sure to request it in the following areas:

- History and physical examination write-ups (e.g., Did I state the history correctly?)
- Physical examinations skills (e.g., Am I locating the spleen correctly?)
- Progress notes and preoperative and postoperative orders (e.g., Were there major omissions?)

- Presentation skills (e.g., Did I present any unnecessary data?)
- Technical skills (e.g., Are my stitches too far apart?)
- Base of knowledge (e.g., What else do I need to know about this patient's problem?)

You may need more feedback in the early part of the clerkship and less as you hone your skills. Recognize your own learning needs, and assert yourself tactfully to get specific feedback when and where you need it.

It is important to self-assess your knowledge, but it is also useful to ask your resident or faculty member, at opportune times, about his or her impressions of your knowledge base (e.g., Do you seem to have a good grasp of the basic sciences related to your patients? Do you understand the pathophysiology of your patients' problem? Can you anticipate possible complications? Do you have a clear understanding of patient management?).

Students and residents commonly make two types of errors[2]:

1. Technical or judgmental errors. These errors are accepted as part of the learning process. If you make a judgmental error, you can expect critical feedback that is intended to be instructive.
2. Normative errors. These errors are not tolerated because they involve a lack of diligence or honesty, failure to reveal mistakes fully, failure to note important findings, inability to function as a team player, or failure to secure cooperation from patients or their families. If you make a normative error, you can expect the worst, and it is not likely to be forgotten.

Some attending physicians and residents have a tendency to come down hard on a learner, regardless of the type of error. Their comments may be demeaning, cutting, and overly severe. Fortunately, these individuals are in the minority. If you experience such comments, you need to adopt a response strategy that is compatible with your own style.

Guidelines for Handling Feedback

- Respond, but do not react. Think before you say anything. An emotional reaction may only make a bad situation worse. Respond in an adult fashion, even if the person who is criticizing you is behaving childishly.
- Repeat aloud what is said to ensure that you understand the key points. Choose your words carefully to avoid sounding defensive.
- If you made a mistake, admit it without making excuses. Apologize, commit to improving, and move on. In these cases, the mistake becomes a lesson. Negative feedback is instructional, and adult learners listen carefully and respond to it. Avoid being defensive or argumentative.

- If the criticism is unwarranted, let the speaker finish before you present your perspective. Do not cut him or her off, but wait until he or she is finished.
- Do not take criticism personally. That is easier said than done, but unless you committed a normative error, most mistakes are forgiven and forgotten. If you do commit a normative error, learn from it, correct your behavior, and move on.
- Control your tone of voice and body language when you receive negative feedback. Remember, your tone of voice sets the tone for the conversation.
- Judge the situation. Sometimes it is better just to listen without saying anything. Ask yourself if responding will be productive. If the answer is "no," just let the speaker vent, and bear it.

Problem Four: I Have No Life, and I Am Stressed to the Max!

Stress Management Principles

- Eat sensibly.
- Take time for your family and friends.
- Commit time to exercise.
- Take time to take care of yourself.
- Find a confidant.

You can do well in a surgery clerkship without compromising every other aspect of your life. In fact, you will perform better if you do not give up everything else. This section will help you to manage your priorities so that you can accomplish tasks faster and with a more positive attitude.

Balancing your work-related responsibilities with your personal needs and those of others takes conscious effort. It is not always easy, and it does not occur overnight. Each day, you should take care of yourself by doing something to meet your physical, social, and emotional needs.[3] You cannot always control how much time you spend at the hospital. The concept is the same, however, regardless of your profession or status. Sources on stress management emphasize several common principles:[4]

Eat Sensibly

- Eat before you go into the operating room in the morning. You cannot be certain how long you will be in there, and some students feel faint when they do not eat something beforehand.
- In case you miss a meal, keep in your pocket or locker healthy snack foods, such as dried fruit, cereal, popcorn (no butter), or other nonperishables with nutritional value.
- Limit caffeine and sugar. (The number of aluminum cans disposed of by medical students over a few days could probably be recycled to

yield enough money for one person's tuition for a semester.)

Take Time for Your Family and Friends

- Talk openly with the people in your life who will be affected by your being busy in a clerkship. Discuss your needs and their needs, and come to an agreement. Some flexibility will be needed on both sides.
- Do your best to plan your studying around the agreed-on plan.
- When you take time for others, give them your full attention. Try to leave your troubles and pressures at the hospital.
- Do not expect others always to play second fiddle to your student-related responsibilities. Yes, you need their support, but they have needs too, and if these needs are consistently ignored, resentment will build and problems will occur.

Use your creativity to devise ways to keep in touch. Some highly scheduled people have themselves videotaped while reading their children's favorite bedtime stories so that the children can watch the tape when Mom or Dad is unavailable. Another idea is to leave a taped message or a note on the kitchen table each morning.

Commit Time to Exercise

A study of medical students showed a significant relation between stress and attitudes toward leisure. Those who did not feel guilty when taking time to exercise reported fewer symptoms of stress and anxiety and an overall more positive attitude toward school.[5] However, exercise should be scheduled during free time; it is inappropriate to take time off during the day unless the rest of the team is exercising as well.

Take Time to Take Care of Yourself

In this fast-paced world, many people find it difficult to stay in touch with themselves. For this reason, it is important to take time at church or another place of worship, in transit to or from work, or before turning out the lights at night to reflect on your life, assess your strengths and weaknesses, and put your activities in perspective. A cup of hot tea, some classical music, and a comfortable chair or warm bath can help you to relax, block out life's complexities, and think about your personal goals. Try to take at least 10 minutes each day to daydream. Envision yourself backpacking in the mountains, golfing under blue skies, or relaxing on the beach—whatever you enjoy. Find a place where you can be alone and comfortable for those few minutes. This technique, called visualization, is advocated by stress management experts as a powerful method of refreshing both mind and attitude.

Some people have a tendency to compare themselves with an ideal image (e.g., the ideal medical student, who knows all and requires no sleep). These compar-

isons ultimately hurt us because there is no ideal, or perfect, student, parent, spouse, or anything else. High achievers set goals, only to set grander ones after the first goals are accomplished. This pattern can cause pressure and stress, and although it is good to have high expectations, it is important to keep this tendency in check. Inner peace is essential to happiness, and it is important to take a step back from time to time to look beyond the many activities that can easily usurp your sense of self.

Find a Confidant

Choose someone to be your sounding board, and be prepared to reciprocate. Air your complaints to a trusted confidant who will maintain your confidences, will not give advice unless asked, and will empathize with you.

Problem Five: How Can I Do Well on the Examination?

Principles for Examination Preparation and Administration

- Study in an environment that is free of distractions.
- Do not procrastinate or deviate from your study schedule.
- Use multiple methods to retain the material (e.g., answer study questions, take practice examinations, teach your peers the material).
- Relate your reading to patients you have encountered.
- Ask yourself, "Why is this important?"

Assisting in the operating room or emergency department or doing procedures is often more interesting (and fun) than reading. Regardless of your specialty preference, the activity of a surgery clerkship can be invigorating, even if it means being up all night. Although being an active member of the surgical team clearly enhances your clinical performance evaluation and your enjoyment of the clerkship, it does not necessarily prepare you for the rigors of the final written examination. Your success in the clerkship will depend in part on your ability to manage the time you spend on clinical activities, to adhere to a steady reading schedule, and to relate your reading material to patients you have encountered.

Whether you take the National Board of Medical Examiners (NBME) shelf examination or an internally generated departmental examination, and whether the test items assess the ability to apply knowledge framed within the context of patient vignettes or written objectives of the clerkship or lectures, you will be held accountable for a basic fund of knowledge that reflects the fundamental principles of surgery. The guidelines for managing reading overload (see Problem Two) will keep you on track throughout your clerkship.

Students who have problems with the final examination typically fall into two categories: (1) those who did not keep up with their reading and (2) those who kept up with their reading superficially, but did not process the information. Students who say, "I didn't keep up with my reading because I was too busy on the service," pose significant problems for surgical educators. Faculty and residents praise their work ethic, interest, and enthusiasm. They reward them by letting them take a more active role in the operating room or clinic. They may tell them that they are among the best students they have ever had and that they have a good working fund of knowledge. What they do not tell them is that they jeopardize their grade in the clerkship because they cannot state what percentage of patients is likely to get a certain disease, what medical and surgical alternatives exist, what percentage of these people will get well because of the treatment, and what percentage will die. You will be held accountable for this type of information on the final written examination, and these are the types of questions in every surgeon's examination-writing armamentarium. Faculty and residents appropriately recognize students who demonstrate a strong work ethic and show personal and professional maturity with patients and the team. However, you must pass the written examination to complete the clerkship, and that means keeping up with reading and reviewing.

If you kept up with the reading, but did not process the information, you must be willing to assess your study practices. First, what was the environment in which you studied? Were you distracted by the television or by activities in the background? Did you study in a setting in which there were significant interruptions? Did you attempt to study while doing another activity? Second, what was your mental and physical status? Did you fall asleep in the middle of each chapter? Did you try to study when your mind was preoccupied with personal problems? Were you physically ill? Third, how well did you read? Did you read actively or passively? Did you take notes on your reading? Did you selectively highlight important points, or did you jaundice the pages by highlighting every word, not discriminating among critical, important, and nice-to-know information? Did you follow a reading schedule? Did you "cram" by trying to cover too much material at one sitting?

If you are completely honest with yourself, a red flag will no doubt rise in response to at least one of these questions. Preparation is the key to performing well on an examination. The following tips may help you.

Pace Yourself

Count how many items are on the test, and calculate how long you have to answer each one. Leave sufficient time to review your answers. Use your watch to keep yourself properly paced. Most examinations allow 1 minute per item. Easier items will take less time, yielding more time for long or difficult questions. Do not spend too much time on one item, however, or you will not have enough time to complete the examination. Needless mistakes are made as a result of poor pacing when students rush through the final items. Even if the test does not have time limits, students often grow fatigued and make mistakes at the end of the examination. To avoid these mistakes, check your pacing quarterly during the examination.

Analyze the Questions in Whole and in Part

Preview the questions, and immediately answer those that you are confident that you know. Then go back to the beginning and complete those that you did not automatically know during the first run-through. Answer the questions that are mostly guesses last. Some students find it helpful to cover the distractors (they are designed to do just that—distract) and mentally answer the question, then uncover the distractors and select the corresponding option. Some students use shorthand in the margins, such as the example below:

L = You are satisfied with your answer and consider the item low priority for reconsideration.
S = You are not entirely confident with your answer, but consider the item second priority for reconsideration.
H = You are completely unsure of the answer and consider the item high priority for reconsideration.

After you complete the examination, check your answers. Make sure that you did not skip any questions or double-mark any items. If you answered questions out of order, verify that you recorded the answers in the correct spaces.

When you read a question, circle the most important words as well as any words that alter the meaning substantially or offer cues for finding the answer (e.g., except, most common, least common, must).

Thorough preparation for an examination is the best way to reduce panic and anxiety; however, pacing, analyzing, and checking can help reduce unnecessary errors.

Problem Six: What Does It Take to Be an Honors Student?

Principles for Achieving Honors

- The honors student clearly understands the criteria that are used to determine honors level performance.
- The honors student uses frequent self-assessment to test his or her fund of knowledge.
- On the ward, the honors student: (1) demonstrates intellectual curiosity; (2) understands the role of a team player; (3) exhibits polished presentation skills; (4) provides the team with information from recent literature; (5) shadows the house officer on call at night; and (6) looks for opportunities to work one-on-one with faculty.

It is safe to assume that every student who is beginning a surgical clerkship is capable of receiving honors as a final grade.

Identify the Criteria for Honors

Understand the emphasis that the clerkship places on test performance versus ward performance. This understanding will help you to allocate your time between reading and involvement in ward activities. Typically, examinations carry significant weight when separating many would-be honors students from honors students. It is important to understand the nature of the final examination and the weight placed on general surgery with respect to the other specialties.

Self-Assess Frequently

If the final examination is a multiple-choice test, your chances for success will be improved by frequently self-testing your knowledge with such resources as *Surgical Secrets* by Abernathy and Harken; the *National Medical Series for Independent Study* (NMS) by Jarrel and Carabasi; *Principles of Surgery: Pretest, Self-Assessment and Review* by Schwartz; and the questions at the end of each chapter in this textbook.[6-8]

Display the Characteristics of Honors Students

The assessment of student ward performance is subjective. However, attending physicians look for certain characteristics in an honors student. These characteristics are described by comparing them with characteristics that are found in the average, or passing, student on the clerkship.

- The passing student reads about his or her patient's problems and is prepared to answer questions during rounds. The honors student demonstrates intellectual curiosity by asking pertinent, probing questions (e.g., after rounds, during breaks) about the etiology, pathophysiology, and natural history of the disease process. These questions can come only from an effort to read for comprehension (i.e., active reading) rather than for memorization.
- The passing student follows through on assigned tasks and enthusiastically provides assistance in the care of his or her assigned patients. The honors student understands the importance of being a team player. In addition to providing excellent care for his or her own patients, the honors student is willing to help with any patient as long as there is an opportunity to learn. This attitude involves avoiding actions that make others (especially other students) look bad. Think in terms of the good of the team and that of every member. Help others, but do not be fawning or obsequious.
- The average, or passing, student makes certain that all pertinent data are presented on rounds

and makes logical and thoughtful assessments based on the data. The honors student does this as well, but also presents the material in a fluent, dynamic, and succinct manner that paints a visual picture for the rest of the team. You can polish your presentation skills by rehearsing, either aloud or mentally, on the way to the hospital, in front of a mirror, or elsewhere. An honors level of presentation results from a great deal of practice and a focus on presentation skills during those early morning hours.

- The average student reads enough from basic texts to achieve a knowledge base that is sufficient to perform patient assessment and daily care. On the other hand, the honors student probes more deeply by using information-seeking skills. For example, each member of a busy surgical team appreciates being provided with a copy of a timely, recent article from the literature, summarizing new diagnostic approaches or management schemes. To provide this information, you must be familiar with the use of MEDLINE and other databases. Most schools have helpful librarians and classes on the use of the library.
- Nights on call provide another setting for the emergence of the honors student. The passing student responds to all requests for assistance from on-call house officers and enthusiastically assists in the emergency room and with new admissions. The honors student shadows the house officer during every waking hour, both to provide assistance and to learn techniques of intern survival on the ward and in the intensive care unit.
- The honors student recognizes the importance of the operating room in the overall scheme of clerkship learning. Textbooks and consultation services will be available throughout a nonsurgeon's practicing career, but there will never be a better opportunity to see surgery "on the inside." The honors student goes to the operating room on cases that are not assigned to him or her when there are opportunities to learn about rare or unfamiliar conditions. When a student shows interest in this type of learning, most faculty members take the time to point out interesting intraoperative findings to make the trip to the operating room worthwhile.
- Finally, the honors student looks for opportunities to work with faculty one-on-one. This experience makes it easier for faculty to provide useful end-rotation evaluation. The clinic may be the best such setting because in many centers, residents are not extensively involved in clinic practice. If these opportunities are available, an honors student arranges his or her daily schedule to allow for participation. In addition to these characteristics, the honors student consistently demonstrates the five qualities addressed under Problem One.

REFERENCES

1. Schwenker JA, Krogull SR, Rudolph JS, Simpson DE. *Mastering Medical Content.* Milwaukee, Wis: Medical College of Wisconsin, 1989.
2. Bosk C. *Forgive and Remember.* Chicago, Ill: University of Chicago Press, 1979.
3. Johnson S. One Minute for Myself. New York, NY: Avon Books, 1987.
4. Calano J, Salzman J. Managing stress and building visibility. In: *Success Shortcuts.* Chicago, Ill: Nightingale-Conant, 1989.
5. Folse L, DaRosa DA, Folse JR. The relationship between stress and attitudes toward leisure among first-year medical students. *J Med Ed* 1985;60:610–617.
6. Abernathy CM, Harken AH. *Surgical Secrets.* Boulder, Colo: University of Colorado Press, 1991.
7. Jarrell BE, Carabasi RA. *The National Medical Series for Independent Study,* 2nd ed. Baltimore, Md: Williams & Wilkins, 1991.
8. Schwartz SI. *Principles of Surgery: Pretest, Self-Assessment and Review,* 5th ed. New York, NY: McGraw-Hill, 1989.

2

Preoperative Medical Evaluation of Surgical Patients

Richard M. Bell, M.D.
Virginia A. Eddy, M.D.

OBJECTIVES

1. Describe the value of the preoperative history, physical examination, and selected diagnostic and screening tests.
2. Describe the important aspects of communication skills.
3. Discuss the elements of a patient's history that are essential in the preoperative evaluation of surgical emergencies.
4. Describe (and perform) the medical history of a patient who is undergoing an elective procedure.
5. Discuss the assessment of pulmonary and cardiac risk.
6. Describe the assessment of coagulation status.
7. Discuss the effect of diabetes, hepatic dysfunction, adrenal insufficiency, and malnutrition on preoperative preparation and postoperative management.
8. Perform a comprehensive physical examination.
9. Discuss the appropriate preoperative screening tests.
10. Document a concise history and physical examination as well as daily progress notes on a surgical patient.

The ability to obtain an adequate history and perform a thorough physical examination is a critical skill for physicians. The importance of this skill lies in the diagnosis of surgical disease, the detection of comorbid factors, the determination of the severity of comorbidity, and an assessment of operative risk. The decision to proceed with an operative procedure is based on an analysis of the risk:benefit ratio. This analysis must begin with an accurate and complete database. Many surgical patients have coexisting medical problems or undiagnosed medical conditions that may affect risk assessment. Surgery and anesthesia profoundly alter the normal physiologic and metabolic states, and estimating the

patient's ability to respond to these stresses in the postoperative period is the challenge of the preoperative evaluation. Perioperative complications are often the result of failure, in the preoperative period, to identify underlying medical conditions, maximize the patient's preoperative health, or accurately assess perioperative risk. Sophisticated laboratory studies and specialized testing are no substitute for a thoughtful and careful history and physical examination. Sophisticated technology has merit primarily in confirming clinical suspicion.

This chapter is not a review of how to perform a history and physical examination. Instead, this discussion is a review of the elements in the patient's history or findings on physical examination that may suggest the need to modify care in the perioperative period. Other chapters discuss the signs and symptoms of specific surgical diagnoses.

Improving Communication

The physician–patient relationship is an essential part of quality care as it relates to patient satisfaction. Good interviewing techniques can help to establish a good physician–patient relationship. One aspect of good interviewing is a genuine concern about people. Another aspect of good interviewing relies on learned skills.

Effective interviewing can be challenging to the surgeon because of the variety of settings in which interviews occur. These settings include the operating room, the surgical intensive care unit, a private office, a hospital bedside, the emergency room, and an outpatient clinic. Each setting has its own requirements to achieve quality communication. To achieve good physician–patient relationships, surgeons adjust their styles to the environment and to each patient's personality and needs. Some basic rules are common to all professional interviews. These include giving adequate attention to personal appearance to present a professional image that inspires confidence; establishing eye contact; communicating interest, warmth, and understanding; listening nonjudgmentally; accepting the patient as a person; listening to the patient's description of his or her problem; and helping the patient feel comfortable in communicating.

11

When the patient is seen in an ambulatory setting, the surgeon spends the first few minutes greeting the patient (using the patient's formal name); shaking hands with the patient; introducing himself or herself and explaining the surgeon's role; attending to patient privacy; adjusting his or her conversational style and level of vocabulary to meet the patient's needs; eliciting the patient's attitude about coming to the clinic; finding out the patient's occupation; and determining what the patient knows about the nature of his or her problem.

The next step involves exploring the problem. To focus the interview, the surgeon moves from open-ended to closed-ended questions. Important techniques include using transitions; asking specific, clear questions; and restating the problem for verification. At this point, it is important to determine whether the patient has any questions. Near the end of the interview, the surgeon explains what the next step will be and when he or she will examine the patient. Last, the surgeon should verify that the patient is comfortable.

Most of the techniques used in the ambulatory setting are also appropriate for inpatient encounters. Usually, more time is spent with the patient in the initial and subsequent interviews than in an outpatient setting. At the initial interview, patients are likely to be in pain, worried about financial problems, and concerned about lack of privacy or unpleasant diets. They may also have difficulty sleeping, be fearful about treatment, or feel helpless. It is important to communicate the purpose of the interview and state how long it will take.

The patient is not only listening, but also is observing the physician's behavior and even attire. The setting also affects the interview. For example, a cramped, noisy, crowded environment can affect the quality of communication. Patients may have negative feelings because of insensitivities on the part of the physician or others. Examples include speaking to the patient from the doorway, giving or taking personal information in a crowded room, speaking about a patient in an elevator or another public space, or speaking to a patient without drawing the curtain in a ward.

Although the same interviewing principles apply in the emergency room as in the outpatient and inpatient settings, the emergency room encounter is tremendously condensed. The role of the student in the emergency room is to discover the patient's chief medical complaint, perform a physical examination, and present the findings to the resident or faculty member. Interviewing a patient in the emergency room requires communicating to the patient who you are and how you fit into the team. The following steps will help you to conduct an effective patient interview:

1. Ask the patient or a family member to describe the problem briefly.
2. Focus on the primary medical problem.
3. Move from general to specific questions.
4. Provide a narrative for the patient.
5. Attend to the patient's privacy.
6. Be careful about expressing nonverbal attitudes about the patient or his or her behavior.

7. When the examination is finished, explain what will happen next and approximately how long the patient will have to wait.
8. After you interview and examine the patient, discuss the patient with the resident or faculty member in a location where the patient and family cannot hear or see you.
9. Finally, guard against any nonprofessional discussion or behavior in the emergency room.

Communication with patients is greatly influenced by both verbal and nonverbal behavior. Attention to these techniques can enhance the surgical student's communication skills and will have a profound influence on the quality of surgical care, particularly as it is perceived by patients.

History

A careful history leads to a differential diagnosis in nearly three-fourths of patients. This observation underscores the advantage of having a working knowledge of the natural history of surgical diseases. The careful physician probes the patient's history to identify preexisting conditions that may indicate the need to modify perioperative management. The next section discusses the systems whose physiology is directly affected by anesthesia and surgery. From this database, the initial steps are taken to determine operative risk.

Surgical Emergencies

Surgical emergencies do not permit leisurely interrogation of the patient to determine the nuances of his or her medical history. However, the urgency of the situation does not preclude obtaining essential information. An emergency situation forces the physician to focus on the critical aspects of the patient's history. An AMPLE history (Allergies, Medications, Past medical history, Last meal, Events preceding the emergency; Table 2-1) provides the important elements that may immediately influence surgical care.

Determining allergies and drug sensitivities is important. The injudicious use of antibiotics or narcotics without an attempt to determine drug sensitivity is ill-advised. Many surgical emergencies, both traumatic and nontraumatic, occur in patients who have preexisting medical conditions. Many of these conditions (e.g., coronary artery disease, chronic obstructive pulmonary disease, diabetes) decrease the patient's physiologic

Table 2-1. AMPLE Medical History

A—Allergies

M—Medications

P—Past medical history

L—Last meal

E—Events preceding the emergency

reserve and are adversely affected by surgery. Most patients with significant medical problems are being treated with medications that may have important implications in perioperative patient management. Some drugs adversely interact with anesthetic agents or alter the normal physiologic response to illness, injury, or the stress of surgery. For example, patients who take beta-blocking agents cannot mount the usual chronotropic response to infection or blood loss. Sudden discontinuation of sympathomimetic medications (e.g., clonidine) may produce a profound catecholamine rebound and reduce coronary perfusion by abruptly increasing myocardial wall tension.

Hyperglycemia is a normal response to the stress of illness or injury. This response may exacerbate diabetes and increase insulin requirements. Patients with prosthetic heart valves, other implanted prosthetic devices, or a history of rheumatic fever should be protected with perioperative antibiotics. Those with chronic congestive heart failure (CHF) or renal insufficiency require meticulous attention to fluid and electrolyte balance.

Information about the timing of the patient's last meal is also important. A full stomach predisposes the patient to aspiration of gastric contents during the induction of anesthesia and increases the risk of postoperative pulmonary complications. A history of recent ingestion of food or drink may force significant modifications in the anesthetic technique used, require steps to decompress the stomach, or in some cases, require postponement of the surgical intervention until gastric emptying occurs.

A history of the events that preceded the accident or onset of illness may give important clues about the etiology of the problem or may help to uncover occult injury or disease. For example, the onset of severe substernal chest pain before the driver of a vehicle struck a bridge abutment may suggest that the hypotension that the driver exhibited in the emergency department may be related to acute cardiac decompensation from a myocardial infarction as well as from blood loss associated with a pelvic fracture. Such a situation might require modification of hemodynamic monitoring and volume restoration. Although such scenarios sound extreme, they are encountered in emergency departments on a daily basis. These historical elements add significantly to the physician's ability to provide optimal patient care.

Elective Surgical Procedures

Most clinical situations provide an adequate opportunity for a careful review of systems. Occasionally, patients cannot provide details of their illness, and the serious investigator must use every available resource, including family, friends, previous medical records, and emergency medical personnel. A specific review of systems, with special emphasis on estimating the patient's ability to respond to the stress of surgery, is imperative. Clinical suspicions are investigated with appropriate laboratory tests or special diagnostic studies. Specialty consultation may be required to determine the degree of

medical illness. Consultants can provide important information about the risk:benefit ratio of a specific surgical procedure or suggest therapies to minimize perioperative risk. Medical consultants cannot "clear" patients for a surgical procedure; their primary value is in helping to define the degree of perioperative risk. Once this risk is determined, the surgical team, in conjunction with the patient or the patient's family, may discuss the advisability of a planned surgical approach to the patient's illness. Postoperative consultation should generally be sought when the patient has unexpected complications or does not respond to initial maneuvers that are commonly employed to address a specific problem. For example, a nephrology consultation is in order for a patient who remains oliguric despite appropriate intravascular volume repletion, particularly if the creatinine level is rising. Likewise, consultation should be obtained from specialists who have expertise in areas that the treating physician does not. For example, a general surgeon would be well advised to obtain consultation from a cardiologist for a patient who had a postoperative myocardial infarction, no matter how benign the myocardial infarction appears.

Pulmonary Evaluation

Postoperative pulmonary complications are the most common cause of postoperative morbidity. For this reason, it is important to understand the factors that place a patient at risk for these problems. Unfortunately, there is no single predictor of increased risk. A careful history and physical examination will indicate which patients are most at risk; specialized testing is reserved for patients who have significant risk factors or who are expected to undergo an operation that carries a relatively high intrinsic risk of pulmonary complications.

Risk Factors

Surgical Factors

The first issue is the type of operation that the patient is to undergo. Obviously, a pneumonectomy carries a higher risk of pulmonary complications than does a hemorrhoidectomy. Elective lung resections carry specific risks, and are considered later in this section. Even among nonpulmonary operations, the risk of pulmonary complications can be stratified by the type of operation. Abdominal operations that require an upper midline incision or involve dissection in the upper abdomen are associated with a much higher pulmonary complication rate than those that are restricted to the lower abdomen. Abdominal incisions are painful and are associated with diminished functional residual capacity. These problems contribute to the higher pulmonary complication rate. Any thoracotomy incision also predisposes the patient to pulmonary complications. Interestingly, the median sternotomy incision is associated with a low incidence of pulmonary complications, probably because it is associated with minimal discomfort during quiet breathing. Longer operations cause greater derangements in pulmonary function than do shorter ones.

Anesthesia Factors

Anesthesia predisposes the patient to pulmonary complications. Simply undergoing general anesthesia produces an 11% reduction in functional residual capacity (FRC). Patients do not cough under anesthesia, and postoperative sedation depresses respiratory drive and inhibits coughing. The lasting effects of neuromuscular blockade can also weaken the coughing effort. Mucociliary clearance is also depressed by anesthetic agents. Anticholinergic drugs commonly thicken the patient's mucus and make it more difficult to mobilize. Tracheal intubation promotes direct colonization of the upper airway by gram-negative organisms and sets the stage for infection.

A significant portion of hospital-acquired infections are caused by iatrogenic induction of nosocomial organisms into the tracheobronchial tree by suction catheters that are passed without attention to aseptic technique.

Gas exchange is directly affected by general anesthesia. Arterial saturation and a decline in PaO_2 occur because of changes in position and ventilation–perfusion (V/Q) mismatching. Even patients who have normal pulmonary function preoperatively may have a decrease in PaO_2 of as much as 33%. High levels of inspired oxygen also compound arterial hypoxemia because of the phenomenon of absorption atelectasis (which occurs when alveoli are filled with gas mixtures that contain high concentrations of oxygen and low concentrations of nitrogen). As oxygen is absorbed into the pulmonary capillaries, less gas is left in the alveoli to maintain FRC. As a result, atelectasis occurs.

It is tempting to assume that regional anesthesia would obviate these problems. In fact, this assumption may be true for procedures on extremities or procedures that can be done with a very specific regional blockade (e.g., axillary block). However, spinal anesthesia is also associated with postoperative pulmonary problems. As a rule, the important factor is not the type of anesthetic agent employed, but the circumstances to which the patient is exposed (e.g., abdominal procedures, loss of periodic hyperinflation by sighing). Positioning, pain, and sedation are not alleviated by spinal anesthesia alone.

Changes in ventilatory patterns also occur after general anesthesia. Within 24 hours, tidal volume is decreased by 20%, but the respiratory rate is increased by 25%. For the patient with normal pulmonary function, the net effect is essentially no change in minute ventilation. These alterations generally return to normal within 1 to 2 weeks. Significant changes in pulmonary compliance also occur; it may be reduced by as much as 33%. The average adult sighs 9 or 10 times per hour. This effort normally hyperinflates the alveoli and prevents atelectasis. Observations in animals and humans indicate that FRC decreases by 10% when hyperinflation by deep breathing is discontinued.

Table 2-2. Risk of Postoperative Pulmonary Complications Associated with Specific Operative Procedures

Procedure	Risk %
Elective thoracic/abdominal surgery	17.5
Elective cholecystectomy	14.8
Coronary artery bypass graft	18.7
Abdominal aortic aneurysm surgery (emergent)	60.0
Laparotomy	23.2
Abdominal aortic surgery (elective)	16.0

The definition of pulmonary complications varies widely in the literature and may account for some of the difference.

Overall, the risk of pulmonary complications varies from approximately 10% to 70% (Table 2-2). Improvements in anesthetic technique and attention to improving pulmonary function preoperatively and postoperatively have reduced the incidence of respiratory problems, but as much as one-third of all postoperative mortality may still be related, directly or indirectly, to pulmonary insufficiency.

Patient Factors

In general, patients who have an obstruction to expiration flow for any reason are in greatest jeopardy. They may need specialized pulmonary function studies preoperatively and vigorous preoperative and postoperative pulmonary care for prophylaxis. The section on nonpulmonary operations in the discussion of evaluating a patient describes specific tests. Table 2-3 lists the categories of conditions that predispose patients to both infectious and noninfectious perioperative deterioration of respiratory function.

There is controversy about whether age itself is a risk factor for pulmonary complications. With increasing age, there is a progressive decline in static lung volume, maximum expiratory flow, and elastic recoil as well as a decrease in PaO_2 because of an increase in the alveolar–arterial oxygen gradient. The net effect is a loss of pulmonary reserve. The confounding factor is that many older persons also have independent risk factors for pulmonary complications. Age itself is not a contraindication to surgical intervention, but the normal changes that occur with the aging process should be kept in mind. However, pulmonary disease is a risk factor. In smokers, the relative risk of pulmonary complications is two to six times greater than that in nonsmokers. Smokers have abnormalities in mucociliary clearance, increased volume of secretions, increased carboxyhemoglobin levels, and a predisposition to atelectasis. Smokers should be asked to stop smoking at least 6 weeks before the procedure; however, compliance with this request is rare.

Chronic obstructive pulmonary disease increases perioperative risk for several reasons. Increased pulmonary secretions, small airway obstruction secondary to mucous plugging, inefficient clearing of secretions,

Table 2-3. General Factors that Predispose Patients to Pulmonary Complications

Cigarette smoking	Chronic bronchitis
Asthma	Occupational lung disease
Neuromuscular disease	Coma
Obesity	Tracheal intubation
Nutritional depletion	Hypotension
Acidosis	Hypoxemia
Chronic obstructive pulmonary disease	Azotemia
	Age > 60 years
Prolonged operative time	Thoracic/abdominal procedure
Hypoalbuminemia	
Extended stay in the hospital (preoperative)	

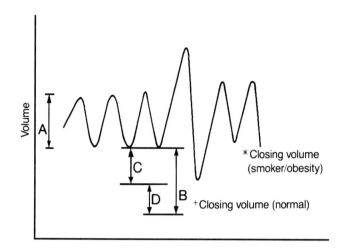

Figure 2-1 Spirometry. **A,** Tidal volume. **B,** Functional residual capacity. **C,** Expiratory reserve volume. **D,** Residual volume. *, Closing volume for smoker/obese patient. †, Closing volume for normal patient.

and a general lack of pulmonary reserve predispose the patient to atelectasis and superimposed infection. Patients with asthma are also at higher risk. Perioperative stress and many medications, including anesthetic agents, can provoke bronchospasm. Compliance with prescribed antiasthma medications and good pulmonary toilet are important in the preoperative phase.

Patients who have a history of occupational exposure to known irritants (e.g., silicone, asbestos, textile components) may have significant restrictive disease and a noticeable reduction in respiratory reserve. Also at high risk are patients who cannot cough or breathe deeply for any reason, such as those with an altered level of consciousness, neuromuscular disease, paraplegia, or weakness as a result of malnutrition.

Obesity contributes directly to the impairment of respiratory function. In simple obesity, FRC and expiratory reserve volume are decreased. As weight increases to 50% above ideal weight, a decrease in other parameters is noted as well. The work of breathing increases dramatically, producing an increase in oxygen consumption and carbon dioxide production. The effect of adipose tissue on the chest wall and the restriction of diaphragmatic excursion by the weight of abdominal contents when the obese patient is supine contribute to the reduction in tidal volume. This reduction results in atelectasis and hypoxemia and contributes to infection. Long-standing obesity may lead to pulmonary hypertension because of the increase in pulmonary blood volume and, later, because of hypoxic vasoconstriction. Eventually, the clinical picture is complicated by hypoxemia (because of a change in V/Q relations secondary to atelectasis and regional redistribution of blood flow and gas) and, ultimately, by hypercapnia (because of hypoventilation).

Evaluating Patients

Nonpulmonary Operations

The pulmonary evaluation of the patient begins with an assessment of his or her functional status. Important historical factors were mentioned earlier, but it is crucial that a careful pulmonary history be obtained. One important question is whether the patient has a history of occupational exposure to known pulmonary irritants. Questions about activities in daily life should also be asked. For example, can the patient shovel snow (or rake the yard)? Is he or she out of breath after walking up a flight of stairs? The patient should be asked about his or her smoking history, sputum production, wheezing, and exertional dyspnea. Physical examination should begin with a general assessment of the patient's habitus. Are there signs of wasting or morbid obesity? Does the patient exhibit pursed lip breathing? Does he or she have clubbing or cyanosis? What is the patient's respiratory pattern? Is there a prolonged expiratory phase, as in obstructive airways disease? What is the anteroposterior dimension of the chest? On auscultation, does the patient wheeze? A patient who cannot climb one flight of steps without dyspnea or blow out a match at 8 inches from the mouth without pursing the lips is a candidate for more sophisticated pulmonary function screening. Another useful bedside test is the loose cough test. A rattle heard through the stethoscope when the patient forcibly coughs is a reliable indicator of underlying pulmonary pathology and warrants investigation, beginning with a chest x-ray, with further studies ordered as appropriate to the patient's history, physical examination findings, and radiography results.

Before the specific elements of pulmonary function tests are discussed, it is useful to review the physiologic definitions of standard lung volumes and capacities. Figure 2-1 shows a standard spirometry curve. Normal tidal ventilation is shown by **A.** At the end of passive tidal exhalation, the patient is said to be at FRC (shown by **B** in Figure 2-1). FRC is equal to the sum of expiratory reserve volume (the amount of air that can be expelled with a forced expiratory maneuver) and residual volume (the volume of air left in the lung after a forced expiration). This volume cannot be exhaled under normal circumstances. There is another volume that is worth considering: closing volume. Closing volume (CV) is the volume below which the alveoli become so structurally unstable that they cannot remain open, even with the benefit of surfactant. In Figure 2-1, normal CV is shown as being slightly lower than residual volume. In a smoker, however, CV requires a much higher volume of air. Consequently, patients with lung pathology tend to have spontaneous atelectasis at much higher volumes than they would otherwise. CV is actually greater than FRC in smokers and obese patients, whereas it is much lower than FRC in normal patients. Because FRC is the volume left in the lung after a passive tidal expiration, it is important to understand that certain lung diseases predispose the patient to atelectasis because CV is actually greater than FRC.

There is no evaluation strategy that precisely defines the pulmonary risk of a given patient. Although it is possible to indicate which patients are likely to fare extremely well or extremely poorly, the middle groups are difficult to stratify. At a minimum, a patient with a preoperative FEV_1 (the amount of air that can be exhaled in 1 second during a forced expiration after the patient inhales to total lung capacity) of less than 1, a PaO_2 of less than 50 mm Hg, or a $PaCO_2$ of greater than 45 mm Hg should have the risks of operation explained in clear terms. These risks include not only death and pneumonia, but also the possibility of long-term ventilator dependence. Because of this possibility, some patients decide against proceeding with the operation.

Any patient who has significant abnormalities in respiratory function on routine history or physical examination may benefit from formal pulmonary function studies. In some patients, such information leads to a decision to postpone or modify the course of therapy. Pulmonary function studies that can potentially uncover or quantitate a condition that can be improved in the preoperative period (thereby lessening the risk of postoperative problems) are cost-effective and justifiable. Pulmonary function tests (PFTs) are often used in combination with arterial blood gas analysis to study the patient who is thought to be at high risk.

The most commonly used PFT is the FEV_1. During the forced vital capacity maneuver (part of obtaining the FEV_1), the patient is evaluated for intrinsic lung disease and also for problems with the ventilatory pump that moves air into and out of the lungs. The American College of Physicians outlined recommendations for preoperative specialized PFTs (Table 2-4).

Pulmonary Operations

Pulmonary resections present the special problem of removal of lung tissue in a patient who is already at risk for postoperative pulmonary complications. These patients are likely to have a significant smoking history. Patients who have a greater than 8–pack-year history are at particular risk for chronic bronchitis. In general, the goal is to leave the patient with an FEV_1 of at least 800 mg postoperatively. If the predicted postoperative FEV_1 is less than 800 mL, the chances are significant that the patient will never wean from the ventilator postoperatively. The predicted postoperative FEV_1 is estimated by a variety of methods, ranging from simple to complex. One of the easiest ways to estimate quickly whether the postoperative FEV_1 will be low is to multiply the preoperative FEV_1 by the percentage of lung tissue that will be left after resection. For example, consider a patient with an FEV_1 of 1.8 L who is scheduled to undergo a right upper lobectomy. The percentage of pulmonary tissue to be removed is one of five total lobes (20% of the total lung tissue). This patient's predicted postoperative FEV_1 is 1.8 L – 80% lung remaining postoperatively = 1.4 L.

In the very high-risk patient who is to undergo pulmonary resection and whose predicted postoperative FEV_1 is less than 1 L, split perfusion radionuclide lung scanning is helpful in predicting the amount of functioning lung that will remain postoperatively. If, after careful study, the patient's predicted postoperative FEV_1 is less than 800 mL, that patient is considered inoperable.

Exercise testing is also useful in the evaluation of these patients and does not require a sophisticated pulmonary laboratory. The stair climb is a simple and reproducible method of assessing pulmonary function. The interested medical student can walk with the patient up stairs. A patient who can climb five flights of stairs can tolerate a pneumonectomy, and one who can climb three flights can usually tolerate a lobectomy.

Table 2-4. American College of Physicians Recommendations for Preoperative Pulmonary Function Testing

Type of Surgery	Spirometry	Blood Gas	Split Function Tests	Exercise Test
Pulmonary resection	All patients	All patients	Some patients	Some patients
Coronary artery bypass surgery	Smokers, history of dyspnea	Smokers, history of dyspnea	No	No
Upper abdominal	Smokers, history of dyspnea	Smokers, history of dyspnea	No	No
Lower abdominal	Suspected lung disease	No	No	No
Head and neck	No	No	No	No
Orthopedic	No	No	No	No

Cardiac Evaluation

Two primary alterations in physiology occur in the postoperative period and impose significant stress on the myocardium. The first is a catecholamine surge that may occur in response to the pain and anxiety associated with the operative procedure or the disease process itself. The result is an increase in the myocardial oxygen requirement secondary to an increase in heart rate and contractility. Concomitantly, myocardial blood flow is reduced by: (1) the vasoconstrictive effect of the α_1-receptor stimulation and (2) the reduced time for blood flow through the myocardium as a result of a reduction in diastolic time (i.e., increased heart rate). The second alteration is suppression of the fibrinolytic system. This suppression predisposes the patient to thrombosis. Myocardial ischemia can result in cardiac segments where blood flow is reduced further by occlusive disease.

In the patient with previous infarction, the risk of postoperative myocardial ischemia is between 5% and 10% overall, with an attendant mortality rate of 50%. This figure contrasts with a risk of less than 0.5% in patients with no history of infarct or clinically evident heart disease. If an elective operative procedure is performed immediately after a recent myocardial infarction, the risk of an additional acute cardiac event or death is approximately 30% within the first 3 months. The risk declines with time, and reaches a plateau of approximately 5% at 6 months. If possible, elective surgery should be postponed for 6 months after a myocardial infarction.

The patient who has unstable angina should avoid surgery, unless it is for coronary artery bypass grafting. Although the patient with stable angina is theoretically at increased risk, no clear answer about the extent of increased postoperative risk is available for this group. In contrast, patients who have undergone coronary artery bypass have a significantly reduced danger of postoperative infarct compared with those who have angina. The risk is estimated at slightly more than 1%, with a similar mortality rate. In a limited study, percutaneous angioplasty conferred myocardial protection in the postoperative period, but studies confirming the value of this procedure are not available. Patients with any cardiac history must be evaluated carefully, and the severity of their disease must be documented. If possible, maximum myocardial performance should be achieved before any operative procedure is undertaken.

The patient who is scheduled to undergo elective surgery should be questioned carefully about the nature, severity, and location of chest pain. Dates and details about infarctions, documented or suspected, should be noted. Additional historical elements of significance include a history of dyspnea on exertion (which may signify underlying cardiac or pulmonary pathology). Other clues to the possibility of coexisting heart disease include syncope, palpitations, and arrhythmia. Patients with a history of rheumatic heart disease require prophylactic antibiotic therapy to prevent endocarditis, even for minor procedures.

A history of diabetes increases the index of suspicion for occult cardiac pathology. Of patients with a documented history of diabetes for 5 to 10 years, 60% have diffuse vascular pathology. After 20 years, nearly all patients with diabetes have some type of vascular abnormality. In addition, the risk of mortality after a cardiac ischemic event for the patient with diabetes is higher than that for people without diabetes. Silent infarctions, or ischemic events without symptoms, have also been reported in the diabetic population. Careful questioning, however, often discloses that these episodes involve some atypical symptoms (e.g., vague pain, breathlessness, syncope, onset of mild congestive heart failure). Therefore, patients with diabetes, especially those with a long-standing history of the disease, should be viewed with suspicion and presumed to have some degree of cardiovascular abnormality.

Special note is taken of the patient's overall status during the physical examination. Vital signs can give important clues about the status of the cardiovascular system (i.e., tachycardia, tachypnea, postural changes in blood pressure). Jugular venous distension at 30°, slow carotid pulse upstroke, bruits, edema, and a laterally displaced point of maximum cardiac impulse all suggest some type of cardiac disease. Auscultatory findings that suggest cardiac problems include rubs, third heart sounds, and systolic murmurs.

Determining which murmurs are clinically significant and which are innocent is perplexing for most medical students. Most innocent murmurs are apical. Innocent murmurs are never associated with a palpable thrill, and there are no innocent diastolic murmurs. Maneuvers that change blood flow (i.e., Valsalva) generally do not change the character or pitch of innocent murmurs. A patient who has hemodynamically significant aortic stenosis usually has a characteristically harsh holosystolic murmur, a slow carotid pulse upstroke, and a displaced primary myocardial impulse that is secondary to left ventricular hypertrophy. This latter finding, as well as poststenotic aortic dilation, may be seen on chest x-ray. Patients who have a history of mitral insufficiency also have an increased risk of postoperative CHF and arrhythmia.

Based on the history, physical findings, and a few simple laboratory studies, efforts have been made to quantify surgical risk. The more commonly used system, the **Dripps-American Surgical Association Classification,** categorizes patients into five groups (Table 2-5). The system offers little guidance, however, for identifying patients who are at risk for postoperative myocardial ischemia.

In 1977, Goldman and associates published a prospective study that attempted to quantitate the perioperative hazards of myocardial infarction based on the history, physical findings, and simple laboratory data. Correlation and regression analysis of multiple recorded factors identified eight specific elements associated with an increased preoperative risk of infarction. Point values were assigned to each variable, and a quantitative estimate of the risk of postoperative

Table 2-5. Dripps-American Surgical Classification

Class I	Healthy patient: limited procedure
Class II	Mild to moderate systemic disturbance
Class III	Severe systemic disturbance
Class IV	Life-threatening disturbance
Class V	Not expected to survive, with or without surgery

Table 2-7. Cardiac Risk Scale

Class	Points	Potentially Fatal Cardiac Complications	Cardiac Death
I	0–5	0.7%	0.2%
II	6–12	5.0%	2.0%
III	13–25	11.0%	2.0%
IV	>26	22.0%	56.0%

Potentially fatal complications include postoperative myocardial infarction, pulmonary edema, and ventricular tachyarrhythmia.

Table 2-6. Assessment of Individual Risk Factors

Factor	Life-Threatening/ Nonfatal Yes	No	Cardiac Death Yes	No	Points	P
3rd heart sound or JVD	14%	3.5%	20.0%	1.2%	11	<0.001
MI in past 6 months	14%	3.7%	23.0%	1.4%	10	<0.001
Rhythm other than sinus	10%	3.0%	9.0%	1.0%	7	<0.001
>5 PVCs/min	16%	3.3%	14.0%	1.4%	7	<0.001
Age > 70 years	6%	3.0%	5.0%	0.4%	5	0.001
Emergency procedure	8%	3.0%	5.0%	1.0%	4	<0.001
Hemodynamically significant aortic stenosis	4%	4.0%	13.0%	1.6%	3	0.007
Aortic, intraabdominal, intrathoracic procedure	7%	1.2%	2.5%	1.4%	3	0.007
Poor general health	7%	2.0%	4.0%	1.0%	3	0.027
Total					53	

Adapted with permission from Goldman L, Caldera DL, Nussbaum SR, et al. Multifactorial index of cardiac risk factor in noncardiac surgical procedures. *N Engl J Med* 1977; 297:845–850. JVD, jugular venous distension. MI, myocardial infarction. PVC, premature ventricular depolarization.

myocardial infarction and death was determined (Tables 2-6 and 2-7).

In this analysis, poor general health is assumed to reflect severe systemic disease, blood gas signs of respiratory insufficiency (PaO_2 < 60 mm Hg or $PaCO_2$ > 50 mm Hg), electrolyte abnormality (K < 3.0 mEq/dL) or metabolic acidosis (HCO_3^- < 20 mEq/dL), acute or chronic renal failure [creatinine > 3.0 mg/dL or blood urea nitrogen (BUN) > 50 mg/dL], or hepatic dysfunction (abnormal transaminase or stigmata of chronic liver disease). Patients who have a combination of risk factors (e.g., chronic renal failure and metabolic acidosis) could be assumed to have additive risk; however, Goldman's work does not address this issue. The danger of nonfatal or fatal postoperative cardiac ischemia is significantly greater if the risk factor is present.

A score of less than 25 total points implies minimal risk; however, the threat of serious, but nonfatal, complications increases more than sevenfold between Class I and Class II and more than twice that between Class II

and Class III. The risk of cardiac death for a patient with any score greater than 5 is increased by a factor of 10. In addition, a score of greater than 26 points suggests that the risk of a fatal coronary event is so great that elective surgery should not be considered. Patients who are categorized as Class II or Class III usually benefit from a period of medical management for several days before elective surgery, if possible, or from coronary angiography to determine the presence of a surgically correctable coronary lesion.

Qualification of Goldman's risk factors should be considered. Age in itself is not a straightforward risk factor. The difference between chronologic age and physiologic age may be substantial. For emergent intrathoracic and intraabdominal procedures, surgical risk is directly related to age. For nonemergent or minor procedures, the relation is less clear.

A reliable indicator of hemodynamic reserve is made by quantitative estimate of the patient's cardiovascular functional class. A useful scale is outlined in

Table 2-8. Energy Expenditure and Metabolic Equivalents

Class	Tasks Patient Can Perform to Completion
I	Activity requiring > 6 METS Carrying 24 lb up 8 steps Carrying objects that weigh 80 lb Performing outdoor work (shoveling snow, spading soil) Participating in recreation (skiing, basketball, squash, handball, jogging/walking at 5 mph)
II	Activities requiring > 4 but not > 6 METS Having sexual intercourse without stopping Walking at 4 mph on level ground Performing outdoor work (gardening, raking, weeding) Participating in recreation (rollerskating, dancing fox trot)
III	Activity requiring > 1 but not > 4 METS Showering, dressing without stopping, stripping and making bed Walking at 2.5 mph on level ground Performing outdoor work (cleaning windows) Participating in recreation (golfing, bowling)
IV	No activity requiring > 1 MET Cannot carry out any of the above activities

Adapted with permission from Paul SD, Eagle KA. A stepwise strategy for coronary risk assessment for noncardiac surgery. *Med Clin North Am* 1995; 79: 1241–1262.
METS, metabolic equivalents.

Table 2-8. Activity is expressed in metabolic equivalents (METs).

Any abnormality seen on routine electrocardiography implies increased risk to the adult patient. Other than acute myocardial infarction or complete heart block, the abnormality rarely requires postponement of surgery, especially in asymptomatic patients.

Mild chronic CHF is not associated with an increased occurrence of perioperative infarction. Patients with cardiomegaly on chest x-ray and even those whose clinical course is effectively managed with diuretics or cardiac glycosides do not represent high-risk groups. However, abnormal third heart sounds or signs of jugular venous distension indicate decompensation of cardiac function. These patients are in jeopardy of serious cardiac complications. Digitalis, however, is a drug with a very narrow therapeutic:toxic ratio. Surgical patients frequently cannot take fluids orally, and often have multiple tubes to remove fluids that are rich in electrolytes. These fluid shifts predispose the patient to electrolyte aberrations (specifically, hypokalemia) and further narrow the therapeutic:toxic ratio.

The patient who has a history of rheumatic fever, a prosthetic heart valve, or other cardiac abnormalities requires preoperative antibiotic prophylaxis to prevent endocarditis before undergoing procedures that may cause transient bacteremia. Antibiotic recommendations for prophylaxis are listed in Table 2-9, although the practice has never been firmly established by prospective, controlled clinical trials. Antibiotic prophylaxis should be given to any patient who has any type of prosthetic device implanted. This recommendation

Table 2-9. Endocarditis Prophylaxis in Surgical Patients with a History of Rheumatic Fever, Cardiac Valvular Disease, or Prosthetic Heart Valve

	Dose for Adults	Dose for Children[a]
Dental and Upper Respiratory Procedures		
Oral[b]		
Amoxicillin[c]	3 g 1 hr before procedure and 1.5 g 6 hr later	50 mg/kg 1 hr before procedure and 25 mg/kg 6 hr later
Penicillin allergy:		
Erythromycin	1 g 2 hr before procedure and 500 mg 6 hr later	20 mg/kg 2 hr before procedure and 10 mg/kg 6 hr later
or		
clindamycin	300 mg 1 hr before procedure and 150 mg 6 hr later	10 mg/kg (300 mg maximum) 1 hr before procedure and 5 mg/kg 6 hr later
Parenteral[b]		
Ampicillin	2 g IM or IV 30 min before procedure	50 mg/kg IM or IV 30 min before procedure
plus gentamicin	1.5 mg/kg IM or IV 30 min before procedure	2 mg/kg IM or IV 30 min before procedure
Gastrointestinal and Genitourinary Procedures		
Oral[b]		
Amoxicillin[c]	3 g 1 hr before procedure and 1.5 g 6 hr later	50 mg/kg 1 hr before procedure and 25 mg/kg 6 hr later
Parenteral[b]		
Ampicillin	2 g IM or IV 30 min before procedure	50 mg/kg IM or IV 30 min before procedure
plus gentamicin	1.5 mg/kg IM or IV 30 min before procedure	2 mg/kg IM or IV 30 min before procedure
Penicillin allergy:		
Vancomycin	1 g IV infused slowly over 1 hr beginning 1 hr before procedure	20 mg/kg IV infused slowly over 1 hr beginning 1 hr before procedure
plus gentamicin	See dose above	See dose above

[a]Dose should not exceed the adult dose.
[b]Oral regimens are safer and more convenient. Parenteral regimens are more likely to be effective and are recommended for patients with prosthetic valves, those with a history of endocarditis previously, or those taking oral penicillin continuously.
[c]Amoxicillin is recommended because of its activity against streptococci and enterococci.
Viridans streptococci are the most common cause of endocarditis after dental or upper respiratory procedures. Enterococci are the most common cause of endocarditis after gastrointestinal or genitourinary procedures.
IM, intramuscular. IV, intravenous.

includes patients with prosthetic joints, vascular grafts, or other hardware implanted for medical reasons.

Evaluation of cardiac function is frequently accomplished with the insertion of a pulmonary artery catheter to monitor hemodynamics and maximize cardiac performance. The use of this tool has theoretical advantages; however, the clinical utility of pulmonary

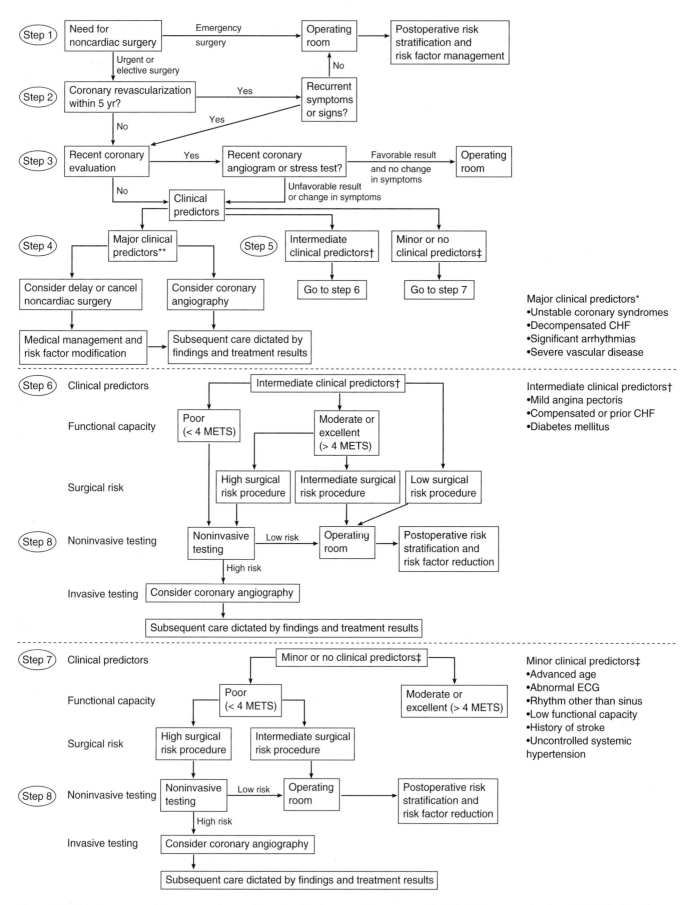

Figure 2-2 Stepwise approach to preoperative cardiac evaluation for noncardiac surgery. (Adapted with permission from Eagle KA, Brundage BW, Chaitman BR. Guidelines for perioperative cardiovascular evaluation for noncardiac surgery: report of the American College of Cardiology/American Heart Association Task Force on Practice Guidelines. *Circulation* 1996;93:1278–1317.)

artery catheters, especially in terms of outcome, is difficult to substantiate in critically ill patients.

The American College of Cardiology and the American Heart Association Task Forces have outlined a logical approach to the preoperative cardiac evaluation of patients who are undergoing noncardiac surgery. The general recommendation is that preoperative testing should be limited to the small subset of patients who are at very high risk, when results will affect patient treatment and, most important, outcome. The algorithm developed by the Task Force on Practice Guidelines (Figure 2-2) shows an eight-step approach to preoperative cardiac assessment. Patients who need emergency noncardiac surgery require operative intervention without extensive preoperative testing. Postoperatively, these patients may require further cardiac evaluation. Step two concerns patients who need urgent or elective operative procedures. Patients who have undergone coronary revascularization within 5 years and who have had no recurring symptoms of myocardial ischemia may proceed to operative intervention without additional cardiac workup. Those who have recurrent signs or symptoms and have not undergone a recent coronary evaluation should be evaluated on the basis of clinical predictors. Patients with major clinical predictors (i.e., unstable coronary syndrome, decompensated congestive heart failure, significant arrhythmia, severe valvular disease) should be evaluated by noninvasive tests of myocardial perfusion. The objective of these noninvasive assessments is to identify patients who would benefit from coronary angiography and subsequent coronary artery bypass grafting before elective surgery. If the patient has only intermediate predictors or if no clinical predictors are present, then assessment for functional capacity can be estimated. Individuals who cannot meet a 4-METS demand are at increased risk for perioperative cardiac ischemia and long-term complications. Those who exceed 4 METS are generally at low risk, and additional preoperative cardiac function testing may not be necessary. Individuals who are at high risk should undergo noninvasive testing and consideration for coronary angiography. Patients who show abnormalities by noninvasive testing and are considered candidates for coronary artery revascularization should undergo coronary angiography and subsequent intervention, as determined by the results of those studies.

Evaluation of Patients with Abnormalities

Coagulation Abnormalities

Most bleeding that occurs during and after surgical procedures is mechanical in nature (i.e., related to the disruption of vessels and failure to achieve surgical hemostasis). Some patients may have potential abnormalities of coagulation that predispose them to excessive blood loss. Examples include chronic anticoagulation for artificial heart valve prophylaxis and the treatment of chronic deep-vein thrombosis. Subtle platelet dysfunction is seen in patients who have degenerative joint disease and are taking large doses of aspirin or nonsteroidal anti-inflammatory agents. A careful history of drug use and an understanding of the adverse side effects of these common medications will identify individuals who are at increased risk for excessive postsurgical bleeding.

The best and most cost-effective screening test for hemostatic abnormality is a careful history. Millions of dollars each year are wasted on needless laboratory determinations of coagulation profiles in healthy patients who are admitted for elective procedures and have no history to suggest a coagulation abnormality. A careful history identifies patients who have excessive bleeding after minor surgical or dental procedures or minor injury. Patients who describe easy bruisability after minor trauma, frequent epistaxis, or a history of chronic excessive alcohol use should be considered for laboratory determination of coagulation status. Coagulopathy that is discovered intraoperatively or postoperatively represents a failure to obtain an adequate history, not a failure to order laboratory tests. Findings on physical examination that suggest potential bleeding disorders include petechiae, joint deformity, generalized lymphadenopathy, hepatosplenomegaly, and severe malnutrition. These findings confirm the suspicions identified in the patient's history. In this setting, laboratory investigation is appropriate. For a more complete discussion of bleeding disorders, see Chapter 5.

The patient who has a family history of a bleeding disorder or who has had menorrhagia or prolonged bleeding after a dental extraction should have screening studies. These studies begin with prothrombin time, partial thromboplastin time, and a complete blood count, specifically to look at cell counts. An early consultation with a hematologist is encouraged in this situation. Screening of prothrombin time, partial thromboplastin time, and platelet count is not necessary unless there is a reason to suspect a defect in the coagulation cascade. Factors that suggest such a defect include an abnormal family history, an abnormal history of bleeding in the patient, a history of malignancy (especially in a patient who recently received chemotherapy), a history of liver disease, or a history of increased bleeding or bruising.

Chronic Renal Disease

In the United States, more than 250,000 patients with end-stage renal disease are maintained on dialysis. An even greater number of patients have renal function that is significantly lower than normal. The metabolic and nutritional consequences of this disease frequently require special preparation of the patient for an elective surgical procedure. Most procedures can be performed with an acceptably low complication rate in patients who have chronic renal failure (CRF), provided that meticulous attention to perioperative care is given. Patients with CRF should not be denied a necessary or beneficial surgical procedure based on a history of renal disease alone.

In CRF, the ability to excrete water and sodium and maintain homeostasis of the intravascular volume is impaired. Excessive preload usually does not appear, however, until renal function deteriorates to less than 10% of normal. Chronic volume depletion is encountered in these patients as frequently as volume overload. These patients often receive potent diuretic agents or have chronic volume contraction associated with hypertension. For this reason, fluid management is dictated by the patient's history and disease process, not by the fact that he or she has CRF. For example, a patient who has end-stage renal disease and is in septic shock because of a perforated sigmoid diverticulum requires crystalloid resuscitation to correct the relative volume deficit, even though he is dependent on dialysis. This patient should not be fluid-restricted. Invasive hemodynamic monitoring can be helpful in this patient group and allows precision in volume replacement. The ability to excrete potassium is also impaired, and patients with impaired renal function do not tolerate sudden changes in potassium level. The risk of malignant hyperkalemia is directly proportional to the serum potassium level before the last dialysis. Serum potassium levels should be less than 5 mEq/L before surgery. Achieving this level may require dialysis or the use of ion-exchange resins. Chronic renal failure is usually accompanied by chronic metabolic acidosis because excretion of fixed acids is reduced. These acids are the by-products of metabolism, and include sulfates, phosphates, and lactate. Respiratory compensation by hyperventilation can maintain the serum pH at an acceptable level that is slightly below normal. The serum bicarbonate level should be greater than 18 mEq/L. Achieving this level may require exogenous bicarbonate administration or dialysis against a bicarbonate bath. Postoperatively, the acid load increases as hydrogen ions are released from damaged cells. Hyperventilation may provide temporary compensation for the metabolic acidosis. However, if $PaCO_2$ increases even slightly, a profound exacerbation of acidosis may occur. This situation is seen in patients who cannot increase minute ventilation, who have increased **dead space,** or who are receiving an excessive carbohydrate caloric load. Aggressive pulmonary toilet to prevent hypoventilation, atelectasis, pneumonitis, and oversedation is prudent.

Another electrolyte abnormality that is often seen in patients with chronic renal failure is hypocalcemia secondary to hyperphosphatemia. Because hypermagnesemia is common, magnesium-containing antacids should be avoided in these patients. Oral phosphate binders and dietary restriction of phosphates may be required as well. Ionized calcium should be followed in these patients and supplemented as needed in the perioperative period.

Most patients with long-standing CRF are malnourished. Anorexia, which results from azotemia and the inability to handle the accumulation of nitrogenous end-products, promotes depletion of both skeletal muscle and visceral protein stores. Malabsorption syndromes are common, as are overt vitamin deficiencies.

Patients who receive long-term peritoneal dialysis may lose as much as 6 to 8 g protein/day, and as a result, may have hypoalbuminemia. Anorexia and a history of weight loss suggest a catabolic state. Aggressive nutritional support should be provided. Patients should not be protein-restricted in the perioperative phase just because they have renal failure. Malnutrition significantly increases the risk of septic complications in the perioperative period.

The normochromic normocytic anemia that is often seen in patients with CRF is usually well tolerated. The added stress and oxygen requirements that follow a surgical procedure, however, may be poorly tolerated. Chronic dialysis is estimated to remove as much as 3 L blood/year, and the reduced production of erythropoietin hampers red blood cell replacement. The life span of red blood cells is also reduced in the uremic state. Immmune responses are deficient, and as a result, the potential for infectious complications may be enhanced. Many patients with CRF are carriers of bloodborne pathogens because of multiple transfusions. Chronic coagulopathy secondary to heparinization during dialysis, or the coagulopathy associated with uremia, may exaggerate blood loss during surgery or in the perioperative period. D-desamino arginine vasopression promotes the release of **von Willebrand's** multimers from endothelial cells. These multimers may be useful in the preoperative preparation of patients with chronic renal disease.

Management of these patients requires careful attention to detail. Daily weighing and accurate intake and output records are essential. Baseline renal function studies should be obtained preoperatively and should include determinations of BUN and creatinine as well as an estimation of glomerular filtration rate. Exacerbation of renal failure is prevented if hypotension is avoided and medications are carefully administered. Most drugs can be nephrotoxic, and doses must be adjusted frequently based on an estimation of the degree of renal function. A coagulation profile may help to identify intrinsic deficiencies, and the anticoagulation effects of heparin may require reversal or time to clear. Patients with renal failure may require modifications in anesthetic techniques. For example, succinylcholine is generally avoided because it may promote or exacerbate hyperkalemia. Also, nondepolarizing neuromuscular blockage agents that are not renally metabolized and excreted should be selected. Atracurium undergoes Hoffman degradation and is often used in the anesthetic management of patients with renal failure. Many other examples of modifications are available in standard textbooks of anesthesiology. Aggressive pulmonary physiotherapy, attention to volume in electrolyte status, and nutritional support can substantially reduce many metabolic sequelae postoperatively. Modification of the timing and type of dialysis may be necessary, and close consultation with a nephrologist is advisable. Despite the formidable spectrum of potential problems faced by the surgical patient who has CRF, elective surgery can be performed safely with a modicum of risk.

Metabolic Abnormalities

Four abnormal metabolic situations may alter the surgical approach to the patient or require extra preoperative preparation: (1) diabetes, (2) hepatic dysfunction, (3) dysfunction of the adrenal cortex, and (4) malnutrition. These situations are discussed in the following sections.

Diabetes

The patient who has diabetes is at increased risk in the perioperative period from a number of perspectives, particularly (1) metabolic (hyperglycemia or hypoglycemia), (2) cardiovascular, and (3) infectious. Those who require insulin to control their diabetes must have their dose adjusted to compensate for periods when food is not allowed or when the hyperglycemic response to the stress of illness, surgery, or trauma is clinically significant. Patients who have diabetes that was previously controlled by diet or oral agents may require insulin in the perioperative period for the reasons mentioned earlier. Infectious etiologies of surgical disease or postoperative infections may promote hyperglycemia and even ketoacidosis. On the other hand, overzealous administration of insulin may lead to hypoglycemia.

The perioperative management of patients with diabetes is approached as follows:

1. Patients who are instructed not to eat or drink after midnight in preparation for an operation the next morning should reduce their morning insulin dose to one-half the usual dose of intermediate- or regular-acting insulin to be taken the morning of the operation.
2. The patient should receive a continuous infusion of 5% dextrose to provide 10 g glucose/hr. Fingerstick glucose levels are monitored intraoperatively and followed postoperatively, at least every 6 hours. The goal is to maintain a glucose level of between 150 and 200 mg/dL. It is generally considered preferable to have the patient at the higher end of this range because of the fearsome consequences of hypoglycemia. Alternatively, continuous intravenous infusion of insulin can be used. This approach is particularly helpful in the brittle diabetic. In the postoperative period, close attention should be paid not only to the patient's blood sugar, but also to the patient's carbohydrate intake. Diabetic ketoacidosis (DKA) can develop in patients with either type I or type II diabetes. DKA is deceptively easy to overlook, because it can mimic postoperative ileus. It may present as nausea, vomiting, abdominal distension, or in association with polyuria (which is commonly mistaken for mobilization of intraoperative fluids). For this reason, patients with type I diabetes (and many with type II diabetes) should have their urinary ketone level monitored by dipstick. This method is faster and much less costly than following serum ketone levels, and it gives a fairly accurate picture of developing ketoacidosis. A glucose level that is less than 250 does not mean that the patient is not at risk for DKA; DKA develops because of the metabolism of fuel in the absence of glucose. Hence, the development of DKA does not depend on a certain level of glucose, but on the absence of insulin. Patients with diabetes are best managed with a continuous infusion of intravenous insulin, usually 1 to 3 units/hr. If a sliding scale is needed, then the subcutaneous route is preferred, except when the subcutaneous tissue is not well perfused.

The cardiac effects of patients with diabetes were discussed previously. The incidence of vascular abnormalities found on physical examination increases with the age of the patient and the duration of the diabetes. Men with diabetes may have twice the risk of cardiovascular mortality as their nondiabetic counterparts. Women have approximately four times the risk. For unexplained reasons, tachycardia may be present in patients with diabetes. Tachycardia is believed to be secondary to autonomic cardiac neuropathy, which is often associated with orthostatic hypotension without an appropriate increase in pulse. These findings are associated with unexplained cardiopulmonary arrest postoperatively.

Gastroparesis, which is also believed to be caused by autonomic neuropathy, may delay gastric emptying and increase the likelihood of aspiration. Gastroparesis is suggested if the patient gives a history of prolonged fullness after eating, or of constipation. A splash of fluid heard with the stethoscope over the stomach at a time when the stomach should be empty may require the placement of a nasogastric tube for decompression.

The risk of infection is substantially greater for the patient with diabetes. Hyperglycemia has an adverse effect on immune function, especially phagocytic activity. The reduced blood flow in patients with vascular disease, especially to the extremities, retards wound healing. Because most peripheral vascular disease in the patient with diabetes is small vessel in nature, palpable pulses are common, even in the face of tissue ischemia. Often the extent of small vessel disease extends deep into the tissue, sparing the skin, much like a cone whose base is directed peripherally and whose apex extends in the central portion of the extremity proximally. For a patient with diabetes, ingrown toenails or minor injuries to the feet are potentially serious problems that can lead to amputation or mortality. Therefore, even minor procedures on the extremities of diabetic patients are approached with utmost caution. Patients with diabetes should always wear shoes.

The surgical patient who has diabetes should be carefully questioned about the duration of the disease, insulin requirements, diet, degree of glucose control, last insulin administration, and peripheral symptoms (i.e., numbness, extremity pain). During the physical examination, special attention is given to the feet, looking for minor injuries, evidence of poor hygiene, inadequate vascular supply, ulcers, or decreased vibratory

Table 2-10. Common Problems in the Cirrhotic Patient

Hepatic Dysfunction	History and Physical Clues	Perioperative Effects or Complications
Drug metabolism	Nonspecific	Sensitivity to narcotics, over sedation, respiratory depression
Protein synthesis	Spider angioma	Abnormalities in coagulation or bleeding
	Petechiae	Reduced factors I, II, V, VII, VIII, IX, X, XI, XIII
	Bruises	Thrombocytopenia
	Changes in sensorium	Exacerbation of encephalopathy, delirium tremens (with Alcohol withdrawal), seizures
	Ascites	Fluid retention/respiratory compromise
	Edema	Intraperitoneal sepsis, potential shifts in intravascular volume, potential electrolyte abnormalities
General nutrition	Weight loss (or weight gain with ascites), anemia, muscle wasting, fever, weakness	Vitamin deficiency (A, B, D, K): poor wound healing, poor handling of glucose, Wernicke's syndrome
	Nausea, anorexia, edema	Magnesium, phosphorus: multiple metabolic abnormalities, arrhythmias, reduced immunocompetence, infection

Table 2-11. Child's Classification of Cirrhosis

Class	Albumin	Bilirubin	Ascites	Encephalopathy	Nutritional State	Mortality Rate (%)
A	> 3.5	< 2.0	Absent	Absent	Good	< 10
B	3.0–3.5	2.0–3.0	Minimal	Minimal	Fair	40
C	< 3.0	> 3.0	Severe	Severe	Poor	> 80

sensation. Patients who have positive findings should give meticulous care to their feet (i.e., daily washing, careful drying, application of softening lotion, protection from minor trauma, avoidance of pressure sores).

Hepatic Dysfunction

Although the liver has an extraordinary amount of reserve as well as the ability to regenerate, a significant number of patients (> 15 million) show evidence of hepatic dysfunction or overt cirrhosis. Usually, the etiology is nutritional and secondary to alcohol abuse, but it may also be secondary to an infectious event or idiopathic. General complications and the risk of impaired liver function are listed in Table 2-10. A careful search should be made for these conditions during the history and physical examination. Child's criteria have long been used to estimate the risk of nonhepatic surgery in the patient with cirrhosis (Table 2-11).

These criteria only quantitate the degree of hepatic impairment as it relates to increased mortality. More frequently, Child's classification is used for the patient who has varices and is a candidate for a portosystemic shunt or a devascularization procedure to treat or prevent the recurrence of gastrointestinal tract hemorrhage. These estimates of mortality are not absolute, and patients may have a significant reduction in risk if hepatic function is improved preoperatively.

The alcoholic patient is protected from withdrawal symptoms by the administration of proper sedatives. The onset of mild withdrawal symptoms can occur anywhere from 1 to 5 days after alcohol is discontinued. Major symptoms generally peak at approximately 3 days, but have occurred as long as 10 days after withdrawal. Benzodiazepines can prevent major withdrawal symptoms if they are instituted prophylactically. Untreated delirium tremens carries a postoperative mortality rate of as high as 50%. This rate is reduced to 10% with proper treatment. The use of intravenous ethanol has also been advocated, but it only postpones withdrawal.

Alcoholics should be given thiamine parenterally before intravenous glucose is administered. Ataxia, ophthalmoplegia, and the severe central nervous system disturbance **Wernicke-Korsakoff syndrome** (i.e., ataxia, ophthalmoplegia, and confusion) may follow if this therapy is not instituted. Magnesium and phosphate deficiencies are common, especially with refeeding, and these elements should be aggressively replaced to prevent abnormalities of glucose metabolism and cardiac arrhythmia.

For a more complete discussion of surgical diseases of the liver, see Chapter 18.

Dysfunction of the Adrenal Cortex

Historically, any patient who received even small doses of glucocorticoid within the 12–month period before surgery was given preoperative glucocorticoid coverage. This practice was based on reports of two patients from more than 40 years ago. These patients had complications that were believed to be caused by steroid-associated adrenal suppression. Recent advances in the understanding of the adverse effects of glucocorticoids, including increased susceptibility to infection, impaired tissue healing, abnormalities of glucose metabolism, and upper gastrointestinal hemorrhage prompted a reconsideration of preoperative glucocorticoid coverage. New recommendations are based on the degree of surgical stress anticipated (i.e., minor, moderate, or major). For minor surgical stress, glucocorticoid replacement is the equivalent of 25-mg hydrocortisone over a 24-hour period. For moderate surgical stress (e.g., open cholecystectomy, colon resection, total joint replacement, hysterectomy), the glucocorticoid replacement is 50- to 75-mg hydrocortisone (or the equivalent) for 24 to 48 hours. For major surgical stress (e.g., cardiopulmonary bypass, esophagogastrectomy, pancreaticoduodenectomy), the glucocortiocoid replacement is approximately 100- to 150-mg hydrocortisone (or the equivalent) for 48 to 72 hours. For comparison, patients with Cushing's syndrome produce the equivalent of 36-mg hydrocortisone/day.

Malnutrition

Poor nutritional status predisposes the patient to operative complications related to wound healing, respiratory insufficiency, and reduced immunocompetence that leads to infection. The mortality rate is substantially higher in patients with poor nutritional status. In some studies, as many as 50% of patients who are admitted to hospitals in the United States have some element of malnutrition. Until recent years, little attention was given to nutritional assessment, and many hospitalized patients with illnesses that lasted longer than 20 to 30 days either starved to death or died of septic complications related to malnutrition. The ability to support patients enterally and parenterally with adequate calories and protein significantly reduced morbidity and mortality rates. Elements in the history that suggest poor nutritional status include anorexia, weight loss, chronic vomiting and diarrhea, and chronic illness. CRF and chronic hepatic dysfunction are frequently associated with malnutrition.

On physical examination, findings of muscle wasting in the temporalis muscle or over the thenar or hypothenar eminence, peripheral edema, or neuropathy suggest possible protein-calorie malnutrition. Glossitis, loss of rugae on the tongue, or smoothing of the edges of the tongue alone suggests vitamin B deficiency. Cheilosis, or scaling and cracking of the vermilion border of the lips or corners of the mouth, likewise suggests vitamin B–complex deficiency.

Several visceral protein markers, albumin, prealbumin, transferrin, retinal binding protein, and carnitine have been used to estimate nutritional deficiency. Delayed sensitivity to recall antigens and total lymphocyte count are sometimes useful to quantitate immune

Table 2-12. Prediction of Morbidity and Mortality on Nutritional Parameters

PNI = 158% − 16.6 (ALB) − 0.78 TSF − 0.2 (TFN) − 5.8 (DH)	HPI = 0.91 (ALB) − 1.0 (DH) − 1.44 (sepsis) + 0.98 (Dx) − 1.09
DH > 5 mm = 2	DH >/0.5 mm = 1 Anergy = 2
DH 1–5 mm = 1 Anergy = 0	Sepsis = 2; no sepsis = 1
	Dx (cancer) = 1; no cancer = 2 HPI = − 3 = 5% HPI = − 2 = 10% HPI = − 1 = 20% HPI = 0 = 50% HPI = + 1 = 74% HPI = + 2 = 88%

PNI, prognostic nutritional index, risk of complication. HPI, hospital prognostic index, probability of survival. ALB, Albumin (g/dl). TSF, triceps skinfold thickness (mm). TFN, transferrin. DH, delayed hypersensitivity. Dx, diagnosis.

function and identify nutritional deficits that are severe enough to affect the outcome of a proposed operation. Anthropomorphic measurements to assess body reserves (e.g., triceps skinfold thickness for body fat) or attempts to estimate body cell mass (e.g., midarm muscle circumference, creatinine–height index) are advocated by some. None of these measurements, singly or in combination, has proved more useful than a careful history.

Attempts have also been made to quantitate the risk of surgical procedures based on nutritional parameters alone. The prognostic nutritional index attempts to define such risk (Table 2–12). In an effort to define mortality in the same way, the Hospital Prognostic Index was developed (see Table 2–12). More important perhaps than specifically identifying the statistical probability of death or of a certain complication, these methods help to identify patients who would benefit from preoperative nutritional support in one form or another. Morbidity and mortality rates can be reduced in nutritionally depleted patients. Waiting until all parameters return to normal is not necessary; it may not be possible to postpone surgical intervention for the many weeks it may take for such a return to normal. For a more complete discussion of the evaluation and treatment of nutritional problems, see Chapter 4.

Physical Examination

Obviously, a complete physical examination should be performed on every preoperative patient. However, certain areas deserve particular emphasis. Vital signs should always be checked and noted in the history and physical examination record. The patient's overall habitus and nutritional status should be assessed. A neurologic examination should be performed to verify that there are no global or focal deficits. The HEENT (*Head, Eyes, Ears, Nose,* and *Throat*) examination should confirm that there is no scleral icterus. Neck masses should be sought, and the neck should be auscultated for bruits, which are actually a stronger marker for coronary artery disease than for significant cerebrovascular disease. The lungs should be auscultated to ensure that there are no wheezes. The heart should also be auscultated to detect murmurs and especially gallops, which could be a sign of CHF. The abdomen should be examined for ascites, auscultated for the quality of bowel sounds, and palpated for masses or organomegaly. Peripheral pulses should be checked and compared with the opposite side. Clearly, depending on the patient's medical history and specific surgical problems, more detailed focused examinations may be appropriate for specific organ systems. See any standard textbook of physical examination for more detail.

Preoperative Screening Tests

Recent interest in hospital cost containment has forced a review of the utility and appropriateness of preoperative screening examinations and diagnostic tests. Routine laboratory or x-ray screening in asymptomatic patients leads to a change in perioperative management in fewer than 1% of cases when an adequate history and physical examination have been performed. Patients who are undergoing procedures of relatively low surgical risk do not require extensive preoperative screening, even in the face of complex medical problems. The determination of baseline laboratory values is generally inappropriate, and is an expensive waste of medical care resources.

Routine screening of hemoglobin concentration is performed only in individuals who are undergoing radical procedures that are associated with an extensive amount of blood loss. Patients with a history of anemia, malignant disease, renal insufficiency, cardiac disease, diabetes mellitus, or pregnancy should have baseline determinations of serum hemoglobin concentration. Individuals who cannot provide a history or who do not have physical findings that suggest anemia should have preoperative baseline hemoglobin determinations.

Evaluation of baseline serum electrolyte concentrations, including serum creatinine, is appropriate in individuals whose history or physical examination suggests chronic medical disease (e.g., diabetes, hypertension, or cardiovascular, renal, or hepatic disease). Patients with the potential for loss of fluids and electrolytes, including those receiving long-term diuretic therapy, those with diabetes, and those with intractable vomiting, should also have preoperative determination of serum electrolytes. The elderly are at substantial risk for chronic dehydration, and testing is appropriate in these patients as well. Although there is no specific age that mandates automatic electrolyte screening, knowledge of the patient's medical history, medications, and systems review should guide decision-making about testing.

Preoperative urinalysis is recommended only for patients who have urinary tract symptoms or a history of chronic urinary tract disease, or in those who are undergoing urologic procedures.

The issue of screening tests for occult coagulopathy was addressed previously.

Screening chest radiography is rarely indicated. Despite the occasional incidental abnormality that is detected with a screening radiograph, these findings rarely receive further investigation and generally do not alter the surgical plans. Screening chest x-ray in asymptomatic elderly patients is also controversial because the usefulness of this diagnostic study in this population is unclear. Chest radiography is recommended for patients who are undergoing intrathoracic procedures and those who have signs and symptoms of active pulmonary disease.

Recommendations for screening electrocardiography are more firm, but likewise, there is a lack of definitive evidence about the utility of the procedure. Men who are older than 45 years of age and women who are older than 55 years of age should have a baseline recording. Patients with symptomatic cardiovascular disease, hypertension, or diabetes are candidates for preoperative electrocardiographic screening. Patients who are undergoing thoracic, intraperitoneal, aortic, or emergency surgery are also candidates for screening examinations.

In summary, laboratory and other diagnostic screening procedures should be performed on patients who are considered to be at risk for specific abnormalities. Neither the laboratory test nor the x-ray is a substitute for taking a careful history, performing a thorough physical examination, or assessing information critically.

The Medical Record

The medical record is a concise, explicit document that chronologically outlines the patient's course of treatment. Careful thought should be given to the information placed in the record; this information must be relevant to the course of treatment or diagnostic workup. The content of the medical record should be limited to a description of the thought process involved in decision-making, the therapeutic or diagnostic interventions employed, and the patient's response to those interventions. Before notes are written, consideration should be given to the following six points.

1. Does the information pertain to patient care? Only information that pertains to the actual care of the patient should be entered into the medical record. The medical record should not be used to relay messages among consulting services. Extraneous information is inappropriate and may generate medicolegal liability. Examples include editorial comments about the appropriateness or inappropriateness of recommendations made by other physicians. If there is genuine disagreement about the appropriate plan of management, then the reasons supporting the plan of management chosen should be doc-

umented in the chart, without editorial comment about the competency of the physicians who have written dissenting opinions.

2. Is the information of value in documenting the treatment course? Little value is obtained in repeating what was previously documented. In teaching institutions, it is common to see history and physical examinations or progress notes recorded by students, house staff, and attending physicians. The delivery of care in an educational environment is by necessity repetitive. Students gain important experience in writing progress notes that reflect careful and thoughtful evaluation of the patient. Students often obtain important medical information, and their notes should be carefully written.

3. What details will be important for the future care of the patient? Operative notes are perhaps the best illustration of the importance of identifying potential needs for future care. For example, recording surgical findings is more important than noting the type of suture used to perform an anastomosis. A careful description of the abdominal organs as they are inspected and palpated may be of value if future review becomes necessary. Information about blood loss, blood and fluid replacement, and operative time is more relevant than many of the technical nuances of the operative procedure. The thought process used in diagnosing an illness or selecting a therapy is often more important than the technical details.

4. Is the information accurate? Extreme care should be taken to ensure the accuracy of information that is entered into the medical record. Confusion may occur when verbal reports of diagnostic studies written into the progress notes do not agree with formal reports, once they are typed, signed, and filed. Erroneous information can lead to disastrous results, and may be more damaging than no information. Every effort should be made to maintain accuracy and consistency in the information that is recorded. In some circumstances, clinical decisions are made based on a verbal report. When this situation occurs, it is appropriate to note it (e.g., "Verbal report of positive blood culture received from the lab; plan removal of central line.").

5. Are suspicions and theories clearly defined as such? An inexperienced physician may not precisely differentiate suspicions, theories, and possibilities from reality. Incorrect documentation leads to distortion of the facts in the record and misconceptions on the part of others who are peripherally involved with the patient's care. Inaccuracy is a powerful deterrent to the quality of patient care at all levels.

6. Does the note serve the best interest of the patient, the physician, and the health care team? The medical record is kept on behalf of the patient to document the events, timing, and thinking relating to the care given during the period of hospitalization. The record is a confidential document and cannot be revealed to anyone who is not directly involved in the care of the patient, nor can it be revealed without the patient's or a responsible agent's written consent. Without this consent, an individual who discloses such information without the patient's consent breaches the ethical contract between patient and physician.

The medical record can be the physician's and the patient's best ally or worst enemy. Documentation of all findings, results, and explanations to the patient, particularly in terms of risks, benefits, anticipated results, and therapeutic alternatives, can protect both the patient and the physician.

The Order Sheet

The physician's order sheet is one of the most crucial components of the patient's medical record. Orders must be entered precisely, with the intent of being followed, not interpreted. Unfortunately, the latter is often the case because of the hasty scribblings of physicians that may be unclear, illegible, or inaccurate. Orders should be written with sufficient detail to eliminate possible misunderstanding. There is no excuse for illegible handwriting or imprecise orders. Every aspect of the patient's life, including diet, level of activity, access to the bathroom—even what the patient is to breathe—is the responsibility of the physician once the patient enters the hospital.

Orders include the elements listed in Table 2-13. Content and format may vary among institutions, but the principles are the same. Usually the first orders written concern general nursing care. Identification of the physician or team who is responsible for the patient is important so that the staff knows whom to contact if problems or questions arise. Listing the working diagnosis or reason for admission gives the staff a general idea of the problem and sets the tone for the delivery of

Table 2-13. General Considerations for Writing Orders

Physician/team responsible

Diagnosis/condition

Immediate plans

Vital signs/special checks/notification parameters

Diet

Level of activity

Special nursing care instructions
  Positioning
  Wound care
  Tubes/drains: management and care

Intake/Output: frequency

Intravenous fluids

Medications: drug, dose, route, frequency
  Routine
  Special

Laboratory orders

Special procedures/x-ray

Miscellaneous

services. The frequency of vital signs is next. Any special nursing evaluations (e.g., neurologic function) are also indicated. If the physician wishes to be notified of any of these assessments (e.g., temperature > 38.5°C), the staff is informed.

Diet specifications or NPO (nothing by mouth) orders are also indicated. Special diets are required by some patients (e.g., those with diabetes, those undergoing special diagnostic procedures). Too frequently, hospitalization is prolonged or expensive procedures must be repeated because of lack of attention to the details of prescribing the appropriate diet. The level of patient activity is specified as well. Such orders are generally considered routine, and some hospitals may have standard protocols. Prudent physicians, however, specifically write their own routine in sufficient detail to ensure that their plans are carefully followed.

Some nursing care functions must also be identified. These include special positioning, turning, pulmonary exercises, and care of wounds or drainage tubes. Foley catheters are placed to gravity drainage, nasogastric tubes to some type of suction apparatus, and wound drains to either suction or dependent drainage. The staff is informed specifically about the management of these drains or tubes. Daily care of the incision site is clearly noted. Retrograde infection from incision sites, especially with urinary catheters and wound drains, is a major contributor to morbidity. Patient positioning is extremely important in preventing pulmonary problems and preventing aspiration of the gastric contents in patients who are receiving enteral tube feedings. Other nursing instructions include the recording of fluid intake or output from urinary catheters and drains; specific instructions for tube care, stripping, or irrigation; and notification of the physician in the event of a specific occurrence (e.g., urine output < 30 mL/hr, chest tube drainage > 100 mL/hr).

The type and rate of intravenous fluid administration are also specified. When multiple intravenous sites are used, it is helpful to specify which fluids are to be infused at which sites.

To prevent potentially fatal medication errors, meticulous attention to detail is mandatory when writing medication orders. The notation sequence is type of drug, dosage, route of administration, and frequency. These orders should be absolutely clear and legible. If a physician is uncertain of the spelling of a drug name, he or she should consult a reference. It is important to use only standard abbreviations. Writing medications on a separate section of the order sheet so that they are not mixed in with nonmedication orders may be advantageous; in this way, confusion and oversights are avoided. Orders for routine medications (e.g., analgesics, laxatives, sleeping pills) are written first, followed by medications for the patient's specific needs. Reviewing the medication lists daily is an excellent habit. Changes in drugs, dosage, or frequency are confusing for both the pharmacy and the nursing staff. If drugs are changed, writing an order to stop the original drug, then ordering the new one is the best approach. In

most institutions, parenteral nutritional products are prepared in the pharmacy; therefore, total parenteral nutrition orders are placed with the medication orders.

Laboratory studies and special diagnostic procedures should be specified as well. Special procedures, such as x-rays, require additional thought. Request slips for these studies should specifically state the presumptive diagnosis and the reason for the test. Personal consultation with the radiologist or technician avoids confusion and prevents delays or unnecessary repetition of procedures. If those who perform the tests are aware of the reason for the testing, the results are nearly always more productive. Some procedures require special preparation of the patient; therefore, these instructions must be included in the orders. "Routine" or "daily" laboratory or radiology orders are wasteful, rarely contribute to care, and should be avoided. In the occasional situation in which serial studies are needed to follow some aspect of the patient's course, a stop time should be specified (e.g., "Please draw hematocrit q 6 hr × 24 hr."). Laboratory and diagnostic studies should be used to confirm clinical suspicions and not as a shotgun approach to reveal a diagnosis.

The miscellaneous category in Table 2-13 is intended for other orders that may be necessary, including requests for consultation, procurement of procedural permits or old records, or admission of a patient to a special study or protocol.

The orders are only as complete as you make them. Clarity and legibility allow for efficient and appropriate delivery of services.

Preoperative Evaluation

A brief preoperative note to summarize the workup and the pertinent physical and diagnostic studies is usually written the day before surgery. These notes serve as a checklist to ensure that the important aspects of preoperative preparation are completed. An example is shown in Table 2-14.

Progress Notes

Progress notes record the patient's clinical course throughout his or her hospital stay. Noting the hospital day number, the postoperative day, or the days after injury is helpful. The format for progress notes varies among hospitals and even among services within the hospital. All notes should be dated, timed, and signed. A brief, handwritten operative note should list the important elements of the operation, with consideration given to recording information that might be important in the immediate perioperative period, before the official typed report is appended to the medical record. These important components are listed in Table 2-15. The important elements of the discharge note are listed in Table 2-16.

In summary, the medical record is a legal document that contains important information about the patient's hospital course and his or her response to diagnostic and therapeutic interventions. It is also a place where

Table 2-14. Sample Preoperative Note

Diagnosis:	Cholelithiasis
Proposed surgery:	Cholecystectomy with operative cholangiogram
History and physical:	Completed (dictated) Grade II/VI systolic murmur at apex Hypertension (controlled)
Laboratory values:	CBC: $\dfrac{14.5}{41.5\%}$ 7,500 Electrolytes: 140 | 4.2 Bun 10 26 | 101 Glu 105 CXR: NAD ECG: NSR-normal Present meds: HCTZ 50 mg qd Blood: type and hold (specimen in blood bank)
Operative permit:	Signed and on chart; risks, rationale, benefits and alternatives have been explained in detail; patient understands and agrees to proceed with the surgical plans
Miscellaneous information:	
	Signature _____

CBC, complete blood count.
BUN, blood urea nitrogen.
GLU, glucose.
CXR, chest x-ray.
NAD, no appreciable disease.
ECG, electrocardiogram.
NSRs, normal sinus rhythm.
HCTZ, hydrochlorothiazide.

Table 2-15. Operative Note

Procedure:	
Findings:	
Surgeons:	Attending surgeon:
Estimated blood loss:	
Crystalloid replaced:	Blood products:
Anethesia:	
Complications:	
Tubes/drains:	
Disposition:	
	Signature:

Table 2-16. Discharge Note

Admission diagnosis:	Date:
Discharge diagnosis:	Date:
Operative procedure:	
Hospitalization course:	
Disposition:	
Home care instructions: Activity Diet Restrictions Wound care Other	
Discharge medications:	
Follow-up instructions:	
Miscellaneous:	

information given to the patient by the health care providers can be documented. Despite the inconvenience involved, the time and effort devoted to thoughtful record-keeping returns many dividends when future review is necessary.

SUGGESTED READINGS

Bronson DL, Halperin AK, Marwick TH. Evaluating cardiac risks in noncardiac surgery patients. *Cleve Clin J Med* 1995;62:391–400.

Constant J. *Essentials of Bedside Cardiology for Students and House Staff.* Boston, Mass: Little, Brown, 1989.

Eagle KA, Brundage BW, Chaitman BR. Guidelines for perioperative cardiovascular evaluation for noncardiac surgery: report of the American College of Cardiology/American Heart Association Task Force on Practice Guidelines. *Circulation* 1996;93:1278–1317.

Hnatiuk OW, Dillard TA, Torrington KG. Adherence to established guidelines for preoperative pulmonary function testing. *Chest* 1995;107:1294–1297.

Jones T, Isaacson JH. Preoperative screening: what tests are necessary? *Cleve Clin J Med* 1995;62:374–378.

Kispert JF, Dazamers A, Roitman L. Preoperative spirometry predicts perioperative pulmonary complications after major vascular surgery. *Am Surg* 1992;58:491–495.

Macario A, Roizen MF, Thisted RA, Kim S, Orkin FK, Phelps C. Reassessment of preoperative laboratory testing has changed test-ordering patterns of physicians. *Surg Gynecol Obstet* 1992;175:539–547.

Paul SD, Eagle KA. A stepwise strategy of coronary risk assessment for noncardiac surgery. *Med Clin North Am* 1995;79:1241–1262.

Roizen MR. Cost-effective preoperative laboratory testing. *JAMA* 1994;271:319–320.

Thomas DR, Ritchie CS. Preoperative assessment of older adults. *J Am Geriatr Soc* 1995;43:811–821.

3

Fluids and Electrolytes

Leigh Neumayer, M.D.
Susan Kaiser, M.D.
David Antonenko, M.D.

OBJECTIVES

1. Know the range of normal values of NA⁺, K⁺, HCO₃⁻, and Cl⁻ in serum, gastric aspirate, bile, and ileostomy aspirate.
2. Understand the contributions that extracellular, intracellular, and intravascular volume make to body weight.
3. List four hormones or substrates that affect renal absorption and excretion of sodium and water.
4. Compare the physical findings or symptoms of dehydration in the young and the elderly.
5. Understand the methods of determining fluid balance.
6. Describe the typical 24-hour fluid and electrolyte needs in the postoperative patient who has no complications.
7. Explain the composition of electrolytes in normal saline, lactated Ringer's solution, and 5% dextrose in water.
8. Given a patient with the condition in the left column, list the direction of change in values and pH for the serum electrolytes observed.

	Na	K	HCO₃	Cl	pH
Excessive gastric losses					
High-volume pancreatic fistula					
Small intestinal fistula					
Biliary fistula					
Diarrhea					
Closed head injury					

9. Given a patient with the condition listed, determine an appropriate replacement fluid.
   a. Pyloric outlet obstruction
   b. Pancreatic fistula
   c. Small bowel fistula
   d. Biliary fistula
   e. Diarrhea

f. Closed head injury
g. Massive blood loss

10. Indicate the direction of change in serum and urine values that might be obtained in patients with each condition listed in the left column.

Serum

	Na	K	HCO₃	Cl	Osmolarity
ATN					
Dehydration					
Inappropriate ADH secretion					
Diabetes insipidus					
Congestive heart failure					

Urine

	Na	K	HCO₃	Cl	Osmolarity
ATN					
Dehydration					
Inappropriate ADH secretion					
Diabetes insipidus					
Congestive heart failure					

11. List the differential diagnosis and treatment for each of the following conditions:
    a. Hypernatremia
    b. Hyponatremia
    c. Hyperkalemia
    d. Hypokalemia
    e. Hyperchloremia
    f. Hypochloremia
    g. Hypercalcemia
    h. Hypocalcemia
    i. Hypermagnesemia
    j. Hypomagnesemia
    k. Hypophosphatemia

12. Indicate the directional change in values expected in patients with each condition listed in the left column:

Arterial Blood
pH PO$_2$ PaCO^2 HCO$_3$ Base Excess

Acute metabolic acidosis _____

Acute respiratory acidosis _____

Chronic respiratory acidosis _____

Compensated metabolic acidosis _____

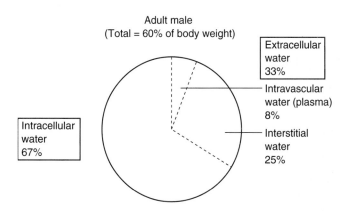

Figure 3-1 Total body water (TBW) in the adult male. (Compartments are expressed as % TBW.)

Table 3-1. Normal Plasma Values

	Concentration (mEq/L)
Cation	
Sodium	135–145
Potassium	3.5–5.0
Calcium	4.0–5.5^a
Magnesium	1.5–2.5
Anion	
Chloride	95–105
Carbon dioxide content	24–30
Phosphate	2.5–4.5
Sulfate	1.0
Organic acids	2.0
Protein	1.6^a

^{a}Values are given in mEq/L; on routine laboratory reports, Ca^{++} and protein levels are usually reported in mg/dL.

Understanding and managing volume, electrolyte, and acid–base status is an integral part of the treatment of a surgical patient. Before discussing specific clinical problems, this chapter provides an overview of fluid, electrolyte, and acid–base balance. This chapter is intended to be an introduction to the subject material; for more complete and comprehensive information, see the many available texts and articles in the literature, some of which are listed at the end of this chapter. A table of normal serum laboratory values is provided in the glossary.

Normal Physiology

Total Body Water and Compartments

Total body water (TBW) in the adult is 45% to 70% of body weight. This value varies as a function of age, sex, and lean body mass. It is lowest in the aged and obese and highest in the very lean and young. TBW is estimated as 60% of body weight in the idealized 70-kg adult male and 50% to 55% in his female counterpart. TBW is partitioned into two main compartments. The intracellular space represents two-thirds of TBW, and the extracellular space one-third, amounting to 40% and 20% of body weight, respectively, in the average adult (Figure 3-1). The extracellular compartment is further divided into the interstitial space (16% TBW) and the intravascular fluid space (4% TBW).

The electrolyte composition of the two subdivisions of the extracellular fluid space is similar. In plasma (Table 3-1), sodium is the chief extracellular cation, with small amounts of potassium, calcium, and magnesium also present. The corresponding anions are chloride, bicarbonate, and smaller amounts of proteins, phos-

phates, sulfates, and organic acids. The ionic composition of the interstitial fluid differs only with respect to its lower concentration of protein and the related minor changes in chloride and bicarbonate levels. In contrast, in the intracellular compartment, the cations potassium and magnesium and the anions phosphates, sulfates, and proteins are the dominant ionic species. The striking differences in intracellular and extracellular electrolyte composition are maintained by the selective permeabilities of cellular membranes. Free diffusion of proteins, chloride, and multivalent ions is limited, and active metabolic "pumps" in the cell wall promote the movement of sodium out of the cell and the passage of potassium into it.

Movement of water from one compartment to another is passive, and is determined by the action of physical forces exerted across the intervening membranes. The capillary membrane that separates the interstitial and intravascular spaces under most circumstances is freely permeable to water, electrolytes, and solutes, but not to proteins. Consequently, the net flow of water between these two spaces is a function of the balance between fluid pressures generated on either side of the membrane and the effective **colloid osmotic pressures** generated by the higher concentrations of nondiffusible protein in the plasma. On the other hand, the exchange of water between the intracellular and interstitial compartments is totally determined by osmotic gradients across the cell membranes. Normally, there is no gradient and no significant net water flow in either direction because the **osmolarity,** or number of osmotically active particles per liter of solution on either side of the membrane, is the same. When extracellular fluid becomes hyposmolar (or hypotonic) relative to normal values, water flows into the cells in which the osmolarity is higher. A new equilibrium is reached, and the osmolarity of both compartments is less than the normal 290 mOsm/L. Similarly, hyperosmolarity (or hypertonicity) develops in both compartments if extracellular osmolarity is increased. In this case, osmotic equilibrium is reached by an egress of water from the cell into the extracellular space. In contrast, isotonic fluid expansion or contraction of the extracellular space, which has no effect on osmolarity, does not include such movements of water between the cells and the interstitial fluid.

Sodium

Total body sodium is estimated as 40 mEq/kg. One-third is fixed in bone, and the other two-thirds, most of which is extracellular, is the exchangeable fraction. Sodium and its related anions represent 97% of the osmotically active particles that are normally present in the extracellular fluid compartments. Extracellular osmolarity is estimated by the formula:

$$Osmolarity = 2 \times [Na]_s + [glucose\ (mg)/dL \div 18] + [BUN \div 2.8]$$

where $[Na]_s$ is serum sodium concentration. If the value approximates 290 ± 10 mOsm/L, it can be reasonably assumed that extracellular osmolarity is within normal limits.

The normal adult sodium requirement is 1 to 2 mEq/kg/day, although the usual intake far exceeds this amount. Fairly constant body sodium content is maintained by normal kidneys that excrete sodium when intake is high and conserve it when intake is low. Renal sodium resorption can be so efficient that nearly none is lost in the urine during maximum conservation. Assuming normal renal perfusion and membrane function, sodium and water are both filtered at the glomerulus. In the proximal tubules, large amounts of each are recovered. Ultimately, however, the determination of renal conservation or excretion of sodium or water depends on selective processes that occur at more distal tubular sites.

Sodium resorption in exchange for potassium and hydrogen ion secretion in the distal tubules is a direct effect of the adrenal cortical hormone **aldosterone.** This action helps to maintain both extracellular volume and osmolarity. Extracellular volume reduction, particularly in the intravascular space, is a potent stimulus for aldosterone release. This response is triggered by a decrease in renal perfusion, which causes the juxtaglomerular apparatus to secrete renin. This secretion, in turn, promotes the secretion of angiotensin I and its conversion to angiotensin II, a potent stimulator of aldosterone secretion. Volume receptors in the right atrium are also present. When activated, these receptors cause aldosterone secretion. The juxtaglomerular apparatus and its renin–angiotensin–mediated aldosterone secretion are also activated by low extracellular fluid sodium concentrations. In addition, aldosterone secretion can be stimulated by an increase in serum potassium levels and by the action of adrenocorticotropic hormone (ACTH). The secretion of aldosterone is suppressed by extracellular volume expansion, increased sodium concentration, and decreased potassium concentration. Aldosterone causes sodium resorption in exchange for potassium and hydrogen ion secretion at the distal tubule. This effect helps to maintain both extracellular volume and osmolarity.

Antidiuretic hormone (ADH) that is released from the posterior pituitary has a potent direct effect on the kidney: it increases tubular resorption of water. This effect and its modulation are important in the regulation of fluid volume and osmolarity in the body. Intracranial osmoreceptors are the sensors that initiate the events that promote ADH secretion when plasma osmolarity increases. They also inhibit ADH secretion when plasma osmolarity decreases. The production and release of ADH also depend on the activity of volume receptors in the right and left atria. Decreased extracellular volume sensed in the right atrium leads to ADH secretion. Increased volume sensed in the left atrium leads to inhibition of ADH release. Volume-dependent responses usually override the effects of the osmoreceptor controlling system when the two are in conflict. ADH acts at the level of the collecting ducts, increasing the permeability of the apical membrane of the cell to water.

Potassium

In the normal adult, total body stores of potassium are approximately 50 to 55 mEq/kg, 98% of which is located intracellularly at a concentration of 150 mEq/L cell water. In the extracellular fluid compartment, a total of 70 mEq (including plasma) is present at a concentration of 3.5 to 5.0 mEq/L. Normal daily intake of potassium averages 100 mEq, 95% of which is excreted in the urine and 5% of which is lost in feces and sweat. In the kidney, most of the filtered potassium is resorbed in the proximal tubular system. Nevertheless, selective secretion or absorption in the distal tubule determines net renal excretion or conservation. Unlike its ability to conserve sodium, the kidney can only decrease potassium excretion to approximately 10 mEq/L. Potassium excretion is directly related to circulating levels of aldosterone, cellular and extracellular potassium content, and tubular urine flow rates. Acid–base disturbances also exert significant influence.

Acid–Base Balance

Acid–base balance is in effect the management of large amounts of hydrogen ion that are produced endogenously each day. There is a 40- to 60-mmol load of fixed nonvolatile organic acids (i.e., sulfuric, phosphoric, and lactic acid), some of which are ingested and some of which are produced by metabolic activity. In addition, 13,000 to 20,000 mmol carbon dioxide constitutes the volatile acid load. Normally, the free hydrogen ion concentration of extracellular body fluids, measured as pH, is maintained at 7.40 ± 0.05. Maintenance at this level is accomplished by the combined action of three mechanisms: (1) buffering systems that are present in body fluids and that immediately offset changes in hydrogen ion concentrations; (2) pulmonary ventilation changes that can promptly adjust the excretion of carbon dioxide; and (3) renal tubular function, which, over time, can contribute by modulating the urinary excretion or conservation of acid or base.

The bicarbonate–carbonic acid buffer system in extracellular fluid is one of the most important factors. Its relation to pH is described by the Henderson-Hasselbalch equation and its modifications:

$$pH = pK^a + \log \frac{[HCO_3^-]}{[H_2CO_3]}$$

$$pH = 6.1 + \log \frac{[HCO_3^-]}{0.03 \times PaCO_2}$$

$$7.4 = 6.1 + \log \frac{24 \text{ mEq/L}}{1.20 \text{ mEq/L}}$$

The value for $[H_2CO_3]$ can be determined as the arithmetic product of a proportionality constant and the $PaCO_2$. In clinical practice, direct measurements of arterial pH and $PaCO_2$ are readily available, and $[HCO_3^-]$ can be calculated or derived from a nomogram. The pH is determined by the ratio $[HCO_3^-]/[H_2CO_3]$, which normally is approximately 20:1. A change in either the numerator or the denominator can alter the ratio and the resulting pH value. In addition, a change of either $[H_2CO_3]$ or $PaCO_2$ can be compensated for by a corresponding change in the same direction of the other, restoring the ratio to 20:1 and the pH to 7.40. Thus, pulmonary regulation of $PaCO_2$ and renal tubular regulation of plasma HCO_3^- are important determinants of extracellular pH.

As effective as the $[HCO_3^-]/[H_2CO_3]$ buffer system is, and as available as its substrates are from metabolic sources, even in combination with all other extracellular buffers, it cannot maintain arterial pH at normal levels in the face of all challenges. Intracellular buffer systems play a major role. As much as 50% of fixed acid loads and 95% of hydrogen ion changes that result from excessive retention or excretion of carbon dioxide are buffered in the cells. The movement of hydrogen into and out of the cell involves cationic exchanges that cause reciprocal shifts of potassium. Thus, **acidosis,** in which hydrogen ions move from an area of high concentration (extracellular) to an area of low concentration (intracellular), causes potassium to move out of the cell. As a result, the concentration of extracellular fluid increases. **Alkalosis,** in which hydrogen ions move from an area of high concentration (intracellular) to one of low concentration (extracellular), causes the opposite movement of potassium into the cell. As a result, the extracellular concentration decreases. Thus, acidosis is associated with hyperkalemia, and alkalosis is associated with hypokalemia. The usual assumption of a direct relation between serum levels and total body stores of potassium is no longer valid. Changes in serum potassium concentration that are induced by acid–base alterations can have significant clinical implications, particularly with regard to myocardial irritability and function.

Fluids and Electrolytes in the Perioperative Period

There are three components of fluid and electrolyte therapy for surgical patients: (1) maintenance, (2) resuscitation, and (3) replacement. The first component involves meeting the requirements for fluid and electrolyte intake that balance daily obligatory losses. The second component involves recognizing and repairing imbalances and deficits that are already present. The third component involves providing for ongoing and additional losses that occur during the course of therapy. Each component must be addressed in the three phases of surgical care (i.e., preoperative, intraoperative, and postoperative).

With no unusual stresses or losses and normal renal function, the fluid and electrolyte balance is maintained by the intake of adequate amounts of water, sodium, potassium, and chloride to balance daily obligatory losses. Intake is calculated to balance outputs of 12 to 15 mL/kg/day urine, 3 mL/kg stool water, 0 to 1.5 mL/kg sweat, 10 mL/kg combined insensible losses from lungs and skin, and an endogenous input of approximately 3 mL/kg water derived from the oxidation of carbohydrate and fat. These estimates apply to adults; more universal guidelines for calculating fluid and electrolyte requirements have also been devised. Probably the most accurate are based on surface area, but they are cumbersome, requiring measurements of height as well as weight and a nomogram for transposing the measurements into a value for surface. For this reason, the common practice is to determine water and electrolyte needs as a function of age and weight. Guidelines for using both methods are shown in Table 3-2. If the entire intake is to be delivered intravenously, 5% dextrose in water is used to meet most of the fluid requirements because the kidney reabsorbs nearly all of the sodium and chloride that the body needs. To replace ongoing losses or existing deficits, 0.45% or 0.9% saline can be given to provide the necessary sodium and chloride. Potassium is added in divided amounts to the various solutions. In this way, its delivery is spread out over time.

Table 3-2. Daily Fluid and Electrolyte Maintenance

Calculated by surface area	
Fluid	1500 mL/m²/day
Sodium	50–75 mEq/m²/day
Potassium	50 mEq/m²/day
Chloride	50–75 mEq/m²/day
Calculated by body weight	
Fluid	
Children > 5 kg to young adulthood	
First 10 kg	100 mL/kg
Second 10 kg	50 mL/kg
Weight > 20 kg	20 mL/kg
Adults	
25–55 yr	35 mL/kg
55–65 yr	30 mL/kg
> 65 yr	25 mL/kg
Sodium	1.0–1.5 mEq/kg
Potassium	0.5–0.75 mEq/kg (~1/2 Na⁺)
Chloride	1.0–1.5 mEq/kg

Overall estimates of daily needs must be adjusted for fever and high ambient temperatures. Insensible skin and pulmonary losses increase with elevations of body temperature (10%–15%/° C, 8%/° F), often requiring an additional 500 mL or more of salt-free water per day in febrile patients. Similar needs for more water because of increased pulmonary insensible losses occur in patients with tracheostomies who are inspiring unhumidified air or gas mixtures, especially with hyperventilation. In a slightly different way, requirements for both salt and water increase when ambient temperatures rise to more than 32° C (85° F). This increase is caused by hypotonic salt losses from sweating. Additional intravenous fluid replacement with 0.45% saline solution is appropriate in this case.

As with all aspects of good surgical care, the management of fluid and electrolyte balance starts with assessment. The surgeon uses the information obtained from a thorough history and physical examination to identify current or potential problems and determine what laboratory data are needed to confirm the problem. In a patient who appears to have no special problems at the time of admission for elective surgery, the initial workup could reveal underlying cardiac, pulmonary, renal, or hepatic disease. These findings may significantly influence the conduct of fluid therapy during and after the operation. In these cases, if stressful surgery is contemplated (e.g., abdominal aortic aneurysmectomy, pulmonary or pancreatic resection), the need for central venous or pulmonary arterial pressure monitoring in the perioperative period becomes apparent. A history of diuretic and digitalis therapy can call attention to the presence of hypokalemia or hyponatremia. Low preoperative serum potassium levels can fall even lower during surgery, particularly in patients who are under general anesthesia, are hyper-

ventilated, and have hypocapnic respiratory alkalosis. If hyponatremia is present on admission, the margin of safety between asymptomatic and symptomatic low serum sodium concentrations is reduced, making even relatively small further decreases potentially hazardous. Depending on the extent of the planned surgery, a patient with chronic pulmonary obstructive disease may need an arterial blood gas evaluation as part of the preoperative workup. Similarly, blood urea nitrogen (BUN), serum creatinine, and electrolyte studies are indicated in a patient who has a history of chronic renal disease. With any of these disorders, any deficits and ongoing needs must be addressed in the preoperative period.

Fluid, electrolyte, and acid–base imbalances must be identified and treated promptly in patients who are acutely ill on admission. This requirement is even more important in patients who need urgent operation. The admitting history and physical examination should clarify the problem. Laboratory data should be obtained immediately. In patients who are vomiting or who have had prolonged gastric drainage, the presence of hypokalemic hypochloremic metabolic alkalosis should be anticipated, rapidly confirmed, and treated with replacement of volume, potassium, and chloride losses. In these circumstances, profound potassium depletion is present if the urine pH is acidic (this **paradoxical aciduria** is explained in more detail later). If emergency surgery is indicated, potassium replacement may need to be given in 10– to 20–mEq/hr boluses and the patient must be monitored electrocardiographically.

Isotonic volume depletion caused by **third-space fluid losses** (i.e., fluid sequestered into extracellular or interstitial space, not available in the intravascular space), is seen with peritonitis (bacterial or chemical), intestinal obstruction, extensive soft tissue inflammation, or trauma. This problem is common. Like hemorrhage, these extracellular fluid losses effectively reduce intravascular volumes, which must be replaced promptly. Balanced salt solutions (lactated Ringer's solution) are used to replace the isotonic losses. The indications of how much to give, however, are not always apparent. In this case, clinical observation of hemodynamic changes (i.e., tachycardia, narrowed pulse pressure, hypotension), decreasing urine output (i.e., < 0.5 mL/kg/hr), and laboratory evidence of isotonic volume contraction (i.e., rising hematocrit, serum BUN to creatinine ratio > 20:1, urine sodium concentrations < 20 mEq/L) make it clear that the losses are significant. With continuous monitoring as intravenous fluid therapy is given, improvements in hemodynamic parameters and hourly urine output indicate when volumes have been restored to more normal levels. To avoid clinically significant dilutional hyponatremia, care must be taken to limit the intravenous administration of hypotonic fluid to patients who need large volumes.

During surgery, attention is focused largely on maintaining circulating volumes and adequate tissue perfusion, as monitored by urine flow rates and central venous or pulmonary arterial pressures. Packed red blood cells and **colloid** and **crystalloid** solutions are used to replace whole blood losses. At least 1 L lactated Ringer's or normal saline solution is used to replace third-space isotonic fluid losses in patients who undergo major abdominal or thoracic surgery. The use of hypotonic intravenous fluid should be limited to the replacement of evaporative water losses. Used freely to replace isotonic losses, these hypotonic fluids lead to dilutional hyponatremia. In patients who have compromised pulmonary function, arterial blood gas and pH studies are performed intraoperatively to monitor gas exchange and acid–base status.

In the immediate postoperative period, the fluid, electrolyte, and acid–base needs of the patient, for the most part, are related to monitoring and maintaining hemodynamic stability and the adequacy of ventilation. In many patients who had relatively unstressful and uncomplicated elective surgical procedures (i.e., inguinal herniorrhaphy, cholecystectomy) and in whom oral intake will be resumed within 48 hours, this process is accomplished simply by physical examination and serial observations of pulse rate, arterial blood pressure, respiratory frequency, and urine output, and by the administration of intravenous fluids as described for maintenance in Table 3-2.

In patients who had more surgically stressful procedures that involved extensive tissue dissection or resection, particularly those with known compromise of cardiac, renal, or pulmonary function, the needs are greater. Additional monitoring with central venous or pulmonary arterial pressure, hourly urine flow collected with an indwelling catheter in the bladder, and serial arterial blood gas and pH measurement may be necessary. Inadequate respiratory gas exchange may require the use of tracheal intubation and mechanical ventilation. Infusions are needed to replace third-space fluid losses that can continue for 48 to 72 hours. In addition to daily maintenance needs, gastric, intestinal, biliary, and pancreatic drainage should be replaced. If these losses are greater than 1000 mL in 24 hours, consideration should be given to replacing them milliliter for milliliter with an appropriate intravenous infusion. The electrolyte content of these infusions generally can be determined by knowing the electrolyte composition of the fluid that is lost. To determine more accurately what must be replaced, fluid samples are analyzed for their electrolyte composition. Daily weights are used to assess fluid volume depletion or retention, recognizing that gains or losses greater than 250 g (approximately 0.5 lb) represent changes in body fluid content. As valuable as it is to monitor extracellular fluid status, weight gains and losses relative to third-space fluid losses and their management must also be considered. During the replacement of third-space losses, weight gains do not represent intravascular volume overload. Rather, they are caused by the replacement of needed extracellular volume to compensate for the volume that was lost or sequestered. Similarly, diuresis and associated weight loss is expected 3 or more days postoperatively, when third-space fluid accumulations are mobilized (i.e.,

moved into intracellular or intravascular compartments). This fluid should be excreted, and not replaced. When this fluid is mobilizing, intravascular volumes are likely to be high, making additional intravenous volume loading undesirable. On the other hand, in patients who are receiving parenteral nutrition with hyperosmolar glucose solutions, increased urine output should not be interpreted simply as appropriate excretion of excess fluids. In fact, the high urine output in these patients is more likely to be caused by osmotic diuresis that is independent of the patient's volume status. This condition requires prompt recognition and correction with intravenous fluids to avoid severe hyperosmolar volume contraction.

The attention to fluid needs continues until the patient's renal and gastrointestinal function returns to normal and all fluid, electrolyte, and nutritional requirements are being met by oral intake. At this point, with the exception of chronically ill patients, who may have ongoing needs, concerns for this aspect of patient care end.

Fluid and Electrolyte Disorders in the Surgical Patient

Disorders of Volume

Volume disorders are common in surgical patients. Patients may lose volume through the loss of blood or gastrointestinal fluid (e.g., vomiting, diarrhea). Conversely, patients may gain excessive volume through volume replacement or physiologic disorders, such as renal failure or **syndrome of inappropriate secretion of antidiuretic hormone** (SIADH).

Volume Depletion
Etiology
Blood lost at the time of surgery may be the most visible type of volume loss. However, gastrointestinal fluid losses, which are common in surgical patients, are related to vomiting, nasogastric suction, diarrhea, and external drainage from enteric, biliary, or pancreatic **fistulas.** For the most part, these losses are isotonic (Table 3-3) and result in extracellular fluid volume depletion. The intracellular compartment is affected only if osmolar concentrations change. Isotonic depletion of functional extracellular fluid volume also occurs with third-space losses. Particularly significant third-space losses occur in burns, crush injuries, long-bone fractures, peritonitis, severe pancreatitis, intestinal obstructions, pleural effusions, and large areas of soft tissue infection. Excessive urinary loss of water and electrolytes also can lead to volume depletion, as seen with diuretic therapy, high-output renal failure, and osmotic diuresis associated with nonelectrolyte hyperosmolar solute loading (e.g., glucose, mannitol, angiographic contrast media). Finally, some volume depletions involve losses of water in excess of solute. These losses include excessive renal free water excretion associated

Table 3-3. Composition of Body Fluids[a]

	[Na⁺]	[K⁺]	[Cl⁻]	[HCO₃⁻]
Plasma	135–150	3.5–5	98–106	22–30
Stomach[b]	10–150	4–12	120–160	0
Bile	120–170	3–12	80–120	30–40
Pancreas	135–150	3.5–5	60–100	35–110
Small intestine[c]	80–150	2–8	70–130	20–40
Colon	50–100	10–30	80–120	25–30
Perspiration	30–50	5	30–50	0
Diarrhea	25–130	10–60	20–90[d]	20–50

[a]Ionic composition varies with rate of secretion for most gastrointestinal sites.
[b][Na⁺] is inversely related to [H⁺].
[c] Differences reflect increased absorption of Na⁺ and Cl⁻ and secretion of K⁺ and HCO₃ in the progression from proximal to distal in the gut.
[d] Higher in small bowel diarrhea versus colon diarrhea.

Table 3-4. Signs of Extracellular Fluid Volume Depletion

10% ECF reduction: threshold changes that can be overlooked
　2% weight loss
　Thirst, mild reduction of urinary output
　Laboratory: slight elevations of hematocrit[a] and urine specific gravity
20% ECF reduction: findings that are always evident
　4% weight loss
　Apathy, drowsiness
　Decreased skin turgor, dry mucous membrane, longitudinal furrowing of the tongue
　Tachycardia, orthostatic hypotension
　Oliguria moderate, with urine output <30 mL/hr
　Laboratory:
　　Hematocrit: elevated[a] (as will be RBC,Hgb, WBC)
　　Urine: Specific gravity 1.020 or higher, osmolarity > 500 mOsm/L, [Na⁺] 10–15 mEq/L or lower
　　BUN/Cr: both values modestly elevated with BUN/Cr ratio > normal 10:1 (as high as 25:1)
30% ECF reduction: findings that are extreme
　6% weight loss
　Stupor or coma
　Skin cool, pale, cyanotic with poor turgor
　Eyes sunken
　Pulse rapid, weak, and thready; hypotension
　Oliguria pronounced, with urine output <10–15 mL/hr
　Laboratory:
　　hematocrit: further elevated[a]
　　Urine: findings as above, except changes indicative of acute tubular necrosis (e.g., [Na⁺] > 20 mEq/L, BUN/Cr ratio falling toward normal value of 10:1, specific gravity and osmolarity decreasing to < 1.020 and 500 mOsm/L, respectively)

[a]Rule of thumb: 1% hematocrit rise for each 500-mL ECF deficit if RBC loss is nil.
ECF, extracellular fluid. RBC, red blood cells. WBC, white blood cells. Hgb, hemoglobin. Bun, blood urea nitrogen. Cr, creatinine.

with primary deficiencies of ADH (i.e., central diabetes insipidus) or nephrogenic causes of diabetes insipidus, increased evaporative losses from burned surfaces, and increased sweating and evaporative losses from the skin and respiratory tract in febrile patients. These hypotonic losses create a hypernatremic hyperosmolar state in the extracellular compartment that draws water from the cell. This repletion of the extracellular space can blunt the clinical picture of volume depletion, which typically reflects extracellular deficits.

Presentation and Diagnosis

Extracellular volume depletion involves equivalent percentage reductions of interstitial and plasma fluid volumes. Signs of an interstitial fluid deficit include decreased tissue turgor, dry skin and mucous membranes, fissuring of the tongue, reduced tongue volume and, if severe, sunken eyes. Signs of plasma volume deficits include reduced tissue perfusion similar to that seen with whole blood loss. The clinical signs and symptoms are directly related to the magnitude and rate at which the deficit occurs (Table 3-4). Further, as shown in Table 3-5, many of these findings are not reliable in elderly or chronically debilitated patients. Body weight can be a valuable measure of extracellular external deficits, but not if third-space sequestration occurs. Neurologic and cardiovascular signs are more prominent with acute losses, whereas tissue signs may not be evident for at least 24 hours. In such acute circumstances, the clinician is more dependent on hemodynamic parameters, elevated hematocrit, **oliguria,** and urinary concentration studies as guidelines. As renal perfusion becomes more restricted and levels of BUN and serum creatinine rise, it is important to verify that these signs are manifestations of prerenal azotemia, and not acute renal failure. Urine sodium concentrations less than 20 mEq/L, BUN to creatinine ratio greater than 20:1, and urine **osmolality** greater than 400 mOsm/L (in the absence of glucosuria or the excretion of other osmotically active particles) are char-

acteristic of prerenal azotemia. With acute renal injury, however, urine sodium increases (usually > 40 mEq/L) as renal tubular resorption of sodium is impaired, BUN to creatinine ratio falls to 10:1 or less (because creatinine starts to rise), and urine osmolality approaches plasma osmolality.

Treatment

Information gathered from the history and physical examination, knowledge of the volume and composition of body fluids lost (see Table 3-3), and appropriate laboratory tests are critical in determining proper fluid therapy. Correction of volume depletion also requires information about the composition of available intravenous fluids (Table 3-6). Treatment of isotonic extracellular volume deficits caused by intestinal, biliary, pancreatic, or third-space losses with intravenous infusion of lactated Ringer's solution or normal saline is usually appropriate. However, lactate-containing solu-

Table 3-5. Signs and Symptoms of Extracellular Fluid Volume Depletion in Young Adults versus the Elderly

Areas Affected	Young Adult Patients <65 yr	Elderly Patients > 65 yr
Vascular volume	Postural hypotension	Common in fit elderly
	Hypotension	May be masked by preexisting hypertension
	Tachycardia	Maximal heart rate response decreases with age
	Reduced pulse volume	Masked by rigid vessels
	Reduced CVP or PaOP	May not reflect left heart function or volume status
	Absence of signs of heart failure or fluid overload	Local causes of ankle edema (e.g., varicose veins) and hypoproteinemia should be excluded
	Oliguria	May be less marked if age-related renal impairment is present
Interstitial volume (tissue changes)	Dry skin and mucous membranes	Common in elderly
	Dry tongue	Unreliable at any age
	Reduced tongue volume	May be useful
	Sunken eyes	Late sign in young and old
	Reduced skin turgor	Questionable validity in elderly
Miscellaneous	Reduced tendon reflexes and distal anesthesia (late signs)	Both may be age- related changes
	Drowsiness, apathy, anorexia	Also casued by infection, medication, hypothyroidism, or depression
	Stupor and coma	Late, nonspecific
	Ileus	Late, nonspecific

Central venous pressure. PaOP, pulmonary artery occlusion pressure.

Table 3-6. Composition of Commonly Used Intravenous Solutions

	Glucose (gm;L)	Na+ (mEq/L)	K+ (mEq/L)	Cl- (mEq/L)	Lactate[a] (mEq/L)	Ca++ (mEq/L)
0.9% Sodium chloride ("normal" saline)		154		154		
Lactated Ringer's solution		130	4.0	109	28	3.0
5% dextrose water	50					
5% dextrose in 0.45% sodium chloride	50	77		77		
3% sodium chloride		513		513		

Converted to bicarbonate.

tions should not be used to replace gastric losses that occur from vomiting or nasogastric suctioning. Inadequate chloride in lactated Ringer's solution plus in vivo conversion of a lactate to bicarbonate does not correct the hypochloremic hypokalemic metabolic alkalosis that occurs in this situation. A solution that more closely approximates the electrolyte composition of gastric fluid (e.g., ½ NS with 20 mEq KCl/L) is a better choice. Glucose solutions should not be used to correct volume deficits that result from an osmotic diuresis that is induced by hyperglycemia. Therapeutic needs are better served by infusion of isotonic crystalloid to restore vascular volume, followed by correction of osmolar and potassium abnormalities. As a rule, the rate of volume correction should be commensurate with the need and the ability of the patient to accept the fluid loads that are being delivered. When the deficits are moderate, complete replacement should be carried

out over at least a 24-hour period. The longer the deficits have taken to occur, the more cautious the clinician should be in replacing them. If deficits are large and the consequences severe, the needs are more urgent. In these cases, the therapeutic priorities are first to correct hemodynamic and perfusion inadequacies as rapidly and safely as possible. Correcting these inadequacies may require rapid infusion of 1 L or more isotonic crystalloid solution to achieve hemodynamic stability. It is also wise to avoid using glucose-containing solutions during rapid correction of such a deficit, because these solutions can lead to an iatrogenic hyperglycemic-induced osmotic diuresis that may cause further fluid loss. The next priority is to correct potassium abnormalities that may be present, after adjusting for the pH effect (see the earlier section on normal physiology). Normalization of glucose and osmolality changes as well as volume correction of interstitial fluid and total body water can be carried out over the next 18 to 24 hours, or as symptoms dictate.

Measurements of weight change and cumulative fluid intake and output provide valuable information over an extended period. However, during vascular volume repletion, repeated physical examination to assess the physiologic response to fluid infusion, central venous or pulmonary artery monitoring (if necessary), and urine output measurements are the mainstay of monitoring the adequacy of replacement therapy. If there is no acute renal failure or significant chronically compromised renal function, osmotic diuresis, use of diuretics, septic-induced polyuria, or hypothermia, urine output at rates greater than 0.5/mL/kg/hr (1.0 mL/kg/hr in children) indicates adequate repletion of vascular volume. Similarly, in the absence of continuing blood loss, declining hemoglobin and hematocrit values signify extracellular volume correction. Reduction of BUN and creatinine toward normal levels is also consistent with restoration of adequate renal perfusion and extracellular volume expansion.

Prognosis

The prognosis for patients with volume depletion depends on the initial amount of depletion and the success of efforts toward volume resuscitation and cessation of ongoing losses. Some patients have such severe volume depletion or shock that, even with apparently adequate fluid resuscitation, the outcome is fatal. Most patients, however, have problems that permit correction and resuscitation (e.g., a patient with a massive gastrointestinal bleed who is given fluid and taken to the operating room, where a bleeding duodenal ulcer is oversewn).

Volume Excess

Etiology

Volume excess for any fluid compartment can be the result of excessive or inappropriate fluids for that compartment, abnormal fluid retention, or a combination of both factors. Excessive intravenous fluid therapy with balanced salt solutions is a common iatrogenic cause of isotonic fluid excess. This therapy causes extracellular expansion. This expansion, in the absence of attendant osmolar changes, is not shared intracellularly. This isotonic extracellular expansion causes both hypervolemia and excess interstitial fluid. These consequences are more likely to occur immediately after surgery or trauma, when maximal hormonal responses to stress (i.e., increases in both ADH and aldosterone) are operating to diminish sodium and water excretion by the kidney. The risk of fluid excess is even greater in the elderly and in patients in whom underlying cardiac, renal, or hepatic disorders contribute to fluid accumulation. Congestive heart failure, oliguric renal failure, and hypoalbuminemia secondary to hepatocellular dysfunction are other recognized causes of extracellular fluid volume expansion.

Hypotonic and hypertonic fluid overloading can also occur. Inappropriate administration of salt-poor solutions to replace isotonic gastrointestinal or third-space fluid loss is a common cause of hyponatremic volume expansion. Enhanced secretion of ADH in surgically stressful situations and inappropriate ADH activity associated with intracranial disorders or ectopic production by malignancies are also causes of selective restriction of water excretion. These conditions can lead to hypotonic fluid expansion. On the other hand, administration of sodium loads that are not balanced by appropriate water intake causes hypernatremic extracellular volume expansion. In this case, water moving out of the cells in response to increased extracellular osmolar concentrations may contribute to intravascular and interstitial fluid overload. The resulting hypervolemic state is even more pronounced when renal tubular excretion of salt or water is compromised. Hypertonic extracellular volume expansion can also be induced by the rapid infusion of nonelectrolyte osmotically active solutes (e.g., glucose, mannitol). This situation, however, is accompanied by hyponatremia, not hypernatremia. Plasma sodium concentration decreases as a result of dilution by the solution that is being infused and the sodium-free water drawn from the cells into the extracellular space in response to the osmolar gradient created by the infused nonelectrolyte solute load.

Presentation and Diagnosis

The clinical picture of extracellular volume excess can vary, depending on the cause, nature, and severity of the challenges. Thus, the signs can range widely. At the lower end of the severity scale are simple weight gain, small decreases of hemoglobin and hematocrit levels (signifying hemodilution), modest elevations of peripheral and **central venous pressure,** and dependent sacral or lower extremity edema. At the other end, there are extreme consequences of vascular and interstitial fluid overload, with frank congestive heart failure, as evidenced by pulmonary edema, pleural effusion, anasarca, and hepatomegaly.

Treatment

Treatment is adjusted according to the severity of fluid compartment changes and related clinical findings. Lesser problems are treated with fluid or sodium restriction. More severe problems require diuresis with loop diuretics as well as replacement of associated potassium losses. Cardiotonic drugs, oxygen therapy, artificial ventilation, or dialysis (if renal insufficiency is present) may also be needed to manage cardiac or respiratory failure. The therapeutic management of related hyponatremic and hypernatremic states is discussed in the next section.

Prognosis

After the volume overload is corrected, most patients do well. The exceptions are patients whose volume overload leads to significant pulmonary edema or adult respiratory distress syndrome (ARDS) and those who have myocardial events associated with the volume overload.

Disorders of Electrolyte Concentrations

Electrolyte imbalances are rarely isolated because the body must maintain electrical neutrality; complex homeostatic and metabolic mechanisms exist to maintain this electrical neutrality. A good history is essential in determining the etiology and proper treatment of electrolyte imbalances. Attempts to correct a low serum level by simple oral or parenteral replacement of an ion may not improve the patient's condition because associated abnormalities are not treated. Although electrolyte abnormalities are corrected easily, if untreated, they may be fatal. Artifactual abnormalities of serum electrolytes may result from improper handling of blood specimens or from obtaining specimens from veins into which solutions are being infused. The range of normal values also varies somewhat from one laboratory to another.

Sodium

Sodium ion is the principal solute that determines extracellular fluid (ECF) osmolarity and volume balance in the body. An increase in extracellular sodium concentration creates an osmotic gradient that draws water across cell membranes and out of cells. A decrease in extracellular sodium concentration does the reverse. These changes in cell volume produce the symptoms of abnormal serum sodium. Disorders of sodium balance are usually associated with disorders of fluid balance.

Hyponatremia

Hyponatremia results from the presence of excess body water relative to body sodium, and the failure of the kidneys to excrete the excess water. The serum sodium concentration does not always reflect true total body sodium content, or even osmolarity. For example, total body sodium may be increased in patients with chronic cardiac, hepatic, or renal disease, but hyponatremia persists because of a proportionally greater increase in water.

Etiology. Hyponatremia may be associated with decreased, increased, or normal ECF volume. The causes of hyponatremia are shown in Table 3-7.

In surgical patients, dilutional hyponatremia occurs most commonly when hypotonic fluids are used to replace isotonic gastrointestinal or third-space losses. Catabolic breakdown of body tissues, which occurs with surgical stress and caloric deprivation, metabolically generates approximately 1 mL sodium-free water for each gram of fat or muscle that is catabolized. Further, the ability of the kidney to excrete excess water in response to decreased serum osmolarity is impaired after surgery or other trauma. Secretion of ADH is increased and uncontrolled by feedback inhibition.

Dilutional hyponatremia may occur with volume deficits if isotonic fluid losses are replaced with hypo-

Table 3-7. Causes of Hyponatremia

Dilution
  Accumulation of excess water
    Hypotonic fluid replacement of isotonic gastrointestinal and third-space fluid losses
    Enhanced metabolic production of free water occuring with surgical stress and caloric deprivation
    Ingestion or infusion of excess free water (e.g., psychogenic polydipsia)
    Retention of excess water secondary to enhanced ADH activity
    Physiologic response to surgical stress or hypovolemia
    Syndrome of inappropriate ADH secretion (SIADH)
    Advanced cardiac, renal, and hepatic disease
Excessive renal loss of sodium
  Thiazide diuretics
  Metabolic alkalosis
  Ketoacidosis
  Adrenal insufficiency
  Salt-wasting nephrophathy
Artifactual
  Hyperlipidemia
  Hyperproteinemia

ADH, antidiuretic hormone.

tonic fluid. It also occurs in patients who have advanced cardiac, renal, or hepatic disease and increased total body sodium, because these patients accumulate proportionally more water.

Artifactually very low serum sodium values are seen in the presence of severe hyperglycemia and hypertriglyceridemia, or after intravenous infusion of lipids. In these cases, the water in the intravascular space is partially replaced, so the concentration of sodium in the total sample is low, even though the proportion of sodium to water may be normal, or even high.

Presentation and Diagnosis. The primary clinical manifestations of hyponatremia are the signs and symptoms of central nervous system dysfunction. Osmotic forces draw water into the cells, and cerebrospinal fluid pressures increase because of cerebral and spinal cord swelling. Neurologic disturbances occur as a result. The severity of these disturbances is directly related to both the degree of the hyponatremia and the rapidity with which it develops. Serum sodium between 130 and 120 mEq/L may cause irritability, weakness, fatigue, increased deep-tendon reflexes, and muscle twitches if the hyponatremia developed rapidly (10–15 mEq/L in < 48 hours, or faster), but the patient may be completely asymptomatic if it developed slowly. Serum sodium levels of less than 120 mEq/L, if untreated, produce seizures, coma, areflexia, and death.

In diagnosing hyponatremia, serum and urine sodium, serum and urine osmolality, and pH are assessed. Blood tests can exclude associated electrolyte abnormalities (e.g., hyperglycemia, liver diseases, acid–base disorders). Volume status should also be assessed.

Treatment. Treatment of hyponatremia depends on the cause, severity, and nature of any associated volume abnormality. Psychogenic polydipsia is treated with water restriction. Most dilutional hyponatremia that is iatrogenically induced in the perioperative period, seen as an asymptomatic decrease in serum sodium along with modest extracellular volume expansion, is readily treated by simple fluid restriction. Thiazide diuretics cause hyponatremia by blocking the resorption of sodium and chloride in the cortical-diluting segment. However, because the resorption of salt in the ascending limb of the loop of Henle is not blocked, excretion of very concentrated urine is possible. This concentration permits the retention of water while sodium, potassium, and chloride are depleted. The best treatment for this condition is discontinuation of the diuretic. In patients who have chronic hyponatremia, even when serum sodium concentration is low, correction of serum sodium is 12 mEq/L/day or less. Treatment of SIADH may require severe fluid restriction to 500 mL/day or less. For patients with chronic SIADH, long-term management options include lithium carbonate and demeclocycline. Both drugs block the effect of ADH on the collecting duct, and both have side effects, but demeclocycline 600 to 1200 mg daily is usually effective and well tolerated. Disorders that involve body sodium excess in addition to disproportionate volume excess are treated by restriction of both sodium and water.

Hyponatremia associated with volume contraction is treated with combined sodium and volume repletion, usually with normal saline or lactated Ringer's solution. The rate of repletion is dictated by the degree of volume deficit. In most cases, rapid restoration of volume and sodium is not only unnecessary, but is also hazardous because it can cause rapid shifts of intracellular water and undesirable neurologic consequences.

Hypertonic 3% saline solutions are indicated only when hyponatremia causes life-threatening neurologic disturbances. To estimate the amount of sodium needed to correct the serum deficit, multiply the decrease in serum sodium (in milliequivalents) by total body water (in liters) as a percentage of total body weight:

$$\text{mEq Na}^+ \text{ needed} = (140 - \text{measured serum Na}^+) \times \text{TBW}$$

where TBW = 0.6 × body weight (kg)

TBW is used because both intracellular and extracellular imbalances must be corrected. No more than one-half of the total calculated amount of sodium is given in the first 12 to 18 hours. The goal is to increase the serum sodium level sufficiently to eliminate the symptoms. Over the next 24 to 48 hours, the remainder of the deficit is corrected with normal saline. Any underlying conditions must also be treated. Responsible drugs should be discontinued, if possible. Rapid correction of chronic hyponatremia (e.g., > 12 mEq/L/day) can cause osmotic demyelination syndrome. The patient usually improves for a day or so, but then deteriorates, with a spectrum of neurologic findings, which can include fluctuating levels of consciousness, seizures, pseudo-bulbar palsy, and paralysis. Some patients improve after several weeks, but others have significant permanent disability.

Prognosis. Once treated, the prognosis of hyponatremia usually depends on the prognosis of the underlying condition. Severe neurologic symptoms may have irreversible sequelae.

Hypernatremia

Hypernatremia results from excess body sodium content relative to body water. Clinically significant hypernatremia, serum sodium greater than 150 mEq/L, is less common than hyponatremia, but it can be just as lethal if it is allowed to progress unchecked.

Etiology. Hypernatremia may result from the loss of water alone (e.g., hypothalamic abnormalities, unreplaced insensible losses); from the loss of water and salt together (e.g., gastrointestinal losses, osmotic diuresis, excessive diuretic use, central or nephrogenic diabetes insipidus, burns, excessive sweating); as a side effect of many drugs (e.g., alcohol, amphotericin B, colchicine, lithium, phenytoin); or from increased sodium without any water loss (e.g., Cushing's syndrome, hyperaldosteronism, ectopic production of ACTH, iatrogenic sodium administration, ingestion of seawater).

When body fluids become hypertonic, thirst is stimulated to compensate. Therefore, severe hypernatremia occurs only in situations in which a person cannot obtain water (e.g., infancy, disability, altered mental states).

Presentation and Diagnosis. The pathophysiologic consequences of hypernatremia reflect both extracellular volume losses and cellular dehydration that result from water shifts in response to osmotic pressure. As with hyponatremia, the severity of the clinical manifestations is directly related to both the degree of the hypernatremia and the rapidity with which it develops. Serum sodium concentrations greater than 160 mEq/L are cause for concern, and may be symptomatic. Signs and symptoms include those of dehydration, including decreased salivation and lacrimation; dry mucous membranes; dry, flushed skin; decreased tissue turgor; oliguria (except when dehydrating renal water loss is the cause); fever; and tachycardia. Signs and symptoms also include those of neuromuscular and neurologic disorders, from twitching, restlessness, and weakness, to delirium, coma, seizures, and death. Intracranial hemorrhage is a common postmortem finding in patients who die of hypernatremia; the hemorrhage is thought to result from cell shrinkage, with associated decreases in brain volume and decreased intracranial pressure, which disrupts the intracranial blood vessels.

In addition to the history and measurement of serum sodium, urine sodium and urine and plasma osmolality should be determined. Hematocrit may be high because of dehydration. The underlying cause should be diagnosed.

Treatment. Treatment of hypernatremia consists of correcting the water deficit, which can be estimated in several ways. The simplest accurate general rule is that for every liter of water deficit, serum sodium rises 3 mEq above the normal value of 140 mEq/L. If deficits are modest, they can be replaced orally or with intravenous 5% dextrose in water. If deficits are more severe, the TBW deficit is calculated as follows:

$$\text{mEq change in serum Na}^+ = (140 - \text{serum Na}^+ \times \text{TBW}$$

where TBW = $0.6 \times$ body weight (kg)

The water deficit (in liters) is equal to the milliequivalent change in serum $Na^+/140$. The water must be replaced slowly, with no more than one-half given over the first 12 to 24 hours. For pure water loss, 5% dextrose is infused intravenously. Therefore, if a 70-kg patient has a serum sodium value of 150, the water deficit is calculated as follows:

$$\text{mEq change in serum Na}^+ = (140 - 150) \times 0.6 \times 70$$
$$= 10 \times 42$$
$$= 420$$
$$\text{Water deficit in liters} = \frac{420}{140} = 3 \text{ L}$$

In patients with associated sodium deficits, if symptoms of dehydration predominate, the volume deficit is initially replaced with normal saline. If neurologic symptoms are more prominent, half-normal saline is used. If the sodium loss is large (e.g., diabetic hyperosmolar coma), the volume is replaced initially with normal saline. The nature of the fluid required may change as different needs become apparent, and the process of reversing hypernatremia requires close monitoring. If water is replaced too rapidly, osmotic shifts can produce cellular edema. Brain cells accumulate intracellular solute slowly in response to slowly developing extracellular hypertonicity; a sudden decrease in extracellular osmolality leads to rapid swelling of brain cells, causing serious neurologic dysfunction.

As with other electrolyte disturbances, underlying problems must also be treated.

Prognosis. The prognosis depends on the severity of symptoms, the correct treatment, and the prognosis of the underlying disorder. Neurologic symptoms, once they develop, may be irreversible.

Potassium

As the principal intracellular cation, potassium is a major determinant of intracellular volume. It is a significant cofactor in cellular metabolism. Extracellular potassium plays an important role in neuromuscular function.

Hypokalemia

Hypokalemia is defined as a serum potassium level less than 3.5 mEq/L. When potassium is deficient, there may also be losses of magnesium and phosphorus. The exact relation between magnesium and potassium is unclear; however, many factors that cause renal potassium wasting also cause renal magnesium wasting (e.g., loop and thiazide diuretic use). The opposite is also true (e.g., potassium and magnesium sparing with amiloride). Hypophosphatemia and hypocalcemia often accompany hypokalemia. Potassium deprivation may impair calcium resorption by the kidney, resulting in a negative calcium balance. This change, in turn, alters phosphorous metabolism.

Etiology. Hypokalemia may reflect potassium deficiency that results from inadequate intake, gastrointestinal tract losses, or renal losses. Hypokalemia may also reflect shifts from the extracellular to the intracellular compartment (e.g., insulin administration).

Gastrointestinal losses (e.g., diarrhea, vomiting, biliary or pancreatic fistulae, villous adenoma, malabsorption) can be major factors in hypokalemia. The highest gastrointestinal concentrations of potassium are found in the colon and rectum. Prolonged vomiting or nasogastric aspiration causes hypokalemia through a combination of factors. In addition to the loss of potassium in the gastric fluid, the loss of hydrogen and chloride ions produces hypochloremic hypokalemic metabolic alkalosis. The increase in extracellular pH causes movement of potassium into the cells, which makes the hypokalemia worse. As a general rule, an increase in pH of 0.1 unit causes a decrease in serum potassium of 0.4 to 0.5 mEq. As the hypokalemia worsens, in the alkalotic state, the kidneys conserve hydrogen ions by excreting potassium. Further, high bicarbonate and low chloride concentrations in the renal tubules cause greater resorption of sodium in the distal tubule, causing additional urinary potassium loss. Finally, extracellular volume deficits stimulate aldosterone activity, which also increases renal potassium excretion. The interaction of these mechanisms, if uncorrected, produces noticeable intracellular and extracellular potassium depletion. At this point, because of the need to conserve potassium, renal tubular hydrogen ion excretion increases. Urinary potassium loss decreases, and paradoxical aciduria appears (i.e., acidic urine in the presence of severe alkalosis).

Renal potassium losses are caused by hyperglycemia, primary or secondary aldosteronism, renal tubular acidosis, elevated ACTH, licorice ingestion, acute leukemia, or corticoid excess. Hypokalemia is often iatrogenic, the result of treatment with thiazides, loop diuretics, or carbonic anhydrase inhibitors. By an unknown mechanism, magnesium deficiency decreases distal renal tubular potassium resorption. If the magnesium deficiency is not corrected, renal losses continue, and it is difficult to correct the hypokalemia.

Presentation and Diagnosis. Hypokalemia rarely becomes clinically significant until serum potassium decreases to less than 3.0 mEq/L. In general, the severity of symptoms is proportional to the degree of deficit and the rapidity with which it develops. Additionally, the consequences of hypokalemia are exacerbated by alkalosis, hypocalcemia, and digoxin therapy. Hypokalemia may cause neuromuscular symptoms that range from skeletal muscle weakness and fatigue to paresthesias, paralysis, and rhabdomyolysis. Deep-tendon reflexes may be diminished or absent. Hypokalemia causes increased production of ammonia in the renal tubules. This increase may worsen hepatic encephalopathy. Other symptoms include anorexia, polyuria, and nausea and vomiting associated with paralytic ileus. Total body potassium depletion produces cellular atrophy and negative nitrogen balance. Renal tubular function is impaired, which may result in polyuria and polydipsia because of decreased concentrating ability.

Cardiac abnormalities are the most important and worrisome consequences of hypokalemia, and in the presence of digoxin, intoxication may appear, even with relatively mild deficits. Progressive electrocardiogram (ECG) abnormalities include low-voltage, flattened, or inverted T-waves, with prominent U waves, depressed S-T segments, prolonged P-R intervals, and (at levels of ≤ 2.0 mEq/L) widened QRS complexes. A rapid decrease in serum potassium may lead to cardiac arrest.

If the deficiency is mild and the cause is clear from the history, serum potassium may be the only test required, with the digoxin level measured if the patient is being treated with this medication. If hypokalemia is more severe or refractory to treatment, other serum electrolytes, including calcium and magnesium, should be measured. An arterial blood gas determination may exclude acid–base disturbances, and urinary electrolytes can be used to exclude renal hyperexcretion. If the hypokalemic patient has normal blood pressure, serum bicarbonate and urine potassium should help distinguish among metabolic causes, gastrointestinal losses, dietary deficiency, and osmotic or drug-induced diuresis. If the patient is hypertensive, plasma renin and aldosterone levels may help identify the cause.

Treatment. Treatment of hypokalemia involves replacing lost potassium and correcting the underlying cause. Whenever possible, potassium is repleted orally, with pills or liquid. Most people find the taste of potassium solutions unpleasant. Enteric-coated tablets should not be used because they can cause small bowel ulceration. In patients with normal kidneys, the oral dose should not exceed 40 mEq/4 hr. If the intravenous route is necessary, the rate should not exceed 10 mEq/hr, with the dose repeated as often as necessary to increase the serum level to within the normal range. Electrocardiographic monitoring is helpful during intravenous potassium repletion, and it is mandatory if a rate higher than 10 mEq/hr is used. Too rapid intravenous administration can cause hyperkalemia and fatal cardiac arrhythmias. Generally, dextrose-containing solutions are not used as the diluent; intravenous dextrose increases endogenous insulin, which induces the movement of potassium into cells and causes the serum level to decrease further, making repletion more diffi-

cult. A serum potassium level lower than 2.9 mEq/L may reflect depletions of the huge intracellular pool and thus require much more supplementation, with closer monitoring.

If hypokalemia is caused by hypomagnesemia, magnesium repletion will correct it. When hypokalemia and hypocalcemia occur together, they must both be treated; treatment of only one may cause the patient to become symptomatic from the other.

Prognosis. Most hypokalemia is moderate and relatively easy to correct. The prognosis depends on the severity of symptoms, correct treatment, and the prognosis of the underlying disorder.

Hyperkalemia

Hyperkalemia is a serum potassium level greater than 5.0 mEq/L.

Etiology. As in hypokalemia, the etiology of hyperkalemia is usually multifactorial. It can be caused by exogenous loading (e.g., from excessive dietary intake in a patient with renal failure or from parenteral sources, such as high-dose penicillin therapy), transfusions of many units of stored banked blood, or too vigorous correction of hypokalemia. Endogenous loading occurs whenever large amounts of intracellular potassium are released into the extracellular space (e.g., crush injuries, hemolysis, lysis and absorption of large hematomata, catabolism of fat and muscle tissue because of stress or starvation, rapid rewarming after severe hypothermia). Hyperkalemia can be caused by decreased renal excretion, which may result from adrenal insufficiency and impaired aldosterone activity, but most often it is caused by intrinsic renal disease. Shifts of potassium from the intracellular to the extracellular compartment also cause hyperkalemia (e.g., acute metabolic or respiratory acidosis, insulin deficiency, therapy with digitalis and related cardiotonic agents). In diabetic ketoacidosis, hyperkalemia may be seen, even with total body potassium deficit.

Numerous drugs cause hyperkalemia. Impaired renal excretion can be caused by diuretics (e.g., spironolactone, triamterene, amiloride) and by nonsteroidal anti-inflammatory drugs, β-adrenergic antagonists, and angiotensin converting enzyme (ACE) inhibitors. Digitalis preparations, arginine, β-adrenergic antagonists, and some poisons, for example, can cause shifts of potassium out of the intracellular compartment.

Artifactually high serum potassium results from hemolysis of the blood specimen, from obtaining a blood specimen from a vein into which potassium is being infused, and occasionally from high platelet or leukocyte counts.

Presentation and Diagnosis. Although hyperkalemia causes peripheral muscle weakness that ultimately progresses to respiratory paralysis, the most important signs and symptoms are cardiac. The first ECG abnormality is peaked T waves, best seen in the precordial leads, at serum concentrations between 6.0 and 7.0 mEq/L. Further elevations produce multiple ECG abnormalities, including flattened P waves, increased P-R intervals, decreased Q-T intervals, widened QRS complexes, depressed S-T segments, and complete heart block with atrial asystole. At elevations of more than 8.0 mEq/L, more widened QRS complexes merge with T waves to produce a sine wave appearance. This change is followed by ventricular fibrillation and cardiac arrest.

Diagnosis is made by measuring serum potassium levels. It is usually relatively simple to determine the cause, but since significant hyperkalemia is uncommon if the kidneys are normal, serum BUN, creatinine, and urine output should be measured. Anuric patients accumulate potassium, but a source must be sought in hyperkalemic nonoliguric patients. Even in the presence of renal insufficiency, medication or excessive dietary intake is often responsible. A 12-lead cardiogram must be performed. If the patient is being treated with digoxin, a digoxin level should be obtained. If the patient had a crush injury, serum and urinary myoglobin should also be measured.

If spurious hyperkalemia is suspected (e.g., from a hemolyzed specimen, from blood drawn above an intravenous site), blood should be redrawn for a serum potassium level measurement or a plasma potassium level ordered. However, treatment of a very high serum potassium level should not be delayed while waiting for results.

Treatment. The primary goal of the treatment of hyperkalemia is to reduce serum potassium to levels that are not life-threatening. In mild hyperkalemia (< 6 mEq/L), the simplest measures are to restrict potassium intake, eliminate causes such as potassium-sparing diuretics, and treat volume or acid–base disorders. Potassium-wasting diuretics may be administered, and hormone deficiencies may be replaced.

For the treatment of potassium levels between 6.5 and 7.5 mEq/L, 10 units insulin is administered intravenously along with 25 g glucose intravenously over 5 minutes. This therapy shifts potassium from the extracellular to the intracellular compartment and may reduce serum potassium by as much as 1 mEq/L. A similar shift may be created by administering a bicarbonate infusion or by injecting 45 mEq sodium bicarbonate intravenously over 5 minutes to induce metabolic alkalosis. These compartment shifts last only a few hours. Sodium polystyrene sulfonate, a cation-exchange resin, administered orally or rectally, actually removes potassium from the body. Each gram of the resin binds approximately 1 mEq potassium. The oral dose is 25 g resin suspended in 50 mL 20% sorbitol solution every 4 to 6 hours. The rectal dose is 50 g in 100 to 200 mL 35% sorbitol given as a retention enema every 4 hours. Patients with potassium levels greater than 6.5 mEq/L are monitored with continuous ECG.

Serum potassium levels greater than 7.5 mEq/L in a patient with evidence of cardiac toxicity should be treated with an intravenous infusion of 10 to 30 mL 10% calcium gluconate given slowly over 5 minutes to reduce cardiac muscle electrical excitability temporarily while other methods are used to rid the body of potassium. Rapid infusion of calcium is dangerous and is justified only when hyperkalemia is severe. Electrocardiographic monitoring is advisable during the treatment of hyperkalemia, and it is mandatory if calcium is being infused.

Hemodialysis and peritoneal dialysis also remove potassium from the body, and may be necessary in patients with renal failure. They may be used along with more rapid methods to reduce serum potassium in moderate to severe hyperkalemia. In treating hyperkalemia with dehydration and acidosis in diabetic ketoacidosis, care must be taken not to allow serum potassium to decrease to subnormal levels.

Prognosis. Hyperkalemia itself does not affect recovery, and it is usually correctable. However, cardiac events caused by hyperkalemia may be fatal if the hyperkalemia and its effects are not promptly treated. The prognosis of patients with hyperkalemia is often related to the underlying cause (e.g., renal failure).

Chloride

Chloride is the major extracellular anion. It is ubiquitous in the diet, absorbed in the small and large intestines, and excreted by the kidneys. Chloride balance usually parallels sodium balance, except when hypochloremia results from the loss of acidic gastric contents. The normal range of serum chloride is 98 to 108 mEq/L. Although no signs or symptoms are specific to abnormalities of chloride balance, changes in extracellular chloride content can significantly affect fluid, electrolyte, and acid–base balance and their management.

Hypochloremia

Hypochloremia is a serum chloride concentration of less than 95 mEq/L. In severe respiratory acidosis, metabolic compensation involves renal tubular resorption of bicarbonate to decrease the extracellular acidosis that is caused by carbon dioxide retention and chloride depletion. As respiratory acidosis resolves and carbon dioxide retention decreases, renal excretion of excess bicarbonate allows the pH to return to normal. Hypochloremia impairs renal bicarbonate excretion, however, and if serum bicarbonate remains high in the presence of decreased carbon dioxide tension, metabolic alkalosis results and persists until the chloride deficit is repleted.

Etiology. Hypochloremia classically results from the loss of acidic gastric contents, either by vomiting or by nasogastric suction. It can result from renal losses caused by diuretics, nonoliguric acute and chronic renal failure, or compensatory renal tubular resorption of bicarbonate in states of respiratory acidosis.

Presentation and Diagnosis. The signs and symptoms are those of the accompanying disorder. The diagnosis is made by measuring serum chloride.

Treatment. In general, hypochloremia is treated with solutions that contain sodium chloride and potassium chloride in a ratio determined by the underlying problem and by serum electrolyte concentrations. Ammonium chloride is not used in patients with advanced liver disease or hepatic failure because it may precipitate or increase encephalopathy. It is important to correct hypochloremia along with other deficits in the treatment of hypochloremic hypokalemic metabolic alkalosis. As noted earlier, hypochloremia must be corrected in the recovery phase after an episode of severe metabolic acidosis.

Prognosis. Hypochloremia has no specific prognostic significance. The prognosis depends on the underlying disorder.

Hyperchloremia

Hyperchloremia is a serum chloride level greater than 115 mEq/L. It is uncommon in surgical patients.

Etiology. Hyperchloremia may occur in association with hypernatremia, in renal tubular acidosis, or after the administration of excess potassium chloride or ammonium chloride. It may be caused by surgical diversion of urine into segments of bowel (e.g., ileal urinary conduits, ureterosigmoidostomy). In these cases, the bowel mucosa absorbs excess chloride in exchange for bicarbonate, especially when evacuation of the urine is delayed.

Presentation and Diagnosis. The signs and symptoms are those of the accompanying disorder. Diagnosis is made by measurement of serum chloride.

Treatment. There is no specific treatment for hyperchloremia. Treatment is directed at the underlying disorder.

Prognosis. Hyperchloremia has no prognostic significance. The prognosis depends on the nature and treatment of the underlying disorder.

Calcium

Calcium is a common divalent cation, almost all of which is found in hydroxyapatite crystals in bone. On the surface of bone, calcium participates in exchange with calcium in the ECF. Of the small amount of calcium in the ECF, approximately 40% is bound to plasma protein and 10% is complexed with bicarbonate, citrate, and phosphate. Only the hormonally regulated ionized portion, the remaining 50%, is physiologically active. This small proportion is of vital importance, however, primarily because of its role in neuromuscular activity. The normal range of total serum calcium is 8.5 to 11.0 mg/dL, and that of ionized calcium is 4.75 to 5.30 mg/dL. Most bound calcium is bound to albumin, and total serum calcium is dependent on serum albumin. Total calcium values may appear artifactually subnor-

mal in hypoalbuminemic patients unless a correction factor, such as the following, is used:

$$\text{Corrected total Ca}^{++} = [0.8 \times (4.0 - \text{patient's albumin})] + \text{patient's total serum Ca}^{++}$$

In this formula, 4.0 represents normal serum albumin. The proportion of calcium bound to proteins is dependent on pH; it is decreased by acidosis, with a concomitant increase in ionized calcium. The level of serum ionized calcium is a more accurate indicator of physiologic activity than total calcium, but it is a more expensive test and is not universally available.

The usual adult dietary intake of calcium is 1 g or more a day. Two-thirds of this calcium passes through the gut and is excreted in stool, and one-third is absorbed in the small intestine, regulated by vitamin D. In normal kidneys, approximately 10% of filtered calcium reaches the distal tubules, where resorption is increased by **parathyroid hormone** (PTH) and metabolic alkalosis, or is decreased by hypophosphatemia and metabolic acidosis. Overall calcium homeostasis, largely regulated by PTH, is the result of intestinal absorption, renal excretion, and calcium exchange between bone and the ECF. Although severe abnormalities of calcium metabolism are uncommon in surgical patients, symptomatic abnormalities are seen.

Hypocalcemia

Hypocalcemia is defined as total serum calcium lower than 8 mg/dL. It is seen in many conditions that are common to surgical patients, several of which are acute problems.

Etiology. Hypocalcemia is often seen in surgical patients (Table 3-8). In acute pancreatitis, the etiology of hypocalcemia is unclear. It probably results from a combination of calcium binding in saponified tissue, PTH deficiency or dysfunction in the kidney and bone, and decreased protein-bound calcium as a result of hypoalbuminemia. Magnesium deficiency decreases PTH

Table 3-8. Causes of Hypocalcemia in Surgical Patients

Artifactual as a result of hypoalbuminemia

Acute pancreatitis

Surgically induced hypoparathyroidism (transient or permanent)

Necrotizing fasciitis

Inadequate intestinal absorption
  Inflammatory bowel disease
  Pancreatic exocrine dysfunction
  Mucosal malabsorptive syndromes

Excessive fluid losses from pancreatic or intestinal fistulae

Chronic diarrhea

Renal insufficiency with impaired calcium resorption

Hypomagnesemia

Hyperphosphatemia

release and activity. Phosphate increases bone deposition of calcium, decreasing the available circulating pool. Inadequate intestinal absorption of calcium may result from inflammatory bowel disease, pancreatic exocrine dysfunction, or malabsorption syndromes. Excessive fluid losses from chronic diarrhea or pancreatic or intestinal fistulas may also seriously deplete extracellular calcium and cause other electrolyte abnormalities. Low serum calcium levels are seen with severe soft tissue infections, such as **necrotizing fasciitis**. Artifactual hypocalcemia is seen when serum albumin is low and total calcium, rather than ionized calcium, is measured. Vitamin D deficiency may result from synthetic failure in renal or hepatic disease, or from conversion to inactive metabolites caused by the anticonvulsants phenytoin and phenobarbital.

Another way to classify hypocalcemia is according to its relation to PTH, which may be: (1) deficient or absent (e.g., hypomagnesemia, any type of true hypoparathyroidism); (2) ineffective (e.g., vitamin D disorders, chronic renal failure, pseudohypoparathyroidism); or (3) overwhelmed (e.g., hyperphosphatemia).

Artifactual hypocalcemia occurs when the serum albumin is low and total calcium, rather than ionized calcium, is measured.

Presentation and Diagnosis. The clinical manifestations of hypocalcemia reflect the role of calcium in neuromuscular activity. Early symptoms of hypocalcemia include circumoral tingling, numbness and tingling of the fingertips, and muscle cramps. Hyperactive deep-tendon reflexes develop, with a Chvostek sign (unilateral facial spasm when the facial nerve on that side is lightly tapped), tetany, and Trousseau's sign (carpopedal spasm), eventually progressing to seizures. The patient may be confused or depressed. Prolonged Q-T intervals are seen on the electrocardiogram.

In acidosis, the ionized fraction of serum calcium increases at the expense of the bound fraction. Because only the ionized fraction is active, symptoms may not appear, even with low total serum calcium. With severe alkalosis, the reverse occurs, and symptoms may appear even when the measured total serum calcium is normal.

Hypocalcemia can occur after blood transfusion, as a result of citrate binding and dilution. However, evidence suggests that at moderate rates of blood transfusion, endogenous release of calcium from bone is adequate to prevent hypocalcemia. Only with massive transfusion and volume replacement at rates of 100 mL/min or higher is there any need to give supplemental calcium.

Diagnosis is made by measuring serum calcium (the ionized portion if possible), along with serum potassium, magnesium, phosphate, and alkaline phosphatase. Other electrolyte abnormalities and acid–base disorders must be excluded. Serum albumin is measured, as well as BUN and creatinine. Measurement of urinary calcium can help assess calcium intake. It may ultimately prove necessary to measure vitamin D levels to help make the diagnosis. The response of urinary cyclic adenosine monophosphate to PTH infusion (increase) may help diagnose idiopathic hypoparathyroidism. During physical examination, a search should be made for a transverse surgical scar on the anterior neck, which would suggest previous thyroidectomy or parathyroidectomy.

Treatment. Treatment of hypocalcemia is directed at correcting the calcium deficit, normalizing the relation between ionized and protein-bound calcium by correcting acid–base disorders, and treating the underlying causes. When the need for correction is urgent (e.g., severe, highly symptomatic hypocalcemia), calcium gluconate or calcium chloride is infused. Hypocalcemia associated with chronic disorders is treated over the long term with oral calcium lactate. Vitamin D supplements may be needed; the high doses required in hypoparathyroidism may be reduced if urinary calcium loss is decreased with thiazide diuretics.

Prognosis. Disorders of calcium balance can be treated with complete resolution of symptoms. Underlying disorders must also be identified and treated.

Hypercalcemia

Hypercalcemia is defined as total serum calcium greater than 11 or 12 g/dL.

Etiology. The causes of hypercalcemia are classified in Table 3-9. In surgical patients, primary and secondary hyperparathyroidism and metastatic breast cancer are among the common causes. In fact, more than 90% of hypercalcemic patients who have no symptoms other than depression and fatigue have primary hyperparathyroidism. Malignancies cause hypercalcemia both by bony involvement and by the secretion of

Table 3-9. Causes of Hypercalcemia

Hyperparathyroidism

Malignancy
   Metastatic cancer
   Lymphoma
   Leukemia

Granulomatous disease
   Sarcoidosis
   Tuberculosis
   Fungal infection

Excessive dietary intake
   Milk-alkali syndrome
   Vitamin A or D intoxication

Thiazide diuretics

Immobilization

Endocrine abnormalities
   Thyrotoxicosis
   Adrenal insufficiency

PTH-like substances that affect calcium metabolism. Malignancies that are sufficiently advanced to cause hypercalcemia are usually symptomatic. Mobilization of calcium from bone in bedridden patients can cause mild, asymptomatic hypercalcemia. The milk-alkali syndrome (i.e., hypercalcemia, alkalosis, and renal failure) results from excessive intake of calcium and absorbable antacids. Rare causes of hypercalcemia include Williams syndrome (a constellation of congenital defects and abnormal sensitivity to vitamin D) and vitamin A intoxication, possibly by increasing bone resorption.

Presentation and Diagnosis. The initial clinical manifestations of hypercalcemia are nonspecific: weakness, fatigue, anorexia, nausea, and vomiting. As serum calcium increases, severe headaches, diffuse musculoskeletal pain, polyuria, and polydipsia develop. The combination of decreased oral intake, vomiting, and polyuria leads to hypovolemia and dehydration, which may become pronounced. The ECG shows shortened Q-T intervals and widened T-waves. With normal or elevated phosphate, calcification may develop in the kidneys as well as in unusual locations (e.g., heart, skin). Pancreatitis and renal failure may develop as well. The renal failure has multiple causes, including volume depletion, nephrocalcinosis, and deposition of nephrotoxic myeloma proteins or light chains. When serum calcium increases to 15 mg/dL and above, confusion and depression progress to somnolence, stupor, and coma. This degree of hypercalcemia results in death unless it is corrected promptly.

Diagnosis is made primarily by a careful history, including all medications, and blood tests. PTH levels are assessed, and imaging procedures are used to locate a tumor. Squamous cell carcinoma of the bronchus and hypernephromas can produce parathyroid hormone–related peptide. A search for bone metastasis in a patient with a known malignancy is indicated.

Treatment. Initially, calcium intake is restricted, hydration status improved, and urinary calcium excretion increased. If the patient is symptomatic or the calcium level is high, the patient is hospitalized. Large volumes of intravenous normal or half-normal saline are infused. Loop diuretics are administered because they enhance calcium excretion. Great care must be taken during this process of vigorous hydration and diuresis, with close monitoring of volume status to avoid overload. Meticulous assessment and replacement of electrolytes are necessary. Hypomagnesemia can develop as a result of forced diuresis.

Oral or intravenous phosphate supplements are sometimes used to form complexes with ionized calcium. Given intravenously, these supplements may produce a precipitous decrease in serum calcium, and resulting tetany, hypotension, and renal failure are reported. Therefore, intravenous phosphate should be given slowly, no faster than 50 mmol/12 hr, and for a limited time, no more than 48 hours if given continuously. Phosphate supplementation should not be used in patients with hyperphosphatemia or renal failure.

Corticosteroids are sometimes used as a longer-term treatment to suppress calcium release from bone in patients with granulomatous disease, vitamin D intoxication, or hematologic malignancies. The usual dose is hydrocortisone 3 mg/kg/day. This treatment may take 1 to 2 weeks to produce an appreciable reduction in serum calcium.

The antineoplastic agent plicamycin (formerly called mithramycin), a DNA-binding antibiotic and an RNA-synthesis inhibitor, acutely reduces serum calcium by an unknown mechanism. It is given in small intravenous doses, 25 µg/kg, for 3 to 4 days. Calcium levels decrease within 48 hours and remain low for several days to weeks. Contraindications include thrombocytopenia, coagulopathy or other bleeding diatheses, and bone marrow suppression from any cause. Plicamycin has significant renal and hepatic toxicity.

Prognosis. If the cause of hypercalcemia is treatable and the hypercalcemia itself is treated before the neurologic symptoms become severe, the patient should recover completely. Many of the causes of hypercalcemia are life-threatening (e.g., metastatic cancer), and this prognosis determines the outcome more than the hypercalcemia itself.

Magnesium

Magnesium plays an important role in metabolism because it is a cofactor for many enzymes. It also affects neuromuscular function. At least one-half of the body's total magnesium is in bone. Most of the remainder is intracellular. Magnesium is the most common intracellular divalent cation, and most intracellular magnesium is bound to adenosine triphosphate. Less than 1% is extracellular. The average daily intake of magnesium is 25 to 30 mEq. Approximately 40% of the magnesium is absorbed, primarily in the jejunum and ileum, and it is excreted primarily by the kidneys. A higher percentage of intake is absorbed if body stores are deficient. The normal range of serum magnesium is 1.5 to 2.5 mg/dL. Normal kidneys conserve magnesium when intake is low, but hypomagnesemia develops if intake remains less than 0.3 mEq/kg/day.

Hypomagnesemia

Hypomagnesemia is common in surgical patients, who are often in a starvation state, experience gastrointestinal losses, or have absorption defects. When magnesium is deficient, losses of potassium and phosphorus, the other two major elements in cells, also occur. These elements are expelled from the cell, and the cells decrease in size to maintain normal intracellular composition. Severe hypomagnesemia also produces severe hypocalcemia by decreasing PTH secretion and by an apparent skeletal resistance and an impaired renal response.

Etiology. The most common cause of hypomagnesemia is dietary deficiency combined with gastrointestinal losses (e.g., diarrhea, nasogastric suction) and deficiencies in other elements. Other causes include chronic alcoholism (especially during withdrawal), malabsorption (especially steatorrhea), acute pancreatitis, improperly constituted hyperalimentation, and endocrine disorders. Hypomagnesemia also occurs as a side effect of many therapeutic drugs, particularly some diuretics, aminoglycosides, amphotericin, cyclosporine, cisplatinum, insulin, and pentamidine. Athletes and pregnant women may be mildly hypomagnesemic.

Presentation and Diagnosis. The effects of magnesium deficiency are not immediate. Like calcium, the body's other major divalent cation, magnesium affects neuromuscular function. Symptoms develop insidiously, first as nonspecific systemic symptoms that include nausea, vomiting, anorexia, weakness, and lethargy, then as neuromuscular symptoms that include muscle cramps, fasciculations, tetany, carpopedal spasm, paresthesias, irritability, inattention and confusion, and cardiac arrhythmias, along with other symptoms of associated hypokalemia and hypocalcemia.

Diagnosis is made by testing serum values. These values may be normal, even in the presence of a deficiency in body magnesium. Volume status should be assessed.

Treatment. Primary attention must be given to correcting the cause. If hypomagnesemia is mild and does not result from an absorptive defect, oral supplements are given. If it is moderate, then it is treated with intravenous magnesium sulfate at a rate of 50 to 100 mEq/day because the oral dose required can cause diarrhea. If symptoms are severe, an intravenous bolus of magnesium sulfate is administered, followed by intravenous infusion at a rate of 1 to 2 mEq/kg/day. Concomitant or resultant deficiencies in other elements must also be corrected, and adequate hydration must be maintained. If the patient is in renal failure, extra care must be taken not to overcorrect the hypomagnesemia.

Prognosis. Recovery from hypomagnesemia may be complete. The prognosis depends on the etiology, the severity of the deficiency and its symptoms, and the promptness of treatment.

Hypermagnesemia

Clinically significant hypermagnesemia is rare, especially if renal function is normal.

Etiology. Hypermagnesemia can result from renal failure; any injury that causes rhabdomyolysis (e.g., crush injuries, severe burns); dehydration; severe metabolic acidosis; adrenal insufficiency; familial benign hypocalciuric hypercalcemia; or overdosage with magnesium salts in cathartics. In addition, in either mother or newborn, it can occur after treatment for eclampsia. It also occurs in patients with renal failure who use magnesium-containing antacids. Renal excretion is decreased in metabolic alkalosis.

Presentation and Diagnosis. Symptomatic hypermagnesemia follows a progressive pattern, with increasing neuromuscular and central nervous system abnormalities as the serum level increases. Initial nausea is superseded by lethargy, weakness, hypoventilation, and decreased deep-tendon reflexes. The condition then progresses to hypotension and bradycardia, skeletal muscle paralysis, respiratory depression, coma, and death. Diagnosis is made by testing serum values.

Treatment. Mild hypermagnesemia is treated with oral hydration and by controlling magnesium intake (e.g., giving patients with renal failure non–magnesium-containing antacids). Severe symptoms are reversed temporarily by intravenous calcium, and the magnesium excess is treated with hydration and diuretics, or hemodialysis.

Prognosis. Recovery from hypermagnesemia may be complete. The prognosis depends on the etiology, the severity of the deficiency and its symptoms, and the promptness of treatment.

Phosphate

Phosphorus is a component of all body tissues, and it participates in virtually all metabolic processes. In a normal adult, approximately 85% of phosphorus is bound in bone and 15% is distributed in other tissues. Less than 1% is extracellular. The intestine, influenced by vitamin D, absorbs approximately 70% of ingested soluble phosphorus, a higher proportion if dietary intake is low. The normal adult phosphorus requirement is 2 to 9 mg/kg/day. The amount of phosphorus excreted by normal kidneys is controlled by PTH and is proportional to the amount absorbed. The normal range of serum phosphatase is 2.4 to 4.7 mg/dL. Circadian variation, mediated by the adrenal cortex, produces the highest serum levels during the afternoon and night and the lowest levels during the morning.

Hypophosphatemia

Hypophosphatemia is common in surgical patients. When phosphorus is deficient, there are also losses of potassium and magnesium, the other two major elements in cells. These elements are expelled from the cell, and the cells decrease in size to maintain normal intracellular composition.

Etiology. The causes of hypophosphatemia are categorized as: (1) inadequate uptake as a result of inadequate dietary intake, malabsorption, gastrointestinal losses, prolonged antacid use, improperly constituted hyperalimentation, or vitamin D deficiency; (2) increased renal excretion as a result of diuretic use, hypervolemia, corticoid therapy, hyperaldosteronism, SIADH, or hyperparathyroidism; or (3) compartmental shifts as a result of hormones, nutrients that stimulate insulin release, treatment of diabetic ketoacidosis, recovery from hypometabolic states, rapidly growing malignancies, or respiratory alkalosis. It is also seen in chronic alcoholism, in burns, and after parathyroidectomy or renal transplantation. Occasionally, hypophosphatemia is the first clue to alcohol withdrawal in a hospitalized patient.

Presentation and Diagnosis. Severe phosphorus deficiency causes anorexia, dizziness, osteomalacia, severe congestive cardiomyopathy, proximal muscle weakness, visual defects, ascending paralysis, hemolytic anemia, and respiratory failure. Leukocyte and erythrocyte malfunction, rhabdomyolysis, hypercalciuria, and severe hypocalcemia are also seen. Central nervous system dysfunction occurs, and can progress to seizures, coma, and death. If the hypophosphatemia is a result of vitamin D deficiency, metabolic acidosis may result from reduced renal hydrogen excretion.

Diagnosis is made by testing serum values, but total body phosphate deficiency may exist, even in the face of elevated serum values. Arterial blood gases, pH, and urine phosphate should be measured, along with serum potassium, calcium, and magnesium.

Treatment. Severe hypophosphatemia should prompt an aggressive search for and treatment of the cause. Phosphate salts may be given orally or intravenously. Other associated electrolyte abnormalities must also be treated. Diuretics may be withdrawn. VIPomas should be surgically removed.

Prognosis. Repletion of phosphorus corrects or decreases most abnormalities. Respiratory failure may not be reversed completely, and the ultimate outcome is likely to depend on the prognosis of the underlying condition.

Hyperphosphatemia

Hyperphosphatemia is relatively common in adults, and is seen even in the presence of total body phosphate deficiency.

Etiology. The causes of hyperphosphatemia are categorized as: (1) decreased renal excretion as a result of renal insufficiency or failure, hyperthyroidism, hypoparathyroidism or pseudohypoparathyroidism, or adrenal insufficiency; (2) increased intestinal absorption as a result of sarcoidosis or tuberculosis (both of which produce vitamin D), or excess phosphate or vitamin D ingestion; (3) iatrogenic, as a result of intravenous infusion of phosphate-containing fluids; or (4) shifts from the intracellular to the extracellular compartment as a result of acidotic states, tumor lysis, hemolytic anemia, thyrotoxicosis, or rhabdomyolysis.

Presentation and Diagnosis. Hyperphosphatemia has no symptoms, although in the presence of severe hypercalcemia, renal failure, or vitamin D intoxication, it may be accompanied by deposition of calcium phosphate in abnormal locations. It is diagnosed by testing serum values. Associated electrolyte abnormalities should also be identified and corrected.

Treatment. Aluminum-based antacids decrease absorption by binding phosphate, and diuretics increase the rate of urinary phosphate excretion. Dialysis is used in patients with renal failure. It is often unnecessary to treat hyperphosphatemia, except by correcting excess intake and addressing associated problems.

Prognosis. The prognosis of hyperphosphatemia depends on its cause.

Disorders of Acid–Base Balance

The management of acid–base disorders depends on prompt recognition and evaluation of the disturbances involved. A history and physical examination alert the physician to the nature and severity of disturbances that can occur in a particular clinical setting. Laboratory data pertinent to fluid and electrolyte status and renal function help to identify alterations that contribute to or result from the underlying disturbance. With the help of this information, the data provided by arterial blood gas and pH determinations are analyzed, an accurate diagnosis is made, and an appropriate course of treatment is defined. The measured arterial pH value (pHa) indicates whether alkalosis (pHa > 7.45) or acidosis (pHa < 7.35) is present. The $PaCO_2$ reflects whether any respiratory component is present. The bicarbonate concentration [HCO_3^-] derived from the Henderson-Hasselbalch equation (pHa = pk + log [HCO_3^-/H_2CO_3]) identifies a metabolic component, assuming that pHa and $PaCO_2$ measurements are reliable. If an error in either measurement is suspected, the test is repeated or correlated with the [HCO_3^-] derived from the carbon dioxide content on the electrolyte measurements. The measured PaO_2 and derived saturation values provide information about pulmonary gas exchange and its possible contribution to the acid–base status.

The need for accurate interpretation of the blood gas data, especially when mixed disturbances are present, prompted the introduction of a variety of methods to facilitate their analysis. Some of these methods are too complex for use at the bedside on a busy surgical service. Others that use rules or guidelines for making simple, quick calculations seem more applicable in that setting. The information that they make available is equivalent to that provided when the Henderson-Hasselbalch equation and its modifications are used. Two rules that can be found in the text used to teach advanced cardiac life support (ACLS) are of particular value in practice. They provide simple means for quantitating the effects of changes of $PaCO_2$ and [HCO_3^-] on pHa. In turn, that information is used to assess the degree to which acidosis or alkalosis is caused by a respiratory or a metabolic disturbance and to quantitate the base excesses or deficits that contribute to the disturbance.

Rule 1. An increase or decrease in $PaCO_2$ of 10 mm Hg is associated with a reciprocal decrease or increase, respectively, of 0.08 pH units.

Rule 2. An increase or decrease in $[HCO_3^-]$ of 10 mEq/L is associated with a directly related increase or decrease, respectively, of 0.15 pH units.

Acidosis

Whether the acidosis has a respiratory or metabolic origin, the consequences of the decreased pHa can be life-threatening. At pHa levels less than 7.2, peripheral vascular and cardiac responsiveness to catecholamines is decreased. Cardiac dysfunction that occurs as a result of direct myocardial depression and arrhythmia can become significant, and even lethal. Ionic exchanges across cell membranes and changes in renal tubular transport of electrolytes induced by acidosis cause extracellular potassium concentrations to increase, at times to clinically symptomatic levels.

Respiratory Acidosis

Etiology. Respiratory acidosis is the result of carbon dioxide retention that occurs because of pulmonary alveolar hypoventilation. It can be acute or chronic. When acute, its causes can be numerous, including respiratory depression as a result of narcotics, sedatives, anesthetic agents, and muscle relaxants; limited ventilatory effort as a result of painful thoracic or upper abdominal incisions, or chest wall and pulmonary parenchymal trauma that interferes with the mechanics of breathing (e.g., fractured ribs, flail chest, hemopneumothorax); abdominal distension and impaired diaphragmatic function; and upper-airway obstruction as a result of tumor, foreign body, edema, laryngospasm, tracheobronchial injury, or improperly positioned endotracheal tubes. On the other hand, chronic respiratory acidosis is most often caused by advanced long-standing disorders of the lungs, especially chronic pulmonary obstructive disease.

Presentation and Diagnosis. The clinical consequences of respiratory acidosis are caused by the effects of hypercapnia and the hypoxia that commonly occurs with it (assuming that the hypoxemia is not masked by increased inhaled oxygen concentrations). Acutely, mild hypertension and restlessness are evident. When $PaCO_2$ levels continue to rise, somnolence, confusion, and ultimately coma (as a result of carbon dioxide narcosis) occur. In combination with hypoxemia, severe hypercapnia is also associated with significant cardiovascular dysfunction, including cardiac arrest. In patients with chronic respiratory acidosis, carbon dioxide narcosis is the major threat, although tolerance to hypercapnia is increased. In part, this increase is related to the compensatory increase in $[HCO_3^-]$ that is caused by the renal conservation of base, a phenomenon that is not apparent in the acute state because of the time needed for it to evolve.

Rules 1 and 2 can be used to determine whether respiratory changes are responsible for an acute acidotic state. According to rule 1, if the magnitude of the $PaCO_2$ increase can account for the pH change, a pure respiratory acidosis exists. If the pH change is greater than can be accounted for, however, a metabolic component of acidosis must also exist. If the pH change is less than the increase in $PaCO_2$ would predict, an element of metabolic alkalosis is present. The use of rule 2 in this case shows the contribution that an elevated $[HCO_3^-]$ makes to the mixed acid–base disturbance. In chronic respiratory acidosis, in contrast to the acute state, this finding is expected as a consequence of compensatory renal retention of bicarbonate.

Treatment. The treatment of respiratory acidosis is directed at removing the cause of the reduced alveolar ventilation while ensuring adequate oxygenation. Inadequate pain control is a common cause of respiratory acidosis. In the acute state, or with acute deterioration of a chronic situation, temporary use of mechanical ventilatory support and oxygen therapy may be necessary. In this case, acute hypercapnea should not be corrected too rapidly. Sudden decreases in $PaCO_2$ cause sudden pH changes and ionic shifts between cellular and extracellular fluids that can produce severe cardiac dysrhythmias, including ventricular arrhythmias. The administration of bicarbonate to improve the buffering capacity of extracellular fluids in respiratory acidosis is not an appropriate treatment option.

Prognosis. In the acute state, once the underlying cause of the decreased alveolar ventilation is treated, the hypercapnia will resolve.

Metabolic Acidosis

Metabolic acidosis (< 7.35) is a decrease in pHa related to a decreased arterial $[HCO_3^-]$. It can be acute or chronic.

Etiology. Metabolic acidosis occurs for two major reasons. The first is the loss of bicarbonate from the extracellular space. This loss occurs acutely with certain gastrointestinal disorders (e.g., diarrhea, external pancreatic fistula) and more chronically with increased urinary bicarbonate losses that occur with renal tubular disorders, ureterointestinal anastomosis, decreased mineralocorticoid activity, and diuresis induced with the carbonic anhydrase inhibitor acetazolamide. The second major cause of metabolic acidosis, most often as an acute process, is an increased metabolic acid load. This increase is seen with lactic **acidemia** secondary to cardiogenic, septic, and hypovolemic low-flow states or ischemia of major tissue beds (e.g., mesenteric infarction), and ketoacidosis.

Presentation and Diagnosis. With both acute and chronic metabolic acidosis, respiratory compensation occurs. Ventilation is stimulated by the increased hydrogen ion concentration in arterial blood, and $PaCO_2$ is reduced. The degree of compensation is determined by the extent of the hypocapnea that is induced and by estimates of its modifying influence on the pHa, as determined by application of rule 1. Similarly, the use of rule 2 to estimate whether measured decreases in $[HCO_3^-]$ can fully account for the measured changes in pHa identifies mixed acid–base disturbances.

Determination of the anion gap can help to distinguish metabolic acidosis caused by a loss of bicarbonate from that caused by an accumulation of a metabolic acid load. The anion gap is the difference between the serum sodium concentration and the sum of the serum bicarbonate and chloride concentrations. With losses of bicarbonate, decreases in the serum concentration of this anion are accompanied by reciprocal increases in chloride ion concentrations. As such, the anion gap remains normal (12 ± 4 mOsm/L). In contrast, with metabolic acid loads, chloride levels do not increase as the bicarbonate levels decrease, and the measured anion gap is greater than normal. Actually, the gap is more apparent than real because unmeasured anions of metabolic acids are present in amounts that account for the differences calculated solely on the basis of measured bicarbonate and chloride values.

Treatment. Treatment of metabolic acidosis involves the correction of the underlying disorder, when possible, and intravenous replacement of bicarbonate as needed. The need to focus attention on the treatment of the underlying cause is critical in the management of metabolic acidosis that is caused by low-flow states. Hypovolemia must be corrected, sepsis must be controlled, and cardiovascular dynamics must be enhanced to improve tissue perfusion and satisfy cellular metabolic needs. Unless these goals are accomplished, no amount of infused bicarbonate by itself will succeed in returning the pHa to normal. Similarly, with diabetic ketoacidosis, treatment of the pHa with bicarbonate is of little value without concomitant administration of insulin and intravenous fluids.

If the patient is compensating fully for the metabolic acidosis by hyperventilating and the pHa is still less than 7.25, then bicarbonate may be used, assuming that the underlying disorder is being corrected. The amount needed to correct the pHa to normal is estimated as follows: (1) Using rule 1, the disparity between the pHa measured and the pHa calculated on the basis of the measured $PaCO_2$ is determined. The difference defines the pHa decrease that is caused by a decrease in $[HCO_3^-]$. (2) Using rule 2, the pHa difference is translated into the decrease in $[HCO_3^-]$ that it represents. With that information and the assumption of a bicarbonate space that is approximately 50% TBW (25%–30% body weight), the amount of bicarbonate needed to correct the total body base deficit is calculated as:

$$mEq\ HCO_3^-\ needed = mEq/L\ [HCO_3^-]\ deficit \times (kg\ wt \times 0.25)$$

In extreme circumstances (e.g., cardiac arrest), when a precipitous and life-threatening decrease in pHa will impair the effectiveness of efforts to resuscitate the patient, bolus administration of 1 mg/kg as an initial dose followed by one-half this dose every 10 minutes until the pHa is greater than 7.25 is justified. Otherwise, when the disturbance is less severe, it is better to proceed at a slower pace to avoid the consequences of overzealous and too rapid administration of intravenous bicarbonate. These consequences include cardiac irregularities, convulsions, metabolic alkalosis, hypokalemia, impairment of the delivery of red blood cell oxygen to tissues, and symptomatic hyperosmolarity as a result of the infusion of excessive amounts of sodium. Usually, it is advisable to replace no more than one-half of the calculated bicarbonate deficit in the first 3 to 4 hours and then, over the next 12 to 24 hours, to administer the remainder until serum bicarbonate and pHa values return to more normal levels. Again, it is imperative to treat the underlying cause of the metabolic acidosis.

Alkalosis

When the pHa rises to more than 7.45, regardless of the cause, alkalosis is present. The nature and importance of alkalosis on fluid and electrolyte balance and oxygen carried by hemoglobin were discussed in the sections on hypokalemia, hypocalcemia, hypomagnesemia, and hypophosphatemia. Alkalosis also has clinical features that are specific to either respiratory or metabolic alkalosis.

Respiratory Alkalosis

When the increase in pHa is related to a decrease in $PaCO_2$, respiratory alkalosis is present. In the surgical patient, this problem is often caused by hyperventilation with short, shallow breaths because of pain.

Etiology. Respiratory alkalosis is the consequence of pulmonary alveolar hyperventilation, which is commonly encountered in surgical patients. Apprehension, pain that does not limit respiratory effort, hypoxia, fever, central nervous system injuries, sepsis, and elevated serum ammonia levels in patients with chronic liver disease can stimulate respiration and cause hypocapnia and respiratory alkalosis. Hyperventilation, causing a decrease in $PaCO_2$, is common in patients who are mechanically ventilated during surgery or perioperatively.

Compensatory mechanisms for acute respiratory alkalosis are relatively ineffective in surgical patients. Renal compensatory efforts occur in the form of distal tubular excretion of bicarbonate. However, hyponatremia and increased aldosterone activity, which are common in surgically stressed patients, limit the effectiveness of this mechanism, which depends on renal excretion of sodium as the accompanying cation. Only with chronic respiratory alkalosis is any notable compensatory decrease in $[HCO_3^-]$ seen.

Presentation and Diagnosis. In addition to the consequences of disturbed potassium, calcium, magnesium, and phosphate metabolism that are seen in all alkalotic states, the low $PaCO_2$ levels that are characteristic of respiratory alkalosis can, by themselves, exert significant pathophysiologic influences. Acute hypocapnia can cause cerebral vasoconstriction, which can reduce blood flow to the brain by as much as 50% (1%–3% for each 1-mm Hg drop in $PaCO_2$). These effects can have particular significance in older patients whose cerebral arterial circulation might also be compromised by atherosclerotic disease.

Treatment. In the artificially ventilated patient, reduction of the amount of ventilation that is being provided can correct both the reasons for and the consequences of respiratory alkalosis. In the absence of mechanical hyperventilation as a cause, however, efforts are directed at treating the underlying conditions that are responsible for hypocapnia.

Metabolic Alkalosis

When an elevated pHa is associated with an elevated $[HCO_3^-]$, metabolic alkalosis is present.

Etiology. The ways in which gastrointestinal and renal losses of potassium and chloride ions can occur and can cause hypochloremic hypokalemic metabolic alkalosis were discussed in the sections dealing with disorders of those ions. The accumulation of exogenously infused excesses of base can also cause metabolic alkalosis in surgical patients. This situation can result from overzealous infusion of bicarbonate in the treatment of metabolic acidosis or the inadvertent administration of large amounts of citrate when multiple transfusions are given. Metabolic alkalosis can also occur through contraction of the extracellular volume from diuretic administration.

In metabolic alkalosis, the retention of carbon dioxide as a result of hypoventilation can help to compensate for the accumulation of base excess. In surgical patients, this mechanism may not be effective. On the other hand, renal tubular excretion of bicarbonate in an alkaline urine may be effective. However, as discussed with paradoxical aciduria that appears in the course of hypochloremic hypokalemic metabolic alkalosis, this mechanism for compensation cannot be sustained as the depletion of electrolytes grows more severe. The urine then becomes acidic as hydrogen ion is secreted and bicarbonate ion is reabsorbed. This situation enhances the severity of the existing metabolic alkalosis.

Presentation and Diagnosis. In general, the clinical problems seen with metabolic alkalosis are most often related to the hypokalemia, hypochloremia, and volume contraction caused by gastrointestinal or renal losses of fluid and electrolytes. Important clinical manifestations of potassium depletion, in particular, include paralytic ileus, digitalis toxicity, and cardiac arrhythmias.

Treatment. The successful treatment of metabolic alkalosis requires control of extrarenal losses of fluid and electrolytes and correction of the fluid volume, potassium, and chloride deficits that are present. Only when all of these issues are successfully addressed can appropriate renal tubular responses be restored and pHa be returned to normal.

Multiple-Choice Questions

1. Which of the following is the best estimate of the volume of total body water in a 25-year-old 75-kg man?
   A. 4 L
   B. 10 L
   C. 15 L
   D. 30 L
   E. 45 L

2. Which of the following is a true statement?
   A. Aldosterone secretion is stimulated mostly by a change in serum osmolality
   B. Antidiuretic hormone secretion can be stimulated by decreased extracellular volume sensed by atrial receptors
   C. Decreased extracellular volume leads to increased stimulation of renin secretion by stimulation of carotid volume receptors
   D. Secretion of aldosterone leads to increased levels of angiotensin II
   E. Adrenocorticotropic hormone (ACTH) is a potent stimulator of aldosterone.

3. Which is the best estimate of plasma osmolality in a patient with the following levels: sodium 140 mEq/L, potassium 4.5 mEq/L, chloride 105 mEq/L, bicarbonate 28 mEq/L, blood sugar 600 mg/dL, and BUN 28 g/dL?
   A. 210 mOsm
   B. 280 mOsm
   C. 320 mOsm
   D. 360 mOsm
   E. 400 mOsm

4. Which of the following events would occur shortly after a rapid intravenous infusion of hypertonic mannitol?
   A. Extracellular fluid osmolarity would increase; intracellular fluid osmolarity would decrease
   B. Intracellular fluid osmolarity would increase; extracellular fluid osmolarity would decrease
   C. Intracellular fluid osmolarity would decrease; extracellular fluid osmolarity would decrease
   D. Intracellular fluid volume would decrease; extracellular fluid osmolarity would increase
   E. Serum sodium concentration would decrease; intracellular fluid osmolarity would decrease.

5. Which of the following is associated with hyperkalemia?
   A. Magnesium deficiency
   B. Insulin administration
   C. Elevated aldosterone secretion
   D. Metabolic alkalosis
   E. Metabolic acidosis

6. The electrolyte disturbance that is most often associated with paralytic ileus and muscular weakness is:
   A. hyponatremia
   B. hypernatremia

C.   hypocalcemia
D.   hypokalemia
E.   hyperchloremia

7. Assuming normal renal function, the most appropriate intravenous solution to use to correct the fluid, electrolyte, and acid–base imbalances associated with gastric outlet obstruction with persistent vomiting is:
A. 0.9% saline solution
B. 0.45% saline solution with 20 to 30 mEq KCl added to each liter
C. Lactated Ringer's solution
D. 5% glucose and 0.15 N hydrochloric acid solution
E. 5% glucose in water

8. Which combination of determinations provides the most information when characterizing an acid–base disturbance?
A. Arterial blood and urine pH
B. Arterial pH and $Paco_2$
C. Arterial and venous blood pH
D. Arterial and venous blood pH
E. Venous blood pH and bicarbonate

9. The correction of persistent metabolic alkalosis is most dependent on the replacement of:
A. sodium
B. potassium
C. magnesium
D. lactate
E. chloride

10. Untreated prolonged and excessive diarrhea usually results in:
A. metabolic acidosis with isotonic extracellular volume contraction
B. metabolic alkalosis with isotonic extracellular volume
C. metabolic acidosis with hypertonic extracellular volume contraction
D. metabolic alkalosis with hypertonic extracellular volume contraction
E. metabolic alkalosis with hypotonic extracellular volume contraction

11. Decreased serum magnesium levels may be associated with all of the following EXCEPT:
A. chronic alcoholism
B. prolonged diarrheal disorders
C. prolonged intravenous fluid therapy
D. hyperparathyroidism
E. long-term use of diuretics

12. A 56-year-old woman with metastatic breast cancer is comatose, with a 3-day history of progressive weakness, anorexia, nausea, vomiting, oliguria, and increasing somnolence. Her serum calcium is 7.5 mEq/L (15 mg/dL). When considering treatment of this patient, which of the following statements is true?

A. This hypercalcemia can safely be treated with oral phosphate supplements
B. She should receive furosemide 40 mg intravenously immediately
C. Insulin and glucose infusions should be given immediately
D. Rapid intravenous administration of phosphate may drop her serum calcium levels precipitously; therefore, it is not the treatment of choice
E. Glucocorticosteroid therapy will have an effect on serum calcium levels within 2 to 4 hours of administration

13. If a patient with pulmonary failure is receiving total parenteral nutrition, difficulty in weaning because of respiratory muscle weakness is most likely to be associated with:
A. hypocalcemia
B. hypochloremia
C. hyponatremia
D. hypomagnesemia
E. hypophosphatemia

14. In a postoperative patient who has oliguria, which of the following would be more diagnostic of acute renal failure than of extracellular volume depletion?
A. Urine output of 20 mL/hr
B. Urine sodium concentration of 70 mEq/L
C. Urine osmolarity of 600 mOsm/L
D. Urine specific gravity of 1.030
E. Blood urea nitrogen:creatinine ratio of 25

15. The most common anion in the interstitial fluid is:
A. phosphate (PO_4)
B. chloride
C. bicarbonate
D. sodium
E. potassium

16. The sodium concentration of lactated Ringer's solution is:
A. 864 mEq/L
B. 154 mEq/L
C. 130 mEq/L
D. 77 mEq/L
E. 34 mEq/L

17. The hormonal response in the early postoperative period causes:
A. an increase in sodium resorption
B. a decrease in sodium excretion
C. an increase in urine sodium levels
D. a decrease in cardiac output
E. an increase in the alveolar water vapor pressure

18. What is the most reliable indicator of the effectiveness of resuscitation efforts in the patient with thermal injury?
A. Central venous pressure
B. Pulmonary capillary wedge pressure

C. Heart rate and blood pressure
D. Hourly urinary output
E. Level of consciousness and body weight

19. A patient is found unconscious in the bathroom after a routine total knee replacement. Initial arterial blood gas measurements are: pH 7.16, Po_2 60 mm Hg, Pco_2 70 mm Hg, and HCO_3 27 mEq/L. Which of the following best characterizes this patient's immediate problem?
    A. Severe hypoxia
    B. Compensated metabolic acidosis
    C. Uncompensated metabolic acidosis
    D. Compensated respiratory acidosis
    E. Uncompensated respiratory acidosis

20. A 60-kg patient arrives at the emergency department after a gunshot wound to the right groin that injured the femoral artery. Paramedics report massive blood loss at the scene and started 3 L lactated Ringer's solution through large-bore intravenous lines. The bleeding is now controlled with pressure. The patient's initial arterial blood gas measurements are: pH 7.20, Po_2 120 mm Hg, Pco_2 32 mm Hg, and HCO_3 10 mEq/L. How much bicarbonate is needed to correct the total body base deficit?
    A. 200 mEq
    B. 225 mEq
    C. 250 mEq
    D. 275 mEq
    E. 300 mEq

Oral Examination Study Questions

CASE 1

A 25-year-old, 70-kg woman is referred to you 4 days after a surgeon in a small, rural hospital performed an emergency laparotomy for a gunshot wound to the abdomen. During the procedure, the surgeon repaired a hole in the proximal jejunum and resected the tail of the pancreas and the spleen. The patient now has a temperature of 104°F, a pulse of 120/min, and blood pressure of 100/70 mm Hg. She also has an obvious area of drainage in her upper midline incision. In addition, she has a 19-gauge scalp vein needle in her hand and a nasogastric tube. How do you manage this patient?

OBJECTIVE 1

The student does the following:

A. Establish two large-bore intravenous lines and start lactated Ringer's solution.

B. Perform a history and physical examination.

C. Request a laboratory examination.

   1. A complete blood count is performed. Hematocrit is 35%, and white blood cell count is 21,000/mm³, with a left shift.

   2. Na^+ is 128 mEq/L, K^+ is 3.3 mEq/L, Cl^- is 100 mEq/L, CO_2 is 18 mEq/L, blood urea nitrogen is 53 mg/dL, and glucose is 201 mg/dL.

   3. Amylase is 300 IU/L.

D. Insert a Foley catheter and culture urine.

E. Perform culture and Gram stain of drainage, blood, and sputum. All are negative.

F. Obtain arterial blood gas measurements. Findings are: Po_2 85 mm Hg on nasal cannula, Pco_2 32 mm Hg, and pH 7.31.

G. Obtain a chest x-ray. Atelectasis is found.

OBJECTIVE 2

The patient's blood pressure responds to the lactated Ringer's solution and is 130/80 mm Hg. Her heart rate drops to 90 beats/min. On physical examination, nothing is unusual, except the drainage, which does not seem purulent. After reviewing the laboratory values, the student takes the following steps.

A. Measure input and output, daily weights, and electrolyte content of the drainage, and establish a central line for pressure monitoring.

B. Rewrite the fluid orders.

   1. Change the intravenous solution to D5 ½ NS with 20 mEq KCl/L at a rate of 125 mL/hr to replace:

      a. Insensible loss of 700 to 1000 mL water plus 7% per degree of fever.

      b. Urine output, which is desirable at 30 to 50 mL/hr.

      c. Drainage loss, which is unknown, but appears significant.

      d. Nasogastric loss, which may contain 75 to 120 mEq Na^+ and 30 mEq K^+/L.

   2. Consider either a pancreatic or a small bowel fistula, and know the electrolyte content expected from drainage: Na^+ 130 to 140 mEq/L, K^+ 5 to 15 mEq/L, Cl^- negligible, HCO_3^- 40 to 80 mEq/L.

   3. Consider ordering "boluses" of KCl initially to replace K^+ losses. Also consider adding bicarbonate to therapy.

   4. Consider beginning total parenteral nutrition (TPN).

Minimum Level of Achievement for Passing

The student recognizes hypovolemic shock, possible septic shock, and metabolic acidosis. The student begins initial therapy. On secondary therapy, the student assesses organic fluid needs and writes orders to correct electrolyte imbalances.

Honors Level of Achievement

The student can discuss the roles of insensible loss, drainage, and nasogastric losses, and knows the approximate volumes and electrolyte contents of each. The student knows to begin TPN.

CASE 2

A 54-year-old homeless man comes to the emergency department with a 3-day history of vomiting partially digested food. His medical history is significant for alcoholism and ulcers. He was taking cimetidine (Tagamet) until he ran out of medication 1 month ago. His temperature is 37.8°C, blood pressure is 130/90 mm Hg, heart rate is 98 beats/min, and respiratory rate is 24 breaths/min. What is the differential diagnosis, and how do you proceed with the diagnosis and management of this patient? What metabolic abnormality would you expect?

OBJECTIVE 1

The student recognizes the following common diagnoses in this type of patient:

A. Peptic ulcer disease and its complications:
  1. Bleeding
  2. Perforation
  3. Obstruction
B. Gastritis
C. Hepatitis (alcoholic)
D. Pancreatitis

OBJECTIVE 2

The student completes the following steps:

A. Take a complete history, and perform a physical examination. On physical examination, the patient has a slightly distended upper abdomen that is dull to percussion. The patient also has a succussion splash.
B. Order laboratory studies. Findings are: Na 133 mEq/L, white blood cell count 10,100/mm³, K 3.1 mEq/L, hematocrit 50.3%, Cl 97 mEq/L, hemoglobin 15.1 g/dL, CO_2 34 mEq/L, and amylase 105 IU/L.
C. Order an abdominal series of x-rays.
  1. No free air is found.
  2. The stomach is dilated.
D. Start an intravenous line. The patient is given D5 1/2 NS, with 20 mEq KCl/L.
E. Place a nasogastric tube.

Minimum Level of Achievement for Passing

The student recognizes common causes of vomiting in alcoholic patients. The student knows that a patient who is vomiting gastric contents has hypochloremic hypokalemic metabolic alkalosis, and the student knows how to treat it.

Honors Level of Achievement

The student can discuss the etiology of the metabolic derangement, including gastric and renal losses. The student can also discuss the electrolyte contents of various intravenous fluids.

CASE 3

A 75-year-old woman undergoes elective colon resection for cancer. On postoperative day 3, she complains of shortness of breath. Her blood pressure is 128/70 mm Hg, heart rate is 75 beats/min, and respiratory rate is 32 breaths/min. How do you manage the patient?

OBJECTIVE 1

The student should:

A. Recognize the common possible etiologies for this patient's shortness of breath.
  1. Pulmonary edema
  2. Myocardial infarction
  3. Preliminary embolism
  4. Pneumonia
B. Perform a physical examination. Bilateral rales are found on auscultation of the chest.
C. Immediately order:
  1. Chest x-ray. Cephalization of pulmonary vasculature is found.
  2. Electrocardiogram. Normal sinus rhythm is found, with no ST segment changes.
  3. Arterial blood gas measurements on room air are: pH 7.47, O_2 saturation 80%, P_{O_2} 50 mm Hg, base excess +0.5, and P_{CO_2} 33 mm Hg.
D. Administer oxygen.
E. Consider diuretic therapy.
F. Consider transfer to the intensive care unit.

OBJECTIVE 2

The student can explain the hormonal changes that occur in the postoperative period.

Minimum Level of Achievement for Passing

The student identifies common causes of postoperative shortness of breath and recognizes the signs and symptoms of pulmonary edema.

Honors Level of Achievement

The student describes the increases and decreases of postoperative hormones, such as antidiuretic hormone (ADH), aldosterone, and cortisol.

SUGGESTED READINGS

Gynn S. Kidney function and fluid balance in the elderly surgical patient. In: Gynn S, ed. *Medical Assessment of the Elderly Surgical Patient.* Rockford, IL: Aspen, 1986:189–223.

Halperin NL, Goldstein MB. *Fluid, Electrolyte and Acid-Base Physiology: A Problem-Based Approach,* 2nd ed. Philadelphia, Pa: WB Saunders, 1994.

Kokko JP, Tannen RL. *Fluids and Electrolytes,* 3rd ed. Philadelphia, Pa: WB Saunders, 1996.

Pestana C. *Fluids and Electrolytes in the Surgical Patient,* 4th ed. Baltimore, Md: Williams & Wilkins, 1989.

Sladen A. Acid-base balance. In: McIntyre KM, Lewis AJ, eds. *Textbook of Advanced Cardiac Life Support.* Dallas, Tex: American Heart Association, 1994.

Valtin H. *Renal Function: Mechanisms Preserving Fluid and Solute Balance in Health,* 3rd ed. Boston, Mass: Little, Brown, 1995.

4

Nutrition

Anthony P. Borzotta, M.D.
Alan B. Marr, M.D.
Anthony L. Imbembo, M.D.

OBJECTIVES

1. List at least four factors in a patient's medical history and physical examination that indicate malnutrition.
2. Discuss the following objective assessments of nutritional status: anthropometric measurements, biochemical blood tests, the urine urea nitrogen test, and indirect calorimetry.
3. Determine a patient's protein and calorie requirements by estimation, with the Harris-Benedict equation, or with specific laboratory tests.
4. List at least four water-soluble vitamins, three fat-soluble vitamins, and four trace elements that must be added to long-term parenteral nutrition.
5. Briefly describe the metabolic changes that occur in short-term and long-term starvation.
6. Discuss the effect of injury or infection on a patient's metabolism, and describe how nutritional support must be altered.
7. List at least five indications each for enteral and parenteral nutritional support.
8. Discuss the factors involved in choosing a route of nutritional support.
9. Describe the risks and benefits of enteral and parenteral nutritional support.
10. List at least four gastrointestinal, four mechanical, and four metabolic complications of enteral therapy, and describe appropriate prevention or treatment of each.
11. List four adverse sequelae of a total parenteral nutrition (TPN) catheter and four metabolic complications of TPN. Describe the appropriate treatment of each.

The surgeon often encounters patients who cannot eat normally, who are nutritionally depleted, or who are at risk for malnutrition. Consequently, surgeons care for patients who need a nutritional support program to maintain or restore normal body weight and composi-

tion. Many major advances in nutritional support were made by surgeons, including the first demonstration that intravenous nutrition alone could support the growth of beagle puppies, reported by Dudrick et al. in 1969.

This chapter describes and defines the current clinical and laboratory techniques for assessing nutritional status; the basic requirements for proteins, carbohydrates, lipids, and micronutrients; and the metabolic patterns found in normal, fasted, and stressed states. The indications for beginning (and the techniques for instituting, maintaining, and monitoring) enteral and parenteral nutritional therapy are outlined. A few surgical conditions are discussed in terms of nutritional support. Finally, some areas of controversy and promise for the future are discussed.

Basic Nutritional Needs

Nutrition is the study of the provision and use of foodstuffs in support of metabolic needs for immediate energy, protein synthesis, circulation and respiration, locomotion, energy storage, and waste product excretion. The supply and use of nutrients interact in a dynamic process. Metabolism varies with the amount of nutrient intake; the proportions of carbohydrate, lipid, and protein; and the homeostatic balance of the organism. This section describes essential substrate needs and how to estimate them.

Protein and Amino Acid Needs

The protein requirement is the amount needed to meet physiologic needs, and is the lowest protein intake at which nitrogen balance can be achieved. Proteins do not exist in storage form: they all have structural, enzymatic, immune, and transport functions. Ingestion of amino acids in excess of needs results not in storage, but in deamination, nitrogen excretion as urea and ammonia, and reuse of the carbon skeletons. When intake is insufficient, functioning protein is mobilized, principally through skeletal muscle proteolysis. As a result, essential amino acids are added to endogenous, nonessential amino acids, and gluconeogenic substrates are provided. Although muscle wasting is the primary site of breakdown, the lungs, heart, kidneys, and white blood cells also contribute. If this self-consumption is unchecked beyond the point at which 50% of lean body mass is lost, death may ensue. The mechanisms of compensation during starvation are discussed later, in the section on metabolic states.

Determining the patient's protein requirement is the first critical step in formulating a nutritional support program. The requirements for a normal, active person are 0.8 to 1.0 g protein/kg body weight daily (6.25 g protein = 1 g nitrogen). Requirements change with the clinical state, decreasing to less than 1 g/kg/day early in refeeding after starvation and increasing from 2 to 2.5 g/kg/day in patients who are burned or severely septic. Total protein intake may need to be limited to 40 to 50 g/day in patients with hepatic failure. A 24-hour urine nitrogen loss measurement provides the most accurate and individualized estimate of nitrogen (protein) needs.

Protein balance cannot be achieved without protein intake, but the provision of nonprotein calories significantly enhances the efficiency of protein use. Protein sparing is maximally achieved with 150 to 200 g (700 kcal) glucose daily. This value is the basis for the hypocaloric, 3% amino acid peripheral vein infusions **(protein-sparing therapy)** that are used by some clinicians in fasting clinical situations, such as repeated nothing by mouth (NPO) status during prolonged diagnostic evaluation, bowel obstruction, or adynamic ileus without previous weight loss. The remaining energy requirements are met by mobilization of fat stores.

Two further concepts should be kept in mind. First, at any fixed level of protein intake, nitrogen balance improves to a maximum as calorie intake increases from inadequate levels to levels that exceed energy requirements. That is, nonprotein calories supply energy to the body, allowing ingested protein to be used for synthetic purposes, rather than being oxidized. Second, even when all energy needs are met by nonprotein calories, the nitrogen balance becomes increasingly negative at a fixed nitrogen intake as catabolism increases in disease states (e.g., burns, peritonitis, multiple trauma).

Several amino acids are of special interest. The branched-chain amino acids (BCAAs; leucine, isoleucine, and valine) are essential amino acids that act as oxidative substrate in skeletal muscle; have protein synthesis–enhancing properties (particularly leucine); and inhibit protein breakdown. Several BCAA-enhanced solutions are available, but they have not proven to clearly improve clinical outcome. Further proof of their benefit is needed before they can be recommended. Glutamine, a nonessential amino acid, is the most abundant in the body, accounting for one-third of the amino acids that are released from muscle during stress. Glutamine is an ammonia donor in the kidney, aiding in acid–base balance; it is a primary fuel for enterocytes and other rapidly proliferating tissues (e.g., fibroblasts, white blood cells); and it is a carbohydrate precursor. It appears to be provisionally essential in catabolic states. Arginine supplements improve immune response in vitro. Two recent studies in trauma patients showed that an arginine-enhanced enteral feeding (with several other potentially positive immunomodulators) significantly reduced septic complications compared with an isocaloric, isonitrogenous formula. To summarize, continuing research shows specific actions by individual amino acids beyond their simple contribution to nitrogen balance.

Energy Needs

Caloric requirements range from 25 to 80 kcal/kg/day, depending on age (greater in childhood) and stress. Glycogen, a carbohydrate storage form that is available for immediate energy needs, is in short supply. The approximately 75 g glycogen in the liver and the 200 to 400 g glycogen in adult muscle lasts only 1 to 2 days without replenishment. After glycolysis, muscle glycogen is released as lactate and pyruvate, which are then transported to the liver to be incorporated into glucose through the Cori cycle. Pyruvate is transaminated in muscle and released as alanine, a major substrate for hepatic gluconeogenesis. Lipolysis in adipose tissue releases triglycerides, which serve immediate energy needs for nonglycolytic tissues. Fat is the largest storehouse of energy, and is the principal energy source during long fasts. Protein, especially from skeletal muscle, can be an energy source, but at the cost of destroying functional proteins. Conservation of protein occurs as a survival mechanism during long fasts.

The energy requirement can be estimated in several ways (Table 4-1). The World Health Organization equations are more precise than the **Harris-Benedict equations,** which overestimate the **resting metabolic expenditure** (RME; the energy needed to lie in bed after a fast) by more than 10%, especially in women. The RME is multiplied by both activity and stress factors to reach a total daily requirement. The factors are: fever, 1.13/1°C; bed rest, 1.15; ambulation, 1.2 to 1.3; major elective surgery, 1.2 to 1.4; trauma and fractures, 1.5 to 1.8; and severe sepsis and burns, 1.8 to 2.5. All of these methods are population-derived estimates and simply approximate needs. Indirect calorimetry is needed to make accurate, individualized determinations.

Nonprotein calories are provided as carbohydrates (dextrose parenterally; monosaccharides, disaccharides, and polysaccharides enterally) and lipids. The energy value of nutrient formulations is described in terms of total kilocalories per milliliter, as total calories per gram nitrogen (TC:N), and as nonprotein calories per gram nitrogen (NPC:N). Energy needs are usually defined in terms of nonprotein calories. The NPC:N ratio varies with the metabolic state. It is higher in well-fed, stable patients, who require relatively more energy than protein (150:1), and lowest in hypercatabolic patients (80:1), who have accelerated proteolysis that is proportionately greater than their increased energy needs. If the daily nitrogen output and metabolic state are known, then the ratio can be applied to estimate energy needs. For example, a patient with pancreatitis (moderately catabolic, assumed ratio 100:1) loses 20 g nitrogen/day (see the later discussion of the urine urea nitrogen test) and requires $20 \times 100 = 2000$ kcal/day.

Table 4-1. Estimating Energy Needs

Harris-Benedict equations for resting metabolic rate (kcal/day)

Men: RME = 66.47 + 13.75 × weight (kg) + 5 × height (cm)
− 6.76 × age (yr)

Women: RME = 665.1 + 9.56 × weight (kg) + 1.85 × height (cm)
− 4.7 × age (yr)

World Health Organization, based on compilation of 11,000
measurements in people of all ages, both sexes, all ethnic groups,
and all body mass indices (kj/24 hr). Convert kilojoules to
kilocalories by dividing by 4.184.

Men: 18 to 30 yr: RME = 64.4 × weight (kg) − 113.0
× height (m) + 3000

30 to 60 yr: RME = 19.2 × weight (kg) + 66.9
× height (m) + 3769

Women: 18 to 30 yr: RME = 55.6 × weight (kg) + 1397.4
× height (m) + 146

30 to 60 yr: RME = 36.4 × weight (kg) − 104.6
× height (m) + 3619

General estimate based on weight alone:

25 to 30 kcal/kg/day in nonobese persons

Increase by 12% after major surgery, by 20% to 50% during sepsis,
and up to 80% with major burns

For obese persons, use ideal body weight

RME, resting metabolic expenditure.

Micronutrients: Vitamins

Vitamins are compounds that are required in minute amounts for normal growth, maintenance, and reproduction. They are not endogenously synthesized. Essential vitamins in humans are the four fat-soluble and nine water-soluble vitamins (Table 4-2). The allowances for normal persons at varying ages are well defined. The American Medical Association (AMA) Nutrition Advisory Group published requirements during total parenteral nutrition (TPN). Needs during stress states are imprecise because of the variability of patient and disease, but have been estimated by the National Academy of Sciences.

The fat-soluble vitamins serve many functions. Vitamin A is an essential component of the visual cycle and preserves the integrity of epithelial membranes by limiting keratinization. Vitamin D enhances gut absorption and resorption from bone of both calcium and phosphorus. Vitamin E is a family of seven tocopherols that have antioxidant properties and indefinite biologic roles. Vitamin K is a cofactor for the synthesis of coagulation factors II, VII, IX, and X. Vitamin K absorption in the jejunum requires the presence of bile salts; hence, the abnormal coagulation times generally associated with bile duct obstruction. The destruction or alteration of colonic microflora by antibiotics also may induce vitamin K deficiency. Patients who are receiving TPN are usually given 10 mg vitamin K intramuscularly once a week, to prevent coagulopathy.

The water-soluble vitamins include the B complex, which contains cofactors of enzymes that are vital to intermediary metabolism, energy supply, and nucleic acid synthesis. Folic acid deficiency is the most common hypovitaminosis in humans; it is often caused by poor nutritional intake, which is common with alcoholism. The B complex or multivitamin formulations must be added to TPN daily and probably should be included once daily in maintenance intravenous fluids.

Micronutrients: Trace Elements

Trace elements are essential minerals: iron, iodine, cobalt, zinc, copper, selenium, and chromium (see Table 4-2). In addition, animal studies indicate important roles for manganese, vanadium, molybdenum, nickel, tin, silicon, fluorine, and arsenic. Zinc plays a key metabolic role in numerous metalloenzymes (e.g., carbonic anhydrase, alcohol dehydrogenase, alkaline phosphatase). Clinically, zinc is required for normal wound healing, normal immunologic function, taste and smell perception, and dark adaptation. In patients who are maintained on TPN without zinc supplements, serial zinc levels usually show progressive decreases. Approximately 60% of the total body zinc content is located within muscle. Therefore, conditions associated with muscle catabolism are associated with marked release of zinc and subsequent increased excretion in the urine. Zinc deficiency can also develop whenever there are protracted losses of gastrointestinal secretions. Acute zinc deficiency is manifested by diarrhea; central nervous system disturbances (including confusion and lethargy); eczematoid dermatitis of the nasolabial area, perineum, elbows, and digits; alopecia; and acute growth arrest in children. Chronic deficiency is more subtle; inability to heal even superficial wounds should raise suspicion. In the stable adult who is receiving TPN, the daily intravenous zinc replacement is 2.5 to 4.0 mg/day. This amount is increased by an additional 2 mg/day in the acutely catabolic patient. In adults with intestinal losses, additional zinc is provided (12 mg/L small bowel fluid lost; 17 mg/kg stool or ileostomy output).

Copper is a component of several important enzyme systems, such as lysoxidase (involved in the maturation of collagen and elastin), ceruloplasmin (involved in iron metabolism), and tyrosinase (involved in melanin synthesis). Acquired copper deficiency is associated with anemia, leukopenia, and bone demineralization. Copper supplementation is usually 0.5 to 1.5 mg/day. Copper replacement is discontinued in the presence of biliary obstruction because copper is primarily excreted in bile.

Chromium is necessary in trace amounts because it acts as a cofactor for insulin. Chromium enhances the initial reaction of insulin with its receptor in insulin-sensitive tissues. Chromium deficiency in patients with prolonged parenteral nutrition without chromium supplementation leads to weight loss, glucose intolerance, and peripheral sensory neuropathy. Selenium is an essential trace element for many animal species, and is

Table 4-2. Micronutrients

Compound	Recommended Daily Amounts			Function	Deficiency States
	Adults Usual to Stressed	**During TPN**	**Intravenous Dosage**		
Vitamins[a–c]					
Fat-soluble vitamins[b–d]					
A, retinol, IU	3300–5000	1300–2900	3300	Retinal pigments; soft tissue and bone growth; functional integrity of epithelium	Xerophthalmia, night blindness, epithelial keratinization, delayed wound healing, anemia
D, cholecalciferol, IU	400	200–400	200 or 5 ug	Mediates bone sensitivity to parathyroid hormones and gut absorption of calcium	Rickets (children); osteomalacia (adults)
E, tocopherol, IU	10–15	2–10	10	Placental implantation; sperm mobility; antioxidant of vitamin A and unsaturated fatty acids	Male and female infertility, vitamin A deficiency, serum deficiencies of phospholipids
K, mg	2–20	2–4 mg/wk	10 once weekly	Cofactor for synthesis of coagulant factors II, VII, IX, X	Bleeding disorders seen in hepatic disease, malabsorption states, certain antibiotic use
Water-soluble vitamins[a–c]					
B_1, thiamine, mg	1.5–10 (0.5 mg/1000 kcal)	1.2–50	3.0	Decarboxylation of pyruvate and ketoacids; coenzyme in carbohydrate metabolism	Beriberi; high-output cardiac failure; Wernicke's encephalopathy
B_2, riboflavin, mg	1.1–1.8	1.8–10	3.6	Cytochrome oxidase cofactors in cellular respiration	Cheilosis, seborrheic dermatitis, magenta tongue of pellagra, angular stomatitis
B_3, niacin, mg	12–20	10–150	40	Cofactor in redox reactions (NAD^+ and $NADP^+$) and energy metabolism	Pellagra; photosensitive dermatitis, diarrhea, gastrointestinal hemorrhage; dementia
B_5, pantothenic acid, mg	7–40	5–25	15	Synthesis of coenzyme A involved in amino acid; carbohydrate and fat metabolism	Malaise, headache, nausea, vomiting (only with a specific antagonist)
B_6, pyridoxine, mg	1.6–2.0	2–15	4	Coenzyme for amino acid deamination, transamination, decarboxylation, transulfuration, and glucose metabolism	CNS (irritation, depression somnolence); skin (seborrheic dermatitis, glossitis); microcytic, hypochromic anemia
Biotin	150–300	100–200	60	Coenzyme in carboxylation reactions of CHO, lipids, and amino acids	Rare; seborrheic dermatitis
B_{12}, cyanocobalamin, mg	2–4	2–50	5	Coenzyme for purine and pyrimidine synthesis	Pernicious anemia; neural lesions

Table 4-2. con't.

Compound	Recommended Daily Amounts			Function	Deficiency States
	Adults Usual to Stressed	During TPN	Intravenous Dosage		
Folic acid, mg	100–300	200–5000	400	Purine and thymine synthesis for DNA	Leukopenia; megaloblastic anemia; steatorrhea secondary to jejunal mucosal atrophy, sprue, glossitis
C, ascorbic acid, mg	45	30–700	100	Anticorbutic; collagen cross-linking; hydroxylation of proline	Defective sulfonated copolysaccharides and chondroitin sulfate with retarded wound healing; scurvy; wound dehiscence; chronic skin ulcers
Trace elements[e]					
Zinc, mg	10–15		2.5–6.0	Metalloenzymes involved in lipid, carbohydrate, protein and nucleic acid metabolism	Hypogonadism; altered hepatic drug metabolism; diminished wound strength and healing rates; anorexia, diarrhea, abnormalities of taste and smell, mental depression, cerebellar dysfunction, alopecia, typical dermatitis of face
Copper, mg	1.2–3.0		0.5–1.5	Metalloenzymes; iron uptake in hemoglobin synthesis; normal CNS function	Anemia; skeletal defects, demyelination; reproductive failure (congenital deficiency); leukopenia
Chromium, µg	50–290		10–15	Insulin cofactor	Hyperglycemia; mental confusion; peripheral sensory neuropathy with ataxia
Iodine, mg	150		1–2 mg/kg	Thyroid hormone synthesis	Hypothroidism; goiter
Iron, mg	10–18		Usefulness questionable	Constituent of hemoglobin, myoglobin, and cytochromes	Hypochromic anemia
Manganese, mg	2.0–5.0		0.15–0.8	Enzyme cofactor in protein and energy metabolism; fat synthesis	Sterility or diminished fertility; glucose intolerance, hypocholesterolemia, growth retardation

[a]Requirements in specific disease states are ill defined.
[b]Recommended daily amounts. 9th ed. Food and Nutrition Board of the National Research Council, National Academy of Science, 1980.
[c]American Medical Association Nutrition Advisory Group. Multivitamin preparations for parenteral use. *J Parent Ent Nutr* 1979; 3:258–262.
[d]Jeppsson B, Gimmon Z. Vitamins. In: Fisher JE, ed. *Surgical nutrition.* Boston: Little, Brown, 1983: 241–281.
[e]AMA Department of Foods and Nutrition. Guidelines for essential trace element preparation for parenteral use: a statement by an expert panel. *JAMA* 1979; 241: 2051–2054.
TPN, total parenteral nutrition.
IU, international unit
NAD^+, oxidized nicotinamide = adenine dinucleotide.
$NADP^+$, oxidized nicotinamide = adenine dinucleotide phosphate.
CHO, carbohydrate.
CNS, central nervous system.

now believed to be required for humans at doses of 50 to 70 µg/day. It is a component of the enzyme glutathione peroxidase in human red blood cells; this enzyme protects against damage from peroxidation of polyunsaturated fats. Occasional case reports of selenium deficiency have appeared; the manifestations include skeletal myopathy or cardiomyopathy. Selenium supplementation in patients who are receiving TPN is generally in the range of 30 to 100 µg/day. Selenium excess can cause central nervous system dysfunction, so serum selenium levels should be monitored when supplementation is given for an extended time.

Clinical trace element deficiency states are rare. In the United States, they appear among food faddists and severe alcoholics. They occur with prolonged TPN (i.e., months) when the trace elements are not routinely added, but are reversible and respond rapidly to supplementation. Parenteral administration bypasses the regulatory gut mucosa, a situation that is exacerbated by renal insufficiency. Monitoring of serum levels may be needed.

Assessment of Nutritional Status

History

Proper history-taking and keen observation usually elicit clinical findings of malnutrition when present. Poverty, alcoholism, and the extremes of age are risk factors for malnutrition. Unplanned weight loss is identified by comparing current with earlier weights and determining whether the skin or clothing has become loose. A recent weight loss of 10% is considered significant, 15% is severe, and 20% may increase operative mortality tenfold.

Malnutrition can develop in a number of ways that can be discovered by taking a careful nutritional history. Diminished intake may occur in people with severely restricted diets; anorexia of depression or illness; psychologic diseases (e.g., bulimia, anorexia nervosa); and dysphagia as a result of esophageal cancer, bulbar palsy after stroke, or breathlessness while eating (e.g., severe obstructive pulmonary disease). Hospitalized patients who are maintained on 5% dextrose solutions are on enforced fasts that may unintentionally become prolonged. Increased losses may occur in malabsorption syndromes or inflammatory bowel disease and from gastrointestinal fistulas or chronically draining wounds. Supranormal nutritional requirements that are unmet by usual feeding habits are seen in trauma, burns, fever, and sepsis. Catabolic medications (e.g., glucocorticoids, immunosuppressants, isoniazid) may alter nutrient requirements, whereas other therapeutic modalities (e.g., cancer chemotherapy, radiation therapy) often have side effects that reduce the appetite or ability to eat.

Many clinicians still rely on subjective global assessment, based on an individual surgeon's clinical experience. When history and physical examination alone were analyzed in comparison with other methods of nutritional assessment, they provided the best combination of sensitivity and specificity for detecting malnutrition (Kinney et al.). This finding indicates two things: (1) the value of close observation and personal clinical experience and (2) the lack of any independent, completely valid measure of nutritional status. The absence of a single standard is a major impediment to the analysis of the effect of nutritional therapy on acute disease.

Many of the techniques described later should be used repeatedly to assess the effectiveness of nutritional therapy. The goals are positive nitrogen balance and repletion of diminished physical and chemical parameters, or their stabilization in the face of elevated metabolic demands.

Anthropometric Measurements

A variety of techniques are used to assess body fuel depots or body composition. The simplest are anthropometric measurements. Height and weight are universally attainable and are compared with standard tables of ideal values adjusted for age and sex. A general guide for ideal weight is adding 5 pounds per inch over 5 feet to 100 pounds for women or 6 pounds per inch over 5 feet to 110 pounds for men. Obesity is defined as a body weight that is greater than 120% of ideal weight, and morbid obesity is greater than 150% of ideal weight. The triceps skinfold is the thickness of a pinch of skin and fat overlying the triceps of the nondominant arm, midway between the acromion and olecranon, measured with skinfold calipers. When compared with standard values, this measurement provides an estimate of subcutaneous fat stores. Skeletal muscle mass, the greatest body protein depot, is assessed with the arm-muscle circumference. This measurement is determined by taking the midarm circumference (in millimeters) minus 0.314 times the triceps skinfold (in millimeters). This measure of skeletal muscle mass, often referred to as somatic protein status, is compared with normal values specific for sex and age.

Measuring function rather than size is more germane to surgical concerns. Muscle strength is related to nutritional status, and is measured by hand-grip or forearm dynamometry. These techniques measure the amount of force that is generated by willed muscle contraction. Age- and sex-related norms in healthy volunteers were recently established. Patients who ranked below the 85% cutoff value had more postoperative complications.

Anthropometric measurements are more useful in population studies and less applicable to individual nutritional assessments, except over long periods of nutritional therapy. Deviation from normal does not reliably predict a malnourished state because the standards poorly account for individual variation in bone size, hydration, or skin compressibility. These measurements respond slowly to changes in nutritional status, and their interpretation may be complicated by simple fluid changes, especially in very ill hospitalized patients.

Biochemical Measurements

Although skeletal muscle mass reflects somatic protein status, concentrations of the plasma transport proteins reflect internal or visceral protein status. Albumin, transferrin, retinol-binding protein, and prealbumin (Table 4-3) are used to assess nutritional status and response to feeding. However, concentrations do not always reflect turnover rates or the production and destruction of a compound. For example, changes in the volume of distribution (e.g., expansion of the extracellular fluid space during a major resuscitation) can decrease the serum albumin level by dilution, regardless of nutritional status. Because of its short half-life, **prealbumin** is the most reliable choice for monitoring visceral protein response to therapy.

The creatinine–height index estimates somatic protein status because creatinine production from creatine is directly related to skeletal muscle mass. The 24-hour urine creatinine excretion divided by the value for a normal individual of the same sex, height, and ideal weight obtained from standardized tables equals the creatinine–height index. The normal creatinine excretion is 23 to 28 mg/kg ideal body weight/day in men and 18 to 21 mg/kg ideal weight in women. These values decrease with age. Creatinine–height indices of 60% to 80% of ideal indicate moderate depletion; indices of 40% to 50% indicate severe depletion of lean body mass.

Accurate measurement of **nitrogen balance** is key to nutritional support practices. Nitrogen balance is nitrogen intake minus nitrogen excretion. Nitrogen intake is determined from dietary history, calorie counts, or the known composition of enteral or parenteral formulations. The clinical standard for measuring nitrogen excretion is a 24-hour urine collection for **urinary urea nitrogen** (UUN) expressed in grams of nitrogen per 24 hours. To compensate for diurnal changes in nitrogen accretion and excretion related to cyclic eating, a 24-hour collection is necessary in the patient who is eating spontaneously. Shorter collection periods of as little as 6 hours are adequate in continuously fed patients. The UUN is 80% to 90% of total urinary nitrogen. The remainder consists of such compounds as ammonia, creatinine, and amino acids. A highly stressed patient loses a greater proportion of nonurea nitrogen compounds than does a stable patient. In these patients, the UUN is increasingly less accurate and should be

replaced by total nitrogen measurements. Customarily, 3 or 4 g is added to the UUN value to account for unmeasured nitrogen losses. A positive nitrogen balance indicates that there is net protein synthesis; a negative balance indicates that more nitrogen is being lost than ingested. Zero, or balance point, varies with the premorbid customary intake, the metabolic state, and the quality of ingested protein. Protein quality is related to the proportions of essential and nonessential amino acids in a foodstuff. Adequate nonprotein calories must be given with protein to prevent excess conversion of ingested protein into oxidative substrate (gluconeogenesis), rather than for new protein synthesis.

Nitrogen losses are roughly proportional to the catabolic state; hence, the following average losses in grams of nitrogen per day: starvation-adapted, 5; stable after elective surgery, 5 to 10; polytrauma, 10 to 15; and sepsis or burns, more than 15. Nitrogen balance measurements are taken before nutritional support is initiated and at least weekly thereafter to assess and assure the adequacy of therapy. For example, a 60-year-old man with esophageal cancer who has limited his food intake because of odynophagia may be in a starvation-adapted state on admission, excreting only 5 g N/day. After esophagectomy the next day, his nitrogen losses double to 10 g N/day, increasing further to 17 g N/day when pneumonia complicates his postoperative course a week later. Throughout this period, his nutritional support provided a steady 10 g N/day. Assuming unmeasured urine nitrogen losses of 3 g/day, his nitrogen balances would be as follows:

Admission, 10 in minus (5 + 3) 8 out, balance +2 g N/day
Postop, 10 in minus (10 + 3) 13 out, balance –3 gN/day
With pneumonia, 10 in minus (17 + 3) 20 out, balance –10 g N/day.

Immunologic Measurements

Nutrition and immunocompetence are closely linked. When entire populations are examined, for example, malnutrition correlates with an increased incidence of tuberculosis, epidemics of contagious diseases, and pneumonia. Malnourished individuals are prey to infectious complications of operations. Hence,

Table 4-3. Visceral Proteins Used in Nutritional Assessment

| Protein | Half-Life (days) | Normal Levels | Malnutrition | | |
			Mild	Moderate	Severe
Albumin	18	3.5–5.5 g/dL	3.0–3.5	2.1–3.0	<2.1
Transferrin	8	200–400 mg/dL	150–190	100–150	<100
Prealbumin	2–4	15.7–29.6 mg/dL	12–15	8–10	<8

Normal ranges may vary according to laboratory.

immunologic functions are used to assess nutritional state. The absolute lymphocyte count reflects visceral protein status in the absence of nonnutritional variables, such as trauma, anesthesia, and chemotherapy, all of which depress the count. Low counts concurrent with hypoalbuminemia are correlated with an increased incidence of postoperative sepsis. The minimum normal level is 1500×10^6 cells/L.

Delayed hypersensitivity skin tests are anamnestic immune responses to a battery of antigens placed intradermally: mumps, purified protein derivative (PPD), streptokinase-streptodornase (SK-SD), *Candida,* and histoplasmin. A normal response is a 5-mm or greater area of induration in response to at least one antigen at 48 hours. Partial responses are smaller, and nonresponders are termed anergic. Response depends on previous exposure, an adequate dose of antigen, and proper technique of injection and measurement. Responses are depressed by malnutrition, infection, trauma, surgery, anesthesia, burns, corticosteroids, malignancy, and renal failure. These tests are not specific measures of nutritional state, but they are applicable in stable patients. They are not of value during acute illness.

Indirect Calorimetry

Energy need can be assessed by measuring energy expenditure. A metabolic cart is a portable instrument that uses **indirect calorimetry** to quantify energy needs. A metabolic cart includes a paramagnetic oxygen analyzer and an infrared CO_2 analyzer to measure the volumes of oxygen consumed and carbon dioxide expired per unit time. The ratio $CO_2{:}O_2$ is the **respiratory quotient** (RQ) and reflects the proportions of different fuels that are being oxidized for energy needs. Carbohydrates produce equal volumes of CO_2 for O_2 consumed, with an RQ of 1.0. Lipids undergo β-oxidation, yielding both ketone bodies and CO_2. Therefore, they are associated with a lower RQ of 0.71, as found during fasting. When calories are supplied beyond the body's energy needs, the excess is converted to fat, and the RQ is greater than 1.0. Indirect calorimetry is more accurate than population-based estimates of energy needs, which often overestimate or underestimate an individual patient's actual needs. However, the equipment is moderately expensive, many technical features must be rigorously observed, and the values measured over 5 to 30 minutes must be extrapolated to 24 hours' worth of activity. The device computes the measured resting energy expenditure (MREE). The resting metabolic expenditure (RME), the energy needed by a fasted, supine patient at rest, must be increased by 20% (or more) for such energy expenditures as activity, digestion, or fever. The greater value is called total energy expenditure (TEE). A metabolic cart study should be ordered at the outset of nutritional support and at least weekly (more often if the patient's metabolic state is changing).

Body Composition Analysis

The measurement of body composition by bioelectrical impedance analysis (BIA) is improving in accuracy and acceptance. This simple, rapid bedside technique uses a tetrapolar electrode array on a hand and a foot to inject an electric current and measure the voltage drop between the sensing electrodes. The measured resistance is combined with height, and sometimes weight, sex, or thigh circumference, into a computation that yields fat-free mass. Fat-free mass is composed of the body cell mass (all of the vital, oxygen-consuming tissues of the body), extracellular fluid, and extracellular solids. BIA-measured fat-free mass compares well with exchangeable Na/K measurements, and with densitometry in well persons, those with acquired immune deficiency syndrome (AIDS), and those who are receiving nutritional support. It is used in both the outpatient and rehabilitation settings. Its precision in hospitalized patients who are experiencing rapid fluid shifts is under study.

Metabolic Patterns That Affect Nutrition

An adequate energy supply is the critical need for living organisms. Metabolic adaptations serve this end; pathologic or iatrogenic maladaptations may subvert it. This section describes energy flux in a variety of nutritional states.

Postprandial

The postprandial state exists after meals, serving immediate energy and synthesis needs as well as laying down stores for the future. Ingested carbohydrates provide glucose for the brain. The human brain consumes 20% of RME, a proportion that is remarkable among mammals. The blood–brain barrier blocks the entry of large free fatty acids (FFA) or chylomicrons, but allows the entry of small water-soluble compounds (e.g., glucose). In other words, the brain has discriminatory energy needs. Other glycolytic tissues are erythrocytes, bone marrow, renal medulla, and peripheral nerves. The remaining tissues oxidize lipids. There is net amino acid uptake into solid organs and lipogenesis in fat (Figure 4-1).

Postabsorptive

The postabsorptive state occurs after an overnight fast. Hepatic glycogenolysis is mildly supplemented by gluconeogenesis from amino acids that are derived from skeletal muscle. Adipose lipolysis releases FFA to fuel liver and muscle, supplemented by products of hepatic ketogenesis that are also used by muscle.

Early Starvation

In early starvation, glycogen stores are depleted in 12 to 24 hours. As blood glucose concentration decreases, insulin levels drop. An elevated glucagon:insulin ratio or an absolute glucagon increase plus chronic sympathetic nerve activity instigates catabolic changes. Glycogenolysis is replaced by gluconeogenesis in the liver, supplied with substrate from enhanced protein breakdown, especially by skeletal muscle. Approxi-

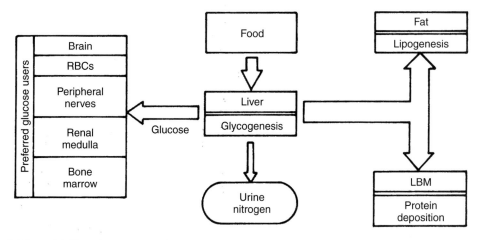

Figure 4-1 Postprandial State. RBCs, red blood cells. LBM, lean body mass (principally skeletal muscle, but includes all viscera).

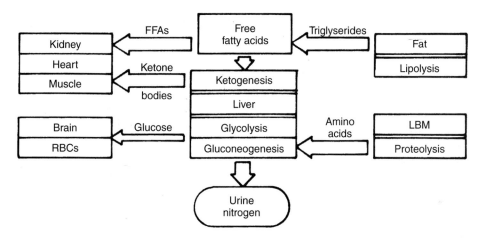

Figure 4-2 The Postabsorptive, or Early Fasting, State. FFAs, free fatty acids. RBCs, red blood cells. LBM, lean body mass.

mately 300 g wet muscle tissue/day is metabolized, and the excess nitrogen is excreted as urea. The UUN is 10 to 12 g/day. Lipolysis increases, and enhanced hepatic ketogenesis occurs. The liver produces ketone bodies (β-hydroxybutyrate and acetoacetate) from the partial oxidation of long-chain fatty acids, which are then used as alternate fuels for extrahepatic tissues. Hepatic ketogenesis reaches a maximum after 2 to 3 days of starvation (Figure 4-2).

Starvation-Adapted

Prolonged starvation leads to the starvation-adapted state, a vital shift that minimizes protein breakdown. Energy expenditure decreases 15% to 25% after 2 weeks of fasting. The peripheral (especially muscle) oxidation of ketone bodies decreases, allowing β-hydroxybutyrate and acetoacetate levels to reach maximal values in 8 to 10 days. Their rising concentrations form a transport gradient into erythrocytes and brain, allowing ketoacids to partially replace glucose as a primary metabolic fuel. After 2 weeks, more than two-thirds of brain oxygen consumption is for ketoacid oxidation. The remainder is for oxidation of glucose derived from glycerol and glu-

coneogenesis. Muscles burn more FFA as declining insulin levels permit enhanced lipolysis. Proteolysis decreases as the need for gluconeogenic substrate decreases; thus, protein is spared (Figure 4-3). The UUN decreases to less than 5 g/day.

Catabolic

A different state of affairs exists in the stressed, hypercatabolic patient. The difference begins with the presence of an injury or infection and the inflammation it evokes. A variety of mediators, including cytokines (e.g., interleukin-1, tumor necrosis factor), bacterial products (e.g., endotoxin), and pain, stimulate catabolic changes, either directly or through the neuroendocrine system. This mediator traffic, which is proportionate to the severity of injury, induces proportional hemodynamic, hormonal, and metabolic alterations. The following changes occur: increased blood flow, hypermetabolism, increased energy expenditure, lean body mass wasting, and abnormal substrate use, lasting 1 to many weeks (Figure 4-4). Resting energy expenditure increases significantly after long bone fracture (10%–30%), sepsis (20%–45%), or burns (40%–100%). Increased metabolic

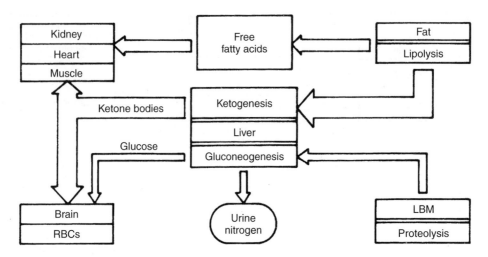

Figure 4-3 Starvation-Adapted State. RBCs, red blood cells. LBM, lean body mass.

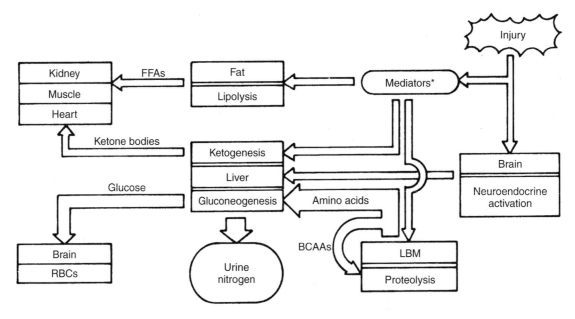

Figure 4-4 Hypercatabolic State. Interleukin-1, prostaglandins, kinins, superoxide radicals, leukotrienes, and pain. FFAs, free fatty acids. RBCs, red blood cells. BCAAs, branched-chain amino acids. LBM, lean body mass.

expenditure is needed for wound healing, synthesis of cellular and humoral immune components, and synthesis of acute-phase reactants until healing is complete. Central thermoregulation is adjusted upward (especially in burns), but increased metabolic expenditure is only slightly abated, even when ambient temperatures are elevated.

Increased catecholamine release is another major catabolic factor. Hypercortisolemia plays a permissive role with the catecholamines. Glucagon concentration rises, increasing proteolysis, gluconeogenesis, and ureagenesis. Unlike in starvation, the anabolic hormone insulin increases, but to a smaller degree than glucagon. The production of glucose is accelerated, and is proportionate to the release of alanine and lactate from skeletal muscle. That is, muscle wasting provides alanine to

meet increased energy needs. The efflux of amino acid from muscle also supplies the raw materials for acute-phase protein synthesis in the liver. The amino acid efflux profile reflects neither the protein composition of muscle nor the composition of newly synthesized protein, which contains disproportionate amounts of glutamine. The fate of the effluxed amino acids is reflected by urine nitrogen losses of more than 20 g/day. Muscle oxidizes BCAA preferentially as an energy source. Ketogenesis is blocked in the liver. Increased lipolysis accelerates the release of FFA and triglyceride, but disposal is impaired, resulting in septic hyperlipidemia. This "auto-cannibalistic" situation continues until infection is controlled or wounds are stabilized by fixation (fractures) or coverage (burns). The late, uncontrolled hypermetabolic state is marked by hepatic failure of gluconeogenesis, hypoglycemia, severe amino acid profile abnormalities, and death.

Techniques of Nutritional Support

Either enteral or parenteral routes of nutritional support will meet a patient's needs. Although parenteral nutrition is well defined, is relatively easy to initiate, and has assured delivery systems, it is costly. Enteral nutrition is less expensive, but more difficult to maintain, and often is less well understood by physicians. During parenteral nutrition, the unused gut shows reduced villus height, enzyme content, and absorptive ability; immunoglobulin E production; and altered bacterial populations, both quantitatively and qualitatively. Combined, these changes may set the stage for transmigration of gut bacteria into the portal system, triggering a catabolic state that precedes multiple organ failure syndrome. A meta-analysis from eight prospective, randomized trials that compared enteral and parenteral support found higher rates of infection and overall complications in patients who were assigned to TPN compared with those who were assigned to enteral feeding. Thus, the advice remains: When the gut is working, use it.

The timing of the onset of nutritional support depends on the disease process. For a fit patient after elective operation, consideration should begin on postoperative day 4 to decide the next day whether the patient will not eat for a more prolonged time. If the patient is not expected to eat, support is begun. Patients with major burns benefit from feedings begun within 24 hours, usually by nasogastric tube. Patients with multiple trauma must first have complete fluid resuscitation, especially before small intestinal feedings begin, because inadequate resuscitation impairs splanchnic perfusion, and food digestion and absorption increase the demands for splanchnic blood flow, potentially causing devastating bowel ischemia.

Enteral Nutritional Support

A variety of enteral formulations are available to satisfy any patient's specialized needs. The products fall into three broad categories based on their composition: (1) polymeric, (2) chemically defined (or elemental), and (3) modular. The products differ in nutrient complexity, osmolarity, caloric density, and viscosity.

Whole food that is blenderized naturally contains intact proteins, fats, polysaccharides, and fiber. Polymeric formulas contain combinations of intact macronutrients. These formulas are high in residue, viscosity, and osmolarity. They are nutritionally complete, and cause few gastrointestinal side effects when delivered into the stomach. Because the feedings are viscous, they may be difficult to deliver through all but a large-bore tube. Energy is supplied as polysaccharides (either milk-based or lactose-free) and lipids, which may be long-chain triglycerides, but also may include medium-chain triglycerides and even short-

chain fatty acids. Protein is derived from whole milk, egg, or soy. Some polymeric formulas are nutritionally complete, but are low in residue, lower in osmolarity, and of only moderate viscosity. Some flavored preparations are palatable and can be administered as oral dietary supplements.

Chemically defined, or **elemental, diets** are characterized by relative chemical simplicity. These products are intended for patients who have impaired digestive capacity or a metabolic state that requires substrate admixtures that are not found in natural foods. These products provide energy as lactose-free polysaccharides. They vary widely in carbohydrate:lipid ratio, and they may include medium-chain triglycerides. Protein is provided as single amino acids or dipeptides, tripeptides, and short polypeptides. Compared with the proportions of amino acids in "ideal" proteins (e.g., albumin), elemental formulas may provide enhanced proportions of BCAAs, glutamine, or arginine. They are also low in residue and nutritionally complete, but are hyperosmolar. They are unpalatable, however, and must be administered through a feeding tube.

Modular products contain only single or a few macronutrients. Protein, fat, and carbohydrate modules are available. By definition, these components cannot provide complete nutrition. They are designed to selectively fulfill special nutritional requirements or to serve as supplements in patients who can tolerate only certain nutrients. Some clinical scenarios illustrate their uses. The willing family of a patient who has head and neck cancer may take a portion of the family meal, blenderize it, and administer it through a gastrostomy tube. A trauma patient would benefit from a high-nitrogen, polymeric formula administered by a continuous infusion pump through a jejunostomy tube. An elderly patient with short-bowel syndrome after resection of ischemic bowel from a mesenteric artery occlusion requires central parenteral nutrition, but may also benefit from an elemental diet given by nasogastric tube, because of the remaining short length of absorptive surface area. Finally, a diabetic patient who is fed with a standard polymeric formulation that worsens hyperglycemia would benefit from a reduced amount of that formula supplemented with a modular product of medium-chain triglycerides to maintain the same total energy supply, but reduce the role of carbohydrate.

Access for Enteral Nutrition

To a large extent, the route chosen for administration of nutritional support depends on a patient's particular circumstances. Patients with adequate appetite and a normally functioning gastrointestinal tract can usually be entirely supported with oral intake. Supplementation with snacks or high-calorie liquids may be appropriate in some patients. In other patients, the gastrointestinal tract is entirely normal, but little or no spontaneous oral intake takes place because of anorexia, depression, inability to swallow, or unconsciousness. Tube feedings permit the use of the functional gastrointestinal system.

Table 4-4. Indications for Enteral Nutritional Support

Preexisting protein-calorie malnutrition because of prolonged
  inadequate intake of nutrients
  Nothing by mouth for 5+ days
  Cancer: oral, esophageal, gastric, pancreatic
  Eating disorders: anorexia, bulimia, severe depression
  AIDS
  Severe chronic obstructive pulmonary disease
  Dietary indiscretion: dietary fads, alcoholism, substance abuse
Sustained inability to eat
  Depressed level of consciousness: stroke, traumatic brain injury,
    metabolic disorders, encephalopathy
  Dysphagia: oropharyngeal cancer operations, advanced
    esophageal motility disorders, pseudobulbar palsy, mandibular
    fractures
  Pulmonary failure requiring prolonged mechanical ventilatory
    support
  Mechanical disability: quadriplegia, severe palsy, spinal cord
    neuropathy
Increased metabolic requirements
  Major burns
  Multiple torso trauma
  Severe brain injury
  Sepsis or systemic inflammatory response syndrome

AIDS, acquired immune deficiency syndrome.

Table 4-5. Enteral Routes for Nutritional Support,
by Site of Nutrient Entry

Oral: Supplements the usual diet or inadequate diet choices by
  increasing calorie or protein intake
Gastric: Also known as prepyloric feeding, therefore dependent on
  the emptying function of the stomach
Nasogastric tube: Passed manually; position must be confirmed by
  chest x-ray (or by aspiration of 10+ mL gastric fluid) to be sure it is
  not in the lungs
Gastrostomy tube (G-tube)
  Tube placed during laparotomy (Stamm, Witzel), by laparoscopy,
    by percutaneous endoscopic gastrostomy (PEG), or by
    fluoroscopy
  Gastrocutaneous fistula (Janeway gastrostomy); often troubled by
    acid erosions at skin level, and largely abandoned
Duodenal: Also known as postpyloric feeding, and dependent mainly
  on how well a tube can be kept in position without reflexing back
  into the stomach
Nasoduodenal tube: Passed manually or with fluoroscopic control,
  often with the help of a dose of metoclopramide; position
  confirmed by abdominal x-ray or pH probe at the tip; often requires
  repeated repositioning
Gastroduodenal tube: Placed during laparotomy to allow
  simultaneous gastric decompression and duodenal feeding
Jejunal: Feedings distal to the ligament of Treitz, with almost no
  chance of reflux of feedings into the stomach (can happen with
  severe ileus, as in peritonitis)
Nasojejunal tube: Passed with fluoroscopic control
Percutaneous endoscopic gastrojejunostomy (PEG/J or PEJ): A
  second, smaller-diameter tube passed within a PEG tube distally
  into the jejunum (allows simultaneous gastric decompression)
Jejunostomy tube (J-tube:) Placed at laparotomy or laparoscopy
Needle catheter jejunostomy: Will accept only elemental diets due to
  its small bore

The essential component of selecting the route for delivery of enteral feeding is choosing which portion of the patient's gastrointestinal tract to access. This decision is influenced by the anticipated duration of feeding and by whether the patient is an operative candidate (Table 4-4). Either the stomach or the small bowel may be used. Delivery of enteral feeding into the stomach **(prepyloric feeding)** ensures exposure to the maximal intestinal absorptive surface available, an important consideration in a patient who has a limited amount of small bowel remaining. In addition, because the stomach is a reservoir where diets are mixed and tonicity is adjusted, greater latitude in the selection of diet and the technique of administration results when intragastric delivery is chosen. The greater ease and flexibility with which intragastric feeding is performed must be weighed against the risks of gastroesophageal reflux, vomiting, and aspiration, especially in the patient who is already debilitated. Instillation of the diet into the small bowel **(postpyloric feeding)** virtually eliminates the problems of gastric retention, reflux, vomiting, and aspiration of feedings, if not of gastric secretions. In addition, jejunal motility is usually not affected by most mechanical and inflammatory processes in the upper abdomen that may inhibit gastric emptying. The parenteral route is necessary when the gastrointestinal tract is nonfunctional or unavailable.

Several means of access to the gastrointestinal tract are available (Table 4-5). Transnasal intubation is the simplest and most widely used method. Although individual differences exist in length and composition, most of the current feeding catheters are manufactured from silicone rubber or polyurethane. Weights incorpo-

rated into the catheter tips facilitate neither introduction nor maintenance in the desired location. Most nasogastric feeding tubes are long enough to allow access to the proximal small bowel. In approximately one-half of ambulatory patients, the feeding catheter spontaneously passes into the small bowel. The proximal small bowel may be successfully cannulated under fluoroscopic control, with the use of a rigid stylet to manipulate the tip of the catheter through the pylorus. Alternatively, the tip of the catheter may be guided into the small bowel with a fiberoptic gastroscope and its snare or biopsy forceps. Gastric or jejunal tubes are easily placed endoscopically (percutaneous endoscopic gastrostomy and percutaneous endoscopic jejunostomy). All of the small, soft, nonreactive nasoenteral catheters are safe for extended use. However, these catheters are generally used for short-term programs because of their propensity to dislodge and cause discomfort. It is essential to confirm the intraabdominal location of the tip of the catheter by x-ray before feeding is instituted. The air insufflation test alone does not protect the patient from inadvertent feeding into the airway as the result of a catheter that is misplaced into a bronchus.

Table 4-6. Schedule for Enteral Nutritional Support

Gastric route
  Adjunctive support to oral diet
    Daytime supplements: One can (250 mL), either orally or through a nasogastric tube, after each meal if < 50% taken
    Nighttime supplements: Continuous feeding from 10:00 PM until 6:00 AM of 30% to 60% of daily needs, based on daytime oral intake
  Complete support
    Continuous: See the jejunal regimen, but advance rates every 24 hours
    Bolus: Through a nasogastric or gastric tube
      Full strength, 100 mL q 3 hours, for 24 hours (800 mL/day)
      Check gastric residual before each feeding: hold for 1 hour if > 100 mL, and recheck. If residuals stay low, then:
      Full strength, 200 mL q 3 hours, for 24 hours (1600 mL/day)
      Check gastric residuals, as above
      Full strength, 300 mL q 4 hours, for 24 hours (1800 mL/day)
      Check gastric residuals, as above
      Full strength, 400–500 mL q 4 to 6 hours (1600–3000) mL/day)
      Check gastric residuals, as above
Jejunal route
  Continuous only (bolus feeding induces cramps, diarrhea, and gastric reflux)
    Full strength, 25 mL/hr[a]
    Advance rate by 25 mL/hr q 12 hours to final rate
    Do not check jejunal residuals
    Flush delivery system with 30 mL tap water at each tube feeding change, and after any medication is given through a tube
    24 hours after final rate is reached, add 300 mL tap water bolus twice a day to four times a day, depending on the patient's volume and electrolyte status

[a]Elderly patients or those whose gut has been unused for some time may not tolerate full-strength feedings. Start at half-strength, increasing to full strength after the final rate is reached.

Table 4-7. Complications of Enteral Therapy

Mechanical
  Pulmonary aspiration
  Esophageal reflux
  Depressed cough
  Parotitis
  Otitis media
  Esophageal erosions
  Tube obstruction
  Inadvertent airway administration
Gastrointestinal
  Diarrhea
  Malabsorption
  Abdominal cramping
  Exacerbation of gastrointestinal disease
  Nausea and vomiting
  Distension
Metabolic
  Prerenal azotemia
  Fluid and electrolyte abnormalities
  Hyperglycemia
  Hyperosmolar dehydration or nonketotic coma
  Inadvertent intravenous administration
  Essential fatty acid deficiency

Operative access to the gastrointestinal tract for feeding can be achieved at a variety of levels. The proximal esophagus, stomach, and jejunum are all sites for operative feeding tube enterostomies. Although placement of a feeding tube may be the primary reason for an operation and general anesthetic, endoscopic procedures are becoming the norm. A feeding tube jejunostomy should be placed during major foregut, biliary, or hepatic operations; during a major trauma laparotomy; after pancreatic surgery; or in nutritionally bankrupt patients. Laparoscopic methods are being developed for the placement of gastric and jejunal tubes.

Implementation and Administration of an Enteral Feeding Program

Table 4-6 shows examples of enteral support programs by various routes. Bolus gastric feeding is advantageous because a pump is not needed, as in continuous feeding, but there may be little difference in nursing time. For intragastric feeding, enteral formulas are initiated at a caloric density of 1 kcal/mL (i.e., full strength). Initially, half-strength feedings may be better tolerated in elderly patients or those whose gut has been unused

for a prolonged period. After the final rate is reached, feedings can be increased to full strength. Patients who are fed intragastrically should be positioned with the head of the bed elevated 30°. These patients should be encouraged to ambulate frequently to minimize the risk of aspiration.

Intrajejunal feeding uses continuous administration by an infusion pump. Too rapid infusion of the diet or excessive caloric density can cause abdominal distension, weakness, sweating, hyperperistalsis, cramps, and diarrhea. The diarrhea can result from several factors: osmotic overload, rapid transit through the small bowel, or incomplete absorption. Because the jejunum lacks the ability of the intact stomach to serve as a reservoir while tonicity is adjusted, there is less flexibility with jejunal feeding than with intragastric feeding.

Complications of Enteral Nutrition

The possible complications of enteral therapy are shown in Table 4-7. Patient interview and examination are the most critical tools for determining gastrointestinal tolerance of a defined-formula diet. Gastrointestinal overload may be signaled by symptoms of fullness, bloating, crampy abdominal pain, and nausea. Hyperactive bowel sounds and abdominal distension may also be noted. Vomiting may follow, particularly with intragastric feeding. Voluminous diarrhea may affect fluid and electrolyte balance. Gastrointestinal side effects occur in 10% to 20% of tube-fed patients. The signs and symptoms of gastrointestinal intolerance are managed by reducing both volume and caloric density until the patient becomes asymptomatic. Alternatively, feedings may be interrupted transiently if symptoms are severe or if the gastric residual is high. Antidiarrheal medications (e.g., paregoric, dilute tincture of opium) may be added directly to the feeding in refractory cases; however, obstipation and distension may occur with these agents. They should not be used if *Clostridium difficile* colitis is present.

Mechanical problems include tube dislodgment; malposition (i.e., into the airway, esophagus, or stomach instead of the duodenum); blockage; nasal sinus obstruction, with consequent sinusitis; and tracheo-esophageal fistula. Operations to place tubes may be complicated by bowel obstruction, wound infection, wound dehiscence, and peritonitis. Metabolic complications are similar to those seen with parenteral nutrition (Table 4-8).

Parenteral Nutritional Support

Formulations

When the gastrointestinal tract is not available for use in providing nutritional support, the parenteral route must be used. Common indications for parenteral nutritional support are shown in Table 4-9. There are three categories of parenteral nutrition. Protein-sparing therapy uses a 3% amino acid solution in 5% dextrose with electrolytes, and is administered through a peripheral vein. This hypocaloric protein source is recommended for the nutritionally fit patient who is undergoing fasting for a week or so. **Peripheral parenteral nutrition** uses a 3% amino acid solution in 10% dextrose with electrolytes, plus a lipid emulsion that supplies as much as 60% of estimated energy needs. It can be given by peripheral vein, but is relatively hyperosmolar. This solution is used to supply all estimated energy needs in nonstressed patients. TPN supplies all energy and nitrogen needs, even in hypercatabolic patients. Because of its hypertonicity, it must be delivered into a central vein (see Table 4-10 and Figure 4-5).

Parenteral caloric requirements are most often met by the administration of dextrose as a 20% to 35% solution, with tonicity ranging from 1000 to 1500 mOsm/L. Parenteral nutritional programs require the administration of nitrogen in the form of pure L-amino acid solutions. Compared with naturally occurring proteins, synthetic amino acid solutions can be selectively enriched by essential amino acids for use in renal failure, or by BCAAs with restricted amounts of aromatic amino acids and methionine for use in hepatic failure. In addition, solutions with an enhanced BCAA content ($\leq$ 45% of protein as BCAA) are available for use in the management of hypercatabolic states. The efficacy of these preparations is limited to the period of hypercatabolism. After the hypercatabolism is resolved, standard amino acid preparations are appropriate. A typical standard solution contains 25% dextrose and 4.25% amino acids, supplying 2700 nonnitrogen calories and 18.75 g nitrogen when 3 L/day is administered.

Electrolytes, vitamins, and trace elements are prescribed as well. Vitamin requirements are shown in Table 4-3. Electrolytes should be monitored frequently, particularly in the face of extraordinary losses. Hypo-

kalemia commonly occurs after parenteral nutritional support is initiated. The use of glucose is associated with intercellular transport of potassium. The administration of carbohydrate and protein may profoundly decrease serum potassium levels if insufficient potassium is administered. Hypophosphatemia can also develop because of intracellular shifts of phosphorus. The usual desired concentrations of electrolytes for TPN are: Na^+, 40 to 50 mEq/L; K^+, 40 mEq/L; Cl^-, 50 mEq/L; Mg^{2+}, 4 to 6 mEq/L; Ca^{2+}, 2.5 to 5.0 mEq/L; HPO^-, 20 to 25 mmol/L; and acetate, 40 to 60 mEq/L.

Access for Parenteral Nutrition

The most commonly used technique for central venous access is percutaneous cannulation of the subclavian or internal jugular vein. With either approach, the tip of the catheter must lie within the superior vena cava before any hypertonic solution is administered. Placement of the catheter under rigidly sterile conditions and a program of regular catheter care will prevent most infectious complications. When the catheter entry site is covered by a sterile occlusive dressing, the dressing should be changed by trained personnel at least three times per week. The transparent dressings may be safely left in place for as long as 3 days. The catheter should be used only to deliver nutrient solutions. Blood should not be withdrawn from or administered through the catheter. Medications and supplemental intravenous infusions are not given through the catheter because they may serve as portals for infections. When multiple-lumen catheters are used, one lumen is used exclusively for nutrition, whereas the other(s) can be used for such procedures as drug delivery and specimen withdrawal. The tubing that is used for parenteral nutrition should be changed daily. The ideal system consists of: (1) a single-solution bottle that is connected to a drip chamber and (2) intravenous tubing that connects directly to the catheter. Infusion pumps keep the solutions running at a steady rate and prevent accidental rapid infusion of large amounts of hypertonic fluid. Volumetric infusion pumps with an occlusion alarm, an infusion-complete alarm, and an air-in-line detector are commonly used.

Once the catheter is properly positioned, the infusion is started slowly, usually at a rate of 40 to 50 mL/hr. Glucose tolerance is assessed by following the patient's urinary and blood sugar levels. If there is no evidence of glucose intolerance, the infusion is increased at the rate of an additional 1 L/day until the desired level is reached. Infusion rates are kept constant through the use of an infusion pump. The patient's weight is measured daily, and urine sugar and serum electrolyte levels, including calcium, phosphorus, and magnesium, are closely monitored. Liver function tests and lipid levels are tested weekly. Transferrin is measured weekly.

Parenteral Nutrition with Lipid Emulsion

An alternate regimen for TPN uses lipid as a prime, or occasionally a supplementary, calorie source. All of the lipid preparations are 10% or 20% emulsions of

Table 4-8. Metabolic Complications of Total Parenteral Nutrition and Their Treatment

Problems	Etiologies	Prevention and Treatment
Glucose metabolism		
Hyperglycemia, glycosuria, osmotic diuresis, hyperosmolar nonketotic dehydration, and coma	Excessive total dose or rate of administration of glucose; inadequate insulin; glucocorticoids; sepsis with insulin resistance	Reduce or stop infusion rate; switch to lipid; add exogenous insulin; control infection (drainage, debridement, antibiotics); free-water resuscitation followed by electrolyte replacement; replace potassium
Ketoacidosis in diabetes mellitus	Inadequate endogenous insulin response; inadequate exogenous insulin therapy	Appropriately increase exogenous insulin; reduce glucose intake
Postinfusion (rebound) hypoglycemia	Persistently elevated islet cell production of insulin; decreased glycogen stores	Taper TPN slowly (over 24–48 hr); always infuse isotonic glucose for several hours after stopping hypertonic infusion
Respiratory failure; unable to wean from mechanical ventilatory support	Conversion of excessive glucose intake into CO_2, especially in patients with chronic obstructive pulmonary disease	Reduce total glucose load or switch to lipid system (40% of total calories as fat emulsion)
Amino acid metabolism		
Hyperchloremic metabolic acidosis	Excessive chloride and monohydrochloride content of crystalline amino acid solutions	Administer Na^+\$ and K^+ as lactate or acetate salts
Serum amino acid imbalance	Nonphysiologic amino acid pattern of the nutrient infusion; differential amino acid uptake in various disorders	Infuse essential amino acid only formulations (renal failure); branched-chain amino acid–enhanced/aromatic amino acid–depleted formulations (sepsis, hepatic failure)
Hyperammonemia (rare)	Arginine, ornithine, aspartic acid, or glutamic acid deficient formulations; primary hepatic disorder	Infuse branched-chain amino acid–enhanced formulations in hepatic encephalopathy; reduce total amino acid intake
Prerenal azotemia	Excessive amino acid infusion; inadequate nonprotein calories	Reduce protein intake; evaluate other causes of prerenal azotemia; increase nonprotein calories-to-nitrogen ratio
Lipid metabolism		
Hyperlipemia	Decreased triglyceride clearance; sepsis	Reduce rate of infusion or discontinue; reassess after bloodstream is cleared of fat
Essential fatty acid deficiency (of phospholipid, linoleic, or arachidonic acids); eczematous, desquamative dermatitis of body folds	Inadequate essential fatty acid administration; inadequate vitamin E administration	Administer linoleic acid twice weekly as 500 mL 10% lipid emulsion; cure by daily lipid emulsion infusion
Calcium and phosphorus metabolism Hypophosphatemia	Inadequate phosphorus administration	Monitor phosphorus levels, especially during repletion of malnourished patients; administer adequate phosphorus
Neuromuscular: weakness, tremor, convulsions, coma, hyporeflexia, death	Decreased central nervous system ATP; inhibition of muscle glycolytic pathways	
Hematologic: hemolytic anemia, decreased oxygen release; decreased leukocyte function; decreased clot retraction and platelet survival	Decreased erythrocyte 2, 3-diphosphoglycerate; decreased cellular ATP; abnormal membrane lipids	
Cardiac: impaired myocardial contractility, congestive cardiomyopathy	Decreased ATP	
Hypocalcemia	Inadequate calcium administration; reciprocal response to phosphorus repletion without calcium; hypoalbuminemia	Add calcium 3 to 4 mEq/kg/ body weight to pediatric TPN; add to base solution as needed in adults
Hypercalcemia	Excessive calcium administration with or without high doses of albumin; excessive vitamin D administration	Withdraw calcium from future infusions; rehydrate; mithramycin, corticosteroids
Miscellaneous		
Hypokalemia	Inadequate potassium intake relative to increased requirements for protein anabolism	Add supplementary potassium to infusion at time of preparation
Hypomagnesemia	Inadequate magnesium intake for increased protein and carbohydrate metabolism	Add supplementary magnesium to infusions at the time of preparation

TPN, total parenteral nutrition.
ATP, adenosine triphosphate.

Table 4-9. Indications for Parenteral Nutritional Support

Gut unavailable
  Prolonged paralytic ileus
  Short-bowel syndrome
  Enterocutaneous and enteroenteral fistulas
  Necrotizing enterocolitis
  Malabsorption syndromes
  Esophageal benign stricture or malignancy
Inadequate oral intake or "bowel rest" indicated
  Acute pancreatitis, hemorrhagic
  Catabolic states: Burns, sepsis, polytrauma
  Extreme prematurity
  Tracheoesophageal fistula (infants; until gastrostomy performed)
  Hyperemesis gravidarum
  Intractable diarrhea
  Wound dehiscence and evisceration
Adjunctive to other therapy
  Cancer chemotherapy
  Cancer radiation therapy
  Inflammatory bowel disease
  Acute hepatitis and hepatic failure
  Perioperative nutritional repletion

Table 4-10. Examples of Parenteral Nutrition Solutions

Standard central formula
  A moderately malnourished patient underwent a major gastric resection 4 days ago, and is not yet capable of eating. He is ordered a standard central formula at a rate of 100 mL/hr. Each day, he will receive 2.4 L fluid; 120 g amino acids (19.2 g nitrogen); 422.4 g dextrose (1436 kcal); and 67.2 g lipids (672 kcal); for a total of 2588 kcal from all sources. There are 2108 nonprotein kcal, for a ratio of 109:1 nonprotein kcal/gram nitrogen (NPC:N); approximately one-third are delivered as lipids.

Standard peripheral formula (PPN)
  A patient whose nutritional state is good has intractable nausea, but has had fluid and electrolyte abnormalities corrected. Peripheral parenteral nutrition is ordered at a rate of 125 mL/hr. Each day, she will receive 3.0 L fluid, 90 g amino acids (14.4 g nitrogen); 300 g dextrose (1020 kcal); and 99 g lipids (990 kcal), for a total of 2370 kcal from all sources. There are 2010 nonprotein kcal, for a ratio of 140:1 nonprotein kcal/g nitrogen, approximately one-half of which are delivered as lipids.

Custom formula
  A 70-kg man has adult respiratory distress syndrome complicating fecal peritonitis from a perforated colon. His nitrogen needs are measured by adding 4 g/day to a recent urine urea nitrogen of 28 g/24 h, for a total of 32 g/day. Although he needs 200 g amino acids/day (32 × 6.25) for nitrogen balance (N_{output} (32) – N_{intake} (32) = N balance), the maximum amount that it is prudent to deliver, even to very catabolic patients, is 2.5 g protein/day, or (70 kg × 2.5 g/kg/day = 175 g amino acids, or 28 N). His energy needs are estimated with an 80:1 ratio of NPC:N, for 2560 kcal/day. One-third will be delivered as lipids (853 kcal ÷ 10 kcal/g = 85 g) and the rest as dextrose (1706 kcal ÷ 3.4 kcal/g = 502 g). His lung disease suggests the need for fluid restriction, so the entire nutritional prescription is to be delivered in a volume administered over 24 hours at 80 mL/hr (1920 mL).

Refer to Figure 4-5, which is an example of preprinted TPN orders. In each example, appropriate electrolytes, vitamins, and trace elements must also be ordered, based on the patient's laboratory tests or particular status each day.

either soybean oil or safflower oil. These oils are mixtures of triglycerides, and they contain predominantly long-chain fatty acids, especially linoleic acid, which is essential in humans. The solutions are relatively isotonic and contain emulsified fat particles that approximate the size of chylomicron (0.5 µm).

In general, fat emulsions make up no more than 60% of total calorie input. Fat intake should not exceed 2.5 g/kg/day in adults and 4 g/kg/day in infants and children, assuming that clearance capacity is normal. The remaining calories are supplied by a 10% to 20% solution of dextrose, primarily to meet the requirements of the central nervous system. Fat emulsions may be infused through a peripheral vein without the rapid development of venous thrombosis, because they are relatively isotonic. To achieve positive nitrogen balance, amino acids are supplied, usually as a 4.25% solution. It is common practice not to mix lipid emulsions with other nutrient solutions, but to administer them through a separate access site or with a Y connector near the point of entry. Single containers that can hold 24 hours' worth of all three nutrients, vitamins, and minerals can be used efficiently when the nutritional prescription is stable.

The use of fat emulsions has the potential advantage of permitting nutritional support through a peripheral vein. Fat emulsions also prevent the development of essential fatty acid deficiency states. A minimum of 500 mL 10% lipid emulsion must be given twice weekly to prevent essential fatty acid deficiency. Essential fatty acid deficiency in humans is caused principally by a lack of linoleic acid. The clinical signs of deficiency are eczematous, desquamative dermatitis of body folds, anemia, thrombocytopenia, and hair loss. Growth retardation can also occur, especially in neonates. Lipid-free solutions can be given for as long as 3 weeks before risking lipid deficiency states. Fat emulsions may be helpful

in patients who have glucose intolerance and in those who require volume restriction because of the greater caloric density of lipid emulsions. Because the metabolism of fat is associated with a lower RQ than the metabolism of carbohydrate, the use of fat emulsions to provide calories may help to wean patients with CO_2 retention from ventilatory support.

Complications of Parenteral Nutrition

The complications of central venous catheterization are shown in Table 4-11. Common complications include technical mishaps, central venous thrombosis, and catheter sepsis. Infusion of a hyperosmolar solution is never started until chest x-rays confirm the correct positioning of the central venous catheter in the superior vena cava and exclude complications secondary to insertion. The overall complication rate of subclavian venous cannulation varies from 3% to 10%. Experience is the major variable. The internal jugular vein can be used as an alternate site for long-term central venous cannulation. Many believe that fewer

LEGACY
Health System

LPH - Adult Parenteral Nutrition
Formula Order Sheet
24 Hour TPN Orders

PRE-PRINTED ORDERS
USE BALL POINT PEN, PRESS FIRMLY

ALL LISTED ORDERS ARE IN EFFECT UNLESS CROSSED OUT. EXCEPTIONS: ORDERS PRECEDED BY A BOX (☐) REQUIRE A (✓) TO INITIATE. ORDERS WITH BLANKS INDICATE ADDITIONAL INFORMATION IS NEEDED.

DATE	TIME:	ORDERS: ANOTHER BRAND OF GENERICALLY EQUIVALENT OR APPROVED THERAPEUTICALLY EQUIVALENT PRODUCT MAY BE ADMINISTERED UNLESS CHECKED.	✓

ALL ORDERS MUST BE WRITTEN BY 1500 TO BE PREPARED AND ADMINISTERED BY 2100. ANY EXCEPTIONS TO THE 2100 START TIME MUST BE COORDINATED WITH THE PHARMACY.

____ **CONTINUOUS**   ____ **CYCLIC**   Bag # ____

TPN SOLUTION CHOICES:

For assistance with TPN orders contact Pharmacist at 34228 (EHHC), 37204 (GSH) or contact Dietitian at 34424 (EHHC), 37084 (GSH)

____ **Standard Central Formula**
Amino Acids   50g/L (Amino Acids 5%)
Dextrose   176g/L (Dextrose 17.6%)
Lipids   28g/L (Lipids 2.8%)
_____
(= approximately 1 Kcal/ml)

NPC:N = 110:1
TC:N = 135:1

____ **Standard Peripheral Formula (PPN)**
Amino Acids   30g/L (Amino Acids 3%)
Dextrose   100g/L (Dextrose 10%)
Lipids   33g/L (Lipids 3.3%)
_____
(= approximately 0.75 Kcal/ml)

____ **Custom Formula****
Protein   ____ g/day x 4.0 = _____ Kcal
Dextrose   ____ g/day x 3.4 = _____ Kcal
*Lipid 20% ____ g/day x 10.0 = _____ Kcal
                TOTAL: _____ Kcal/24 hours

____ **Specialty Formula****
(Check one)
____ BCAA   ____ Hepatic   ____ Renal

NOTE:
* Lipids will be dispensed separately if not compatible.
** See reverse side for instructions and description of Custom & Specialty Formulas.
** BCAA and Hepatic Formula use must have prior approval of attending physician.

ADDITIVES / 24 HOURS:

____ Standard Formulation	____ Extra Additives	____ Other Additives	____ Custom Made Formulation
100 mEq NaCl	____ mEq NaCl	____ u Reg. Human Insulin	____ mEq NaCl
40 mEq K Acetate	____ mEq Na Acetate	____ mg Zinc	____ mEq Na Acetate
20 mEq K Phos	____ mEq Na Phos	____ mg Vit. C	____ mEq Na Phos
9 mEq Ca Gluconate	____ mEq KCl	____ mg Folic acid	____ mEq KCl
10 mEq MgSO$_4$	____ mEq K Acetate	____ Cimetidine	____ mEq K Acetate
1 vial 10 ml MVI	____ mEq K Phos	Other:	____ mEq K Phos
1 vial Trace Elements	____ mEq MgSO$_4$	_____	____ mEq MgSO$_4$
*** 1000 u/L Heparin	____ mEq Ca Gluconate	_____	____ mEq Ca Gluconate
VIT K 10mg q Monday	(✓)____ vial 10ml MVI	_____	(✓)____ vial 10ml MVI
	(✓)____ vial TR Elements	_____	(✓)____ vial TR Elements
			(✓)____ 1000 u/L Heparin

*** Unless otherwise ordered, 1000 units heparin will be added to each liter of TPN.

CONTINUOUS RATE

CPN: Day one infusion rate: Start Infusion at (i.e. 50% final rate) _____ ml/hr for _____ hr, then _____ ml/hr for _____ hours, then final infusion rate: _____.

Continuous Infusion Rate: _____ ml/hr.   NOTE: Substrate amounts must be adjusted proportionally (e.g. Kcal/24 hours) for rate changes.

PPN: Administration Rate: _____ ml/hr.

CYCLIC RATE:

Taper up _____ ml/hr for _____ hr, _____ ml/hr for _____ hr.
Taper down _____ ml/hr for _____ hr, _____ ml/hr for _____ hr.

INFUSE CYCLIC TPN
from _____ hours to _____ hours.

OTHER INSTRUCTIONS:

I. Initiate "Inpatient Nutrition Support Orders" - Nutritional Assessment Orders, Parenteral Route Orders.
II. Hang TPN bags at 2100 unless otherwise specified and coordinated with the Pharmacy.

Physician's or Credentialed Provider's Signature_____

All Pre-Printed Orders must have a Physician/Credentialed Provider's signature to initiate.

105133 (12/95)   Original - Chart • Canary - Pharmacy • Pink - IV

Figure 4-5 Example of Preprinted Total Parenteral Nutrition (TPN) Orders.

Table 4-11. Complications of Central Venous Catheterization

Upon Insertion	During Maintenance
Pneumothorax	Infection or sepsis
Tension pneumothorax	Central vein thrombosis
Subcutaneous emphysema	Thromboembolism
Subclavian or carotid artery injury	Hydrothorax
Subclavian hematoma	Hydromediastinum
Hemothorax	Cardiac tamponade
Caval or cardiac perforation	Endocarditis
Thoracic duct injury	Arteriovenous fistula
Brachial plexus injury	Air embolus
Horner's syndrome	
Phrenic nerve injury	
Improper position	

technical complications occur with internal jugular venous cannulation; however, it is more difficult to stabilize and secure this catheter, and as a result, the rate of infectious morbidity is slightly increased.

Sepsis is one of the most serious complications of nutritional support with a central venous catheter. Solution contamination is rare. Catheter sepsis, defined as positive blood cultures along with identical microbial growth from the cultured catheter, is a much more common problem. When a rigid aseptic protocol is followed for catheter insertion and maintenance, the incidence is 3% to 5%. The infusion line is used only for parenteral nutrition (or one port of a multilumen device is assigned the role), dressings are changed regularly, and skin care is provided at the entry site. The appearance of fever during TPN is an urgent problem because of the possibility of catheter sepsis. A thorough workup to identify the source of fever should be performed expeditiously. If no explanation for the fever is found, the catheter is considered suspect, removed, and cultured. Suspect catheters should be replaced at a new site. In some patients, venous access is difficult, and the TPN catheter may be salvaged by interrupting the flow of nutrients for a day and using an antibiotic solution instead of a heparin solution to "lock" the catheter. Catheter-related sepsis usually resolves within 24 to 48 hours after removal, and antibiotic therapy is often unnecessary.

The metabolic complications of TPN and their treatment are detailed in Table 4-8.

Home Parenteral Nutrition

Home parenteral nutrition is provided for patients who cannot meet their nutritional needs through their gastrointestinal tract and, after careful evaluation, are determined able to manage the complexities of home TPN. Home TPN is used in patients with short-bowel syndrome, inflammatory bowel disease, AIDS, and certain types of cancer. In the hospital, the patient's nutritional needs are established, and a consistent formulation is prescribed. The patient is then discharged on

1.5 times his or her basal energy expenditure (RME), 1 to 2 g/kg/day protein, and the appropriate electrolytes, vitamins, and trace elements. These are mixed in a 2- to 3-L solution that is infused over a 12-hour period while the patient sleeps. This regimen is considered the least disruptive to the patient's lifestyle. These patients need permanent central venous access, either tunneled and cuffed catheters (e.g., Hickman, Groshong) or completely implanted devices. Visiting nurse support is essential.

Nutritional Support in Selected Surgical Situations

Cancer

Protein-calorie malnutrition often occurs in patients with cancer, partly because of the presence of tumors that cause metabolic abnormalities. These abnormalities include inefficient energy metabolism, abnormal carbohydrate metabolism (including glucose intolerance), accelerated breakdown of body fat, abnormal protein metabolism causing host nitrogen depletion, decreased muscle protein synthesis, and increased muscle protein breakdown. Compounded by the associated stresses and side effects of surgery, chemotherapy, and radiation therapy, the patient's nutritional status is further compromised. Malnutrition and weight loss have long been known to predict increased morbidity. However, nutritional support in surgical oncology patients has not significantly reduced morbidity rates in objective clinical trials.

The Veterans Administration (VA) Total Parenteral Nutrition Cooperative Study showed that preoperative TPN benefited only cancer patients who were considered severely malnourished. Well-nourished or moderately malnourished patients did not experience a benefit, but had an increased risk of catheter-related infection. Patients who are not expected to have oral intake for more than 5 days may be helped by postoperative TPN. Patients who have postoperative complications need support. Although chemotherapy and radiation therapy place additional stresses on the patient, clinical trials showed no difference in response to therapy with the addition of nutritional support. There is a trend toward fewer side effects, and this trend alone may allow more patients to undergo or complete full courses of treatment.

The role of nutritional support in cancer therapy is controversial. Formulations with specific amino acid modifications may help to suppress tumor growth, but some research suggests that nutritional support accelerates tumor growth. Further study of the role of nutritional support in better defined subsets of cancer patients is needed.

Inflammatory Bowel Disorders

Patients with Crohn's disease and ulcerative colitis are often malnourished, and have weight and micronutrient depletion. Pubescent patients frequently exhibit growth failure because of deficient intake of nutrients or decreased absorption from diseased bowel. Acute exacerbations can lead to significant loss of body protein and physiologic impairment, but the increase in protein synthesis and breakdown rates is moderate, with an average combined fecal and urine nitrogen excretion of 15 g/day. Steroid therapy sharply increases nitrogen excretion.

The nutritional state of patients with inflammatory bowel disorders can be improved by nutritional support. This support has no primary therapeutic benefit in ulcerative colitis, but in Crohn's disease, individual diet counseling decreases disease activity, improves remission rates, and decreases the need for drug therapy, rehospitalization, and lost work days. Elemental diets have primary therapeutic efficacy in acute Crohn's disease, but randomized trials do not show them to be more effective than polymeric formulations. Several studies confirmed that an elemental diet is equal to or more effective than steroids in inducing remission in acute disease. The benefits of long-term diet supplementation are less clear.

TPN improves the general nutritional state, but is not useful as a primary therapy. Its main role is in managing fistula, intestinal obstruction, and short-bowel syndrome. A controlled, randomized trial of patients who were given postoperative TPN compared with standard intravenous fluids did not show a reduction in complication rate. Home TPN is effective in active Crohn's disease that is unresponsive to conventional medical management.

Short-Bowel Syndrome

Short-bowel syndrome is a serious consequence of massive bowel removal or dysfunction. When a large segment of the small bowel is removed, the ability of the intestine to absorb nutrients, fluids, and electrolytes is impeded. The result is known as short-bowel syndrome. Short bowel syndrome causes a variety of complications, many of which are secondary to the lack of absorption of food and nutrients. These patients commonly experience protein-calorie malnutrition. They also have diarrhea, with or without steatorrhea, and often become dehydrated.

Therapy focuses on electrolyte and fluid replacement, early institution of enteral and parenteral nutrition, and symptomatic control of complications. Enteral feedings, even in the smallest amount, should begin as early as possible to prevent the remaining small bowel mucosa from degenerating. Once fluid and electrolyte balance is stabilized and nutrition is repleted, treatment consists of assisting the dietary intake and modifying it as needed. Patients need frequent nutritional assessments with the appropriate therapy. Weaning from TPN is attempted when the patient can tolerate oral feedings. If, after 1 year, the patient remains dependent on TPN, surgery may be considered. Restoration of continuity to lengths of bowel that are out of the enteral stream, construction of mucosal valves, reversed peristalsis of

bowel segments to prolong bowel transit time, longitudinal splitting of lengths of remaining bowel to increase length, and small bowel transplantation have been described. These options, however, are controversial. Surgical intervention is experimental, and until recently, has not produced good results. Small bowel transplantation appears more promising.

Frontiers and Controversies

This section discusses areas of active investigation and preliminary clinical use.

The role of anabolic steroid hormones as an adjunct to nutritional support is under investigation. Nandrolone decanoate reduces nitrogen loss, but increases total plasma amino acid levels; it also may enhance protein synthesis. Stanozolol improves nitrogen balance in postcolectomy patients who are given amino acids only, but provides no additional benefit to patients who are receiving amino acids, lipids, and carbohydrates.

Growth hormone (GH) has been studied as an adjunct to nutritional therapy since 1956. Recombinant human GH enhances nitrogen retention in patients who are receiving TPN and in those who have burns, chronic obstructive pulmonary disease, cancer, or other critical illnesses. Several investigations suggested that this effect occurs secondary to improved conservation of skeletal muscle protein mass and enhanced lipolysis. GH acts in a complex interrelation with insulin-like growth factor-1, and this factor may be a more effective anabolic agent in critical illness. Although GH accelerates protein gain and reduces fat and extracellular water gain during TPN, its influence on patient outcome is still in the early stages of definition.

Internationally, diets vary in their content of polyunsaturated fatty acids, either omega-6 (vegetable oils) or omega-3 (fish oils). Their effect on cardiovascular disease is an area of intense epidemiologic study. Some investigators are using TPN to treat plaque regression in patients with premature atherosclerosis.

Alternative sources of energy are sought for use in clinical conditions that are marked by insulin resistance, hyperlipidemia, and carnitine deficiency. Long-chain fatty acids (e.g., the essential lipid linoleic acid) require carnitine to enter mitochondria for oxidation. Medium-chain triglycerides, however, do not. Consequently, much work is underway to define medium-chain triglyceride absorption, uptake into organs, and interaction with long-chain triglycerides, as well as their role in nutritional therapy. Xylitol is metabolized through the pentose phosphate pathway. In combination with long-chain triglycerides, it is more effective than glucose in improving nitrogen retention in septic rats. Azelaic acid is a dicarboxylic acid that undergoes β-oxidation through carnitine-independent pathways. These acids are being studied in carnitine-deficient states of sepsis, cirrhosis, prematurity, and hemodialysis.

Multiple-Choice Questions

1. The technique that is LEAST useful in assessing nutritional status is:
   A. Delayed hypersensitivity skin tests
   B. Serum transferrin concentration
   C. Anthropometric measurements
   D. Serum alkaline phosphatase concentration
   E. Nitrogen balance study

2. The "stressed," or hypercatabolic, state of metabolism is best characterized by:
   A. Increased levels of catecholamines and decreased gluconeogenesis
   B. Mediators from inflammatory sites that promote a catabolic response
   C. Preferential use of fatty acids with minimal protein breakdown
   D. A shift to peripheral oxidation of glutamine and alanine
   E. A decreased resting metabolic expenditure and urine urea nitrogen excretion

3. Nutritional support should be considered or provided for each of the following patients EXCEPT:
   A. A ventilator-dependent 8-year-old with multiple fractures and pneumonia
   B. A patient who is in a coma 1 week after a stroke
   C. A 16-year-old girl with gangrenous appendicitis
   D. A patient with esophageal cancer and a recent 18% weight loss
   E. A patient with high-output enterocutaneous fistula from Crohn's disease

4. Metabolic complications of parenteral nutrition include all of the following EXCEPT:
   A. Hypokalemic, hypochloremic metabolic alkalosis
   B. Hypophosphatemia
   C. Hypoglycemia
   D. Hypermagnesemia
   E. Nonketotic hyperglycemic coma

5. Either the parenteral or the enteral route for nutritional support can be used in all of the following cases EXCEPT:
   A. A proximal enteroenteral or enterocutaneous fistula
   B. Diabetes mellitus requiring insulin therapy
   C. Major burn of the anterior trunk
   D. Anorexia associated with depression or malignancy
   E. Pancreatic abscess requiring operative drainage

6. The frequency of catheter-related sepsis in intravenous parenteral nutrition is reduced by:
   A. Meticulous aseptic care of the catheter insertion site
   B. The use of heparin-containing solutions
   C. The prophylactic use of systemic antibiotics
   D. Increasing the amount of glucose in the solutions
   E. The size of the catheter used

7. In chronically and critically ill patients, zinc deficiency:
   A. Reduces the synthesis of high-energy organic bonds
   B. Causes diarrhea, confusion, and failure to heal wounds
   C. Creates microcytic anemia
   D. Significantly alters the effects of insulin on glucose metabolism
   E. Has no clinical significance

8. The most sensitive measure of an acute change in nutritional status is:
   A. Serum albumin level
   B. Creatinine-height index
   C. Nitrogen balance
   D. Serum prealbumin
   E. 3-Methylhistidine excretion

9. In a patient with severe sepsis, the resting metabolic expenditure calculated by the Harris-Benedict equation must be multiplied by which of the following stress factors to best estimate total energy needs:
   A. 0.9
   B. 1.24
   C. 1.75
   D. 2.0
   E. 2.8

10. Essential fatty acid deficiency in humans is caused principally by a deficiency of:
    A. Linolenic acid
    B. Glycerol
    C. Palmitoleic acid
    D. Linoleic acid
    E. Oleic acid

11. The amino acid that is primarily used for gluconeogenesis in the liver is:
    A. Alanine
    B. Arginine
    C. Isoleucine
    D. Tyrosine
    E. Valine

12. Potential advantages of using a lipid emulsion to meet approximately 40% of a patient's caloric needs include all of the following EXCEPT:
    A. Avoids the development of essential fatty acid deficiency
    B. Decreases the risk of hyperosmolar nonketotic coma
    C. May facilitate weaning from mechanical ventilatory support
    D. Facilitates volume restriction
    E. Decreases the risk of hyperchloremic metabolic acidosis

13. Hypophosphatemia as a result of inadequate provision of phosphate during total parenteral nutrition can cause each of the following EXCEPT:
    A. Congestive heart failure
    B. Seizures

C. Hemolytic anemia
D. Bone pain
E. Impaired granulocyte function

14. Diarrhea after the institution of enteral feeding in a patient with a functionally intact gastrointestinal tract may be caused by all of the following EXCEPT:
   A. Excessively high infusion rate
   B. Use of milk solid–based feedings in a patient with lactase deficiency
   C. Excessively high fat content of the preparation
   D. Excessively hypertonic feeding
   E. Bacterial contamination of the feeding

15. The greatest energy depot in the body is best assessed by:
   A. Bioimpedance assessment
   B. Arm-muscle circumference
   C. Indirect calorimetry
   D. Nitrogen balance studies
   E. Liver biopsy for glycogen stores

16. The daily protein requirement for a normal active man is approximately:
   A. 0.5 g protein/kg/day
   B. 1.5 g protein/kg/day
   C. 2.0 g protein/kg/day
   D. 2.5 g protein/kg/day
   E. 3.0 g protein/kg/day

17. Tissues that require glucose to meet energy requirements include all of the following EXCEPT:
   A. Bone marrow
   B. Brain
   C. Erythrocytes
   D. Peripheral nerves
   E. Intestinal epithelium

18. Body protein sparing is greatest in association with:
   A. Early starvation
   B. Prolonged starvation
   C. Sepsis
   D. Trauma
   E. Burns

19. All of the following are true relative to chemically defined, or "elemental," enteral diets EXCEPT:
   A. They contain no lactose
   B. Carbohydrates are in the form of monosaccharides
   C. Protein is in the form of amino acids or oligo-peptides
   D. Fat content is high
   E. Minimal digestion is required

20. The major disadvantage of nasogastric administration of an enteral diet is:
   A. Diarrhea
   B. Aspiration pneumonitis

C. Patient discomfort
D. The need for a chemically defined (elemental) diet
E. Erosion of the esophageal wall

21. Anemia and leukopenia may develop secondary to chronic deficiency of:
   A. Zinc
   B. Copper
   C. Chromium
   D. Selenium
   E. Magnesium

22. Enteral nutritional support is appropriate in each of the following situations EXCEPT:
   A. Adynamic ileus
   B. Prolonged coma as a result of head injury
   C. Severe dysphagia secondary to a bulbar stroke
   D. Acute exacerbation of Crohn's disease
   E. Postoperative pancreaticocutaneous fistula

23. The caloric requirement calculated by the Harris-Benedict or World Health Organization equation for resting metabolic rate adjusted for actual daily needs is modified by each of the following EXCEPT:
   A. Age
   B. Sex
   C. Activity
   D. Weight
   E. Body habitus

24. After a long course of total parenteral nutrition (TPN), one unit of whole blood is administered through the central line before it is removed. Two hours after the start of transfusion, a nurse finds the patient comatose and hypotensive. The most likely cause is:
   A. Hypokalemia
   B. Hypoglycemia
   C. Transfusion reaction
   D. Bacteremia from catheter contamination
   E. Air embolus

25. Nutritional support of the traumatized or burned patient should include:
   A. Supplying more than 50% of nonprotein calories as fat
   B. A marked reduction of arginine
   C. The immediate use of the gastrointestinal tract
   D. Total parenteral nutrition (TPN) for 10 to 14 days
   E. A decrease in the amount of protein supplied to avoid increases in blood and urine urea nitrogen concentration

26. The maximum number of calories that should be offered to a patient with a thermal injury is:
   A. 100% of the calculated resting energy expenditure
   B. 150% of the calculated resting energy expenditure
   C. 200% of the calculated resting energy expenditure
   D. 250% of the calculated resting energy expenditure
   E. 300% of the calculated resting energy expenditure

Oral Examination Study Questions

CASE 1

A 75-year-old man is admitted to your service. He has a large abdominal aortic aneurysm that should be addressed operatively. However, the patient is severely malnourished because of chronic anorexia, refusal to eat, and mental confusion. Preoperative nutritional support is indicated to improve the patient's ability to tolerate the procedure and have a smooth postoperative course.

OBJECTIVE 1

The student outlines the ways in which chronic malnutrition is assessed.

A. History of weight loss (30 lb)

B. Dietary history (long history of poor intake)

C. Anthropometric measurements: triceps skinfold and arm-muscle circumference (below normal); hand grip or forearm dynamometry

D. Serum albumin (< 2.1 g/dL) or transferrin (< 100 mg/dL) level

E. Creatinine-height index (40%–50%)

F. Nitrogen balance

G. Absolute lymphocyte count (< 1500 cells/mm^3) or delayed cutaneous hypersensitivity skin tests (absent response)

OBJECTIVE 2

The student outlines the preferred method of nutritional support, the type of formula, the methods of institution, and the necessary precautions.

A. Enteral nutrition is provided through the placement of a thin nasogastric or nasoduodenal tube.

B. Polymeric formula is preferred because the gastrointestinal tract has normal digestive and absorptive capacity.

C. The feeding is started at 50 mL/hr, with constant infusion preferred. A caloric density of 1 kcal/mL is used. The rate of feeding is increased every 24 hours in increments of 25 to 50 mL/hr until the desired level is reached.

D. Gastric residuals are determined every 4 hours, and feeding is discontinued if they are greater than 100 mL.

E. The head of the bed is elevated 30°, and the patient is encouraged to ambulate frequently to prevent aspiration.

OBJECTIVE 3

The student discusses the reasons for the development of diarrhea during enteral nutritional support and suggests therapy for this complication.

A. Diarrhea may be caused by too rapid an infusion rate, excessive caloric load, or excessive solute load.

B. Treatment may consist of interrupting feedings until the diarrhea resolves and reinstituting the diet in a diluted form at a slower infusion rate.

C. Antidiarrheal medications may be used cautiously, with care taken to avoid the development of obstipation and abdominal distension.

OBJECTIVE 1

Minimum Level of Achievement for Passing

A. The student recognizes the importance of the history of weight loss and poor intake.

B. The student names three objective techniques that are used to assess chronic malnutrition (e.g., ideal weight, triceps skinfold, arm-muscle circumference, function dynamometry, albumin, transferrin, prealbumin, creatinine-height index, 24-hour creatinine excretion, immunologic measurements).

Honors Level of Achievement

A. The student gives values that reflect severe depletion for these assessment techniques.

B. The student discusses special assessment techniques (e.g., nitrogen balance, indirect calorimetry, body composition analysis).

OBJECTIVE 2

Minimum Level of Achievement for Passing

A. The student recognizes that enteral nutrition is the only appropriate choice.

B. The student writes initial orders for infusion and states the precautions for gastric residual and the steps to avoid aspiration.

Honors Level of Achievement

A. The student can discuss the differences between polymeric and chemically defined (elemental) formulas.

OBJECTIVE 3

Minimum Level of Achievement for Passing

A. The student states at least one reason why diarrhea develops during enteral support.

B. The student suggests either temporary cessation of feeding or dilution of the diet with decreased infusion rate as therapeutic steps.

CASE 2

A 40-year-old man is admitted to the hospital for severe blunt trauma. He has fractures of both femurs and the pelvis. At exploratory laparotomy, a ruptured spleen is removed. A tear of the distal ileum is repaired, and a minor hepatic hematoma is drained. The patient needs ventilator support because he has a pulmonary contusion. Nutritional support is believed to be indicated.

OBJECTIVE 1

The student outlines the potential methods of nutritional support and the general nutritional requirements of the patient.

A. Either enteral or parenteral nutrition can be used. The operating team places a jejunal feeding tube, even with a distal small bowel repair. Small intestinal motility and absorptive function are maintained with early enteral feeding, even after abdominal trauma. If a jejunal tube was forgotten, parenteral nutrition is required. Neither begins until hemodynamic stability is achieved.

B. Caloric needs are estimated by the Harris-Benedict equation, with a multiplier of 1.8 for trauma and fractures. Alternatively, the base of 25 kcal/kg/day can be used, incremented by 50% to 80% because of trauma and hypercatabolism.

C. Protein needs are estimated at 1.5 to 2.0 g/kg/day, but can be confirmed by a urine urea nitrogen test.

OBJECTIVE 2

The student outlines the basic components of a total parenteral nutrition (TPN) solution.

A. The calorie source is hypertonic dextrose (20%–35%), with or without a lipid emulsion (10%–20%). If combined, the ratio of dextrose- to lipid-derived calories may range from 95:5 to 60:40.

B. The protein source is L-amino acid solution.

C. The special electrolyte requirements include:

1. Potassium, because of an intracellular shift of potassium with glucose use

2. Phosphorus, because of an intracellular shift with glucose use

3. Acetate, to prevent the development of hyperchloremic metabolic acidosis secondary to amino acid solution

D. The trace element requirements include:

1. Zinc, to prevent a zinc deficiency state, which can cause wet dermatitis and alopecia and can impair wound healing

2. Copper, to prevent a deficiency state characterized by anemia and leukopenia

E. Multivitamins are also needed.

OBJECTIVE 3

The student describes the enteral and parenteral routes of administration and compares the rationale for either choice and the potential major complications that are associated with each access route.

A. Either enteral or parenteral access can be used.

1. Parenteral support is given by central venous access because of the hypertonic nature of the solution. This access is achieved by cannulation of either the subclavian or the internal jugular vein.

2. Enteral support is given through a jejunal tube placed at exploratory laparotomy, a percuta-neous endoscopic jejunostomy tube placed later, or a nasoduodenal tube. Nasogastric tube feeding will likely be delayed by postoperative gastric atony.

B. Parenteral nutritional support is always given in the patient who has multiple injuries, but it should bypass the gut, leading to intestinal mucosal atrophy and possibly enhancing bacterial translocation. Enteral support can be given, even with moderate abdominal injuries, but it requires postpyloric access and careful observation of tolerance. It is associated with decreased septic complication in trauma patients.

C. Complications are related to the selected route.

1. The most common complication of central venous access is pneumothorax. Longer-term complications include catheter sepsis and subclavian vein or superior vena cava thrombosis.

2. The risks of enteral feeding include gastric aspiration and pneumonia, abdominal distension, diarrhea, and possible delayed or inadequate delivery of needed nutrients.

OBJECTIVE 1

Minimum Level of Achievement for Passing

A. The student recognizes that either parenteral or enteral nutritional support is possible.

B. The student describes the principles by which calorie and protein requirements are estimated.

Honors Level of Achievement

A. The student discusses the Harris-Benedict equation in detail or describes the use of indirect calorimetry versus estimation of needs.

B. The student appropriately estimates the patient's protein needs.

OBJECTIVE 2

Minimum Level of Achievement for Passing

A. The student realizes that calories, protein, vitamins, and trace elements are needed in a nutritional support program.

B. The student lists the special electrolyte requirements for a patient who is receiving TPN.

Honors Level of Achievement

A. The student explains why potassium, phosphorus, and acetate are needed by patients who are receiving parenteral nutrition with hypertonic dextrose and amino acids.

B. The student discusses the consequences of zinc and copper deficiencies.

OBJECTIVE 3

Minimum Level of Achievement for Passing

A. The student can explain why parenteral nutrition is preferred, describe the central venous access routes, and describe the risks of pneumothorax and catheter sepsis.

B. The student can discuss several methods of gaining enteral access and describe the risks of aspiration with prepyloric feeding, distension, diarrhea, or inadequate nutritional support.

Honors Level of Achievement

A. The student discusses the consequences of prolonged nonuse of the gastrointestinal tract and the diminished risks of sepsis from all sources in trauma patients who are fed enterally.

CASE 3

A 43-year-old woman has extensive Crohn's disease of the small intestine. Four weeks ago, she underwent small bowel resection, but had an enterocutaneous fistula postoperatively. It was managed conservatively. She received TPN with hypertonic dextrose and amino acids. She tolerated this regimen with minimal glucosuria and blood sugar levels of approximately 200 mg/dL.

OBJECTIVE 1

The student can discuss the reasons why the patient might suddenly become hyperglycemic (with a blood sugar level of 800 mg/dL), confused, and lethargic (i.e., sepsis, inadvertent high-volume administration, diabetes mellitus). The student can also discuss the management of this complication (i.e., change the line, perform cultures; temporarily change the infusion to D_5W, insulin and antibiotics; treat the source of sepsis).

A. The patient has a hyperosmolar, nonketotic hyperglycemic coma. This coma may be the result of too rapid infusion of hypertonic dextrose or the sudden development of glucose intolerance, possibly because of latent sepsis. Hyperglycemia causes glucosuria, osmotic diuresis, dehydration, and coma.

B. Treatment consists of discontinuing the glucose, vigorous rehydration, cautious administration of insulin, and monitoring for the possible development of hypokalemia.

OBJECTIVE 2

The student discusses why the patient might have exfoliative desquamative dermatitis, beginning in the skinfolds, and suggests therapy.

A. This complication is most likely a manifestation of essential fatty acid deficiency syndrome, largely because of a deficiency of linoleic acid. It develops because parenteral nutritional support is based on a lipid-free program.

B. Therapy consists of the addition of 500 mL 10% or 20% lipid emulsion daily, for 7 to 10 days. The deficiency state is prevented by the administration of 500-mL lipid emulsion twice weekly.

OBJECTIVE 1

Minimum Level of Achievement for Passing

The student recognizes the existence of hyperosmolar coma and discusses the pathophysiology of this condition.

Honors Level of Achievement

The student provides a detailed management program.

OBJECTIVE 2

Minimum Level of Achievement for Passing

The student recognizes the existence of essential fatty acid deficiency syndrome and suggests treatment.

Honors Level of Achievement

The student can discuss the potential advantages of the use of lipid emulsions as a calorie source in parenteral nutrition.

SUGGESTED READINGS

Burzstein S, Elwyn DH, Askanazi J, Kinney JM. Energy metabolism, indirect calorimetry, and nutrition. Baltimore, Md: Williams & Wilkins, 1989.

Hill, GL. Body composition research: implications for the practice of clinical nutrition. *J Parenter Enter Nutr* 1992;16:197–218.

Kinney JM, Jeejeebhoy KN, Hill GL, Owen OE, eds. *Nutrition and Metabolism in Patient Care*. Philadelphia, Pa: WB Saunders, 1988.

Moore FA, Feliciano DV, Andrassy RJ, et al. Early enteral feeding, compared with parenteral, reduces postoperative septic complications: the results of a meta-analysis. *Ann Surg* 1992;216:172–183.

Pellett PL. Food energy requirements in humans. *Am J Clin Nutr* 1990;51:711–722.

Pellett PL. Protein requirements in humans. *Am J Clin Nutr* 1990;51:727–737.

Siegel JH, Cerra FB, Coleman B, et al. Physiological and metabolic correlations in human sepsis. *Surgery* 1979;86:163–193.

5

Surgical Bleeding and Blood Replacement

Hollis W. Merrick, III, M.D.
Mary R. Smith, M.D.
Bruce V. MacFadyen, Jr., M.D.

OBJECTIVES

1. Using a patient's physical examination and medical history, determine the likelihood and etiology of possible bleeding disorders.
2. Name five major etiologic factors that may lead to bleeding disorders.
3. Describe the common laboratory tests that are used to assess coagulation status, and explain how these tests apply to the diagnosis of the conditions discussed in Objective 2.
4. Identify the acute etiologic factors that might be responsible for extensive bleeding in a patient who has received massive transfusions.
5. Name the conditions that might lead to disseminated intravascular coagulation (DIC).
6. Describe the recommended component replacement therapy for the etiologic categories named in Objective 2, as well as the definitive treatment for the underlying cause of each.
7. Describe the process of obtaining and transfusing blood, the symptoms of a transfusion reaction, and the diagnosis and appropriate management of the different types of transfusion reactions.

Bleeding is an accepted occurrence in most surgical procedures. Although the volume of blood lost is usually not large enough to create a major problem, certain operations are invariably associated with large blood losses that may impair the normal hemostatic process. Additionally, some patients with congenital or acquired clotting disorders require elective or emergency surgery. Therefore, surgeons must be prepared for significant blood losses that may have an adverse effect on patient recovery, and they must be able to manage blood loss in their patients. In addition, surgeons must be knowledgeable about common bleeding and clotting disorders, the components of blood replacement, and the problems associated with the transfusion of blood products.

The Hemostatic Process

The hemostatic process involves an interaction among the blood vessel wall, the platelets, and the coagulation pathways. After injury, hemostasis begins with a brief period of **vasoconstriction** by the vessels that have muscular layers in their walls. This vasoconstriction in the region of injury only controls blood loss for a brief time and cannot offer significant control of bleeding.

The next step is mediated by **platelets,** which **adhere,** or stick, to areas of vascular injury or to exposed subendothelial structures (Figure 5-1). Platelets also adhere to structures other than platelets. After adhesion, the platelets extrude their contents, the most important of which is adenosine diphosphate. As a result, platelet **aggregation** occurs. This platelet-to-platelet sticking causes the initial **thrombus.** The process from initial injury to the white (platelet) thrombus occurs independently of the coagulation pathways; hemophiliacs, for example, can generate a normal white thrombus. However, a more permanent thrombus is required for control of bleeding and eventual healing. This thrombus is accomplished through the formation of **fibrin.**

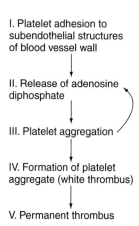

Platelets in the Control of Bleeding

I. Platelet adhesion to subendothelial structures of blood vessel wall

II. Release of adenosine diphosphate

III. Platelet aggregation

IV. Formation of platelet aggregate (white thrombus)

V. Permanent thrombus

Figure 5-1 Platelets in the Control of Bleeding.

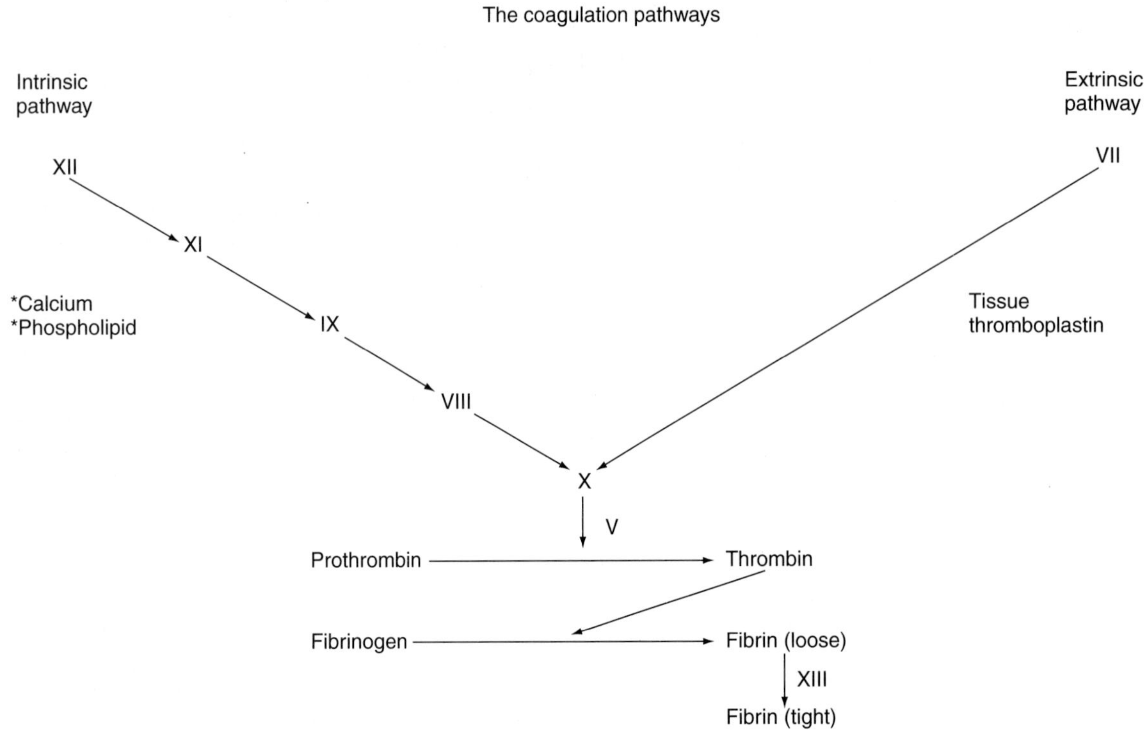

The coagulation pathways

Intrinsic
pathway

XII

XI

*Calcium
*Phospholipid

IX

VIII

X

V

Prothrombin ——————————————→ Thrombin

Fibrinogen ——————————————→ Fibrin (loose)

XIII

Fibrin (tight)

Extrinsic
pathway

VII

Tissue
thromboplastin

Figure 5-2 The Coagulation Pathways. *Calcium and phospholipid from platelets are needed to permit the coagulation pathways to proceed at optimum rates. Activated factor XI in turn activates factor IX to become factor IXa. Factor IXa, in the presence of factor VIII, platelet phospholipid, and calcium, activates factor X. The rate of this reaction is greatly increased by the presence of the platelet phospholipid.

The coagulation pathways use various **coagulation factors** to generate fibrin, which stabilizes the white thrombus (Figure 5-2). The **extrinsic coagulation pathway** begins with tissue thromboplastin, which interacts with factor VII to convert factor X to factor X^a and initiates the common pathway. The **intrinsic coagulation pathway** requires factors XII, XI, IX, and VIII to interact and eventually convert factor X to factor X^a. The **common coagulation pathway** involves factors X, V, II (prothrombin), and I **(fibrinogen).** The end-product of coagulation is fibrin, which has a weak clot-stabilizing ability. Factor XIII (fibrin-stabilizing factor) is required to create fibrin of optimal strength (see Figure 5-2).

Bleeding may occur in the presence of a deficiency of any of the factors of the coagulation pathways, except factor XII. Additionally, although normal hemostasis requires calcium, hypocalcemia does not cause bleeding.

Evaluation of the Patient

Detecting and correcting bleeding disorders before surgery is the best way to avoid major bleeding problems during and after surgery. Therefore, a careful screening for bleeding risks is an essential part of the preoperative evaluation (Table 5-1).

History

Obtaining a detailed **bleeding history** is one of the most important steps in evaluating patients for possible

Table 5-1. Preoperative Evaluation for Bleeding and Clotting Disorders

Study	When Performed
History, physical examination	In all patients as part of routine preoperative evaluation
Laboratory studies: PT, APTT, platelet count	In all patients as part of routine preoperative evaluation
Bleeding time, thrombin time	In patients with evidence of bleeding disorders or in whom excessive bleeding is anticipated because of the nature of the surgery

PT, prothrombin time.
APTT, activated partial thromboplastin time.

bleeding problems. Patients should be asked if they have had prolonged bleeding after dental extractions, minor cuts, or previous operations; if they have prolonged or frequent menses; or if they have experienced bruising after minor injury. A history of "bleeders" in the family is also important to obtain. For the individual patient, a history of bleeding problems is the most important preoperative information that predicts unexpected bleeding complications. This information is even more reliable than laboratory tests.

Physical Examination

The physical examination is less helpful than the history in assessing bleeding risk, because most patients with mild to moderate bleeding disorders do not have physical signs. The examiner should seek signs of blood disorders, splenomegaly, hepatomegaly, hemarthroses, petechiae, or ecchymoses, which can be associated with bleeding disorders. Petechiae are typical of platelet disorders, whereas ecchymoses are more typical of abnormalities in the coagulation pathways.

Tests to Evaluate Hemostasis

Platelet count, prothrombin time (PT), and **activated partial thromboplastin time** (APTT) should be determined in all patients as part of the routine preoperative evaluation to exclude thrombocytopenia, a coagulation factor deficiency, or an acquired coagulation factor inhibitor. Certain other screening tests, such as bleeding time, or **thrombin,** are indicated when the history or physical examination suggests a bleeding or clotting disorder, or if major bleeding is expected because of the nature of the planned surgery. These studies should be carried out in all patients as a part of preoperative screening unless there has been a recent significant challenge to the patient's hemostatic competence. Acquired bleeding disorders (e.g., thrombocytopenia) or acquired inhibitors against clotting factors can lead to a bleeding disorder in a previously hemostatically healthy person.

These tests are relatively inexpensive (< $100 in most laboratories) and may potentially avoid unexpected bleeding and the ensuing urgent need for transfusion of blood products.

Platelet Count

The platelet count verifies that an adequate number of platelets are available in the circulation. Platelet counts are done by automated methods in most institutions. However, automated counters may not be accurate at platelet counts of less than 40,000. For this reason, very low platelet counts may need to be confirmed by manual methods. Review of the peripheral blood smear provides a reasonable estimate of platelet numbers.

Platelets may be present in adequate numbers and yet may not function appropriately (e.g., von Willebrand's disease, qualitative platelet defects). In this case, bleeding time is prolonged.

Prothrombin Time

The PT measures the ability of the blood to form stable thrombi. It evaluates the extrinsic coagulation pathway and the common pathway. In other words, it evaluates the adequacy of factors VII, X, and V; prothrombin; and fibrinogen (Figure 5-3). Its most common use is to monitor oral anticoagulation with warfarin (Coumadin). Today, PT is reported with the International Normalized Ratio (INR). The INR permits the use

Tests of the coagulation pathways

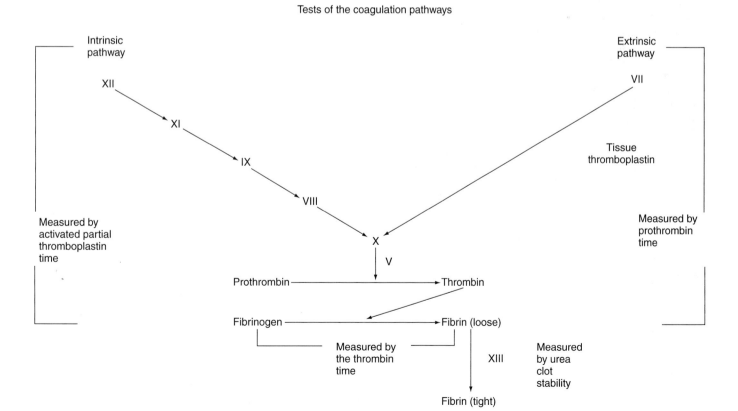

Figure 5-3   Tests of the Coagulation Pathways.

of data from multiple laboratories to manage a patient's anticoagulation therapy. The INR also permits comparison of research studies performed in different sites. Mastery of the use of the INR as a tool for anticoagulation therapy is important for physicians. Although most patients are adequately anticoagulated when the INR is between 2.0 and 2.5, certain patients require more intense therapy that results in an INR of 3.0 or more.

Activated Partial Thromboplastin Time

The APTT evaluates the adequacy of fibrinogen, prothrombin, and factors V, VIII, IX, X, XI, and XII in the intrinsic and common pathways (see Figure 5-3). It is the most commonly used test to monitor the effectiveness of heparin therapy. The APTT is normal in patients with factor VII deficiency, but it is elevated during Coumadin therapy because of reductions in factors II, IX, and X.

Bleeding Time

The **bleeding time test** is conducted by making two standard wounds (6 mm long, 1 mm deep) in the forearm of the patient with a spring-loaded lancet. The time from injury until the cessation of bleeding from both wounds is measured. A normal bleeding time requires adequate numbers and function of platelets and normal blood vessel walls. A normal bleeding time range (in minutes) is established by each laboratory. The usual range is 5 to 10 minutes, but small variations are found from laboratory to laboratory. A mild prolongation of bleeding time may be caused by aging skin or long-term corticosteroid therapy. In both cases, senile ecchymoses may be seen, especially on the patient's forearms.

A prolonged bleeding time is often associated with significant bleeding at surgery. Bleeding time may be prolonged by certain drugs [e.g., aspirin, other nonsteroidal anti-inflammatory drugs (NSAIDs), ticlopidine]. An abnormal bleeding time in a patient without a history of associated drug use indicates a potential bleeding disorder. A newly found prolonged bleeding time may be caused by any of the following disorders:

1. Thrombocytopenia
2. Abnormal platelet function because of:
   A. Medication (e.g., aspirin)
   B. Dense granular disorders of platelets
3. Von Willebrand's disease (congenital or acquired)

Thrombin Time

The thrombin time evaluates fibrinogen-to-fibrin conversion with an external source of thrombin. Prolongation of thrombin time can be caused by: (1) low fibrinogen levels (hypofibrinogenemia), (2) abnormal fibrinogen (dysfibrinogenemia), (3) fibrin and fibrinogen split products, or (4) heparin (see Figure 5-3). Thrombin time is used to evaluate disseminated intravascular coagulation (DIC) and chronic liver disease.

Causes of Excessive Surgical Bleeding

Most patients are hemostatically normal before they enter the operating room. They have no bleeding history or evidence of bleeding by physical examination, and the results of their coagulation screening tests are normal. However, in some patients with large blood losses, generalized oozing is noted after a certain period. In addition, some operations (e.g., cardiopulmonary bypass, liver transplant surgery, prostate surgery, placement of portacaval shunts) are frequently associated with large blood losses.

Preexisting Hemostatic Defects

When abnormal bleeding begins within the first 30 minutes of the operative period, a preexisting bleeding disorder is suspected. Preexisting hemostatic defects are most readily identified through an accurate patient history.

Congenital Bleeding Disorders

Congenital bleeding disorders, such as hemophilia and **von Willebrand's disease,** are fairly uncommon. Mildly affected patients may be asymptomatic. **Type A hemophilia** and von Willebrand's disease are both characterized by deficiencies of factor VIII clotting activity (VIII_c), but there are differences in the two disease processes. Hemophilia is seen almost exclusively in males, and platelet function is normal. Von Willebrand's disease affects people of both sexes. In addition to factor VIII_c deficiency, von Willebrand's disease is associated with platelet dysfunction, which is diagnosed by decreased aggregation in response to ristocetin and is corrected by normal **plasma.** Deficiency of von Willebrand activity is corrected with cryoprecipitate infusions or desmopressin (DDAVP) therapy. Cryoprecipitate is a fraction of plasma that contains von Willebrand's factor, factor VIII clotting activity, and fibrinogen. DDAVP is given as an intravenous infusion or as nasal "snuff." DDAVP is a hormone that, in addition to other properties, leads to the release of von Willebrand's factor from its endothelial cell storage sites.

Congenital platelet function disorders are uncommon and usually occur in patients who have a history of mucous membrane bleeding and easy bruising. Factor IX deficiency (e.g., Christmas disease, hemophilia B) is seen only in males and is less common than type A hemophilia. Type A hemophilia is treated with purified factor VIII concentrates. Factor XI deficiency is found almost exclusively in Jewish patients.

Acquired Bleeding Disorders

Acquired bleeding disorders are more common than congenital bleeding disorders and may have a variety of causes. Liver disease is a common cause of coagulation abnormalities. Inability of the liver to synthesize proteins leads to decreased levels of prothrombin and factors V, VII, and X (but not VIII), which may cause prolonged PT and APTT. Alcohol ingestion may result in acute thrombocytopenia. Hypersplenism may depress the platelet count moderately. Obstructive jaundice may lead to clotting factor deficiencies, which can usually be corrected with parenteral vitamin K. Cirrhosis may also cause clotting factor deficiencies. These respond less well to vitamin K. However, gastrointestinal bleeding in the patient who has cirrhosis is usually caused by varices or gastritis rather than by a coagulation defect.

Anticoagulant therapy with heparin or oral anticoagulants (e.g., Coumadin) leads to acquired bleeding disorders. Coumadin causes depression of the clotting activity of four coagulation factors (II, VII, IX, and X). Because both the intrinsic and extrinsic pathways are affected by Coumadin, both PT and APTT are prolonged. Heparin prolongs both APTT and thrombin time. Heparin (high–molecular-weight, or native, heparin) works by increasing the speed with which antithrombin III binds to and neutralizes factors IXa, Xa, XIa, XIIa, and thrombin. Low–molecular-weight heparins, which are less than 18 residues long, can bind with antithrombin III and neutralize factor Xa, but not thrombin. Low–molecular-weight heparins that have more than 18 residues retain their effect against thrombin. It is important to recognize the specifics of various low–molecular-weight preparations when selecting an agent for clinical use.

Acquired thrombocytopenia is caused by four mechanisms: (1) decreased platelet production in the bone marrow (e.g., aplastic anemia); (2) increased destruction of platelets in the peripheral blood [e.g., idiopathic thrombocytopenia purpura (ITP) or DIC]; (3) splenic pooling in an enlarged spleen (e.g., cirrhosis); or (4) any combination of these disorders (e.g., alcoholic liver failure).

Platelet function disorders are usually associated with drugs (e.g., aspirin, other NSAIDs). Unlike other NSAIDs, however, aspirin induces a defect that does not reverse; thus, patients should be instructed to avoid aspirin for 1 full week before elective surgery.

A second important cause of acquired platelet dysfunction is uremia. Patients who are uremic and are bleeding require dialysis before surgery to correct their platelet dysfunction.

Intraoperative Complications

Several common conditions contribute to bleeding during a surgical procedure. Shock may cause or aggravate DIC. Extensive trauma is also associated with DIC. Massive transfusion of stored packed red blood cells may lead to bleeding. This bleeding occurs after rapid transfusion of 10 units or more of stored blood over a 4- to 6-hour period. It is caused by low numbers of platelets and by dilution of the clotting factors as a result of the infusion of nonplasma fluids for volume support.

Acute hemolytic blood transfusion reactions may lead to DIC. When a patient is under general anesthesia, there may be no clues that incompatible blood has been infused until the onset of generalized bleeding as a result of DIC. The usual symptoms of an incompatible

blood transfusion (e.g., agitation, back pain) do not occur under general anesthesia. Hemoglobinuria and oliguria provide additional clinical evidence of DIC.

Postoperative Bleeding

Fifty percent of postoperative bleeding is caused by inadequate hemostasis during surgery. Other causes of postoperative bleeding include:

1. Circulating heparin that remains after bypass surgery.
2. Shock that results in DIC.
3. Altered liver function after partial hepatectomy. If a large portion of the liver is removed, the remaining liver may need 3 to 5 days to increase its production of clotting factors sufficiently to support hemostasis.
4. Acquired deficiency of the vitamin K-dependent clotting factors (II, VII, IX, and X). This deficiency may develop in patients who are poorly nourished and are receiving antibiotics.
5. Factor XIII deficiency. In this case, bleeding occurs 3 to 5 days after surgery. The diagnosis of factor XIII deficiency is confirmed with a urea clot stability test, which evaluates the ability of a clot to remain intact. If the clot dissolves rapidly, it suggests a deficiency of factor XIII, which is an uncommon cause of postsurgical bleeding.
6. DIC and fibrinolysis.

Common Bleeding Disorders in the Surgical Patient

Disseminated Intravascular Coagulation (Consumptive Coagulopathy)

As the name suggests, **disseminated intravascular coagulation**, or DIC, is characterized by intravascular coagulation and thrombosis that is diffuse rather than localized at the site of injury. This process results in the systemic deposition of platelet-fibrin microthrombi that cause diffuse tissue injury. Some clotting factors may be consumed in sufficient amounts to eventually lead to diffuse bleeding. DIC may be acute or clinically asymptomatic and chronic.

Etiology

The etiology of DIC may be any of the following: (1) the release of tissue debris into the bloodstream after trauma or an obstetric catastrophe; (2) the introduction of intravascular aggregations of platelets as a result of the activation of platelets by various materials, including adenosine diphosphate and thrombin (which may explain the occurrence of DIC in patients with severe septicemia or immune complex disease); (3) extensive endothelial damage, which denudes the vascular wall and stimulates coagulation and platelet adhesion (as seen in patients with widespread burns or vasculitis); (4) hypotension that leads to stasis and prevents the normal circulating inhibitors of coagulation from reaching the sites of the microthrombi; (5) blockage of the reticuloendothelial system; (6) some types of operations that involve the prostate, lung, or malignant tumors; (7) severe liver disease.

Diagnostic Studies

The diagnosis of DIC is established by the detection of diminished levels of coagulation factors and platelets. The following laboratory results may be useful in diagnosing DIC: (1) prolonged APTT, (2) prolonged PT, (3) hypofibrinogenemia, (4) thrombocytopenia, (5) the presence of fibrin and fibrinogen split [(f)D-dimer] products. The presence of fibrin and fibrinogen split products is caused by activation of the fibrolytic pathway in response to activation of the clotting pathway.

Treatment

The most important aspect of the treatment of DIC is to remove the precipitating factors (e.g., treating septicemia). If DIC is severe, replacement of coagulation factors is required to correct the coagulation defect. Cryoprecipitate is the best method to replace a profound fibrinogen deficit. Platelet transfusions may also be required. **Fresh frozen plasma** is useful to replace other deficits that are identified, but it must be used judiciously if volume overload is a potential problem. In rare cases, the coagulation pathway must be inhibited with heparin or with drug therapy to prevent platelet aggregation.

The use of heparin to treat DIC is controversial. There is no conclusive evidence that using heparin alters the outcome of DIC. Because antithrombin III is consumed during DIC, the use of heparin as an anticoagulant may be severely compromised. Large trials are underway to evaluate the benefit of using antithrombin III concentrates as part of the treatment of DIC. Preliminary data from some trials are promising.

Bleeding Disorders Caused by Increased Fibrinolysis

Primary Fibrinolysis

Primary fibrinolysis is a disorder that occurs most commonly after fibrinolytic therapy with drugs such as streptokinase or urokinase, which are used to lyse coronary artery or peripheral artery thromboses. Primary fibrinolysis is also seen in conjunction with surgical procedures on the prostate gland, which is rich in urokinase. It also occurs in patients with severe liver failure. Very rare disorders of inhibitors of the fibrinolytic pathway (e.g., congenital deficiencies of α_2-antiplasmin) can also cause primary fibrinolysis. Treatment of these disorders is best accomplished by eliminating the precipitating cause.

If primary fibrinolysis becomes severe, ε-amino caproic acid can be used for therapy. This drug must be used cautiously because it blocks the fibrinolytic pathway and may predispose the patient to thrombotic events.

Secondary Fibrinolysis

Secondary fibrinolysis is most often seen in response to DIC. The coagulation pathway is activated, followed by the fibrinolytic pathway. Manifestations of this activation in laboratory tests include hypofibrinogenemia and the presence of fibrin split products. As the DIC is corrected, the secondary fibrinolysis resolves.

Hypercoagulable States in the Surgical Patient

Thromboembolism may occur for a number of reasons during the course of surgery and in the postoperative period. Both congenital and acquired disorders can put surgical patients at risk for thromboembolism.

Etiology

Congenital Disorders

The most common cause of congenital hypercoagulable states is activated protein C resistance (APCR). The most common cause of APCR is factor V Leiden. Activated protein C binds to and neutralizes factors VIII and V, thus acting to regulate the rate at which the intrinsic and common pathways proceed. Genetically abnormal factor V (factor V Leiden) lacks the binding site for activated protein C; thus, it cannot be neutralized. Patients with factor V Leiden abnormality are predisposed to thromboembolic events. Additional causes of congenital hypercoagulable states include deficiencies of antithrombin III and proteins C and S. Protein C is present in the plasma in an inactive form. When thrombin is attached to thrombomodulin on the endothelial cell surface, protein C is activated. Protein S functions as a catalyst to this activation. Activated protein C has two functions: (1) as an anticoagulant (as described earlier) and (2) as an inducer of fibrinolysis.

A careful medical history and family history can often suggest the presence of a hypercoagulable state. Of particular note is the need to define the age of onset of thromboembolism. Events that occur in the 40s or younger should raise suspicion of an inherited hypercoagulable state.

Acquired Hypercoagulable States

Acquired hypercoagulable states may result from:

1. Decreased production of naturally occurring anticoagulants (e.g., liver failure).
2. Ineffective fibrinolysis secondary to reduced or defective plasminogen.
3. Very high levels of clotting factors, especially fibrinogen, which may occur in response to the stress of severe illness or trauma.
4. Platelet counts greater than $1000 \times 10^3/mm^3$ ($1000 \times 10^9/L$).
5. The antiphospholipid syndromes (e.g., lupus anticoagulant phenomenon).
6. Some cases of chronic DIC.

Diagnostic Laboratory Studies

The following laboratory studies should be considered when a patient is evaluated for a possible hypercoagulable state: (1) activated protein C resistance test; (2) antithrombin III activity assay; (3) proteins C and S activity assay; and (4) assay for antiphospholipid antibody (especially if the patient had an arterial thromboembolism).

Management of Hypercoagulable States

Therapy for hypercoagulable states is primarily directed at the following: (1) interfering with the coagulation pathways (with heparin, Coumadin, or both) and (2) interfering with platelet function (with aspirin, ticlopidine, or other platelet-inhibiting drugs). Therapy must be individualized both to the patient and to the site and severity of the thromboembolism. The duration of therapy requires careful consideration; the risks and benefits of protracted anticoagulation therapy must be weighed.

During the perioperative period, therapy for patients with a history of thromboembolism and a documented hypercoagulable state must be planned carefully by both the surgeon and the hematologist. Low-dose heparin provides adequate protection from thromboembolism for short periods without compromising surgical hemostasis. For patients with a documented hematologic risk factor for thrombosis (e.g., activated protein C resistance) who have never had a thromboembolic event, prophylaxis with pneumatic compression boots or low-dose heparin is adequate.

Blood Replacement Therapy

Collection and Storage of Blood and Blood Products

Whole blood is collected into plastic reservoir bags that contain an anticoagulant solution that binds to plasma calcium and prevents activation of the coagulation pathways. Whole blood is usually separated into four major components: (1) plasma, (2) platelets, (3) **white blood cells,** and (4) **red blood cells.** Administering only the specific components that are deficient in the patient is the preferred approach to therapy.

Packed red blood cells may be stored at 4°C for as long as 5 weeks. During storage at 4°C, platelets and leukocytes become nonfunctional within hours. A gradual reduction in red cell viability also occurs with prolonged storage. Red blood cells that are stored for 5 weeks have a mean recovery of approximately 70%. Cellular metabolism during storage leads to progressive increases in plasma potassium and an increase in hydrogen ion concentration. The result is a lowered pH.

Platelet-rich plasma is obtained by gentle centrifugation of whole blood. The resulting suspension is rich in platelets and has a volume of 200 mL. Platelet concentrate is obtained by recentrifugation of platelet-rich plasma. Platelet concentrates contain approximately 6×10^{10} platelets and can be stored for 3 to 5 days in plastic containers at 22°C. They should not be refrigerated.

Platelet-poor plasma may be frozen and stored as fresh frozen plasma, or it may be fractionated into cryoprecipitate and other plasma fractions. A single 200-mL plastic bag of fresh frozen plasma contains all of the coagulation factors and can be stored for as long as 12 months at ‾30°C. A unit of cryoprecipitate measures 5 to 30 mL in a single plastic bag. It is rich in factor VIII, fibrinogen, and fibronectin, and can be stored for 12 months at ‾30°C. Stored plasma, which is available from some blood banking centers, contains coagulation factors other than factors V and VIII, and can be stored for 5 weeks at 4°C or for 2 years at ‾30°C.

Blood Component Therapy

The major indication for the administration of fresh whole blood is the replacement of massive blood losses. The use of fresh whole blood for transfusion is limited to selected operations in small children. Otherwise, specific blood components are used. Blood components that carry oxygen include: (1) red cell concentrates, (2) leukocyte-poor blood, (3) frozen and thawed red blood cells, and (4) whole blood (no longer readily available in most centers). Platelet-containing components include: (1) platelet-rich plasma and (2) platelet concentrates.

The major blood groups are A, B, and O, and the major blood types are Rhesus (Rh)-positive and Rh-negative. There are also numerous minor groups that generally do not complicate transfusion. The universal donor red cells are O-negative red blood cells, but the plasma from type O donors is not universal donor plasma. Plasma from patients who are type O-negative contains varying levels of anti-A and anti-B antibodies. This plasma can cause some degree of hemolysis if it is given to individuals who are blood type A, B, or AB. In all but the most life-threatening emergency states, at least type-specific blood, or blood that has been crossmatched, must be given.

If transfusion of blood is expected during surgery or within 48 hours postoperatively, the patient is typed and crossmatched preoperatively. If the probability of transfusion is low, a "type and screen" is usually sufficient. In a type and screen, the patient's ABO group and Rh type are determined, and an antibody screen is carried out. Patients who have a positive antibody screen must have blood crossmatched to minimize the risk of hemolytic transfusion reactions.

Transfusion reactions occur frequently, and their management depends on their type and severity. Febrile transfusion reactions are the most common adverse reaction to the transfusion of blood products. They can be controlled with antipyretics and antihistamines. Repeated transfusion of blood products increases the possibility of a transfusion reaction. The removal of white cell debris from red cell, platelet, and plasma fraction transfusions may significantly reduce the risk of febrile transfusion reactions. If a patient has a febrile transfusion reaction, the use of antipyretics before future transfusions may prevent or reduce the severity of febrile transfusion reactions. If a major hemolytic transfusion reaction occurs, the administration of blood is stopped immediately, and the blood is returned to the laboratory for a repeated crossmatch. Hemolytic transfusion reactions require: (1) support of blood pressure, (2) maintenance of renal perfusion, and (3) management of DIC. Aggressive fluid support, diuretics, and renal dialysis may also be needed.

Many hospitals now allow appropriate patients to donate their own blood before elective surgery for possible use during the procedure (the safest blood transfusion practice). A healthy patient can bank two to three units of his or her own blood preoperatively.

Transfusion of Red Blood Cells

The transfusion of red blood cells is indicated when red cell mass is decreased, compromising oxygen transport and delivery to tissues. The decision to transfuse a patient with red blood cells must be individualized to the patient. The important considerations are as follows:

1. The patient's age
2. The presence of hemodynamic instability
3. Underlying medical conditions (e.g., cardiac, pulmonary, or cerebrovascular disease)
4. The etiology, degree, and time course of the patient's anemia.

Acute hemorrhage, with loss of 30% of blood volume, requires volume support and possibly red blood cell transfusion. Patients who have chronic anemia do not require red blood cell transfusions until the anemia causes systemic effects (as a result of the hypoxia that occurs secondary to the reduced oxygen-carrying capacity). Blood group and type must be considered when red cell transfusions are given.

Estimating Red Blood Cell Transfusion Needs

The formulas shown in Table 5-2 are used to calculate the number of units of red cell concentrate needed to raise the hematocrit to 40% (the normal value).

Table 5-2. Formula for Calculating Red Blood Cell Transfusion Needs

1. Calculate total blood volume (TBV) [mL]:	Patients weight (kg) × 7% × 1000 = TBV
2. Determine amount of increase (INC) in patient's hematocrit (Hct) from 1 unit of RBC concentrate:	$\dfrac{200\text{ mL}}{\text{TBV}} = \text{INC}$
3. Calculate number of units needed based on patient's current Hct:	40% (normal value) − Hct = Y%; $\dfrac{Y\,\%}{\text{INC}}$ = units needed

RBC, red blood cell.

The total blood volume is calculated by multiplying the patient's weight by 7%, or 0.07. For example, in the case of a person who weighs 70 kg:

$$70 \times 0.07 = 4900 \text{ mL (4.9 L)}$$

One unit of red blood cell concentrate contains approximately 200 mL red blood cells. At transfusion, this concentrate is distributed throughout the total blood volume. Thus, administering one unit of red blood cell concentrate raises the hematocrit by 4%:

$$200 \text{ mL} \div 4900 \text{ mL} = 0.04, \text{ or } 4\%$$

This hypothetical patient had a hematocrit of 15%. Therefore, to raise the hematocrit from 15% to 40% (i.e., 25%), the patient must receive seven units of red blood cell concentrate:

$$25 \div 4 = 6.25, \text{ or 7 full units}$$

Plasma Component Therapy

Fresh frozen plasma can be used to correct all clotting factor deficiencies. Plasma products do not require crossmatch before use, but should be ABO-compatible with the patient.

Coagulation factor concentrates are also a part of plasma component therapy. Cryoprecipitate is used primarily to treat hemophilia A and von Willebrand's disease. There is a small risk of hepatitis and human immunodeficiency virus (HIV) transmission when cryoprecipitate is given. Monoclonal factor VIII concentrates have the advantage of being storable at 4°C. Factor VIII concentrates can be used in the treatment of hemophilia A, but not all are useful in the treatment of von Willebrand's disease. The level of von Willebrand's factor in factor VIII concentrates may not be adequate to support the patient's needs. A pasteurized intermediate-purity factor VIII concentrate (Humate-P) contains some high–molecular-weight von Willebrand's multimers, and has been used successfully to treat some patients with von Willebrand's disease. Other intermediate-purity factor VIII concentrates contain only intermediate– and low–molecular-weight multimers. These preparations increase the factor VIII level, but may not correct the bleeding time abnormality. High-purity plasma factor VIII concentrates and recombinant factor VIII concentrates contain little or no von Willebrand's factor.

Estimating Factor VIII Transfusion Requirements

The formulas shown in Table 5-3 are used to calculate factor VIII transfusion requirements. Again, a 70-kg patient is used as an example.

The plasma volume in the body is equal to 4% of the total body weight. Therefore, in a 70-kg person, the plasma volume is 2.8 L:

$$70 \times 0.04 = 2.8 \text{ L, or 2800 mL}$$

A clotting unit of a coagulation factor is the amount of that factor (arbitrarily called 100%) in 1 mL normal plasma. To calculate the number of clotting units needed to raise the patient's level to 50% (which

Table 5-3. Formula for Calculating Factor VIII Transfusion Needs

1. Calculate total plasma volume (TPV) [mL]:	Patient's weight (kg) × 4% × 1000 = TPV
2. Determine number of units needed:	(0.50 − Factor VIII level) × TPV = Y
3. Calculate number of bags of cryoprecipitate needed, based on 80 units per bag:	$\dfrac{Y}{80}$ = units needed

controls most bleeding), the baseline level in the patient's blood is subtracted from 50%. The result is multiplied by the patient's plasma volume. For example, in a 70-kg patient who has a factor VIII level of 3% (as measured by an APTT-based testing method):

$$(0.50 - 0.03) \times 2800 \text{ mL} = 1316 \text{ units}$$

One bag of cryoprecipitate contains 80 clotting units of factor VIII. Therefore, the patient should receive 17 bags of cryoprecipitate:

$$1316 \div 80 = 16.45, \text{ or } 17 \text{ bags}$$

The amount of von Willebrand's factor in each bag of cryoprecipitate is similar to the amount of factor VIII clotting activity.

Management of Hemophilia

Hemophilia is an inherited bleeding disorder that affects males almost exclusively. It is caused by a reduction in factor VIII clotting activity. Recommended levels of factor VIII for the management of hemophilia type A have been established for minor and major trauma. After minor trauma or during the healing period after surgery, 15% to 20% activity of factor VIII should be maintained. After major trauma, major surgery, or bleeding at a dangerous site (e.g., intracranial bleed), 50% to 60% activity should be maintained. In the management of type A hemophilia, cryoprecipitate or monoclonal factor VIII is transfused every 12 hours to maintain the desired factor VIII level.

Management of von Willebrand's Disease

Von Willebrand's disease is a complex coagulopathy that is characterized by prolonged bleeding time and low levels of factor VIII$_c$. Factor VIII clotting activity increases slowly, reaching its maximum 6 to 12 hours after infusion. However, all transfused factor VIII is cleared from the patient's circulation within 48 hours after transfusion. The bleeding time is often shortened after transfusion with factor VIII-containing material, but the interval of this shortening is difficult to predict, and may be only 2 to 3 hours. Therefore, transfusion support must be individualized for patients with von Willebrand's disease. Transfusion with cryoprecipitate may be required as often as every 2 to 3 hours or as infrequently as every 24 hours. NSAIDs should be avoided during therapy for von Willebrand's disease because they aggravate coagulopathy. To avoid the use of blood products, DDAVP therapy is used in many

patients with von Willebrand's disease. If the use of DDAVP is being considered to protect a patient during surgery, a test dose of DDAVP is given 1 to 2 weeks before surgery to ensure that bleeding time and APTT are corrected. On the day of surgery, DDAVP is given 1 hour preoperatively as a 30-minute infusion. (The dose of DDAVP is 0.3 µg/kg.) A repeat dose of DDAVP is given 12 hours later if needed. Repeated doses, however, will not elicit desired responses. An interval of 2 to 3 days between doses usually permits good correction of bleeding time and APTT deficits in patients with von Willebrand's disease.

Other Indications for Plasma Component Use

Factor IX concentrates are used primarily to treat factor IX-deficient hemophilia or factor VIII-deficient hemophilia with severe factor VIII inhibitors. The major side effects of factor IX concentrates are hepatitis and HIV contamination. Some recipients may have DIC because of activated factors in the concentrate.

Albumin is prepared from whole plasma by ethanol fractionation. There is no risk of transmitting hepatitis with albumin transfusion. The primary role of albumin is as an oncotic agent.

Transfusion Safety

To ensure that blood transfusion products are as safe as possible, every effort must be made to avoid: (1) immunologic transfusion reactions, (2) transmission of infections, and (3) fluid overload.

Immunologic Transfusion Reactions

Immunologic transfusion reactions include hemolytic transfusion reactions, febrile transfusion reactions, posttransfusion thrombocytopenia, anaphylactic shock, urticaria, and graft-versus-host disease. Symptoms of immediate hemolytic transfusion reactions include fever, constrictive sensation in the chest, and pain in the lumbar region of the back. Signs include fever, hypotension, hemoglobinuria, bleeding as a result of DIC, and renal failure. Acute hemolytic reactions occur when A and B alloantibodies in the patient's plasma bind to antigens on the transfused donor red blood cells.

If a hemolytic transfusion reaction is suspected, the transfusion is stopped immediately, but the intravenous line is left in place. All of the documentation and other clerical information about the transfusion is checked to ensure that the blood that the patient is receiving is correctly crossmatched. Blood samples are taken from the patient to recheck the ABO blood group and Rh type and also to check for free-plasma hemoglobin. The crossmatch and Coombs' test are repeated. The investigator then retypes all donor units of blood for this patient, cultures the transfused blood to exclude bacterial infection, cultures the patient's blood, examines the patient for DIC caused by microaggregates and immune complexes, and initiates close monitoring of renal function.

Treatment of acute hemolytic transfusion reaction initially involves management of hypotension with volume expanders (e.g., lactated Ringer's solution) and vasoactive drugs. Good renal function is maintained with diuretic therapy (e.g., furosemide, mannitol). Bicarbonate is given to alkalinize the urine, and any depleted coagulation factor or platelets are replaced. Heparinization is rarely indicated, and dialysis is used only if acute renal failure develops.

Transmission of Infection

The transmission of infection through blood transfusion therapy is uncommon, but both patients and physicians have significant concerns about this possibility. There is a small possibility of transmitting a number of different types of infections. These include viral infections (e.g., viral hepatitis A, B, and C); HIV; cytomegalovirus; and human T-lymphotropic retrovirus (HTLV-I and HTLV-II). All blood is screened for hepatitis and HIV. Transmission of bacterial infections is rare. Parasitic infections, such as malaria and *Trypanosoma cruzi* (the cause of Chagas' disease), may also be transmitted through transfusion.

Careful screening of blood and blood donors has reduced the risk of transmission of infection to very low levels. Despite continuing improvement in the screening and handling of blood products, however, the risk of transmission is not zero, and this risk must always be weighed against the benefit of a planned transfusion.

Fluid Overload

Fluid overload associated with blood transfusion usually occurs with plasma or plasma fraction therapy. These products contain proteins that hold or draw fluid into the vascular space and may cause fluid overload. Transfusion with packed red blood cells is less often associated with fluid overload. Careful planning of therapy and monitoring of the patient's cardiovascular status during transfusion therapy should identify fluid overload (e.g., dyspnea, orthopnea, hypoxia) promptly and lead to therapy with diuretics to avoid harm to the patient.

Conclusion

Surgeons should be able to perform preoperative screening evaluations for bleeding and clotting disorders, and they must be prepared to handle surgical hemostatic emergencies. However, a patient whose history or screening examination indicates a possible bleeding problem should also be evaluated preoperatively by a qualified hematologist. If a hemostatic disorder is found, the surgeon and hematologist should work in cooperation to manage the problem, thereby optimizing the patient's safety and well-being in the perioperative period.

Multiple-Choice Questions

1. The extrinsic coagulation pathway begins with:
   A. The interaction of factor VII with tissue thromboplastin
   B. Factor XII forming a clot
   C. Activation of factor XIII
   D. Activation that can be measured by the thrombin time (PT)
   E. Dysfibrinogenemia

2. An increased bleeding time occurs in:
   A. Disorders of the extrinsic system
   B. Disorders of the intrinsic system
   C. Disorders of platelet number or function
   D. Plasminogen deficiencies
   E. Increased factors V, VII, and X

3. The prothrombin time (PT) measures the adequacy of:
   A. Factors XII, VIII, IX, and XI
   B. Von Willebrand's factor
   C. Platelet function
   D. Factors V, VII, and X, and prothrombin and fibrinogen
   E. Protein C

4. The activated partial thromboplastin time (APTT) measures:
   A. Factors V, VIII, IX, X, XI, XII, and prothrombin and fibrinogen
   B. Tissue thromboplastin
   C. Platelet function
   D. Factors V, VII, and X
   E. Protein S

5. The pharmacologic effect of warfarin (Coumadin):
   A. Causes depression of factors V, VII, VIII, and IX
   B. Causes prolongation of prothrombin time (PT) and activated partial thromboplastin time (APTT)
   C. Causes prolongation of APTT and thrombin time
   D. Is calcium-dependent
   E. Is antithrombin III-dependent

6. A 40-year-old man undergoes a right colectomy for Dukes' Stage A carcinoma of the colon. During the procedure, he receives two units of blood. Near the end of the procedure, the surgeon notices generalized oozing. The anesthesiologist reports that urine output has ceased. The most likely diagnosis is:
   A. Hemolytic transfusion reaction
   B. Thrombotic thrombocytopenia
   C. Dilution of clotting factors
   D. Occult von Willebrand's disease
   E. Fibrinolysis secondary to cancer

7. Disseminated intravascular coagulation (DIC) is commonly associated with all of the following EXCEPT:
   A. Shock
   B. Extensive trauma
   C. Sepsis
   D. Acute hemolytic blood transfusion reaction
   E. Immunosuppression

8. The most common cause of postoperative bleeding is:
   A. Disseminated intravascular coagulation
   B. Von Willebrand's disease

C. Antithrombin III deficiency
D. An unligated vessel
E. Acquired vitamin K deficiency

9. Disseminated intravascular coagulation (DIC) is best treated by:
A. Warfarin (Coumadin)
B. Removal of all precipitating causes
C. Factor VIII
D. Red blood cell transfusions
E. Cryoprecipitate

10. Symptomatically severe primary fibrinolysis is best treated by:
A. Whole blood transfusion
B. Cryoprecipitative plasma
C. Factor IX concentrate
D. Platelet concentrate
E. ε-Amino caproic acid

11. Platelet concentrates:
A. Contain 1,000,000 platelets/bag
B. May be stored for 3 to 5 days at 22°C
C. Must be refrigerated at 10° to 15°C
D. Are usually cryopreserved by control rate freezing
E. Are usually preserved in glycerin or dimethyl sulfoxide

12. Cryoprecipitate is used to treat all of the following EXCEPT:
A. Hypofibrinogenemia
B. Disseminated intravascular coagulopathy
C. Von Willebrand's disease
D. Hemophilia A
E. Volume loss

13. Approximately how many units of red cell concentrate are needed to raise the hematocrit of a 70-kg man from 15% to 40%?
A. 2
B. 4
C. 7
D. 10
E. 12

14. Match the following phrase with the single best response. Number and function of platelets:
A. Bleeding time
B. Prothrombin time (PT)
C. Activated partial thromboplastin time (APTT)
D. Thrombin time
E. Fibrin split products

15. Match the following phrase with the single best response. Factors V, VIII, IX, X, XI, XII
A. Bleeding time
B. Prothrombin time (PT)
C. Activated partial thromboplastin time (APTT)
D. Thrombin time
E. Fibrin split products

16. Match the following phrase with the single best response. Fibrinogen-to-fibrin conversion:
A. Bleeding time
B. Prothrombin time (PT)
C. Activated partial thromboplastin time (APTT)
D. Thrombin time
E. Fibrin split products

17. Match the following phrase with the single best response. Factors V, VII, and X
A. Bleeding time
B. Prothrombin time (PT)
C. Activated partial thromboplastin time (APTT)
D. Thrombin time
E. Fibrin split products

18. Match the following phrase with the single best response. Vessel wall integrity:
A. Bleeding time
B. Prothrombin time (PT)
C. Activated partial thromboplastin time (APTT)
D. Thrombin time
E. Fibrin split products

19. Banked blood, compared with fresh blood, has all of the following EXCEPT:
A. Increased red blood cell viability
B. Decreased platelet function
C. Increased potassium concentration
D. Increased hydrogen ion concentration
E. Decreased coagulation factors

20. The abnormality that is NOT associated with liver failure is:
A. Partial thromboplastim time
B. Prothrombin time (PT)
C. Factor VII level
D. Platelet deficiency
E. Factor VIII level

Oral Examination Study Questions

CASE 1

You are a general surgeon in a mid-sized community hospital, and you are performing a colectomy for carcinoma of the colon. The procedure is bloody, and the anesthesiologist is administering one unit of packed red blood cells. After approximately one-half the unit is administered, you notice spontaneous oozing from the incision, and the anesthesiologist reports that the patient is hypotensive.

OBJECTIVE 1

The student elicits the following information.
A. Ask the time of onset and the degree of hypotension.

B. Ask the anesthesiologist to evaluate the patient for other causes of hypotension, such as cardiac-induced or drug-induced.

C. Look for the presence of hemoglobinuria.

D. Check urinary output.

OBJECTIVE 2

The student can discuss these differential diagnoses:

A. Causes of hypotension: cardiac, volume depletion, loss of vascular tone as a result of anesthetic drug administration

B. Causes of sudden onset of oozing from incision (Why is it not a congenital disorder?)

C. Causes of intraoperative bleeding

D. Disseminated intravascular coagulation (DIC): its causes, its effects, and the cause of the problem

OBJECTIVE 3

The student requests the following:

A. Immediate discontinuation of the transfusion and a recheck of the unit of blood to verify unit labeling and patient identification numbers

B. Return of the unit of blood to the blood bank for repeat crossmatch

C. Drawing of blood samples to recheck A, B, and O blood group and Rh type as well as free plasma hemoglobin

D. Repeated crossmatch and Coombs' test

E. Type and crossmatch of all of the donor units of blood for this patient as well as culture of the transfused blood and the patient's blood

OBJECTIVE 4

The student makes the following therapeutic responses based on the presumptive diagnosis of a transfusion reaction.

A. Investigate the patient for DIC. Order a complete blood count with platelet count, prothrombin time (PT), partial thromboplastin time, fibrinogen, and fibrin split products.

B. Initiate a close monitoring of urinary output.

C. On finding that the patient is oliguric, attempt a trial of an osmotic diuretic, such as mannitol, to maintain urine output. A test dose of 12.5 g mannitol (1 ampule) is administered over a 5-minute period. Volume is replaced with lactated Ringer's solution to correct hypotension; vasoactive drugs are used if necessary. The urine is alkalinized by giving intravenous bicarbonate, and urinary output of approximately 50 mL/hr is sought. Coagulation factors and platelets are replaced as necessary.

D. The surgical management is determined by the severity of the transfusion reaction. The procedure is completed as rapidly as possible, and the patient is transferred to the surgical intensive care unit.

Minimum Level of Achievement for Passing

The student recognizes the occurrence of a transfusion reaction under general anesthesia.

Honors Level of Achievement

The student not only recognizes the transfusion reaction, but also handles this complication rapidly by discontinuing the transfusion and aggressively treating the secondary effects of oliguria, bleeding, and hypotension.

CASE 2

You are an emergency department physician in a community in the upper peninsula of Michigan. On a sunny winter Sunday afternoon, a 22-year-old female college student comes to the emergency department with severe pain in the right knee radiating both up and down the leg. The pain started suddenly after she had a twisting fall while skiing. It is relieved somewhat by flexing the knee, but is not totally abated by application of either heat or cold. The patient describes herself as bruising easily. Her mother confirms that, as a child, the patient had more bruises than her older sister. Initial vital signs include blood pressure of 128/75 mm Hg, temperature of 98.7°F, pulse rate of 110 beats/min, and respiration rate of 16 breaths/min.

OBJECTIVE 1

The student elicits the following history and physical findings:

A. There is a history of two previous episodes of unusually severe bleeding, both of which were trauma-related.

B. The patient reports that her menstrual periods occur at normal intervals, but seem longer than those of her friends, lasting 7 to 8 days, with the first 2 days being very heavy.

C. The patient has had anemia since the age of 10 years and has been receiving iron supplementation since that time.

D. The patient's mother and maternal grandfather are reported to be "bleeders."

E. Examination of the right leg shows swelling around the joint, with marked tenderness, but no redness or heat.

F. The patient is most comfortable with the joint held in a slightly flexed position. There is no specific tenderness in the muscle masses of the thigh or calf region. The patient can move her ankle joint normally, and has no swelling of that joint.

OBJECTIVE 2

The student recognizes that the problem is acute, almost certainly noninflammatory, and probably related to a sudden event involving the left knee (e.g., hemorrhage into the joint). The student differentiates this condition from chronic joint disorders.

A. Inflammatory arthritis. This condition is characterized by redness, somewhat slower progression of pain, and fever associated with joint pain. Predisposing historic factors include a history of bleeding, both trauma-related and associated with menses, and a family history of bleeding.

B. Fracture. A history of bleeding does not exclude fracture. However, the sudden swelling of the joint, associated with a twisting injury, suggests an intrajoint phenomenon as opposed to a fracture.

C. Chronic arthritis. The age of the patient and the suddenness of the development of the symptoms make this diagnosis unlikely.

D. Acute systemic arthralgia or arthritis. There is no other joint involvement, and there are no systemic symptoms (e.g., fever, malaise).

OBJECTIVE 3

The student makes a definitive diagnosis of an acute joint bleed and requests the following studies:

A. A complete blood count. Hemoglobin is 11.2 g/dL, hematocrit is 32%, and white blood cell count is 9000/mm^3, with 68% polymorphonuclear leukocytes, 0 bands, and 32% lymphocytes.

B. Screening coagulation tests, including a platelet count of 280,000/mm^3 (normal), a PT of 11.2 seconds (normal), a partial thromboplastin time of 52 seconds (prolonged), and a bleeding time greater than 20 minutes (prolonged).

C. Bone films of the right knee area, which show no bony destruction, but do show increased fluid within the joint.

D. A tap of the joint, which shows bright red blood. When the blood is removed from the joint, the patient's symptoms are markedly improved.

OBJECTIVE 4

The student makes a rapid differential diagnosis.

Possible diagnoses in this patient with an apparently significant medical history and an acute history of bleeding include von Willebrand's disease and other abnormalities, either congenital or acquired. Specific studies to order include factor VIII, both clotting and von Willebrand factor activity, and platelet aggregation. Factor VIII clotting activity is low, 8%. Factor VIII von Willebrand activity is also low, 11%. Platelet aggregation is consistent with von Willebrand's disease, showing marked reduction in response to ristocetin. This reduction is corrected by the addition of 50% normal pooled plasma.

OBJECTIVE 5

The student can discuss the management of this injury.

A. The most appropriate management is cryoprecipitate administration based on the patient's weight, using the same calculations that are used to treat type A hemophilia. The patient's joint is briefly immobilized, packed in ice, and strapped with a pressure bandage to prevent reaccumulation of blood.

B. Cryoprecipitate is given as frequently as needed, usually at least once every 24 hours, to maintain a partial thromboplastin time within the normal range and to correct the bleeding time abnormality. The duration of therapy is approximately 5 to 10 days, as indicated by the symptoms. Medications to be avoided during the treatment period include nonsteroidal anti-inflammatory drugs (NSAIDs), because these, specifically aspirin, aggravate coagulopathy. Remobilization begins after the coagulopathy is corrected.

Minimum Level of Achievement for Passing

The student recognizes that the problem is bleeding rather than infection and can differentiate the causes of an acute bleeding event caused by an inherited disorder.

Honors Level of Achievement

The student makes the specific diagnosis of von Willebrand's disease and formulates a treatment plan. The student recognizes the importance of the use of cryoprecipitate in the management of this case and understands the need to avoid NSAIDs.

CASE 3

You are the surgery resident in the emergency department when a 24-year-old man is "life-flighted" into the department after being struck by a car traveling at a high speed on the freeway. On-site resuscitation included 2 L intravenous fluids, placement of a cervical collar, and bracing of the left leg, which was believed to be fractured. On presentation to the emergency department, the patient is unconscious, and has a blood pressure of 90/40, pulse rate of 140, respiratory rate of 24 breaths/min, and temperature of 99°F. He is pale, his extremities are cool, and his abdomen is "board-like" on examination.

OBJECTIVE 1

The student elicits the following information:

A. The degree of anemia, by obtaining hemoglobin and hematocrit.

B. The presence or absence of free air in the abdomen, by obtaining an "acute abdomen" series of x-rays.

C. Evidence of possible liver or spleen injury by obtaining a computed tomography (CT) scan of the abdomen.

OBJECTIVE 2

The student can discuss the differential diagnosis of:

A. Hypotension occurring after severe trauma

B. A board-like abdomen

The student can outline the steps in the initial resuscitation of a trauma patient.

OBJECTIVE 3

The student should:

A. Request immediate fluid resuscitation

B. Request urgent type and crossmatch for four units of packed red blood cells

C. Notify the operating room to be prepared for emergency laparotomy

Minimum Level of Achievement for Passing

The student recognizes the occurrence of a ruptured viscus as a cause of board-like abdomen.

Honors Level of Achievement

The student describes the steps in the emergency management of acute abdominal injury.

SUGGESTED READINGS

Lumadue JA, Ness PM. Current approaches to red blood cell transfusion. *Semin Hematol* 1996;33(4):277–289.

Rosenberg RD. Biochemistry and pharmacology of low molecular weight heparin. *Semin Hematol* 1997;34(4):2–8.

Rosendaal FR. Risk factors for venous thrombosis: prevalence, risk, and interaction. *Semin Hematol* 1997;34(3):171–187.

Schuster H-P. Epilogue: disseminated intravascular coagulation and antithrombin III in intensive care medicine: pathophysiological insights and therapeutic hopes. *Semin Thromb Hemost* 1998; 24(1):81–83.

6

Shock

Kenneth W. Burchard, M.D.

OBJECTIVES

1. Define shock, and list the two primary mechanisms that may cause cellular malfunction consistent with shock.
2. List the etiologies of these primary mechanisms that are responsible for shock.
3. List the clinical information (i.e., history, physical examination, diagnostic tests, hemodynamic parameters) that helps to determine which of the two primary mechanisms is the predominant cause of shock in an individual patient.
4. Describe the interrelation between the two primary mechanisms of shock as a cause of cellular injury.
5. Describe the general principles of management that diminish cellular injury from the primary mechanisms of shock.

Traditional descriptions of **shock** often use systolic hypotension (< 90 mm Hg) as the defining variable. According to this criterion, classification schemes that use categories such as hypovolemic, septic, cardiogenic, and neurogenic shock are common. However, certain etiologies of hypotension (i.e., neurogenic vasodilation after spinal cord injury) do not necessarily cause significant cellular or organ injury. In addition, cellular and organ injury may develop without hypotension reaching 90 mm Hg. Therefore, definitions of shock based on systolic blood pressure are potentially misleading and narrow in scope.

A broader definition of shock is a condition in which total body cellular metabolism is malfunctional. When treated aggressively, this cellular metabolic dysfunction is reversible. When allowed to continue, however, shock results in cellular death, organ damage, and eventual death.

During the 20th century, many theories were developed to explain this cellular injury and death (i.e., disorders of the circulation, disorders of the nervous system, toxemia). By 1950, two competing theories were predominant: (1) shock is secondary to inadequate oxygen delivery; (2) shock is secondary to a toxic cellular insult that can progress even when sufficient oxygen is delivered. Such conditions as severe hemorrhage and cardiac malfunction were recognized throughout the century as etiologies of inadequate oxygen delivery. The recognition that the primary toxins of cellular injury are endogenous (the products of tissue injury or the consequent inflammatory response) rather than exogenous (endotoxin) emerged primarily over the last two decades. Tissue injury and the associated inflammatory response result in the production or activation of cellular molecules (i.e., cytokines, superoxide radicals, prostaglandins, adhesion factors) that promote local cellular activation, tissue repair, and host defenses. However, sometimes this local response incites similar responses in cells that are distant from the primary insult. The result is systemic **inflammation** that can cause organ malfunction and shock.

Simultaneously, during the last two decades, experimental and clinical studies showed that these two mechanisms of cellular injury are not competitive or exclusive, but are most often additive during shock states. Simply stated, hypoperfusion begets inflammation, and inflammation begets hypoperfusion. The clinician must be alert to this association and must approach each patient who has the manifestations of total body cellular malfunction with the dual goals of carefully assessing the circulation for oxygen delivery and carefully assessing the state of inflammation for cell toxicity. Restoring excellent circulation and treating severe inflammation are the primary tenets for managing the patient with shock.

This chapter describes the pathophysiology that links **hypoperfusion** with inflammation and provides clinical guidelines for recognizing hypoperfusion and **severe inflammation** and managing these two mechanisms of cellular injury.

Normal Physiology of the Circulation and of Inflammation

The main function of the circulation is to deliver oxygen to the capillaries. The determinants of total body oxygen delivery are listed with other commonly measured or calculated hemodynamic variables in Table 6-1. As the formula for oxygen delivery shows, the pulmonary component is limited to providing adequate

Table 6-1. Hemodynamic and Oxygen Delivery Variables

Item	Definition	Normal
CVP	Central venous pressure; CVP = RAP; in the absence of tricuspid valve disease, CVP = RVEDP	5–15 mm Hg
LAP	Left atrial pressure; in the absence of mitral valve disease, LAP = LVEDP	5–15 mm Hg
PCWP	Pulmonary capillary wedge pressure; PCWP = LAP, except sometimes with high PEEP levels	5–15 mm Hg
MAP	Mean arterial pressure, mm Hg; MAP = DP + 1/3 (SP − DP)	80–90 mm Hg
CT	Cardiac index; CI = CO/m² BSA	2.5–3.5 L/min/m² BSA
SI	Stroke index; SI = SV/m² BSA	35–40 mL/beat/m²
SVR	Systemic vascular resistance; $SVR = \dfrac{(MAP - CVP) \times 80}{CO}$	1000–1500 dyne-sec/cm⁵
PVR	Pulmonary vascular resistance; $PVR = \dfrac{(MAP - PAOP) \times 80}{CO}$	100–400 dyne-sec/cm⁵
CaO_2	Arterial oxygen content (vol %); $CaO_2 = 1.39 \times Hgb\ SaO_2 + (PaO_2 \times 0.0031)$	20 vol %
CvO_2	Mixed venous oxygen content (vol %); $C\bar{v}O = 1.39 \times Hgb \times S\bar{v}O_2 + (P\bar{v}O_2 \times 0.0031)$	15 vol %
$C(a - \bar{v})O_2$	Arterial venous O_2 content difference; $C(a - \bar{v})O_2 = CaO_2 - C\bar{v}O_2$ (vol %)	3.5–4.5 vol %
O_2D	O_2 delivery; $O_2D = CO \times CaO_2 \times 10$; 10 = factor to convert mL O_2/100 mL blood to mL O_2/L blood	900–1200 mL/min
O_2C	O_2 consumption; $O_2C = (CaO_2 - C\bar{v}O_2) \times CO \times 10$	250 mL/min 130–160 mL/min/m²

BSA, body surface area (m²). CO, cardiac output. DP, diastolic pressure. LVEDP, left ventricular end-diastolic pressure. PaO_2, PAOP, pulmonary artery occlusion pressure. PEEP, positive end = expiratory pressure, arterial PO_2 (mm Hg). $P\bar{v}O_2$, mixed venous PO_2. RAP, right atrial pressure. RVEDP, right ventricular end-diastolic pressure. SaO_2, arterial oxygen saturation (%). $S\bar{v}O_2$, mixed venous oxygen saturation. SP, systolic pressure. SV, stroke volume.

arterial oxygen saturation (≥ 90% saturation is usually present when PaO_2 ≥ 60 mm Hg). This goal is usually readily achieved with modern respiratory therapy. Hemoglobin is frequently increased with transfusion. Usually, the most difficult component to treat is **cardiac output.** The determinants of cardiac output are organized by both the variables that affect ventricular function and the variables that affect **venous return.** Depending on clinical circumstances, sometimes it is more useful to use the logic associated with alterations in ventricular physiology to enhance the circulation,

Table 6-2. Determinants of Ventricular Function

Preload
Afterload
Contractility
Heart rate

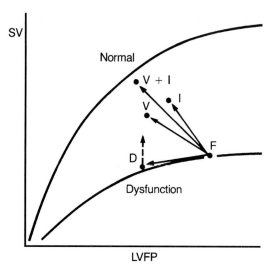

Figure 6-1 Expected hemodynamic response in severe left ventricular dysfunction to administration of diuretics (D), inotropic drugs (I), vasodilators (V), and a combination of vasodilators and inotropics (V + I). SV, stroke volume. LVFP, left ventricular filling pressure. F, failure.

and sometimes it is more useful to use the logic associated with alterations in venous return physiology. This logical application of one circulatory physiology versus another (physio-logic) is described in more detail in the hypoperfusion section.

Ventricular Physiology

The major determinants of ventricular performance are listed in Table 6-2. **Preload** is the magnitude of myocardial stretch, the stimulus to muscle contraction that is described by the Frank-Starling mechanism (Figure 6-1), whereby increased stretch leads to increased contraction until the muscle is overstretched (commonly recognized clinically as congestive heart failure; see the hypoperfusion section). Preload is most appropriately measured as end-diastolic volume. Because volume is not easily measured clinically, the direct proportion between ventricular volume and ventricular end-diastolic pressure allows the measurement of pressure [measured as central venous pressure (CVP) for the right side of the heart and pulmonary capillary wedge or pulmonary artery occlusion pressure (PAOP) for the left side of the heart] to estimate volume.

Ventricular afterload is determined primarily by the resistance to ventricular ejection that is present in either

Table 6-3. Factors That Affect Myocardial Contractility

Increased	Decreased
Catecholamines	Catecholamine depletion and receptor malfunction
Inotropic drugs	Alpha and beta blockers Calcium channel blockers
Increased preload	Decreased preload Overstretching of myocardium
Decreased afterload	Increased afterload Severe inflammation and ischemia

the pulmonary (pulmonary vascular resistance) or systemic arterial tree (systemic vascular resistance). With constant preload, increased afterload diminishes ventricular ejection, and decreased afterload augments ejection (see Figure 6-1).

Contractility is the force of contraction under conditions of a predetermined preload or afterload. Factors that increase and decrease contractility are listed in Table 6-3. A change in contractility, like a change in afterload, results in a different cardiac function curve (see Figure 6-1).

The combined influence of increasing contractility and decreasing afterload to improve ventricular function is also shown in Figure 6-1.

Heart rate is directly proportional to cardiac output (not to cardiac muscle mechanics) until rapid rates diminish ventricular filling during diastole.

Venous Return

Venous return is described by the following formula:

$$VR = \frac{MSP - CVP}{RV + RA/19}$$

where MSP = mean systemic pressure, CVP = central venous pressure (right atrial pressure), RV = venous resistance, and RA = arterial resistance.

The division of arterial resistance by 19 was formulated by Guyton in 1973 using both calculations and empirical observation. As might be expected, alterations in arterial resistance have much less effect on venous return than alterations in venous resistance, as indicated in the formula.

Mean systemic pressure (MSP) is not the same as mean arterial pressure. MSP is the pressure in small veins and venules. This pressure must be higher than CVP in the periphery so that blood can flow from the periphery to the thorax. Venous resistance occurs primarily in the large veins in the abdomen and thorax. Arterial resistance occurs mostly in the arterioles.

Factors that alter venous return variables are listed in Table 6-4. Surgical patients frequently have diseases or therapeutic interventions that may inhibit venous return.

Table 6-4. Factors That Alter Venous Return Variables

Increased venous return
  Increased MSP
    Increased vascular volume
    Increased vascular tone
    External compression
    Trendelenburg position (increased MSP in lower extremities and abdomen)
  Decreased CVP
    Hypovolemia
    Negative pressure respiration
  Decreased venous resistance
    Decreased venous constriction
    Negative pressure respiration
Diminished venous return
  Decreased MSP
    Hypovolemia
    Vasodilation
  Increased CVP
    Intracardiac
      Congestive heart failure
      Cardiogenic shock
      Tricuspid regurgitation
      Right heart failure
    Extracardiac
      Positive pressure respiration
      PEEP
      Tension pneumothorax
      Cardiac tamponade
      Increased abdominal pressure
  Increased venous resistance
    Increased thoracic pressure
    Positive pressure respiration
    PEEP
    Increased abdominal pressure
    Tension pneumothorax
  Increased abdominal pressure
    Ascites
    Bowel distension
    Tension pneumoperitoneum
    Intraabdominal hemorrhage
    Retroperitoneal hemorrhage

MSP, mean systemic pressure. CVP, central venous pressure. PEEP, positive end-expiratory pressure.

Physiology of Inflammation

The normal response to tissue injury is essential for restoring normal tissue function and wound healing. The initial response to tissue damage by trauma is bleeding and coagulation. This response is less likely, but not impossible, with tissue damage from ischemia or infection. Platelet activation results in the release of important chemoattractants [i.e., platelet-derived growth factor (PDGF), transforming growth factor-β (TGF-β)].

Damaged blood vessels initially vasoconstrict, but this constriction is soon followed by vasodilation and increased capillary permeability secondary to the action of agents such as prostaglandin E_2, prostacyclin, histamine, serotonin, and kinins. When blood flow is present, this vascular response results in the accumulation of protein-rich edema fluid (exudate). White cells adhere to these damaged, leaky vessels.

Attracted by chemoattractants (e.g., PDGF), polymorphonuclear cells (PMNs) are the first white cells to migrate to the inflammatory site (within minutes if the circulation is good). PMNs phagocytize dead tissue and foreign objects. Opsonins and preformed antibodies may assist in the removal of bacteria. PMNs produce proteases and intracellular oxygen radicals that are critical for beneficial PMN activity. Besides proteases and oxygen radicals, PMNs can also release interleukin-1 (IL-1), or endogenous pyrogen. IL-1 mediates temperature elevation through the thermoregulatory center and also stimulates other inflammatory activity (e.g., migration of macrophages). Another cytokine, interleukin-8 (IL-8), is a potent PMN attractant that is produced by many cell types after incubation with IL-1 and the cytokine tumor necrosis factor (TNF). Incubation involves the in vitro juxtaposition of cells with a substance of interest in a physiologic environment that supports cell survival. If the cells respond to the substance, then the effect can be assayed in this controlled, isolated milieu. The PMNs last only for a period of hours.

Within hours, tissue macrophages and circulating monocytes are attracted by such substances as PDGF, TGF-β, and IL-1; they migrate into the injured area, and last for days to weeks. The continuing inflammatory process is largely regulated by macrophages through such mediators as IL-1, TNF, PDGF, TGF-β, TGF-α, and fibroblast growth factor.

For instance, fibroblast migration and angiogenesis begin next. Fibroblasts are influenced by IL-1, TNF, PDGF, TGF-β, TGF-α, insulin-like growth factor, and epidermal growth factor (EGF). Angiogenesis is influenced by TNF, TGF-β, TGF-α, and EGF. The combined process of fibroblast proliferation and capillary budding produces granulation tissue that is friable and bleeds easily.

Fibroblasts produce collagen. This process usually accelerates 5 days after tissue damage occurs. Collagen synthesis is influenced by IL-1, TNF, PDGF, TGF-β, and EGF.

A summary of cellular activity in inflammation is shown in Tables 6-5 and 6-6.

Hypoperfusion States

Hypoperfusion is a decrease in total body or regional blood flow that is sufficient to result in cellular malfunction or death. Hypoperfusion is the primary mechanism that is responsible for inadequate oxygen delivery; the immediate effects of hypoperfusion on cell viability are secondary to the interruption of oxidative metabolism.

The Neurohumoral Response to Hypoperfusion

Total body hypoperfusion usually manifests as a reduction in cardiac output. The most frequently studied models of total body hypoperfusion cause a reduction in cardiac output from loss of volume (hypovolemic hypoperfusion) or loss of cardiac function (cardiogenic hypoperfusion). Either of these etiologies may result in the neurohumoral response shown in Table 6-7.

The clinically apparent effects of this neurohumoral response are tachycardia (epinephrine, norepinephrine, dopamine), vasoconstriction (norepinephrine, arginine

Table 6-5. Normal Inflammation

Event	Cells Responsible
Coagulation	Platelets
Early inflammation	Polymorphonuclear leukocytes (first few hours)
Later inflammation	Monocytes (days) macrophages
Collagen and mucopolysaccharide	Fibroblasts (maximum deposition 7–10 days)
Capillary budding	Endothelial cells (maximum 7–10 days)

Table 6-6. Functions of Inflammatory Cells

Cells	Function
Platelets	Coagulation, release PDGF, IL-1
Polymorphonuclear leukocytes	Phagocytosis, especially microbes, release IL-1, IL-8
Macrophage	Phagocytosis; stimulate fibroblast migration and growth; stimulate endothelial cell migration and growth; release FGF, PDGF, IL-1, TNF, TFG-β, TGF-α
Fibroblast	Collagen deposition
Endothelial cells	Capillary budding

PDGF, platelet-derived growth factor. IL, interleukin. FGF, fibroblast growth factor. TNF, tumor necrosis factor. TGF, transforming growth factor.

Table 6-7. Neurohumoral Response to Hypoperfusion

Increased	Decreased
Epinephrine	Insulin
Norepinephrine	Thyroxine
Dopamine	Triiodothyronine
Glucagon	Luteinizing hormone
Renin	Testosterone
Angiotensin	Estrogen
Arginine vasopressin	Follicle-stimulating hormone
Adrenocorticotropic hormone	
Cortisol	
Aldosterone	
Growth hormone	

vasopressin, angiotensin), diaphoresis (norepinephrine), oliguria with sodium and water conservation [adrenocorticotropic hormone (ACTH), cortisol, aldosterone, arginine vasopressin], and hyperglycemia (epinephrine, glucagon, cortisol, insufficient insulin). This activation of the neuroendocrine system may preserve blood flow to vital organs (heart, lungs, brain) while diminishing flow to less vital organs (kidneys, gastrointestinal tract). In this way, it preserves or increases intravascular volume by limiting urine output. This response is more homeostatic under conditions of hypovolemic hypoperfusion compared with cardiogenic hypoperfusion, in which tachycardia, vasoconstriction, and sodium and water retention may aggravate rather than diminish hypoperfusion by decreasing ventricular filling time, increasing afterload, and increasing myocardial stretch, respectively.

The Effects of Hypoperfusion on Inflammation

The most clearly documented association of hypoperfusion with inflammation is the effect of **ischemia followed by reperfusion.** Clinically, this effect is most obvious in patients with isolated limb ischemia (compartment syndrome) and in some patients with localized intestinal ischemia. However, severe systemic hypoperfusion may cause a similar response in many tissues, particularly the gastrointestinal tract.

The mechanism that is responsible for ischemia reperfusion injury appears to require both local and systemic factors. A complex interaction of oxygen free radicals, thromboxane, leukotrienes, phospholipase A_2, and leukocytes participates in both regional and total body alterations in capillary permeability and organ function. Anatomic and physiologic damage to the intestine, limb, kidney, liver, and lung may occur after reperfusion, even when a specific organ (i.e., lung) was not initially hypoperfused. Because PMNs are potent producers of oxygen free radicals, these cells are central to this pathophysiology.

The potential for severe inflammation to develop during, rather than after, hypoperfusion is less well documented and more controversial. Some experimental studies showed an increase in inflammatory mediators and cellular activity during hemorrhagic hypoperfusion. Others did not show this increase.

In clinical hypoperfusion, particularly with trauma, it is difficult to separate tissue injury that is secondary only to hypoperfusion from damage from other mechanisms (e.g., a direct blow). Again, whatever the cause, hypoperfusion and inflammation commonly occur together.

The Effects of Hypoperfusion on Cellular Metabolism

The classic effect of hypoperfusion on cellular metabolism is anaerobic metabolism caused by an oxygen deficit. The reduction in adenosine triphosphate (ATP) production that occurs secondary to the loss of mitochondrial function can result in inadequate energy to meet cellular needs, with cell death as a consequence.

Elevated levels of lactic acid, with low pyruvate levels, characterize anaerobic gylcolysis as the primary means of ATP production in anaerobic states.

Besides an elevation in lactic acid, cell membrane function may be impaired by decreased intracellular ATP production and from a circulating protein that can depolarize cell membranes. Possibly as a result of such cell membrane alterations, sodium and calcium can move into cells, with water following the sodium. Sequestration of water in cells can cause a deficit in extracellular fluid, which may accentuate the fluid requirements during resuscitation.

Etiologies, Diagnosis, and Management of Hypoperfusion States

The primary etiologies of hypoperfusion states in surgical patients are decreased venous return and decreased myocardial function (Table 6-8).

Decreased Venous Return: Hypovolemia

Hypovolemia is the most common etiology of decreased venous return secondary to decreased MSP. Common etiologies of hypovolemia are listed in Table 6-9. Hypovolemia is the most common cause of hypotension.

Table 6-8. Etiologies of Hypoperfusion

Decreased venous return
  Hypovolemia
  Pericardial tamponade
  Tension pneumothorax
  Increased abdominal pressure
    Bowel obstruction
    Tension pneumoperitoneum
    Massive bleeding
    Diagnostic laparoscopy
    Pneumatic antishock garment
    Ascites
Positive end-expiratory pressure
Decreased myocardial function
  Congestive heart failure
  Cardiogenic shock

Table 6-9. Common Etiologies of Hypovolemia

Hemorrhage
Severe inflammation or infection
Trauma
Pancreatitis or other causes of peritonitis
Burns
Vomiting or other intestinal losses
Excess diuresis
Inadequate oral intake

Severe hypoperfusion secondary to hypovolemia (i.e., hypovolemic shock) was studied most frequently in experimental and clinical hemorrhage. Hemorrhagic shock not only diminishes venous return, but also may cause cardiovascular alterations (Table 6-10). Cellular effects (other than lactic acidosis from anaerobic glycolysis) are listed in Table 6-11. As mentioned earlier, ischemia-induced local and systemic inflammation have also been described.

The metabolic and toxic phenomena associated with hypovolemic shock, even without severe inflammation, result in loss of plasma and interstitial volume beyond what is accounted for by the primary disease process (i.e., hemorrhage, vomiting). Migration of interstitial fluid into cells and increased capillary permeability are implicated as mechanisms.

Physical Examination in Hypovolemic Hypoperfusion

In the patient who has hypovolemia, vital signs and physical findings show evidence of hypoperfusion roughly in proportion to the degree of hypovolemia. A

Table 6-10. Cardiovascular Effects of Hemorrhagic Shock

Decreased venous return

Increased systemic vascular resistance

Decreased ventricular contractility

Decreased ventricular compliance

Increased atrial contractility

Transcapillary refill of water to restore plasma volume

Intravascular protein replenishment from preformed extravascular protein

Table 6-11. Cellular Effects of Hemorrhagic Shock

Diminished transmembrane potential difference

Increased intracellular sodium

Decreased intracellular adenosine triphophate

10% loss of blood volume (560 mL, approximately the amount donated for transfusion) produces little, if any, disturbance. A 20% loss may cause tachycardia and orthostatic hypotension. A 30% loss may produce hypotension while the patient is supine. However, a patient may be normotensive when supine, even with greater loss of blood volume (Table 6-12).

Agitation, tachypnea, and peripheral vasoconstriction are common with any etiology of hypoperfusion. Hypotension, however, most commonly occurs secondary to hypovolemia. Hypotension as a result of disruption of intrinsic cardiac function (cardiogenic shock) is much less common (discussed later). Congestive heart failure, a distinct clinical entity from cardiogenic shock, frequently causes increased blood pressure.

The neck veins are not distended unless hypovolemia is accompanied by an extracardiac increase in central venous pressure (tension pneumothorax, pericardial tamponade, severe effort during expiration, increased abdominal pressure). An S_3 gallop is not usually present. An etiology of hypovolemia may also be apparent (open wound with hemorrhage, distended abdomen, femur and pelvic fractures).

Common Laboratory Aids

Hypovolemic hypoperfusion that is severe enough to cause hypotension is associated with metabolic acidosis that is recognized either from serum electrolytes or, more precisely, arterial blood gases. Elevated serum blood urea nitrogen (BUN) and creatinine levels that are indicative of renal malfunction are common. CVP and PAOP are low, as are cardiac index and oxygen delivery.

Other tests (e.g., hemoglobin level, other serum chemistries, radiographic studies) are usually used to determine the etiology of hypovolemic hypoperfusion rather than to document the severity of the perfusion deficits.

Treatment of Hypovolemia

In the patient who has severe hypovolemic hypoperfusion, the circulation must be restored simultaneously with diagnostic and therapeutic interventions to correct

Table 6-12. Hemodynamic Effects of Intravascular Volume Loss in Supine Subjects

Amount	Rate	Blood Pressure	Pulse	Mentation	Skin Vasoconstriction	Urine Output
≤ 10%	5 min	NL	NL	NL	NL	NL
≤ 10%	1 hr	NL	NL	NL	NL	NL
20%	5 min	↓	↑	NL	↑	↓
20%	1 hr	NL	↑	NL	NL	↓
30%	5 min	↓↓	↑↑	↓	↑↑	↓↓
30%	1 hr	↓	↑	↓	↑	↓
50%	5 min	↓↓↓	↑↑↑	↓↓	↑↑↑	↓↓↓
50%	1 hr	↓↓	↑↑	↓↓	↑↑	↓↓

NL, normal.

the underlying cause of the hypovolemic state. The circulatory, metabolic, and toxic effects of hypovolemic hypoperfusion are best treated by rapid (within minutes) restoration of intravascular volume, thereby increasing MSP, venous return, and oxygen delivery. In general, two types of fluid, **crystalloid** and **colloid,** are used for volume replacement (Table 6-13). Red blood cells are effective when needed. After hemorrhage is arrested, the administration of red cells causes increased cardiac output, increased oxygen-carrying capacity, and little, if any, leakage of red cells into the interstitium, even in the face of increased capillary permeability. The primary disadvantage of red cell transfusion is the rare risk of infection with a transmissible disease (e.g., hepatitis C, human immunodeficiency virus). Also rare is an incompatible red cell hemolytic transfusion reaction. Febrile episodes that do not represent true transfusion incompatibility are more common, and are most often secondary to antibodies to the small numbers of white cells that remain in the packed red cell unit. Potential advantages and disadvantages of various resuscitation fluids other than red cells are shown in Tables 6-14 and 6-15.

Fresh frozen plasma (FFP) should not be used primarily as a colloid. Only when hypovolemia is accompanied by bleeding and a deficiency in intrinsic or extrinsic coagulation (partial thromboplastin time > 1.5 × control, prothrombin time < 50%) should FFP be used. In general, red blood cells are used to replace lost red cells and are administered until the serum hemoglobin approaches 10 g/100 mL. Little advantage is documented for increasing the hemoglobin to greater than 10 g/100 mL, even in patients with little ability to increase cardiac output. Although hemoglobin concentrations of as low as 7 g/100 mL are now considered acceptable for some acute illnesses, cautious assessment of oxygen delivery and consumption variables is recommended if a plan to avoid red cell transfusion for such concentrations is considered advantageous (see section on endpoints of resuscitation of the circulation).

Much more controversial than the appropriate use of FFP and red blood cells are the advantages and disadvantages of the various crystalloid and colloid solutions previously listed. Most investigators agree that colloid administration results in less sodium administration compared with crystalloid solutions and less water administration compared with isotonic crystalloid solutions. In addition, plasma oncotic pressure is higher after the administration of colloids. Still debated is whether increased total body sodium and water gain are detrimental to organ function after resuscitation of the circulation.

When a patient who has hypovolemia is receiving large volumes of crystalloid or colloid and is not responding well to therapy (most often seen in severe septic shock), dopamine administration is a logical adjunct. Dopamine increases left ventricular filling pressures as it increases cardiac output, probably as a result of constriction of the veins and decreased venous capacitance. This increase may occur at the expense of increasing myocardial oxygen demands. After adequate vascular volume is attained, the dopamine can usually be discontinued.

Decreased Venous Return: Pericardial Tamponade

The primary mechanism for decreased venous return during pericardial tamponade is an extracavitary increase in CVP. The etiologies of tamponade are most

---

Table 6-13. Fluids for Hypovolemia Resuscitation

Crystalloid
  Isotonic
    Ringer's lactate
    0.9% saline
  Hypertonic saline
Colloid
  Red blood cells
  Fresh frozen plasma
  Albumin
  Processed human protein
  Low–molecular-weight dextran
  Hydroxyethyl starch

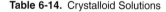

Table 6-14. Crystalloid Solutions

Isotonic solution advantages
  Inexpensive
  Readily available
  Replenishes epidermal growth factor
  Freely mobile across capillaries
  No increase in lung water
Isotonic solution disadvantages
  Rapid equilibration with interstitial fluid
  Lowers serum oncotic pressure
  No oxygen carrying capacity
  Increase in systemically perfused interstitial fluid

Table 6-15. Colloid Solutions (Other than Red Cells)

Advantages
  Less water administered (more resuscitation per milliliter)
  Less sodium administered
  Less decrease in oncotic pressure
  Acid buffer (fresh frozen plasma)
Disadvantages
  Expensive (albumin, fresh frozen plasma)
  Transmissible disease (fresh frozen plasma)
  Increased interstitial oncotic pressure
  Depressed myocardial function (albumin:50% reduction in left
    ventricular stroke work index at a pulmonary capillary occlusion
    pressure of 15 mm Hg)
  Depressed immunologic function (albumin: decreased
    immunoglobulins, decreased response to tetanus toxoid)
  Delayed resolution of interstitial edema
  Coagulopathy: infrequent in low doses (low–molecular-weight
    dextran: platelet malfunction; hydroxyethyl starch: decreased
    factor VIII:c concentrations; albumin: decreased fibrinogen,
    decreased prothrombin, decreased factor VIII)

commonly chest trauma (penetrating and blunt) and bleeding after cardiac surgery. Physical examination usually shows evidence of hypoperfusion, along with distended neck veins, muffled heart sounds, and an increased paradoxical pulse (> 15 mm Hg). The electrocardiogram may show low voltage, the CVP is often elevated, and a chest x-ray may show an enlarging heart. With severe hypovolemia, the CVP may be normal despite tamponade, and may become elevated only after fluid resuscitation. An echocardiogram shows fluid surrounding the heart, with diminished ventricular volumes.

It is important to distinguish this etiology of hypoperfusion from congestive heart failure (CHF) or cardiogenic shock because reducing fluid intake and administering a diuretic would reduce venous return further in tamponade. As stated, CHF usually results in normal or elevated blood pressure. Severe tamponade results in hypotension. Therefore, tamponade simulates cardiogenic shock more closely than CHF. Because cardiogenic shock requires a major insult to myocardial function (see later), hypotension with elevated CVP should increase suspicion of tamponade or a tension pneumothorax unless obvious evidence of severe myocardial malfunction is found.

The incidence of cardiac tamponade in surgical patients is low, and it is most often seen in patients with chest trauma or in those undergoing cardiac surgery. Removal of the fluid surrounding the heart (pericardiocentesis) is the most effective therapy, and it can result in a dramatic improvement in cardiac output. However, venous return also improves as a result of increasing MSP with intravenous fluid. Therefore, vigorous fluid administration should be provided despite elevated CVP.

Decreased Venous Return: Tension Pneumothorax

Tension pneumothorax reduces venous return by producing an extracavitary increase in CVP and by increasing venous resistance in the chest. Tension pneumothorax may occur spontaneously from rupture of a bleb or, more commonly, after penetrating or blunt trauma. Physical examination shows evidence of decreased perfusion, along with decreased breath sounds over the affected thorax, tracheal deviation away from the affected thorax, and distended neck veins. A chest x-ray may be the first clue to a tension pneumothorax, but most often, the diagnosis is made at the beside without radiologic assistance.

Treatment consists of emergently releasing the tension (e.g., placing a 14-gauge needle into the chest, placing a finger in a large penetrating injury), followed by closed thoracostomy. Administration of intravenous fluid to increase MSP is also beneficial, and neck vein distension may not be evident with severe hypovolemia.

Decreased Venous Return: Increased Abdominal Pressure

Increased abdominal pressure (> 20 mm Hg) diminishes venous return by increasing intrathoracic pressure, producing an extracavitary increase in CVP, and increasing venous resistance in abdominal veins. Increased abdominal pressure may be particularly detrimental to renal blood flow, but it can cause marked total body hypoperfusion despite a well-maintained mean arterial blood pressure from increased systemic vascular resistance.

Abdominal pressure is increased by a variety of mechanisms (see Table 6-4). It is most easily measured with a bladder catheter: 50 to 100 mL fluid is inserted into the bladder through the fluid sampling port on a Foley catheter; the catheter is clamped distal to the sampling port; and pressure is measured by connecting the needle in the sampling port to standard hemodynamic monitoring tubing, using the pubis as the zero pressure level.

Physical examination often shows evidence of hypoperfusion along with a tensely distended abdomen and possibly distended neck veins. The most effective treatment is to relieve the pressure. However, aggressive fluid management to increase MSP may be the only option in some cases where, for instance, exploration of the abdomen is considered prohibitively risky. When hemodynamics and respiratory function are severely impaired by increased abdominal pressure, then opening the abdomen and closing it with a prosthesis or leaving it packed open may be the best alternative.

Cardiogenic Hypoperfusion and Cardiogenic Shock

To cause cardiogenic shock, or hypotension, on a cardiac basis, cardiac function must be severely disrupted (cardiac index < 2.2 L/min/m^2) from etiologies such as those listed in Table 6-16. Hypoperfusion of this magnitude, especially when it is secondary to myocardial infarction, is associated with a high mortality rate. Cardiogenic shock is a clinical entity distinct from CHF. In CHF, arterial blood pressure is characteristically well maintained or increases. This characteristic distinguishes cardiogenic shock (the term applied to significant reductions in systolic pressure) from CHF.

In general, the diseases listed in Table 6-16 are not subtle and do not cause gradual alterations in cardiac

Table 6-16. Etiologies of Cardiogenic Shock

Acute ischemia
  Ventricular wall infarct
  Papillary muscle infarct
  Ventricular septal defect
Acute valvular disease; mitral, tricuspid, or aortic regurgitation
Arrhythmias
  Rapid supraventricular
  Bradycardia
  Ventricular tachycardia
Miscellaneous
  End-stage cardiomyopathy
  Severe myocardial contusion
  Severe myocarditis
  Severe left ventricular outflow obstruction
  Severe left ventricular inflow obstruction

function. Hypotension is more often a disease of hypovolemia than a disease of severe impairment of cardiac function. When a clinician decides not to administer fluid to a hypotensive patient, he or she is actually making a diagnosis of cardiogenic shock. Cardiogenic shock is the only major circulatory deficit that can be worsened by the administration of fluid. Because cardiogenic shock is secondary to severe, usually obvious, cardiac disease, the clinician should be able to document the occurrence of a marked insult to cardiac function. Without such documentation and the associated recognition of a disease that requires aggressive monitoring and management in a critical care setting, the clinician should consider the hypotensive patient to be hypovolemic and not in cardiogenic shock.

Physical Examination

Physical examination shows hypotension, tachycardia, tachypnea, peripheral vasoconstriction, distended neck veins, agitation, and confusion. An S_3 gallop may be apparent, and when valvular dysfunction is present, associated murmurs may be auscultated.

Laboratory Aids

Cardiogenic shock is associated with chest x-ray evidence of pulmonary edema, metabolic acidosis (lactic acidosis), increased CVP and PAOP, and increased BUN and creatinine. A cardiogram often shows evidence of acute ischemia, infarct, or arrhythmias. An echocardiogram can provide information about ventricular wall motion and valve function. The cardiac index is low (< 2.2 L/min/m^2), and both systemic and pulmonary vascular resistance are high.

Treatment

As always, treatment is based on the etiology. Arrhythmias are usually the most readily treated etiology of severe cardiac impairment. Arrhythmias are diagnosed and treated as described in textbooks that cover advanced cardiac life support. When the etiology is not an arrhythmia, the same sequence of interventions used to increase cardiac output in CHF may be used for cardiogenic shock (Tables 6-17 and 6-18). However, hypotension (often < 90 mm Hg systolic) makes the use of vasodilators alone less attractive. Therefore, a combination of **inotropic drug support** and vasodilation is frequently used. Mechanical support of the heart with an intraaortic balloon pump (IABP) increases cardiac output while reducing preload and afterload. IABP may be more successful than high-dose dobutamine in supporting patients during severe cardiac impairment. IABP may be adequate to support a patient until cardiac function improves, or may be required until surgery (e.g., replacement of the aortic valve, coronary revascularization) is performed. Complications of IABP are listed in Table 6-19.

Endpoints for Resuscitation of the Circulation

Endpoints for resuscitation of the circulation depend on such variables as the primary etiology of the circulatory deficit, the underlying state of the patient's circulation, and the magnitude of cellular and organ malfunction recognized during the hypoperfusion insult. However, for most clinical conditions, bedside recognition of normal circulation is adequate for assessing the outcome of resuscitation. Such variables as normal (the designation of normal depends on knowledge of the patient's premorbid blood pressure) or increasing blood pressure, pulse rate of less than 100/min, normal or improved mental status, urine output greater than 0.5 mL/kg/hr,

Table 6-17. Treatment of Cardiogenic Shock

Reversal of underlying disease
  Coronary artery bypass
  Valve replacement
  Rx myopathy
  Repair ventricular septal defect
Reduce preload
  Decrease water intake
  Diuretics
  Venous dilation
    Nitroglycerin
    Calcium channel blockers
    Narcotics
Reduce afterload
  Nitroprusside
  Antihypertensives
  Diuretics
  Narcotics
Increase contractility
  Intravenous inotropes
Increase arterial oxygen
  Supplemental O_2
  Mechanical ventilation

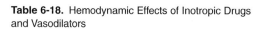

Table 6-18. Hemodynamic Effects of Inotropic Drugs and Vasodilators

	Hemodynamic Parameters			
	Heart Rate	Contractility	Preload	Afterload
Dopamine	↑↑	↑	↑	↑ or NC
Dobutamine	↑	↑↑	↓	NC or ↓
Isoproterenol	↑↑	↑↑	↓	↓
Nitroprusside	±	NC	↓	↓↓
Nitroglycerin	±	NC	↓↓	↓

NC, no change.

Table 6-19. Complications of the Intraaortic Balloon Pump

Injury to femoral vessels
Ischemic extremity
Hemolysis or thrombocytopenia
Infection

warm extremities, and resolution of metabolic acidosis usually suffice.

However, patients who have had a severe cellular insult may require more complicated hemodynamic monitoring and adjustment of the circulation. Certainly, patients who are in cardiogenic shock require precise hemodynamic monitoring (i.e., pulmonary artery catheterization, echocardiogram, cardiac catheterization) to make the proper diagnosis and adjust therapy. In such cases, return of the cardiac index from low (< 2.2 L/min/m²) to normal (2.5–3.5 L/min/m²), along with normal amounts of oxygen delivery (400 mL/min/m²) and consumption (130 mL/min/m²), may allow cellular and organ function to recover. A normal cardiac index may also be adequate in patients with underlying heart disease who have a further reduction in cardiac function from noncardiac causes and then undergo resuscitation of their circulation close to baseline. Unfortunately, despite the achievement of normal cardiac index and oxygen parameters, patients with or without severe acute or chronic heart disease commonly continue to have cellular malfunction that progresses to organ failure and death after a severe hypoperfusion insult.

The recognition that normal circulation, oxygen delivery, and oxygen consumption may be inadequate for cellular and organ recovery after severe hypoperfusion was inferred from epidemiologic data that associated an increase in these parameters (cardiac index > 4.5 L/min/m²; oxygen delivery > 600 mL/min/m²; oxygen consumption > 170 mL/min/m²) with eventual survival. In patients who achieve these endpoints, metabolic acidosis usually resolves. This situation also portends a favorable outcome. Therefore, several investigators champion the use of fluids, inotropes, and sometimes vasodilators to push for these hemodynamic endpoints in every critically ill patient. The results of such management remain controversial, with some studies supporting these endeavors and others finding an increase in mortality rates.

Severe Inflammatory States

Inflammation is a normal response to tissue injury, and it is necessary for tissue repair and wound healing. However, although localized inflammation in response to an insult is usually beneficial, severe tissue injury from a variety of causes (Table 6-20) can result in inflammation distant from the original disease (sys-

temic inflammation). This inflammation may cause cellular malfunction and death in remote organs. In the **systemic inflammatory response syndrome (SIRS)**, many disease states cause systemic inflammation, probably as a result of the activation of cellular mediators of inflammation at remote sites.

To meet the definition of SIRS, a patient must have two or more of the following conditions: (1) temperature greater than 38.5° C or less than 36° C; (2) heart rate greater than 90 beats/min; (3) respiratory rate greater than 20 breaths/min or $Paco_2$ less than 32 torr; and (4) total leukocyte count greater than 12,000 cells/mm, less than 4000 cells/mm³, or greater than 10% immature forms. Many patients with systemic inflammation, but without evidence of significant cellular and organ malfunction (i.e., not in shock) may meet the definition of SIRS. The SIRS variables of hypothermia (< 36° C) and leukopenia (< 4000 cells/mm³) are associated with more severe inflammation, as are systolic hypotension and evidence of organ malfunction (e.g., elevated BUN and creatinine, oliguria, altered mental status, decreased arterial oxygenation, increased bilirubin, decreased platelets). These patients are in shock, even if infection is not present and the term sepsis cannot strictly be applied. Therefore, the traditional concept of septic shock is too narrow. Patients with severe systemic inflammation are in shock. When infection is the cause of severe systemic inflammation, then septic shock can be considered the diagnosis.

Effects of Severe Inflammation on the Circulation

Severe systemic inflammation is associated with alterations in both total body and regional perfusion. Mechanisms that reduce cardiac output during systemic inflammation are listed in Table 6-21.

The most common etiology of inadequate cardiac output during inflammation is decreased venous return, which results from both loss of intravascular fluid and vasodilation. Intravascular volume decreases as plasma exudes into the primary focus of inflammation (area of

Table 6-20. Etiologies of Systemic Inflammation (Partial List)

Infection (meets definition of sepsis)

Trauma

Burns

Ischemia or reperfusion: regional or total body

Pancreatitis

Drug reactions

Hemolytic transfusion reactions

Table 6-21. Circulatory Disorders in Severe Inflammation: Reduced Cardiac Output

Hypovolemia
    Peripheral vasodilation
    Increased capillary permeability, local or total body
    Intracellular migration of fluid
    Sequestration in gastrointestinal tract lumen
Myocardial depression
Increased pulmonary vascular resistance
    Hypoxia
    Platelet emboli
    Thromboxane release
    Serotonin release
    White blood cell aggregation
Deficits in the microcirculation
    Gastrointestinal tract
    Renal

injury or infection). When systemic inflammation develops in response to the primary focus of inflammation, plasma may also exude into some or all of the other tissues. Such exudation causes an increase in interstitial fluid, which becomes protein-rich compared with normal. In general, interstitial fluid is maintained in the extracellular space by active cellular processes that maintain cell membrane integrity and perform such functions as sodium-potassium exchange, which keeps potassium in the cell and sodium out of the cell. Severe inflammation may interfere with active cell membrane function, decrease ion-exchange capabilities, and allow more interstitial water and solutes to enter cells. Depletion of interstitial fluid is another mechanism that aggravates plasma volume loss.

Ileus is common during severe inflammation, regardless of the location of the primary focus. Ileus can cause fluid to accumulate in the lumen of the gastrointestinal tract, which can be as voluminous as that sequestered during bowel obstruction.

Collectively, the exudation of plasma volume into inflammatory foci, the accumulation of fluid in the gastrointestinal tract, and the migration of fluid into cells is known as the third space, to distinguish it from normal plasma and interstitial fluid spaces. The magnitude of the third space effect is roughly proportional to the magnitude of tissue injury or infection that is present. The primary effect of **third-space fluid accumulation** is to deplete intravascular volume and impair venous return.

Vasodilation of the systemic veins and arterioles is characteristic of severe inflammation, and several inflammatory mediators are implicated as causative (e.g., histamine, kinins, prostacyclin, nitric oxide). Increasing the capacitance of veins decreases MSP and may decrease venous return, especially if CVP (discussed previously and in the section on venous return) does not decrease proportionally because of increased pulmonary vascular resistance.

Severe inflammation may directly depress the function of previously normal myocardial cells. Less severe inflammation may result in augmented malfunction of previously abnormal cardiac tissue. Therefore, cardiac output may be impaired and result in a physiology that is consistent with an excess, rather than a deficit, of intravascular volume (i.e., CHF, cardiogenic shock physiology). Recognition of such **cardiogenic states** of hypoperfusion during inflammation is important for proper therapeutic intervention (see later).

Severe inflammation is associated with increased pulmonary vascular resistance. This increase in right ventricular afterload may cause dilation of the right ventricle, decreased right ventricular ejection, and impaired filling of the left ventricle. Right atrial pressure may increase and impair venous return.

In addition to the recognized effects on cardiac function and cardiac output, which can reduce total body perfusion, severe inflammation may cause deficits in the microcirculation, which in turn can result in regional ischemia to organs or within organs. This ischemia will accentuate cell and organ injury. The gastrointestinal tract and kidneys appear to be particularly prone to such alterations.

Effects of Severe Inflammation on Cellular Function

Severe inflammation can result in alterations of cellular metabolism that are independent of inflammation-induced reductions in oxygen delivery, but similar to abnormalities recognized with hypoperfusion. In fact, the neuroendocrine response to severe inflammation is similar to that described for severe hypoperfusion, and can result in such common alterations as elevated levels of blood glucose and lactic acid. However, the elevation in lactic acid level that is associated with severe inflammation is not necessarily secondary to cellular anaerobic metabolism. Increased lactic acid production can also develop secondary to alterations in glucose metabolism that are associated with increased pyruvate production or decreased pyruvate metabolism without mitochondrial malfunction (i.e., aerobic glycolysis). Therefore, an elevated lactic acid level does not necessarily support the conclusion that a patient has inadequate oxygen delivery. In addition, the same cell-depolarizing molecule that appears in the circulation after hypovolemic hypoperfusion is present after inflammatory insults. Further, a decrease in serum ionized calcium is common in both hypoperfusion and inflammatory states. This decrease, shown experimentally to be associated with increased intracellular calcium, is also likely a marker for cell membrane malfunction.

Diagnosis and Management of Severe Inflammation

The clinical manifestations of severe systemic inflammation (Table 6-22) are as potentially varied as the many organs that may manifest malfunction. Most patients have hemodynamic alterations, but sometimes abnormal lung, central nervous system, hematologic, or other organ function is the primary evidence of inflammation, rather than hemodynamic changes. Therefore, a high index of suspicion of the patient at risk, aug-

Table 6-22. Common Clinical Manifestations of Severe Inflammation

Vital signs
  Temperature elevation, hypothermia
  Tachycardia
  Tachypnea
  Hypotension with warm or cold extremities
Change in mental status
Respiratory insufficiency
Ileus
Oliguria, increased urine protein
Elevated hemoglobin, thrombocytopenia, leukocytosis, leukopenia
Increased serum glucose, decreased ionized calcium

mented by evidence gathered during physical examination and with selected laboratory tests, supports the diagnosis of significant inflammation.

The Patient at Risk

The first category of risk is a patient who recently acquired a disease (e.g., severe pancreatitis) or had an injury (e.g., unstable pelvic fracture with ruptured spleen) that is characterized by severe inflammation. The second category of risk is a patient who has an underlying condition (e.g., immunosuppression after liver transplantation) or who recently underwent a procedure (e.g., elective colon resection for carcinoma) that makes systemic inflammation, particularly from infection, more likely. Any patient who has had a significant episode of hypoperfusion (e.g., cardiogenic shock after an acute myocardial infarction, upper gastrointestinal hemorrhage sufficient to result in hypotension) is also at risk for systemic inflammation, either at the time of the hypoperfusion or days later.

Physical Examination
Outward Manifestations

The patient is usually restless and may have alterations in mental status ranging from delirium to coma. In fact, mental status changes may precede obvious hemodynamic or respiratory findings. These alterations sometimes lead the clinician to a misdirected evaluation (i.e., computed tomography of the brain). Such alterations in central nervous system function are rarely focal and are most consistent with a metabolic encephalopathy.

If intravascular volume is decreased, the skin is cool and possibly mottled, with vasoconstriction most often evident in both the upper and lower extremities. Capillary refill time is also decreased.

Vital Signs

Usually, severe systemic inflammation is seen as a decrease in blood pressure, an increase in heart rate, an increase in respiratory rate, and elevated temperature. Patients who have underlying cardiac disease may have hemodynamics that are more consistent with congestive heart failure (i.e., elevated blood pressure, tachycardia). Hypothermia may be present in the most severe cases.

Lung Examination

At lung examination, the lungs may be clear, even when acute respiratory distress syndrome (ARDS) is present. However, rales, rhonchi, and bronchospasm may be found. Examination findings consistent with consolidation (e.g., tubular or tubulovesicular breath sounds, egophony) may assist in locating an inflammatory process, but they are clearly not specific to systemic inflammation. The lung examination is not sufficiently specific to permit a diagnosis of systemic inflammation or other etiology of diffuse pulmonary malfunction.

Cardiovascular Examination

Hypotension and tachycardia are usually present, along with crisp heart tones. After intravascular volume is restored, the extremities are warm, demonstrating good capillary refill. Hypotension with warm hands and feet usually represents the response to inflammation, although anaphylaxis and a high spinal cord injury can produce similar findings. Jugular venous pressure is low by clinical examination.

As a result of plasma exudation and the other causes of plasma volume loss, the patient usually is sequestering fluid. This sequestration can be sudden or, if the patient has been monitored in a hospital setting, the positive fluid balance and an increase in weight may have been documented for several days before acute deterioration is noted.

Myocardial depression from inflammation might cause elevated jugular venous pressure, hypertension, and an S_3 gallop. Myocardial depression that is severe enough to result in hypotension and a clinical picture identical to cardiogenic shock is possible. However, such myocardial malfunction is much less common than are circulatory deficiencies secondary to hypovolemia. The clinician must be careful to distinguish the fluid sequestration and positive fluid balance associated with severe inflammation (which is universal) from the same phenomena seen with cardiogenic states. Treating hypovolemia with fluid restriction and diuretics causes further circulatory embarrassment.

Fluid administration is directed at restoring and maintaining the plasma and blood volume that is threatened by the fluid sequestration associated with severe inflammation. Thus, the primary reason for fluid administration is to support the circulation. Often the circulation is assessed with urine output. Decreased urine output secondary to severe inflammation is most often caused by inadequate cardiac output. Therefore, it is a marker of inadequate circulation.

Laboratory Studies
Hematologic Studies

An increase in total white blood cell count, particularly young PMNs, is most common. Leukopenia denotes more severe disease and consists mostly of immature PMNs. The platelet count usually falls, and evidence of consumption of coagulation proteins, with breakdown of fibrinogen (increased prothrombin time, increased partial thromboplastin time, and increased fibrin split products or D-dimer), denotes more severe disease. Hemoglobin may increase as plasma exudes into inflammatory sites. This increase indicates hemoconcentration, and may be a useful tool in assessing intravascular volume resuscitation because plasma volume is likely to be inadequate until the hemoglobin returns to the patient's baseline value.

Lung Studies

A decrease in arterial P_{O_2} and P_{CO_2} is characteristic of severe systemic inflammation as well as many other lung disease states. The increase in physiologic shunt, which results in a decrease in arterial P_{O_2}, is associated with stimuli that increase minute ventilation and decrease arterial P_{CO_2}. A chest x-ray may be clear or may demonstrate loss of lung volume as well as evidence of pulmonary fluid accumulation, most often from a noncardiogenic pathophysiology (i.e., ARDS). The clinician should recognize that respiratory signs and symptoms and laboratory data during severe inflammation (shortness of breath, tachypnea, crackles, wheezing, decreased arterial P_{O_2}, chest x-ray showing increased lung water) may be indistinguishable from those seen with CHF. In addition, he or she should recognize the dangers of misdiagnosing the effects of severe lung inflammation as CHF.

Urine Studies

Oliguria is common during severe inflammation, and is most often secondary to low intravascular volume and inadequate circulation. It causes laboratory test results that are consistent with a prerenal state (e.g., elevated urine specific gravity, low urine sodium, increased urine osmolality, elevated BUN:creatinine ratio).

Serum Chemistries

An elevated blood glucose level is common during inflammation from such alterations as increased gluconeogenesis, glycogen lysis, and relative insulin resistance.

For many years, decreased total serum calcium has been recognized as associated with one particular severe inflammatory disease, pancreatitis. The amount of decrease correlates with the severity of disease. Ionized calcium is the calcium that is not bound to albumin. Therefore, it is not affected by albumin concentrations, which can change significantly during critical illness. Ionized calcium is also better correlated with parathyroid hormone release compared with total calcium.

Ionized calcium decreases with any disease that causes either severe hypoperfusion or inflammation. This decrease is not secondary to inadequate parathormone secretion. Several recent studies showed an increase in intracellular calcium during or after hypoperfusion or inflammatory states. In addition, the magnitude of the decrease correlates with the severity of disease. Although it is not specific for inflammation, ongoing severe inflammation must be considered in any patient who has decreased ionized calcium. In contrast, a normal ionized calcium level is unusual during severe inflammation or hypoperfusion. Therefore, a normal value suggests that a severe acute systemic insult is not present.

The combination of electrolyte or arterial blood gas levels that are consistent with metabolic acidosis and an elevated lactic acid level is often seen in severe inflammation. An elevated lactic acid level may develop secondary to anaerobic metabolism, suggesting hypoperfusion as the cause. However, an elevated lactic acid level can also result from metabolic alterations associated with inflammation in the presence of normal oxygen concentrations. Therefore, like ionized calcium, these abnormalities do not distinguish severe inflammation from a decrease in either regional or global perfusion. Persistent metabolic acidosis could mean that either disease is present and should prompt further diagnostic and, possibly, therapeutic efforts.

Treatment

Treating the Underlying Cause

Once severe inflammation is recognized, the first principle of treatment is to determine the underlying cause and initiate appropriate therapy (Table 6-23). Infection and infection-like processes (i.e., infusion of endotoxin) are the most commonly considered etiologies of severe inflammation. However, reactions to drugs or transfusions and tissue injury without infection (i.e., early severe pancreatitis) can also cause severe systemic inflammation that is indistinguishable from that seen with the invasion of microorganisms.

While the search for the primary disease is underway and therapy is initiated, vital organ function must be supported until the primary process is under control. Unfortunately, systemic inflammation may continue despite adequate resolution of the initiating insult. In some patients, inflammation appears to become self-sustaining, as though a positive feedback system developed in one or more of the organs with systemic inflammation. For instance, ARDS initiated by an inflammatory process in the abdomen causes inflammatory cells to accumulate in the lungs. The inflammation caused by these pulmonary cells usually, but not always, subsides when the underlying illness is effectively treated. Sometimes the lung inflammation becomes chronic despite resolution of the first inflammatory focus.

As discussed later, novel therapies that focus on interrupting various steps in the inflammatory process are being studied to determine whether they can ameliorate the adverse effects of severe inflammation and improve clinical outcome. In addition, therapies designed to enhance immunologic function may prevent subsequent inflammatory insults from infection or microbiologic by-products.

Supporting Organ Function: Cardiovascular and Pulmonary

Support of the circulation usually starts with treatment of hypovolemia. The result is usually an increase

Table 6-23. Treatment of Severe Inflammation

Control etiology
  Drug or transfusion reaction
  Tissue injury
  Infection
Support organ function
Antagonize inflammatory and metabolic mediators

in cardiac output such that hypotension is alleviated, if not completely reversed. The temperature of the extremities also changes from cool to warm. For most patients, the combination of restoration of intravascular volume, peripheral vasodilation, and the neurohumoral response to inflammation produces a hyperdynamic (cardiac index > normal) circulatory state. Urine output and mental status usually improve. Unfortunately, pulmonary function does not characteristically improve dramatically with treatment of hypovolemia alone. Ionized calcium alterations and metabolic acidosis may or may not improve as a result of simple improvement in the circulation.

Red blood cell transfusion is reserved for patients who have ongoing hemorrhage or hemoglobin levels of less than 10 g/100 mL and who have abnormalities that are consistent with inadequate oxygen delivery. For patients with hemoglobin levels of more than 10 g/100 mL, simply increasing hemoglobin does not appear to significantly improve oxygen consumption.

Dopamine, usually in low, or "renal," concentrations, is commonly administered during severe inflammation. Because dopamine, even at these low doses, tends to increase left ventricular end-diastolic pressure as cardiac output increases, this drug has a physiologic effect that is similar to fluid infusion, and is most useful when hypovolemia is the primary abnormality.

The diagnosis and treatment of a cardiogenic state usually requires more complicated monitoring than simply recording blood pressure, pulse, skin color, mental status, urine output, and electrolyte concentrations. Insertion of a pulmonary artery catheter (PAC) allows more precise measurement of cardiac filling pressures and the response to inotropic and vasodilator manipulations.

The primary advantage of PAC insertion is the ability to acquire hemodynamic data to assist in hemodynamic diagnostic and therapeutic decision-making. Given the evidence that achieving excellent circulation is associated with improved outcome in patients who have severe hypoperfusion or inflammation, using technologic devices (which might include echocardiography) to evaluate the circulation and possibly avoid continuing hypoperfusion clearly appears beneficial. This argument is not supported by data accrued during routine use of PACs, however, because critical assessment of the circulation is not likely to be crucial for any common illness or surgical intervention (e.g., major vascular surgery). Likewise, it may be difficult to discern a survival advantage to using such equipment in large groups of patients in the intensive care unit. However, an individual patient may achieve a distinct advantage, especially when a therapeutic intervention that reverses hypoperfusion is documented.

The disadvantages of PAC insertion include complications related to central venous access (e.g., pneumothorax, central venous thrombosis) as well as those associated with the cardiac location (e.g., ventricular arrhythmias, damage to the tricuspid or pulmonic valves, rupture of the pulmonary artery). Ventricular arrhythmias are usually not sustained, and anatomic injuries are rare. Despite the relatively low risk, PAC insertion should be used when the potential advantage, as described earlier, is considered worth the risk.

During severe inflammation, myocardial depression may be a manifestation of decreased function of the myocardial catecholamine receptors. Phosphodiesterase inhibitor drugs (e.g., amrinone), which do not require this receptor function for action, may be particularly useful inotropic agents during severe inflammation.

In a patient who is hyperdynamic, has elevated cardiac output, and has low systemic resistance states, the use of an alpha agent (e.g., norepinephrine, neosynephrine) may be indicated, especially when certain vessels with fixed stenoses (e.g., atherosclerotic plaques in renal, carotid, or coronary arteries) are likely to require higher mean arterial pressure for adequate perfusion. Under these circumstances, the use of such vasoconstrictors (with simultaneous documentation of no significant reduction in cardiac output) may increase mean arterial pressure and provide evidence of better organ perfusion (e.g., increased urine output).

Endpoints for resuscitation of the circulation during severe inflammation are as controversial as those described in the hypoperfusion section. Because severe inflammation commonly increases cardiac index, one indicator that inflammation is resolving may be a decrease in cardiac index (e.g., from 5.0 to 3.5 L/min/m²) and an increase in systemic resistance (e.g., from 350 to 900 dynes-sec/cm⁵).

Support of pulmonary function often requires mechanical ventilation and various associated techniques of ventilator management. Such management is sufficient when arterial oxygen saturation is greater than 90%.

Achieving a Balance in the Effects of Inflammation

Much experimental and clinical research has evaluated the antagonism of inflammatory and metabolic mediators in severe inflammatory states (Table 6-24). Many studies show promise, but none has become standard therapy.

As previously stated, inflammation has beneficial effects (e.g., wound healing, defense against invasive organisms) that are important for survival during critical illness. Therefore, a successful outcome depends significantly on a balance between the beneficial and the detrimental effects of inflammation. Therapy that aggressively suppresses inflammation (i.e., pharmacologic doses of anti-inflammatory steroids) may provide short-term benefits (e.g., improvement in hemodynamic and pulmonary function), but the loss of the beneficial effects of inflammation may result in death secondary to recurrent infection or wound breakdown.

For all of the therapies listed in Table 6-24, this balance must be considered. The benefits of inflammation are primarily local (i.e., at the focus of tissue injury or infection). The detrimental effects are primarily systemic (e.g., alterations in circulation or pulmonary function). Therapies that allow local inflammation to continue while the systemic inflammation is suppressed may allow the proper inflammatory balance.

In general, these therapies are most helpful in patients who appear to have severe systemic inflammation despite usually adequate therapy for the underlying illness. For instance, consider a 65-year-old previously healthy woman who has perforated diverticulitis and undergoes a sigmoid resection with end-sigmoid colostomy. Ordinarily, fluid resuscitation, surgery, and antibiotics are sufficient to reverse the detrimental effects of this severe inflammatory illness and support the proper balance between the beneficial and detrimental effects of inflammation. However, if organ malfunction (e.g., ARDS, hyperdynamic circulation, impaired renal function) consistent with ongoing severe inflammation is still present 3 to 4 days later, then one possible explanation is that the inflammation stimulated in other organs by the perforated diverticulitis is responsible for the lack of resolution, despite therapy that is often sufficient. In other words, the detrimental and beneficial effects of severe inflammation are out of balance. Under such circumstances, therapy directed at the systemic inflammation may be warranted.

A Practical Guide to the Patient in Shock

Once a patient is recognized to be in shock, the guiding principles are to: (1) provide an excellent circulation and (2) treat severe inflammation.

Recognize the Patient in Shock

Clearly, the first step in the evaluation and management of the patient who is in shock is to recognize that a deficit in total body cellular function is present. The history is the first clue to the patient who is at risk (Table 6-25). Next, bedside examination can provide clues, but severe hypotension and marked tachycardia may not always accompany other evidence of shock (Table 6-26). Next come common laboratory data, which are frequently abnormal during shock (Table 6-27).

Provide an Excellent Circulation

An accurate diagnosis of the state of the circulation is critical (see the section on hypoperfusion states).

The patient who is in cardiogenic shock requires aggressive hemodynamic monitoring as well as

Table 6-24. Antagonism of Inflammatory and Metabolic Mediators

Interference with effects of endotoxin
  Clear endotoxin from the circulation
    Antiendotoxin antibody
    Bind toxin to membrane
    Filter toxin out
    Interfere with binding of endotoxin to effector cells (i.e., bactericidal
      or permeability-increasing protein)
Interference with the activation of proinflammatory cytokines
  Steroids
  Nonsteroidal anti-inflammatory agents
  Inhibition of IL-1–converting enzyme
Interference with the activity of increased pro-inflammatory cytokines
  Anti-TNF, anti-IL-1 antibodies
  Binding of TNF and IL-1 with excess receptors
  Blocking of effector cell receptors (i.e., administration of IL-1
    receptor antagonist)
  Continuous blood filtration
Administration of anti-inflammatory cytokines
Interference with superoxide activity
  Decrease production
  Increase scavenging
Interference with secondary mediators
  Cyclooxygenase system
  Nitric oxide system
  Complement
  Histamine, serotonin, kinin system
  Coagulation system
Interference with inflammatory cell activation by blocking activation
  receptors (i.e., inhibition of leukocyte integrin and selectin)

IL, interleukin. TNF, tumor necrosis factor.

Table 6-25. Characteristics of the Patient Who Is at Risk for Shock

Trauma or burn
Vascular catastrophe
Acute cardiac disease
Acute abdominal disease
Severe extraabdominal infection
Drug exposure

Table 6-26. Bedside Examination Indicators of Shock

Hypotension
Tachycardia
Tachypnea
Hyperthermia or hypothermia
Peripheral vasoconstriction and cool extremities
Hypotension with warm extremities
Agitation and altered mental status
Oliguria

Table 6-27. Common Laboratory Abnormalities With Shock

Metabolic acidosis
Elevated blood urea nitrogen and creatinine
Leukocytosis or leukopenia
Elevated blood glucose
Decreased platelet count
Decreased ionized calcium

pharmacologic and possibly mechanical assistance of the circulation (see earlier sections). This level of care clearly requires a critical care environment and physician expertise. The decision may be made to perform emergency cardiac catheterization or cardiac surgery.

The hypotensive supine adult who does not have a cardiogenic process most often has lost at least 30% of intravascular volume (approximately 1500 mL in a 70-kg person). Replacement with crystalloid requires a 3:1 ratio as the crystalloid distributes throughout the extracellular space. Therefore, 4500 mL crystalloid solution is required to begin plasma volume restitution in this patient. Because there is no organ in the body that is improved by hypoperfusion, and because prolonged hypoperfusion induces or aggravates tissue inflammation, restitution of an adequate circulation should be accomplished rapidly (within minutes, if possible, with two large-bore intravenous lines wide open).

When decreased venous return (most often as a result of hypovolemia) is the cause of hypoperfusion, a diagnostic evaluation of the etiology of impaired venous return must occur simultaneously with restoration of the circulation. Venous return can improve with fluid infusion, regardless of the underlying etiology of the decrease (e.g., hypovolemia vs pericardial tamponade).

As described in previous sections, the circulatory parameters that indicate an excellent circulation may vary from patient to patient, but general bedside guidelines are listed in Table 6-28. More sophisticated indicators of an excellent circulation have been proposed, and may be of particular value when evidence of organ malfunction is present, despite bedside indicators that the circulation is adequate (i.e., BUN and creatinine levels are increasing when the blood pressure and pulse are normal; Table 6-29).

Table 6-28. Bedside Indicators of an Excellent Circulation

Normal blood pressure and pulse for the individual
Normal mental status
Warm extremities
Urine output ≥ 0.5 mL/kg/hr
Resolution of metabolic acidosis

Table 6-29. Monitors of Circulation Status

Cardiac index	> 4.5 L/min/m²
Mixed venous O₂ saturation	≥ 75%
Oxygen delivery	> 600 mL/min/m²
Oxygen consumption	> 170 mL/min/m²
Gastric mucosal pH (tonometer measurement)	> 7.35
Right ventricular end diastolic volume index	> 100 mL/m²

Ideal values indicate a good prognosis.

Treat Severe Inflammation

Treating severe inflammation requires recognition that an inflammatory disease is present (see discussion of severe inflammatory states). Next, the focus of severe inflammation must be localized and treated (e.g., antibiotics for pneumonia, colon resection for perforated diverticulitis). Usually, these interventions suffice. Occasionally, the other methods described in the section on severe inflammatory states are used to diminish the effects of severe inflammation.

Hypoperfusion can cause inflammation or aggravate established inflammation. Therefore, providing an excellent circulation is as much a treatment of inflammation as is the use of antibiotics or surgery. As a corollary, because inflammation can induce both total body and regional hypoperfusion, treating inflammation improves the circulation.

Conclusion

Total body cellular malfunction (i.e., shock) can result from various insults that may be broadly categorized as severe hypoperfusion or severe inflammatory disturbances. Almost invariably, hypoperfusion and inflammation coexist in patients who have shock. Restoring an excellent circulation and treating severe inflammation are the keys to preserving cellular and organ function and preventing death from shock.

Multiple-Choice Questions

1. The most common cause of severe hypovolemic hypoperfusion is:
   A. Peritonitis
   B. Burns
   C. Hemorrhage
   D. Sepsis
   E. Spinal cord injury

2. The major component of a decrease in cardiac output in hypovolemia is:
   A. Increased systemic vascular resistance
   B. Decreased venous return
   C. Myocardial ischemia
   D. Increased pulmonary vascular resistance
   E. Low hemoglobin

3. In a 70-kg man who has a 20% loss of intravascular volume, the volume of isotonic electrolyte solution required to return the vascular volume to normal is:
   A. 500 mL
   B. 1500 mL
   C. 3000 mL
   D. 4500 mL
   E. 6000 mL

4. A 45-year-old man is admitted to the hospital with hematemesis. His blood pressure is 90/60 mm Hg,

his pulse rate is 120/min, and he is diaphoretic and restless. The best therapy for his restlessness is:
A. Intravenous diazepam
B. Rapid intravenous fluid administration
C. Intramuscular chlordiazepoxide (Librium) administration
D. Nasal oxygen
E. Restraints

5. The most practical, objective bedside monitor of the adequacy of volume resuscitation in states of severe hypovolemic hypoperfusion is determination of:
A. Serial lactate levels
B. Mental status
C. Urinary output
D. Blood pressure
E. Arterial blood gases

6. As severe inflammation progresses to cardiogenic hypoperfusion:
A. Cardiac output increases
B. Pulmonary artery occlusion pressure decreases
C. Arterial lactate level decreases
D. Oxygen delivery decreases
E. Respiratory rate decreases

7. The first therapeutic measure to improve blood pressure and cardiac output in severe inflammation is:
A. Dopamine administration
B. Dobutamine administration
C. Nitroprusside administration
D. Steroid administration
E. Intravenous fluid administration

8. Which of the following hemodynamic variables is within the normal range?
A. Systemic vascular resistance of 2500 dynes-sec/cm^{-5}
B. Cardiac index of 3.3 L/min/m^2
C. Pulmonary artery pressure of 70/50 mm Hg
D. Pulmonary vascular resistance of 480 dynes-sec/cm^{-5}
E. Oxygen consumption of 80 to 100 mL/min

9. Cardiogenic shock is distinguished from severe hypovolemic hypoperfusion by:
A. The depression in cardiac output in hypovolemic states
B. The degree of vasoconstriction
C. Oliguria
D. Mental obtundation
E. Right and left ventricular filling pressure measurements

10. Match the following phrase with the best single response. Acute hemorrhage:
A. Elevated arterial lactate
B. Elevated blood sugar
C. Both
D. Neither

11. Match the following phrase with the best single response. Response to catecholamine elevation:
A. Elevated arterial lactate
B. Elevated blood sugar
C. Both
D. Neither

12. Match the following phrase with the best single response. Necessary to make the diagnosis of severe hypovolemic hypoperfusion:
A. Elevated arterial lactate
B. Elevated blood sugar
C. Both
D. Neither

13. After intravascular volume restitution, the hyperdynamic response to severe inflammation is characterized by:
A. Decreased oxygen consumption
B. Decreased intrapulmonary shunt
C. Increased peripheral vascular resistance
D. Increased cardiac output
E. The universally beneficial application of the vasoactive drugs norepinephrine and epinephrine

14. The hormones that affect hemodynamic parameters the most during severe hypovolemic hypoperfusion are:
A. Epinephrine and norepinephrine
B. Insulin and glucagon
C. Glucocorticoids
D. Mineralocorticoids
E. Antidiuretic hormones

15. The biochemical effects of severe hypovolemic hypoperfusion and severe inflammation are characterized by:
A. Decreased gluconeogenesis
B. Decreased glucocorticoid release
C. Decreased muscle breakdown
D. Increased glycogen stores
E. Elevated blood glucose

16. The normal usage of oxygen at rest is:
A. 250 mL/min
B. 100 mL/min
C. 500 mL/min
D. 2500 mL/min
E. 1500 mL/min

17. The most accurate predictor of oxygen consumption is:
A. Central venous pressure
B. Mixed venous oxygen content
C. Arterial oxygen saturation
D. Arteriovenous oxygen difference
E. Pulmonary capillary wedge pressure

18. Of the following, the most important principle for treating patients who have severe inflammation is to:
    A. Maximize oxygen delivery and consumption
    B. Diagnose and treat the primary disease process
    C. Maintain urine output
    D. Provide anti-inflammatory steroids
    E. Use vasconstricting drugs judiciously

19. Severe inflammation can produce all of the following alterations in the circulation EXCEPT:
    A. Decreased venous return from hypovolemia
    B. Myocardial depression
    C. Microcirculation deficits
    D. Decreased venous return from increased intrathoracic pressure
    E. Increased pulmonary vascular resistance

20. Severe hypoperfusion begets inflammation primarily as a result of:
    A. Ischemia and reperfusion pathophysiology
    B. Translocation of organisms across the gastrointestinal tract
    C. Lactic acid stimulation of inflammatory cells
    D. Activation of the coagulation cascade
    E. Macrophage activation by ischemia

Oral Examination Study Questions

CASE 1

You are the only attending physician in a small community emergency department. Paramedics arrive with a 25-year-old man who, when leaving a tavern, stepped off of the sidewalk and into the path of an oncoming motor vehicle. He is conscious and breathing spontaneously, and has a heavy odor of alcohol on his breath. On arrival, his vital signs are: temperature 97.6° F, pulse 120/min, blood pressure 90/70 mm Hg, and respiratory rate 34 breaths/min. Pulse oximetry of his left ear shows 95% saturation. There are no obvious areas of ecchymosis over the upper abdomen or thorax. He is agitated and combative, and has cool, cyanotic extremities. He has bilateral breath sounds and crisp heart tones. There is no jugular venous distension. How would you assess and manage this patient's circulation?

OBJECTIVE 1

To evaluate the circulation in this patient, the student considers all diagnoses of severe hypoperfusion that are related to trauma: severe hypovolemia from hemorrhage, tension pneumothorax, and pericardial tamponade. Based on the information given, the student hones in on the diagnosis of hemorrhagic hypoperfusion.

OBJECTIVE 2

The student outlines the treatment intervention for a patient with hemorrhagic hypoperfusion.
    A. The student recognizes the need for two large-bore intravenous lines, the need for crystalloid

resuscitation, and the probable need for packed red blood cells.
    B. The student initially estimates the amount of blood loss in this patient, based on hypotension in the average-sized man. The student recognizes that at least 30% of intravascular blood volume was lost.
    C. The student recognizes the need for a bladder catheter to measure urine output and the need for laboratory tests to assess the degree of circulatory deficit and inflammation. Laboratory tests should include: complete blood count with white cell differential; arterial blood gases, especially to measure arterial pH; serum electrolytes, blood urea nitrogen, and creatinine; platelet count; coagulation studies; and blood glucose.

OBJECTIVE 3

After resuscitation begins, the student can describe the methods of evaluating where blood loss has occurred.

The student recommends further examination to evaluate the chest, abdomen, and extremities for evidence of blood loss (e.g., fractures, abdominal tenderness, pelvic instability, displacement of the prostate).

Minimum Level of Achievement for Passing

    A. The student recognizes that hemorrhage is the most likely etiology of the hypoperfusion.
    B. The student knows the minimum requirements for fluid resuscitation in a patient with hemorrhagic shock.
    C. The student recognizes that performing the basic clinical examination will lead to the recognition of suspicious areas for blood loss.

Honors Level of Achievement

    A. The student can describe the possibility of tension pneumothorax or pericardial tamponade in the patient with traumatic injury.
    B. The student can differentiate tension pneumothorax or pericardial tamponade from hemorrhagic shock.
    C. The student can describe how much blood loss may occur in occult sites (e.g., abdomen, pelvis).
    D. The student can describe the appropriate laboratory tests and the expected values, comparing mild with severe circulatory alterations.

CASE 2

You are a surgeon who is called to see a 60-year-old man who arrived in the emergency room with severe abdominal pain, fever, and chills of 4 days' duration. His blood pressure is 60/40 mm Hg, pulse is 130/min, respiratory rate is 30 breaths/min, and temperature is 102° F. He is agitated, his chest is clear, and findings at cardiac examination are unremarkable. He has no jugular venous distension. Abdominal examination shows diffuse abdominal tenderness with diffuse involuntary guarding. Rectal examination is negative. His extremities are cool and vasoconstricted. An electrocardiogram shows a sinus tachycardia.

How would you assess and manage this patient's circulation deficit?

OBJECTIVE 1

The student realizes that the patient requires rapid resuscitation of the circulation. The student also realizes that this patient most likely has severe hypovolemic hypoperfusion, probably from severe inflammation rather than cardiogenic shock. The student recommends:

A. Rapid administration of intravenous fluids. The student can describe the volume of crystalloid required to resuscitate a patient who is hypotensive. For a 70-kg man, it is the volume of crystalloid required to replace approximately 30% of blood volume (1500 mL blood/4500 mL crystalloid).

B. Insertion of nasogastric tube because of an acute abdominal process

C. Insertion of a bladder catheter to monitor resuscitation

D. Blood tests, including complete blood count, electrolytes, blood gases (to assess the degree of acidosis or respiratory complications), and blood cultures

E. No use of inotropes before aggressive fluid resuscitation unless severe shock unresponsive to fluid resuscitation is present

OBJECTIVE 2

The student attempts to make a diagnosis of the cause of shock, including the following steps:

A. Obtain a more detailed history, particularly a gastrointestinal history related to such previous diseases as ulcer disease, biliary tract disease, and diverticulosis.

B. If vital signs improve, obtain x-rays of the chest and abdomen.

OBJECTIVE 3

The student describes further management of the patient once resuscitation is complete, based on the various possible etiologies of severe inflammation from an intraabdominal source.

A. The student describes the various potential etiologies of this degree of inflammation from an abdominal process (i.e., cholangitis, pancreatitis, perforated peptic ulcer, perforated diverticulitis, ischemic bowel).

B. The student describes the processes that require emergency surgery for management: cholangitis, perforated peptic ulcer, perforated diverticulitis, and ischemia.

Minimum Level of Achievement for Passing

A. The student recognizes that the patient requires resuscitation with large volumes of intravenous fluid.

B. The student recognizes that hypoperfusion of this magnitude from an intraabdominal inflammatory process commonly requires surgery.

Honors Level of Achievement

A. The student can describe the various etiologies of severe intraabdominal inflammation

B. The student can describe the systemic inflammatory response syndrome (SIRS) and explain how this patient may fit this clinical entity.

C. The student can describe the fundamental principles of managing the patient with severe SIRS. These principles include achievement of an excellent circulation and eradication of the severe inflammatory process.

ADDITIONAL QUESTIONS

1. What are the most common sites of infection that cause SIRS and inflammation-induced hypoperfusion? The student should consider, most commonly, urinary tract infection, pneumonia, peritonitis, and intraabdominal abscess.

2. What are the etiologies of hypoperfusion from severe inflammation? The student should describe the causes of hypovolemia (vasodilation, exudation of fluid into the area of inflammation as well as into other regions of the body, intracellular fluid migration). In addition, the student should describe the possibility of myocardial depression as well as right-sided heart failure from increased pulmonary vascular resistance.

3. How much fluid is usually required to correct the hypovolemia that is seen with septic shock that is caused by peritonitis? The student should recognize that frequently 5 to 10 L crystalloid solution is required to resuscitate hypovolemic patients who are in septic shock.

4. Why is the central venous pressure (CVP) high in some hypovolemic patients who have septic shock? The student should recognize that increasing pulmonary vascular resistance in patients with sepsis may be of a magnitude that will cause right ventricular dysfunction and elevation of venous pressure.

5. What should be done at the time of surgery for an intraabdominal process that produces septic shock? The student should describe the need to obtain smears and cultures of what appears to be infected fluid in the abdominal cavity and should recognize that correcting the primary underlying disease is indicated (e.g., perform definitive ulcer surgery or sigmoid resection for perforated diverticulitis). The student should also describe irrigation of the abdomen to remove as much contamination as possible.

CASE 3

You are the resident on the surgical intensive care unit. One of your patients is a 65-year-old man with known coronary artery disease. He recently underwent repair of a ruptured abdominal aortic aneurysm. During the operation, the patient's blood pressure fell to 60 mm Hg systolic several times, for a total duration of 30 minutes. Urine output over the 3-hour operation was 45 mL, despite administration of a diuretic and mannitol. The last arterial blood pH obtained in the operating room, 15 minutes before the patient was transferred to the intensive care unit, was 7.3, with Po_2 of 120 mm Hg, Fio_2 of 50%, Pco_2 of 30 mm Hg, and Tco_2 of 20 mm Hg. On arrival in the surgical intensive care unit, his blood pressure was 80/60 mm Hg, pulse was 120 beats/min, respiration rate was 16 breaths/min, and temperature was 96° F. He received narcotic anesthesia and is still unconscious. His neck veins are not visible; he has a central venous catheter in his right internal jugular vein, with marked edema above the clavicles; his chest is clear; his heart sounds are distant; and his carotid, radial, and femoral pulses are palpable at 1+. No pulses are palpated below the femoral arteries. He is severely vasoconstricted.

OBJECTIVE 1

The student realizes that this patient requires rapid evaluation of and resuscitation from the severe hypoperfusion state. The student also realizes that hypovolemic shock is much more likely than cardiogenic shock, but is alert to the second possibility. The student begins evaluation and resuscitation with an algorithm similar to the following one:

A. Obtain an electrocardiogram and compare it with previous cardiograms to evaluate the possibility of a myocardial infarction. If the finding is negative, fluids are administered rapidly.

B. Recognize that CVP monitoring alone will likely be inadequate because it does not provide information about the left side of the heart or the cardiac index. Therefore, insertion of a pulmonary artery catheter is more helpful.

C. Obtain other laboratory studies: hemoglobin, electrolytes, and blood gases.

D. Avoid vasoconstricting drugs, even if clear evidence of cardiac insult is present.

E. If the electrocardiogram shows an acute myocardial infarction, the student realizes that the management principles may be distinctly different if the patient is in cardiogenic shock. The student can describe the hemodynamic parameters that are typical of cardiogenic shock.

OBJECTIVE 2

The student can describe the continuing efforts to treat shock in patients with hypovolemia or cardiogenic shock.

A. If hypovolemic shock is present, the student realizes that the patient has at least a 30% reduction in intravascular volume.

B. The student realizes that hypothermia contributed to the intense vasoconstriction and that, if the patient is hypovolemic, he requires further repletion of vascular volume as the hypothermia is corrected.

C. The student can describe the therapeutic options available for the patient who is in cardiogenic shock:
   1. Inotropic therapy: dobutamine
   2. Vasodilator therapy: nitroglycerin or nitroprusside
   3. Intraaortic balloon pump insertion

D. The student can describe the benefits and deleterious effects of each of the therapies provided for cardiogenic shock.

Minimum Level of Achievement for Passing

The student recognizes that the patient is in a state of severe hypoperfusion, that hypovolemic hypoperfusion is much more likely than cardiogenic shock, and that vasoconstrictors are not used in the initial therapy for either hypovolemic or cardiogenic shock.

Honors Level of Achievement

A. The student demonstrates a clear understanding of the volume of resuscitation needed for the hypotensive, vasoconstricted, hypothermic patient who is in severe hypovolemic hypoperfusion.

B. The student can describe the effects of drugs and the intraaortic balloon pump on myocardial oxygen consumption and the relation of this value to the treatment of cardiogenic shock.

C. The student can discuss the potential etiologies of cardiogenic shock other than myocardial infarction.

D. The student demonstrates knowledge of the normal pressures as measured with central venous pressure or pulmonary capillary wedge pressures.

SUGGESTED READINGS

Baue AE. MOF/MODS, SIRS: an update. *Shock* 1996;6:S1–S5.
Burchard KW, Gann DS, Wiles CE. *The Clinical Handbook for Surgical Critical Care.* New York, NY: Parthenon, 1999.
Califf RM, Bengtson JR. Cardiogenic shock [review]. *N Engl J Med* 1994;330:1724–1730.
Eastridge BJ, Darlington DN, Evans JA, Gann DS. A circulating shock protein depolarizes cells in hemorrhage and sepsis. *Ann Surg* 1994;219:298–305.
Livingston DH, Mosenthal AC, Deitch EA. Sepsis and multiple organ dysfunction syndrome: a clinical-mechanistic overview. *N Horizons* 1995;3:257–266.
Pricolo VE, Demaria EJ, Burchard KW. Venous return: physiology, monitoring, and manipulation. I and II. *Surg Rounds* 1993; Sept:703–707; Oct:775–782.

7 Wounds and Wound Healing

David J. Smith, Jr., M.D.
Kevin C. Chung, M.D.
Martin C. Robson, M.D.

OBJECTIVES

1. Define a wound, and describe the sequence and approximate time frame of the phases of wound healing.
2. Describe the three types of wound healing and the elements of each. Describe the phases of wound healing that are distinct to each type of wound.
3. Describe the essential elements and significance of granulation tissue.
4. Describe the clinical factors that decrease collagen synthesis and retard wound healing.
5. Describe the rationale for the uses of absorbable and nonabsorbable sutures.
6. Discuss the functions of a dressing.
7. Define clean, contaminated, and infected wounds, and describe the management of each type.

A wound, in the broadest sense, is a disruption of normal anatomic relations as a result of an injury. The injury may be intentional (e.g., elective surgical incision) or unintentional (e.g., trauma). Regardless of the cause of injury, the biochemical and physiologic processes of healing are identical, although their time course and intensity may vary. The closure of wounds is classified into three distinct types: (1) primary, (2) secondary, and (3) tertiary, based on the timing of replacement of the epithelium over the wound. Wound healing is also divided by physiologic process into three stages, or phases: (1) **substrate,** (2) **proliferative,** and (3) **remodeling.** These biochemical and physiologic events are correlated with gross morphologic changes in the wound. A knowledge of these events and changes allows the physician to maximize the chances of successful healing and minimize scarring.

Physiology of Wound Healing

Inflammation is the basic physiologic process that is common to all wounds. Clinically, inflammation is iden-

tified by the cardinal signs of redness (rubor), heat (calor), swelling (tumor), pain (dolor), and loss of function. These signs of inflammation are also seen in wound infections, which ultimately may cause wound disruption. They differ only in degree and time course from the primary sequence of events that leads to normal wound healing. The physiology underlying these clinical signs is a complex amalgam of biochemical and cellular events.

Biochemical Aspects

Trauma activates a cascade of chemoattractants and mitogens that recruit phagocytes, fibroblasts, and endothelial cells. These chemoattractants, which include platelet-derived growth factors and complement peptide (C5A), are produced during the clotting of blood by degradation of the surrounding tissue and by cells entering the wound. The first cells that enter the wound are platelets, which come into contact with the damaged **collagen** at the time of injury. The platelets degranulate and release alpha granules that contain multiple growth factors, including platelet-derived growth factor (PDGF) and transforming growth factor-β (TGF-β). These factors influence the subsequent wound healing process by attracting inflammatory cells and fibroblasts into the wound (chemoattractants), stimulating the formation of new blood vessels (angiogenesis), and modulating responses in the surrounding cells (cytokines).

Many types of growth factors have been identified: epidermal growth factors, PDGF, transforming growth factors, and fibroblast growth factors (FGFs). These factors are grouped based on their cellular origins, functions, and structural similarities. At the time of injury, when the platelet plug is in place, several growth factors are released that are chemotactic and mitogenic (promote mitosis) for inflammatory cells. Two such factors are PDGF and TGF-β, which mediate the chemotaxis of neutrophils, monocytes, and macrophages into the wound. PDGF is more important during the period of inflammation: it is responsible for the directed and sequential migration of neutrophils, macrophages, and fibroblasts into the wound over the first several days after injury. PDGF and another growth factor, β-FGF, are also produced by the injured cells. β-FGF binds to heparin in the extracellular matrix, and it is rapidly available to participate in the wound healing process. Arachidonic acid is contained in the walls of the cells. It is released when the cells are injured. The degradation of arachidonic acid into prostanoid derivatives of prostaglandins and thromboxanes causes a number of responses associated with the inflammatory response, including vasodilation, swelling, and pain.

Physiologic Aspects

At the same time that these biochemical events are developing, leukocytes are marginating, sticking to vessel walls, and migrating through the walls toward the site of injury. In addition, venules are dilating, and lymphatics are being blocked. This inflammatory response in the wound occurs for a variable period, depending on local tissue and host factors. Some of these factors are responsive to manipulation by the knowledgeable physician.

Phases of Wound Healing

Understanding the phases of wound healing is important in treating conditions and diseases that affect various stages of the healing cascade (e.g., diabetes mellitus, malnutrition, immunodeficiency). The three phases of wound healing are: (1) substrate, (2) proliferative, and (3) maturation. The second and third phases are relatively constant, regardless of the type of wound healing. These phases begin only when the wound is covered by epithelium.

Substrate Phase

The substrate phase is also known as the inflammatory phase, lag phase, or exudative phase. The main cells involved in this process are polymorphonuclear leukocytes (PMNs) and macrophages. Shortly after a wound occurs, PMNs appear and remain the predominant cell for approximately 48 hours. These leukocytes may be the origin of many inflammatory mediators, including complement and kallikrein. Small numbers of bacteria are handled by the macrophages that are present in the wound. However, large numbers of bacteria cannot be controlled; in the neutropenic state, they lead to a clinical wound infection.

The neutrophil is not crucial for normal wound healing, but the macrophage is. Monocytes enter the wound after the PMNs, reaching maximum numbers approximately 24 hours later. They evolve into macrophages, which are the main cells involved in wound **debridement.** Experimental wounds that are depleted of macrophages and monocytes show marked inhibition of fibroblast migration, proliferation, and loss of collagen production. Macrophages, which can secrete more than 100 different molecules, are an important producer of growth factors. Some of these factors are TGF-β, which stimulates the proliferation of fibroblasts, and interleukin-1 (IL-1), which is partially responsible for regulating the repair of damaged tissue. IL-1 is an important growth factor in the regulation of many processes in the inflammatory response; it may induce fever, promote hemostasis by interacting with endothelial cells, enhance fibroblast proliferation, and activate T-cells.

At the time that clot, debris, and bacteria are being removed, substrates for collagen synthesis are being arranged. In primary wound healing (discussed later), the substrate phase occurs over approximately a 4-day period. The wound is edematous and erythematous. This normal process may be difficult to distinguish from early signs of wound infection. In healing by secondary or tertiary intention (discussed later), this phase continues indefinitely until the wound surface is closed by ectodermal elements (i.e., epithelium for skin, mucosa in the gut).

Proliferative Phase

The second and third phases of wound healing are relatively constant, regardless of the type of wound healing. These phases begin only when the wound is covered by epithelium. The proliferative phase is the second stage of healing. It is characterized by the production of collagen in the wound. The wound appears less edematous and inflamed than before, but the wound scar may be raised, red, and hard. The primary cell in this phase is the cell that produces collagen, the fibroblast.

Collagen is the principal structural protein of the body and is ubiquitous through all of its varied tissues. It has a complex, three-dimensional structure. Collagen synthesis begins with the production of amino acid chains in the cytoplasm of the fibroblast. These α-chains are unique in that each third amino acid is glycine (Gly-x-y). Two amino acids, hydroxyproline and hydroxylysine, are found only in collagen, and require hydroxylation in their synthesis by specific enzymes. Important cofactors involved in the hydroxylation process are ferrous ion, α-ketoglutarate, and ascorbic acid. Insufficient consumption of one of the cofactors can lead to an interruption of the proliferative phase. For example, scurvy is caused by vitamin C deficiency. The absence of ascorbic acid leads to the production of defective, unhydroxylated collagen, which leads to wound breakdown.

Maturation Phase

The third, and final, phase of wound healing is the remodeling, or maturation, phase. It is characterized by the maturation of collagen by intermolecular cross-linking. The wound scar gradually flattens and becomes less prominent and more pale and supple. This phase is a time of great metabolic activity, although there is no net collagen production. The maturation process clinically corresponds to the flattening of the scar. It requires approximately 9 months in the adult. The proliferative and maturation phases of wound healing are divided into categories to describe the predominant physiologic process that occurs at a particular time.

Classification of Healing Wounds

Wounds are often classified as acute or chronic. One way to understand this classification is to consider the concepts of order and time. Orderliness refers to a sequence of biologic events in wound healing: control of infection, resolution of inflammation, angiogenesis, restoration of a functional connective matrix, contraction, resurfacing, differentiation, and remodeling. Timeliness is relative; it is affected by wound severity and the patient's medical condition. Therefore, an acute wound is one in which the reparative processes occur in an orderly and timely fashion, culminating in a sustained restoration of the anatomic and functional integrity of the tissues (Figure 7-1). In contrast, a chronic wound is one in which these processes do not occur in an orderly and timely sequence. Consequently, a chronic wound is one in which the wound healing process is interrupted and delayed.

Primary Healing

In **primary healing** (healing by first intention), the wound is closed by direct approximation of the wound edges. In larger defects, pedicled flaps or skin grafts are used to close the wound. This process is still primary wound healing because the healing occurs by immediate coverage with epithelial elements in some form.

Secondary Healing

In **secondary healing** (spontaneous wound closure), the wound is left open and allowed to heal spontaneously. Spontaneous wound closure is a bimodal process of wound contraction and epithelialization (Figure 7-2). Normal contraction occurs by a centripetal force from the margin of the wound. This centripetal force, which may be initiated by the myofibroblasts, draws the margins of the wound together to achieve closure.

Epithelialization is the other component of healing by secondary intention. The epithelium proliferates from the wound margins to the center at the approximate rate of 1 mm/day. This proliferation occurs only in a wound that is not infected (see the discussion of managing contaminated and infected wounds).

In the middle of an open wound that is healing by secondary intention, the inflammatory phase continues unabated. The product of this prolonged inflammatory process is granulation tissue. Granulation tissue consists of inflammatory cells and a proliferation of capillaries. This tissue is the "proud flesh" that our surgical forefathers welcomed as a sign of healthy wound healing. The modern surgeon should view the appearance

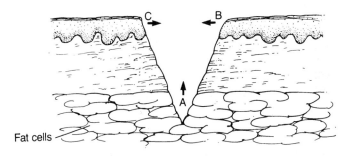

Figure 7-2 Wounds that heal by secondary intention. **A,** Granulation tissue forms at the base. **B,** The wound margins contract. **C,** The epithelium migrates.

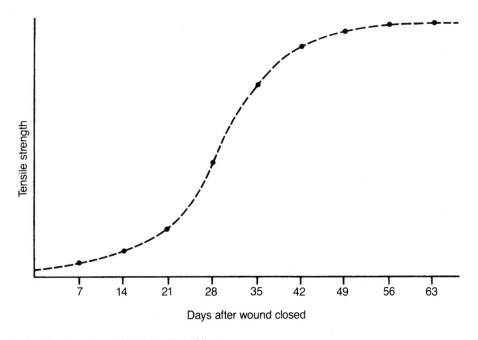

Figure 7-1 Strength of primarily closed wound as a function of time.

of this tissue merely as a prolonged inflammatory phase in a wound that is in need of closure. There are a number of options in the management of most of these granulating wounds. The informed physician will choose among these options, and may elect to excise all of the wound granulation and perform a delayed primary (tertiary) closure. Another option is to allow healing by secondary intention to proceed. A third option is to close the wound with a skin graft.

Tertiary Healing

In **tertiary healing** (healing by third intention), the wound is closed by active means after a delay of days to weeks. This process occurs when a granulating, open wound is closed with sutures or sterile tape before it has healed. The process of closing the wound interrupts the secondary healing process. Delayed closure should be performed only in wounds that have a quantitative bacterial count of less than 10^5 (see the discussion of managing contaminated and infected wounds).

Factors That Affect Wound Healing

Proper wound closure is the sine qua non of successful wound management. The goal of all wound closure is expedient, precise, and definitive tissue approximation without the complications of infection, fibrosis, and secondary deformities (wound contracture). The ability of the surgeon to achieve this goal depends on his or her knowledge of local and systemic factors that affect this process and his or her willingness and ability to control them.

Several local factors are extremely important, and should be considered each time the physician treats a patient who has a wound problem.

1. The amount of tissue trauma caused by the wound is extremely important. A **laceration** with a knife is minimally damaging to any tissue except the tissue that is directly in the wound margin. Crush or **avulsion** injuries are much more difficult to evaluate and manage successfully. In a crush injury, large areas of tissue adjacent to the wound are ischemic, and viability may be difficult to assess.
2. Hematoma is the bane of unimpeded wound healing. A collection of clot in the wound does not permit orderly removal of debris and laying down of collagen. In addition, the hematoma is a perfect medium for promoting bacterial proliferation and fostering clinical wound infection.
3. Bacterial contamination and wound infection are important factors in local control and proper closure of the wound. All wounds contain some bacteria. A relation exists between the bacteria in the wound and the patient who is wounded; this relation can best be described as a biologic balance (or equilibrium). A number of factors affect this equilibrium: blood supply to the wound, amount of necrotic debris present, local wound care require-

ments, and the use of systemic or topical antimicrobial agents. A wound can usually tolerate contamination with fewer than 10^5 organisms/g tissue and still be closed successfully without infection developing. If more than 10^5 bacteria/g are present, however, closure will lead to clinical wound infection. A quantitative bacterial count may be useful in judging whether a wound can be closed. Streptococci are the only exception. The presence of streptococci in the wound in any quantity is a contraindication to wound closure.

Proper wound management depends on a number of factors, including the type of injury, the degree of contamination, the time from injury to treatment, and the patient's host defense mechanisms. A careful history reveals much about the nature of a wound and the amount of contamination present. Proper assessment of the contamination dictates the subsequent care and ultimate success of wound management.

In addition to assessing contamination with common pathogens, the student should be aware of the possibility of *Clostridium tetani* in many wounds. Tetanus prophylaxis is an important consideration in all wounds. The best means to prevent tetanus is toxoid immunization combined with thorough cleansing and debridement. The Committee on Trauma of the American College of Surgeons has published guidelines that should be carefully reviewed (see Chapter 9).

General Management of the Clean Wound

A **clean wound** is one that is relatively new (< 12 hr) and has minimal contamination. Clean wounds are classified according to presentation and method of injury.

Classification of Clean Wounds

An **abrasion** is a superficial loss of epithelial elements, with much of the dermis and deeper structures intact. Usually, only cleansing of the wound is required because the remaining epithelial cells regenerate and migrate to close the wound. Careful cleansing is critical to prevent traumatic tattoos. Traumatic tattooing occurs when dirt particles are trapped beneath newly regenerated epithelial cells. A surgical scrub brush is often helpful in removing debris. For large abrasions with traumatic tattooing, general anesthesia is often required to adequately scrub and care for the wound. Epithelial migration occurs most rapidly in a moist environment. Therefore, desiccation of an abrasion should be avoided by applying a layer of antibacterial ointment (e.g., bacitracin, Neosporin).

A **contusion** is an area of soft tissue swelling and hemorrhage without violation of the skin elements. Evacuation of a hematoma with aspiration may be required. Otherwise, management consists of the application of cold compresses early (< 2 hr after injury) to minimize swelling, followed by the application of warm, moist compresses to provide comfort and speed the absorption of blood.

A **laceration** is the classic wound. It is managed with debridement of ragged edges and devitalized tissue, followed by atraumatic suture closure.

An **avulsion** injury is more difficult to manage than a simple laceration because of the extensive undermining that creates a flap. Partial avulsions are debrided and sutured into place, if viable. Total avulsions are generally not replaceable, except as a skin graft after the fat is removed. If the avulsed part contains an adequate single artery and a vein (> 0.5 mm), sometimes it can be replanted microsurgically.

Puncture wounds generally do not require closure. Management consists of assessment of the damage to underlying vital structures and examination for a foreign body. X-rays are often helpful in assessing the presence of a foreign body.

Crush injuries are often accompanied by the loss of significant amounts of tissue that may initially appear viable. The extent of injury may be evaluated with intravenous fluorescein, which diffuses into the interstitial tissue from patent capillaries in the immediate area. Fluorescence under an ultraviolet lamp indicates blood flow in the area and predicts tissue survival. Nonviable wound tissue is debrided, and the wound is closed with either skin graft or flaps.

Technique of Wound Debridement and Closure

Treatment requires debriding the wound and approximating the tissue in physiologic and anatomic order. Almost all nonmilitary wounds can be managed by primary closure if they are prepared properly (Table 7-1). Sedation of the patient may help to allay anxiety; however, sedation should be done only after any possible central nervous system injury is assessed.

Anesthesia and Wound Cleaning

The wounded area is prepared by washing with an antibacterial solution. If the wound is extensive, local anesthetic may be required before this step to reduce patient discomfort. An adequate working area must be prepared around the wound to prevent contamination of suture material and instruments. Sterile gloves are worn, and the physician frequently wears a surgical mask and gown as well. Sterile towels are draped around the wound to provide a sterile field. Some

Table 7-1. Steps in Wound Care

1. Sterile preparation and draping
2. Administration of local anesthetic
3. Hemostasis
4. Irrigation and debridement
5. Closure in layers
6. Dressing and bandage

wounds require ingenuity in draping, particularly in areas that are difficult to reach. It is helpful to take a few extra minutes to consider draping plans to ensure that the drapes do not cover the patient's face, interfere with breathing, or confine the patient and promote a sensation of claustrophobia. This consideration is particularly important if closure may take some time. Patients may become restless, frightened, or uncooperative, making the situation difficult for the patient and frustrating for the physician. Particular thought should be given when preparing a child for wound closure. In children, adequate sedation and monitoring are essential.

Local anesthesia is generally adequate for small wounds. Patients should be questioned about known sensitivity or adverse reactions to anesthetic agents. Xylocaine 1% or 0.5% is usually sufficient. Marcaine, an anesthetic agent with longer action, is occasionally useful. A new vial of anesthetic agent should be opened. Agents that contain epinephrine should be used with caution. Although chemical vasoconstriction is often helpful in tissue with a rich blood supply, it may cause detrimental ischemia in other areas (e.g., digital blocks of fingers or toes). The agent is injected slowly, with as small a needle as is practical (23–26 gauge). The patient should be told what is being done and what he or she can anticipate, such as the stick and the burning sensation with the injection. The difference between a good and a poor local anesthetic is 5 minutes. It is important to allow time for the drug to work. The toxic dose of lidocaine is approximately 7 mg/kg. A 1% solution contains 10 mg/mL, a 0.5% solution contains 5 mg/mL, and so on. A 10-mL dose of 1% Xylocaine in a 20-kg child approaches the toxic dose.

Wound Debridement and Closure

The best way to cleanse the wound is sharp debridement to remove clot, debris, and necrotic tissue, followed by irrigation with a physiologic saline solution. A 20-mL syringe with a 19-gauge needle is ideal (Figure 7-3). Hematoma is evacuated, and all active bleeding is controlled. Hemostasis is achieved with cauterization or absorbable ligature. Wound closure is undertaken in layers, with **absorbable sutures** placed in the layers that provide the greatest strength (i.e., dermis, fascia). The epithelium is approximated with superficial placement of nonabsorbable, monofilament sutures to seal the wound (Figure 7-4). Closure of "dead space" is usually not necessary, given proper closure of the strong layers of the wound, skin, or fascia. Sutures placed in the subcutaneous layer only necrose fat cells and introduce a foreign body that promotes infection. Handling of the tissue with atraumatic technique aids wound healing. Proper atraumatic technique involves using instruments that grasp, but do not crush, the tissues.

Suture Material

Great emphasis is often placed on the suture material that is used for closure, but the suture material is less important than attention to adequate debridement and

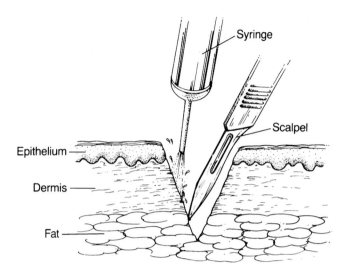

Figure 7-3 Sharp debridement and saline lavage to prepare the wound for closure.

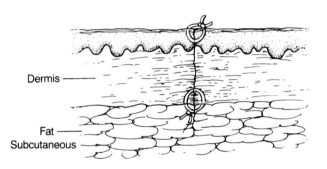

Figure 7-4 The dermis is approximated for strength, and the epidermis is closed to seal the wound and align the surface cells.

hemostasis. Suture material is classified as synthetic or biologic, absorbable or nonabsorbable, and monofilament or multifilament. Gut sutures, which are usually derived from sheep intestine, are examples of biologic sutures. These sutures last 7 to 10 days and are absorbed by proteolysis and phagocytic action. Because they cause an inflammatory reaction in the tissue, they are not usually used for skin closure.

Newer absorbable sutures are made of polyglycolic acid (e.g., Dexon, Vicryl). These polyfilament sutures are absorbed by hydrolysis and are useful for reapproximation of tissue below the skin surface. Because these sutures are braided, they are less desirable for skin closure.

Nylon is an excellent example of synthetic suture material. It is usually monofilament, but may be woven or braided. Because nylon is biologically inert, it cannot be broken down or absorbed. Monofilament nylon induces little inflammatory reaction; for this reason, it is useful for skin closure.

Suture size is graded by the number of zeros (0). The more zeros, the smaller the suture (i.e., 0 is very large; 0000 (4-0) is smaller). Number 1 suture is even larger. A 3-0 or 4-0 suture is used for skin on the extremities or torso, whereas a 5-0 or 6-0 suture is appropriate for the more delicate tissues of the face. A 2-0 to 4-0 suture is appropriate for closure of deeper tissues.

Suture material, size, and type should be chosen based on the type of reapproximation that is needed. Usually, absorbable synthetic suture (e.g., Vicryl) is preferred for closure of the deep layers. Muscle is very friable and does not hold sutures; therefore, the fascial covering of the muscle must be used for approximation. Subdermal tissue is closed, then skin. Wound drains are not required for simple closure. The need for drainage usually suggests the need for better hemostasis. Small monofilament sutures are ideal for the skin. Knots should be tight, and the suture should be tied to approximate, not strangulate, the tissue. Swelling of the tissue occurs over 24 to 48 hours; this swelling tightens the suture naturally. Excessive tension produces ischemia of the wound edge and additional inflammation. This inflammation exaggerates the suture marks across the wound and accounts for the "railroad track" appearance of the scar. Although cosmesis is the last element to consider in wound closure, avoiding excessive tension produces a better result. If the wound will not close without excessive tension, another management plan (e.g., rotational flaps, skin graft) should be considered.

Dressings

A dressing is usually placed over the closed wound. The dressing has many functions. To be maximally functional, the dressing should: (1) protect the wound, (2) immobilize the area, (3) compress the area evenly, (4) absorb any secretions, and (5) be aesthetically acceptable. Proper wound dressing should fulfill all of these criteria. The dressing should provide sufficient bulk to afford protection from inadvertent trauma. The bulk provided by fluffed gauze and gauze pads allows for adequate absorption of wound secretions and helps to immobilize the area. Further immobilization may be provided by a plaster splint or cast. An outer layer of firmly wrapped, rolled gauze and a loosely, but evenly, applied elastic roll can provide even compression and an aesthetic appearance.

Suture Removal

Sutures used for skin closure are removed when they have done the job for which they were placed. Skin layers with the greatest strength in wound closure are the dermis and fascia. Therefore, if dermal sutures are placed properly, the epidermal sutures may be removed within several days of placement. If skin is closed in a single layer, the sutures may not be removed for 7 to 10 days. Sterile forceps and fine scissors are the basic instruments that are used to remove sutures. The use of sterilized supplies is important for infection control. The suture is grasped with forceps and cut, then gently removed.

Management of the Contaminated and Infected Wound

The Contaminated Wound

All wounds are **contaminated** to a greater or lesser extent. Even the wounds that are considered clean have a bacterial inoculum that is much greater than expected. Proper wound care, with debridement and adequate lavage, can markedly diminish the inoculum and result in successful primary wound healing. Exceptions to the primary closure of these contaminated wounds include a very high bacterial inoculum (e.g., human bite, farm injury), a long time lapse since the initial injury, and a severe crush injury. In these instances, delayed closure is the preferred management.

The contaminated wound is closed by keeping buried sutures to a minimum. Monofilament skin sutures are used to reduce the possibility of wound infection. If the surgeon has doubts about the extent of contamination or the safety of the closure, delay is the judicious approach to wound management. Delay allows time for further debridement and reduction of the bacterial count to 10^5 or fewer bacteria/g tissue. Follow-up within 48 hours is the rule to detect early signs of clinical infection.

The Infected Wound

Infected wounds are sometimes difficult to assess. Proper management begins with identifying the truly infected wound. Any layperson can observe **pus** exuding from a severely inflamed wound and tell that the wound is infected. On the other hand, the most experienced surgeon will have no better chance than the flip of a coin in identifying the level of bacterial contamination in a chronically granulating wound.

The number of bacteria that can be tolerated and still allow successful wound closure is the most precise definition of an infected wound. This level of contamination has a distinct number: greater than 10^5 organisms/g tissue. The proper management of the infected wound is to decrease the bacterial count to 10^5 or fewer organisms/g tissue so that the wound may be closed. Debridement is the most important technique to decrease the bacterial count. Frequent dressing changes (every 4 hr) can also decrease the bacterial count. Systemic antibiotics are of little use in local bacterial control because they do not penetrate the granulating wound bed. However, topical antibacterials (e.g., mafenide acetate, silver sulfadiazine) are effective and may be used. Because of possible corneal irritation, mafenide acetate or silver sulfadiazine should not be used near the face. Biologic dressings (e.g., allograft, amniotic membrane) also decrease the bacterial level. Successful adherence of a biologic dressing indicates a reduced bacterial count and accurately predicts success with either wound closure or autograft.

Successful wound management requires diligent preoperative, intraoperative, and postoperative care as well as meticulous surgical technique. Proper handling of tissues, adequate debridement, physiologic placement of sutures, and bacteriologic knowledge of the wound are critical steps in wound closure.

Multiple-Choice Questions

1. A wound:
   A. Is not a puncture
   B. Is a disruption of normal anatomic relations as the result of an injury
   C. Is usually infected
   D. Is a laceration, but not an abrasion
   E. Always requires suturing

2. Granulation tissue consists of:
   A. Mature collagen fibers
   B. Fibroblasts, bacteria, capillaries, and inflammatory cells
   C. Epithelial cells and skin appendages
   D. Bacteria only
   E. Fibroblasts only

3. Match the following phrase with the best single response. Maturation phase:
   A. No collagen; macrophages and polymorphonuclear leukocytes (PMNs) are present
   B. No net collagen production; collagen cross-linking occurs
   C. High collagen production
   D. High collagen destruction
   E. High collagen production; many macrophages are present

4. A clean wound:
   A. Has fewer than 100,000 organisms/g tissue
   B. Will not take a skin graft
   C. Is more than 12 hours old
   D. Has beefy, red granulation tissue
   E. Has no bacteria

5. The inflammatory phase of wound repair is characterized by:
   A. No collagen; macrophages and polymorphonuclear leukocytes (PMNs) are present
   B. No net collagen production; collagen cross-linking occurs
   C. High collagen production
   D. High collagen destruction
   E. High collagen production; many macrophages are present

6. An infected granulating wound:
   A. Should not be treated with delayed primary closure
   B. Will take a skin graft

C. Usually has multiple organisms
D. Should be treated with systemic antibiotics
E. Looks purulent

7. Functions of a dressing include all EXCEPT:
A. Compression of the wound
B. Immobilization of the area
C. Protection of the wound
D. Decreased bacterial growth
E. Absorption of exudate

8. The proliferative phase of wound repair is characterized by:
A. Raised, red scar
B. Edema, erythema, and warmth
C. Flat, more supple scar
D. Moist, edematous, supple scar
E. Decreased polymorphonuclear infiltrate

9. The best time to remove skin sutures from a wound is:
A. After 7 days
B. After 20 days
C. Within a few days if dermal sutures were placed separately
D. After the inflammatory phase of wound healing
E. After the proliferative phase of wound healing

10. To provide maximum wound strength, the most important layers of a wound to close are the:
A. Subcutaneous fat–fascia
B. Fascia–epidermis
C. Dermis–fascia
D. Epidermis–subcutaneous fat
E. Dermis–subcutaneous fat

11. Factors that affect the bacterial balance of a wound include all of the following EXCEPT:
A. Blood supply
B. Systemic antibiotics
C. Debris in the wound
D. Granulation tissue
E. Dead space

12. Gut suture is:
A. Polyfilament and absorbable
B. Monofilament and absorbable
C. Polyfilament and nonabsorbable
D. Monofilament and nonabsorbable
E. Biologic and absorbable

13. Silk suture is:
A. Polyfilament and absorbable
B. Monofilament and absorbable
C. Polyfilament and nonabsorbable
D. Monofilament and nonabsorbable
E. Biologic and absorbable

14. Nylon suture is:
A. Polyfilament and absorbable
B. Monofilament and absorbable

C. Polyfilament and nonabsorbable
D. Monofilament and nonabsorbable
E. Biologic and absorbable

15. Polyglycolic suture (e.g., Dexon, Vicryl) is:
A. Polyfilament and absorbable
B. Monofilament and absorbable
C. Polyfilament and nonabsorbable
D. Monofilament and nonabsorbable
E. Biologic and absorbable

16. The maturation phase of wound healing is characterized by:
A. Raised, red scar
B. Edema, erythema, and warmth
C. Flat, more supple scar
D. Moist, edematous, supple scar
E. Many polymorphonuclear lymphocytes

17. Select the true statement regarding suture.
A. A 0 suture is smaller than a 0000 suture.
B. Polyfilament suture is most desirable for skin.
C. Absorbable suture is most desirable for skin closure.
D. Sutures that are placed deep in the skin should be absorbable so they need not be removed.
E. Monofilament suture is better to use in a contaminated wound than is polyfilament suture.

18. When wounds are allowed to heal by spontaneous contracture of the granulation tissue:
A. It is a primary intention closure
B. It is a delayed primary closure
C. It is a secondary intention closure
D. Antibiotics are required until epithelialization
E. Daily debridement is necessary

19. The proliferation phase of wound healing is characterized by:
A. No collagen; macrophages and polymorphonuclear leukocytes (PMNs) are present
B. No net collagen production; collagen cross-linking occurs
C. High collagen production
D. High collagen destruction
E. High collagen production; many macrophages are present

20. The best method to minimize postoperative wound infection after removal of a perforated appendix with pus in the peritoneal cavity is:
A. Betadine irrigation of the wound with tight primary closure of the skin
B. Closure of the wound on the second postoperative day
C. Closure of the wound on the fifth postoperative day
D. Antibiotic irrigation with loose approximation of the skin
E. Placement of a subcutaneous drain and tight wound closure

Oral Examination Study Questions

CASE 1

You are an attending physician in an emergency room in a small community. A man is brought to the emergency room by paramedics after he is involved in an automobile accident. He is awake and alert, and has a large laceration on his right lateral calf. He denies loss of consciousness at the time of the accident.

OBJECTIVE 1

The student does not miss an intracranial, intrathoracic, or intraabdominal injury and does not focus immediately on the bleeding laceration.

A. The student applies a pressure dressing to stop the bleeding and enumerates the "ABCs" of resuscitation.

B. The student describes the basic maneuvers to exclude serious injuries, including auscultation, percussion, and palpation of the organ cavities.

C. The student orders routine laboratory and x-ray studies. Hematocrit and x-rays of the injured part are also taken.

D. The student obtains a history of tetanus prophylaxis.

OBJECTIVE 2

After a more serious injury is excluded, attention is turned to the laceration and the specific management strategies of a clean, acute laceration.

A. Hemostasis: control of bleeding with ligation of the bleeding points

B. Wound debridement

C. Irrigation of the wound to decrease the bacterial count and remove debris

D. Layered closure of the wound to provide strength, approximate edges, and maximize aesthetic appearance

E. Tetanus prophylaxis

F. Discussion of when, how, and why sutures are removed

ADDITIONAL QUESTIONS

1. Under what circumstances would this wound not be closed? These circumstances include the presence of streptococci, more serious injury, long interval since injury, severe crush, and the assessment that there are more than 10^5 organisms/g tissue.

2. How would you approach this wound of a delayed primary closure at 72 hours?

OBJECTIVE 1

Minimum Level of Achievement for Passing

A. The student outlines the technical aspects of wound closure and gives the physiologic reason for each step.

1. Hemostasis to avoid hematoma
2. Irrigation to decrease bacterial inoculum
3. Layered closure of wound with particular attention given to the dermis as the layer of strength in the wound

B. The student outlines the phases of wound healing (substrate, proliferative, maturation).

C. The student discusses the appropriate use of quantitative bacteriologic studies in planning wound closure and mentions 10^5 organisms/g tissue as the critical number.

D. The student outlines the appropriate technical steps for proper wound closure.

E. The student knows the guidelines for tetanus prevention.

Honors Level of Achievement

A. The student recognizes that this wound is of relatively little importance if the patient is otherwise severely injured. The student discusses the principle of delayed primary closure of a wound in a patient who is critically ill.

B. The student can draw a wound-healing curve and show the phases of wound healing as they appear on the curve.

C. The student states that *Streptococcus* organisms are an exception to the 10^5 rule.

D. The student describes alternatives to wound closure (e.g., local flap, skin graft).

CASE 2

A 45-year-old woman comes to your office with an open wound over her right upper arm. She injured herself several days ago, but procrastinated about seeing a physician.

OBJECTIVE 1

The student knows the physiology of an open neglected wound.

This wound is in the inflammatory phase of wound healing. The student outlines the phases of wound healing and describes how this wound is behaving physiologically.

1. Substrate (inflammatory) phase
2. Proliferative phase
3. Maturation phase

OBJECTIVE 2

The student outlines the proper management of this type of wound.

A. The student describes the management of the wound to obtain bacterial balance and close the wound by delayed primary closure rather than allowing the wound to heal by secondary intention. Appropriate management could include frequent saline dressing changes or the use of topical antimicrobial agents (e.g., silver sulfadiazine). A quantitative biopsy of the wound is appropriate before wound closure is attempted.

B. The student knows that in wounds that are more than 24 hours old, the patient is given both tetanus toxoid and human antibody.

OBJECTIVE 1

Minimum Level of Achievement for Passing

A. The student describes the inflammatory phase of wound healing.

B. The student describes the components of granulation tissue: white blood cells, fibroblasts, bacteria, and capillaries (essentially no collagen).

Honors Level of Achievement

The student describes the means by which this wound enters the proliferative phase of wound healing and recognizes that the essential elements are bacterial balance and epithelial coverage.

OBJECTIVE 2

Minimum Level of Achievement for Passing

A. The student outlines the difference between allowing the wound to heal by secondary intention and closing the wound by delayed primary closure.

B. The student names two means of decreasing the bacterial count in an open wound.
   1. High-pressure lavage with saline
   2. Topical antimicrobials
   3. Frequent saline dressing changes

Honors Level of Achievement

A. The student names an exception to the 10^5 bacteria/g tissue rule for bacterial balance: *Streptococcus*.

B. The student briefly describes another means of closing this wound: flap or skin graft.

CASE 3

You are in the operating room during an elective colon operation with a preoperative bowel preparation. The operating surgeon passes out. He is resuscitated, but cannot continue the surgery. The midline abdominal wound must be closed, and you must do it.

OBJECTIVE 1

The student discusses the possible causes of contamination of this wound and the proper management of wound closure.

1. Closure with adequate bowel preparation
2. Emergency colon surgery with unprepared bowel

OBJECTIVE 2

The student discusses the closure of a midline abdominal wound and states which layers provide the ultimate strength of this wound.

1. Fascia
2. Dermis

OBJECTIVE 1

Minimum Level of Achievement for Passing

A. The student describes the differences among clean, contaminated, and infected wounds.

B. The student discusses the physiologic basis for closing the wound with the bowel preparation area and leaving the wound open during surgery with an unprepared bowel.

Honors Level of Achievement

The student enumerates the bacterial count of unprepared colon and colon with accepted preoperative bowel preparation.

OBJECTIVE 2

Minimum Level of Achievement for Passing

A. The student discusses wound healing in terms of the wound strength of the fascia and the dermis.

B. The student identifies the fascia as the most important layer of wound in this case.

Honors Level of Achievement

The student discusses the consequences of skin and fascia dehiscence.

SUGGESTED READINGS

Babion BM. Oxygen-dependent microbicidal killing of phagocytes. *N Engl J Med* 1978;298:659.

Burke JF. The physiology of wound infection. In: Hunt TK, ed. Wound healing and wound infection. New York, NY: Appleton-Century-Crofts, 1980:242–247.

Cohen IK, Diegelmann RF, Lindblad WJ. *Wound healing: Biochemical and Clinical Aspects*, 1st ed. Philadelphia, Pa: WB Saunders, 1992.

Covino BG. Comparative clinical pharmacology of local anesthetic agents. *Anesthesiology* 1971;35:158–167.

Guber S, Rudolph R. The myofibroblast. *Surg Gynecol Obstet* 1978;146:641–649.

Hamer MI, Robson MC, Krizek TJ, et al. Quantitative bacterial analysis of comparative wound irrigations. *Ann Surg* 1975;181:819–822.

Mulliken JB, Heale NA. Pathogenesis of skin flap necrosis from an underlying hematoma. *Plast Reconstr Surg* 1979;63:540–545.

Peacock EE. *Wound Repair*, 3rd ed. Philadelphia, Pa: WB Saunders, 1984.

Robson MC, Krizek TJ, Heggers JP. Biology of surgical infection. *Curr Probl Surg* March 1973; 1–62.

8

Surgical Infections

Richard N. Garrison, M.D.
Donald E. Fry, M.D.

OBJECTIVES

1. List the factors that contribute to infection after a surgical procedure.
2. List the four classes of surgical wounds and the frequency with which each type becomes infected.
3. Describe the principles of prophylactic antibiotic use.
4. List the clinical variables that affect antibiotic sensitivity when compared with in vitro tests.
5. Describe the events that lead to antibiotic resistance in a surgical patient who has an infection.
6. Discuss four common hand infections, and describe the treatment of each.
7. List the clinical variables that contribute to foot infections in patients with diabetes.
8. Identify the most likely bacterial species encountered initially with infection from a dog bite, from acute cholecystitis, and from acute perforated appendicitis, and infection found 2 hours after a perforated duodenal ulcer.
9. List three viruses that pose an occupational hazard for surgeons, and discuss methods to protect against infection.
10. List the causes of postoperative fever, and discuss the diagnostic steps for evaluation.

Treatment of the diverse surgical infections that a surgeon encounters requires an understanding of the etiology of the invading organism, the physiologic response of the host, and the mechanism of the treatment objectives. Currently, the limiting factor in advanced surgical care is the inability to control infectious processes that are ubiquitous. As surgical care has advanced, the wholesale use of antibiotics has caused the emergence of virulent bacteria, fungi, and viruses that are resistant to standard methods of treatment. Similarly, the surgical host has become more vulnerable as such factors as aging, transplantations, tumor therapies, foreign body implants, and prolonged intensive care have weakened both the immune system and the ability of the host to respond. Thus, the surgeon must be familiar with both the simple and the complex infectious challenges of modern surgical care. This chapter describes the diagnostic characteristics and the therapy indicated for common infections that are encountered by the surgeon and introduces some of the complex issues of **sepsis** that are prominent within surgical intensive care units.

Pathogenesis of Infection

Planned surgical procedures, traumatic injury, and nontraumatic local invasion can lead to severe bacterial insult. Regardless of the anatomic site, bacterial soilage of host tissues initiates well-defined processes of host defense. Potent mediators of the inflammatory response (e.g., kinins, histamine) are released from mast cells and fixed granulocytes, altering capillary permeability in the area of injury and contamination. Plasma proteins, such as **complement,** fibrinogen, and specific or nonspecific **opsonins,** are delivered into the area of the bacterial invaders. Circulating neutrophils then "marginate" at the capillary site of the alteration in vascular permeability and, through the process of diapedesis, move out of the intravascular compartment and into the interstitium. Neutrophils are directed toward the site by chemoattractants from tissue macrophages, platelets, and vascular endothelial cells, which include complement cleavage products, leukotrienes, kinins, and others. Neutrophils subsequently make contact with the foreign particles or bacteria. Opsonins bind to the foreign particle and facilitate adherence to the neutrophil plasma membrane, where phagocytosis is initiated. The engulfed organism or foreign particle is then surrounded within the phagosome, and intracellular killing and digestion are initiated by the release of lysosomal enzymes, hydrolases, superoxide compounds, and other enzymes into the surrounding vacuole. Ingestion of microorganisms in excess of the ability of the neutrophil to achieve intracellular killing results in death and dissolution of the phagocytic cell. Dead phagocytic cells, fibrin, opsonic proteins, densities of both dead and viable microorganisms, and bacterial products are the essential components of **pus.** The microenvironment that develops is relatively hypoxic

Table 8-1. Factors That Increase the Incidence of Surgical Infection

Local
　Wound hematoma
　Necrotic tissue
　Foreign body
　Obesity
Systemic
　Advanced age
　Shock (hypoxia, acidosis)
　Diabetes mellitus
　Protein-calorie malnutrition
　Acute and chronic alcoholism
　Corticosteroid drug therapy
　Cancer chemotherapy
　Transplant immunosuppression

and acidotic. As a result, cellular and enzyme function is inhibited. Thus, the primary determinant of infection for a given level of contamination is the density of bacteria present versus the efficiency and effectiveness of the host in disposing of the organisms.

Numerous adjuvants affect either bacterial virulence or cellular host response and thus may alter the host–pathogen interaction in favor of the bacteria (Table 8-1). Hemoglobin potentiates bacterial virulence because ferric iron may enhance bacterial growth, and hemoglobin diminishes the efficiency of the neutrophil in eradicating the microorganism. Therefore, it is advisable to rid the wound of blood before closure. Likewise, dead tissue and foreign bodies are potent adjuvants. Dead tissue is not readily penetrated by host defense mechanisms, and it provides a haven for bacterial proliferation. Thus, effective wound debridement and cleansing are essential for healing. Foreign bodies in surgery are numerous, and regardless of whether they are suture material in the surgical wound, Foley catheters in the urinary bladder, or intravenous cannulae, they protect bacteria against the host response.

Systemic factors (e.g., shock, hypovolemia, hypoxia) cause systemic acidosis and weaken host defense. Hemorrhagic shock causes tissue hypoperfusion and increases septic complications in patients who have traumatic injury or who have undergone surgical procedures. Oxygen is an essential metabolic component of phagocytosis and intracellular killing. Inadequate oxygenation results in acidosis at the site of contamination and significantly enhances the likelihood of subsequent infection.

Other coexisting systemic variables within the host also diminish host response. Patients with diabetes have impaired neutrophil mobility. Obesity facilitates local wound infection because the blood supply to adipose tissue is poor. Starvation with protein-calorie malnutrition increases the vulnerability of the host to infection, and acute or chronic alcoholism impairs host response. Systemic drug therapy with corticosteroids, cancer chemotherapeutic agents, and immunosuppression

during transplantation also increases vulnerability to invasive infection.

The systemic response to the initial injury and subsequent locally infected microenvironment is mediated by several factors. Tissue macrophages are stimulated to produce cytokines that have profound stimulatory effects on other systemic cellular and humoral cascades. The best characterized of these cytokines is tumor necrosis factor. When produced in excess, this factor is associated with tissue destruction and a hypermetabolic state. Similarly, the endothelial cell, whether injured or stimulated, causes local changes in blood flow, coagulation, and (through the release of vasoactive substances) a systemic vascular response.

In summary, the interaction between the pathogen and the host determines whether contamination has no sequelae or clinical infection occurs. Numerous local and systemic variables swing the biologic balance of power in favor of the bacterial invaders and determine whether the infection remains local or causes a systemic inflammatory state. The objective of surgical therapy is to reduce the bacterial concentration and alter the tissue environment so that supremacy of the host defense is established.

Prevention of Surgical Infection

Preventing infection in patients who are injured or undergo elective surgical procedures is essential for quality surgical care. Numerous soft tissue local adjuvant factors must be managed mechanically to avoid infection. Mandatory steps include debridement of nonviable tissue, irrigation to remove bacteria-laden clot and fibrin, control of bleeding, and meticulous removal of dirt and other foreign bodies. The wound can then be closed with a reasonable prospect for uncomplicated healing. Preservation of systemic oxygenation and tissue perfusion is important in the prevention of infection.

Surgical wounds are at different degrees of risk for infection. Infection in these wounds is primarily a consequence of contamination and adjuvant factors that are present in the wound at the time of closure. These different degrees of risk are organized into several classification schemes to allow stratification of similar operations. Only when operative wounds at similar risk are examined can the effect of different preventive measures be assessed. The classification system that is most commonly used for surgical wounds is shown in Table 8-2.

Surgical Asepsis

In clean procedures, surgical asepsis is of paramount importance in the prevention of operative site infection. The frequency of **clean wound** infection is the most sensitive indicator and is a surveillance tool that is used to judge overall sterile technique in the operating room. Certain techniques are used to obtain a low rate of infection. Preoperative hospitalization should be limited to avoid colonization of the patient with antibiotic-resistant, hospital-acquired bacteria. Preoperative

Table 8-2. Classification of Surgical Wounds

Wound	Bacterial Contaminants	Source of Contamination	Infection Frequency	Examples
Clean	Gram-positive	Operating room environment, surgical team, patient's skin	3%	Inguinal hernia, thyroidectomy, mastectomy, aortic graft
Clean-contaminated	Polymicrobial	Endogenous colonization of the patient	5%–15%	Common duct exploration, elective colon resection, gastrectomy
Contaminated	Polymicrobial	Gross contamination	15%–40%	"Spill" during elective gastrointestinal surgery, perforated gastric ulcer
Dirty	Polymicrobial	Established infection	40%	Drainage of intraabdominal abscess, resection of infarcted intestine

showers with specific cleansing of the proposed operative site are useful. Hair removal should be performed immediately before the procedure in the operating room to avoid colonization of small razor nicks and cuts. Adhesive plastic skin drapes actually increase clean wound rates of infection. Reducing the operative time is associated with a lower wound infection rate. Operations that last more than 2 hours have a 40% greater infection rate than those that last less than 1 hour. A careful preoperative examination of all patients who are about to undergo an elective procedure should include a search for areas of existing cutaneous infection (e.g., boil, furuncle). These sources of infection should be treated before the surgeon performs the procedure to avoid endogenous wound contamination.

Intraoperative efforts should minimize the introduction of bacteria and reduce adjuvant factors. Hemostasis is important, but excessive use of suture material and the indiscriminate use of electrocautery, which may leave large areas of devitalized tissue, should be avoided. Wound drains are seldom indicated, but when needed, they should be closed-suction drains that have a separate stab wound to exit the subcutaneous space. The purpose of drains is to remove adjuvant material (e.g., blood), and they should be used only when they are actively removing debris or fluid. At the time of wound closure, the patient's fate is sealed with respect to wound infection. A postoperative dressing is generally applied, but it does not prevent wound infection after the first few hours.

Although most surgical infections stem directly from the patient's endogenous microflora and the degree of contamination present at the time of the procedure, the operating room environment also contributes to wound infection. Personnel (i.e., surgeons, anesthetists, nurses, students) are a common source of bacterial contamination in this setting. Respiration and mouth secretions, along with the bacteria shed from exposed skin and hair, are measurable threats to clean incisions. Operating room attire is designed to minimize this source of contamination. Scrubbing of the hands and arms with an antiseptic solution and donning of sterile gowns and gloves are the last barriers against contamination. When infections occur after clean operative procedures, a break in this routine should be suspected. Appropriate scrubbing and the maintenance of a sterile environment are necessary for all procedures performed within the operating room. Other expensive devices (e.g., ultraviolet irradiation, laminar flow air-handling systems, space suit attire for operating room personnel) have been used, most often when the patient requires implantation of a permanent foreign body, such as an orthopedic joint or a vascular graft. However, the efficacy of such techniques is not proven.

Perioperative Antibiotics

Since their introduction in the 1940s, antibiotics have been used to prevent infection in patients who are undergoing elective operations. Studies show that **prophylactic antibiotics** must be present in the tissue at the time of bacterial contamination to be effective. Antibiotics that are given after contamination occurs are not effective. Clinical studies show the effectiveness of preoperative systemic antibiotics in reducing the incidence of tissue infection, especially in **clean-contaminated** and **contaminated** wounds. Few studies support the use of antibiotic prophylaxis for clean operative procedures. In these cases, the risk from the antibiotic is greater than the minimal benefit that could be obtained. For clean procedures in which a foreign body is implanted (e.g., aortic graft, total hip replacement), prophylaxis is used because a septic complication, although infrequent, is a morbid event. The important issues in surgical prophylaxis with antibiotics, regardless of the clinical setting, are to give the drug preoperatively and to select a drug that is active against the anticipated pathogens. Antibiotics that have a long half-life are preferable to those that have a short half-life; they should be given as close to the time of incision as possible, and again 4 to 6 hours later. Antibiotics used in a perioperative prophylactic manner should not be continued past two postoperative doses to avoid the emergence of resistant bacteria.

Because elective colon surgery is associated with high rates of wound infection, it is considered a special area for antibiotic prophylaxis. Orally administered, poorly absorbed antibiotics reduce the numbers of aerobic and anaerobic species that reside in the bowel and can ultimately contaminate the surgical wound during colon resection. Oral antibiotics are effective in reducing wound infection rates to less than 10% for elective colon resections. Oral neomycin–erythromycin base antibiotics are most commonly used, along with a mechanical bowel preparation. Whether prophylactic systemic antibiotics and preoperative oral neomycin–erythromycin base antibiotics used together are superior to either type used individually remains controversial.

For grossly contaminated wounds or dirty procedures, the risk of a wound infection exceeds 15% to 20%. Therefore, many surgeons close only the fascial layers, with the skin and subcutaneous tissues left open. The open wound can then be managed with wet-to-dry saline dressings, and may be closed by delayed primary closure on postoperative day 4 or 5. Small open wounds rarely become infected when the underlying tissue is viable, although the wound surface may become colonized. Prolonged postoperative systemic antibiotics do not facilitate the process of delayed primary closure.

Management of Established Infection

Established surgical infections are organized into community-acquired infections and hospital-acquired, postoperative (nosocomial) infections. Community-acquired infections are active processes that were initiated before the patient presented for treatment. Hospital-acquired infections include all infections that occur after surgical procedures. Thus, **peritonitis** is usually a community-acquired infection, but intraperitoneal abscess is most commonly a postoperative problem. Potential choices for antibiotic selection for each type of infection are shown in Table 8-3.

Several caveats must be considered in choosing a **therapeutic antibiotic.** Antibiotic sensitivity to an identified organism should always be determined for serious invasive infections and, if necessary, the antibiotic should be switched. However, because of the arbitrary testing environment of the laboratory, in vitro sensitivity does not indicate clinical responsiveness. Factors that must be considered in choosing an appropriate agent include bacterial counts, tissue environment (e.g., pH, tissue hypoxia), antibiotic concentration, function of organs that either metabolize or excrete the drug, and inherent toxicity of the agent. Regardless of the drug used, an ongoing daily assessment of the response of the host to the therapy is an essential component of care for surgical infections. If therapy is effective, that course of action should be sustained; however, if there is little or no sign of effectiveness, both the drugs used and the infection source that is being treated should be reevaluated.

Antibiotic resistance is a prominent concern in the treatment of surgical infection. Resistance means that a structural or functional change within the microorganism enables formerly sensitive bacteria to resist the antimicrobial effects of specific antibiotics. The bacterial changes may be mediated primarily by acquired genetic material (through plasmid transfer from other organisms) or by

Table 8-3. Antibiotic Selections for Common Infections

Infection Site	Anticipated Organism	Antibiotic Choice
Soft tissue cellulitis	Group A *Streptococcus,*	Nafcillin/oxacillin
Breast abscess	*Staphylococcus*	Nafcillin/oxacillin
Synthetic vascular graft	Usually *Staphylococcus*	Nafcillin/oxacillin
Hip prosthesis		
Heart/valve prosthesis	*Staphylococcus, Streptococcus viridans, Enterococcus, etc.*	Specific sensitivity needed
Biliary tract infection	*Escherichia* coli, Klebsiella, Enterococcus[a]	Aztreonam, cefazolin
Peritonitis; intraabdominal abscess	*E. coli,* other *Enterobacteriaceae, Bacteroides fragilis,* other obligate aerobes	*Clindamycin/aminoglycoside, metronidazole/ aminoglycoside, third- generation cephalosporin*[b]
Hospital-acquired pneumonia	*Pseudomonas, Serratia,* resistant Enterobacteriaceae	Ciprofloxacin, amikacin (or expanded-spectrum penicillin)
Catheter-associated bacteremia	*Staphylococcus,* Enterobacteriaceae	Specific sensitivities (beware methicillin-resistant *Staphylococcus epidermidis*)
Urinary tract (postcatheterization)	*Pseudomonas, Serratia,* Enterobacteriaceae	Specific sensitivity
Candidiasis	*Candida*	Amphotericin, ketoconazole
Pneumocystis	*Pneumocystis carinii*	Trimethoprim/sulfamethoxazole

[a]*Enterococcus* is not specifically covered primarily—either in the biliary tract or in intraabdominal infection. Consideration for treatment should be given when *Enterococcus* emerges as a secondary pathogen or when it is isolated in blood culture.
[b]Includes cefotaxime, cefoperazone, moxalactam, ceftizoxime, and ceftriaxone.

spontaneous chromosomal mutation. Once genetic changes are established within a given bacterial population, sustained use of the antibiotic preferentially promotes the resistant organisms by effectively eliminating the sensitive microbial population. Although this resistance is an evolutionary process and new techniques and drugs with different mechanisms of action have outpaced the surge of resistance, clinical practice concerning antibiotic selection and use is of utmost importance. Antibiotic therapy should be initiated only when there is clear evidence that an infection that is amenable to that form of therapy is present. Most surgical infections require drainage or debridement, and antibiotics should be used as an adjuvant to mechanical treatment. Finally, with the exception of only a few narrow indications, antibiotic therapy should not be used to prevent infection over an extended period. Application of these principles will at least forestall the development of resistant strains of microorganisms within both the individual patient and the surgical unit.

Community-Acquired Infections

Skin and Soft Tissue Infections

Soft tissue infection, usually after a minor cut or puncture, ordinarily presents with spreading cellulitis. The blanching erythema of cellulitis is usually caused by group A streptococci and responds to penicillin therapy. Staphylococci may also be the cause of cellulitis, particularly if gross suppuration (pus) is present at the injury site. Common soft tissue infections are listed in Table 8-4.

Necrotizing streptococcal gangrene is rarely seen in these patients. These infections are characterized by nonblanching erythema, with blisters and frank necrosis of the skin. Nonblanching erythema indicates subdermal thrombosis of the nutrient blood supply of the skin. Extensive surgical debridement of the affected area, in combination with high-dose penicillin, is the appropriate treatment. Many surgeons add clindamycin as a second antibiotic for these infections. A Gram stain of blister fluid is useful in differentiating this infection from other necrotizing infections of the skin and subcutaneous tissue.

Severe staphylococcal soft tissue infections are usually identified by Gram stain of the pus. Nafcillin and oxacillin are first-line antibiotics that are used in addition to surgical drainage and debridement of the primary focus of infection. Because staphylococci are readily passed to other patients by health care personnel or by objects passed between patients, sterile isolation techniques must be used for any patient contact or treatment. Sensitivity data are important to confirm that methicillin-resistant staphylococci are not present.

Isolation is applied to bacterial (e.g., staphylococcal) infections and selected viral infections (e.g., hepatitis A) to prevent the organism from being carried out of the room or treatment area. Gowns and gloves are worn and then removed on leaving the patient's room, and traffic into the patient's room is restricted. The objective is to prevent nurses and physicians from serving as vectors in transmission of the organism to others. Isolation is contrasted with reverse isolation, where the objective is to prevent pathogens from being introduced into contact with severely immunosuppressed patients. In this situation, nurses, physicians, and others who attend these patients wear masks to prevent airborne organisms from being introduced into the controlled environment.

Table 8-4. Common Soft Tissue Infections

	Etiology	Usual Organism	Physical Findings	Treatment
Cellulitis	Break in skin barrier	Streptococcus	Diffuse nonblanching erythema, tenderness	Systemic antibiotics usually, local wound cleansing
Furuncle, carbuncle	Bacterial growth within skin glands and crypts	Staphylococcus	Localized induration, erythema, tenderness, swelling, creamy pus fomation	1 + D, systemic antibiotics for carbuncle
Hidradenitis suppurativa	Bacterial growth within apocrine sweat glands	Staphylococcus	Multiple abscesses, drainage, thick pus from axilla and groin regions	1 + D of small lesions, wide debridement, excision and grafting of large areas
Lymphangitis	Infection within lymphatics	Streptococcus	Swelling and erythema of distal extremity, inflamed streaks along involved lymphatic channels	Local wound cleansing, removal of any foreign body, systemic antibiotics
Gangrene	Destruction of healthy tissue by virulent microbial enzymes	Synergistic Streptococcus/ Staphylococcus, mixed aerobic–anaerobic organisms, Clostridium	Necrotic skin/fascia, extremity swelling, grayish liquid discharge, crepitation/gas formation within tissue planes	Radical debridement of involved tissues, parenteral antibiotics

I & D, irrigation and debridement.

Breast Abscess

Breast abscess is a common staphylococcal soft tissue infection. Postpartum women with galactoceles are particularly at risk for this infection. These abscesses are characterized by localized pain, swelling, and redness associated with a mass that may or may not be fluctuant. Aspiration with a needle is helpful to confirm the presence of purulent material; however, the treatment requires incision and drainage. Antibiotics alone will not suffice, and a delay in surgical drainage while awaiting unrealistic results from antibiotics may result in necrosis of large amounts of breast tissue.

Perirectal Abscess

These abscesses result from infection within the crypts of the anorectal canal that subsequently suppurate; they are identified as tender masses in the perianal area. Because both perirectal and breast abscesses are exquisitely tender, they usually must be drained under general anesthesia. Antibiotics for the patient with a perirectal abscess are usually broad-spectrum for both anaerobes and aerobes, but are probably necessary only to protect the patient from the **bacteremia** that is associated with drainage, which is the mandated treatment. Perianal infection and resultant subcutaneous tissue necrosis can be extensive if drainage is not adequate. In this instance, fecal diversion should be considered to avoid further soilage to the area.

Gas Gangrene

Clostridial soft tissue infections include both cellulitis and myonecrosis. This combination is referred to as gas gangrene. These infections occur after soft tissue wounds with contaminated objects (e.g., nail puncture to the foot). These infections commonly cause a brown, watery drainage from the wound site and are associated with marked tenderness. Palpable crepitance is commonly present, but may be subtle when the myonecrosis extends along the subfascial plane. Roentgenograms may show soft tissue gas.

Tetanus toxoid immunization, along with adequate surgical debridement without primary wound closure, prevents clostridial myonecrosis or cellulitis in most patients who are at risk. Tetanus antitoxin is administered to patients with high-risk wounds who have an uncertain history of immunization. When clostridial gas gangrene is diagnosed, immediate radical surgical debridement is necessary. Massive doses of penicillin are necessary to kill the organism *Clostridium perfringens,* but penicillin is not useful in the absence of aggressive debridement of the affected tissue. Metronidazole and clindamycin are alternative antibiotic choices when penicillin cannot be used because of an allergic history. Hyperbaric oxygen is an unproved, but often employed treatment in these patients.

Tetanus

Tetanus (lockjaw) is caused by the exotoxin produced by the organism *Clostridium tetani.* After an incubation period of 2 days to several weeks, a prodromal symptom complex of restlessness, headache, stiffness of the jaw muscles, and muscular contractions in the area of the wound evolves. Violent generalized tonic muscle spasms usually follow within 24 hours, and respiratory arrest occurs. The keystone of management is the prevention of endotoxin production by debridement and cleansing of all wounds in which devitalized, contaminated tissue is present, along with a program of immunization. All patients who have traumatic wounds should receive tetanus prophylaxis in accordance with the recommendations of the Committee on Trauma of the American College of Surgeons (Tables 8-5 and 8-6). Patients with tetanus-prone wounds should be given tetanus toxoid. The only contraindication to the use of tetanus toxoid is a history of a neurologic or hypersensitivity reaction to a previous dose. Patients who have not been immunized within 10 years should receive additional therapy with tetanus immune globulin (human). The use of systemic antibiotics specific for clostridia (e.g., penicillin) should be considered for all tetanus-prone wounds to eliminate residual tetanus bacilli.

Hand Infections

Hand infections are common. They are described in Table 8-7. Although they are not life-threatening, hand

Table 8-5. Wound Classification

	Tetanus Prone	Nontetanus Prone
Age	> 6 hr	< 6 hr
Type	Crush Avulsion Extensive abrasion Burn or frostbite	Sharp/clean
Contaminants (soil, saliva)	Present	Absent

Table 8-6. Immunization Recommendations

History of Immunization	Tenatus Prone		Nontetanus Prone	
	Tetanus Toxoid	Tetanus Immune Globulin	Tetanus Toxoid	Tetanus Immune Globulin
Unknown or incomplete	0.5 mL[a]	250 units	0.5 mL[a]	No
Complete, last booster > 5 yr ago	0.5 mL	No	No[b]	No
Complete, last booster < 5 yr ago	No	No	No	No

[a]In unimmunized children, DT (diphtheria, tetanus) or DPT (diphtheria, pertussis, tetanus) is used. Completion of immunizations is necessary.
[b]Yes, if booster > 10 yr ago.

infections can lead to severe morbidity because of the loss of hand function. **Paronychia** is usually a staphylococcal infection of the proximal fingernail that ordinarily points in the sulcus at the nail border. Simple drainage and hot soaks are usually adequate therapy for these infections. **Felons** are deep infections of the pulp space of the terminal phalanx. These infections usually occur after penetrating injuries of the distal phalanx and are treated by drainage. A subungual abscess is the extension of a deep paronychia. It is identified by fluctuance beneath the nail. Removal of the nail is usually necessary to permit adequate drainage. Neglected infections of the fingers may result in **tenosynovitis,** an infection that extends along the tendon sheath of the finger. Drainage requires opening the sheath along its entire length to prevent necrosis of the tendon, with its functional implications.

Penetrating trauma or spread from a contiguous fascial compartment can result in an infection in one of three **deep-space compartments** in the hand. A thenar space infection causes swelling and pain directly over the thenar prominence. The thumb is held in abduction. Loss of normal concavity as a result of tense, painful swelling of the palm is characteristic of a midpalmar space abscess. Rarely, the hypothenar space presents in a similar fashion, with swelling and painful movement. In all cases, incision and drainage are urgently required, and antibiotics are empirically initiated and then continued, based on culture and sensitivity reports, for at least 10 days.

Human bites of the hand are common, but their potential infectious nature should not be underestimated. These infections are caused by contamination with **polymicrobial** aerobic and anaerobic mouth flora. Deep-space infections, including tenosynovitis, may be consequences of these bites. Copious irrigation, debridement, hand elevation, and systemic antibiotics are required initially to prevent infection. Human bites are the only penetrating injury of the hand in which primary closure is not employed. The hand is often injured by animal bites as well. Debridement and irrigation are required (as for human bites), but the pathogens involved are more likely to be aerobic *Pasteurella* species.

Foot Infections

Foot infections result from direct trauma or, more commonly, from mechanical and metabolic derangements that occur in patients with diabetes. Trauma-related infections are best prevented by adequate wound cleansing at the time of injury. Established infections raise concern that a foreign body or osteomyelitis is present. Radiographs and bone scans, along with aggressive debridement and cultures, should establish the extent of the infection and identify the organisms involved.

Foot infections in patients with diabetes are a common problem because of neuropathy, the resultant bone deformities, and the vascular compromise that occurs in this population. A thorough examination of the infected foot should determine the extent of vascular and neurologic impairment. Cultures should always be obtained, followed by specific broad-spectrum antibiotic therapy, debridement, and drainage. In addition, mechanical external support devices can be fitted to relieve pressure points and provide protection. All efforts should focus on limb salvage in these patients because amputation is a frequent morbid consequence of these complex infections.

Biliary Tract Infections

Biliary tract infections are usually a consequence of obstruction within the biliary tree, involving either the cystic or the common bile duct. The bacteria that are likely to be involved include *Escherichia coli, Klebsiella* species, and the enterococci. Anaerobes are not commonly encountered. Antibiotics to cover these anticipated organisms are usually used, but surgical intervention in the biliary tract is often necessary for effective drainage and resolution.

Acute cholecystitis is the most common inflammatory process in the biliary tract. It begins as a nonspecific

Table 8-7. Common Hand Infections

	Location	Signs	Treatment
Felon	Pulp space of digits	Swollen, indurated, tense, throbbing distal finger; point tenderness	1 + D over length of phalanx along side of finger
Paronychia	Skin over mantle of nail and lateral nail folds	Swelling/induration of nail folds, point tenderness, purulent drainage	1 + D at base of nail; removal of nail if infection beneath nail
Tenosynovitis	Tendon sheath	Throbbing, pain with movement, entire finger swollen, tenderness over sheath, finger held semiflexed	1 + D over length of sheath and bursa; systemic antibiotics ususally indicated
Fascial space	Spaces of hand/thenar regions	Tenderness of involved space, swelling over region involved, limited motion	1 + D along surface lines of projection; systemic antibiotics indicated
Human bites	Point of skin penetration and underlying regions	Injury site wound, induration and swelling, purulent drainage, limited motion	Wide debridement and irrigation; systemic antibiotics and tetanus immunization indicated

I & D, irrigation and debridement.

inflammatory process secondary to obstruction of the cystic duct. Entrapped bacteria may give an invasive infectious character to the process. Empyema of the gallbladder occurs when infection in the gallbladder is undrained, leading to purulent distension and, often, severe systemic sepsis. Increased intraluminal pressure combined with invasive bacterial infection may impede the blood supply of the gallbladder, resulting in gangrene and perforation. Prevention of these complications can best be achieved by early operation.

Infection proximal to a common duct obstruction causes ascending cholangitis. Patients have fulminant fever, leukocytosis, and jaundice. These patients are usually toxic and often have hemodynamic instability. Prompt surgical intervention is imperative. At operation, or by percutaneous radiologic methods, the common duct must be drained, usually with a T-tube placed during operative intervention. Endoscopic drainage of the common duct through the ampulla provides adequate drainage in selected patients.

Acute Peritonitis

Acute peritonitis occurs when bacteria are present within the peritoneal cavity after mechanical perforation of a hollow viscus. Primary peritonitis may occur without a perforation, but it is uncommon, and is usually seen in alcoholics with ascites or in immunocompromised patients. Peritonitis causes acute abdominal pain, usually accompanied by fever and leukocytosis. Palpation of the abdomen usually shows marked tenderness with rebound and also may show a board-like rigidity. An upright chest roentgenogram commonly shows free air beneath the diaphragm from the perforated viscus.

Peritonitis is variable in severity. Different segments of the intestine that may perforate have different bacterial and chemical compositions and microorganism densities; therefore, it is probably inappropriate to consider all of the illnesses that are classified as peritonitis as a single disease entity.

Perforated gastroduodenal ulcers usually occur as precipitous events with acute abdominal pain. Approximately 80% of patients have free air on an upright chest film (Figure 8-1). Patients may or may not have antecedent symptoms of ulcer disease. The peritonitis may be entirely chemical, with no bacteria culturable from the peritoneal cavity in the first 12 hours. If the perforation persists for longer than 12 hours, however, bacterial infection becomes increasingly severe. Operative repair of the perforation, usually with a definitive ulcer operation (e.g., vagotomy and pyloroplasty), is the treatment of choice. Antibiotics for common Gram-negative bacteria are usually used, but provide minimal benefit, except in patients with delayed operation.

A perforated appendix is another common cause of peritonitis that starts as acute appendicitis. In the absence of an appropriate operation, perforation may occur after 24 hours of symptoms. Patients usually have diffuse tenderness and generalized rebound tenderness. Antibiotic therapy is directed against both aerobic

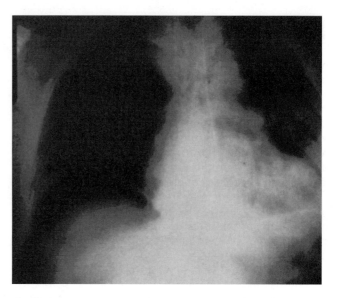

Figure 8-1 A large amount of free air is seen in this patient who has a perforated duodenal ulcer of 12 hours' duration.

(E. coli) and anaerobic *(Bacteroides fragilis)* enteric organisms. Treatment requires appendectomy and drainage of any right lower quadrant abscesses. When a localized abscess is identified, external drainage is indicated. External drainage is unnecessary and ineffective for diffuse peritoneal spillage in the absence of a localized abscess.

Colonic perforation from either carcinoma or diverticular disease is the most virulent cause of peritonitis. Colonic microflora have high densities of both aerobic and anaerobic bacteria. Patients usually have marked peritoneal signs and are systemically toxic. After volume resuscitation and the initiation of broad-spectrum systemic antibiotics, operation is required to manage the perforation, drainage (of pus), and debridement of nonviable tissue within the peritoneal cavity. Left colon perforations usually require diversion of the fecal stream as part of their management.

Peritonitis can occur from other sources as well. If sufficient physical findings are present (e.g., diffuse rebound tenderness), a celiotomy (laparotomy) is justified. It is important to diagnose peritonitis and not to delay operative intervention while radiologic studies are performed to define the offending organ system. Exploration will define the specific diagnosis.

Viral Infections

The diagnosis and treatment of viral infections is not usually the province of the surgeon, except in cases of severely immunosuppressed patients, in whom invasive infection may mimic a bacterial etiology. However, occupational exposure of health care workers to patients who are infected with hepatitis or human immunodeficiency virus (HIV) requires an understanding of the route of transmission so that preventive measures can be taken.

The DNA virus hepatitis B is the pathogen of greatest concern for surgeons because blood or body fluid is the primary route of transmission. In 5% to 10% of infected patients, a chronic carrier state develops. Many of these chronic carriers progress to end-stage liver disease or hepatocellular carcinoma. An acute infection often results in hepatic failure and death. Once an infection is established, effective therapy is limited; however, a highly effective hepatitis B vaccine is available. All health care workers who are at risk should undergo vaccination, with follow-up antibody titers determined to assure protection.

Hepatitis C, an RNA virus, poses a similar risk because it is also transmitted by blood and body fluids. Although acute infection from hepatitis C virus is usually mild or occult, the chronic carrier state occurs in approximately 60% of patients. In these patients, chronic active hepatitis and cirrhosis eventually develop. Because there is no vaccine and because 3.5 million people in the United States have chronic hepatitis C, it is important that health care workers exercise universal precautions in all patient contacts.

Infections secondary to the retrovirus HIV have been a recent focus of public concern. Although our understanding of this viral disease and its treatment continues to evolve, it is clear that blood and body fluid exposure is the primary mode of transmission. Therefore, the disease presents a potential risk to surgical care providers. With few exceptions, HIV infection appears to progress to clinical acquired immunodeficiency syndrome (AIDS), a fatal illness. The only strategy to combat HIV is prevention; therapy is currently limited to protease inhibitors, which appear to delay the progression to clinical AIDS. Modification of professional behavior, with universal precautions and strict limits on contact exposure by workers (e.g., physicians, nurses, students), is mandatory.

Hospital-Acquired Infections

The discussion of hospital-acquired infections in surgical patients is by definition a discussion of postoperative fever. The onset of fever usually heralds an evolving infectious problem. The student of surgery should understand the pathogenesis of fever and its many causes.

Fever is a consequence of the synthesis and release of the endogenous pyrogens, of which interleukin-1 is the most notable. Macrophages come into contact with foreign particles (usually bacteria), and stimulate the synthesis of interleukin-1. Interleukin-1 is released into the inflammatory environment and transported by the circulation to the hypothalamus, which then acts to increase body temperature. This temperature increase is accompanied by neutrophilia, hypoferremia, hypozincemia, hypercupremia, and the synthesis of acute-phase proteins by the liver (e.g., C-reactive protein). All acute responses that are mediated by interleukin-1 are adaptive responses mediated by the host, presumably to bolster defenses against evolving infections. To manage fever in surgical patients, the source of the pathogen–macrophage interaction must be identified. Empiric use of antibiotics as an initial response to fever should not be a customary practice. The primary focus of surgical infection must be identified and then disrupted, usually by mechanical means (e.g., drainage of infected sites), before or during the administration of systemic antibiotics.

Pulmonary Infection

Pulmonary infection in the postoperative patient may have three pathologically distinct causes. First, non–respirator-associated **pneumonia** results from atelectasis. Poor postoperative tidal volumes as a result of anesthesia, analgesia, and painful abdominal or thoracic incisions can cause small airways to collapse. Entrapped organisms plus alveolar macrophages cause fever, usually within the first 48 hours after operation. Early ambulation, coughing, deep breathing, and even nasotracheal suctioning (in refractory cases) of postoperative patients can prevent and manage atelectasis. Various incentive spirometers are expensive, and probably less effective, alternatives to the prevention and management of atelectasis. When a new fever and suspected atelectasis are present in the first 48 hours after surgery, laboratory and radiographic studies are usually unnecessary. If fever persists despite aggressive pulmonary chest physical therapy, a chest roentgenogram is often informative. When infiltrates are identified on chest roentgenograms and leukocytosis evolves, then invasive infection has occurred and systemic antibiotics are warranted. Drug selection requires culture and sensitivity data. Organisms in this setting may be either Gram-positive or Gram-negative.

Second, postoperative pneumonitis may be respirator-associated. Critically ill patients are very vulnerable to infection while they are receiving ventilatory support. In these patients, the lung has usually been assaulted by large volumes of intravenously administered fluids. The endotracheal tube is a foreign body that injures tracheal mucosa and permits bacterial proliferation. The ventilator then serves as a reservoir to "shower" the vulnerable pulmonary tissues with multiresistant hospital-acquired microflora. Weaning the patient from the ventilator promptly is the most important preventive measure. When infection occurs in this setting, opportunistic Gram-negative species endogenous to the hospital unit (e.g., *Pseudomonas, Serratia*) predominate. These patients require systemic antibiotics directed toward culture results obtained by endotracheal sampling. In some cases, pulmonary cultures are obtained by bronchoscopy with bronchoalveolar lavage or protected-brush sampling. In addition, frequent suction through the endotracheal tube removes purulent material and retained secretions.

Third, aspiration is an ever-present risk in the postoperative patient. The patient who is at risk for aspiration usually has gastric distension and altered mental status. Patients who have a head injury or are elderly are particularly at risk. Gastric decompression does not totally obviate the risks of aspiration, but certainly reduces the probabilities. After aspiration occurs, bronchoscopy is diagnostic and may also permit evacuation of particulate matter from the tracheobronchial tree. If hypoxemia is present after aspiration, bronchoscopy must be approached cautiously to avoid causing cardiopulmonary arrest. Management of aspiration requires support of systemic oxygenation. Antibiotics are withheld until clinical and culture evidence identifies an organism for specific therapy. Systemic corticosteroid therapy has no role in aspiration.

Urinary Tract Infection

Postoperative **urinary tract infections** are usually consequences of an antecedent indwelling Foley catheter. These catheters traumatize the bladder and urethral tissues and provide ready access for pathogens. To-and-fro movements of the catheter provide a "sump" effect to translocate catheter and urethral microorganisms into the bladder. Prevention requires aseptic placement of the catheter, firm fixation after placement, maintenance of the closed drainage system, daily catheter care, and removal of the catheter as soon as it serves its purpose. Although systemic antibiotics do not prevent postoperative urinary tract infection, they modify the microflora that are potential pathogens.

The diagnosis of postoperative urinary tract infection has traditionally been made with a quantitative bacterial culture. When more than 100,000 organisms/mL urine are identified, surgeons should not assume that the source of postoperative fever has been located. Bacteriuria does not indicate invasive urinary tract sepsis, and it does not cause fever. In most cases, cultures that are positive after Foley catheterization clear with removal of the catheter and an adequate "flush" by volume-induced diuresis. Systemic bacteremia from the urinary tract is uncommon in surgical patients who do not have functional or anatomic obstruction to urine flow. Significant postoperative fever from the urinary tract is always a presumption, even with positive cultures. Constant surveillance for other sources of fever must be pursued.

Urinary infections that develop after catheterization are not caused by the usual urinary tract pathogens (e.g., *E. coli*). They are usually caused by *Pseudomonas, Serratia,* and other resistant Gram-negative organisms. Treatment almost always requires culture and sensitivity data. *Candida* and enterococci are being cultured from the urinary tract in more and more patients. Systemic treatment for these presumed urinary tract pathogens should be deferred in the absence of positive blood cultures.

Wound Infections

Postoperative fever should alert the clinician to look where "the hands of man" have been. The wound is always a prime suspect, especially when tenderness, redness, heat, or a mass effect is noted when inspecting the wound. The discharge of pus from the wound is definitive. The absence of a "healing ridge" in one portion of the incision is also a useful clinical sign of wound infection.

A wound infection requires the wound to be opened. Pus is evacuated, fibrin is debrided, and subcutaneous suture material is removed. Systemic antibiotics are not an alternative to drainage. Antibiotics are necessary only for patients who have severe or progressive cellulitis or necrotizing infection. In the latter case, frequent wound debridement is an essential component of management.

Intraabdominal Infection

Postoperative intraabdominal infection generally occurs in two settings. First, complications of elective gastrointestinal or biliary surgery may result in postoperative peritonitis or abscess. Major dehiscence of anastomoses is usually associated with florid sepsis, and reoperation for management of this complication is usually based on clinical criteria. Abdominal tenderness and pain, fever, leukocytosis, and the toxic septic state (rather than roentgenograms, contrast studies, or other sophisticated diagnostic methods) are the most important indicators of the need for reoperation. Patients who underwent an initial laparotomy for infection or penetrating trauma often have a degree of bacterial contamination that makes a subsequent abdominal abscess a common event. Most postoperative intraabdominal infectious complications are abscesses.

Intraabdominal abscess is difficult to diagnose. Physical examination is significantly compromised by the painful abdominal incision of a previous procedure. Localized tenderness is a useful indicator in only approximately one-third of patients, and palpable masses are helpful in fewer than 10% of patients with abscess. Rectal examination is a particularly valuable method of diagnosis when pelvic abscess is a concern.

Roentgenograms of the abdomen are helpful in the few cases in which positive findings are identified. An abdominal series is occasionally ordered, but is useful in fewer than 20% of patients (Figure 8-2).

Upper or lower gastrointestinal studies with Gastrografin may show filling defects or intestinal leaks (Figure 8-3), but may be undesirable in patients who underwent recent construction of anastomoses. Under fluoroscopic guidance, installation of water-soluble contrast agents through drain sites may also help to identify undrained collections within the abdomen.

Ultrasound is also used to identify intraabdominal abscesses. It is inexpensive, it allows for immediate interpretation, and the equipment can be taken to the bedside (which eliminates the need to transport critically ill patients to another area of the hospital for evaluation). However, the receiver surface must make direct contact with the skin of the abdomen. For this reason, ultrasound may not provide a complete examination in patients with dressings, open wounds, or stomas. Ultrasound provides poor anatomic detail, and intestinal gas, which is commonly encountered in septic postoperative patients, leads to limited anatomic detail and outline of abscesses.

With an accuracy rate of more than 90%, computed tomography (CT) is the fastest and most useful

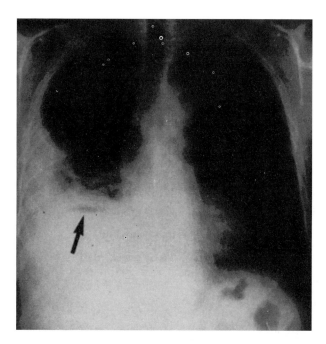

Figure 8-2 An upright chest x-ray showing an air-fluid level below the right hemidiaphragm and a reactive pleural effusion in a patient with a subphrenic abscess (arrow).

diagnostic study for suspected intraabdominal abscess (Figure 8-4). A water-soluble contrast agent can be given orally and intravenously to help distinguish abscesses and fluid collections from gastrointestinal, vascular, and urinary structures. However, when adynamic ileus prevents filling of the gastrointestinal tract, the contrast agent is contraindicated. In addition, when the patient has ascites (making identification of specific fluid collections difficult), CT results are frequently equivocal. In these cases, diagnosis can be made by radionuclide scanning after the injection of indium-111-labeled autologous leukocytes. Total body scanning can be done within 1 day after injection, and all sites of infection can be shown. If indium-111 leukocyte scanning is added to CT in equivocal cases, abdominal abscess can be diagnosed accurately in nearly all instances.

Drainage is the primary treatment of an intraabdominal abscess. Drainage allows removal of the bacteria, fibrin, and debris that fuel the septic process. After the abscess is precisely located in a patient who is tolerating the septic process, localized drainage with CT or other radiologically guided percutaneous methods or a limited operative procedure is justified. However, patients who have severe metabolic and physiologic decompensation as a result of the septic process, particularly those with associated organ failure, must undergo comprehensive reexploration to ensure complete surgical drainage and debridement.

Infection in the peritoneal cavity is usually polymicrobial. These infections usually have lipopolysaccharide-laden organisms (e.g., *E. coli*) and obligate anaerobes (e.g., *B. fragilis*). These organisms appear to have a complex synergistic relation. Conventional antibiotic cover-

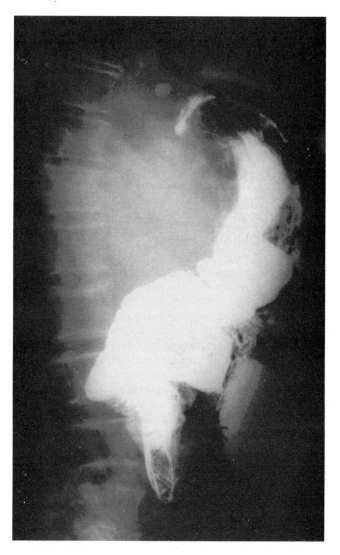

Figure 8-3 A large retrogastric filling defect noted on the upper gastrointestinal barium study represents a lesser sac abscess after a penetrating injury to the abdomen.

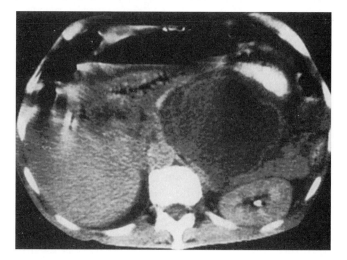

Figure 8-4 A large lesser sac abscess is noted on the abdominal computed tomography (CT) scan of a patient who has severe pancreatitis.

age for patients with peritonitis or intraabdominal abscess requires coverage of both halves of the synergistic pair. Regardless of the antibiotic used, treatment of intraabdominal infection is destined to failure without adequate surgical drainage, intestinal diversion or exteriorization, and debridement of the infected soft tissues that surround the focus of infection.

Pleural Empyema

Empyema may be a complication in the postoperative period after thoracotomy or chest tube placement. Occasionally, it occurs spontaneously in association with a pneumonic process. Endogenous flora from pulmonary or esophageal resection or from technical failures of these resections may cause empyema. Chest tubes are "two-way" streets that may allow blood and fluid to exit the pleural space, but may also allow exogenous bacteria to enter this space. Roentgenograms show an effusion, usually in the dependent portion of the pleural space. Because patients may be lying down most of the time, a loculated empyema cavity may be posterior. Thus, a lateral chest film, CT, or ultrasound may be helpful in the diagnosis. CT is particularly useful for distinguishing among loculated empyema, lung abscess, and combinations thereof. The diagnosis of empyema is confirmed by aspiration of pus by needle thoracentesis. Ultrasound guidance during needle placement is helpful. CT guidance is invaluable to depict the anatomy when multiple loculations require tube drainage.

Pathogens in an empyema are highly variable, and Gram stain of the pus is useful for selecting antibiotics. In patients with empyema after previous placement of a chest tube, Gram-positive staphylococcal organisms predominate. Antibiotic failure in patients with appropriate coverage usually reflects inadequate drainage. In this case, rib resection to marsupialize the empyema may be necessary.

Foreign Body–Associated Infection

Surgical patients are inundated with invasive intravascular catheters and devices. Peripheral intravenous cannulae, Swan-Ganz catheters, percutaneous pacemakers, and arterial lines are only a few of the devices that are used in patients in the intensive care unit. These portals of entry into the intravascular compartment are being recognized with increasing frequency as sources of postoperative nosocomial bacteremia. Indwelling lines permit organisms to migrate from the skin level into the intravascular compartment of the device. Bacteremia then occurs from the catheter. Intimal injury, with localized clot formation, may provide an additional growth medium for bacteria. Newly designed subcutaneous implanted infusion ports decrease the chance of contamination through the skin entrance site, but are still a potential source of infection because of pericatheter clot formation. To prevent this complication, all percutaneous peripheral intravenous cannulae, central venous catheters, and monitor devices (e.g., Swan-Ganz catheters, arterial lines) must be placed with sterile technique and removed or replaced within 72 hours. Only alimentation catheters should be maintained for longer periods, and they must be handled with meticulous sterile technique. Asepsis must be exercised in the care of all intravascular devices.

The diagnosis of intravascular device bacteremia is suspected in any postoperative patient who has positive blood cultures, particularly when either *Staphylococcus aureus* or *Staphylococcus epidermidis* is recovered. A semiquantitative culture of the suspected catheter tip may help to confirm the diagnosis. The essential component of treatment of intravascular device–associated bacteremia is removal of the foreign body. The patient's clinical response to removal usually confirms the diagnosis. Persistent fever, leukocytosis, and bacteremia suggest suppurative thrombophlebitis; therefore, the sites of previous intravascular devices must be examined carefully. Local incision and drainage to identify pus within the vein dictate excision of the entire length of involved vein. Antibiotics specific to the bacteremic organisms are used until clinical resolution occurs. Longer courses of antibiotics (e.g., 14 days) are recommended for patients with *S. aureus* bacteremia to prevent the complications of bacterial endocarditis.

Fortunately, infection of implanted vascular grafts, orthopedic joints, or other permanent devices occurs infrequently; however, when infection of these implants does occur, the device must be surgically removed for therapy to be effective. In most cases, removal of these devices requires alternate prosthetic implants (e.g., extraanatomic vascular bypass for an infected aortofemoral graft). Management of these complex clinical problems dictates the prolonged use of culture-specific systemic antibiotics. Recently, antibiotic-impregnated beads have been used adjacent to the infected site to permit the delivery of higher doses of antibiotic to the area. This technique had dramatic effects in selected anecdotal cases.

Fungal Infections

Fungal infections are being identified with increasing frequency in surgical patients. The use of antibiotics with an expanded scope of coverage has caused the ubiquitous fungi to become opportunistic pathogens. Patients who are immunosuppressed, are undergoing advanced cancer chemotherapy, or are older and have chronic debility have provided an abundance of susceptible hosts for these fungi. Most of these fungi can be isolated from the patient or environment routinely because they are part of the natural microbial milieu. It is only under selected environmental conditions that fungi cause clinical invasive infection. The most common of these microbes seen in the clinical setting is the *Candida* species. Because of the ubiquitous and, at times, subtle nature of most fungi, systemic or invasive infection must be documented by blood or tissue culture to confirm the diagnosis. Therapy consists of debridement of infected tissue when applicable, along with prolonged systemic antifungal chemotherapy. Amphotericin B is the mainstay of therapy for most invasive infections, but careful dosing is needed because of the toxicity of the drug. Fluconazole is another widely used antifungal, but it is unclear whether this less toxic drug is clinically comparable to amphotericin B.

Multiple-Organ Failure

The clinical events of surgical infection are most often resolved at the local site of inflammation; however, when proinflammatory products of inflammation are sustained or extensive, systemic exposure occurs and a generalized septic state is created. This physiologic state is characterized by an increase in cardiac output; a reduction in peripheral vascular resistance; a narrowed arteriovenous oxygen difference; hypermetabolism, with increased gluconeogenesis and ureagenesis; and sustained lactic acidemia. If left unabated, this heightened state causes dysfunction of both metabolic and vascular processes in vital organ systems. The affected organs fail in a sequential pattern that culminates in death of the host.

This syndrome of **multiple organ system failure** (MOSF) is a common scenario for death in most surgical intensive care units. The treatment of MOSF requires assessment of all potential causes of systemic inflammation; however, once it begins, the process often continues despite control of the principal infection. Current management entails both organ system support (e.g., renal dialysis) and nutritional support to avoid metabolic collapse.

The Future of Surgical Infection

The character of the pathogen in surgical infection has undergone a constant evolution since the introduction of antibiotics. All evidence suggests that this evolution is continuing. Instead of bacterial pathogens, the organisms that are now commonly identified are fungi, viruses, and protozoans. Because critically ill patients are sustained for longer periods in the contemporary intensive care unit, the host is vulnerable to all manner of microorganisms. The pattern of bacteria and other organisms to adapt to various types of antimicrobial chemotherapy suggests that other treatment modalities (e.g., immune augmentation, cytokine inhibition) will be tried. The results of these strategies to date have been disappointing. MSOF remains an area for intensive investigation, and effective therapy awaits the identification of uniform etiologies. Until that time, the common thread of treatment of all infections in surgical patients is to ensure that local mechanical treatment is optimized and that antibiotic therapy is timely and appropriate.

Multiple-Choice Questions

1. Prophylactic antibiotics should be used in:
   A. Insertion of a vascular prosthesis
   B. Elective herniorrhaphy on a diabetic patient
   C. Cases where all surgical postoperative drainage is contraindicated
   D. Patients who are younger than 2 years of age or older than 65 years of age
   E. Incision and drainage of a pelvic abscess

2. Which one of the following most effectively contributes to maintaining a low wound infection rate in clean operations?
   A. Preoperative antibiotics
   B. Laminar flow operative room
   C. Prolonged preoperative workup in the hospital
   D. Short operative time
   E. Preoperative shaving of the surgical area

3. The most common hospital-acquired (nosocomial) infection is:
   A. Pneumonia
   B. Wound infection
   C. Urinary tract infection
   D. Laryngitis
   E. Suppurative phlebitis

4. A 25-year-old man has a fiery red, tender, inflammatory area on his back. It is well demarcated, with a raised serpiginous border. The appropriate management of this problem is:
   A. Intravenous hydrocortisone
   B. Intravenous antihistamine
   C. Intravenous antibiotics
   D. Topical antifungal agent
   E. Surgical incision and drainage

5. The main difference between a paronychia and a felon is that the:
   A. Primary treatment of a felon is medical
   B. Paronychia involves the fingernail
   C. Felon has a potential for abscess development
   D. Felon can spread into the synovial space
   E. Paronychia has the potential for invasive sepsis

6. Necrotizing fasciitis:
   A. Requires radical debridement of tissue
   B. Is nearly always fatal
   C. Is associated with beta-hemolytic streptococci in 90% of cases
   D. Most often occurs after surgical procedures on the abdomen
   E. Requires hyperbaric oxygen therapy

7. Fever on the third postoperative day occurs in a patient who had a splenectomy for idiopathic thrombocytopenic purpura. The first radiographic test that you would perform on this patient is:
   A. Chest x-ray
   B. Flat and upright x-rays of the abdomen
   C. Computed tomography (CT) scan of the abdomen
   D. Intravenous pyelogram
   E. Venogram

8. The evaluation of a postoperative patient for intraabdominal sepsis does NOT include:
   A. Review of the type of operative procedures
   B. Complete blood count and urinalysis
   C. Plain and upright x-rays of the abdomen
   D. Upper gastrointestinal series
   E. Physical examination

9. To localize the source of intraabdominal sepsis, the most accurate diagnostic study is:
   A. Flat and upright x-rays of the abdomen
   B. Abdominal sonogram
   C. Abdominal computed tomography (CT) scan
   D. Upper gastrointestinal series with Gastrografin
   E. Intravenous pyelogram

10. The preoperative antibiotic coverage in an 85-year-old woman with known diverticulitis and proven pneumoperitoneum is:
    A. None
    B. Routine preoperative antibiotic prophylaxis
    C. Oral antibiotics to reduce the bowel flora
    D. Combination antibiotics to cover Gram-positive, Gram-negative, and *Bacteroides* species
    E. Oral antibiotics to reduce bowel flora with intravenous prophylactic antibiotics

11. Antibiotics used to prevent wound infection should:
    A. Have a short half-life of 3 to 5 days
    B. Be used in most operations
    C. Be given until the wound is 4 to 5 days old
    D. Be initiated in the recovery room
    E. Be directed toward specific pathogens

12. An increased risk of infection is associated with all of the following EXCEPT:
    A. Protein-calorie malnutrition
    B. Patients younger than 2 years of age
    C. Obesity
    D. Shock
    E. Diabetes mellitus

13. The principal method to prevent infection in soft tissue injuries is:
    A. Antibiotics
    B. Antibacterial dressings
    C. Adequate debridement
    D. Primary closure of the wound
    E. Topical antibiotics

14. The most common cause of rapidly spreading cellulitis that occurs 48 hours after a minor laceration is:
    A. *Staphylococcus aureus*
    B. Beta-hemolytic *Streptococcus* A
    C. *Escherichia coli*
    D. *Clostridium welchii*
    E. *Streptococcus faecalis*

15. Primary treatment of synergistic gangrene of the foot that is caused by *Escherichia coli* and microaerophilic streptococci includes:
    A. Hyperbaric oxygen
    B. Clostridial-specific antitoxins
    C. Intravenous penicillin only
    D. Debridement of the involved tissue
    E. Immediate amputation of the foot

16. The infection that causes fever, bacteremia, and leukocytosis is:
    A. Suppurative thrombophlebitis
    B. Impetigo
    C. Atelectasis
    D. Furuncle
    E. Hashimoto's thyroiditis

17. Match the following phrase with the best single response. Adequately treated with intravenous antibiotics without other intervention:
    A. Suppurative thrombophlebitis
    B. Intravascular device–associated bacteremia
    C. Both
    D. Neither

18. The most important step in the treatment of an intraabdominal abscess is:
    A. Local hot soaks
    B. Drainage
    C. Broad-spectrum antibiotics
    D. Elevation
    E. Immobilization

19. The presence of multiple abscesses in the groin is called:
    A. Hidradenitis
    B. Sebaceous cyst
    C. Felon
    D. Furuncle
    E. Pilonidal cyst

20. An effective vaccine is available for which virus that is potentially transmitted from the patient to the surgeon during an operative procedure:
    A. Human immunodeficiency virus (HIV)
    B. Hepatitis C
    C. Hepatitis B
    D. Cytomegalovirus
    E. Hepatitis A

Oral Examination Study Questions

CASE 1

A 60-year-old man is scheduled to undergo an iliac endarterectomy in the morning for an isolated occlusion that was nondistensible by angioplasty today. Discuss what preparations, if any, will decrease his risk of infection and whether he should receive prophylactic antibiotics.

OBJECTIVE 1

The student should have some knowledge of the types of operation and which types require prophylactic antibiotics.

A. Clean operations (e.g., vascular operations, mastectomy) do not require prophylaxis. However, if a medical device is to be implanted, such as a prosthetic vascular graft (if the endarterectomy cannot be completed successfully) or a silicone breast implant, the antibiotics are standard. Antibiotics should be effective against *Staphylococcus epidermidis*.

B. Clean-contaminated operations (e.g., gastrointestinal surgery have a decreased risk of postoperative infectious complications if one preoperative dose and two postoperative doses of cephazolin are given.

C. Contaminated and dirty procedures (e.g., gunshot wounds to the large bowel, intraabdominal abscess) require treatment that should be initiated preoperatively.

OBJECTIVE 2

The student knows that certain events are associated with increased or decreased risk of postoperative infection and should be included in operative planning.

A. Preoperative showering with antibiotic soap decreases the infection rate for clean wounds by 50%. Patients who have their skin shaved immediately before surgery for clean operations have only one-half as many wound infections as patients who are shaved the night before.

B. The length of the operation affects the infection rate. Patients who have operations that last longer than 2 hours have four times as many infections as patients who have operations that require less than 1 hour.

C. Preoperative stay also influences infection rates. Patients who are in the hospital for more than 2 weeks before their operation have four times the infection rate of patients who are operated on in the first 24 hours.

OBJECTIVE 3

The student can identify a group of patients who have an increased risk of postoperative infection that must be accepted in most circumstances.

A. Elderly patients and patients with diabetes have an increased infection rate that must be accepted.

B. Patients who are obese, malnourished, or receiving steroids also have an increased infection rate. If any of these conditions can be reversed before elective surgery is required, the infection rate is decreased.

Minimum Level of Achievement for Passing

The student knows that the risk of postoperative infection can be manipulated by physician and patient behavior. The student also understands that prophylaxis is not appropriate for all operations.

Honors Level of Achievement

The student can identify the four types of operations and the requirements for antibiotic usage for each type. Also, the student can provide correct responses to objectives 2 and 3.

CASE 2

One day after the ruptured appendix of a 17-year-old girl is removed, she has a fever of 101.5° F. What condition might be developing? What should be done? Does it matter that the fever started on postoperative day 1 versus day 3, 6, or 9? What factors may contribute to the development of fever on these particular days?

OBJECTIVE 1

The student realizes that, in the 48 hours immediately after surgery, atelectasis and other pulmonary problems that may be related to aspiration at the time of surgery are the primary cause of the fever. The student can also spontaneously discuss most of the following points.

A. The more the patient smoked preoperatively, the more the patient can be expected to have postoperative atelectasis.

B. Upper abdominal and thoracic procedures probably cause more pain and interfere with breathing more significantly than extremity or lower abdominal procedures.

C. Atelectasis is usually prevented by encouraging deep breathing, which requires adequate pain control. At times, a patient can be encouraged to breathe deeply only by noxious stimulus (e.g., nasotracheal suctioning). Voluntary deep inspirations are preferable.

D. If the character of the sputum has changed, culture and Gram stain are obtained. On auscultation, if there are decreased breath sounds that seem to be localized at the base of each lung, the culture may be more expensive than it is worth.

OBJECTIVE 2

Fevers that develop only after the first 48-hour period are less likely to be pulmonary. The student knows that, at this point, an infected urinary tract is the most common cause of fever, especially if the patient was catheterized. The student can discuss the following points.

A. Postoperative fluid management influences the development of urinary tract infections, especially if a Foley catheter is in place. Good urine output helps to wash out the urinary tract. Proper catheter care decreases the incidence of infection. It is especially important to avoid contaminating the urinary drainage system by fixing the catheter securely and never disconnecting the Foley catheter from the urinary drainage bag at any point after the catheter is placed.

B. Any preoperative or postoperative cause of obstruction also increases the rate of urinary tract infection. An elderly man with prostatism has a higher incidence of urinary tract infection than a young man with no obstructive symptoms.

C. Any manipulation of the urinary tract during surgery may also increase the rate of infection. This manipulation includes inserting a ureteral catheter or manipulating the kidney or ureters at operation to the point at which they are traumatized and the number of red blood cells in the urine increases.

OBJECTIVE 3

The student realizes that by the fifth to sixth postoperative day, the most common cause of fever is wound infection. Important points include the following:

A. Operations are divided into four classes, and each class has a different grade of wound infection.

B. By the fifth or sixth postoperative day, most wounds are stuck together and are not leaking fluids, so any evidence of fluid exudation from the wound suggests infection. Any postoperative seroma or hematoma that forms in the wound increases the chance of wound infection.

OBJECTIVE 4

After hospital discharge, or if the patient remains in the hospital for a prolonged period because of complications, unusual causes of fever include phlebitis or reactions to drugs introduced after the operation. Significant points include the following:

A. Phlebitis can be accurately diagnosed by duplex ultrasound or venogram, and this route should be pursued if there is any suggestion of tenderness in the leg on walking or to palpation.

B. Any drug that was introduced that the patient did not receive before can cause a drug fever. Discontinuing the drug rapidly reverses these symptoms.

Minimum Level of Achievement for Passing

The student realizes that fevers are caused by distinctly different events at different times postoperatively. The student can list at least three potential causes and can discuss precipitating events with minimal prompting.

Honors Level of Achievement

The honors student lists all of these objectives without prompting.

CASE 3

A 21-year-old farmer comes to the emergency room with swelling and pain in the left hand 3 days after he has a pitchfork injury to the palm. Explain how your examination can identify which type of hand infections the farmer might have, and describe the appropriate therapy.

OBJECTIVE 1

The student describes how to examine the hand to differentiate among the four major types of infection. This patient has a palmar space infection on the ulnar side of the vertical septum (i.e., midpalmar space infection).

A. The student can eliminate the diagnoses of felon, acute suppurative arthritis, and nonspecific tenosynovitis. This patient does not have a felon, which is an infection of the digital pulp at the end of the digit. Acute suppurative arthritis is excluded by the patient's young age. Nonspecific tenosynovitis is out of the question because of the specific puncture wound associated with the onset of symptoms.

B. The student then differentiates between bacterial tenosynovitis and a palmar space infection. The student identifies this infection as a palmar space infection by determining that the swelling in the palm is localized to the midpalmar space, with redness and tenderness to palpation. This condition is differentiated from bacterial tenosynovitis by flexing the fingers, which in this case should not increase pain, because the tendon sheath is not involved.

OBJECTIVE 2

The student realizes that a farm injury could introduce clostridia and gram-negative organisms and requires both surgical drainage and broad-spectrum antibiotics. Important points for the student to realize are as follows:

A. The palmar spaces are divided into the thenar space and the midpalmar space, so any surgical incision should not cross the vertical septum between the palmar fascia and the third metacarpal. The incision to enter the midpalmar space can be made in a variety of ways, as long as it does not cross areas of flexion.

B. Because of the time that elapsed since the initial injury and because of the bacteria that can be associated with barnyard injuries, a combination of clindamycin and high-dose penicillin is the treatment of choice. Any broad-spectrum antibiotics could initially be used, as long as cultures are obtained and antibiotics adjusted if the cultures show untreated or resistant organisms.

C. The student realizes that pain is a serious symptom. Increasing pain is associated with greater degrees of infection. If pain was present but then disappeared, the hand may not be salvageable.

Minimum Level of Achievement for Passing

The student realizes that the hand is a common site of injury. Because of its functional importance, the hand must be treated aggressively. Because of the large number of avascular tendons it contains, the hand is often the site of disastrous infection. In addition, unlike other areas of the body, it cannot localize and destroy bacteria. The student also realizes that the various types of infection travel within the various spaces created. The student also realizes that there are tendon sheaths and spaces between the tendon sheaths. Also, not all of these sheaths are interconnected, and the spread of infection depends on the initial area of injury. The student realizes that gangrene is a possibility in a hand injury, just as it is in any soft tissue infection, and senses the urgency with which this patient should be treated.

Honors Level of Achievement

The student identifies the types of sheaths, including the ulnar and the radial bursas as well as the separate tendon sheaths for the second, third, and fourth digits. The student can also rapidly identify, without prompting, the different palmar spaces, the thenar space, and the midpalmar spaces. The student also realizes that arthritis causes symptoms similar to those of hand infections and includes it in the differential diagnosis.

SUGGESTED READINGS

American College of Chest Physicians/Society of Critical Care Medicine Consensus Conference. Definition for sepsis and organ failure and guidelines for the use of innovative therapies in sepsis. *Crit Care Med* 1992;20:864.

Asher EF, Oliver BG, Fry DE. Urinary tract infection in the surgical patient. *Am Surg* 1988;54:466.

Bohnen JMA, Solomkin JS, Dellinger EP, et al. Guidelines for clinical care: anti-infective agents for intra-abdominal infection. *Arch Surg* 1992;127:83.

Fry DE. Occupational risks for surgeons: hepatitis. In: Fry DE, ed. *Surgical Infections*. Boston, Mass: Little, Brown, 1995:657–668.

Galandiuk S, Polk HC Jr, Jagelman OG, et al. Re-emphasis of priorities in surgical antibiotic prophylaxis. *Surg Gynecol Obstet* 1989;169:219.

Garrison RN, Wilson MA. Intravenous and central catheter infections. *Surg Clin North Am* 1994;74:557.

Gold HS, Moellering RC. Antimicrobial-drug resistance. *N Engl J Med* 1996;335:1445.

Hausman MR, Lisser SP. Hand infections. *Orthop Clin North Am* 1992;23:171.

Jimenez P, Torres A, Rodriguez-Roisin R, et al. Incidence and etiology of pneumonia acquired during mechanical ventilation. *Crit Care Med* 1989:17:882.

9

Trauma

Delford G. Williams, III, M.D.
Charles D. Hanf, M.D.
Virginia A. Eddy, M.D.

OBJECTIVES

1. Outline the steps that must be followed to assess the patient who has multiple injuries.
2. Describe the principles and methods that are used in the initial resuscitation and definitive care phase of trauma management.
3. Define shock, discuss its pathophysiology, and outline the management of hemorrhagic shock.
4. Describe the pathophysiology and initial treatment of both immediately life-threatening and potentially life-threatening thoracic injuries.
5. Describe the diagnostic and therapeutic procedures that pertain to abdominal trauma, including the indications, contraindications, and limitations of peritoneal lavage.
6. Outline the initial management of the unconscious patient who has a traumatic injury, and discuss the complications that can develop after head injury.
7. Define the Glasgow Coma Scale, and describe its point scale and its prediction of neurologic recovery.
8. Describe the therapeutic interventions that reverse or delay the consequences of increased intracranial pressure.
9. Outline the management of a patient with a suspected spine or spinal cord injury, including proper immobilization techniques.
10. List the types of extremity injuries, and prioritize their assessment and management.
11. Describe the issues involved in the transportation or transfer of injured patients.

Overview and Epidemiology

Trauma is the number one cause of death in the first four decades of life (ages 1–44 years). It is the third leading cause of death in all age-groups, surpassed only by heart disease and cancer. In 1996, the Centers for Disease Control and Prevention reported that, in 1993, a total of 151,061 people died of accidents, suicides, and homicides. Of these deaths, motor vehicle accidents and firearms accounted for 28% (41,893) and 26% (39,595), respectively. Overall, the age-adjusted death rates for accidents and firearms increased approximately 3% and 5%, respectively, from the previous year. Trauma-related costs are estimated at more than $100 billion annually. This monumental figure is approximately 40% of the health care dollar. The real cost of trauma, however, is not measured in dollars, but in lives lost. Trauma robs society of its youngest and, conceivably, most productive members. For the most part, trauma is a preventable problem that involves controversial social issues. Until society deals with the issues of gun control, illicit drugs, and drunk drivers, the need will continue to train physicians in managing the associated trauma.

This chapter describes the principles of the Advanced Trauma Life Support (ATLS) program and describes the care of the patient with multiple injuries. The ATLS program was developed by the American College of Surgeons to save the lives of patients who would otherwise die an early death, defined as one occurring in the minutes to hours after injury.

Trimodal Distribution

The time of death from trauma has a trimodal distribution. The first peak includes immediate deaths that occur within seconds to minutes of injury: patients die of lacerations to the brain, brain stem, spinal cord, heart, or major blood vessels. Most of these patients die before they reach the hospital. The second peak includes early deaths that occur within minutes to hours of injury: patients die of major hemorrhage of the head, chest, or abdomen, or of multiple injuries that cause significant blood loss. Most of these injuries can be treated if the patient is rapidly assessed and resuscitated according to the ATLS program within the first hour after injury. The third peak includes deaths caused by sepsis and multiple organ failure that occur several days to weeks after injury. The outcome of this third group of patients is related to their initial care. If proper care is delivered during the "golden hour," the number of early and late trauma deaths will be decreased.

Algorithm

The management of trauma is based on a logical sequence of steps. Conceptually, the process is organized into four phases: (1) **primary survey**, (2) **resuscitation**, (3) **secondary survey**, and (4) **definitive care**. The ongoing care of the injured patient requires frequent repetition of the primary and secondary surveys to confirm the patient's response to therapy. In practice, these activities occur in parallel or are often done simultaneously. The following discussion describes the logical steps of trauma care. This algorithm provides the physician with a method to mentally check and recheck the management of the injured patient.

The primary survey involves the diagnosis and treatment of all immediately life-threatening injuries. This process is the essence of the ABCDE algorithm of trauma management. In a sequential fashion, the physician protects the cervical spine while assessing the *Ai*rway, *B*reathing, *C*irculation, and neurologic *D*isability of the injured patient. *E*xposure of the patient, by removing all clothing, and the prevention of hypothermia, by keeping the patient warm with blankets, are the last steps of this phase. The physician treats all immediately life-threatening injuries in sequence before proceeding to the next phase.

The neurologic disability assessment establishes the patient's level of consciousness, pupillary size and reaction, and motor response to stimuli. The level of consciousness is assessed quickly with the mnemonic **AVPU**. Is the patient *A*lert, responsive to *V*ocal stimuli, responsive to *P*ainful stimuli, or *U*nresponsive? A more detailed quantitative neurologic evaluation is performed with the **Glasgow Coma Scale** (GCS), which is explained later.

Resuscitation is begun simultaneously with the primary survey. The **airway** is secured, ventilation is assured, and oxygen is administered. External blood loss is controlled with direct pressure. Intravenous lines are established, and a balanced electrolyte solution is administered (lactated Ringer's solution is preferred). High-flow fluid warmers are used to combat hypothermia. Aspiration and gastric distension are reduced with the placement of a gastric tube. The patient's **pulse oximetry,** blood pressure, electrocardiogram reading, and urine output are monitored during the resuscitation phase.

The secondary survey follows the initiation of resuscitation and a reassessment of the primary survey. A detailed head-to-toe evaluation, including an **AMPLE history** and a physical examination, is undertaken to identify all injuries: *A*llergies, *M*edications, *P*ast illnesses, *L*ast meal, and the *E*vents surrounding the injury are noted. Tubes or fingers are placed in every orifice. Baseline laboratory studies are drawn at this time if they were not drawn when the intravenous lines were started. Portable x-rays are taken at this time, but should not interrupt resuscitation efforts. Three essential x-ray views are the lateral cervical spine, anteroposterior (AP) chest, and AP pelvis. Special procedures (e.g., peritoneal lavage) are also performed during this phase.

The definitive care phase follows the secondary survey. The patient is reevaluated, and all injuries are prioritized. The care plan is based on the mechanism of injury, the patient's physiologic status, anatomic injuries, and concomitant disease conditions that may affect the patient's survival. During this phase, blood is administered and surgical procedures are performed, if indicated.

This algorithm forms the basis for the early care of the injured patient. Later sections describe the management of specific injuries that are common to the trauma patient.

Airway and Breathing

The physician's first priority in managing an injured patient is to assess the airway. For this discussion, the term airway is used interchangeably with airway management, which refers to maintaining patency of the upper airway, specifically the mouth, oropharynx, larynx, and trachea. Because patients die rapidly if they are deprived of oxygenated blood, every injured patient should be given supplemental oxygen. One common cause of preventable death is failure to recognize the need for an adequate airway. Other causes are esophageal intubation, aspiration of the gastric contents, and failure to provide adequate ventilation. Patients at particular risk are those who are unconscious or who have sustained injures to the head, face, neck, or chest. Those who are intoxicated with alcohol or other drugs are also at risk of **airway compromise.**

Airway Obstruction

The physician who arrives at the side of the trauma patient must rapidly determine whether the patient is unconscious. The physician should listen and feel for air movement from the victim's mouth. The physician should touch the patient and say, "Are you OK?" When the patient's response is appropriate and his or her voice is normal, the *talking patient* informs the astute physician that the airway is patent, the brain is perfused, and ventilation is adequate. However, when there is airway compromise, the physician may hear abnormal sounds coming from the mouth. The presence of stridor, snoring, or gurgling suggests a supraglottic problem. Dysphonia, hoarseness, or pain when speaking suggests a laryngeal problem. Other signs to look for are tachypnea, agitation, cyanosis, and the use of the accessory muscles of ventilation. Agitation suggests hypoxia, and obtundation suggests hypercarbia. The agitated, abusive, or belligerent patient is considered hypoxic until proven otherwise, regardless of whether the patient is intoxicated with alcohol or other drugs. In the worst case, there is no air movement from the mouth and the patient is unconscious. In this situation, an adequate airway must be provided immediately. Patients who are involved in motor vehicle, diving, or falling accidents frequently strike their heads. These types of deceleration injuries can cause hyperextension or hyperflexion of the cervical spine, with injury to the bony and ligamentous elements of the cervical spine. Movement of the unstable cervical spine can sever the cervical spinal cord. Therefore, it is imperative to stabilize the cervical spine while opening the airway. The head and neck are held in the neutral position by the physician or another health care provider who is positioned at the head of the stretcher. This maneuver is called in-line immobilization of the cervical spine. It cannot be accomplished with a soft or rigid cervical collar alone because these types of collars do not assure complete stabilization of the cervical spine. A cervical collar can also hide the trachea and hinder frequent visual inspection and palpation. Patients are often brought to a trauma center immobilized on a backboard, with a cervical collar in place. Adequate immobilization of the spine for transport requires immobilization of the entire patient. An adequately transported patient has a cervical collar in place and is secured to a rigid backboard with straps and tape. The patient's head, neck, and shoulders are bolstered to prevent movement of the cervical spine. If the patient is lying supine on a stretcher, immobilization of the neck while the airway is assessed is best accomplished by designating an individual to kneel at the head of the stretcher and grasp the patient's shoulders with both hands while immobilizing the neck and head with both forearms (Figure 9-1). Next, the mouth is opened with a **jaw-thrust** or **chin-lift maneuver.** In the unconscious supine patient, the relaxed muscles cause the jaw to fall posteriorly. The tongue can then prolapse into the hypopharynx and obstruct the airway. The **jaw-thrust** is accomplished by standing behind the patient's head, placing one's fingers behind the angle of the jaw, grasping it on both sides, and lifting the jaw forward. The thumbs are used to open the mouth by drawing the mouth and chin downward, revealing the oral cavity for inspection. The disadvantage of this maneuver is that it requires the use of both hands; therefore, an assistant is needed to suction or remove any foreign objects (Figures 9-1 and 9-2). The **chin-lift** is accomplished by placing the fingers of the left hand under the chin while placing the thumb anteriorly below the lips. The chin is grasped and lifted forward and downward, opening the mouth for inspection. A more secure grip on the jaw can be accomplished by placing the thumb inside the mouth and behind the lower incisors (Figure 9-3). The disadvantage of this maneuver is that in the semiconscious patient, the thumb can be bitten. The jaw-thrust and chin-lift maneuvers must be done carefully to avoid extending the neck and moving the cervical spine.

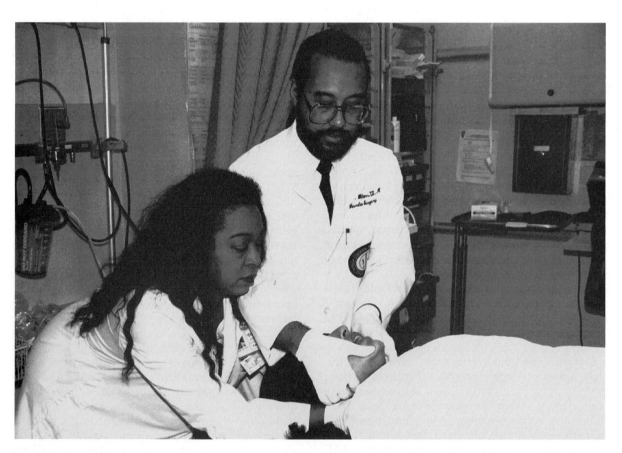

Figure 9-1 In-line immobilization of the cervical spine and opening the airway with the jaw-thrust maneuver. The nurse at the head of the bed has her hands placed on the patient's shoulders at the base of the neck. The nurse's wrist and forearm prevent the patient's head from moving while the physician opens the mouth with the jaw-thrust maneuver.

Next, the oral cavity is illuminated, inspected, and suctioned. Any foreign objects are removed. A rigid (Yankauer) sucker (Figure 9-4F) is preferred because it can be controlled better than a soft, flexible suction catheter. After excess secretions are removed, the airway can be maintained with an **oropharyngeal (oral) airway** or a **nasopharyngeal (nasal) airway**. The **oropharyngeal airway** is made of plastic. It is inserted into the mouth over and behind the tongue. A tongue blade is used to depress the tongue to allow airway insertion. An alternate method of insertion involves putting the airway in upside down so that the concave side is up. When the soft palate is reached, the oral airway is rotated 180° into the proper position (Figures 9-4E and 9-5). The oropharyngeal airway, if inserted improperly, can push the tongue backward and block the entrance to the larynx. This airway should not be used in the conscious patient who has an intact gag reflex because it can cause gagging, vomiting, and possible aspiration. The **nasopharyngeal airway** is a soft, flexible tube that has a trumpet-like flange on one end. It is commonly made of rubber (Figure 9-4D). The **nasal airway** is well lubricated and passed gently through one of the nostrils into the hypopharynx. This airway is well tolerated in patients who have an intact gag reflex.

Tracheal Intubation: The Definitive Airway

If the patient's airway cannot be secured by an oropharyngeal or nasopharyngeal airway, then he or she needs a definitive airway provided by a cuffed tube placed in the trachea. There are several ways to provide definitive airways: orotracheal intubation, nasotracheal intubation, surgical **cricothyroidotomy**, needle cricothyroidotomy, and tracheostomy. Emergency surgical airways include the surgical cricothyroidotomy and needle cricothyroidotomy. Because a tracheostomy is a more complex procedure than a cricothyroidotomy, it is not considered an emergency surgical airway. A tracheostomy is normally performed in the operating room because of the anatomic position of the thyroid gland, its generous blood supply, and its relation to the trachea.

Indications for a definitive airway are based on the physician's knowledge of the mechanism of injury and concern that the patient will need mechanical ventilation, may aspirate blood or gastric contents, or may obstruct the airway because of edema or expanding hematoma. Mechanical ventilation is needed in cases of apnea, hypoxia despite supplemental oxygen by face mask, hypercarbia, and head injury that requires controlled ventilation. Before a definitive airway is

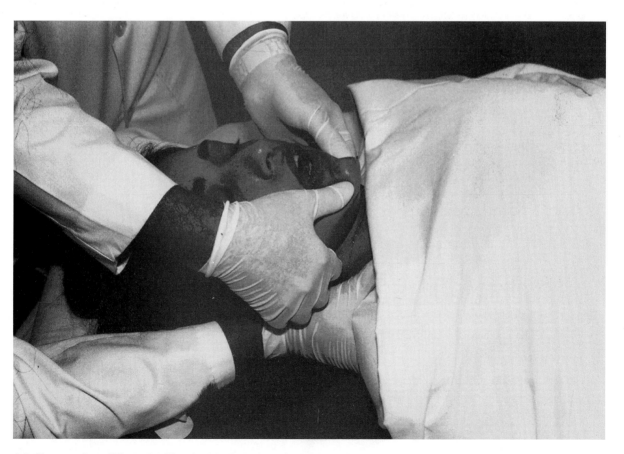

Figure 9-2 Close-up view of Figure 9-1. The physician's thumbs are placed on the patient's chin, and the physician's fingers are placed behind the angle of the mandible. The nurse's thumbs are placed on top of the patient's shoulder, and her fingers are placed underneath the shoulder. The nurse's forearms are placed against the patient's head.

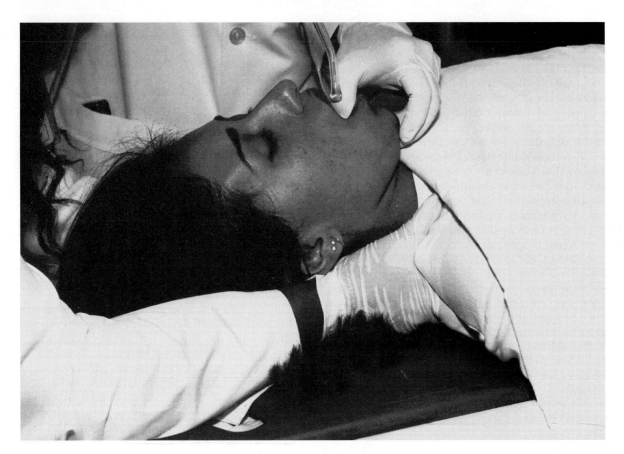

Figure 9-3 Chin-lift maneuver. The physician's thumb is placed behind the patient's lower incisors to securely lift the jaw and open the mouth for suctioning with a rigid (Yankauer) sucker. The nurse's hands are stabilizing the cervical spine.

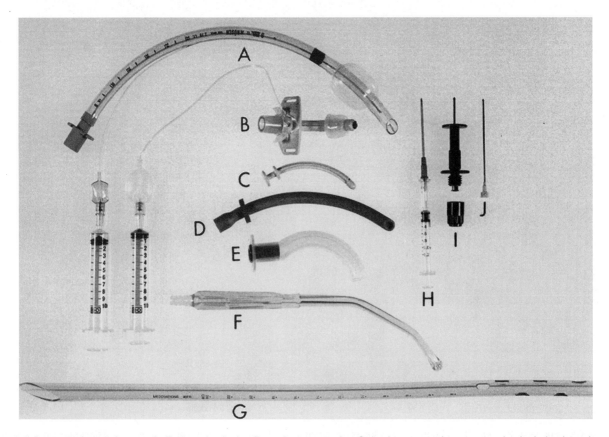

Figure 9-4 Resuscitation equipment. **A,** Endotracheal tube; **B,** tracheostomy tube; **C,** tracheostomy obturator, used only during insertion; **D,** nasopharyngeal airway; **E,** oropharyngeal airway; **F,** rigid sucker; **G,** chest tube; **H,** over-the-needle catheter with syringe; **I,** intraosseous infusion needle; and **J,** intraosseous infusion needle stylet, used only during insertion.

144

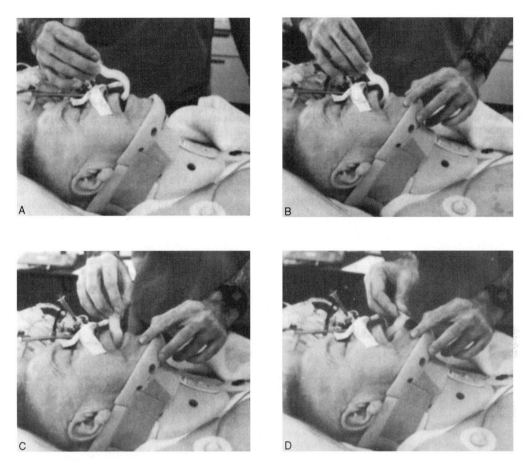

Figure 9-5 Insertion of an oral airway. **A** and **B,** Airway inserted upside down over the tongue. **C** and **D,** Once over the tongue, the airway is rotated 180°. The cervical spine is immobilized with a rigid collar.

inserted, supplemental oxygen must be provide by face mask or bag-valve-mask device, and the physician must inspect and palpate the neck to determine whether the trachea is in the midline, the larynx or the trachea is fractured, or the neck veins are distended. The significance of these conditions is discussed later.

Orotracheal intubation is performed under direct visualization of the vocal cords (Figures 9-6 and 9-7). The patient is maintained in in-line cervical immobilization. Then the laryngoscope is inserted, the vocal cords are visualized, and an endotracheal tube (Figure 9-4A) is inserted through the cords, approximately 1 to 2.5 cm beyond the cuff. The tip of the endotracheal tube is placed midway between the vocal cords and the carina. The cuff is inflated, and the endotracheal tube is attached to a bag-valve device, which allows the patient to be ventilated with oxygen. As the bag is squeezed, the patient's chest is inspected for movement. Auscultation is performed over the lateral aspect of the right and left sides of the chest, in the midaxillary line, and over the epigastrium. The presence of breath sounds bilaterally confirms proper intubation. End-tidal carbon dioxide can be measured to confirm proper ventilation and tube placement. The presence of gurgling in the epigastrium confirms an esophageal intubation; in this case, the tube should be removed immediately. Before

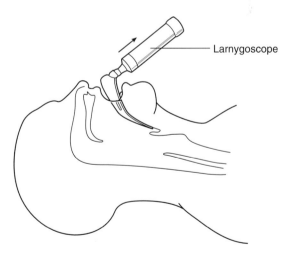

Larnygoscope

Figure 9-6 Visualization of the vocal cords for oral tracheal intubation with a laryngoscope that is fitted with a curved blade. The epiglottis is displaced anteriorly by upward traction on the laryngoscope while the tip of the blade is placed in the epiglottic vallecula. In the trauma patient, the neck is not extended during this procedure.

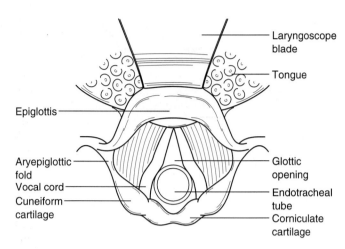

Figure 9-7 Laryngoscopic view of the vocal cords with the endotracheal tube in place.

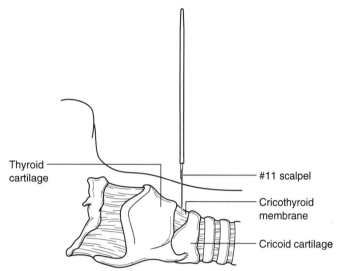

Figure 9-8 Surgical cricothyroidotomy. With the patient in the supine position, a 2-cm transverse incision is made through the skin and cricothyroid membrane. The incision is made in a single stabbing motion with a #11 scalpel blade. The scalpel blade is kept perpendicular to the skin. The cutting edge of the blade is swept upward as it is removed, making the transverse incision.

another attempt at intubation is made, the patient should be ventilated and oxygenated with a bag-valve-mask device. Absent or decreased breath sounds on the left side of the chest may indicate a right main stem bronchus intubation, in which case the tube should be pulled back a few centimeters. However, absent or decreased breath sounds on either side of the chest can suggest **pneumothorax** or **hemothorax.**

Nasotracheal intubation is performed in the breathing adult patient. It is contraindicated in apneic patients and in children because of the acute angle between the nasopharynx and the glottis. In the conscious patient, the nasal canal is sprayed with an anesthetic and a vasoconstrictor (to shrink the nasal mucous membranes). An endotracheal tube is well lubricated with anesthetic jelly and passed gently through a nostril without a stylet. It is then guided into the pharynx. At this point, airflow can be heard coming from the end of the tube. The tube is then advanced slowly until the sound of airflow is maximal. At the point of inhalation, the tube is quickly advanced into the trachea. Successful intubation is confirmed with a rush of air, water vapor frosting in the tube, or expulsion of respiratory secretions from the end of the tube. Finally, the cuff is inflated, and the patient is ventilated with oxygen.

Emergency Surgical Airway

When it is impossible to insert an orotracheal or a nasotracheal tube, an emergency surgical airway is required. This type of airway is usually necessary in patients with massive facial trauma with no recognizable normal anatomy or when the vocal cords cannot be visualized because of bleeding, glottic edema, or laryngeal fracture. In this situation, there are two options: surgical cricothyroidotomy or needle cricothyroidotomy. Surgical cricothyroidotomy is performed by first locating the cricothyroid membrane. The index finger is placed in the sternal notch and moved up the trachea. As the finger moves cephalad, the tracheal rings are palpated. The cricoid cartilage is more prominent than

the first tracheal ring, and as the finger passes over this distinctive cartilage, it falls into a depression, the cricothyroid membrane. This membrane is located just below the thyroid cartilage. Next, the cricoid cartilage is stabilized between the thumb and index finger. The skin is held taut to occlude any subcutaneous veins. A 2-cm transverse incision is made through the skin and cricothyroid membrane in a single stabbing motion with a #11 scalpel blade. The scalpel blade is kept perpendicular to the skin. The cutting edge of the blade is swept upward as it is removed, making the transverse incision. The trapezoid-shaped cricothyroid space averages 0.9 × 3 cm. The knife handle is then inserted through the incision and rotated 90° to allow insertion of a small #4 (8.5 mm outside diameter) tracheostomy tube (Figures 9-4B, 9-8, and 9-9). The cuff on the tube is inflated. The patient is allowed to ventilate spontaneously or, if necessary, is manually or mechanically ventilated. This procedure is not recommended for children younger than 12 years of age because of potential damage to the cricoid cartilage and the small size of the trachea.

Needle cricothyroidotomy is performed similarly to surgical cricothyroidotomy, except that the cricothyroid membrane is pierced with an over-the-needle catheter, which is a standard intravenous catheter also known as an Angiocath (Figure 9-4H). In adults, a 12- to 14-gauge (16–18 gauge in children), 5-cm-long, over-the-needle catheter attached to a 3- to 10-mL syringe is used to pierce the cricothyroid membrane. The catheter is inserted at 45° caudally while aspirating on the syringe. Aspiration of air confirms entry into the trachea. The needle is removed while the catheter is advanced. The catheter is then attached to wall oxygen at 15 L/min

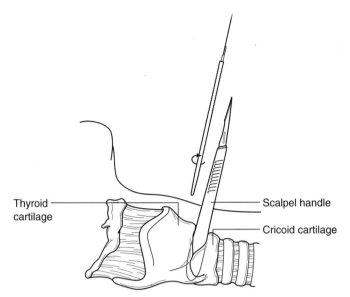

Figure 9-9 Surgical cricothyroidotomy. After the cricothyroid membrane is cut, the handle of the scalpel is inserted through the incision and rotated 90° to allow insertion of a small tracheostomy tube.

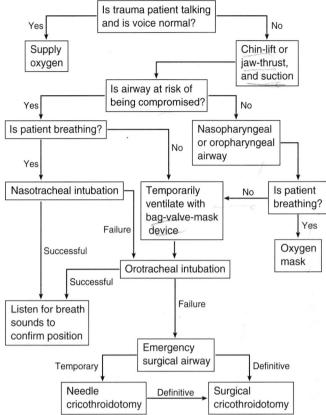

Figure 9-10 Airway algorithm.

through tubing with a side hole cut into it. Intermittent insufflation is accomplished by placing the thumb over the side hole for 1 second and releasing it for 4 seconds. An alternate method is placing a Y-connector between the oxygen source and the catheter. Intermittent insufflation is then accomplished by placing the thumb over the free hole of the Y-connector for 1 second and releasing it for 4 seconds. Adequate oxygenation can be maintained for approximately 30 to 45 minutes. However, because exhalation is inadequate, hypercarbia can occur. Needle cricothyroidotomy is the emergency surgical airway of choice in children who are younger than 12 years of age. In adults and children, this method provides a rapid, temporary airway that allows time to place another type of definitive airway, including a tracheostomy.

Breathing

Breathing is the "B" component of the trauma ABCDE algorithm. The physician must assess the patient's ability to breathe. Is the patient breathing spontaneously? Is air moving in and out of the mouth? These questions are answered by assessing the airway. After the cervical spine is stabilized, the chin-lift or jaw-thrust maneuver is executed. The mouth is inspected and cleared of any foreign objects, secretions, or blood. The neck is inspected and palpated to determine whether the trachea is in the midline, the larynx or trachea is fractured, or the neck veins are distended. After these steps, the physician knows whether air is moving in and out of the mouth spontaneously. However, the next step in assessing breathing is answering the question, "Is air moving in and out of both lungs equally?" This question is answered by auscultation of the right and left sides of the chest, a crucial maneuver that must

be repeated often during the evaluation of the injured patient. Specifically, it should be repeated after any therapeutic maneuver that can affect pulmonary function. These maneuvers include, but are not limited to, the placement of a definitive airway, a chest tube, and a subclavian central venous pressure (CVP) line. The airway algorithm is summarized in Figure 9-10.

Circulation

After ventilation is confirmed by the presence of bilateral breath sounds, the next logical step is to listen to the heart. The quality, rate, rhythm, and location of heart sounds can provide vital information about the patient's circulation. Initial management of the circulation involves controlling obvious hemorrhage with direct pressure, assessing tissue perfusion, and administering intravenous fluids. External hemorrhage is best managed by placing a dressing on the wound and applying direct pressure. Application of a tourniquet is not recommended because it crushes the tissue beneath it and makes the distal extremity ischemic by occluding collaterals. Tissue perfusion is assessed by the patient's pulse, skin color, and level of consciousness. Pulse quality, rate, and rhythm provide an estimate of stroke volume and cardiac output: a weak, rapid pulse denotes a narrow pulse pressure and low cardiac output; a palpable radial pulse indicates a systolic blood pressure that is usually at least 80 mm Hg; a palpable femoral pulse typically means that the systolic blood pressure is at least 70 mm Hg; and a carotid pulse that is not palpable indicates a systolic blood pressure that is less than 60 mm Hg. The patient who is ashen gray with pale nailbeds is severely hypovolemic. As blood volume decreases, so does cerebral perfusion, resulting in a progressive change in mental status. First the patient displays anxiety, then confusion, then lethargy, and finally unconsciousness.

Hemorrhagic Shock

The management of trauma requires a thorough knowledge of **shock,** which is inadequate organ perfusion. The first step in managing shock is to recognize it. The second step is to identify its cause. In trauma, shock is directly related to the mechanism of injury. The most common cause is hypovolemia secondary to hemorrhage. Organ perfusion is directly related to cardiac function. Preload is based on intravascular volume and venous capacitance. Afterload is determined by systemic vascular resistance (SVR), or the degree of vasoconstriction. In hemorrhagic shock, treatment is directed at stopping the bleeding and restoring intravascular volume. Therapy should not be directed at merely restoring the patient's blood pressure. It is not appropriate to use vasoconstrictors in patients with hemorrhagic shock because these drugs increase afterload, which in turn increases myocardial oxygen consumption. Vasoconstrictors also promote ongoing ischemia to the kidneys and splanchnic viscera, which can contribute to the progression of the shock state until it becomes irreversible.

Pathophysiology of Blood Loss

The pathophysiology of blood loss is a compensatory progressive vasoconstriction to preserve oxygen delivery to the brain and heart. A generalized adrenergic response to hemorrhage causes elevated plasma catecholamine levels. The skin becomes cool and clammy (moist) as a result of vasoconstriction and stimulation of the sweat glands by a generalized sympathetic discharge. The degree of vasoconstriction or perfusion of the extremities can be measured by capillary refill time. The patient's fingernail is depressed and released; the interval until the normal color returns is timed. Normal capillary refill time is approximately 2 seconds, or the time it takes to say "capillary refill." This test is unreliable in the hypothermic patient. Tachycardia (heart rate > 100 beats/min) is the earliest response to hemorrhage. Cells that are inadequately perfused switch to an anaerobic metabolism and the formation of lactic acid. Intracellular adenosine triphosphate (ATP) stores become depleted, the sodium potassium ATPase pump is inhibited, and membrane potentials approach neutrality. Cell membrane dysfunction occurs, leading to an influx of fluid into the cell and concomitant cellular swelling. The administration of intravenous lactated Ringer's solution fights this process by restoring intravascular volume and increasing tissue perfusion. Resuscitation is often accompanied by interstitial edema, which is the result of vascular endothelial injury that allows electrolytes, water, and protein to leak out of the capillaries. This capillary leak usually causes larger volumes of resuscitation fluid to be used than initially predicted.

Classification of Blood Loss

The human response to hemorrhage is directly related to the volume of blood loss (Table 9-1). In the 70-kg adult, blood volume is approximately 7% of body weight, or approximately 5000 mL. A class I hemorrhage is defined as blood loss of less than 15%, or 750 mL in a 70-kg person. When a person donates blood, the donation is usually approximately 10% of blood volume, or approximately 450 to 500 mL. If a blood donation is roughly equal to a class I hemorrhage, then it is easy to understand the hemodynamics of this category of hemorrhage. Heart rate is less than 100 beats/min, and there is no measurable change in blood pressure, pulse pressure, or respiratory rate.

Table 9-1. Classification of Hemorrhage

	Class I	Class II	Class III	Class IV
Blood loss (mL) 70–kg person	< 750	750–1500	1500–2000	> 2000
Blood volume loss (%)	< 15	15–30	30–40	> 40
Heart rate	< 100	> 100	> 120	> 140
Blood pressure	Normal	Normal	Decreased	Decreased
Pulse pressure	Normal	Decreased	Decreased	Decreased
Respiratory rate	14–20	20–30	30–40	> 35
Urine output (mL/hr)	> 30	20–30	5–15	Negligible
Capillary refill (sec)	Normal	> 2	> 2	> 2
Mental status	Slight anxiety	Mild anxiety	Anxious/confused	Confused/lethargic
Fluid management	Crystalloid	Crystalloid	Crystalloid and blood	Crystalloid and blood

Urine output is normal at greater than 30 mL/hr. Slight anxiety may be present. Capillary refill time is normal. Treatment is administration of crystalloid solution (lactated Ringer's solution is preferred). A class II hemorrhage is defined as blood loss of 15% to 30%, or 750 to 1500 mL in a 70-kg person. Tachycardia is present, with a heart rate greater than 100 beats/min. Blood pressure is normal. Pulse pressure (systolic minus diastolic pressure) is decreased because systolic pressure is unchanged, but diastolic pressure is elevated as a result of catecholamine-induced vasoconstriction. Tachypnea is present, with a respiratory rate of 20 to 30 breaths/min. Urine output is 20 to 30 mL/hr. The patient has mild anxiety that may be expressed as fear or hostility. Capillary refill time is greater than 2 seconds. Treatment is also administration of crystalloid solution. A class III hemorrhage is defined as blood loss of 30% to 40%, or 1500 to 2000 mL in a 70-kg person. Heart rate is greater than 120 beats/min, and blood pressure is definitely decreased. Pulse pressure is also decreased, and tachypnea is present, with a respiratory rate of 30 to 40 breaths/min. Urine output is low at 5 to 15 mL/hr. The patient is very anxious and confused. Capillary refill time is greater than 2 seconds. Treatment is administration of lactated Ringer's solution; blood transfusions are typically required as well. Class IV hemorrhage is defined as a blood loss of more than 40%, or 2000 mL in a 70-kg person. This magnitude of exsanguination is immediately life-threatening. Heart rate is greater than 140 beats/min, and blood pressure is markedly decreased. Often, it cannot be obtained with a standard sphygmomanometer. Pulse pressure is very narrow and often unobtainable. Respiratory rate is greater than 35 breaths/min, and urine output is almost nonexistent. The patient is confused and lethargic. Capillary refill time is greater than 2 seconds. Treatment is administration of lactated Ringer's solution and blood transfusions.

Treatment of Hemorrhagic Shock

The initial management of hemorrhagic shock involves rapid diagnosis, replacement of intravascular volume, and control of obvious external hemorrhage. A minimum of two large-bore (minimum of 16 gauge) peripheral intravenous catheters should be established and infused with lactated Ringer's solution. These lines should be placed in uninjured extremities using percutaneous techniques. However, in patients with class IV hemorrhage, the peripheral veins are often collapsed, and the only way to gain access is through venous cutdown. The saphenous vein at the ankle is suitable for this procedure. The femoral vein can also be accessed percutaneously or through cutdown. The subclavian and internal jugular veins should not be used immediately for vascular access. They are often collapsed in severely injured patients, and a result, the risk of arterial puncture and hydrothorax is increased. However, in the definitive care phase, when intravascular volume is adequate for safe placement, these sites are used to monitor CVP or to place a Swan-Ganz catheter.

Lactated Ringer's solution is the resuscitation fluid of choice. Normal saline is the second choice because massive amounts may cause hyperchloremic acidosis. This potential is increased if the patient has impaired renal function. Normal saline, 0.9%, has an electrolyte content as follows: Na^+ = 154 mEq/L, Cl^- = 154 mEq/L. Lactated Ringer's solution has an electrolyte content as follows: Na^+ = 130 mEq/L, K^+ = 4 mEq/L, Ca^{++} = 3 mEq/L, Cl^- = 109 mEq/L, lactate = 28 mEq/L.

The amount of fluid and blood needed to resuscitate a given trauma patient is difficult to predict. However, a rough estimate can be made based on the patient's clinical presentation. A general rule of thumb is that it takes 3 mL of crystalloid fluid to replace 1 mL of blood loss. This 3:1 ratio allows for the redistribution of crystalloid into the interstitial and intracellular spaces. For example, if a 70-kg patient loses 30% of blood volume, or 1500 mL, it will take 4500 mL of crystalloid to replace it. It is not unusual to give this amount of crystalloid in the first hour of resuscitation.

The patient's initial response to fluid is the best guide to subsequent fluid therapy. When a patient with hypotensive trauma comes to the emergency room, two large-bore intravenous lines are started and a 1-L bag of lactated Ringer's solution is attached to each line. The fluid is allowed to run in as rapidly as possible (≤ 10 minutes if the fluid is pumped in manually). This method of letting fluid run in as rapidly as possible is called a fluid bolus, or fluid challenge. The initial fluid bolus in adults is usually 1000 to 2000 mL; in children, it is 20 mL/kg body weight. After the initial bolus, the patient's vital signs and urine output are measured. Practically speaking, these measurements are taken before the bags run dry (when there is approximately 250 mL left in each bag, or approximately 1500 mL has been infused). If the patient does not respond to the first bolus, a second bolus is given. In general, if the hemodynamic response after the second bolus is inadequate, then type-specific or O-negative blood is transfused, along with more crystalloid. The response to this initial fluid challenge identifies patients who have greater blood loss than expected or those who continue to bleed. The hemodynamically normal patient has normal vital signs, urine output, and arterial blood gases. The hemodynamically stable patient has normal blood pressure, but is persistently tachycardic, tachypneic, and oliguric. Arterial blood gas measurements may show metabolic acidosis. The hemodynamically unstable patient never achieves normal blood pressure, despite crystalloid and blood transfusions. Arterial blood gas measurements show persistent metabolic (lactic) acidosis. The rapid responder becomes hemodynamically normal after the initial fluid bolus, and fluid rates can be set to maintenance levels. The transient responder's blood pressure increases to normal, but additional boluses of crystalloid and blood are required to maintain blood pressure. This type of patient is hemodynamically stable as long as fluid and blood are infused. The minimal responder or the nonresponder does not achieve normal blood pressure despite the administration of large volumes of crystalloid and blood. This type of patient is obviously hemodynamically unstable, and requires an immediate operation to prevent exsanguination.

The pneumatic antishock garment (PASG), or Military Antishock Trousers (MAST) suit, is an inflatable garment that is sometimes used as an adjunct to fluid resuscitation. It has three compartments and is wrapped around each leg and the abdomen (Figure 9-11). The garment is inflated to a pressure that increases the patient's systolic blood pressure to 90 mm Hg. Inflation of the garment raises the systolic blood pressure by increasing SVR and left ventricular afterload. The clinical role of this garment is controversial. Hypovolemia and the adrenergic response to hemorrhage appear to empty the venous capacitance vessels in the early stages of shock, resulting in displacement of little additional blood by inflation of the garment. It is compression of the arterioles of the lower extremities that increases SVR. Inflation of the abdominal compartment of the PASG can compress the inferior vena cava and elevate the diaphragm, impeding venous return to the heart and compromising ventilation of the lungs. The major

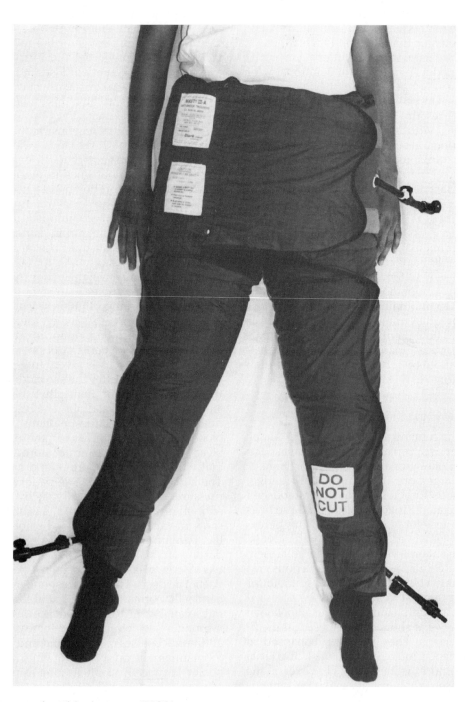

Figure 9-11 Inflated pneumatic antishock garment (PASG).

indication for its use is in patients with pelvic fractures who have ongoing bleeding and hypotension. The PASG splints and stabilizes the pelvic fractures and also controls hemorrhage. Another possible indication is in patients with intraabdominal trauma and severe hypovolemia who are en route to the operating room or another hospital. Contraindications to the PASG include pulmonary edema, diaphragmatic rupture, or uncontrolled bleeding outside the confines of the garment (i.e., chest, face, arms).

Nonhemorrhagic Shock

Nonhemorrhagic causes of shock include cardiogenic shock, **tension pneumothorax,** neurogenic shock, septic shock, and hypoadrenal shock. The patient's initial response to therapy usually allows recognition and management of all forms of shock.

Cardiogenic shock in the trauma patient is myocardial dysfunction that usually occurs as a result of cardiac contusion, **cardiac tamponade,** air embolus or, rarely, myocardial infarction.

Tension pneumothorax produces shock by impeding venous return. Cardiac tamponade and tension pneumothorax are discussed in more detail later. Classically, these patients have hypotension and distended neck veins or elevated CVP. When the cause is primarily myocardial, therapy is based on increasing contractility, adjusting preload and afterload, controlling arrhythmias, and providing mechanical support as needed.

Neurogenic shock results from injury to the descending sympathetic pathways in the spinal cord. It is caused by high thoracic and cervical spinal cord injuries. Patients who are in neurogenic shock are hypotensive without tachycardia. Loss of sympathetic vasomotor tone causes hypotension secondary to vasodilation and intravascular pooling of blood. Loss of sympathetic innervation to the heart produces bradycardia. Primary treatment involves the administration of intravenous fluids to restore intravascular volume. Vasopressors (e.g., phenylephrine) can be used as an adjunct to fluid therapy. Atropine can be used to counteract bradycardia in these patients. Management can be challenging when neurogenic shock is combined with hemorrhagic shock in the patient with multiple injuries. Neurogenic shock is not caused by isolated closed head injuries.

Septic shock is not common immediately after injury. It occurs in patients for whom definitive care is delayed (e.g., a patient who has a penetrating abdominal injury and does not arrive at a trauma center until 6 hours after injury). Septic patients who are hypovolemic resemble patients who are in hypovolemic shock. Normovolemic septic patients have warm extremities, wide pulse pressures, and elevated cardiac outputs. Treatment consists of intravenous fluid, antibiotics, and eradication of the source of infection.

Hypoadrenal shock is caused by adrenal insufficiency. Patients who are taking exogenous therapeutic corticosteroids are at particular risk because the exogenous steroids cause adrenal suppression. Circulatory collapse can be triggered by the stress of injury. The hypotension can be onerous, despite the administration of large volumes of crystalloid and inotropic agents. No specific findings may suggest the diagnosis, except the lack of response to conventional therapy. The diagnosis can be made early, or the condition can even be prevented, if the patient gives a history of taking steroids. Therapy requires the administration of stress doses of hydrocortisone (100 mg every 6–8 hours).

Thoracic Trauma

Thoracic trauma accounts for one-fourth of trauma deaths and is second only to head trauma as the most common type of fatal injury. Although some of these injuries are immediately or rapidly fatal, others can be treated with simple interventions if they are recognized. Knowing the signs and symptoms of these injuries and having a high index of suspicion is the key to early recognition. Of thoracic injuries, 85% can be treated with simple maneuvers that are taught in medical school. The other 15% usually require operative intervention. It is convenient to divide these injuries into groups according to their severity (Table 9-2).

Immediately Lethal Thoracic Injuries

Airway obstruction, the first entity in this category, was previously discussed. Tension pneumothorax, the second type, occurs when there is a continuous build-up of air in the pleural space, with no means of escape. As the intrapleural pressure rises, the ipsilateral lung collapses, the mediastinum is displaced to the opposite side, and the contralateral lung is compressed. On the injured side, the intrapleural pressure becomes positive relative to the uninjured side, and can exceed ambient pressure. The mediastinum and trachea are pushed to the contralateral side. As a result, compression, distortion, and kinking of the superior and inferior vena cavae occur. Venous return to the heart is significantly

Table 9-2. Categories of Thoracic Trauma

Immediately Lethal Injuries	Potentially Lethal Injuries	Nonlethal Injuries
Airway obstruction	Pulmonary contusion	Simple pneumothorax
Tension pneumothorax	Myocardial contusion	Simple hemothorax
Open pneumothorax	Traumatic aortic rupture	Scapula and rib fractures
Massive hemothorax	Traumatic diaphragmatic rupture	
Flail chest	Tracheobronchial tree disruption	
Cardiac tamponade	Esophageal injury	

decreased, and as a result, oxygen delivery is compromised. Unless this condition is rapidly treated, death ensues. Tension pneumothorax should never be diagnosed by chest x-ray; it is a clinical diagnosis that is made by physical examination. Waiting for x-ray confirmation may lead to the patient's death. Physical signs include respiratory distress, tachycardia, hypotension, jugular venous distension, and contralateral tracheal deviation. On the injured side, breath sounds are absent or markedly decreased, with hyperresonance (tympany) to percussion (Table 9-3). If tension pneumothorax is suspected, rapid decompression with a needle is indicated. A 14-gauge (or larger), 5-cm-long, over-the-needle catheter is inserted into the pleural cavity through the second intercostal space (just over the top of the third rib) in the midclavicular line. A rush of air from the needle signifies decompression of the tension. The needle is removed, but the catheter is left in place to prevent recurrence. Needle decompression is a rapid, temporary treatment that converts a tension pneumothorax into a simple pneumothorax.

Definitive treatment requires a chest tube thoracostomy, placement of a polyethylene tube into the pleural cavity, often through the fifth intercostal space in the midaxillary line (Figure 9-4G). The tube is placed to establish a closed intercostal drainage system to remove air, fluid, and blood from the pleural space, thus allowing the lung to expand. The external end of the chest tube is attached to a water seal, which acts as a one-way valve that lets air escape from the pleural cavity. Suction is commonly applied to the water seal to ensure adequate evacuation of the pleural cavity and expansion of the lung. The suction pressure is commonly set at $^-$20 cm H_2O.

Open pneumothorax, or a sucking chest wound, occurs when a large chest wall defect permits equilibration of intrapleural and atmospheric pressures. This situation leads to lung collapse. As the patient breathes, air is heard or seen bubbling from the wound. If the size of the opening in the chest wall is two-thirds the diameter of the trachea or larger, resistance to flow is lower through the injury than through the trachea. Air then moves preferentially in and out of the pleural space instead of into the trachea, thus preventing effective ventilation. Therefore, this wound is immediately life-threatening. The fastest and easiest way to stop this abnormal air movement is to cover the wound with an impermeable dressing (e.g., Vaseline gauze, plastic wrap), taped on three sides, to create a one-way flap valve. During expiration, as pressure in the pleural space increases, air can escape under the open side of the dressing. During inspiration, as pressure in the pleural space decreases, the dressing is sucked down, occluding the wound and preventing air from entering the pleural space. It is crucial not to tape the dressing on all four sides because doing so might convert an open pneumothorax to a tension pneumothorax. Definitive care involves placement of a chest tube and closure of the chest wall defect.

Massive hemothorax is the rapid loss of more than 1500 mL blood into the thoracic cavity. It is a class III or greater hemorrhage into the chest. Diagnosis is made when a hypotensive patient has decreased or absent breath sounds and dullness to percussion on one side of the chest. Initial management is the same as that of any patient who is in hemorrhagic shock. A portable supine chest x-ray usually shows complete opacification on the injured side. Treatment typically begins with the insertion of a large (#36–40 French) chest tube. An autotransfusion device should be set up, if available. If 1500 mL blood is immediately evacuated, the patient will probably require an emergent thoracotomy. If less than 1500 mL blood is initially evacuated and bleeding continues at a rate of 200 mL/hr or more, thoracotomy may still be required. Sometimes, there is no further significant blood loss from the chest tube, and thoracotomy is avoided. A post–chest tube chest radiograph should be obtained to verify complete drainage of the hemothorax.

Flail chest occurs when consecutive ribs are fractured in multiple places (i.e., each rib is fractured in at least two places). This free-floating, or flail, segment of the chest wall moves paradoxically with inspiration and expiration. Paradoxical motion occurs because the flail segment is not in bony continuity with the rest of the thoracic cage. As the patient inhales, the ribs rise and the diaphragm descends, creating negative pressure in the pleural space. The uninjured chest wall expands, but the flail segment, responding to the negative intrapleural pressure, moves inward. Similarly, as the patient exhales, the normal ribs retract, but the flail segment moves outward. Seeing or palpating this paradoxical motion makes the diagnosis. The ventilatory insufficiency that is seen in flail chest is not simply caused by the abnormal chest wall motion. What is more important is the underlying lung injury in combination with hypoventilation. A significant amount of force is required to break multiple ribs in multiple places. Some of this energy is transmitted through the chest wall into the underlying lung, causing a **pulmonary contusion,** which involves extensive intraparenchymal hemorrhage and alveolar collapse. As a result, a ventilation–perfusion mismatch occurs and results in hypoxemia.

Table 9-3. Signs of Tension Pneumothorax and Cardiac Tamponade

Tension Pneumothorax	Cardiac Tamponade
Respiratory distress	Respiratory distress
Tachycardia	Tachycardia
Hypotension	Hypotension
Jugular venous distension (elevated CVP)[a]	Jugular venous distension (elevated CVP)[a]
Ipsilateral absent or markedly decreased breath sounds	Muffled or distant heart sounds
Ipsilateral hyperresonance to percussion (tympany)	Pulsus paradoxus > 10 mm Hg
Contralateral tracheal deviation	

[a]In the hypovolemic patient, this sign may not be present.
CVP, central venous pressure.

The pain associated with multiple rib fractures causes the patient to splint the injured chest wall by inhibiting its movement during ventilation. Hypoventilation is the consequence. Patients with significant ventilatory impairment need mechanical ventilation to prevent hypoxia and hypercarbia. Positive end-expiratory pressure (PEEP) may also be required to maintain adequate oxygenation. Optimization of intravascular volume and myocardial performance often requires placement of a central venous or pulmonary artery catheter. Definitive treatment requires reexpansion of the lung, adequate oxygenation, judicious use of fluids, and adequate analgesia to improve ventilation.

Cardiac tamponade as a result of trauma occurs when blood accumulates within the pericardial sac and compresses the heart. It is associated with blunt and penetrating injuries to the heart (e.g., a car accident that thrusts the driver's sternum into the steering wheel). Even isolated injuries to the small pericardial and coronary vessels can cause tamponade. In blunt trauma, the site that is most likely to be injured has the thinnest wall, the right atrial appendage. However, rupture of other cardiac chambers, including the great vessel, can also occur. When blood leaks into the fibrous, nondistensible pericardium, it compresses the cardiac chambers and restricts ventricular filling in diastole. As a result, stroke volume and cardiac output decrease. The increased pressure within the pericardial sac is transmitted to each cardiac chamber, resulting in equalization of the right atrial, right ventricular diastolic, pulmonary artery diastolic, pulmonary capillary wedge, left atrial, left ventricular diastolic, and intrapericardial pressures. Three classic clinical signs, known as **Beck's triad,** are related to these hemodynamics: (1) muffled (distant) heart sounds; (2) elevated central venous pressure (jugular venous distension); and (3) hypotension. Other signs include **pulsus paradoxus** (a decrease of > 10 mm Hg in systolic blood pressure during inspiration) and **Kussmaul's sign** (an increase in CVP with inspiration). Muffled heart sounds and pulsus paradoxus may be difficult to elicit in a noisy emergency department. Distended neck veins associated with elevated CVP may not be present in the hypovolemic patient. Cardiac tamponade and tension pneumothorax are included in the differential diagnosis in patients who are pulseless, but have cardiac electric activity (see Table 9-3).

The initial treatment of a patient who is suspected of having cardiac tamponade is administration of intravenous fluids. Raising CVP higher than the intrapericardial pressure temporarily increases cardiac output, allowing time to prepare for definitive therapy. Measuring CVP after placement of a central venous catheter and setting up bedside echocardiography are helpful steps in confirming the clinical diagnosis. However, **pericardiocentesis** should not be delayed for these diagnostic adjuncts. A 16- to 18-gauge, 15-cm-long, over-the-needle catheter attached to a 30- to 60-mL syringe is used for the procedure. The patient's electrocardiogram (ECG) reading is monitored with standard leads or a precordial lead that can be attached to the needle with a sterile alligator clip. The needle is inserted 1 to 2 cm to the left and inferior to the xiphochondral junction at a 45° angle to the skin. The needle is directed toward the tip of the left scapula and slowly advanced while the syringe is aspirated. Return of blood into the syringe signifies entry into the pericardium. Removal of as little as 10 mL blood can significantly improve cardiac function. The catheter (not the needle) is advanced into the pericardial sac, the needle is withdrawn, and the catheter is anchored in place and capped with a three-way stopcock to allow for repeat aspirations, if necessary. Pericardiocentesis can be negative if the blood is clotted. If the needle enters the heart, the ECG reading will show an injury pattern (i.e., ST-T wave changes, QRS widens and enlarges). If a precordial ECG lead is attached to the needle, the tracing inverts when the epicardium is entered. Pericardiocentesis is a temporizing maneuver. Definitive therapy requires opening the pericardium, finding the source of bleeding, and repairing it. This repair requires a qualified surgeon. If one is available, then it becomes a clinical decision as to whether to first perform the pericardiocentesis followed by operative exposure of the heart or to proceed directly to the operating room without pericardiocentesis. In extreme cases, there may not be time to go to the operating room, and a left anterior thoracotomy must be done in the emergency room.

Potentially Lethal Thoracic Injuries

Pulmonary contusion is an injury to the lung parenchyma that causes interstitial hemorrhage, alveolar collapse, and extravasation of blood and plasma into alveoli. It causes a ventilation–perfusion mismatch that results in hypoxemia. Physical examination may show a blunt or penetrating injury to the chest. Blunt injuries are associated with chest wall contusions, rib fractures, sternal fractures, and flail chest. The radiographic appearance is that of a poorly defined infiltrate that develops over time. These findings on chest x-ray are usually present within 1 hour of injury, but may take as long as 6 hours to become visible. Treatment includes observation, supplemental oxygen, or mechanical ventilation in patients who have pulmonary insufficiency.

Myocardial contusion is a difficult diagnosis to make. The diagnosis of blunt cardiac injury requires a high index of suspicion, especially in patients who have had deceleration or crush injuries to the anterior chest. These injuries are associated with motor vehicle accidents that involve the driver's sternum being propelled into the steering wheel. Fractures of the sternum or ribs may be present. The anterior myocardium (right ventricle) is primarily involved, and when severely injured, may lead to right-sided heart failure, hypotension, arrhythmia, and rarely, myocardial rupture. Management of this type of severe injury requires ECG monitoring, creatine kinase isoenzymes, echocardiography, and CVP monitoring. Making the diagnosis by ECG is often difficult because the weaker right ventricular electric activity is overshadowed by the stronger left ventricle. However, ECG changes (i.e., depression or elevation of the ST segment) or elevation of the creatine kinase myocardial band (CK-MB) fraction to greater than 6% of the total CK can be helpful in identifying patients with significant injury. Myocardial contusion should be considered in any patient who has blunt chest trauma and subsequently has arrhythmia. Echocardiography may show abnormal ventricular wall motion. Cardiac monitoring for 24 hours is usually all that is necessary in the susceptible, but asymptomatic patient. Longer monitoring is essential for patients who have arrhythmia, heart failure, elevated CK-MB, or abnormal ventricular wall motion.

Traumatic aortic rupture is a common cause of immediate death in abrupt deceleration injuries associated with motor vehicle accidents or falls from great heights. For survivors, salvage is possible with early diagnosis and treatment. Shear forces work on the aorta at sites of anatomic fixation. Common sites are just distal to the origin of the left subclavian at the ligamentum arteriosum, at the root of the aorta near the aortic valve, and at the diaphragmatic hiatus. The mechanical forces associated with this type of injury work on the aorta at sites of anatomic fixation. In a horizontal deceleration, seen in motor vehicle accidents, the heart and aortic arch continue to move forward, while motion of the descending aorta is limited because of its posterior attachments. In a vertical deceleration, seen in falls from great heights, the heart, weighted with blood, moves rapidly downward, stretching the aortic arch and causing injury in this location. Anterior-posterior compression of the chest and abdomen can also result in fracture or dislocation of the lower thoracic spine, which can injure the aorta at the diaphragmatic hiatus. The forces involved in these types of injury are complex and interrelated. For example, in motor vehicle accidents, the body moves forward, the heart and aortic arch decelerate at a different rate than the descending aorta, the chest hits the steering wheel (causing anterior-posterior compression, and the heart is displaced caudally and to the left. As a result, the aorta is exposed to shearing, bending, and torsion stresses that are beyond its ability to maintain structural integrity. If the initial tear involves the intima and media, the aortic blood is contained by the aortic adventitia and a pseudoaneurysm forms. If the initial tear involves all three layers of the aortic wall, the patient exsanguinates into the chest. Ruptures at the aortic root carry a high mortality rate; those at the diaphragmatic hiatus are rare. Of the survivors, most have injuries at the ligamentum arteriosum. Specific symptoms include severe chest or back pain. Radiographic signs that suggest aortic disruption are listed in Table 9-4. Often, however, there are no specific symptoms or signs. Having a high index of suspicion in patients with deceleration trauma may be the only indication for further evaluation. Arteriography is the diagnostic procedure of choice. Computed tomography (CT) is not an optimal study to diagnose this condition. More useful diagnostic studies include transesophageal echocardiography and spiral CT scan arteriography. Rapid operative repair is necessary if these patients are to survive. Preoperative preparation includes control of blood pressure. Hypotension

Table 9-4. Radiographic Signs That Suggest Aortic Disruption

Widened mediastinum (> 8 cm at the aortic knob)

Fracture of the first and second ribs

Obliteration of the aortic knob

Deviation of the trachea or endotracheal tube to the right

Deviation of the esophagus or nasogastric tube to the right

Presence of a left pleural apical cap

Depression of the left main stem bronchus more than 140° from the trachea

Elevation and rightward shift of the right main stem bronchus

Obliteration of the space between the aorta and pulmonary artery

is treated with intravenous fluids or blood, whereas hypertension must be controlled pharmacologically to avoid free rupture before surgical repair.

Traumatic diaphragmatic rupture is associated with blunt trauma to the lower chest and abdomen. The rupture can occur at any site on the diaphragm, but 90% of cases involve the left hemidiaphragm. The pressure gradient between the pleural and peritoneal cavities of 5 to 10 cm of water favors the movement of abdominal viscera into the chest. Blunt trauma produces large radial tears that can permit the stomach, spleen, colon, or small bowel to herniate into the thorax. Physical examination may show bowel sounds in the chest. The chest x-ray may be misinterpreted as showing elevated left hemidiaphragm, gastric dilation, loculated pneumothorax, pleural effusion, or subpulmonic hematoma. If diaphragmatic rupture is suspected, a nasogastric (NG) tube should be inserted to decompress the stomach. In such cases, chest x-ray shows the NG tube curling up into the chest. This finding is diagnostic of diaphragmatic rupture, and no further diagnostic studies are needed (Figure 9-12). If the diagnosis is still in question after an NG tube is inserted, then an upper gastrointestinal contrast study can be performed. On the right side, the liver usually prevents the abdominal contents from entering the thorax. As a result, making the diagnosis of a right diaphragmatic laceration may be difficult. Penetrating trauma may produce small holes in the diaphragm that may take years to develop into a diaphragmatic hernia. Treatment of acute diaphragmatic rupture is direct repair from an abdominal approach. The high incidence of associated intraabdominal injuries makes exploratory laparotomy mandatory.

Disruption of the tracheobronchial tree is an uncommon injury. However, because of the high mortality rate associated with airway obstruction, subtle signs must be investigated thoroughly. Laryngeal and tracheal injuries may cause hoarseness, subcutaneous emphysema, palpable fracture **crepitus,** hemoptysis, and respiratory distress. Severe anteroposterior crush injuries to the chest cause lateral deformation to the thorax, which can result in a traction injury to the trachea and main stem bronchi. Such injuries to the main stem bronchi usually occur within 2 cm of the carina. These patients may have hemoptysis, subcutaneous emphysema,

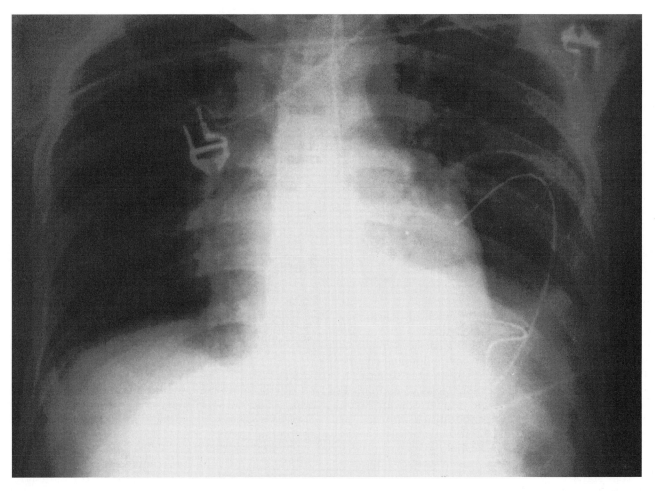

Figure 9-12 Chest x-ray of a patient with a traumatic diaphragmatic rupture. The nasogastric tube is curling up into the chest. This finding is diagnostic of diaphragmatic rupture.

pneumothorax, or pneumomediastinum. The diagnosis is confirmed by bronchoscopy. Treatment may require only airway maintenance with an endotracheal tube. Major disruptions demand operative repair.

Esophageal injury is usually caused by penetrating trauma. If the potential path of a penetrating object is near the esophagus, this injury should be suspected. Blunt injury to the esophagus is rare, but can result from a severe blow to the lower sternum or upper abdomen, which causes a forceful eruption of gastric contents into the esophagus. A linear tear is produced through the left posterior wall of the esophagus. Symptoms associated with esophageal trauma are severe epigastric or left-sided chest pain, dysphagia, hematemesis, left pleural effusion, subcutaneous emphysema, pneumothorax, and pneumomediastinum. A chest tube thoracostomy may show food particles in the chest. The diagnosis can be confirmed with an esophagogram or esophagoscopy. Acute perforations are treated with operative repair and drainage. Patients with missed injuries are usually septic; treatment usually requires wide drainage and esophageal exclusion, including proximal diversion with a cervical esophagostomy, gastrostomy, and feeding jejunostomy. Mediastinitis is often fatal.

Nonlethal Thoracic Injuries

Simple pneumothorax is caused by a lung laceration or a chest wound that extends into the pleural space. Breath sounds may be decreased or normal. Diagnosis is made by chest x-ray. An expiratory chest x-ray can make a small pneumothorax more visible. A simple pneumothorax may become a tension pneumothorax and therefore should be treated with a chest tube.

Simple hemothorax is the presence of less than 1500 mL blood in the pleural cavity. It is caused by laceration of the lung or intrathoracic blood vessels. Blood in the pleural cavity can lead to restrictive lung disease if it is not evacuated. Placement of a chest tube is not only a means to evacuate the chest but also a means to monitor blood loss from the chest. The bleeding is often self-limited, and no further therapy is needed.

Rib fractures are the most common injury in patients with blunt thoracic trauma. Pain with movement causes the patient to splint the chest wall. As a result, ventilation is reduced, and the clearance of respiratory secretions is impeded. Fractured ribs are characteristically diagnosed by physical examination with findings of localized pain, tenderness, and crepitus. A chest radiograph is appropriate to exclude pneumothorax or other thoracic injuries. The upper ribs and scapula are protected by the shoulder girdle and clavicle. Fractures of the scapula and upper ribs 1 to 3 require significant force. As a result, these fractures are associated with major injuries to the head, neck, cervical spine, lung, and aorta and its major branches. Fractures of ribs 9 through 12 are associated with injuries to the spleen and liver. Treatment of isolated rib fractures is supportive. Intercostal nerve blocks may be necessary if oral or parenteral analgesics do not control pain adequately. Analgesics allow the patient to cough and breathe deeply, thus preventing atelectasis by clearing respiratory secretions. Binders or rib belts should not be used to treat rib fractures because they promote atelectasis.

Abdominal Trauma

Abdominal Evaluation

Abdominal evaluation occurs during the secondary survey. In trauma patients, unrecognized intraabdominal hemorrhage is one of the leading causes of preventable deaths. Patients with significant abdominal trauma often have no significant physical findings to indicate intraabdominal injury. The classic signs of abdominal pain, tenderness, and rebound tenderness are often camouflaged by other extraabdominal injuries or masked by an altered level of consciousness as a result of head trauma, drugs, or alcohol. In patients with hypotensive trauma, normal breath sounds, and no external signs of blood loss, the abdomen is a likely source of occult hemorrhage. As many as 20% of patients with acute intraperitoneal hemorrhage have a normal abdominal examination. For this reason, the astute physician must have a high index of suspicion when managing patients who have deceleration injuries or penetrating trauma to the torso. In evaluating abdominal trauma, the goal is to determine whether a significant intraabdominal injury exists, not to determine which organ is injured. If a significant injury is identified, an exploratory laparotomy is performed: a midline incision is made from the xiphoid process to the symphysis pubis. Through this incision, all intraabdominal organs are examined and all injuries are treated.

The abdominal cavity extends from the diaphragm to the pelvic floor. It is divided into four zones: (1) upper abdomen, (2) lower abdomen, (3) pelvis, and (4) retroperitoneum. The upper, or intrathoracic, abdomen is confined by the rib cage. During expiration, the diaphragm is elevated to as high as the fourth intercostal space anteriorly (the male nipple line) and the seventh intercostal space, or the tip of the scapula, posteriorly. The upper abdomen is at risk for lower thoracic injuries. Organs located in the upper abdomen include the liver, spleen, stomach, transverse colon, and diaphragm. The lower abdomen contains the small bowel and the residual portions of the intraperitoneal colon. Pelvic organs include the bladder, rectum, iliac vessels, and in females, the uterus and ovaries. The

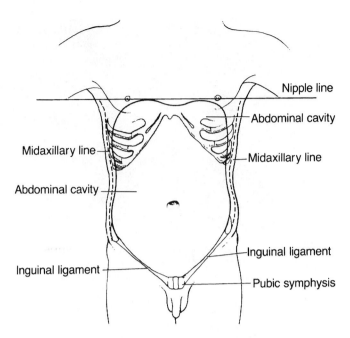

Figure 9-13 Surface landmarks of the abdominal cavity.

retroperitoneum contains the kidneys, ureters, duodenum, pancreas, aorta, vena cava, and parts of the colon. Figure 9-13 shows the surface landmarks that define the abdominal cavity.

Physical examination of the abdomen begins with inspection, auscultation, percussion, and palpation. Inspection of the abdomen begins with the patient fully undressed. A careful inspection of the anterior, lateral, and posterior surfaces of the torso is made, looking specifically for abrasions, contusions, lacerations, and penetrating wounds. When the possibility of a spine injury exists, the patient is cautiously logrolled to reveal the dorsum. Other clues to injury come from noting whether the abdomen is scaphoid, flat, or distended. Auscultation of the abdomen in a noisy emergency department is often difficult. The absence of bowel sounds implies ileus. A search should be made for vascular bruits. If any are found, a specific note should be made about their relation to the cardiac cycle. A continuous bruit implies a left-to-right shunt or, more precisely, an arteriovenous fistula. For example, a loud supraumbilical continuous bruit can be caused by an **aortocaval fistula.** Percussion can elicit subtle signs of peritoneal irritation, and it is another way to test for rebound tenderness. It can also detect gastric distension when there is tympany in the left upper quadrant. Normally, there is dullness to percussion over the liver; however, the absence of this sign or the presence of tympany in the right upper quadrant may indicate free air in the abdomen. Palpation of the abdomen is crucial to the evaluation of the trauma patient. Gentle palpation may show tenderness, guarding, or the presence of an abnormal mass. Voluntary muscle guarding usually indicates a fear of pain, whereas involuntary muscle guarding means significant peritoneal inflammation.

Analogously, rebound tenderness is an unequivocal sign of peritonitis. Evaluation of the abdomen also includes palpation of the iliac crests and symphysis pubis. Manual compression of the iliac wings, inward and outward, may show abnormal movement that indicates pelvic fracture.

Perineal and rectal examinations are essential to the complete abdominal evaluation. Inspection of the perineum begins with gentle separation of the thighs and buttocks. The presence of blood at the urethral meatus or a scrotal hematoma suggests significant lower genitourinary tract injury. Digital rectal examination is mandatory in all trauma patients. Abnormal sphincter tone implies a neurologic injury. A boggy, spongy, or soft prostate may indicate periurethral bleeding, and a floating prostate or one that is found more superiorly than normal may indicate a urethral transection. Blood in the rectum indicates a rectal injury until proven otherwise. Proctosigmoidoscopy is usually required to identify the location of the injury. In female trauma patients, a bimanual pelvic examination should be performed. Vaginal lacerations are easily overlooked in patients with pelvic fracture or penetrating injuries. Speculum examination of the vagina is often required to identify these injuries.

Gastric and Bladder Catheters

NG and bladder intubations are integral to the management of the injured patient. The placement of an NG tube is both diagnostic and therapeutic. When placed with low continuous suction, it removes air and gastric contents. The presence of blood in the NG aspirate may represent oropharyngeal injury (swallowed blood), traumatic insertion of the tube, or distinct injury to the esophagus, stomach, or duodenum. An NG tube reduces the risk of vomiting and aspiration. It also prevents acute gastric dilation that is associated with aerophagia and assisted ventilation with a bag-valve-mask device. Air can be forced down the esophagus almost as easily as it can be forced down the trachea with a bag-valve-mask device. Acute gastric dilation may cause a vasovagal reaction that can lead to hypotension and bradycardia. The outcome of a vasovagal reaction in a hypotensive trauma patient can be cardiac arrest. Caution must be exercised in patients with severe facial fractures because these injuries are associated with fractures of the cribriform plate. In these cases, the NG tube should be inserted orally to avoid inadvertent insertion of the tube through the cribriform plate fracture and into the brain.

Bladder (Foley) catheter insertion serves several purposes: (1) it decompresses the bladder, and (2) it provides a means to monitor urine output, both in color and in volume. Hematuria (red urine) implies genitourinary trauma. Myoglobinuria (red-brown urine) is associated with severe muscle trauma. Concentrated (dark yellow) urine means hypovolemia. Urine output provides an index of tissue perfusion and is the best way to assure that resuscitation is adequate. Appropriate resuscitation should produce urine output of approximately 50 mL/hr in adults, 1 mL/kg/hr in children, or 2 mL/kg/hr in infants younger than 1 year old. In general, urine output less than 0.5 mL/kg/hr (30 mL/hr in adults) causes acute tubular necrosis unless intravascular volume is restored. Before a transurethral bladder catheter is inserted, the perineum and rectum must be examined. The presence of blood at the urethral meatus, a perineal hematoma, or an abnormal finding on prostate examination requires that a retrograde urethrogram be performed to assure continuity of the urethra. A suprapubic bladder catheter is normally required if the urethra is injured. Urethral injuries are commonly associated with pelvic fractures in men. In women, urethral injury is rare because the urethra is short.

Diagnostic Evaluation

Physical examination of the abdomen is unreliable in patients who are unconscious, intoxicated, or insensate below the nipple line. Lower rib fractures may imitate abdominal pain when the bony ends move with palpation of the upper abdomen. In these situations, a more accurate method to evaluate the abdomen is required. Abdominal ultrasonography and peritoneal lavage are two rapid methods. Bedside abdominal ultrasound in the emergency department can be used to search for the presence of intraabdominal fluid, which is equivalent to blood in the trauma patient. Ultrasound is operator-dependent and limited by bowel gas, large wounds, and dressings. It is also limited in its ability to detect hollow viscous injury.

Diagnostic peritoneal lavage (DPL) is an effective method of evaluating the critically injured patient. It is 98% sensitive for intraperitoneal hemorrhage and takes approximately 5 to 10 minutes to perform. In comparison, an abdominal CT scan takes approximately 1 hour to perform, including transport time from the emergency department to the radiology department. The major disadvantage of abdominal CT scan is that the patient must be moved from the resuscitation area. Therefore, CT scan is reserved for hemodynamically stable patients. CT scan plays an important role in the evaluation of retroperitoneal organs and has greater specificity than the DPL.

DPL is an operative procedure that is performed to determine whether an intraperitoneal injury exists. A positive DPL finding is an indication for exploratory laparotomy. The procedure begins after the stomach and bladder are decompressed, a critical step to avoid injury to these organs. Therefore, the patient must have a gastric tube and a bladder catheter in place before the procedure begins. After the abdomen is cleansed with antiseptic solution, the DPL typically is performed through a midline incision just below the umbilicus (except in cases of suspected pelvic fracture, as explained later). The area is infiltrated with a local anesthetic (e.g., 1% lidocaine with epinephrine 1:100,000). Epinephrine is needed to maintain hemostasis and prevent contamination of the peritoneal cavity by blood from the incision. A small (2–5 cm) vertical midline incision is made and carried down through the skin and subcutaneous tissue to the linea alba. The linea alba is incised, and the peritoneum is identified and grasped with forceps. A small hole is made in the peritoneum, and through it, a peritoneal catheter is advanced into the peritoneal cavity and into the pelvis. The other end is attached to a syringe. If 10 mL gross blood is aspirated, the procedure is terminated and the patient is taken to the operating room for laparotomy. Otherwise, 10 mL/kg ($\leq$ 1 L in adults) warmed lactated Ringer's solution or normal saline is infused through the catheter. The lavage fluid is retrieved after 5 to 10 minutes by gravity siphon technique, with the empty fluid bag placed on the floor. A 50-mL sample of the lavage fluid is sent to the laboratory for microscopic analysis, cell count, bile, and amylase analysis. Positive findings for blunt trauma are 100,000 red blood cells/mm^3 or more; greater than 500 white blood cells/mm^3; the presence of bacteria, bile, or food particles; or amylase greater than serum amylase. A negative finding does not exclude retroperitoneal injury to the duodenum, pancreas, kidneys, diaphragm, aorta, or vena cava. Specific indications for DPL in blunt trauma are listed in Table 9-5. An absolute contraindication to DPL is an existing indication for laparotomy (Table 9-6). Relative contraindications include previous abdominal operations (because of adhesions), morbid obesity, advanced cirrhosis (because of portal hypertension and the risk of bleeding), and preexisting coagulopathy. Complications of DPL include bleeding; perforation of the stomach, intestines, or bladder; injury to

retroperitoneal organs or vessels; and insertion-site wound infections.

In penetrating abdominal trauma, the use of DPL is controversial. DPL is not customarily used in the management of abdominal gunshot wounds because these wounds have a high incidence of significant intraabdominal injury. Therefore, prompt laparotomy is required. However, in abdominal stab wounds, mandatory exploratory laparotomy is associated with a negative or nontherapeutic exploratory laparotomy rate of as high as 65%. In an attempt to decrease the number of negative or nontherapeutic laparotomies, many surgeons use a selective approach to the management of abdominal stab wounds. The first step in the hemodynamically stable patient involves determining whether the wound is superficial or deep. In many cases, this determination requires local wound exploration. Superficial wounds that are limited to the subcutaneous tissue require nothing more than local wound care. Deep wounds that penetrate the anterior fascia require further evaluation or observation, with frequent repeat physical examinations. Many surgeons use DPL to help determine whether a patient has a significant intraabdominal injury. The real question is whether the risk of a missed injury is more important than the consequences of a nontherapeutic laparotomy. To address this issue, some investigators advocate lowering the criteria for a positive DPL to greater than 1000 red blood cells/mm^3, whereas others use greater than 100,000 red blood cells/mm^3. Still others observe all patients with abdominal stab wounds. The decision to perform an exploratory laparotomy should not rest on a single test (e.g., DPL), but should be individualized and based on all available information about the injury and the patient's physical condition. Figure 9-14 summarizes the management of abdominal trauma.

Pelvic Fractures

Pelvic fractures are associated with high energy forces (e.g., motor vehicle accidents, falls from great heights). The large bones of the pelvis have an abundant blood supply, and when fractured, the ends of the bones bleed. Forces that injure the pelvis can also rip the sacral venous plexus and cause lacerations to branches of the internal iliac artery. Ongoing bleeding causes the blood to dissect in the retroperitoneal and preperitoneal spaces, forming a pelvic hematoma. As expected, hemorrhage can be massive. Management of a hypotensive patient with pelvic fracture is challenging. After initial fluid resuscitation is begun, a search for unrecognized blood loss must be made, despite obvious identification of a pelvic fracture. If a force is great enough to fracture the pelvis, it can also injure the intraabdominal viscera. If there are significant associated intraabdominal injuries, a laparotomy is required.

As mentioned, DPL is useful in assessing the peritoneal cavity for associated injuries. In patients with pelvic fractures, DPL is performed through a supraumbilical incision rather than through the usual infraumbilical incision to avoid entering a concomitant pelvic

Table 9-5. Indications for Diagnostic Peritoneal Lavage in Patients with Blunt Trauma

Hypotension with evidence of abdominal injury

Multiple injuries and unexplained shock

Potential abdominal injury in patients who are unconscious, intoxicated, or paraplegic

Equivocal physical findings in patients who have sustained high-energy forces to the torso

Potential abdominal injury in patients who will undergo prolonged general anesthesia for another injury, making continued reevaluation of the abdomen impractical or impossible

Table 9-6. Indications for Laparotomy and Contraindications to Diagnostic Peritoneal Lavage

Peritonitis

Positive diagnostic peritoneal lavage

Gunshot wound

Injured diaphragm

Extraluminal air by x-ray

Significant intraabdominal injury by computed tomography scan

Intraperitoneal perforation of the bladder by cystography

Stab wounds associated with hemorrhagic shock or evisceration

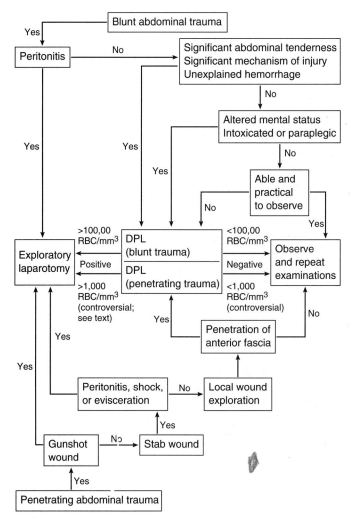

Figure 9-14 Abdominal trauma algorithm.

hematoma. From a surgical standpoint, it is important to avoid entering a pelvic hematoma because attempting to control a bleeding pelvic fracture surgically is extremely difficult. Therefore, management centers around stabilizing the pelvis and permitting the closed retroperitoneum to tamponade. Most of the time, the bleeding is low-pressure hemorrhage from the fracture sites, venous plexus, and contiguous tissues. However, in major crush injuries to the pelvis in which the iliac wings, sacrum, and pubic rami are fractured, the patient can lose more than 5 L blood into the retroperitoneum. Bleeding can be temporarily controlled with the PASG (described earlier). The best method is to stabilize the pelvic fracture with external pelvic fixation (a metal C-clamp or vise-type mechanical device that is applied externally to the pelvis). If external fixation does not control the bleeding, arteriography should be performed to identify any arterial bleeding that can be treated with embolization.

Genitourinary tract injuries are associated with both pelvic fracture and abdominal trauma. Hematuria, whether gross or microscopic, is a sensitive clinical indi-

cator of genitourinary trauma. Patients with blunt trauma to the genitourinary tract and microscopic hematuria usually have renal contusion. Those with penetrating trauma to the genitourinary tract usually have hematuria, but may not. Urethral injuries, suspected when blood is found at the urethral meatus, are diagnosed with a urethrogram; bladder injuries are diagnosed with a cystogram; kidney and ureteral injuries are diagnosed with an intravenous pyelogram (IVP) or a CT scan. An advantage of IVP is that it can be performed in the emergency department.

Head Injury

Head injury is the most common cause of trauma-related mortality, accounting for approximately one-half of all deaths and more than 60% of motor vehicular deaths. Head injury is also the leading cause of disability in trauma patients. Primary injury to the brain can be caused by either penetrating or blunt trauma. Blunt trauma may injure the brain by direct transmission of energy at the point of impact, or at a point distant from impact because the brain rebounds against the inner surface of the skull (i.e., contrecoup injury). Regardless of the mechanism, primary injuries to the brain include lacerations, contusions, and shear injuries. Although primary brain injury is difficult to treat, secondary brain injury is preventable or treatable and, thus, is the focus of head trauma management. Secondary brain injury occurs when local processes within the skull or systemic processes worsen the initial brain injury and cause further damage. Local processes include intracranial hematomas and local or diffuse brain swelling, which can increase intracranial pressure and decrease cerebral perfusion. Systemic processes that can worsen the primary injury include hypoxia, hypotension, and anemia. Hypotension in a patient with a head injury should prompt a search for hemorrhage. Isolated closed head injuries do not cause hypotension.

Cerebral Anatomy and Physiology

A review of the anatomy and physiology of the cranium is essential to understanding the issues involved in the management of head trauma. The mnemonic **SCALP** is useful in recalling the five layers of the scalp: *S*kin, sub*C*utaneous tissue, galea *A*poneurotica, *L*oose areolar tissue, and *P*eriosteum (pericranium). Dense connective tissue within the subcutaneous tissue accounts for the firm attachment of the first three layers, allowing them to move together in wrinkling the scalp. Blood vessels are held securely by the dense subcutaneous connective tissue and are prevented from retracting when severed. For this reason, scalp laceration can cause major hemorrhage, especially in children. This problem occurs with superficial lacerations into the subcutaneous tissue as well as with deep lacerations through the galea. The galea is attached anteriorly to the frontalis muscle and posteriorly to the occipitalis muscle. When the galea is lacerated, these muscles pull the galea in opposite directions. Consequently, the wound is held open, which perpetuates bleeding. The irregular surface of the base of the skull can cause damage to the brain if the brain moves inside the cranium during acceleration or deceleration. The dura mater is a thick, dense fibrous layer that encloses the brain and spinal cord. It forms the dural venous sinuses, diaphragm sellae, falx cerebri, falx cerebelli, and tentorium cerebelli. Cerebral venous blood flows into the dural sinuses through bridging veins, such as the superior cerebral veins that terminate in the superior sagittal sinus. These bridging veins can be torn and are, along with cerebral lacerations, a cause of subdural hemorrhage. The meningeal artery lies between the skull and the dura. Nondisplaced linear fractures in the temporoparietal region that cross the middle meningeal artery can lacerate this artery and cause an epidural hematoma. Beneath the dura is the arachnoid, and cerebrospinal fluid circulates in the subarachnoid space. The vascular pia mater is the final covering of the brain. Injuries to the blood vessels of the pia as well as the underlying brain can cause subarachnoid hemorrhage.

The brain and spinal cord are housed within a rigid bony case, the skull and vertebral column. Changes of pressure within this bony case are transmitted to its contents and affect blood flow into the case. The skull and vertebral column can be compared with a funnel with a long tube attached. The cerebrum is in the mouth of the funnel, the brain stem is in the neck of the funnel, and the spinal cord is in the tube. The brain stem enters the neck of the funnel through the incisura of the unyielding tentorium cerebelli. Within this opening, the oculomotor nerve exits the midbrain and enters the superior orbital fissure. An increase in supratentorial pressure, from hemorrhage or brain edema, pushes, or herniates, the brain through the neck of funnel. The temporal lobe uncus is easily herniated through the tentorial incisura. This herniation compresses the oculomotor nerve and causes the ipsilateral pupil to become fixed and dilated. As herniation progresses, the corticospinal (pyramidal) tract in the cerebral peduncle can be compressed on either side, but the side ipsilateral to the injury is usually jeopardized, causing contralateral spastic weakness and a positive Babinski sign. Further compression can cause dysfunction of the cardiorespiratory centers that reside in the medulla. The hypotension and bradycardia that follow constitute a terminal event. The reticular activating system is essential for the alert state of wakefulness, and is located in the midbrain and upper pons. Altered consciousness can result from decreased cerebral perfusion, increased intracranial pressure, injury to the cerebral cortex, or injury to the reticular activating system.

Cerebral blood flow (CBF) is affected by many factors, including cerebral vascular resistance (CVR) and intracranial pressure (ICP). CBF is **cerebral perfusion pressure** (CPP) divided by CVR:

$$CBF = CPP/CVR$$

Under normal circumstances, CBF is constant over a wide range of CPP (approximately 50–150 mm Hg), and

is autoregulated by CVR. After a brain injury, autoregulation is usually disrupted; in such cases, a clinically acceptable CPP is approximately 70 mm Hg in adults. CPP is the difference between mean arterial pressure (MAP) and ICP:

$$CPP = MAP - ICP$$

Normal ICP is usually less than 10 mm Hg. Generally, an ICP of greater than 20 mm Hg requires treatment to prevent herniation or cerebral ischemia. When ICP rises, the body attempts to maintain CPP by increasing the systemic blood pressure. This early response to increased ICP is known as the **Cushing reflex.** In addition to hypertension, this reflex is associated with bradycardia and a decreased respiratory rate. Brain death occurs as ICP approaches MAP and CPP decreases to less than 50 mm Hg.

Carbon dioxide is a potent cerebral vasodilator that decreases CVR and increases CBF. Conversely, low CO_2 levels increase CVR and decrease CBF. The effect of CO_2 on CBF is linear in the $Paco_2$ range of 20 to 80 mm Hg. These changes in CBF are mediated primarily by changes in interstitial cerebral pH associated with rapid diffusion of CO_2 across the blood–brain barrier. Changes in CBF produced by changes in $Paco_2$ are relatively short-lived because of the brain's ability to restore the interstitial pH toward normal. In patients with head injury, hyperventilation can decrease ICP, but it carries the risk of cerebral ischemia. CBF is also influenced by sympathetic tone.

Neurologic Evaluation

Important information that is obtained from an AMPLE history includes the patient's neurologic status at the scene. Was the patient initially alert, with a later loss of consciousness? Was the patient moving all four extremities? Did the patient have any seizures? In the primary survey, the state of consciousness is assessed with the AVPU mnemonic. In the secondary survey, a complete neurologic examination is performed that focuses on the level of consciousness, pupillary function, and the presence of lateralizing extremity weakness. The neurologic evaluation is repeated periodically to detect deterioration. Hypotension in a patient with a head injury indicates blood loss until proven otherwise. Hypertension, bradycardia, and a slow respiratory rate signify increased ICP. Hypertension, either alone or with hyperthermia, can indicate central autonomic dysfunction. Abnormal respiration [e.g., periods of apnea separated by equal periods of hyperventilation (Cheyne-Stokes respiration) and periods of rapid, deep breathing (central neurogenic hyperventilation)] is associated with herniation.

The GCS is a widely accepted and reproducible method that is used to quantitatively assess the patient's level of consciousness. This rapidly performed assessment assigns scores for eye opening (E), verbal response (V), and best motor response (M). The sum total of the E, V, and M scores is the GCS score (Table 9-7). A normal person has a GCS score of 15; a

Table 9-7. Glasgow Coma Scale (GCS)[a]

Test	Response	Points
Eye opening (E score range 1–4)	Spontaneous	4
	To verbal command	3
	To painful stimuli	2
	No response	1
Best verbal response (V score range 1–5)	Oriented conversation to person, place, and time	5
	Disoriented, confused conversation	4
	Inappropriate words without sustained conversation	3
	Incomprehensible sounds, moans, and groans	2
	No response	1
	Intubated	1T
Best motor response (M score range 1–6)	Follows verbal commands (moves extremity as directed)	6
	Localizes pain (reaches for the painful site)	5
	Withdraws from pain (moves away from painful stimulus)	4
	Abnormal flexor posturing to pain (exhibits decorticate rigidity)	3
	Abnormal extensor posturing to pain (exhibits decerebrate rigidity)	2
	No response	1
GCS score range	Extubated	3–15
	Intubated	3–11T

[a]GCS score = E score + V score + M score. Head injury severity = severe GCS < 9, moderate GCS 9–12, minor GCS > 12.

comatose person has a score of less than 9; and a dead person has a score of 3. It is important to memorize the GCS so that the evaluation can be performed quickly. The GCS score is a prognostic indicator that is closely correlated with outcome, especially in the early stages of coma. It is a useful indicator of the severity of head injury. A score of 3 to 4 is associated with a probability of mortality or a vegetative state of approximately 97%. A score of 5 to 6 corresponds with a probability of death of approximately 65%, and a score of 7 or 8 has a mortality rate of approximately 28%.

The patient's pupils are assessed for equality, size, and briskness of response to light. Differences of greater than 1 mm are abnormal. Extremity weakness is identified by observing spontaneous movements and response to painful stimuli. Neurologic deterioration is recognized on repeat examination by a decrease in the GCS score of 2 points or more, increased severity of headache, increased size of one pupil, or the development of unilateral weakness.

In the secondary survey, the patient's scalp is inspected for lacerations and the skull is palpated. With the examiner wearing sterile gloves, wounds are palpated for step-offs that indicate depressed skull fractures. Bleeding is controlled first with direct pressure. Periorbital ecchymoses (raccoon eyes), perimastoid ecchymoses (Battle's sign), hemotympanum, and leakage of cerebrospinal fluid (CSF) from the nose or ear are signs of a basal skull fracture. In basal skull fractures, blood from the fracture site tracks along the base of the skull, becoming visible as ecchymoses. Cribriform plate fractures are associated with raccoon eyes; their presence alerts the astute physician to the dangers of inserting an NG tube into the cranium. CSF otorrhea and rhinorrhea are difficult to detect when there is bleeding. Placing a drop of the bloody fluid on filter paper and looking for the **ring sign,** or **target sign,** helps to make the diagnosis. Standard laboratory filter paper works best, but if it is not readily available, then a paper towel or bedsheet may be used. CSF diffuses more quickly than blood, and as a result, the blood remains in the center, and one or more concentric rings of clearer (pink) fluid forms around the central red spot.

CT is enormously useful and should be obtained in any patient who is suspected of having a head injury. The CT scan can show intracranial hematomas, areas of swelling in the brain, midline shift, and skull fractures. Plain radiography of the skull adds little to the evaluation in view of the information provided by CT scan, and is usually not necessary. Although recognizing a skull fracture is important, recognizing a brain injury is more important. Brain injuries can occur with or without skull fractures, and vice versa. Occult cervical spine injuries are found in as many as 15% of patients with head injury. For this reason, cervical spine radiographs should be obtained for all patients with head injuries. Table 9-8 summarizes the clinical findings associated with common types of brain injuries.

Management of Head Injuries

The management of head injury begins with the ABCDE algorithm of the primary survey. The rates of morbidity and mortality for head trauma are profoundly affected by resuscitation. The National Institute of Neurological Diseases and Stroke conducted a prospective, multicenter study of 717 patients with severe head injuries. This study showed that the presence of hypoxia, hypotension, or both, at the time of arrival at the emergency room was associated with, respectively, a mortality rate of 33.3%, 60.2%, and 75.0%. Therefore, it is imperative for the trauma surgeon to establish respiratory and hemodynamic stability rapidly in patients with head injuries.

Patients with significant nonoperative head injuries are admitted to the intensive care unit and usually require tracheal intubation and ICP monitoring. There are several methods of ICP monitoring. The ventricular catheter method consists of placing a catheter into the lateral ventricle of the brain through a hole drilled into the skull. The catheter is connected to a transducer that allows continuous ICP monitoring as well as withdrawal of CSF as indicated to reduce ICP. Many neurosurgeons consider the ventricular catheter the "gold standard" of ICP monitoring. A second method is placement of a subarachnoid bolt. With this technique, a bolt is screwed into a hole drilled into the skull and

Table 9-8. Types of Brain Injury

Injury	Clinical Findings
Diffuse brain injuries	
Concussion	A diffuse brain injury associated with brief loss of neurologic function with little or no apparent cerebral tissue damage. This injury is exceedingly common. Unconsciousness is usually short (minutes) and usually disappears before the patient gets to the hospital. There is usually some degree of posttraumatic amnesia. It represents approximately 59 % of head injuries.
Diffuse axonal injury (DAI)	A diffuse brain injury caused by microscopic damage distributed throughout the brain. It is often referred to as a closed head injury, or brain stem injury. Coma is present for days or weeks. The mortality rate can be as high as 50 %. CT scan shows no mass lesion. Treatment is mainly nonsurgical, with control of intracranial pressure. It represents approximately 44% of severe (GCS < 9) head injuries.
Focal brain injuries	
Contusion	A focal injury that is directly related to the site of impact (coup contusion) or an area remotely related to the point of impact (contrecoup contusion). The tips of the frontal and temporal lobes are frequently involved. Focal deficits, confusion, obtundation, and coma can be seen. It represents approximately 15% of head injuries.
Acute hemorrhage	
Epidural hemorrhage	Usually results from a tear in the middle meningeal artery. Classical signs are loss of consciousness (concussion) followed by a lucid interval, then depressed consciousness and contralateral hemiparesis. The prognosis is usually excellent because there is minimal underlying brain injury. Treatment is evacuation of the hematoma. It represents 0.5% of head injuries.
Subdural hemorrhage	Caused by ruptured bridging veins, tears in cortical arteries, or cerebral laceration. Clinical problems are caused by severe underlying brain injury as well as mass effect. It accounts for approximately 30% of head injuries.
Subarachnoid hemorrhage	The most common intracranial hemorrhage. It is caused by injury to vessels in the pia that bleed into the cerebrospinal fluid, producing meningeal irritation (headache, stiff neck). It has little surgical significance by itself because the blood distributes throughout the subarachnoid space and no mass effect is produced.
Intracerebral hemorrhage	Severe brain injury. It is commonly associated with DAI, cerebral lacerations, and gunshot wounds.

CT, computed tomography. GCS, Glasgow Coma Scale.

positioned in the subarachnoid space. The bolt is connected to a transducer for ICP monitoring. This method is used when there is no need for ventricular drainage or when the ventricles cannot be cannulated. A third technique involves placement of a fiberoptic transducer into the epidural space, subdural space, or lateral ventricle. The appropriate method for a specific patient should be left to the judgment and experience of the neurosurgeon.

Care of the patient with head trauma focuses on supporting CPP and preventing elevation of ICP. If it is not contraindicated by cervical spine injury, elevation of the head to 30°, in the neutral position, facilitates venous drainage and helps to decrease ICP. Other methods that lower ICP include sedation, hyperventilation, prudent fluid administration, and diuretics. Sedation with narcotics or paralyzation with appropriate nondepolarizing neuromuscular-blocking agents (e.g., pancuronium) reduce posturing and combative behavior, both of which increase ICP. Moderate hyperventilation to a $Paco_2$ of 30 to 35 mm Hg lowers ICP in most cases without causing cerebral ischemia. Intravenous fluids are administered judiciously to ensure filling pressures that preserve adequate cardiac output. This goal can be accomplished by monitoring CVP, pulmonary capillary wedge pressure, and urine output. Mannitol is a free-radical scavenger and a hyperosmolar osmotic diuretic that effectively reduces brain swelling and lowers ICP. Patients must be monitored for an unreasonable increase in CVP during intravenous infusion of mannitol and later for a decrease in CVP secondary to hypovolemia caused by excessive urine output. Sometimes loop diuretics are given in an attempt to reduce brain edema, but they must be used with caution. Hypovolemia is best avoided in patients with multiple injuries, who may already have volume deficits, because hypotension increases both secondary brain injury and mortality. Patients with head injuries should be closely observed for seizures and treated appropriately when they occur. Diazepam is a common first-line therapy; when it is unsuccessful, longer-acting phenytoin may be used. Nutritional support is important and should be instituted early, enterally if possible.

Other Trauma

Penetrating Neck Injuries

Penetrating injuries to the neck are associated with injuries to the trachea, esophagus, great vessels, and spinal cord. Spinal cord injuries are discussed in the next section. To evaluate penetrating neck injuries, the anterior neck is divided into three zones. Zone I is the base of the neck. It extends from the head of the clavicles inferiorly in one classification, and in another, from the sternal notch to the cricoid cartilage. The latter classification is shown in Figure 9-15. Injuries in this area carry a high mortality rate because of major vascular and tracheal injuries. Zone II is the central portion of the neck. It

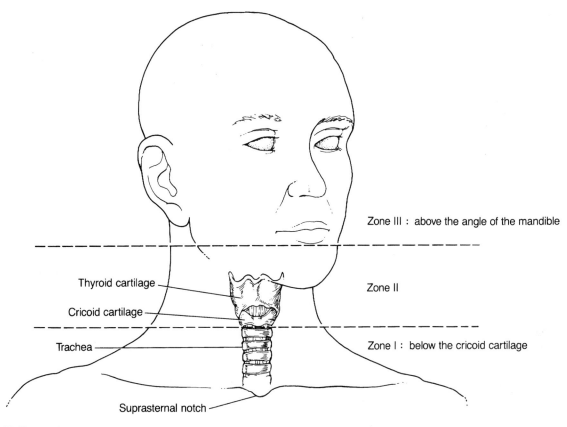

Zone III : above the angle of the mandible

Thyroid cartilage

Cricoid cartilage

Zone II

Trachea

Zone I : below the cricoid cartilage

Suprasternal notch

Figure 9-15 Zones of the neck.

extends from the top of zone I to the angle of the mandible. Injuries in zone II carry a lower mortality rate because they are obvious and operative exposure is not difficult. Zone III is the distal portion of the neck. It extends from the angle of the mandible to the base of the skull. Operative exposure in this region can be difficult.

The student should not be overly concerned about the differences between the two classifications of zone I injuries. The key to understanding zone I injuries is to remember that when the neck is in the neutral position, the bottom of the cricoid cartilage is basically at the same level as the top of the clavicular heads. When the neck is extended, the cricoid cartilage is clearly above the clavicular heads. The real issue is whether a penetrating injury to the neck has entered the tissues below the clavicles. If it has, operative exposure of an injury to the great vessels, trachea, or esophagus requires median sternotomy or thoracotomy in addition to a neck incision.

Differentiating between selective and mandatory operative exploration of penetrating neck injuries requires surgical experience and clinical judgment. Zone II injuries can be explored without further evaluation. Injuries in zones I and III usually require further evaluation. Diagnostic evaluation of zone I penetrating injuries is advisable because the great vessels are located in this area. Zone III penetrating injuries need further study because gaining control of the distal internal carotid can be arduous. Preoperative diagnostic studies include arteriography, esophagography, and endoscopy. Endoscopic evaluation often involves laryngoscopy, bronchoscopy, and esophagoscopy.

Spine and Spinal Cord Injury

Any patient who has significant multiple injuries should be assumed to have a potential vertebral spine injury. In these patients, the entire spine is immobilized with a rigid cervical collar and a long spine board. Spinal injury precautions continue until the spine is radiographically and clinically evaluated and fractures and dislocations are excluded. Patients with injury above the clavicles should be considered to have a cervical spine injury until proven otherwise. As many as 10% of patients who are unconscious on presentation have an associated cervical spine injury.

Physical examination begins with assessment of the vital signs. Hypotension associated with bradycardia suggests neurogenic shock, especially in high thoracic and cervical cord injuries (usually above the T-5 level). Other findings that suggest cervical spine injury include flaccid areflexia; diaphragmatic breathing; the ability to flex, but not extend the elbow (in which case the injury involves the C-7 nerve root, which supplies the triceps); grimaces to pain above, but not below, the clavicles; and priapism. Spinal injury is commonly associated with local pain and tenderness. Patients with these symptoms require careful evaluation. Less frequently, an anatomic deformity is palpated. Examination requires the patient to be carefully log-rolled: while in-line vertebral immobilization is maintained, the back is inspected and the spine is palpated from the base of the skull to the tip of the coccyx. The unconscious patient should be considered to have an occult spine injury until proven otherwise. A patient who is mentally alert, sober, and normal neurologically; has no neck pain; and can actively move his or her neck through a complete range of motion usually does not have a cervical spine injury.

Motor and sensory function is assessed, and based on this assessment, the diagnosis of complete or incomplete cord lesion is made. In a complete spinal cord transection, there is no motor or sensory function below the injury. This situation has a dismal prognosis, with minimal recovery, if any. Patients with incomplete cord injury have some sensory or motor function and are more likely to have significant recovery. The corticospinal tract is located in the posterolateral portion of the cord and is involved in motor function on the same side of the body. Pain and temperature are transmitted by the lateral spinothalamic tract, which is located in the anterolateral portion of the cord. Proprioception, deep touch, two-point discrimination, and vibration are carried in the posterior columns. Light touch is often preserved in incomplete cord injuries because it is conveyed by both the lateral spinothalamic tract and the posterior columns. Sparing of the sacral dermatomes is also seen in incomplete spinal lesions. Preservation of rectal tone and the bulbocavernosus reflex are signs of sacral sparing.

Spinal shock is a neurologic condition that occurs after spinal cord injury. It is caused by acute loss of stimulation from higher levels. This shock, or stun, to the injured cord makes the cord appear functionless. There is complete flaccidity and areflexia instead of the predicted spasticity, hyperreflexia, and positive Babinski sign that are seen in the classic upper motor neuron lesion. Spinal shock may last days to weeks after injury. As it abates, motor tone becomes spastic, reflexes are accentuated, and the Babinski sign becomes positive. Spinal shock is not synonymous with neurogenic shock.

Radiologic assessment of vertebral injury usually begins during resuscitation. In most cases, lateral cervical spine, AP chest, and AP pelvis x-rays are taken first. An acceptable lateral cervical spine x-ray is required to show the base of the skull, seven cervical vertebrae, and the superior aspect of the first thoracic vertebra (T-1). If the top of T-1 is not visualized, then a "swimmer's view" is taken (i.e., x-ray through the axilla of the lower cervical and upper thoracic spine). During the secondary survey, other x-rays are obtained, including an open-mouth odontoid view, an AP cervical view, two oblique cervical views, and an AP thoracolumbar view.

Initial management focuses on the ABCDE algorithm and on vertebral spine immobilization. Hypotension is first managed with intravenous fluids (described earlier). In clinical trials, patients who received high-dose methylprednisolone sodium succinate within 8 hours of spinal cord injury had improved neurologic recovery.

Based on this evidence, many neurosurgeons treat blunt spinal cord injuries with 30 mg/kg methylprednisolone, followed by an infusion of 5.4 mg/kg/hr for 23 hours. For this therapy to be effective, it must be started within the first 8 hours after injury. Definitive care involves spinal stabilization followed by rehabilitation, which is an important part of long-term management.

Pediatric Trauma

Trauma is the leading cause of death in the pediatric population. Although the resuscitation priorities (ABCDE algorithm) are the same for children as for adults, anatomic differences require modifications to the approach. Because of their greater surface area to body mass ratio, children lose heat more quickly. For this reason, care must be taken to keep the child warm. Airway management also differs because the child's larynx is more cranial and anterior, and the trachea is shorter. Orotracheal intubation is the preferred route. Nasotracheal intubation is contraindicated because of anatomic factors that increase the risk of injury to the nasopharynx as well as the risk of penetration into the calvarium. Uncuffed endotracheal tubes are used because, in a child, the cricoid is the narrowest part of the airway, and it forms a natural seal around the tube. Tube size can be estimated by the diameter of the child's fifth finger or external nares. In a child, as in an adult, the first response to hypovolemia is tachycardia. However, because tachycardia can also be caused by fear or pain, it is important to monitor other signs of organ perfusion (e.g., urine output). Children have an enormous physiologic reserve and usually do not become hypotensive until they lose more than 45% of their blood volume. At this point, tachycardia can quickly convert to bradycardia, and unless the child is resuscitated rapidly, circulatory arrest occurs. Normal systolic blood pressure for a child is approximately 80 mm Hg plus twice the child's age in years, and diastolic pressure is two-thirds (67%) of the systolic blood pressure. Therefore, a 10-year-old child's systolic blood pressure should be 80 + 2 (10) = 100 mm Hg, and the diastolic blood pressure should be 100 (0.67) = 67 mm Hg.

Management priorities are the same for children as for adults. Volume resuscitation begins with the placement of two peripheral intravenous lines. If percutaneous access fails after at least two attempts in a child who is younger than 6 years of age, an intraosseous infusion needle (Figure 9-4I) can be inserted into the tibia for bone marrow infusion of crystalloid solution. In children who are 6 years of age or older, a venous cutdown may be necessary if percutaneous access is not possible. Common femoral lines should be avoided in infants and children because of the high incidence of venous thrombosis and limb ischemia from iatrogenic arterial injury. Warm, lactated Ringer's solution is used for resuscitation, beginning with an initial bolus of 20 mL/kg. If there is no improvement, a second bolus is given. If, after two boluses, the child shows minimal or no improvement, a third bolus is given. If the patient remains hemodynamically unstable, a transfusion of 10 mL/kg of packed red blood cells is promptly instituted. It is important to remember that a child's blood volume is approximately 8% of body weight, or 80 mL/kg.

Because a child's skeleton is softer and more pliable than an adult's, a child's bones can take a great deal of force without breaking. Therefore, in a child, a broken bone is evidence of injury from a massive force. However, the absence of broken bones does not exclude serious injury. Child abuse should be suspected when a child has repeated episodes of injury, when there is a delay in seeking medical attention, when parental response is inappropriate, or when there are discrepancies between the history and the degree of injury. Certain types of injuries suggest abuse: multiple old scars or fractures, scars that resemble cigarette or rope burns, long bone fractures in children younger than 3 years of age, genital or perineal injuries, perioral trauma, internal injuries without a history of trauma, multiple subdural hematomas, and retinal hemorrhage. Health care personnel are required by law to report suspected child abuse to local authorities.

Trauma in Women

Domestic violence is the leading cause of death in women 15 to 44 years old. Trauma is now the leading cause of death in pregnant women. The most important principle in managing the pregnant trauma victim is that resuscitating the mother will resuscitate the fetus. Once obvious shock develops in the mother, the chances of saving the fetus are approximately 20%. The uterine vascular bed is a passive, low-resistance system, without autoregulation. Thus, uterine blood flow is dependent on uterine perfusion pressure. Significant maternal hemorrhage causes uterine artery vasoconstriction, which reduces uterine blood flow. Uterine perfusion can decrease by as much as 20% before changes in the mother's vital signs are seen. If low uterine perfusion is uncorrected, the fetus becomes hypoxic and ultimately bradycardic. Maternal hypotension is best managed with vigorous resuscitation with lactated Ringer's solution. The use of vasopressors to support blood pressure is contraindicated because these drugs further decrease uterine perfusion and increase fetal distress.

Several important physiologic changes occur during pregnancy. Plasma volume expands by 40% to 50% and is proportionately greater than the expanded red blood cell mass. This expansion causes a decrease in hematocrit and accounts for the physiologic anemia that is seen in pregnancy. Systolic and diastolic blood pressure decrease by 5 to 15 mm Hg because of decreased SVR. Auscultation of the heart may show grade I to II systolic flow murmurs and S3 heart sounds. ECG may show left axis deviation. Cardiac output is increased by 1 to 1.5 L/min. Compression of the vena cava by the uterus can significantly decrease cardiac output by 30% to 40%, especially in the last trimester. Therefore, unless contraindicated by an assumed spinal injury, appropriate management of the pregnant woman demands that she be placed in the left lateral decubitus position. If she cannot be turned, then the right hip should be elevated and flexed to relieve vena cava compression. Appropriate spinal precautions are maintained during these maneuvers.

The respiratory system is affected by the size of the uterus. Upward displacement of the diaphragm causes a decrease in residual volume and increases the patient's susceptibility to atelectasis. Progesterone stimulates hyperventilation, with an increase in minute ventilation and tidal volume. Hypocapnia is common with $PaCO_2$ of approximately 30 mm Hg. Impaired function of the lower esophageal sphincter, delayed gastric emptying, and decreased intestinal motility predispose these patients to aspiration. Early NG tube placement is therefore indicated. The white blood cell count is commonly 10,000 to 12,000 cells/mm^3, and may increase to 20,000 cells/mm^3 in late pregnancy.

Management of the injured pregnant patient is basically the same as that of the nonpregnant patient. The major difference is that two or more lives are at risk. Because of their physiologically expanded blood volume, pregnant women can lose 30% to 35% of their blood volume before becoming hypotensive. In addition, some effort should be made to limit exposure to x-rays and anesthesia to minimize the teratogenic risk to the fetus. Evaluation of the pregnant trauma patient includes an obstetric history and physical examination. Important information includes the date of the last menses, the expected date of confinement, the number and outcome of past pregnancies, and the most recent fetal movement. Abruptio placentae is associated with uterine tenderness and contraction, with or without vaginal bleeding. Ruptured chorioamniotic membranes are associated with excess vaginal fluid with a pH of 7 to 7.5.

Fetal evaluation consists of assessing the uterus and fundal height and documenting fetal heart tones, heart rate, and movement. The normal fetal heart rate is 120 to 160 beats/min. A heart rate of less than 100 beats/min indicates bradycardia. The Doppler ultrasonic cardioscope is the best method of monitoring fetal heart rate and rhythm. Early decelerations of heart rate associated with uterine contractions are not considered significant; however, late decelerations that occur after uterine contractions imply fetal hypoxia. In Rh-negative women, the Kleihauer-Betke test can detect fetomaternal hemorrhage, and the administration of Rh immunoglobulin can prevent Rh alloimmunization of the mother and subsequent erythroblastosis fetalis.

Medically indicated radiographic studies should not be avoided simply to spare the fetus possible exposure to ionizing radiation. The greatest period of risk for radiation-induced anomalies is during the first 16 weeks of gestational life. This risk also appears to be directly proportional to the amount of exposure. In general, a fetal dose of less than 10 rad is believed to be reasonably safe. Low-dose exposure is defined as less than 1 rad, or 1000 mrad. A standard chest x-ray delivers approximately 10 mrad to the chest, and with proper shielding, it delivers negligible amounts of radiation to the fetus (< 1 mrad). An AP view of the abdomen delivers approximately 220 mrad to the skin and 70 mrad to the fetus.

When there is a concern about intraabdominal injury, ultrasound or DPL can be used to further evaluate the patient. Ultrasound is an excellent choice because, in addition to providing information about the presence of intraperitoneal fluid or blood, it can provide information about the fetus, placenta, and uterus. Indications for DPL in a pregnant woman are the same as those in a nonpregnant patient. However, the incision is properly made above the apex of the uterine fundus.

Extremity Trauma

Extremity injuries are usually not immediately life-threatening, except in the case of uncontrolled hemorrhage. Potentially life-threatening injuries are major crush injuries, severe open fractures, proximal amputations, and multiple fractures. Limb-threatening injuries are vascular injuries, **compartment syndromes,** open fractures, crush injuries, and major dislocations. In the primary survey, proper management includes controlling obvious hemorrhage with direct pressure. A tourniquet is applied only as a last resort because it crushes the tissue beneath it and makes the distal extremity ischemic by occluding collaterals. In the secondary survey, the limbs are thoroughly examined and appropriate x-rays are taken. Early care involves alignment and splinting of the extremity, restoration of perfusion, wound care, and tetanus prophylaxis.

The physical examination begins with exposure of the extremities. Inspection of the limbs involves noting the color and looking for wounds, deformities, and swelling. Palpation begins with an assessment of temperature, tenderness, crepitation, capillary fill, and quality of the pulses. Every long bone is palpated. Sensory and motor function is tested. An injury to a major blood vessel is likely if there are hard signs of vascular injury (e.g., history of significant blood loss at the scene, brisk bleeding from the wound, expanding hematoma, bruits, thrills, abnormal pulses). A vascular injury is possible if the injury is near a major blood vessel, especially in the case of gunshot and stab wounds. In these cases, the circulation to the extremity is assessed with a continuous-wave Doppler flow probe. Doppler pressures are taken by placing an appropriately sized blood pressure cuff around the extremity distal to the suspected injury. The recorded blood pressure of an artery is based on the location of the blood pressure cuff, not the location of the Doppler. It is useful to compare the pressures in all four extremities. When the Doppler ankle pressure is compared with the Doppler brachial pressure, it is called an ankle–brachial index (ABI). Pressures in the legs are normally higher than in the arms, so the ABI is greater than 1. Normally, pressures are equal between segments in the same extremity. Any deviation from the norm implies a traumatic, flow-restricting lesion until proven otherwise. For example, arterial injuries that cause vessel transection, thrombo-sis, intimal flap, or vasospasm are flow-restricting lesions. Other injuries that cause a pseudoaneurysm (hole in the arterial wall) or an arteriovenous fistula may not be flow-restricting. As a result, pulses and Doppler pressures may be normal.

Vascular injuries can be obvious or occult. Transmural arterial wall injuries rarely heal spontaneously, and if they are not treated appropriately, may cause gangrene, stroke, or bleeding. Because missed arterial injuries can produce serious complications hours to years after injury, early diagnosis and treatment is essential. Diagnostic vascular imaging is often necessary to completely evaluate the structural integrity of the vascular system. These studies are used to augment the physical and Doppler examination, to exclude the presence of an injury, to locate an injury exactly, and to identify anatomic features that may affect operative management. Arteriography is considered the gold standard. However, other less invasive modalities (e.g., duplex scan, spiral CT angiography, magnetic resonance angiography) are also useful.

The management of blunt and penetrating injuries to the extremities requires a thorough knowledge of vascular anatomy. Supracondylar fractures of the humerus, severely displaced fractures of the knee, and knee dislocations are frequently associated with significant injuries to the brachial and popliteal arteries, respectively. Arteriography is usually indicated in these injuries, despite the lack of any clinical signs of vascular injury. Gunshot and stab wounds that are in close proximity to major blood vessels require close scrutiny. Arterial and venous injuries can be occult. In the absence of abnormal Doppler pressures and other clinical signs of vascular injury, these extremities may require diagnostic vascular imaging. Determining whether contrast arteriography, duplex scan, or spiral CT angiography is necessary requires the expertise of a surgeon who has a solid knowledge of three-dimensional vascular anatomy.

Traumatic amputations, especially of the proximal limb, are severe open wounds that carry significant risk to life and limb. These amputations can be complete or incomplete. When the amputated part has been crushed and there is severe soft tissue damage, there is little hope for replantation. However, when the ends have been sharply severed, with minimal distal soft tissue injury, there is potential for replantation. The more distal the amputation, the better the prognosis for replantation. The amputated part should be cleansed of gross dirt, wrapped in a saline-moistened sterile towel, placed in a sterile plastic bag, sealed, and transported in an insulated container filled with crushed ice and water. Keeping the part cold, but not allowing it to freeze, is essential for successful replantation.

Wounds are inspected to determine the extent of tissue injury. All wounds are irrigated with saline and debrided of foreign material and devitalized tissue. Depending on the extent of injury and degree of contamination, wounds may be closed primarily with sutures, left open to be closed later (delayed primary closure), or left open to be closed by secondary intention. Wounds may also be skin grafted, or closed with a cutaneous or myocutaneous flap. Tetanus prophylaxis is essential and is given based on established criteria. The risk of infection is considered, and appropriate antibiotics are given as indicated.

Fractures can cause significant blood loss. For example, a femur fracture can account for the loss of 1500 mL blood into the thigh. The larger the number of fractures, the greater the associated blood loss and the greater the risk of hemorrhagic shock. Dislocations should be reduced as soon as possible. The longer the delay in reducing a dislocated hip, the greater the risk of avascular necrosis of the femoral head. If a wound is associated with a fracture, then it is assumed that the wound communicates with the fracture. Therefore, this type of fracture is treated as an open fracture. An open fracture is, by definition, contaminated, and it requires immediate treatment to avoid infection. The administration of an intravenous broad-spectrum antibiotic that is effective against staphylococcus and streptococcus is an integral part of the management of an open fracture.

Compartment syndrome is associated with conditions that increase fascial compartmental pressure. This increase, in turn, causes interstitial tissue pressure to become higher than capillary perfusion pressure. The result is ischemia of the muscles and nerves within the fascial compartment. The syndrome usually takes hours to develop, but may develop rapidly (e.g., when there is an arterial bleed into a compartment). It typically occurs in the calf and forearm, but can also occur in the thigh, arm, foot, and hand. Muscular swelling and compartmental bleeding are the usual etiologic factors. Initiating events include arterial injuries, crush injuries, fractures, prolonged compression, and restoration of blood flow to a previously ischemic extremity. An early sign is decreased sensation, caused by neural ischemia, in the distribution of the compartmental nerves. Other signs and symptoms include pain, especially pain that is exacerbated by passive stretch of the involved muscles, a tense swollen compartment, and weakness of the involved muscle. Decreased pulses and capillary filling are not reliable findings because they usually do not occur until late in the evolution of this condition. The diagnosis is usually made clinically; however, compartmental pressures can be measured whenever there is a question about the diagnosis. Compartmental pressures greater than 35 to 40 mm Hg confirm the diagnosis. Treatment is surgical **fasciotomy.** With reestablishment of capillary blood flow, there is a general outpouring of acidic blood, potassium, myoglobin, and other cellular metabolites into the systemic circulation. Adequate renal function is necessary to clear these ischemic by-products from the circulation. Myoglobin-induced acute renal failure is of great concern whenever there is severe muscle injury. Myoglobin exerts its toxicity in acid urine through direct tubular cell injury and through precipitation, which causes obstruction of the renal tubules. Treatment requires the maintenance of a high urine output (100 mL/hr or 1 mL/kg/hr) and alkalinization of the urine (pH > 7.0).

Transfer of the Injured Patient

Outcome is enhanced when patients are cared for at regional trauma centers. It is no longer appropriate for trauma patients to be taken to the closest hospital; instead, they should be taken to the closest appropriate trauma center. In most major metropolitan areas, trauma patients are transported by emergency medical services to designated trauma facilities. However, it is not unusual for a trauma victim to be taken to the nearest hospital by friends or family. In rural areas, the patient initially may need to be taken to the closest hospital. Therefore, it is essential for the physicians involved in initial management to recognize patients whose needs exceed the capability of the institution and to arrange for early transfer to a regional trauma center. Before transfer is considered, the physician should complete the primary and secondary surveys and initiate resuscitation. If the decision is made to transfer a patient to another hospital, direct physician-to-physician communication is necessary before the transfer occurs. Satisfactory transfers are based on the principle of "do no further harm." In other words, the patient's level of care should never decline from one step to the next.

Summary

Care of the injured patient begins with the primary survey. Identifying and treating all immediately life-threatening injuries is the first priority. Resuscitation is begun simultaneously with the primary survey. The secondary survey follows the rapid initial evaluation and involves a detailed head-to-toe assessment. In the definitive care phase, all injuries are prioritized and treated. The patient's ultimate outcome is directly related to the length of time between injury and definitive care.

Multiple-Choice Questions

1. You are called to see a 60-year-old man who was involved in a head-on motor vehicle accident. Your first priority is to:
   A. Start a Foley catheter
   B. Diagnose and treat all immediately life-threatening injuries
   C. Perform a complete physical examination
   D. Order an electrocardiogram
   E. Draw baseline laboratory values, and obtain x-rays of the cervical spine, chest, and pelvis

2. Your father is on a ladder painting his house and falls 30 feet to the pavement. You hear him fall and rush immediately to the scene. Your first step is to:
   A. Perform a head-to-toe physical examination
   B. Assess his level of consciousness
   C. Listen for breath sounds
   D. Protect his cervical spine while you assess his airway
   E. Check for a carotid pulse

3. You perform the jaw-thrust maneuver on an intoxicated, lethargic man who was involved in a motor vehicle accident. During suctioning of the mouth, the patient gags. The oral cavity is free of any obstruction, and the flow of air into and out of the mouth is more than adequate. The larynx and trachea are not injured. The trachea is in the midline. When you remove your hands from the jaw, the patient begins to snore and gurgle. You perform the jaw-thrust maneuver again, and the abnormal sounds stop. Your next step is to:
   A. Intubate with an orotracheal tube
   B. Perform the chin-lift maneuver
   C. Insert a nasotracheal tube
   D. Insert an oropharyngeal airway
   E. Insert a nasopharyngeal airway

4. A 25-year-old woman has a stab wound to the anterior triangle of the left side of the neck. Beneath the wound is a rapidly expanding pulsatile hematoma. The patient is alert and oriented, with a normal voice and normal breath sounds bilaterally. She can move all four extremities. Her blood pressure is 120/80 mm Hg, her pulse rate is 90/min, and her respiratory rate is 18/min. Before she goes to the operating room, the patient should have:
   A. An orotracheal tube placed under direct vision
   B. A nasotracheal tube placed blindly
   C. A 100% oxygen mask
   D. A cricothyroidotomy
   E. An oropharyngeal airway

5. A 40-year-old, 70-kg man has a gunshot wound to the abdomen. His blood pressure is 90/70 mm Hg, and his pulse rate is 130/min. What is this patient's anticipated blood loss?
   A. < 750 mL
   B. 750–1500 mL
   C. 1500–2000 mL
   D. > 2000 mL
   E. Need to know the hematocrit to make this calculation

6. A 30-year-old woman falls through a plate-glass window. Paramedics estimate blood loss of 1500 mL at the scene. Dressings are applied to the wounds, and the bleeding stops. If there is no more hemorrhage, the amount of crystalloid needed to replace the volume of blood loss is:
   A. 1500 mL
   B. 2500 mL
   C. 3500 mL
   D. 4500 mL
   E. 5500 mL

7. A 45-year-old homeless woman is hit by a bus. She has a major pelvic fracture and bilateral femur fractures. Diagnostic peritoneal lavage is negative, and her chest x-ray is normal. Over the first 90 minutes, she is given 6000 mL Ringer's lactate solution and six units of blood. She has a transient response to the initial fluid boluses. Her blood pressure is now approximately 80 mm Hg systolic, and the decision is made to place her in a pneumatic antishock garment (PASG). With inflation of all three compartments, her blood pressure increases to 90 mm Hg systolic and stabilizes within 15 minutes at 100 mm Hg systolic. This increase in blood pressure is caused by:
   A. Displacement of blood from the legs into the central circulation
   B. Increased venous return to the heart
   C. Increased pulmonary vascular resistance
   D. Decreased systemic vascular resistance
   E. Stabilization of the fractures and increased systemic vascular resistance

8. A 27-year-old man is brought to the emergency department after he is involved in a motor vehicle accident. He was the unrestrained driver of a car that struck a telephone pole, head on. Both the steering wheel and the windshield were broken by the impact of his body. At the scene, he was conscious and complained of chest pain. Paramedics immobilized him with a cervical collar and long spine board. You assess his airway. The aroma of alcohol is clearly on his breath. The oral cavity is patent, with poor air movement; the neck veins are distended; the trachea is displaced 0.5 cm to the right; and the left side of the chest is hyperresonant to percussion. The nurse tells you that his vital signs are: blood pressure 80 mm Hg systolic, pulse rate 130/min, and respiratory rate 40/min. You immediately perform a:
   A. Left needle thoracostomy followed by a left chest tube thoracostomy
   B. Right needle thoracostomy followed by a right chest tube thoracostomy
   C. Left needle thoracostomy only
   D. Pericardiocentesis
   E. Supine chest x-ray, then place a left chest tube

9. A 60-year-old man is brought to your hospital after he is involved in a motor vehicle accident. He was driving his family to church when he swerved to avoid hitting a bicyclist. His car went over a 50-foot cliff. He is the only survivor. Chest x-ray shows fracture of the left clavicle, first rib, second rib, and scapula, but no pneumothorax or hemothorax. The trachea is in the midline. The mediastinum measures 7.8 cm at the aortic knob, and there is a left pleural cap. Which of the following do you obtain during the definitive care phase of management?
   A. Esophagram
   B. Pulmonary arteriogram
   C. Computed tomography (CT) scan of the chest
   D. Arteriogram of the thoracic aorta and its branches
   E. Repeat chest x-ray in 24 hours to look for a delayed pneumothorax

10. A 25-year-old man is injured when a 1000-lb steel beam falls across his abdomen. His abdomen is distended and diffusely tender, with rebound tenderness. There are no bowel sounds. Physical examina-

tion shows abnormal movement of the iliac wings with manual compression, scrotal hematoma, and blood at the urethral meatus. The following is contraindicated in this patient:
A. Foley catheter
B. Nasogastric tube
C. Retrograde urethrogram
D. Arterial line
E. Rectal examination

11. A 21-year-old, 70-kg man is drinking with a friend at a local bar. He leaves the bar at 2:00 AM and is hit by a car when he stumbles off the curb. On arrival at your hospital, his blood pressure is 84 mm Hg systolic, his pulse rate is 135/min, and his respiratory rate is 35/min. The patient is agitated, has no external signs of blood loss, and moves all four extremities. The lungs have normal breath sounds bilaterally, and the abdomen is soft and nontender. The extremities have no gross deformity. Cervical spine, chest, and pelvis x-rays are all within normal limits. The initial hematocrit is 35%, with a blood alcohol level of 450 mg/dL. Over the first 30 minutes, the patient required 4500 mL Ringer's lactate; now his vital signs are: blood pressure 90/60 mm Hg, pulse rate 130/min, respiratory rate 30/min, and urine output 10 mL/30 min. To further manage this patient, you should do the following:
A. Obtain spiral computed tomography (CT) scan of the chest
B. Perform diagnostic peritoneal lavage
C. Decrease the intravenous fluid rate to prevent fluid overload
D. Obtain an arteriogram of the abdominal aorta
E. Perform an exploratory laparotomy

12. A 28-year-old, 90-kg woman is brought to your hospital after sustaining a gunshot wound to the abdomen. She is alert and oriented. The abdomen has a 1-cm gunshot wound 2 cm above the umbilicus in the midline. Breath sounds are normal bilaterally, and the abdomen is obese, soft, and mildly tender. There are no other gunshot wounds or injuries over her entire body. Vital signs are: blood pressure 110/80 mm Hg, pulse rate 90/min, and respiratory rate 20/min. Her urine is pale yellow and negative for blood. Intravenous lines are started, laboratory samples drawn, and x-rays ordered immediately. After the chest x-ray and abdominal x-ray are completed, the patient should have:
A. A computed tomography (CT) scan of the abdomen
B. A diagnostic peritoneal lavage
C. An intravenous pyelogram
D. An abdominal ultrasound
E. An exploratory laparotomy

13. A 56-year-old man slipped on the ice while walking home. According to his wife, he was unconscious for approximately 15 minutes and then woke up and appeared to be normal. He walked 100 feet to his house without assistance. Six hours later, his wife noticed that he was restless, incoherent, and unable to move his right arm. From this history, the most likely diagnosis is:
A. A stroke
B. An acute epidural hematoma
C. A subarachnoid hemorrhage
D. A subdural hematoma
E. An intracerebral bleed

14. An 18-year-old man is the unrestrained driver in a motor vehicle crash. He was intubated in the field. On arrival in the emergency department, his blood pressure is 80/50 mm Hg, his heart rate is 150/min, and his neck veins are flat. He is unconscious, with extensor (decerebrate) posturing and a fixed and dilated left pupil. The most likely cause of his shock is:
A. Septic shock
B. Spinal cord injury
C. Brain injury
D. Hemorrhage
E. Cardiac injury

15. You are asked to see a 55-year-old unconscious man. Vital signs are: blood pressure 190/110 mm Hg, pulse rate 50/min, and respiratory rate 10/min. It appears that he was beaten with a blunt instrument. He has ecchymoses around the eyes, behind the ears, and on the left arm, chest, abdomen, and thighs. He responds to painful stimuli by withdrawal, but does not open his eyes or make any sounds. This patient has the following:
A. Intracranial pressure > 20
B. Neurogenic shock
C. Hypoadrenal shock
D. Intracranial pressure < 10 mm Hg
E. Increased intrathoracic pressure in the right or left side of the chest

16. A 16-year-old, 60-kg boy is brought in by paramedics with a through-and-through gunshot wound to the neck. He is alert, oriented, and moves all four extremities. His voice is hoarse, but it appears to clear after he coughs up some blood-tinged sputum. Vital signs are: blood pressure 115/75 mm Hg, pulse rate 95/min, and respiratory rate 22/min. Physical examination reveals two gunshot wounds to the neck. There is a 0.5-cm wound 4 cm below the right mandible and a 1-cm wound 3 cm below the left mandible. Both wounds are anterior to the sternocleidomastoid muscle, and there is no hematoma. Neck x-ray shows subcutaneous emphysema confined to the neck. Chest x-ray is normal. The following is true about this patient:
A. He has a zone I injury that requires a carotid arteriogram
B. He has a zone II injury and may be taken to the operating room without further delay
C. He has a zone III injury that requires a computed tomography (CT) scan of the neck and chest

D. If laryngoscopy, bronchoscopy, and esophagoscopy are normal, then nothing further needs to
   be done
E. The only concern is a laryngeal injury

17. A 16-year-old boy dives into a shallow pool and
    strikes his head on the bottom. He is immediately
    retrieved from the pool. On arrival in the emergency
    department, his blood pressure is 80/40 mm Hg, his
    pulse rate is 60/min, his neck veins are flat, and he
    has priapism. The most likely cause of shock is:
    A. Sepsis
    B. Brain injury
    C. Spinal cord injury
    D. Hemorrhage
    E. Cardiac injury

18. A 3-year-old boy is brought to the emergency depart-
    ment after he is severely bitten on the face and left
    arm by a neighbor's dog. He is sitting on the stretcher
    quietly, asking for his father. He weighs 15 kg. His
    pulse rate is 160/min, and his blood pressure is 70/50
    mm Hg. The findings of physical examination are
    notable for near-complete amputation of the left arm
    and multiple bite marks over the left cheek. Which of
    the following methods of airway management is con-
    traindicated in an injured child?
    A. Orotracheal intubation
    B. Bag-valve-mask ventilation
    C. Jaw-thrust maneuver
    D. Oxygen mask
    E. Nasotracheal intubation

19. A 21-year-old woman who is 22 weeks' pregnant is
    the restrained passenger in a motor vehicle crash. She
    is alert, and complains of abdominal pain. Her pulse
    rate is 90/min, with a blood pressure of 100/65 mm
    Hg. Her examination is notable for mild tenderness in
    the left upper quadrant of the abdomen. The follow-
    ing method would be most appropriate to evaluate
    her for intraabdominal injury:
    A. Diagnostic peritoneal lavage
    B. Flat and upright abdominal radiographs
    C. Abdominal ultrasound
    D. Arteriography
    E. Serial physical examinations

20. A 15-year-old boy is brought to your office 24 hours
    after he is injured with a target arrow. He and a friend
    were in a field shooting arrows at a target, and some-
    how an arrow missed the target, ricocheted, and
    stabbed him in the right leg. He pulled the arrow out
    immediately, as he had seen done in western movies.
    The wound bled, so he covered it with a handkerchief
    and secured it with his belt. He did not tell his mother
    until the next morning, when his leg hurt as he tried
    to walk on it. On examination, you find a single,
    nonerythematous, 1-cm wound in the middle one-
    third of the calf, lateral to the tibia and medial to the
    fibula. The leg is warm, pedal pulses are palpable,
    and the lower leg muscles feel firm to palpation.

There is pain with passive movement of the toes, and
sensation is decreased and abnormal over the entire
foot. You make the diagnosis and recommend that the
patient have:
A. A computed tomography (CT) scan
B. A four-compartment fasciotomy
C. An amputation
D. Leg elevation and intravenous antibiotics
E. An electromyogram with nerve conduction

Oral Examination Study Questions

CASE 1

You are a physician at a trauma center. Paramedics
bring in a 20-year-old man who was the restrained
driver of a motor vehicle that collided head-on with a
brick wall. The patient smells of alcohol and is groan-
ing. His vital signs are: blood pressure 85/60 mm Hg,
pulse rate 130/min, and respiratory rate 35 breaths/
min.

OBJECTIVE 1

The student performs the primary and secondary
surveys, elicits the following physical findings, and
intervenes accordingly. The student should:

A. Protect the cervical spine and assess the airway.
   The jaw-thrust maneuver shows good air movement into and out of the mouth, with no obstruction. The patient gags when suctioned. When the
   jaw-thrust is released, the patient snores and
   gurgles.

B. Assess the breathing. There are decreased breath
   sounds and tender ribs on the left.

C. Assess the circulation. The heart rate is 130
   beats/min, with regular rhythm and no murmurs. Look for obvious signs of blood loss. Capillary refill is greater than 2 seconds, and pulses are
   weak.

D. Assess the patient's neurologic disability. The
   patient responds to painful stimuli.

E. Expose the patient, and begin the secondary
   survey with a head-to-toe examination. The
   abdomen shows mild distension and no bowel
   sounds. It is tympanic to percussion in the left
   upper quadrant, and soft and nontender. The perineum and rectum are normal. The extremities are
   cool, with no obvious fractures.

F. Order essential laboratory tests and x-rays.
   Hematocrit is 40%. Cervical spine x-rays are normal. Chest x-ray shows that ribs 6 through 10 are
   fractured on the left. There is no hemothorax or
   pneumothorax. Pelvic x-ray is normal.

OBJECTIVE 2

Thirty minutes after arrival, the patient received
4500 mL Ringer's lactate solution. His vital signs are:
blood pressure 100/60 mm Hg, pulse rate 120/min,

respiratory rate 25 breaths/min, and urine output 10 mL/30 min. The student should:

A. Continue resuscitation, consider blood transfusion, and reevaluate the patient.

B. Further evaluate the abdomen as a site of unrecognized blood loss.

C. Perform diagnostic peritoneal lavage, which is positive for 10 mL gross blood. Alternatively, the student could perform an abdominal bedside ultrasound, which is positive for fluid in the pelvis and around the spleen.

OBJECTIVE 1

Minimum Level of Achievement for Passing

A. The student recognizes the importance of cervical spine stabilization and uses a nasopharyngeal airway to secure the airway in a patient with an intact gag reflex.

B. The student performs inspection, palpation, auscultation, and percussion of the chest.

C. The student listens for heart sounds, looks for obvious signs of blood loss, and checks the pulses. The student hangs Ringer's lactate solution and uses 16-gauge or greater intravenous catheters placed in the arms to administer this solution as a 2000-mL bolus.

D. The student knows the AVPU mnemonic.

E. The student removes all of the patient's clothing, performs a systemic head-to-toe physical examination, and inserts a nasogastric tube and a Foley catheter.

F. The student orders the following laboratory tests: complete blood count, electrolytes, blood urea nitrogen, creatinine, glucose, amylase, type and crossmatch for six units of packed red blood cells, and urinalysis.

G. The student orders x-rays of the cervical spine, chest, and pelvis.

Honors Level of Achievement

A. The student administers 100% oxygen, palpates the trachea to determine whether it is in the midline, looks for jugular venous distension, and discusses the techniques for securing the airway.

B. The student runs the intravenous lines at a wide-open rate and draws blood for laboratory tests, including type and crossmatch when the intravenous lines are started.

C. The student orders an arterial blood gas evaluation.

D. The student knows the Glasgow Coma Scale.

OBJECTIVE 2

Minimum Level of Achievement for Passing

A. The student recognizes that the patient is not fully resuscitated and will need blood.

B. The student indicates the need for a diagnostic peritoneal lavage or abdominal ultrasound to look for a source of blood loss.

C. The student knows that the patient must go to the operating room.

Honors Level of Achievement

A. The student knows the technique of diagnostic peritoneal lavage and the criteria for a positive finding.

B. The student knows why diagnostic peritoneal lavage and abdominal ultrasound are preferred over computed tomography (CT) scan in the evaluation of blunt abdominal trauma.

CASE 2

You are a physician at a trauma center. Paramedics bring in a 45-year-old man with a single gunshot wound to left side of the chest in the fifth intercostal space, midaxillary line. The patient's face is dark blue-purple, and his neck veins are distended.

OBJECTIVE 1

The student begins the primary survey, elicits the following physical findings, and intervenes accordingly. The student should:

A. Protect the cervical spine and assess the airway. The patient is not breathing, and the trachea is deviated to the right.

B. Assess the patient's response to ventilation with a bag-valve-mask device or placement of an endotracheal tube. The left side of the chest is hyperresonant to percussion, and there are no breath sounds on the left.

C. Perform needle thoracostomy (which produces a small gush of air) and chest tube insertion (which produces a large gush of air and 500 mL blood). The patient does not respond to the pain caused by needle thoracostomy and chest tube insertion.

OBJECTIVE 2

After appropriate intervention, the student continues the primary survey and intervenes accordingly. The student should:

A. Assess the circulation. Heart sounds are difficult to hear (muffled), the heart rate is 140 beats/min, there is no carotid pulse, and the neck veins are still distended.

B. Perform pericardiocentesis; 20 mL blood is removed. The patient now has a carotid pulse.

C. Assess neurologic disability. The patient does not respond to painful stimuli.

D. Expose the patient, and begin the secondary survey. No other wounds are found.

OBJECTIVE 1

Minimum Level of Achievement for Passing

A. The student recognizes the importance of cervical spine stabilization and orally intubates the patient.

B. The student diagnoses tension pneumothorax and treats it with a needle thoracostomy, followed by chest tube insertion.

C. The student reassesses the chest after each intervention.

Honors Level of Achievement

A. The student emphasizes that, in the primary survey, all immediately life-threatening injuries are treated when they are identified.

B. The student performs needle thoracostomy before or at the same time as intubation.

C. The student describes the technique of needle thoracostomy and uses at least a 14-gauge over-the-needle catheter.

D. The student describes the technique of intubation and bags the patient with 100% oxygen.

E. The student describes the technique of chest tube insertion.

OBJECTIVE 2

Minimum Level of Achievement for Passing

A. The student listens for heart sounds, looks for obvious signs of blood loss, checks pulses, uses 16-gauge or greater intravenous catheters placed in the arms, and hangs Ringer's lactate solution, wide open, as a 2000-mL bolus.

B. The student recognizes cardiac tamponade and treats it with pericardiocentesis.

C. The student reassesses the pulses and blood pressure.

D. The student exposes the patient and looks for other wounds.

Honors Level of Achievement

A. The student recognizes cardiac tamponade and treats it with thoracotomy. If the student treats the cardiac tamponade with pericardiocentesis, he or she recognizes that cardiac tamponade requires a thoracotomy for definitive treatment.

B. The student can describe the technique of pericardiocentesis.

C. The student can discuss the prevention of hypothermia.

CASE 3

A 19-year-old man crashes his motorcycle at a high rate of speed. His eyes are swollen shut, and his midface is grossly unstable. His respirations are noisy and labored. His pulse is 110/min, and his blood pressure is 160/90 mm Hg. He shows extensor (decerebrate) posturing to painful stimulation.

OBJECTIVE 1

A. The student verbalizes the primary survey. The student finds distorted anatomy in the oral cavity. Breath sounds are equal after cricothyroidotomy.

B. The student recognizes the presence of a severe head injury.

OBJECTIVE 2

After the appropriate initial maneuvers, the patient has a heart rate of 140 beats/min and blood pressure of 95/60 mm Hg.

A. The student recognizes the presence of hemorrhagic shock and starts fluid resuscitation.

B. The student outlines the step needed to determine the cause of the hemorrhagic shock.

OBJECTIVE 1

Minimum Level of Achievement for Passing

A. The student names the different techniques for securing the airway while maintaining cervical spine protection. The student indicates the need to perform a cricothyroidotomy and initiate ventilation.

B. The student looks for obvious signs of blood loss, checks pulses, uses 16-gauge or greater intravenous catheters placed in the arms, and hangs Ringer's lactate solution.

C. The student performs an abbreviated neurologic examination, using the AVPU mnemonic, and exposes the patient.

D. The student performs a thorough secondary survey, including a neurologic examination.

E. The student verbalizes the three components of the Glasgow Coma Scale score.

Honors Level of Achievement

A. The student describes the technique of cricothyroidotomy.

B. The student verbalizes the three components of the Glasgow Coma Scale score and calculates that this patient has a score of 4.

C. The student can describe the findings that will affect the patient's cerebral perfusion.

OBJECTIVE 2

Minimum Level of Achievement for Passing

A. The student begins fluid resuscitation with a 2000-mL bolus of Ringer's lactate solution.

B. The student recognizes the abdomen as a potential source of blood loss.

C. The student can name methods to identify the source of blood loss.

Honors Level of Achievement

A. The student identifies factors other than hemorrhage that can cause sudden hypotension and tachycardia in this patient.

B. The student can discuss the relative strengths and weaknesses of diagnostic peritoneal lavage, abdominal ultrasound, and CT scan to evaluate intraabdominal blood loss.

SUGGESTED READINGS

Alexander RH, Proctor HJ, et al. *ATLS: Advanced Trauma Life Support Program for Physicians.* Chicago, Ill: American College of Surgeons, 1993.

American College of Surgeons. *Advanced Trauma Life Support Program for Doctors.* Chicago, Ill: American College of Surgeons, 1997.

Bell RM. *ATLS: Advanced Trauma Life Support Compendium of Changes.* Chicago, Ill: American College of Surgeons, 1997.

Bracken MB, Collins WF, et al. A randomized, controlled trial of methylprednisolone or naloxone in the treatment of spinal cord injury: results of the Second National Spinal Cord Injury Study. *N Engl J Med* 1990;322:1405–1411.

Chambers IR, Kane PJ, Choksey MS, Mendelow AD. An evaluation of the camino ventricular bolt system in clinical practice. *Neurosurgery* 1993;33:866–868.

Chestnut RM, Marshall LF, Klauber MR, et al. The role of secondary brain injury in determining outcome from severe head injury. *J Trauma* 1993;34:216-222.

Eddy VA, Morris J, Rozycki G. Trauma and pregnancy. In: Ivatury R, Cayten C, eds. *The Textbook of Penetrating Trauma.* Media, Pa: Williams & Wilkins, 1996.

Feliciano DV, Moore EE, Mattox KL. *Trauma.* Stamford, Conn: Appleton & Lange, 1996.

Gardner P, Hudson BL. Advance report of final mortality statistics, 1993. Monthly Vital Statistics Report. Center for Disease Control and Prevention/National Center for Health Statistics 1996;44:1-84.

Greendyke RM. Traumatic rupture of the aorta. *JAMA* 1966;195:119-122.

Greenfield LJ, et al. *Surgery: Scientific Principles and Practice.* Philadelphia, Pa: Lippincott-Raven, 1997.

Kraus J, Black M, et al. The incidence of acute brain injury and serious impairment in a defined population. *Am J Epidemiol* 1984;119:186-201.

Kraus JF, Sorenson SB. Epidemiology. In: Silver JM, Yudofsky SC, Halea RE, eds. *Neuropsychiatry of Traumatic Brain Injury.* Washington, DC: American Psychiatric Press, 1994:3-41.

Meyer JP, Barrett JA, Schuler JJ, Flanigan DP. Mandatory vs selective exploration for penetrating neck trauma. *Arch Surg* 1987;122;592-597.

Narayan RK, Wilberger JE, Povlishock JT. *Neurotrauma.* New York, NY: McGraw-Hill, 1996.

Oreskovich MR, Carrico JC. Stab wounds of the anterior abdomen. *Ann Surg* 1983;198:411-419.

Roon AJ, Christensen N. Evaluation and treatment of penetrating cervical injuries. *J Trauma* 1979;19:391-397.

Ward JD. Intracranial pressure monitoring. In: Champion HR, Robbs JV, Trunkey DD, eds. *Rob and Smith's Operative Surgery: Trauma Surgery. Part 1.* London, England: Butterworths, 1989:217-223.

Wilmore DW, Cheung LY, Harken AH, Holcroft JW, Meakins JL. *Scientific American Surgery.* New York, NY: Scientific American, 1988-1998.

Wilson RF, Walt AJ. *Management of Trauma Pitfalls and Practice.* Baltimore, Md: Williams & Wilkins, 1996.

10 Burns

Jeffrey R. Saffle, M.D.

OBJECTIVES

1. List the classification of burns by depth of injury, and indicate the anatomic and pathophysiologic differences between these injuries.
2. List the initial steps in the acute care of the patient with a burn injury.
3. List three types of inhalation injury, and describe their pathophysiology.
4. List the general indications for referral of a patient to a burn center.
5. Define burn shock, and outline its treatment.
6. List the advantages and disadvantages of fascial and tangential excision of burn wounds.
7. In addition to fluid resuscitation and surgery, list three other general areas of care that are important in the management of patients with burns.

Major burns hold a unique position in the public imagination as the most horrifying of all injuries, a perception that is often correct. To patients, acute burns are the "ultimate agony," and their long-term consequences present enormous psychological, social, and physical challenges to meaningful recovery. To the treatment team, burns are labor-intensive injuries that involve every facet of surgical care. Major burns are often used as paradigms for the most severe physiologic derangements that accompany trauma.

Burns are a major public health problem as well. In the United States, approximately 1.25 million patients sought medical attention for burns in 1992. More than 5500 people die each year of burn-related injuries, primarily from house fires, and approximately 51,000 patients are hospitalized. This chapter describes the basic pathophysiology of burns and provides practical guidelines for their treatment.

Pathophysiology of Burn Injury

The skin can be burned by a variety of agents, including direct heat from flames or scalding liquids, contact with hot objects or corrosive chemicals, and electrical current. Burns are classified according to the depth of injury. Figure 10-1 shows these injuries in relation to the structures of the skin. This knowledge provides a basic understanding of both the physiologic effects of burns of various depths and the findings seen on examination.

Epidermal Burns

Epidermal burns ("first-degree burns") involve only the epidermis. Within minutes of injury, dermal capillaries dilate. As a result, these burns are red, moderately painful areas that blanch with direct pressure. Blistering is absent from true epidermal injuries. Epidermal burn injuries have limited physiologic effects, and even extensive burns usually require only supportive care. This care usually consists of pain control (i.e., oral analgesics), adequate oral fluid intake, and application of a soothing topical compound (e.g., Neosporin ointment). Healing occurs within a few days as the injured epidermis peels off, revealing new skin. Because scarring occurs in the dermis, epidermal burns do not form scar tissue. Figure 10-2 shows a patient with primarily epidermal burns and some superficial dermal burns.

Partial-Thickness Burns

Partial-thickness burns ("second-degree burns") extend into, but not through, the dermis. These injuries vary greatly in both appearance and significance, depending on their exact depth. Superficial partial-thickness burns (see Figure 10-2) typically are reddened areas of skin. These burns form distended blisters, which consist of epidermis filled with proteinaceous fluid that escapes from damaged capillaries. The underlying dermis is moist, blanches on direct pressure, and is usually very painful because the cutaneous nerves, which reside in the deeper dermis, are intact. During the first 24 to 48 hours after the burn occurs, a coating of dead tissue, coagulated serum, and debris develops. This coating is called **eschar.** The appearance of the wound changes dramatically as eschar develops; it changes again as eschar separates during wound healing. In superficial partial-thickness burns, eschar usually separates within 10 to 14 days. As this separation occurs, punctate areas of new epidermal growth, called skin "buds," develop from the epidermal lining of hair follicles and sweat glands (Figure 10-3).

Deep partial-thickness injuries look very different from more superficial burns. Coagulation necrosis of

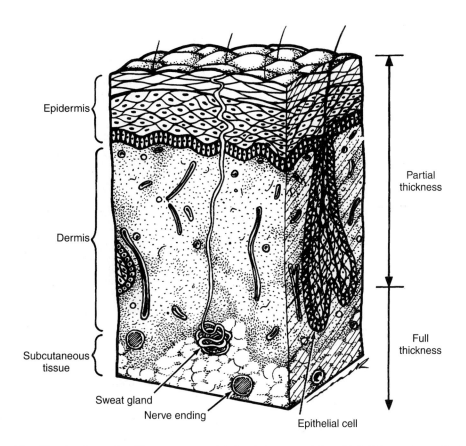

Figure 10-1 Anatomy of the skin, showing major skin structures and their relation to partial- and full-thickness burns. Epithelial cells make up the lining of hair follicles, and these structures penetrate deeply within the dermis. Even very deep partial-thickness burns can heal if these "epidermal appendages" survive. Dermal capillaries and nerve endings also reside in the deep dermis and survive most partial-thickness burns.

the upper dermis gives these wounds a dry, leathery texture. Erythema is usually absent, and the wounds may be a variety of colors, most often waxy white. Because epidermal appendages penetrate far into, and sometimes through, the dermis, even a very deep dermal burn can heal if it is followed long enough. These wounds also vary in the amount of pain that they produce; very deep wounds cause destruction of many dermal nerve endings and are less painful than more superficial injuries. Such wounds heal badly, however, because damaged dermis does not regenerate; instead, it is replaced by scar tissue that is often rigid, tender, and friable. For this reason, many deep dermal burns are best treated with excision of the burned tissue and skin grafting. The exact depth of partial-thickness burns is often difficult to judge, particularly after eschar forms. Burns of "indeterminate" depth (those that have some features of both partial- and full-thickness injuries) can be treated conservatively for 10 to 14 days; wounds that remain unhealed should undergo grafting. Figure 10-4 shows this type of burn.

Full-Thickness Burns

Full-thickness burns ("third-degree burns") occur when all layers of the skin are destroyed (Figure 10-5). These wounds are usually covered with dry, avascular coagulum that is relatively insensate, because nerve endings have been destroyed. The wound surface may be almost any color, from waxy white (chemical burns) to completely black and charred (flame injury). In addition, as dermal proteins are coagulated, they contract, often forming a tight, tourniquet-like constriction that can cause circulatory compromise in the extremities. Very small full-thickness burns can heal by contraction, but larger injuries require skin grafting because even the deepest epidermal appendages are destroyed.

Initial Care of the Patient With Burns

Patients with burn injuries should be considered victims of multiple trauma, and many of the same treatment priorities and algorithms apply to their care. Familiarity with the principles of Advanced Trauma Life Support (see Chapter 9) is essential. This chapter focuses on the aspects of care that are unique to burn injuries.

Stop the Burning Process

A special problem associated with burn trauma is the tendency for burns to continue to produce tissue damage for minutes to hours after the initial burn occurs.

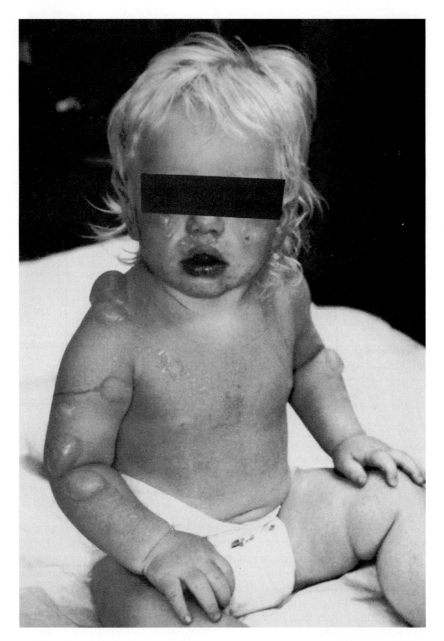

Figure 10-2 Superficial burn wounds. This child had extensive sunburn as a result of playing outdoors unattended. Most of his wounds are reddened, blanch easily, and show no blistering. These are epidermal, or first-degree, burns. Some areas on the right shoulder, right arm, and face show elevated blisters filled with fluid. They are characteristic of a superficial partial-thickness, or second-degree, burn. Although this child required only supportive care, this figure serves as a reminder that sunburns can be deep and serious injuries.

This process can further injure the patient as well as endanger medical personnel. For example, if an oxygen mask is placed on a victim of flame injury, smoldering clothing may reignite. For this reason, it is critically important to stop the burning process before proceeding with any other measures. Flame burns should be extinguished completely by dousing with water, smothering, or rolling patients on the ground. Hot liquids, especially viscous liquids (e.g., tar, plastic), can remain hot enough to burn for some time; they should be cooled immediately with cool water or moist compresses. Once cooled, these compounds can be left in place on the patient if necessary. Caustic chemicals must be diluted immediately and completely with large amounts of water. Victims of electrocution can conduct current to rescue workers. These patients cannot be approached until the source of current is removed.

Primary Survey

The primary survey is a quick examination that is designed to detect and treat immediately life-threatening conditions. It begins with evaluation of the patient's airway, breathing, and circulation (the "ABCs"

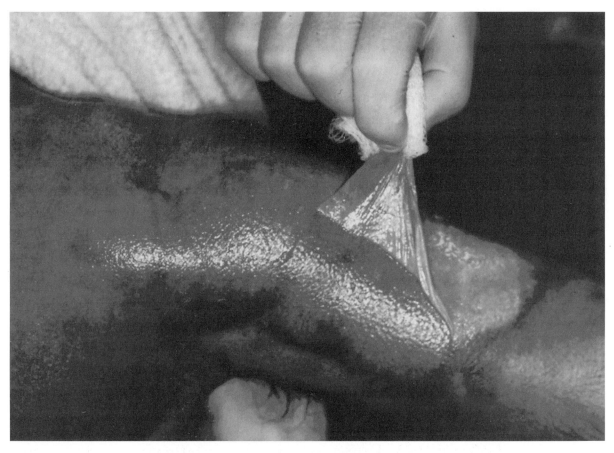

Figure 10-3 Separation of eschar in a superficial partial-thickness burn, approximately 5 days after injury. The yellowish, filmy eschar separates easily with gentle debridement, revealing an irregular surface of epidermal buds. Formation of an overlying eschar complicates the diagnosis of burn depth, but once eschar separates, the depth of injury can be determined accurately. This type of gentle debridement is performed at least twice daily on all open burn wounds.

of resuscitation). When the primary survey is performed on burn victims, special attention is paid to the possibility of smoke **inhalation injury,** which is a major source of both immediate and long-term morbidity and mortality. Inhalation injury should be suspected whenever the patient has been exposed to smoke. Table 10-1 lists the major types of inhalation injury and their treatment. The most common killer of victims of house fires is carbon monoxide, which displaces oxygen from hemoglobin and causes severe tissue hypoxemia. Smoke inhalation also produces airway swelling and obstruction or severe pulmonary edema. Even in the absence of smoke exposure, patients with severe facial burns can have massive swelling that leads to obstruction of the supraglottic airway. Because edema is progressive, signs of airway compromise may be absent for several hours after injury. Patients should be followed and reexamined regularly to detect this complication. Also during the primary survey, the examiner should note evidence of circulatory compromise in the extremities, which can be caused by severe edema and constricting burn wounds. Chapter 22 provides a more detailed review of the signs and symptoms of vascular compromise.

Resuscitation

The initial resuscitation of burn victims is similar to that of other patients. If injuries appear to be major, two large-bore intravenous lines are secured. A Foley catheter is placed to aid in resuscitation, and blood is drawn for laboratory studies. Formal calculation of fluid requirements is not performed, however, until the secondary survey is completed. Fluid resuscitation is an important, ongoing part of the definitive treatment of burn injuries, and is discussed in detail later.

Secondary Survey

Often, the presence of a dramatic burn wound distracts the examiner from detecting other, more urgent injuries. In addition, the swelling, discoloration, and pain that accompany burns can obscure underlying abdominal tenderness, extremity fractures, or cyanosis. For these reasons, it is imperative that a comprehensive, head-to-toe examination of every burn patient be conducted. Only after the secondary survey is completed should burns be debrided by removing blistered skin and washing the burn wound thoroughly. The location, extent, and depth of burn wounds should be documented with a

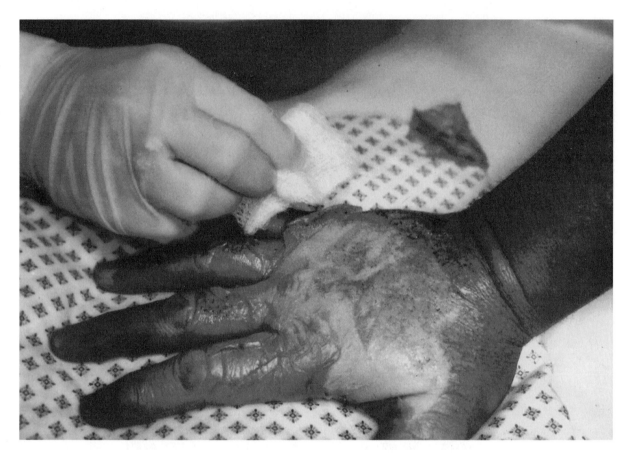

Figure 10-4 Deep partial-thickness burn. This man burned his hand with hot grease while cooking bacon. Loose, blistered skin is seen on the dorsal hand and fingers, but there is very little fluid beneath the blisters because of coagulation of the upper dermis. As the wound is debrided, a dry, pale, relatively insensate dermis is revealed. Although this wound has a deceptively unimpressive appearance, it is actually a far more serious injury than the wound shown in Figure 10-2.

diagram such as the Lund and Browder chart (Figure 10-6). This chart is used to calculate the total burn size, which is expressed as percentage of total body surface area (% TBSA). Only partial-thickness (second-degree) and full-thickness (third-degree) burn wounds are included in this estimate of burn size. This estimate is used to guide fluid resuscitation, nutrition, and other aspects of care. Wounds should not be dressed with antibiotic creams or ointments, or wrapped with dressings, until secondary assessment is completed and the burn is evaluated.

Burn Center Referral

Over the last 50 years, specialized burn care facilities have been developed to treat patients with serious burns. The American Burn Association and the American College of Surgeons have defined criteria for **burn centers,** similar to those developed for trauma centers. These criteria require that institutions maintain significant, multidisciplinary expertise in all phases of burn treatment. They also must commit space, resources, and personnel to the care of patients with burns. In addition, specific guidelines for the referral of patients to burn centers have been developed (Table 10-2). These guidelines are not absolute, but are widely used as standards

for treatment. As a general rule, surgeons who do not work in burn centers should treat only patients with burn injuries that they are experienced in treating. They should consult a burn center with any questions about patient management.

Definitive Care of Burn Injuries

After the initial assessment, patients with burn injuries require treatment for a number of physiologic consequences of injury. Support for several different problems may be required simultaneously, although the importance and magnitude of these problems may change. To help in organizing treatment priorities and protocols, many physicians divide burn care into three periods: (1) resuscitation, (2) wound closure, and (3) rehabilitation. These distinctions are somewhat artificial, however, and many aspects of care overlap these periods. Careful attention to the individual patient's needs is essential at all stages of treatment.

Resuscitation Period

This period lasts for the first 24 to 48 hours after injury. After an acutely burned patient is evaluated and

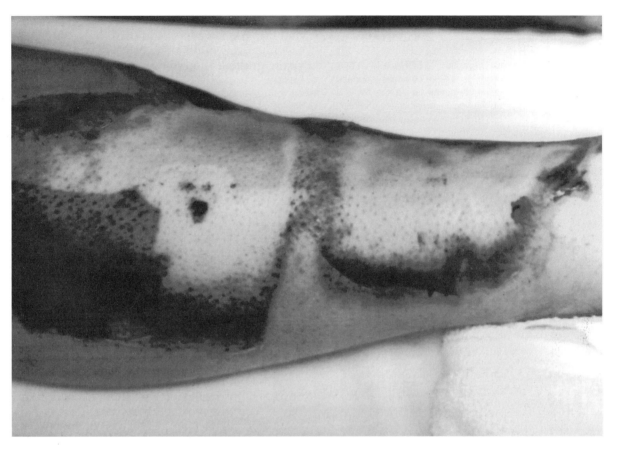

Figure 10-5 Full-thickness burn on the leg of a man whose pants caught fire while he was burning weeds. After debridement, the entire wound is dry, leathery, and painless. The wound is a variety of colors–white, brown, red, and black–because of areas of scorching of the dermis. When viewed tangentially, the contracture produced by coagulation of dermal proteins is seen. There is no need to follow a burn this deep conservatively; this wound was skin-grafted the day after the patient's admission.

stabilized as described previously, fluid resuscitation is the most important goal of initial treatment. Burn injury produces a loss of capillary integrity, which results in edema formation. With large ($\geq$ 15%–20% TBSA) injuries, capillary leakage becomes systemic, producing total body edema and severely depleting circulating volume, a phenomenon known as **burn shock.** All patients who have burns of 10% to 15% TBSA or greater require formal fluid resuscitation. Remarkable amounts of fluid may be required for successful resuscitation of patients with very large burn injuries.

Many algorithms have been developed for burn resuscitation, but most successful regimens share several basic concepts. These are shown in Table 10-3 by the **Parkland formula,** a widely used, simple, and relatively generous resuscitation formula. It calls for isotonic crystalloid fluid (lactated Ringer's solution) to be given at an initial rate that is determined from burn size and body weight. Edema formation occurs throughout the first 24 hours postburn, but because it is most pronounced during the first 8 hours, one-half of the total fluid is given during that period. However, inhalation injury, multiple trauma, and other factors can influence an individual's fluid requirements. For this reason, regimens such as the Parkland formula really only indicate

where to begin resuscitation, which should be guided thereafter by frequent and repeated evaluation of the patient. Maintenance of adequate urine output (> 30 mL/hr in adults; 1–2 mL/kg/hr in children) is an indicator of appropriate fluid intake and an important goal of treatment. The infusion rate is adjusted according to urine output. It is gradually decreased until a maintenance rate is reached. Vital signs, hematocrit, and other laboratory test results are carefully monitored as well.

Fluid resuscitation does not stop the leakage of fluid into the interstitium; it is intended only to keep up with ongoing losses, which decrease over time. As resuscitation proceeds, therefore, so does tissue swelling. Fluid accumulating beneath the constricted eschar of a deep burn increases tissue hydrostatic pressure, sometimes to the point at which circulation is compromised. Frequent evaluation of extremity pulses, sensory and motor function, and pain is essential to the diagnosis of progressive ischemia. The treatment of this problem is **escharotomy,** an incision made through the rigid, leathery eschar to relieve the compression that is produced by ongoing edema and, thus, to restore distal circulation. Compression by edema can also affect the chest and abdomen, resulting in respiratory compromise and even arrest. Escharotomies can be performed on the torso and should

Table 10-1. Types of Inhalation Injury

Carbon Monoxide Poisoning
  Presentation: Immediately after exposure to flames and smoke.
  Pathophysiology: Carbon monoxide (CO), a colorless, odorless gas, is a by-product of *incomplete* combustion. It acts by displacing oxygen bound to hemoglobin molecules, producing carboxyhemoglobin (COHb) and causing tissue hypoxemia.
  Diagnosis: Patients may have cherry-red coloration. Neurologic dysfunction is common, progressing from headache to confusion to coma. CO poisoning should be *strongly suspected* in any patient who is found unconscious at a fire scene or is trapped in a smoke-filled enclosure. Definitive diagnosis requires measurement of blood COHb levels, but treatment should not be postponed while the diagnosis is confirmed.
  Treatment: Because oxygen competes with CO for hemoglobin binding, anyone who is suspected of having CO poisoning should be treated *immediately* with high-flow oxygen. Unconscious patients should be intubated. Hyperbaric oxygen helps to clear COHb more quickly, but should not supersede more immediate treatment. *Note:* CO does not affect arterial oxygen tension. PO_2 is usually normal, but SaO_2 is greatly affected by CO poisoning.

Upper-Airway Obstruction
  Presentation: Immediately up to 24 hours postburn.
  Pathophysiology: Smoke contains hot gases, particulate matter, and chemicals, all of which can damage the oropharyngeal mucosa. This damage causes edema, mucosal sloughing, and gradual airway obstruction.
  Diagnosis: Patients with burns of the mouth, nose, or pharynx may display singeing of nasal hairs or eyebrows, carbonaceous material on the lips or tongue, and blistering on the palate. Hoarseness, cough, and increasing stridor signal impending loss of airway.
  Treatment: Early endotracheal intubation, high-flow oxygen, and meticulous pulmonary toilet (coughing, suctioning, and clearing of secretions). *Note:* Edema increases during the first 24 hours after injury, so airway obstruction can develop hours after the burn event, even in patients with no burns of the face or exposure to smoke.

Pulmonary Injury (True Inhalation Injury)
  Presentation: Can be immediate, but symptoms may be entirely absent until days after injury.
  Pathophysiology: Smoke contains a host of toxic chemicals, including formaldehyde, formic and hydrochloric acids, and acrolein, which are activated on contact with moist airways. The resulting damage causes mucosal sloughing, airway collapse, bronchiectasis, and hypoxemia, and predisposes damaged segments to the development of pneumonia.
  Diagnosis: Patients present with hypoxia, respiratory distress, and infiltrates on chest x-ray. The most important clue to diagnosis is a history of prolonged exposure to smoke. Other signs and symptoms that are suggestive (but not diagnostic) of inhalation injury include burns of the face, nose, or lips; singeing of the nasal hairs or eyebrows; carbonaceous sputum or saliva; hoarseness or "crowing" respirations; bronchorrhea; and tachypnea. Bronchoscopic findings of carbonaceous deposition, swelling or erythema of the tracheobronchial tree are diagnostic.
  Treatment: Early, elective intubation should be considered. Patients should be treated with high-flow, moisturized oxygen and given meticulous pulmonary toilet, as described previously. Pneumonia should be sought and treated immediately, but prophylactic antibiotics have not proven helpful. *Note:* All three types of inhalation injury—CO poisoning, upper-airway obstruction, and "true" pulmonary injury—can occur individually or may be present simultaneously.

provide immediate relief (Figure 10-7). Because escharotomies are always made within surrounding burn wounds, they are repaired during wound excision and skin grafting, and they usually leave no additional scars.

Wound Coverage Period

This phase of treatment begins immediately after fluid resuscitation and lasts for days to weeks, until the burn wound either heals primarily or is successfully replaced with skin grafts. This period constitutes most of the patient's hospital care, and is the period of most intensive treatment. Patients who attain successful wound closure usually survive, although they may face prolonged rehabilitation.

Excision and Skin Grafting

Deeply burned skin is a great liability to the patient. Burn eschar serves as a site for infection. In addition, the loss of skin integrity causes increased evaporative fluid losses, severe pain, and an intense inflammatory response that can escalate, leading to multiple organ failure and death. If followed conservatively, deep eschar eventually separates spontaneously, but this process can take weeks. During this time, the patient is exposed to ongoing stress and risk of infection. For these reasons, most burn centers now employ **early excision,** in which burned skin is cut off of the underlying tissue. Two techniques are used: **fascial** and **tangential excision.** In fascial excision, the scalpel or cautery is used to excise the entire skin and subcutaneous tissue, usually to the level of the underlying fascia. This procedure is easy to perform, is relatively bloodless, and permits good skin graft "take." Fascial excision is disfiguring, however, and the removal of subcutaneous fat leads to joint stiffness and poor mobility. During the last two decades, the technique of "layered," or tangential, excision has gained popularity. With this technique, sequential thin slices of skin are removed with a dermatome until viable tissue is encountered. This technique requires skill, and it produces significant bleeding. However, the cosmetic and functional results of grafting this type of wound are often superior to those of fascial excision. Tangential excision of deep partial-thickness burns permits salvaging of intact dermal elements, which improves the results of skin grafting. To permit stabilization of cardiovascular function and intravascular volume (which can be further compromised by surgical blood loss), most surgeons wait until fluid resuscitation is completed before they begin excisional therapy. Limited burns of mixed or indeterminate depth can be followed for 10 to 14 days before the decision to proceed with surgery must be made.

Skin grafting is usually performed at the same time as excision. Currently, permanent coverage of an excised wound can be achieved only with the patient's own skin **(autograft).** Autografting can be performed with **full-thickness** or **split-thickness grafts.** Full-thickness grafts are obtained by excising an ellipse of skin from the groin or flank, which is closed with sutures. Split-thickness

BURN ESTIMATE AND DIAGRAM
AGE vs AREA

Area	Birth 1 yr.	1-4 yr.	5-9 yr.	10-14 yr.	15 yr.	Adult	2⁰	3⁰	Total	Donor Areas
Head	19	17	13	11	9	7				
Neck	2	2	2	2	2	2				
Ant. Trunk	13	13	13	13	13	13				
Post. Trunk	13	13	13	13	13	13				
R. Buttock	2½	2½	2½	2½	2½	2½				
L. Buttock	2½	2½	2½	2½	2½	2½				
Genitalia	1	1	1	1	1	1				
R. U. Arm	4	4	4	4	4	4				
L. U. Arm	4	4	4	4	4	4				
R. L. Arm	3	3	3	3	3	3				
L. L. Arm	3	3	3	3	3	3				
R. Hand	2½	2½	2½	2½	2½	2½				
L. Hand	2½	2½	2½	2½	2½	2½				
R. Thigh	5½	6½	8	8½	9	9½				
L. Thigh	5½	6½	8	8½	9	9½				
R. Leg	5	5	5½	6	6½	7				
L. Leg	5	5	5½	6	6½	7				
R. Foot	3½	3½	3½	3½	3½	3½				
L. Foot	3½	3½	3½	3½	3½	3½				
						TOTAL				

Cause of Burn_____

Date of Burn_____

Time of Burn_____

Age_____

Sex_____

Weight_____

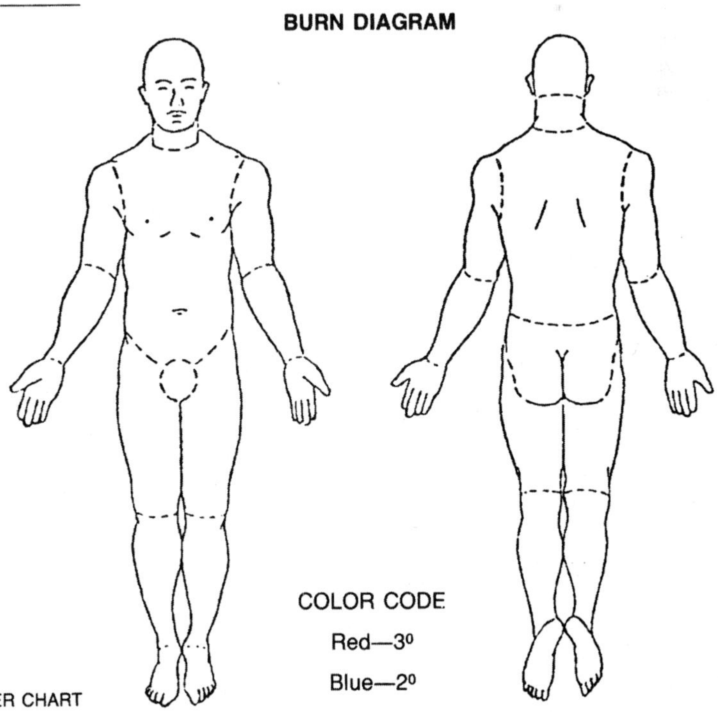

BURN DIAGRAM

COLOR CODE

Red—3⁰

Blue—2⁰

LUND AND BROWDER CHART

Figure 10-6 Lund and Browder chart. This chart is used to diagram the location and extent of burn wounds. The chart divides the body into its component parts and indicates the size of each part, expressed as percentage of total body surface area (% TBSA). Burned areas are indicated and also expressed as % TBSA. Accuracy is increased if burns are charted after the initial cleansing and debridement. The estimate of total burn size is used to guide initial fluid resuscitation, nutritional support, and surgical treatment. (Reprinted from Lund CC, Browder NC. The estimation of areas of burns. *Surg Gynecol Obstet* 1944;79:352–358).

Table 10-2. Criteria for Referral to a Burn Center

Total burn size
  Partial and full-thickness burns ≥ 10% TBSA in patients < 10 yr or > 50 yr.
  Partial and full-thickness burns ≥ 20% TBSA in patients 10–50 yr.
Full-thickness burns: Full-thickness burns > 5% TBSA in any age-group.
"Special care" areas: Partial or full-thickness burns that involve the face, hands, feet, genitalia, perineum, or major joints.
Electric burns, including lightning injury.
Chemical burns.
Inhalation injury.
Preexisting medical problems: Burn injury in patients with preexisting conditions that could complicate management, prolong recovery, or affect mortality (e.g., diabetes, AIDS).
Burns and trauma: Patients with burns and concomitant trauma in which the burn injury poses the greatest risk of morbidity or mortality. If the trauma poses the greater risk, the patient may be treated initially in a trauma center until he is stable before being transferred to a burn center. Physician judgment is necessary in such situations.
Pediatric burns: Hospitals without qualified personnel or equipment for the care of children should transfer children with burns to a burn center with these capabilities.
Special care: Burn injury in patients who require special social, emotional, or long-term rehabilitative support, including suspected child abuse or substance abuse.

Adapted with permission from Committee on Trauma, American College of Surgeons. Resources for the optimal care of the injured patient, 1993; and Burn Care Rehab 1995; 16:1
TBSA, total body surface area.
AIDS, acquired immune deficiency syndrome.

Table 10-3. Principles of Fluid Resuscitation for Burns: The Parkland Formula

Principles
Resuscitation should use primarily isotonic crystalloid solution because it is inexpensive, readily available, and can be given in large quantities without harmful side effects. Because injured capillaries are porous to proteins for the first several hours after injury, colloid-containing fluids are not used during this period.
Resuscitation requirements are proportional to burn size and patient's body weight.
Edema formation is most rapid during the first 8 hours postburn. It continues for 24 hours.
Resuscitation must be guided by patient response (e.g., urine output, vital signs, mental status).
Practice: The Parkland Formula
The formula:
  4 mL lactated Ringer's × Body weight (kg) × % TBSA burned
    = Total fluid for 24 hr
First 8 hours postinjury: Give one-half the calculated total.
Second 8 hours postinjury: Give one-fourth the calculated total.
Third 8 hours postinjury: Give one-fourth the calculated total.
Example:
  A 220-lb (100-kg) man is burned while filling the gas tank on his boat. He is wearing a swimming suit and is burned over all of both legs, his chest, and both arms. Calculated burn size is 65% TBSA.
Calculated fluid requirements:
  Total 4 mL lactated Ringer's × 100 kg × 65% TBSA burned
    = 26,000 mL in 24 hr.
First 8 hours = 13,000 mL or 1625 mL/hr
Second 8 hours = 6500 mL or 812 mL/hr
Third 8 hours = 6500 mL or 812 mL/hr

TBSA, total body surface area.

grafts use a dermatome to harvest intact skin at the level of the superficial dermis, typically 0.0004 to 0.015 inch deep. This process yields a graft with sufficient dermis to provide secure coverage of the excised burn, and leaves a wound that is superficial enough to heal spontaneously in 7 to 14 days. Figure 10-8 shows tangential excision and split-thickness skin grafting of a burned hand. In the treatment of very large burns, the urgency to remove eschar often requires that excision be performed, even if no donor sites are available for grafting. When insufficient autograft is available, several techniques are used to obtain skin coverage. First, skin can be expanded by meshing, or cutting multiple small slits in the skin. Widely meshed autografts cover larger areas, although the interstices of the mesh are prone to desiccation. For this reason, widely meshed autografts are usually covered with one of several skin substitutes, which can also be used alone to attain temporary closure of burn wounds. The most widely used skin substitute is cadaver **allograft** skin, obtained from tissue banks. Other skin substitutes include freeze-dried pig's skin, human amniotic membrane, and various synthetic materials. In recent years, considerable research has been devoted to the development of a man-made "artificial dermis," which could be taken off the shelf and used to cover large burn wounds. A number of products are undergoing clinical testing, but it is too early to predict how effective they will be. Finally, it is possible to grow a patient's own epidermal cells in culture. These cultured epidermal allografts are expensive, fragile, and easily lost as a result of infection. Nonetheless, they have proved life-saving in some patients with massive burns.

Infection Control

Immediately after burning, the skin surface is virtually sterile for 24 to 48 hours. Then it gradually becomes repopulated with bacteria. Burn eschar, especially the thick, avascular eschar of deep burns, is an ideal culture medium for bacteria, which multiply rapidly on such a surface. These bacteria may colonize burn eschar harmlessly. On the other hand, by penetrating through the burn wound, they may invade intact tissues and overwhelm local defenses, producing an invasive infection known as **burn wound sepsis.** Infection is also favored by the immunosuppression that accompanies severe burn injury. Burn wound sepsis is frequently fatal and, until recently, was the most common cause of death in hospitalized burn victims. With modern methods of wound management, however, it is now an uncommon occurrence in burn centers.

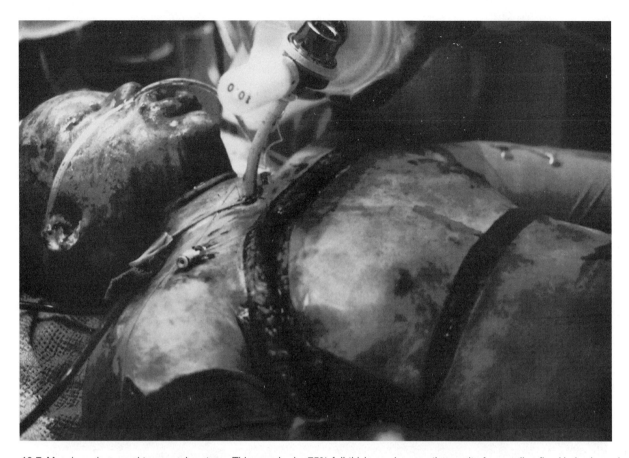

Figure 10-7 Massive edema and torso escharotomy. This man had a 75% full-thickness burn as the result of a gasoline fire. He is shown here approximately 24 hours after injury. Massive facial edema made oral intubation impossible; the patient required emergent cricothyroidotomy because of airway obstruction. As fluid resuscitation proceeded, edema accumulating beneath the rigid eschar of the torso created progressive compression and compromised ventilation. Chest escharotomy relieved this compression and improved ventilation. The escharotomy wound spread apart with progressive swelling.

Much of the increased survival in patients with burns achieved in the last 50 years is the result of improved understanding and treatment of burn wound infections. Beginning in the 1940s, systemic antibiotics (e.g., penicillin) as well as many topical agents were used to control microbial contamination of burn wounds. The first widely used topical antimicrobial, silver nitrate solution, proved particularly effective in controlling infections caused by *Staphylococcus* and *Streptococcus* species. A variety of gram-negative infections began to predominate as causes of burn wound infection. In the 1960s, the development of two powerful topical agents, mafenide acetate (Sulfamylon), and **silver sulfadiazene** (Silvadene, Thermazene, and SSD, among others), helped to control many gram-negative bacteria, which were then replaced by resistant *Pseudomonas* as a leading cause of infection. More recently, a host of powerful systemic antibiotics and numerous other topical agents have helped to control *Pseudomonas* infections. This success has been followed by (and, to some extent, caused) the emergence of multiply resistant bacteria (e.g., methicillin-resistant *Staphylococcus aureus*, *Acinetobacter*, and vancomycin-resistant *Enterococcus*), as well as fungi and other exotic organisms, as important clinical pathogens in burn victims. This problem is multiplied by the development in many burn centers of entrenched, endemic microbial populations that are difficult to eradicate. Thus, as the medical community has developed increasingly powerful antimicrobials for burn care, the microbial fauna has adapted and continued to present new problems.

The most effective technique in the battle against burn wound infection is early burn excision and skin grafting (discussed previously). Meticulous wound care also remains an essential part of burn treatment during the repair phase. Beginning immediately postburn, wounds must be washed regularly and debrided carefully of old topical creams and ointments, dried serum, and bits of loose eschar (see Figure 10-3). Topical antimicrobials are effective for only a few hours, and most experts agree that their replacement, as well as regular and thorough **debridement,** should be performed at least twice daily. These requirements also apply to freshly grafted burn wounds and to skin graft donor sites. Detailed information about burn wound care and the many products and protocols in current use can be found in Saffle and Schnebley (see Suggested Readings).

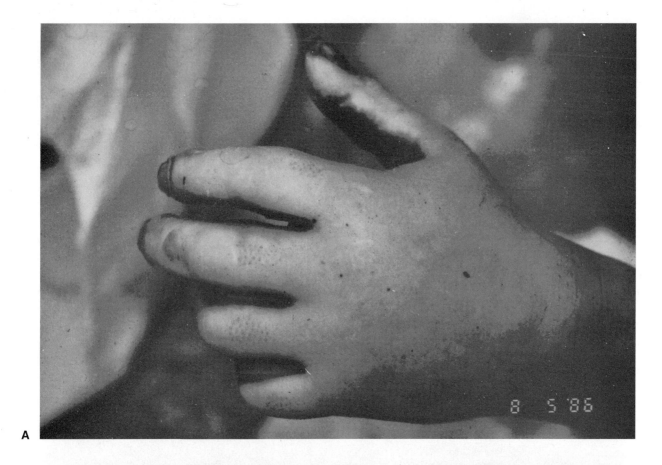

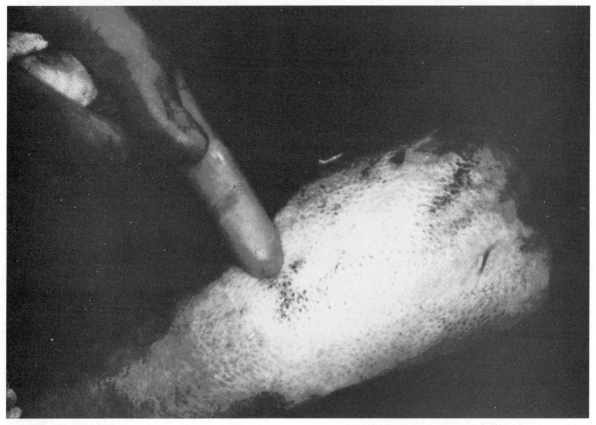

Figure 10-8 Excision and skin grafting. **A,** A 36-year old man had a deep partial-thickness burn of the dorsal hand and fingers. **B,** Under tourniquet control, the eschar is excised until only pale, intact dermis is seen. An area of residual discoloration is shown, indicating damaged tissue; this tissue will also be excised.

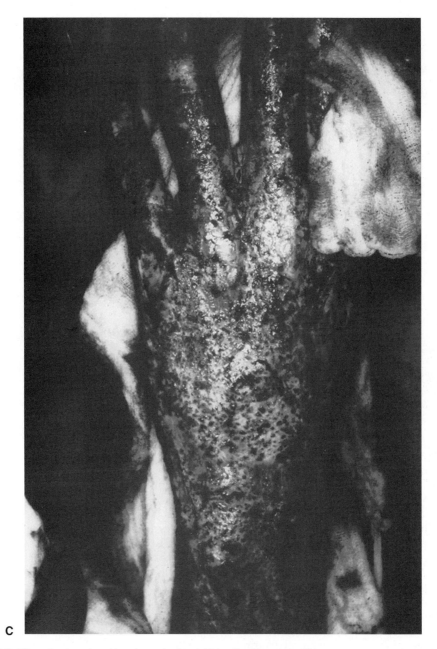

Figure 10-8 *continued.* **C,** When the tourniquet is released, pinpoint bleeding is seen in all areas.

As the prevention and treatment of burn wound infection has become more successful, other problems have gained prominence as causes of morbidity and mortality in burn victims. In particular, pneumonia has emerged as the most common, and often the most troublesome, infection seen in burn patients. As outlined in Table 10-2, smoke inhalation causes chemical injury to the small airways of the lung, leading to bronchiectasis and mucous plugging. These effects permit infections to develop and render them difficult to clear. Pneumonia, in turn, often serves as a stimulus for systemic inflammation and infection, leading to the development of multiple organ failure. A host of other infectious complications can occur in burn victims. Septic thrombophlebitis can occur in veins that are cannulated for vascular access. When central veins are involved, systemic sepsis, endocarditis, and death can result. Localized infections can also develop in exposed bone or cartilage, the urinary tract, salivary glands, gallbladder, and other areas. Happily, these complications are rarely seen in burn treatment.

Nutritional Support

As part of the hormonal response to burn trauma, the metabolic rate rises dramatically. It can exceed twice the normal rate for prolonged periods, with a corresponding increase in nitrogen excretion. This change is the most severe metabolic response seen with any type of illness or injury, and the resulting catabolism can cause

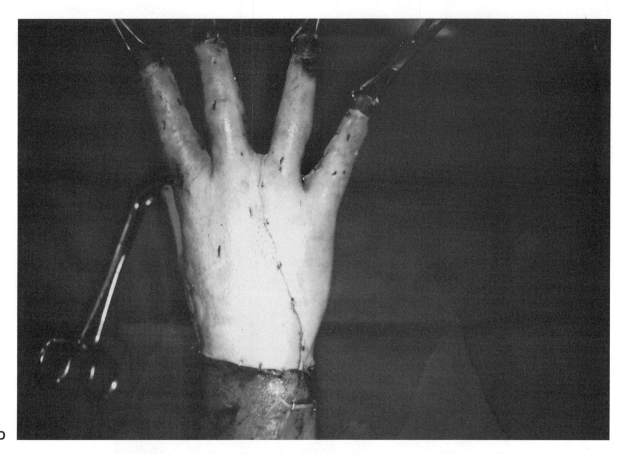

D

Figure 10-8 *continued.* **D,** The hand is suspended with towel clips to facilitate placement of a split-thickness skin graft harvested from the patient's back. The graft is secured with skin staples and sutures.

a fatal degree of inanition within a few weeks. In these patients, protein malnutrition causes both wasting of respiratory muscles and immune compromise, with resulting pulmonary infection and death. For this reason, burn patients require aggressive nutritional support and close monitoring throughout the wound closure phase of treatment, and sometimes longer. Enteral feeding is clearly superior to intravenous nutrition in burn victims. For this reason, patients with large injuries should undergo placement of enteral feeding tubes as soon as possible. A high-protein liquid diet should be infused until oral intake is adequate. Various formulas have been used to predict the caloric requirements of burn patients. None are entirely satisfactory, however, partially because of the wide variation seen among individuals and the fluctuations in energy expenditure that occur during the postburn course. Many experts recommend the routine measurement of energy expenditure with indirect calorimetry and measurement of protein use with nitrogen-balance determinations, at least weekly. The technique of indirect calorimetry calculates the energy requirements of an individual by measuring the oxygen consumed during normal breathing. In recent years, improved understanding of the role of nutrition in trauma management has led to the development of "customized" nutritional products aimed at the specific needs of burn and trauma

patients. The advantages of these products remain to be proven; a basic high-protein diet (1.5–2.0 g protein/kg body weight daily), in quantities sufficient to satisfy caloric requirements, is the most important principle in the nutritional management of these patients.

Rehabilitation Period

After burn wounds are closed, major emphasis is shifted to rehabilitation. However, it is incorrect to infer that rehabilitation should await wound closure. In practice, rehabilitation begins at the time of injury. As burn wounds heal, they contract because of the presence of myofibroblasts that begin to accumulate within wounds shortly after injury and continue to proliferate within scar tissue. If unopposed, burn scar contractures can immobilize extremities completely and produce hideous disfigurement. Much of the therapy provided during burn rehabilitation is aimed at preventing and correcting contractures. This therapy is more effective if it is begun quickly, while the scar tissue is still pliable, and before it can "set" into significant contractures. Scar tissue remains inflamed and continues to remodel and reshape itself for at least a year after injury. Burn patients are usually followed for at least that long. In addition to motion and stretching exercises, tight-fitting

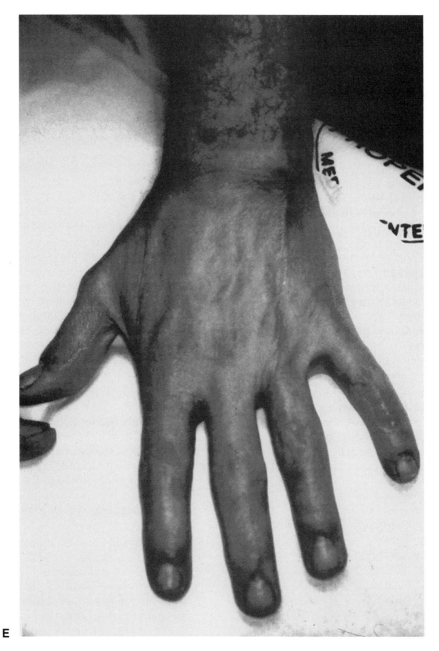

Figure 10-8 *continued.* **E,** The hand several months later. The cosmetic result is excellent, and function is perfect. This result is far superior to the result expected with spontaneous healing.

antiburn scar garments are frequently used to retard the growth of hypertrophic scars. These custom-made garments are worn until the scar tissue softens and erythema fades. The process of recovering completely from a major burn is long and labor-intensive, but most burn victims can return to active and useful lives with appropriate therapy. Most patients return to work or school, even after burns of 70% TBSA or greater.

Reconstructive surgery may be needed to correct particularly difficult contractures, resurface areas of unstable wound coverage, or improve cosmetic appearance. This surgery is usually postponed until the burn scars mature and soften. However, many reconstructive pro-

cedures can be avoided with early and continued application of physical therapy and other rehabilitative techniques.

Multiple-Choice Questions

1. A 27-year-old man is sprayed with concentrated sulfuric acid while working in an oil refinery. He has burns to his face, hands, and forearms. He is immediately brought to the emergency room. On initial examination, he is awake and in pain. His clothes are soaked with acid. The first step in management is to:

A. Debride his burns and complete a Lund and Browder chart
B. Immediately place the patient in a decontamination shower, with appropriate protection for all health care workers
C. Perform a secondary survey
D. Begin fluid resuscitation
E. None of the above

2. A 48-year-old alcoholic man passes out while smoking and sets his sofa on fire. Paramedics drag the man from the building. He is brought to the emergency room unconscious, and the primary survey shows singed nasal hairs, carbonaceous debris in the nose and mouth, facial burns, and respiratory stridor. The next step in management is to:
   A. Perform immediate intubation and ventilation with high-flow oxygen
   B. Complete the primary survey, begin resuscitation, and complete the secondary survey
   C. Obtain a chest x-ray
   D. Order a head computed tomography (CT) scan to evaluate his coma
   E. Perform burn wound excision and skin grafting

3. A 19-year-old woman who is working at a fast food restaurant slips and falls, immersing her entire left hand and forearm in hot grease. On evaluation, the burned hand is tightly swollen, cool, dry, and waxy white. She cannot move her fingers, and complains of deep, throbbing pain. You cannot feel a radial pulse. Management includes:
   A. Evaluation for inhalation injury
   B. Evaluation for a fracture of the arm
   C. Evaluation for escharotomy to relieve ischemic compression
   D. Referral to a plastic surgeon for skin grafting
   E. Enteral nutrition

4. Full-thickness, or "third-degree," burns usually require skin grafting because:
   A. They are too painful to be left to heal spontaneously
   B. The dermis will regenerate, but epidermis cannot
   C. They cannot form an adequate layer of scar tissue as well as more superficial injuries
   D. Fluid resuscitation requirements will be less
   E. They destroy deep epidermal appendages from which healing must occur

5. The edema that accumulates beneath burned skin:
   A. Can be prevented with appropriate fluid resuscitation
   B. Is usually worst within minutes of injury
   C. Can always be adequately treated with the Parkland formula
   D. Can lead to life-threatening loss of intravascular volume
   E. Is worst with first-degree burns

6. A 6-year-old girl is rescued by firefighters from a burning house. She is initially unconscious, but responds to oxygen and stimulation. In the emergency room, she is awake and alert. Blood gas measurements show normal oxygenation, and the chest x-ray is clear. A diagnosis of inhalation injury:
   A. Can be excluded, given her normal chest x-ray
   B. Must be considered despite normal oxygenation
   C. Requires the finding of facial burns or singed nasal hair
   D. Is unnecessary; she clearly requires endotracheal intubation
   E. All of the above

7. Invasive infection that develops within a burn wound, known as burn wound sepsis:
   A. Is prevented by the dry, impenetrable eschar that forms on full-thickness burn wounds
   B. Has been eradicated by the use of topical antibiotics (e.g., silver sulfadiazene)
   C. Results in the penetration of bacteria through eschar into viable tissue and blood vessels
   D. Is rarely fatal
   E. Is increased by excision and skin grafting

8. Early excision and skin grafting of extensive, deep burns:
   A. Is rarely performed because of the prohibitive blood loss and pain produced by the surgery
   B. Promotes the development of burn wound sepsis
   C. Is usually performed within 24 hours of injury
   D. Is always performed to the level of muscle fascia
   E. Shortens the exposure to infection and metabolic stress associated with a major burn

9. A 25-year-old man is injured when he falls asleep while driving. His car rolls over repeatedly and explodes. He is brought to the emergency room with extensive flame burns of the upper body, arms, and face. Firefighters at the scene extinguished the fire, and paramedics performed endotracheal intubation before transport. He is conscious and oxygenating well, and has good breath sounds. Two intravenous lines were started and are running lactated Ringer's solution. The next important step in his treatment is:
   A. Calculating fluid requirements with the Parkland formula
   B. Beginning enteral nutrition
   C. Evaluating him for extremity escharotomy
   D. Performing a thorough head-to-toe physical examination to look for evidence of other trauma
   E. Excision of burn wounds

10. A 3-year-old girl is injured while playing with matches. She has a 75% total body surface area burn and significant inhalation injury. She arrives intubated, and is treated with fluid resuscitation. Two days after the injury, she is taken to the operating room for the first of several excision and skin grafting

procedures. An important part of her ongoing care should include:
A. Administration of prophylactic broad-spectrum antibiotics
B. Placement of an enteral feeding tube and institution of aggressive nutritional support
C. Administration of systemic corticosteroids to treat inhalation injury
D. Placement of a central venous line and institution of total parenteral nutrition
E. All of the above

11. An 82-year-old woman is burned when her dress catches fire while she is cooking. She is brought to a small local hospital emergency room, where her total burn size is estimated at 64% total body surface area, 35% full-thickness injury, involving the hands, feet, face, trunk, and all of both arms. She has evidence of inhalation injury and is intubated. She has a history of steroid-dependent rheumatoid arthritis. She is referred to a burn center for definitive care because:
A. She has burns of the "special care" areas: hands, joints, face, and feet
B. She has full-thickness burns of greater than 5% total body surface area
C. She has concomitant medical problems that are likely to complicate treatment
D. She has inhalation injury
E. All of the above

12. In the treatment of a small (1% total body surface area) burn of the palm of the hand, physical therapy consultation should be considered:
A. As soon as possible after the initial evaluation
B. After skin grafting is performed
C. 6 months after injury, when scar tissue formation is resolving
D. Never
E. If the wound is followed for 10 to 14 days and shows no evidence of eschar separation

13. Organisms that commonly infect burn wounds include:
A. *Staphylococcus* species, especially methicillin-resistant *Staphylococcus aureus*
B. *Pseudomonas* species
C. Yeast
D. Multiply resistant gram-negative organisms
E. All of the above

14. Inhalation injury significantly increases the mortality rate of patients with major burns mostly because of:
A. Increased metabolic rate and protein-calorie malnutrition
B. Persistent pulmonary infection and eventual development of multiple organ failure
C. Hypoxia
D. Airway obstruction
E. None of the above

15. A 19-year-old man is injured in a high-speed collision with a tree. His car catches fire. He is not wearing a seat belt, and he is ejected from the vehicle. He arrives in the emergency room alert and with a patent airway approximately 20 minutes after his injury. His blood pressure is 75/40 mm Hg, and his heart rate is 140 beats/min. His breath sounds are equal bilaterally. Arterial blood gas measurements are: Pao_2 140, Sao_2 98%, $Paco_2$ 34, and pH 7.33. He has burns of approximately 15% total body surface area, involving the anterior trunk and legs. His abdomen is covered with burns, but appears distended; tenderness is hard to determine because of painful burn wounds. His hypotension is probably caused by:
A. Smoke inhalation injury
B. Burn shock
C. Intraabdominal hemorrhage
D. Ethanol intoxication
E. Closed head injury

Oral Examination Study Questions

CASE 1

A 60-year-old woman is burned in a house fire. She is found unconscious and tachypneic, with a blood pressure of 120/80 mm Hg and a heart rate of 110 beats/min. She is brought by paramedics to your emergency room. She has partial- and full-thickness burns to her entire anterior torso, face, neck, arms, and hands, totaling 50% total body surface area (TBSA).

OBJECTIVE 1

The student outlines the initial management of the burned patient.
A. The student evaluates the potential for airway obstruction and inhalation injury during the primary survey.
B. The student performs appropriate primary and secondary surveys.

OBJECTIVE 2

The student outlines the fluid requirements for resuscitation.

Minimum Level of Achievement for Passing
A. The student indicates that the primary survey is the same as that for any trauma victim.
   1. Outline the primary survey.
   2. Identify the potential for airway obstruction and inhalation injury.
B. The student begins initial resuscitation in a manner identical to that for any trauma patient.
C. The student performs a detailed secondary survey, followed by an evaluation of the extent and depth of the burn injury.
D. The student calculates fluid resuscitation requirements based on the Parkland formula.

Honors Level of Achievement

A. The student indicates the possibility of carbon monoxide poisoning and outlines its pathophysiology.

B. The student identifies the criteria for referring the patient to a burn center.

C. The student outlines the three phases of patient care: resuscitation, wound coverage, and rehabilitation.

CASE 2

A 3-year-old girl is camping with her parents. While running in the campground, she falls and places her entire right forearm, from fingertips to elbow, into a burning campfire. She has dry, tight, leathery eschar covering the entire area. She has no pulses in her wrist on the right side and no apparent pain.

OBJECTIVE 1

The student outlines the initial management of the burned patient.

OBJECTIVE 2

The student determines that the patient has full-thickness burn wounds.

OBJECTIVE 3

The student evaluates the potential for circulatory compromise of the extremity.

OBJECTIVE 4

The student states the indications for referral to a burn center.

Minimum Level of Achievement for Passing

A. The student indicates that the primary survey is the same as that for any trauma victim, and outlines the primary survey.

B. The student performs a detailed secondary survey.
1. The student evaluates the extent and depth of the burn injury.
2. The student identifies the potential for circulatory compromise of the extremity.

C. The student knows that the patient fulfills the indications for referral to a burn center.

Honors Level of Achievement

A. The student describes the physical features of full-thickness burns.

B. The student lists the signs and symptoms of vascular compromise of the extremity.

C. The student identifies as many criteria as possible for referring the patient to a burn center.

D. The student outlines the three phases of patient care: resuscitation, wound coverage, and rehabilitation.

CASE 3

A 29-year-old man is working in an oil refinery when he is accidentally sprayed with a concentrated solution of sulfuric acid. He is immediately brought to the emergency room. When he is first seen, he is still dressed in cotton coveralls, which are smoking slightly and have an acrid smell. The skin of his hands, legs, and feet appears blistered.

OBJECTIVE 1

The student outlines the initial management of the burned patient.

OBJECTIVE 2

The student indicates the danger to health care workers of chemical contamination and lists the appropriate techniques for neutralizing chemicals.

OBJECTIVE 3

The student performs appropriate primary and secondary surveys.

OBJECTIVE 4

The student outlines the fluid requirements for resuscitation.

Minimum Level of Achievement for Passing

A. The student indicates that the primary survey is the same as that for any trauma victim.
1. Outline the primary survey.
2. Identify the potential for chemical contamination and the need to stop the burning process by washing the patient with large amounts of water before other care is delivered.

B. The student begins initial resuscitation in a manner identical to that for any trauma patient.

C. The student performs a detailed secondary survey. The student also evaluates the extent and depth of the burn injury and indicates the potential for deep burns from strong acid solutions.

D. The student calculates the fluid resuscitation requirements based on the Parkland formula.

Honors Level of Achievement

A. The student indicates the possibility of inhalation injury from caustic chemicals.

B. The student identifies the criteria for referring the patient to a burn center.

C. The student outlines the three phases of patient care: resuscitation, wound coverage, and rehabilitation.

SUGGESTED READINGS

Goodwin CW. Metabolism and nutrition in thermally injured patients. *Crit Care Clin* 1985;1:97–117.

Herndon DN, ed. *Total Burn Care.* Philadelphia, Pa: WB Saunders, 1996.

Monafo WW. Current concepts: initial management of burns. *N Engl J Med* 1996;225:1581–1586.

Pruitt BA, McManus AT. The changing epidemiology of infection in burn patients. *World J Surg* 1992;16:57–67.

Saffle JR, Schnebley WA. Burn wound care. In: Richard RL, Staley MJ, eds. *Burn Care and Rehabilitation: Principles and Practice.* Philadelphia, Pa: FA Davis, 1994.

Sharar SR, Heimbach DM. Inhalation injury: current concepts and controversies. *Adv Trauma Crit Care* 1986;6:213–230.

Warden GD. Burn shock resuscitation. *World J Surg* 1992;16:16–23.

11

Abdominal Wall, Including Hernia

D. Byron McGregor, M.D.
L. Beaty Pemberton, M.D.
Richard A. Bomberger, M.D.
Todd R. Arcomano, M.D.

OBJECTIVES

1. Know the relations of the layers of the abdominal wall and their pertinent reflections into the groin.
2. Define indirect inguinal hernia, direct inguinal hernia, and femoral hernia.
3. List the factors that predispose to the development of inguinal hernias.
4. Define and discuss the relative frequency of indirect, direct, and femoral hernias by age and sex.
5. Define incarcerated inguinal hernia, strangulated hernia, sliding hernia, and Richter's hernia.
6. Outline the principles of management for patients with groin hernias, including the surgical treatments for repair and the indications for their use.
7. Discuss the appropriate use of prosthetic materials in hernia repair.
8. Discuss the embryology of an umbilical hernia.

The abdominal wall is of obvious importance in keeping our insides inside. Knowledge of its anatomy is vital to plan transgressions for access to the enclosed viscera and to understand the common clinical problem of groin **hernias.** These hernias are the most common clinical problem addressed by surgeons, with more than 700,000 repairs performed annually. As many as 10% of these hernias eventually recur and require additional therapy. This chapter emphasizes anatomy and embryologic development because only with that knowledge can the surgeon plan structural changes to correct symptomatic defects. The chapter reviews the pertinent anatomy and discusses the most common hernias and their repair.

Anatomy of the Abdominal Wall

Surface Relations

The abdominal wall has few anatomic landmarks. Only the costal margins, anterior superior iliac spines, and umbilicus break the otherwise flat plane. Where anatomy failed, verbiage was substituted. Hypochondriacal (below the ribs), periumbilical (around the belly button), and epigastric (high abdominal) are examples of colorful, but imprecise, terms. Other attempts were made to define abdominal regions by drawing imaginary lines across the abdominal wall. Thus, the abdomen was halved, trisected, and even divided into as many as nine imaginary compartments in attempts to provide reliable topographic characteristics. The most useful of these is the creation of simple vertical and horizontal lines through the umbilicus, dividing the abdomen into four imaginary quadrants (Figure 11-1). In this format, the right upper quadrant covers such symptom-prone intraabdominal organs as the gallbladder, duodenum, right pleura, and liver. The left upper quadrant protects the spleen, stomach, left pleura, and the tail of the pancreas. The left lower quadrant obscures the sigmoid colon and left ureter. The right lower quadrant overlies the right ureter, cecum, Meckel's diverticulum, and that paradigm of right lower quadrant pain, the appendix.

Cutaneous Nerves

Sensory innervation of the anterior abdominal wall is supplied by the sensory branches of the lower intercostal nerves down through L-1. They appear first on the anterior abdominal wall as the lateral cutaneous nerves seen at the anterior axillary line. They proceed anteriorly, dividing into anterior and posterior branches, and supply the anterior and posterior abdominal walls in a dermatome-like fashion, with a relatively transverse distribution in the upper abdomen and a more oblique pattern in the groin (Figure 11-2A). The intercostal nerves also provide the anterior cutaneous branches that run in the anterior abdominal wall, between the transversus abdominus muscle and the

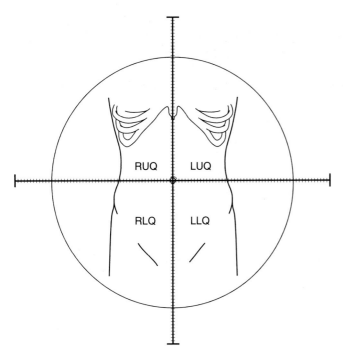

Figure 11-1 View of the anterior abdominal wall defining the descriptive sectors of anatomy. *RUQ* = right upper quadrant; *LUQ* = left upper quadrant; *RLQ* = right lower quadrant; *LLQ* = left lower quadrant.

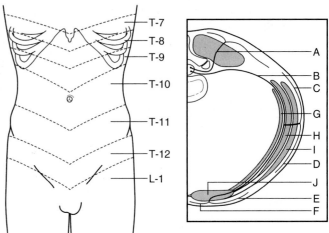

Figure 11-2 *Left,* Cutaneous nerve distribution to the anterior abdominal wall. *Right,* Schema of the cutaneous nerves. **A,** Posterior primary division. **B,** Anterior primary division. **C,** Posterior division of the lateral cutaneous nerve. **D,** Anterior division of the lateral cutaneous nerve. **E,** Lateral division of the anterior cutaneous nerve. **F,** Medial division of the anterior cutaneous nerve. **G,** Transversus abdominus muscle. **H,** Internal oblique muscle. **I,** External oblique muscle. **J,** Rectus abdominus muscle.

internal oblique muscle, toward the midline. There, they pierce the rectus sheath, supply the rectus muscle, and proceed anteriorly to innervate the midline and contribute to the segmental pattern started by the lateral cutaneous branches (see Figure 11–2*B*). The result of this rich cutaneous innervation is a series of dermatome-related clues to intraabdominal diagnoses. For example, visceral afferent fibers from the appendix follow the same nerve distribution as the small intestine, back to their T-10 origins. Therefore, early in its course, appendicitis causes central abdominal pain in the T-10 dermatome distribution. Later in the course of the disease, if the inflammatory process from the appendix develops anteriorly and irritates the peritoneum beneath the right lower quadrant of the abdomen, this irritation is sensed by somatic afferent fibers of the T-12 nerve route. It is reflected back in the appropriate lower cutaneous distribution as hyperesthesia. The disease can be well described by abdominal wall findings alone. Despite this apparent degree of segmental precision, considerable overlap of cutaneous nerves exists. Because of this overlap, the sacrifice of any single cutaneous nerve usually causes no permanent sensory loss. This safety factor is less pronounced in the lower sensory nerves (ilioinguinal and iliohypogastric). Injury to these nerves can leave permanent numbness in the groin, scrotum, and anterior thigh.

Layers of the Abdominal Wall

A brief review of the seven individual layers that make up the abdominal wall is helpful before any dis-

cussion of the use of these layers to explain surgical disease or design surgical repairs. The following discussion describes the anatomy of the seven individual layers, with particular attention to the origins and reflections of fascial continuity for each. The most notable reflection occurs in the groin, where all of the layers of the abdominal wall are reflected into the scrotum, much as the layers of a shirt, jacket, and overcoat are reflected off the chest wall and onto a sleeve, while maintaining constant relation to each other.

Skin

As elsewhere, the skin over the abdominal wall is transgressed by Langer's lines of cleavage. These lines of skin tension are produced by the course of fibrous bundles and the disposition of elastin fibers in the corium. Across the anterior abdominal walls, these lines are dispersed transversely. In the lower abdomen, like the cutaneous nerves, Langer's lines assume a slightly more oblique pattern as they course into the groins. The skin, its cleavage lines, and its superficial cutaneous innervation all are continuous onto the scrotum in the male and the labia in the female.

Superficial Fascia

The superficial fascia of the abdominal wall has two layers. The more superficial and fatty of the two is Camper's fascia. The deeper, more fibrous, denser layer is Scarpa's fascia. There is considerable disagreement about the precise definition and fascial connection of these two adipose layers. In general, they can be incised in any plane, with little adverse effect. They are generally considered to be contiguous into the perineum as the superficial perineal fascia of Colles of the penis and the tunica dartos of the scrotum. It is from this fascial continuity that infections and urinary extravasations proceed out of the perineum and into the abdominal wall.

External Oblique Muscle

The major functioning muscles of the abdominal wall are broad, flat constricting layers. In general, these layers overlap throughout their course and join symmetrically in the midline. The most superficial of these is the external abdominal oblique muscle. This muscle arises broadly from the lower six ribs and interdigitations of the serratus anterior muscle. In the flank, it forms a thick, broad muscle whose fibers run obliquely downward. However, as it courses over the anterior aspect of the abdominal wall, the fibers of its **aponeurosis** run essentially transversely. High in the abdomen, this aponeurosis fuses with half of the aponeurosis of the internal oblique muscle at the lateral margin of the rectus abdominus muscle to form the anterior rectus sheath (Figure 11-3). Lower in the abdomen, this fusion occurs near the midline.

In the groin, the aponeurotic fibers of the external oblique muscle angle downward, taking the direction of your fingers if they are placed comfortably in your jeans. Further laterally, this aponeurosis rolls on itself to form the inguinal ligament. This ligament is a free margin suspended between the anterior superior iliac spine and the pubic tubercle, with no muscular origins or insertions. Medially, the fibers of the inguinal ligament rotate and attach onto the most medial portion of **Cooper's ligament** as the lacunar ligament, which forms the final medial containment of a femoral hernia. The external oblique aponeurosis is contiguous into the scrotum as the external spermatic fascia and onto the anterior thigh as the fascia lata. Finally, near the medial attachment of the external oblique aponeurosis onto the pubic tubercle, the aponeurosis divides, forming a triangular orifice through which the spermatic cord and testicle descend. This aperture persists as the external or superficial inguinal ring.

Internal Oblique Muscle

The internal oblique muscle also arises broadly from the iliac crest, lumbodorsal fascia, and psoas fascia, as well as from continuity with its homologue, the internal intercostal muscles of the lower chest wall. Its fibers are directed obliquely upward in the high flank, transversely in the midflank, and obliquely downward in the low flank. Like the external oblique muscle, the internal oblique forms a broad aponeurosis that fuses into the midline and contributes to the anterior rectus sheath throughout the abdomen as well as the posterior rectus sheath in the upper abdomen (see Figure 11–3). The internal oblique remains muscular in the groin, where it has no attachments, and its fibers continue into the spermatic cord as the cremasteric muscle.

Transversus Muscle

The transversus abdominus muscle, the deepest of the three muscular layers, has similar origins and attach

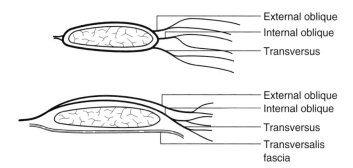

Figure 11-3 Midline fascial relations above *(top)* and below *(bottom)* the semicircular line of Douglas.

ments to the internal oblique, arising from the lower six ribs, the thoracolumbar fascia, and the iliac crest. It fuses medially to form the rectus sheaths and the linea alba. The fibers of its aponeurosis again run transversely, except in the groin, where they curve medially and downward to attach onto the pubic tubercle, the pectineal (Cooper's) ligament, and continue down the thigh as the anterior femoral sheath. In the groin, the aponeurosis of the transversus abdominus is fused to the underlying transversalis fascia to form the posterior inguinal wall. The spermatic cord descends through this wall (through its triangular orifice, the "abdominal," "deep," or "internal" inguinal ring). It is through this layer that all groin hernia pathology develops.

Transversalis Fascia

The transversalis fascia forms a complete, uninterrupted envelope of fascia around the interior of the abdominal cavity. Because it is a true fascial layer, it has little intrinsic strength, but through its fusion to aponeurotic layers, it establishes continuity among such seemingly unrelated areas as the diaphragm, the obturator internus, and the aforementioned layers of the anterior abdominal wall. It is separated from the underlying peritoneum by a variable layer of preperitoneal connective tissue and fat. With the descent of the testicle, the transversalis fascia establishes continuity with the internal spermatic fascia of the spermatic cord.

Peritoneum

The peritoneum is a serous membrane that lines the entire peritoneal cavity and invests the intraabdominal structures. Details of the intraabdominal reflections of the peritoneum and the formation of the greater and lesser peritoneal sacs are discussed in Chapters 13, 14, and 15. The peritoneum is best described here as only the exquisitely sensitive final lining layer of the anterior abdominal wall. With the descent of the testicle, a portion of the peritoneum is also advanced into the scrotum (Figure 11-4). With complete development, this peritoneal remnant remains as the tunica vaginalis of the testicle. In normal development, the remainder of the peritoneal connection is obliterated and the peritoneal cavity is once again a sealed space within the abdominal cavity (with the exception of the fallopian

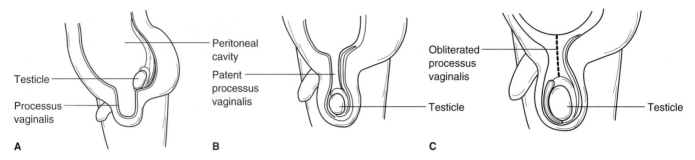

Figure 11-4 Peritoneal accompaniment of testicular descent. **A,** Before descent. **B,** Full patency of the processus vaginalis after descent. **C,** Patent remnant or noncommunicating hydrocele.

tube orifices). If this obliteration process is not completed, the result is varying degrees of persistence of an open communication between the peritoneal cavity and the tunica vaginalis. These varying degrees of patency result in either a communicating or a noncommunicating hydrocele, or a mere persistent patency of the processus vaginalis, inviting herniation.

Midline Structures

All of the layers of the abdominal wall are continuous across the anterior midline. The skin, subcutaneous tissues, transversalis fascia, and peritoneum are simple continuations, but the fusions and attachments of the abdominal muscles, umbilicus, and umbilical cord remnants deserve special attention.

To understand these midline structures, the sheaths and locations of the rectus abdominus muscles must be described. In comparison to the other abdominal muscles, these are narrow, thick bands of muscle that parallel the midline from the costal cartilages to the pubic symphysis. Each muscle is divided along its course by a variable number of tendinous inscriptions that essentially divide the muscle into a series of interconnected muscles. They are separated in the midline, above the umbilicus, by a condensation of the aponeuroses of the other abdominal muscles (linea alba). The formation of the linea alba and of the rectus sheaths is of some anatomic interest and surgical importance (see Figure 11–3). Approximately midway between the umbilicus and the symphysis pubis is an anatomic landmark, the semicircular line of Douglas. Above this line, the anterior sheath is formed by fusion of the external oblique aponeurosis and the anterior leaf of the internal oblique aponeurosis. The posterior sheath in this position is formed by fusion of the posterior leaf of the internal oblique aponeurosis and the aponeurosis of the transversus. Below the semicircular line, all three aponeuroses cross anterior to the rectus muscle, leaving only the peritoneum and the transversalis fascia between the rectus muscles and the abdominal contents. Below the semicircular line, the exact point of fusion of the aponeurotic layers to form the rectus sheath is variable. The external oblique usually joins far medially. The internal oblique and transversus fuse near the lateral edge of the rectus muscle. Wherever the latter fusion occurs,

the anterior rectus sheath is born. No fusion of these layers occurs along the inguinal canal, so the often mentioned, but seldom present, "conjoint tendon" normally (95% of cases) does not exist.

Umbilicus

By the start of the second trimester, the omphalomesenteric duct disappears, the gut rotates and reenters the peritoneal cavity, and the body walls form, with the exception of a ring of variable size in the middle of the abdomen. Through this ring pass the umbilical arteries, left umbilical vein, and allantois, a tubular diverticulum of the embryonic hindgut. At birth, these three atrophy into fibrous cords. With healing of the transected cord, the force of retraction of those vessels modifies the formation of the umbilical ring scar. These forces result in weak portions of the scar, usually at the superior portion of the umbilical defect, where later herniations can develop.

Remnants of this physiologic closure yield structures that are of occasional surgical interest. The left umbilical vein persists as the ligamentum teres of the liver, coursing in the falciform ligament from the umbilicus to the hepatic margin. Although it physiologically closes and fibroses after birth, this vessel is frequently available for cannulation in the newborn (and even occasionally in the adult) for venous access. Remnants of the omphalomesenteric duct persist as vitelline duct cysts, duct patency with stooling at the umbilicus, or Meckel's diverticulum. Finally, failure of allantois closure may result in urachal cysts or total urachal fistula, with urinary soiling at the umbilicus.

Abdominal Incisions

Access through the abdominal wall is obtained by surgical incisions. The ideal incision provides adequate access to the intraabdominal organ under investigation, reestablishes the strength and form of the abdominal wall postoperatively, and leaves a cosmetically acceptable surgical scar. The commonly used surgical incisions are few (Figure 11-5), but they deserve individual mention.

Vertical incisions are the most widely used. They are directed through the fused aponeurotic midline, anywhere from the xiphoid to the pubic tubercle. This inci-

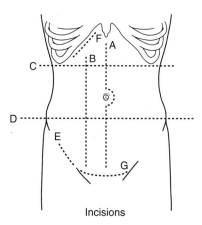

Incisions

Figure 11-5 Common incisions across the anterior abdominal wall. **A,** Midline incision. **B,** Paramedian incision. **C** and **D,** Two of the multiple planes of transverse incisions. **E,** Rocky-Davis incision. **F,** Subcostal incision. **G,** Pfannenstiel incision.

sion has multiple advantages, including the speed at which it can be made (because no vascular structures cross the midline), its ability to provide access to all portions of the abdomen, and its extendibility. It is the incision of choice in trauma or when lack of a preoperative diagnosis requires exposure of all portions of the abdomen.

Transverse incisions are preferred by some surgeons as being more "physiologic." The skin incisions are made in line with Langer's lines, resulting in more cosmetic scars. More important, they are made in line with the direction of muscle tension, so postoperative coughing or exercise tends to close the incision rather than open it (as occurs in vertical incisions). As a result, the incidence of wound dehiscence and late herniation is minimized. Transection of the rectus abdominus muscle is not a significant problem because a fibrous union that is the equivalent of an additional tendinous inscription results. However, intraabdominal exposure is compromised by transverse incisions. Misdiagnosis can result in awkward, cumbersome exposure, or it may necessitate the creation of a second appropriate incision after the diagnosis is made.

Paramedian incisions fell into disrepute in recent years. They add very little to the exposure provided through a midline vertical incision. In addition, they have several disadvantages: (1) they are time-consuming to create and close; (2) they may denervate medial portions of the rectus muscle and overlying skin; and (3) because of their inherent weakness, they are the most prone to herniation or disruption. The farther lateral a paramedian incision is fashioned, the more detrimental it is.

Subcostal incisions are advocated because they improve visibility for certain diseases in the upper abdomen. Although they combine some of the better features of the previous incisions, they offer the disadvantages of both. Lines of muscular pull, cutaneous innervation, and skin tension are all traversed, as with a vertical incision, whereas the possibility of extension in

the case of misdiagnosis is compromised, as with a horizontal incision.

Specific incisions are occasionally useful for specific diseases. The best example is the right lower quadrant Rocky-Davis incision for approach to the appendix. When a localized preoperative diagnosis is made, all of the benefits of this well-planned surgical incision can be realized. The transverse skin incision is in line with Langer's lines, and none of the cutaneous nerves, including the ilioinguinal and iliohypogastric, are disturbed. The precise location of McBurney's point, two-thirds of the distance from the umbilicus to the anterior iliac spine, allows the placement of a small incision immediately over the disease. The muscle layers are divided bluntly in line with their direction of pull, so herniation and disruption are rare. Once the peritoneum is closed, some claim that no further approximation of soft tissues is necessary for strong and cosmetic healing. Similarly, the Pfannenstiel incision, commonly used in gynecologic procedures, provides the strength of a transverse incision with the added cosmetic benefit of placement of the skin incision in the pubic hairline.

Hernias

A hernia is the protrusion of any organ, structure, or portion thereof through its normal anatomic confines. In the abdominal wall, a hernia is the protrusion of all or part of any intraabdominal structure through any congenital, acquired, or iatrogenic defect.

Inguinal Hernias

Indirect Inguinal Hernia

Anatomy and Pathophysiology

An indirect inguinal hernia occurs when bowel, omentum, or another intraabdominal organ protrudes through the abdominal ring within the continuous peritoneal coverage of a patent processus vaginalis (Figure 11-6). An indirect inguinal hernia is a congenital lesion; if the processus vaginalis does not remain patent, an **indirect hernia** cannot develop. Because 20% of male cadaver specimens retain some degree of processus vaginalis patency, patency of the processus vaginalis is necessary, but not sufficient, for hernia development. The medical history often yields the immediate reason for herniation.

The indirect hernia has two close cousins in the groin, the hydroceles. The communicating hydrocele differs from the indirect hernia only in that no bowel has yet protruded into the groin. Instead, serous peritoneal fluid fills this peritoneal peninsula to whatever level the patency exists. Because there is free communication between the hydrocele and the peritoneal cavity, the fluid collection is greater after standing and less after recumbency, and it is significantly augmented by pathologic formation of ascites within the abdominal cavity. The noncommunicating hydrocele occurs when a small portion of the processus vaginalis adjacent to the testicle

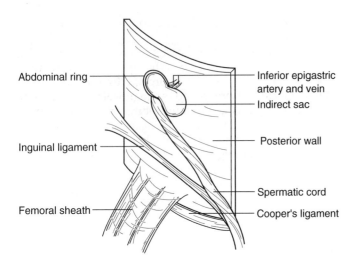

Figure 11-6 Indirect inguinal hernia. The posterior inguinal wall is intact. A hernia develops in the patent processus vaginalis (sac) on the anteromedial aspect of the cord. (In this figure and in Figures 11-7 and 11-8, the external oblique and internal oblique layers are not shown because they have no role in the development or repair of inguinal hernias.)

Table 11-1. Approximate Relative Incidence of Hernia Type

	Direct	Indirect	Femoral
Men	40%	50%	10%
Women	Rare	70%	30%
Children	Rare	All	Rare

is not obliterated, but the remainder of the processus vaginalis between it and the peritoneal cavity is obliterated (see Figure 11–4).

Clinical Presentation

Indirect hernias usually cause a bulge in the groin, typically with increased abdominal pressure. A 20-year-old workman hoisting a refrigerator has adequate cause for increased intraabdominal pressure, but it is equally valid to ask of a 60-year-old man, who has had a congenital patency since birth, why this congenital lesion would appear at this late date. Often, chronic coughing from bronchial carcinoma, straining at micturition from prostatism, or straining at defecation from a sigmoid obstruction causes an inguinal hernia. Still, most authors believe that extensive invasive investigation of these organ systems at the time of hernia diagnosis is inappropriate in the absence of related symptoms. Indirect hernias are the most common hernias in both sexes and all age groups (Table 11-1). They occur more commonly on the right because of delayed descent of that testicle.

Because indirect inguinal hernias originate through a relatively small aperture in the posterior inguinal wall (abdominal ring), there is a significant risk that bowel that slips easily into the processus vaginalis may become swollen, edematous, engorged, and finally entrapped outside of the abdominal cavity. This process, known as **incarceration,** is the most common cause of bowel obstruction in people who have not had previous abdominal surgery. It is the second most common cause of small bowel obstruction (see Chapters 18 and 19). This entrapment can become so severe that the blood supply to or from the bowel is compromised **(strangulation).** The result is bowel necrosis. Although

omentum or even loops of bowel can remain incarcerated outside the abdominal wall for months or years without proceeding to strangulation, surgeons seek to prevent this complication by recommending hernia repair whenever the diagnosis is made. With time, repeated protrusion of abdominal organs sufficiently dilates the abdominal ring, and incarceration and strangulation become less likely. This process, however, also implies greater destruction of the posterior inguinal wall, which is more difficult to repair, and a greater likelihood of recurrence.

Treatment

Indirect hernias are not amenable to medical therapy, although palliation is sometimes sought with the use of a truss. A truss is a fist-sized ball of leather, rubber, or fabric that is positioned by the patient over the protruding hernia bulge and strapped in place with variously designed belts and straps. Hernia defects never close spontaneously, and the use of a truss only increases scarring and the risk of incarceration. These two facts emphasize the importance of early diagnosis and surgical treatment of all hernias. Despite this caution, some patients are at such high risk for complications from any invasive procedure that a truss may be the best approach.

When an incarceration is encountered, a few gentle manual attempts at reduction (i.e., returning the entrapped organ to the confines of the abdominal cavity) are warranted. Although these attempts are successful in only 60% to 70% of cases and are associated with some risk to the entrapped structure, they are justified by the potential benefits of patient comfort, relief of obstruction, and prevention of strangulation, and by the diagnostic information obtained.

The surgical repair of indirect hernias is conceptually simple: (1) reduce any abdominal viscus to the abdominal cavity; (2) obliterate the processus vaginalis at a point high against the abdominal wall; and (3) reform a snug abdominal ring around the spermatic cord by anchoring the nondiseased remnants of the posterior wall or its replacement to their normal anatomic insertions onto Cooper's ligament and the anterior femoral sheath. This simple concept took anatomists and surgeons 100 combative years to develop, and is still in evolution (discussed later).

Direct Inguinal Hernia

Anatomy and Pathophysiology

Unlike the serpentine course of the indirect hernia, the direct inguinal hernia proceeds directly through the

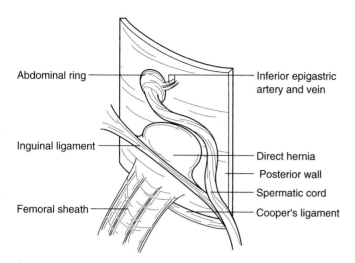

Figure 11-7 Direct inguinal hernia. The abdominal ring is intact. A hernia defect is a diffuse bulge in the posterior inguinal wall medial to the inferior epigastric vessels.

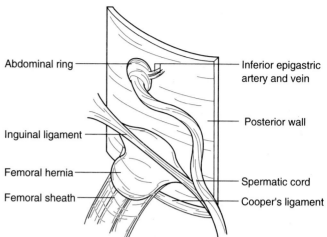

Figure 11-8 Femoral hernia. The defect is through the femoral canal, but otherwise involves similar structures and insertions as a direct inguinal hernia.

posterior inguinal wall (Figure 11–7). As opposed to indirect hernias, **direct hernias** protrude medial to the inferior epigastric vessels and are not associated with the processus vaginalis. Because there is no sac, they tend not to protrude with the cord into the scrotum and are generally believed to be acquired lesions, although there is considerable congenital variation in the strength of the posterior walls. Because they are acquired lesions, they are more common in older men. They occur over time as a result of pressure and tension on the muscle and fascia.

Clinical Presentation

Direct hernias, like indirect hernias, cause bulges in the groin. A spectrum of abnormality exists from very small-necked pedunculated herniations of preperitoneal fat (diverticular direct hernias) to large, bulging protrusions that destroy the entire posterior inguinal wall.

Treatment

Because of the lower incidence of incarceration and strangulation associated with direct hernias, a more relaxed approach to their repair is tolerated. However, because larger anatomic areas are frequently involved, more complex repairs are often required. The same procedures are employed as in the repair of indirect hernias, but with no attention needed to a (nonexistent) hernia sac.

Femoral Hernia

Anatomy and Pathophysiology

The third category of herniation in the groin is the **femoral hernia.** Like the direct hernia, it is an acquired lesion and has no hernia sac. Its etiology lies in a short medial attachment of the transversus abdominus muscle onto Cooper's ligament that results in an enlarged femoral ring that invites herniation (Figure 11-8).

Clinical Presentation

On physical examination, these hernias cause bulges much lower in the groin than other hernias (below the inguinal ring and onto the anterior thigh). Despite maximal dilation from repeated protrusion, the femoral hernia ring is finally limited by rigid structures (the inguinal ligament, its lacunar attachments, and Cooper's ligament). Therefore, this hernia is very susceptible to incarceration and strangulation.

Treatment

Despite its different anatomic location, a femoral hernia is repaired similarly to other groin hernias. The herniated contents are returned to their usual location, and abdominal wall continuity is restored.

Repair of Inguinal Hernias

In addition to the material described later in this chapter, see Chapter 26.

Classic Repairs

Marcy Repair. The Marcy repair is popular in very small or early indirect hernias. Because these hernias represent only a dilation of the abdominal ring, the Marcy repair simply snugs that aperture by sewing the transversus aponeurosis on the lateral side of the ring to the transversus aponeurosis on the medial side of the ring until that layer is snug around the cord.

McVay (Cooper's Ligament) Repair. The McVay procedure is an anatomic repair, like the Marcy operation, that is used for larger indirect hernias and direct hernias. The principle of this repair is that when the posterior inguinal wall is destroyed by the hernia, the surgical repair of that wall should be as close as possible to the original anatomy. Any remaining strong transversus aponeurosis is sewn to that tendon's natural lateral insertions, Cooper's ligament and the anterior femoral sheath.

Bassini Repair. The Bassini repair is a more superficial repair in which margins of transversus and internal oblique muscles are anchored laterally to the inguinal ligament.

Shouldice Repair. The Shouldice repair incorporates a series of four running suture lines that approximate and imbricate the transversus aponeurosis to several lateral structures. In a sense, this procedure combines a deep repair similar to McVay's with a superficial repair similar to Bassini's.

Newer Repairs

After nearly half a century of relative complacency, in the last decade, a series of changes revolutionized the surgical approach to the hernia. These changes are both commercial (e.g., expanded use of local anesthesia, increased use of the outpatient venue) and more fundamental (e.g., use of prosthetic meshes to replace attenuated aponeuroses, use of the laparoscope).

Mesh Repairs. The use of sheets of synthetic materials, usually polypropylene (Marlex) or polytetrafluoroethylene (PTFE; Gore-Tex), is increasingly popular. Because of their space-filling properties, these materials not only provide strength to the repair but also release tissue tension on anatomic structures. Available as plugs, patches, or in customized patterns to surround the spermatic cord, these materials do not alter the anatomic features of the repair, but their use permits the creation of tension-free repairs with remarkably low rates of recurrence. Caution is warranted, however. Although the infection rate does not seem to be increased, an infection that involves these materials can be severe.

Laparoscopic Repairs. Three basic laparoscopic approaches are used to repair an inguinal hernia: the transabdominal preperitoneal repair (TAPP), the totally extraperitoneal repair (TEP), and the intraperitoneal onlay mesh approach (IPOM).

With TAPP, the laparoscope is inserted into the peritoneal cavity through an infraumbilical incision, and the peritoneum of the groin is incised from within. Indirect, direct, and femoral hernias can all be approached with direct visualization where they transgress the transversalis fascia. A sheet of mesh is placed over the entire area to cover the femoral opening, direct space, and internal ring. Metallic staples or tacks are used to secure the mesh to the posterior abdominal wall, and the peritoneum is returned to line the repair.

TEP involves the use of a balloon insufflated in the preperitoneal space to push the peritoneum posteriorly. The balloon produces a space into which the laparoscope can be inserted. The aponeurotic mesh repair is similar, but the peritoneum is not entered, eliminating the risk of injury to peritoneal structures as well as subsequent adhesive complications.

The IPOM technique is less popular. Diagnostic laparoscopy is performed, and a piece of synthetic mesh is stapled over the visible defect without dissecting the peritoneum or identifying the borders of the defect. Direct and indirect hernias can be quickly repaired, but the risk of subsequent adhesion of intestinal content to the mesh is real. Similarly, laparoscopic methods of inguinal hernia repair that used only mesh plugs were uniformly unsuccessful, with high recurrence rates and migration of the mesh plugs.

Advantages of the laparoscopic approach include a low recurrence rate, diminished pain, and an earlier return to work. The drawbacks include the need for either regional or general anesthesia and the expense of instrumentation.

Umbilical Hernias

Anatomy and Pathophysiology

Like groin hernias, **umbilical hernias** are of three types. By far the most common is fortunately of least significance and threat to the patient. It is the small (usually < 1 cm) defect in the abdominal wall that results from incomplete umbilical closure. Through this fascial defect can protrude small portions of omentum, bowel, or other intraabdominal organs. In adults, even if umbilical closure occurred, the umbilical scar is subject to stretching and defects that can enlarge and produce a hernia. The other two types of abdominal wall herniation are much more severe, affect only the newborn and, fortunately, are very uncommon. An omphalocele occurs when, after incomplete closure of the abdominal wall by the time of birth, a portion of the abdominal contents herniates into the base of the umbilical cord. Unlike the simple umbilical hernia, which is covered by skin, in omphalocele, the abdominal contents are separated from the outside world by only a thin membrane of peritoneum and the amnion. Gastroschisis is an even more severe failure of abdominal wall closure. It causes a full-thickness abdominal wall defect lateral to the umbilicus. The hernia of gastroschisis is into the amniotic cavity, so there is no sac. There is no covering of any kind over the intestinal contents, which protrude from the lateral edge of the umbilicus.

Clinical Presentation

Because the developmental process of the abdominal wall continues into extrauterine life, small protrusions of this type are very common in infants. Unless incarceration occurs, they are best ignored until the preschool years, and most resolve spontaneously. Despite their innocuous nature in infancy, however, umbilical hernias are some threat in adulthood. The rigid surrounding walls of the linea alba predispose the patient to strangulation and incarceration of protruded organs. Omphaloceles and gastroschisis, however, are perinatal emergencies that require immediate surgical attention.

Treatment

Commonly used folk remedies (e.g., stuffing cotton balls into the umbilicus, taping coins over it to prevent protrusion) only delay developmental closure or complicate the hernia with necrosis of the overlying skin.

The treatment of umbilical hernia is as straightforward in concept as that of groin hernia: (1) reduce the abdominal contents, and (2) establish the continuity of the abdominal wall. The surgical procedures for a simple umbilical hernia are as straightforward in execution as they are in concept. By necessity, surgical therapy for omphalocele and gastroschisis is intricate and complex, including bowel resection and the formation of extraanatomic compartments fashioned of prosthetic materials. Despite these efforts, the mortality rate for these lesions remains high.

Other Hernias

Spigelian Hernia

Spigelian hernias are herniations through the semilunar line, which is the lateral margin of the rectus muscle, at or just below the junction with the semicircular line of Douglas. Unlike groin hernias, these hernias lie cephalad to the inferior epigastric vessels. The tight aponeurotic defect predisposes them to incarceration.

Grynfelt's Hernia

Grynfelt's hernia is a wide-mouthed hernia that protrudes through the superior lumbar triangle, which is bounded by the sacrospinalis muscle, the internal oblique muscle, and the inferior margin of the twelfth rib. Diagnosis is hampered by the protrusion of these hernias under the latissimus dorsi muscle.

Petit's Hernia

Petit's hernia protrudes through the inferior lumbar triangle, which is bounded by the lateral margin of the latissimus dorsi, the medial margin of the external oblique, and the iliac crest. Like the superior lumbar hernia, these hernias are broad, bulging hernias that usually do not incarcerate.

Richter's Hernia

Richter's hernia is a hernia at any site through which only a portion of the circumference of a bowel wall, usually the jejunum, incarcerates or strangulates. Because the entire lumen is not compromised, symptoms of bowel obstruction can be absent, despite gangrene of the strangulated portion.

Littre's Hernia

Any groin hernia that contains Meckel's diverticulum is Littre's hernia. This type of hernia is usually incarcerated or strangulated.

Obturator Hernia

Obturator hernias are deceptive hernias, often of Richter's type, that protrude through the obturator canal. They are much more common in women and usually occur in the seventh and eighth decades. An obturator hernia is classically diagnosed by the symptoms of intermittent bowel obstruction and paresthesias on the anteromedial aspect of the thigh as a result of compression of the obturator nerve (Howship-Romberg sign).

Hesselbach's Hernia

Like a femoral hernia, Hesselbach's hernia protrudes onto the thigh beneath the inguinal ligament, but courses lateral to the femoral vessels. The portion of the posterior inguinal wall through which direct herniation occurs is **Hesselbach's triangle.** Its classic boundaries are the rectus sheath, inferior epigastric vessels, and inguinal ligament. Because the inguinal ligament has no attachments to the posterior wall, it is increasingly popular to define the lateral margin as Cooper's ligament.

Pantaloon Hernia

The pantaloon hernia is the simultaneous occurrence of a direct and an indirect hernia. The pantaloon hernia causes two bulges that straddle the inferior epigastric vessels.

Sliding Hernia

A **sliding hernia** is any hernia in which a portion of the wall of the protruding peritoneal sac is made up of some intraabdominal organ (usually sigmoid, cecum, ovary, or bladder). As the sac expands, the organ is drawn out, into the hernia. Its repair involves the careful return of the organ to the abdominal cavity, followed by the traditional sequence of obliteration of the sac and closure of the fascial defect.

Incisional Hernia

The protrusion of abdominal contents through a defect acquired from incomplete closure of a previous abdominal incision is an incisional hernia. Although the orientation of the incision, the suture materials chosen, and various technical details can be implicated, the most common reason for the formation of an iatrogenic hernia is the development of an infection in the previous wound.

Multiple-Choice Questions

1. A simple indirect inguinal hernia is characterized by:
   A. An enlarged external ring
   B. Protrusion of abdominal contents through an epigastric defect
   C. A mass caudal to the inguinal ligament
   D. Difficulty in reduction of a groin mass
   E. Protrusion of intraabdominal contents through the internal ring

2. Which of the following hernias is LEAST likely to incarcerate?
   A. Femoral hernia
   B. Richter's hernia
   C. Umbilical hernia
   D. Direct inguinal hernia
   E. Spigelian hernia

3. Operative repair is indicated in umbilical hernia:
   A. In all infants younger than 2 years of age
   B. As soon as the diagnosis is made
   C. When it is nonreducible
   D. In all patients after a coin is taped over the protrusion for 6 months
   E. In adult patients who have hepatomegaly

4. The most common cause of an incisional hernia is:
   A. Obesity
   B. The use of a transverse incision
   C. The surgical technique used during wound closure
   D. Wound infection
   E. Early ambulation

5. A hernia in which a part of the wall of the protruding peritoneal sac is formed by an intraabdominal structure is called a:
   A. Littre's hernia
   B. Sliding hernia
   C. Richter's hernia
   D. Spigelian hernia
   E. Pantaloon hernia

6. Which of these structures forms the external inguinal ring?
   A. Conjoined tendon
   B. Inguinal ligament
   C. Internal oblique muscle and aponeurosis
   D. Cooper's ligament
   E. External oblique aponeurosis

7. The normal remnant of the peritoneum within the scrotum of an adult is the:
   A. Internal spermatic fascia
   B. Tunica vaginalis
   C. Linea alba
   D. External spermatic fascia
   E. Vas deferens

8. Below the semicircular line of Douglas, the posterior rectus sheath:
   A. Is absent
   B. Arises from the internal oblique muscle only
   C. Arises from the transverse abdominal muscle fascia only
   D. Is formed by the fusion of the aponeuroses of the external and internal oblique fascia
   E. Is formed by the posterior leaflet of the internal oblique muscle and the transversalis fascia

9. The hernia that is most likely to incarcerate is:
   A. Direct inguinal hernia
   B. Ventral hernia
   C. Indirect inguinal hernia
   D. Umbilical hernia
   E. Femoral hernia

10. The advantage of a midline vertical incision over a transverse abdominal incision is:
    A. Reduced postoperative pain
    B. The speed of making the incision
    C. A low incidence of incisional hernias
    D. A low incidence of dehiscence
    E. Alignment with the direction of muscle contraction

11. The majority of adult umbilical hernias:
    A. Close spontaneously
    B. Are caused by cord infections
    C. Occur in white men
    D. Result from a stretching or defect of the umbilical scar
    E. Are covered by the rectus sheath, fascia, and skin

12. Whether the patient is a child or an adult, an indirect inguinal hernia has:
    A. An infectious cause from a variety of organisms
    B. An acquired etiology
    C. A secondary etiology from coughing or straining
    D. A congenital etiology
    E. A neoplastic cause

13. Gastroschisis:
    A. Is a full-thickness abdominal wall defect lateral to the umbilicus
    B. Protrudes from the middle portion of the umbilicus
    C. Contains only the stomach
    D. Is covered by the amniotic membrane
    E. Is produced by malrotation of the intestine, with a left abdominal wall defect

14. An omphalocele is covered by:
    A. All layers of the abdominal wall
    B. Skin only
    C. Peritoneum only
    D. Peritoneum and amnion
    E. Peritoneum and skin

15. The inferior, or lower, border of Hesselbach's triangle in the groin is the:
    A. Transversalis fascia
    B. Inferior epigastric artery and vein
    C. Lateral margin of the rectus sheath
    D. External inguinal ring
    E. Inguinal ligament

16. What is the best definition of an abdominal wall hernia?
    A. A collection of fluid in a sac in the skin or the subcutaneous layers of the abdomen
    B. The protrusion of an intraabdominal structure through an abdominal wall defect
    C. Distension of the abdomen by air, fluid, neoplasm, or infection
    D. Any painful mass in the abdominal wall or scrotum
    E. Distension of any part of the gastrointestinal tract with air, fluid, or feces that causes a bulge in the abdominal wall

17. The hernia that is more common in older men than in younger men is:
    A. Femoral hernia
    B. Indirect inguinal hernia
    C. Direct inguinal hernia
    D. Incarcerated hernia
    E. Strangulated hernia

18. An inguinal hernia that cannot be reduced is called:
    A. Indirect
    B. Scrotal
    C. Direct
    D. Incarcerated
    E. Sliding

19. Match the following phrase with the single best response. Incarceration is a complication in:
    A. Indirect inguinal hernia
    B. Direct inguinal hernia
    C. Both
    D. Neither

20. Match the following phrase with the single best response. Diagnosed without a bulge:
    A. Indirect inguinal hernia
    B. Direct inguinal hernia
    C. Both
    D. Neither

21. Match the following phrase with the single best response. Has a true hernia sac:
    A. Indirect inguinal hernia
    B. Direct inguinal hernia
    C. Both
    D. Neither

22. Match the following phrase with the single best response. Occurs in infants:
    A. Indirect inguinal hernia
    B. Direct inguinal hernia
    C. Both
    D. Neither

23. Match the following phrase with the single best response. Frequently closes spontaneously:
    A. Indirect inguinal hernia
    B. Umbilical hernia
    C. Both
    D. Neither

24. Which of these hernias presents as a bulge below the inguinal ligament?
    A. Direct inguinal hernia
    B. Femoral hernia
    C. Indirect inguinal hernia
    D. Richter's hernia
    E. Spigelian hernia

25. A true fascial layer that forms a complete uninterrupted envelope of fascia external to the peritoneum of the abdominal cavity is called:
    A. Rectus sheaths and linea alba
    B. Scarpa's fascia
    C. Transversalis fascia
    D. External oblique aponeurosis
    E. Transversus muscle aponeurosis

26. Match the following phrase with the single best response. Truss application obliterates the sac:
    A. Direct inguinal hernia
    B. Indirect inguinal hernia
    C. Both
    D. Neither

27. Which phrase best describes the site of the protrusion in the abdominal wall for a direct inguinal hernia?
    A. A previous abdominal incision
    B. The inferior lumbar triangle bounded by the lateral margin of the latissimus, the medial border of the external oblique, and the iliac crest
    C. The internal ring through a patent processus vaginalis
    D. The lateral margin of the rectus muscle at the junction of the semicircular line of Douglas
    E. The posterior inguinal wall, through the floor of Hesselbach's triangle

28. An inguinal hernia with localized bowel swelling and gangrene that eventually causes perforation is a:
    A. Strangulated hernia
    B. Spigelian hernia
    C. Littre's hernia
    D. Sliding hernia
    E. Incarcerated hernia

Oral Examination Study Questions

CASE 1
You are the sole practitioner in an ambulatory care clinic in a medium-sized community with all available medical specialists nearby. A 52-year-old construction worker comes for his scheduled appointment. He has a recurring sensation of a bulge in his left groin. His vital signs are normal, and he appears generally healthy.

OBJECTIVE 1
The student elicits the following history.
    A. There is no previous serious medical history.
    B. The patient's only previous operation was a right-sided hernia repair as a child.
    C. The sensation of a bulge occurred at the time of physical exertion.

D. The patient has no other sources of increased abdominal pressure, specifically:
   1. No cough or new wheezing
   2. No urinary symptoms of prostatism
   3. No change in bowel habits
E. The student specifically elicits the lack of history of incarceration episodes.

OBJECTIVE 2

The student elicits physical findings consistent with simple indirect inguinal hernia.

A. The bulge is located above the inguinal ligament (to differentiate from femoral).
B. The bulge tends to appear at the abdominal ring and follows the course of the cord with any Valsalva maneuver of the student's choice.
C. The physical examination, including a rectal examination, is normal.
D. There is no other instance of similar bulge on the opposite (previously operated) side.

OBJECTIVE 3

The student describes the groin anatomy pertinent to angina hernias. The components are:

A. The attachments of the abdominal wall layers in the groin
B. The location and margins of the abdominal ring
C. The location and margins of the external ring
D. The location and margins of the femoral ring
E. The definition of Hesselbach's triangle
F. The congenital nature of the processus vaginalis
G. The sites of the various types of hernia

OBJECTIVE 4

The student explains the treatment options, including:

A. Observation, with counseling about the potential complications and risks of incarceration and strangulation
B. Truss, with a discussion of its purpose, use, and potential value
C. Surgical intervention, which is the only potential "cure" for this lesion

Minimum Level of Achievement for Passing

The student gives satisfactory presentations of the history and the physical and anatomic findings.

Honors Level of Achievement

A. The student extrapolates from the history and physical examination more advanced concepts (e.g., increased incidence because of the previous contralateral repair).
B. The student expands on the anatomic details to include surgically important concepts (e.g., anatomy of a sliding hernia, definition of the iliopubic tract).

C. The student offers a spontaneous explanation of common surgical techniques for repair based on the anatomic principles.

CASE 2

You are a board-certified general surgeon covering night call for a 200-bed general hospital in a town of 15,000 people. At 9:00 PM, you are called by an emergency room physician to see a 46-year-old woman who came to the emergency room with a 2-day history of progressively severe crampy abdominal pain, repeated episodes of vomiting, and a sensation of fever. The emergency room physician reports that her temperature is 39°C. Her pulse is 110/min, her blood pressure is 110/80 mm Hg, and her abdomen is extremely tender to palpation.

OBJECTIVE 1

The student recognizes this potential surgical emergency that requires on-site surgical evaluation. Temporizing by the student (e.g., x-rays, laboratory studies) should prompt the interviewer to present a rapidly deteriorating patient.

OBJECTIVE 2

The student elicits a history and a physical examination consistent with acute mechanical small bowel obstruction.

A. The patient has no significant medical history.
B. The patient had a previous paramedian incision for cholecystectomy, but no other previous operations.
C. Physical examination shows abdominal tenderness and voluntary guarding, but no peritoneal signs. The student performs auscultation and detects the high-pitched, tinkling bowel sounds of mechanical obstruction.
D. A firm, nonreducible mass is found at the lower pole of the surgical incision.

OBJECTIVE 3

The student provides a differential diagnosis.
A. Small bowel obstruction
B. Adhesions
C. Herniation

OBJECTIVE 4

The student digresses and discusses the anatomy of the various abdominal incisions and their relative surgical merits.

A. The student describes the layers of the abdominal wall that are traversed by the incisions.
B. The student describes one advantage and one disadvantage of each common abdominal incision, to include:

1. Ease of performance
2. Location with regard to the suspected organ operated on
3. Anatomic strength
4. Extendibility
5. Cosmetic considerations

OBJECTIVE 5

The student describes incarceration and strangulation, recognizes that they are urgent conditions, and describes a course of treatment that reflects that urgency.

Minimum Level of Achievement for Passing

The student shows an understanding of the anatomy of the abdominal wall and its incisions as well as an appreciation for the usually elective, but occasionally emergent, nature of incisional herniation.

Honors Level of Achievement

The student spontaneously explains more advanced concepts of physiology, such as the metabolic alkalosis of upper gastrointestinal fluid loss as a basis for urgency, aponeurotic fiber orientation as a basis for the choice of incision, and advanced wound closure techniques (e.g., rotation flaps, synthetic screen materials for hernia closure).

SUGGESTED READINGS

Anson BJ, McVay CB. The anatomy of the inguinal region. *Surg Gynecol Obstet* 1960;111:707.

Bassini E. Sulla cura radicale dell'ernia inguinale. *Arch Soc Ital Chir* 1887a;4:380. [Summarized by G Lusena in *La Societa Italiana di Chirurgia Nei Suio 30 Congressi (1883–1923).* Rome, Italy: Manuzio, 1934:284.]

Lichtenstein IL, Shulmen AG, Amid PK, Montillor MM. The tension-free hernioplasty. *Am J Surg* 1989;157(3):188–193.

McVay CB, Chapp JD. Inguinal and femoral hernioplasty: the evaluation of a basic concept. *Ann Surg* 1958;148:499.

Shouldice EE. Surgical treatment of hernia. *Ont Med Rev* 1945;4:43.

Stoker DL, Spiegelhalter DJ, Singh R, Wellwood JM. Laparoscopic versus open hernia repair. *Lancet* 1994;343:1243.

Toy F, Smoot R. Laparoscopic hernioplasty update. *J Laparoendosc Surg* 1992;2(5):197–205.

12

Esophagus

Hiram C. Polk, Jr., M.D.
Mary C. Mancini, M.D.
James McCoy, M.D.

OBJECTIVES

1. Describe the anatomic and physiologic factors that predispose people to reflux esophagitis.
2. Describe the techniques for examining the esophagus.
3. Describe esophageal hiatal hernia with regard to anatomic type (sliding and paraesophageal) and the need for treatment.
4. Describe the symptoms of reflux esophagitis, and discuss the diagnostic procedures used to confirm the diagnosis.
5. List the indications for operative management of esophageal reflux. Discuss the physiologic basis for the antireflux procedure used.
6. Describe the pathophysiology and clinical symptoms associated with achalasia of the esophagus. Briefly outline the management options.
7. Describe the radiologic findings that characterize motility disorders of the esophagus, including achalasia. Discuss manometric evaluation of the lower esophageal sphincter.
8. List the common esophageal diverticula in terms of their location, symptoms, and pathogenesis.
9. Differentiate the etiologic factors associated with pulsion and traction diverticula of the esophagus.
10. List the common types of benign esophageal neoplasms, and briefly describe how they are differentiated from malignant lesions.
11. List the two major cell types of esophageal neoplasms.
12. List the known etiologic factors for esophageal neoplasms.
13. List the symptoms that suggest esophageal malignancy.
14. Describe the natural history of a malignant lesion of the esophagus, and list the treatment options in order of preference.
15. Outline a plan for the diagnostic evaluation of a patient with a suspected esophageal tumor.
16. List the diagnostic modalities that are helpful in staging esophageal neoplasm.
17. Describe the etiology and presentation of traumatic perforation of the esophagus and the physical findings that occur early and late after this type of injury.

The esophagus provides a muscular conduit for the passage of orally ingested material from the mouth, through the negatively pressurized thorax, and into the upper stomach. An important secondary function is to permit emesis of material, either because it is toxic or because the distal alimentary tract cannot provide for timely prograde passage. The esophagus also provides a conduit for endoscopic evaluation of the upper alimentary tract, including the biliary and pancreatic ducts. It also allows evaluation of the heart and thoracic aorta by transesophageal ultrasound and transesophageal echocardiography. Common problems that affect the esophagus and require a physician's attention are hiatal hernia and **reflux esophagitis,** esophageal motility disorders, cancer, and occasional esophageal disruption.

Anatomy

The esophagus is a muscular tube that originates at the cricoid cartilage and pharynx in the neck. It traverses the posterior mediastinum behind the aortic arch and left mainstem bronchus to enter the abdominal cavity through the esophageal hiatus of the diaphragm. In most adults, a very short (< 3 cm) segment of true esophagus lies within the celomic cavity before it joins with the fundus of the stomach (Figure 12-1).

The esophagus has a mucosal layer, which consists of stratified squamous epithelium and occasional mucous glands, and two muscular layers. The inner muscular layer is oriented in a circular fashion, and the outer layer is oriented longitudinally. In contrast to the remainder of the gastrointestinal tract, there is no

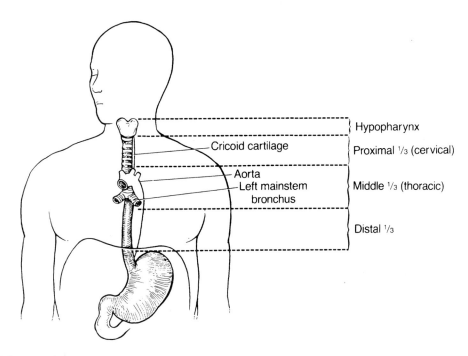

Figure 12-1 Clinical divisions of the esophagus.

serosal layer. The significance of this anatomic relation is apparent when considering the extension of neoplasms that originate in the esophagus, the relative ease with which the esophagus can be perforated during instrumentation, and the difficulty associated with surgical reconstruction after resection. The musculature of the upper one-third of the esophagus is skeletal, and that of the lower two-thirds is smooth muscle. Although the division between striated and smooth muscle cannot be determined precisely by histologic examination, the entire esophagus functions in a coordinated fashion. One physiologic sphincter is located in the neck (upper esophageal sphincter). Another is located at the level of the diaphragm **(lower esophageal sphincter).** Distinct muscle fibers with specialized sphincter function cannot be identified at this lower position. However, the peritoneal reflection that surrounds the esophageal hiatus and the phrenoesophageal ligament function together to produce an area of relatively high pressure with respect to the remainder of the esophagus and the stomach, which is located just distally.

Physiology

The motility of the distal esophageal sphincter is being studied increasingly, and the understanding of this physiology is growing rapidly. The esophagus is an active organ rather than a passive tube. When food enters the upper esophagus, it is propelled down the esophagus by a peristaltic wave. Figure 12-2 shows the coordination of contraction and relaxation in the esophagus. The lower esophageal sphincter relaxes in anticipation of the food bolus, allowing the food to enter the

stomach. The lower esophageal sphincter then returns to its normal high resting pressure of 15 to 25 cm H_2O greater than the pressure in the stomach to prevent reflux. Normally, swallowing a bolus of food causes a primary **peristaltic wave.** Secondary waves occur if the food is not cleared from the esophagus. Tertiary waves are abnormal and represent nonpropulsive "fibrillation" of the esophagus (Figure 12-3).

Pathophysiology

Like all sphincter mechanisms in the gastrointestinal tract, the purpose of the lower esophageal sphincter is to prevent the reflux of gastric content. However, unlike other sphincter mechanisms with well-defined circular muscle fibers (e.g., pylorus), this sphincter relies on a unique anatomic relation to accomplish this goal. Disturbances of this precarious relation allow for the reflux of acid gastric content onto a very sensitive, unprotected epithelial surface that is rich in sensory innervation. Failure of this lower sphincter to "relax" appropriately can result in proximal dilation of this muscular tube, which is not confined by a serosal layer, and can result in disordered contractility.

Clinical Presentation and Evaluation

Detecting esophageal disorders requires meticulous attention to the symptoms described by the patient because they may be manifestations of disease in other organ systems (e.g., heart, lungs) or signs of a systemic problem (e.g., collagen vascular disease, neurologic

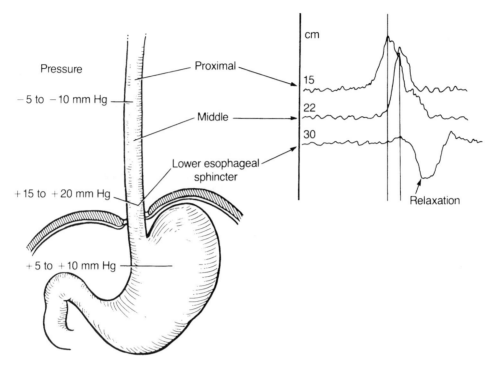

Figure 12-2 Manometry of a normal swallow. Note the progression of the primary peristaltic wave and the appropriate "relaxation" of the lower esophageal sphincter.

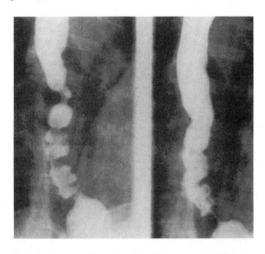

Figure 12-3 Barium swallow showing severe esophageal dysmotility with tertiary contractions in association with a sliding hiatal hernia.

disorder). To better assess the patient, the student should become familiar with several terms.

Difficulty with the transition of ingested substances from the mouth to the stomach is called **dysphagia.** The patient usually complains that food becomes "stuck" and may be able to define the point of obstruction. Dysphagia occurs with both liquids and solids, and pain is usually not a component of the process. **Odynophagia** is painful swallowing. It may occur secondary to esophageal infection (e.g., *Candida* esophagitis, cytomegalovirus, or herpesvirus infection), a foreign body in the esophagus, or injury to the esophagus. **Globus hystericus** is a "lump in the throat." These

patients must be evaluated carefully because the sensation may represent a mass lesion and not a psychological symptom.

Heartburn is known as **pyrosis** or **water brash.** It is associated with gastroesophageal reflux disease (GERD), achalasia, and esophageal strictures. In exploring the diagnosis of GERD, it is best to allow patients to describe their symptom complex in their own words. Heartburn that spontaneously disappears over a period of months without therapy may be a sign of a severe disease process (e.g., esophageal stricture, carcinoma).

Regurgitation is the passive return of ingested material into the oropharynx. **Vomiting** is the active return of stomach contents to the oropharynx.

Recurrent episodes of bronchitis or pneumonia, particularly in the very young and the elderly, may be signs of recurrent aspiration of esophageal or gastric contents because of esophageal obstruction, congenital malformation, diverticula, or esophageal motility disorders. Esophageal disease must also be considered in the differential diagnosis of anemia and bleeding. Ulcerative esophagitis is the most common cause of esophageal bleeding and usually causes occult blood in the stool.

Hiccup, or **singultus,** is a sign of diaphragmatic irritation and may indicate a diaphragmatic hernia or subendocardial myocardial infarction.

Esophageal disease may cause signs and symptoms that are often indistinguishable from those of angina pectoris. Some historical features may help to differentiate between the two disease processes. Symptoms related to the esophagus are aggravated by changes in body position, particularly bending over. The symptoms are relieved by belching and only marginally

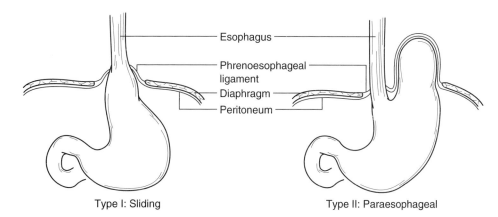

Esophagus

Phrenoesophageal
ligament

Diaphragm

Peritoneum

Type I: Sliding   Type II: Paraesophageal

Figure 12-4 The two most common types of hiatal hernia. Note the relation of each to the phrenoesophageal ligament and peritoneum.

relieved by nitroglycerin. Nitroglycerin relieves the symptoms of diffuse esophageal spasm. Usually, other symptoms related to the esophagus can be elicited from the patient. In any case, cardiac and esophageal evaluation must proceed simultaneously when the history is unclear.

Examination of the Esophagus

After a careful history is obtained, a physical examination is performed. Particular attention is paid to the oropharynx, neck, and supraclavicular regions. The stool is checked for occult blood. Subsequent diagnostic studies are directed by the patient's symptoms and the differential diagnosis. Posteroanterior and lateral chest radiographs are obtained to eliminate other thoracic pathology. Contrast studies with barium (e.g., barium swallow, cine-esophagogram) are safe, cost-effective, and efficient methods for evaluating esophageal anatomy and function. Computerized axial tomography (CT) scan of the chest is useful in examining the esophagus in relation to other anatomic structures in the thorax and in assessing the status of the mediastinum, particularly in esophageal cancer. Magnetic resonance imaging (MRI) provides no advantage over CT imaging in esophageal disease. Esophagoscopy allows for direct visualization of the esophageal lumen and is an indispensable diagnostic and therapeutic tool. With esophagoscopy, tumor specimens may be obtained for biopsy and varices may be occluded with sclerosing agents.

Manometry and fluoroscopy are used to diagnose uncommon abnormalities in esophageal motility. Esophageal manometry measures changes in pressure of the upper and lower esophageal sphincters as well as in the body of the esophagus, providing a quantitative assessment of esophageal motility. In addition to assessing peristalsis, manometry can identify the normal cricopharyngeal and lower esophageal sphincters and determine whether they function normally. To determine the chemical basis of GERD, pH monitoring may be used, but it is seldom needed clinically.

Hiatal Hernia and Gastroesophageal Reflux Disease

There are two major types of hiatal hernia: type I, "sliding," and type II, paraesophageal, or "rolling" (Figure 12-4). Sliding hiatal hernias are 100 times more common than paraesophageal hernias. A sliding hernia allows the gastroesophageal junction and a portion of the stomach to "slide" into the mediastinum. A true sliding hernia involves the retroperitoneal portion of the proximal stomach. This type of hernia is physiologically significant only when it is associated with the reflux of gastric acid into the lower esophagus. With a paraesophageal hiatal hernia, the esophagogastric junction is in a normal position, and reflux is uncommon. The portion of the gastric fundus that herniates alongside the esophagus is prone to **incarceration** or **strangulation,** much like inguinal hernias. Like a true **hernia,** the fundus of the stomach is inside a sac of peritoneum. The medical treatment or surgical repair of a type I hiatal hernia depends on the degree of acid reflux and the resulting symptoms. In contrast, like any other hernia, a paraesophageal (type II) hiatal hernia should be surgically repaired on discovery to preclude incarceration or strangulation. A type III hiatal hernia is a combination of the elements of types I and II. It is usually a very large defect in the esophageal hiatus. Other abdominal organs may be found in the mediastinum with the stomach. These organs require surgical repair to preclude necrosis.

In Western society, hiatal hernia occurs predominantly in women who have been pregnant and in men and women with increased intraabdominal pressure. Type I hiatal hernia with reflux is often found in patients who are overweight. Most investigators believe that increased intraabdominal pressure predisposes patients to reflux of gastric acid into the distal esophagus.

Although it is tempting to ascribe reflux to the presence of hiatal hernia, they are truly separate conditions. Although 80% of patients with reflux have hiatal hernia, some do not. Qualitative investigation of reflux and the quantitation of its severity are relatively sophisticated processes that require several independent invasive tests. These tests include prolonged pH monitoring of the distal esophagus, with correlations of patient symptoms and delays in acid clearance (Figure 12-5). These tests are expensive and are seldom needed in the case of the typical patient. Their use should be the exception rather than the rule. These investigations suggest that the symptoms of reflux are not exclusively related to an acidic environment and that alkaline reflux may occur as well. Pressures are recorded manometrically from three positions. Perfusion of the distal esophagus with hydrochloric acid alternating with normal saline is correlated with the patient's symptoms. Acid reflux is assessed by injecting a 15-mL bolus of hydrochloric acid into the midesophagus and monitoring pH levels 5 cm above the high-pressure zone. Additionally, the rate of clearance of acid from the esophagus can be measured. A normal individual restores the pH to normal with fewer than 10 swallows. Manometry and pH testing are of value when barium studies show abnormal peristalsis, when periodic dysphagia occurs, or when esophagi-

tis is not confirmed on endoscopy. Other uses may not be cost-effective.

Pathophysiology

The loss of the anatomic relation between the diaphragmatic hiatus and the esophagus disrupts the mechanism of the lower esophageal sphincter, rendering it incompetent. Reflux of acid gastric juice produces a chemical burn of the susceptible esophageal mucosa. The degree of mucosal injury is a function of the duration of acid contact, not a product of excessive gastric acidity. It is caused by normal acid in the wrong place. Continued inflammation of the distal esophagus may cause mucosal erosion, ulceration, and eventually scarring and stricture.

The subject of acid reflux into the lower esophagus deserves special comment because an understanding of the concept began to emerge only recently. The length of the intraabdominal segment of the esophagus may play a significant role in limiting reflux. A shortened intraab-

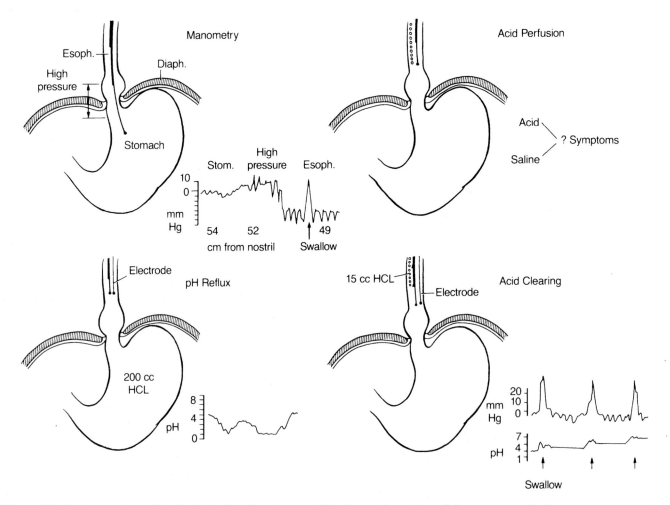

Figure 12-5 Various esophageal function tests. Catheters are passed into the esophagus through the nose or mouth. Pressure measurements are then made, or the catheters are used to infuse hydrochloric acid or saline to reproduce the symptoms of acid reflux. To determine the presence of endogenous acid reflux, pH electrodes can also be inserted. (Reprinted with permission from Skinner DB, Booth DJ. *Ann Surg* 1970;172:627–637.)

dominal segment (the distance between the insertion of the phrenoesophageal membrane into the wall of the esophagus to the flare of the gastric pouch) correlates with symptomatic reflux. Further, after surgical antireflux procedures or esophageal replacement with reversed gastric tubes or colonic segments, a high-pressure zone can be measured that functions, both quantitatively and qualitatively, as the normal distal esophagus. Basic physical laws, specifically, the law of Laplace, may have some bearing on reflux. Simply stated, the pressure required to distend a pliable tube is inversely related to the diameter of the tube. Applied to the problem of reflux, it is easy to see how the larger-diameter stomach distends more than the small esophagus in response to pressure, unless the anatomic relation is altered. Consider this difference in view of the anatomic relations shown in Figures 12-2 and 12-6. Other considerations in the pathophysiology of reflux include other anatomic relations involving the angle of His and gastric mucosal folds, and a role for gastric emptying. Figure 12-6 shows a summary of these mechanisms.

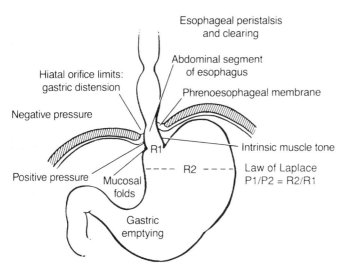

Figure 12-6 A summary of the anatomic and physiologic factors that are thought to prevent reflux of gastric content into the lower esophagus. (From Skinner DB. Pathophysiology of gastroesophageal reflux. *Ann Surg* 1985;202:553.)

Clinical Presentation

Many patients with type I hiatal hernia have no symptoms. Those with significant reflux classically have burning epigastric or substernal pain or tightness. Usually, the pain does not radiate. It may be described as tightness in the chest and can be confused with the pain of myocardial ischemia. The intensity of the pain is positional, becoming worse when the patient is supine or leaning over. Antacid therapy often improves the symptoms. Patients may also complain of a lump or a feeling that food is stuck beneath the xiphoid. This sensation is generally caused by muscular spasm of the esophagus. All common gastric irritants and stimulants (e.g., alcohol, aspirin, tobacco, caffeine) exacerbate the symptoms. Occasionally, the only indication of reflux is chronic aspiration pneumonitis. Late symptoms of dysphagia and vomiting usually suggest stricture formation. Even in this case, nearly all patients have reflux symptoms before the onset of dysphagia. Type II hernias generally produce few symptoms until they incarcerate and become ischemic. Dysphagia, bleeding and, occasionally, respiratory distress are the presenting symptoms.

Diagnosis

The diagnosis of hiatal hernia and reflux esophagitis can be confirmed by fluoroscopy during a barium swallow (Figure 12-7). Sometimes barium reflux from the stomach into the distal esophagus is not observed radiographically, but is inferred by the presence of other anatomic abnormalities (e.g., dysmotility, stricture, ulceration). In addition, local signs of esophageal irritation or ulceration are often present. The diagnosis of reflux esophagitis is usually suspected based on the patient's history. Physical examination is generally unrewarding, unless weight loss is a feature because of distal esophageal stricture and resultant nutritional depletion. The diagnosis of reflux esophagitis can also be made by esophagogastric endoscopy and biopsy of the inflamed esophagus. Most experienced endoscopists recognize esophagitis visually, and biopsy is seldom necessary to confirm the clinical findings. The basic evaluation for most patients is barium swallow and esophagoscopy. Esophagoscopy can be deferred if the response to nonoperative therapy is satisfactory.

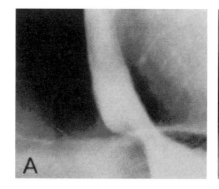
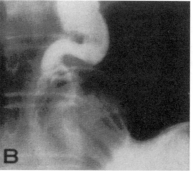

Figure 12-7 A, Normal distal esophagus shown by barium swallow. **B,** Small sliding hiatal hernia shown by barium swallow.

The symptoms of GERD may be nonspecific and may mimic those of other disease processes (Table 12-1). Angina of cardiac origin must be evaluated if the patient has a sensation of substernal pressure that is not relieved by belching or antacids. Occult blood in the stool may be secondary to erosive esophagitis, but peptic ulcer disease and colon cancer must be included in the differential diagnosis. Dysphagia may be a sign of oropharyngeal carcinoma or esophageal motility disorders secondary to collagen vascular disease or stroke. A history of recurrent pneumonia may point to advanced GERD accompanied by distal esophageal stricture. In immunocompromised patients, the symptoms of GERD may indicate *Candida* esophagitis, cytomegalovirus, or herpesvirus infection.

Treatment

Approximately 80% of patients respond to medical treatment, and half of them respond so completely that surgery is unnecessary. Approximately 20% of patients do not respond to initial medical treatment, and half of those who initially respond ultimately relapse and require surgery.

Medical Treatment

Primary treatment for esophagitis is medical and includes all of the following:

1. Avoidance of gastric stimulants (e.g., coffee, tobacco, alcohol, chocolate)
2. Elimination of tight garments that raise intraabdominal pressure (e.g., girdles, abdominal binders)
3. Regular use of antacids, particularly those that coat the esophagus (e.g., Gaviscon), as well as the use of antacid mints (e.g., Tums, Rolaids) to provide a steady stream of protection. H$_2$ blockers may also be beneficial because they increase the pH of the refluxed gastric juice. In selected cases, metoclopramide is helpful when poor gastric emptying is a component of the symptom complex.
4. Abstinence from drinking or eating within several hours of sleeping
5. Sleeping with the head of the bed elevated at least 6 inches to reduce nocturnal reflux
6. Weight loss in obese patients

With the advent and popularity of ion, or proton pump, inhibitors, second-line medicinal therapy has been altered. Omeprazole (Prilosec), ideally in combination with the measures described earlier, is effective in reversing severely symptomatic reflux esophagitis, but it is dose-dependent, is effective relatively briefly (i.e., < 6 months), and has some alleged carcinogenicity (carcinoid tumors in some animal models). This treatment is both popular and expensive.

Surgical Treatment

The principles of surgical treatment are relatively straightforward: to correct the anatomic defect and prevent the reflux of gastric acid into the lower esophagus by reconstruction of a valve mechanism (Figure 12-8). There are several eponyms for the common surgical procedures for reflux esophagitis (Nissen, Hill, Belsey). Each one has its advocates, and each varies in its approach to repairing the defect and creating the valve. However, all procedures combine these two principles. The route of repair is important: it may be accomplished with a transthoracic or a transabdominal approach. The abdominal approach is much more common and allows access to other intraabdominal pathology that might require repair at the same time. On the other hand, esophageal shortening is best approached with a transthoracic exposure.

The advent of laparoscopic techniques for transabdominal **fundoplication** altered the face of surgical care in the United States. Clearly, this procedure can now be done reasonably simply and with an acceptable learning curve for the laparoscopically skilled surgeon. Significantly shorter hospital stays and convalescent periods are offset by the greater operating room expense of laparoscopy. Relaxation of the indications for surgery led to a rapid increase in antireflux surgery in the United States. The best overall course of care remains to be determined.

Table 12-1. Gastroesophageal Reflux Disease: Symptoms, Diagnosis, and Therapy

Symptoms	Diagnosis	Pathology	Therapy	Follow-up
Heartburn	Endoscopy	Erythema with or without ulcers	Eliminate coffee, tobacco, alcohol; administer antacids, H$_2$ blockers; elevate head of bed	Repeat endoscopy after 6–8 wks
Heartburn, odynophagia angina	Endoscopy, barium study, cardiac workup	Linear ulceration	Medical therapy as above	Repeat endoscopy after 6–8 wks; if unimproved, consider surgery
Cessation of symptoms, aspiration	Barium study, endoscopy with biopsy	Stricture, carcinoma	Benign biopsy findings; biopsy equivocal or positive for cancer	Dilation and antireflux; resection

Complications

Postoperative complications include the inability to belch or vomit **(gas-bloat syndrome).** This complication is generally caused by overtightening of the valve and is minimized by the use of intraoperative calibration of the size of the gastroesophageal junction with a mercury bougie. Chewable simethicone tablets minimize gas bloating in the early postoperative period. Another complication, dysphagia, may result from making the gastroesophageal junction too narrow. Disruption of the repair with recurrent symptoms, intraabdominal infection, and esophageal perforation are also complications. Finally, splenic injury is always a possibility for procedures in this area.

Prognosis

The common surgical procedures relieve symptoms in more than 90% of patients. The surgical mortality rate is less than 1%, and the morbidity rate is typical for clean, major abdominal procedures. The abdominal procedure has slightly less morbidity than the transthoracic approach. With the laparoscopic approach, symptoms appear to be controlled at short-term follow-up. Many patients who were operated on laparoscopically also seemed to have less severe esophagitis initially, reflecting an almost palpable decrease in the extent of esophagitis required to justify an operation.

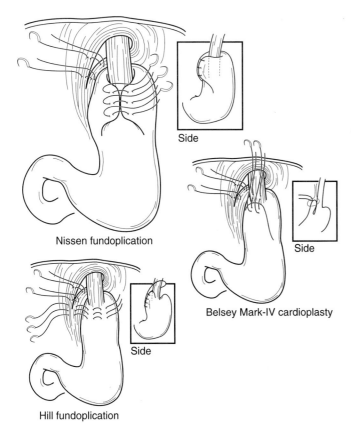

Figure 12-8 Three common hiatal hernia repairs. In each case, the defect at the esophageal hiatus is repaired and a valve mechanism is constructed with all or part of the gastric fundus.

Esophageal Motility Disorders

Esophageal motility disorders occur because of abnormalities of peristalsis at various levels in the esophagus. They may also lead to other disorders (e.g., diverticula) as a result of distal obstruction.

Achalasia

The most common motility disorder affecting the esophagus is **achalasia,** which literally means "failure to relax."

Pathophysiology

The pathophysiology of achalasia is located at the distal esophageal circular muscle segment. Contrary to common belief, it is not caused by spasm, but rather by failure of the high-pressure zone sphincter to relax. The result is painless dysphagia and slow, progressive dilation of the proximal esophagus. The precise mechanism for the distal circular muscle abnormality is not known.

Clinical Presentation and Evaluation

Dysphagia, regurgitation of undigested food, and weight loss are the classic symptoms of achalasia. Unlike reflux esophagitis, achalasia is seldom accompanied by pain. Patients often report consuming large quantities of liquids to force their food down. Aspiration pneumonia is common. Patients frequently complain of spitting up foul-smelling secretions when they simply lean forward.

The diagnosis of achalasia is generally first confirmed roentgenographically by contrast studies of the esophagus, frequently with cineradiography. Dilation of the proximal esophagus is a classic sign, and **esophageal diverticula** may occur at any level. Although endoscopy is frequently performed, it is important to avoid diverticular perforation because it is sometimes easier to pass the endoscope into the diverticulum than into the main channel of the esophagus. In complicated cases, esophageal manometry may be extremely helpful, particularly in patients who have undergone previous operations. The manometric pressures are characteristic, showing tertiary waves with diffuse spasm and evidence of hypertonic activity of the esophagus at the high-pressure zone of the distal esophagus.

Treatment

Medical treatment is generally not helpful, although calcium channel blockers have not been adequately studied in proper trials. Surgical treatment is the most reliable, and more than 95% of patients have complete relief of symptoms.

Medical Treatment

Medical treatment involves an invasive endoscopic procedure in which a balloon is placed at the region of high pressure in the esophagogastric junction. The balloon is rapidly inflated ("forceful dilation") to rupture the distal esophageal circular muscle, without rupturing the full thickness of the mucosa. The response to forceful dilation is variable. Approximately 80% of patients are cured by this procedure, but the complications, when they occur, are severe. The procedure is neither widely practiced nor readily learned.

Surgical Treatment

Esophageal myotomy is carried out over the distal 2 inches of the esophagus and extended 1 cm onto the stomach, producing the same result as forceful dilation. The procedure, which can now be performed thoracoscopically, involves a surgical incision in the muscular layer of the lower esophagus (myotomy). Its only disadvantage is the occasional development of reflux as a result of an overly lengthy myotomy. Consequently, some surgeons accompany the myotomy with a modified **fundoplication**. A complete 360° wrap of the lower esophagus occasionally exacerbates dysphagia and therefore should be avoided.

Esophageal Diverticula

The second most common manifestation of esophageal motility disorders is the development of **diverticula** (outpouching of all or part of the wall of the organ). Diverticula are classified as either pulsion or traction, depending on the mechanism that leads to their development.

Pathophysiology

Cervical diverticula and Zenker's diverticula (Figure 12-9) are classified as pulsion diverticula. They are closely related to dysfunction of the cricopharyngeal muscle, although the precise abnormality of motility is unknown. Anatomically, they occur between the oblique fibers of the thyropharyngeal muscle and the more horizontal fibers of the cricopharyngeus, an area of potential weakness.

Pulsion diverticula of the distal one-third of the esophagus are generally associated with dysfunction of the esophagogastric junction. They are caused by chronic stricture from acid reflux, antireflux surgical procedures, achalasia, or other uncommon disorders.

Middle-third esophageal diverticula are almost always traction diverticula and therefore are not related to an intrinsic abnormality in esophageal motility. They are usually caused by mediastinal inflammation (usually inflammatory nodal disease from tuberculosis or sarcoidosis) or histoplasmosis. This inflammation results in scar formation and subsequent contracture that places traction on the esophagus.

Clinical Presentation and Evaluation

Patients with symptomatic Zenker's diverticula have regurgitation of recently swallowed food or pills, choking, or a putrid breath odor. Patients with traction diverticula are usually asymptomatic and do not require treatment.

Treatment

Patients with Zenker's diverticula are best treated by excision of the diverticulum and myotomy of the cricopharyngeal muscle. Patients with diverticula of the distal third of the esophagus should also have the diverticula excised and the underlying pathologic process

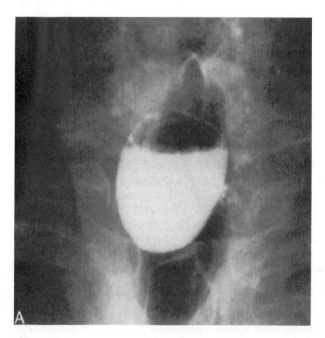
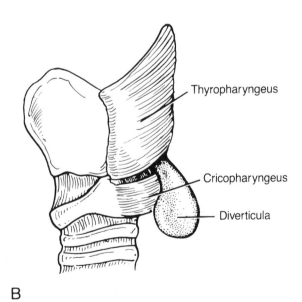

Figure 12-9 A, Barium retained after barium swallow shows a large pharyngealesophageal diverticulum, also known as Zenker's diverticulum. **B,** A diverticulum is a mucosal hernia between the two muscles of the pharyngeal constrictor mechanism. The diverticulum is false because it does not contain all of the layers of the esophagus, only mucosa.

corrected. This therapy relieves symptoms in more than 90% of patients, with surgical morbidity and mortality rates of less than 1%.

Other Disorders

Esophageal motility disorders are commonly found in association with a number of collagen vascular diseases, most notably scleroderma, a disease in which systemic smooth muscle is replaced by fibrosis. Although the etiology of scleroderma is not understood, its diagnosis depends in large part on the determination of esophageal abnormalities because as many as 70% of patients with scleroderma have esophageal involvement. Patients show marked abnormalities of esophageal motility, with a progressive decline in muscular contractility toward the lower esophageal sphincter. At this level, ineffective, poorly coordinated simultaneous contractions are recorded. These findings occur before the classic changes are noted by standard barium swallow radiographs. Patients have the constitutional symptoms of general malaise and fatigue and, if the esophagus is involved, may also have dysphagia or may need to force down their food with large volumes of liquids. With progressive reflux, extensive ulceration of the distal esophagus may occur. Medical therapy with antacids and H$_2$ blockers may offer only partial relief. **Stricture** formation is common. Although there is no known cure for the disease, surgical therapy to relieve severe esophageal symptoms may offer significant palliation.

Esophageal Neoplasms

Benign tumors of the esophagus are exceedingly rare and are mentioned only for the sake of completeness. Malignant tumors affect 2.6 per 100,000 population in the United States, with an increased incidence among African-American men. Squamous cell carcinoma is three to four times more common in African-American men than in white men, but it has the same dismal prognosis. The male:female ratio is 3 to 4:1 for both races. Worldwide, the incidence of esophageal cancer varies tremendously, from an extremely low incidence in many western societies to endemic proportions in certain regions of China.

Benign Tumors

Benign tumors of the esophagus arise from the various anatomic layers of this organ. They are most common in the middle and distal thirds. Leiomyomas are the most common intramural tumors, and the potential for malignant degeneration appears quite low. They have a characteristic smooth surface that is seen to indent the lumen of the esophagus on contrast radiography. Although the tumors are usually asymptomatic, many surgeons recommend excision because they tend to grow progressively and cause dysphagia, and to exclude the possibility of malignancy.

Malignant Tumors

Squamous cell carcinoma makes up approximately 85% of all primary esophageal neoplasms. Adenocarcinoma is seen in approximately 10% of esophageal cancers. Malignant melanoma, arising primarily in the esophagus, makes up less than 1% of esophageal tumors. Adenoid cystic tumors occur in 1 in 10,000 esophageal neoplasms. Sarcomas account for 0.8% of all esophageal tumors. Primary esophageal lymphoma is rare, but potentially curable. Tumors of the amine precursor uptake and decarboxylation system (APUDomas) make up 0.8% to 2.4% and usually have metastatic spread on initial presentation.

Epidemiology

The high incidence of esophageal cancer in various geographic areas (i.e., Coastal South Carolina; Washington, DC; Linxian County, China; Transkei, South Africa) suggests that environmental factors are important in the etiology. For example, low dietary levels of ascorbic acid, alpha-tocopherol, retinol, and riboflavin, and high levels of nitrosamines in fungus-infected food are associated with endemic areas of esophageal cancer in Linxian County, China. In the United States and other western countries, alcohol, tobacco, achalasia, **Barrett's esophagus,** and caustic esophageal injury all play a role in the pathogenesis of esophageal cancer.

In the high-risk areas of the United States, tobacco and alcohol were identified as major risk factors for esophageal cancer, particularly when the daily consumption of alcohol is equivalent to greater than 9 g ethanol (1 fl oz beer = 1.1 g ethanol; 1 fl oz wine = 2.9 g; 1 fl oz hard liquor = 9.4 g) and when the patient smokes more than 20 cigarettes per day. In other parts of the world, the etiology is related to diet, vitamin deficiency, poor oral hygiene, surgical procedures, and a number of premalignant conditions (e.g., caustic burns, Barrett's esophagus, radiation, Plummer-Vinson syndrome, esophageal diverticula).

Adenocarcinoma develops in approximately 10% of patients with Barrett's esophagus. Tylosis, an autosomal dominant disorder characterized by hyperkeratosis of the palms and soles, is the only verified genetic disorder associated with esophageal cancer. It is estimated that affected family members have a 95% chance of esophageal cancer if they live long enough.

Pathophysiology

Carcinoma of the esophagus usually arises from the squamous epithelium. Occasionally, adenocarcinoma occurs in the esophagus, but more commonly, these tumors originate in the fundus of the stomach and extend upward into the esophagus. Submucosal extension is common and frequently occurs over an extended distance. Because there is no serosal layer, invasion of adjacent structures is common. Adenocarcinomas may be the result of malignant transformation of the columnar epithelium that replaces the normal squamous lining of the distal esophagus as a result of chronic acid reflux. This metaplasia is known as Barrett's esophagus.

Clinical Presentation and Evaluation

Unfortunately, the symptoms of esophageal malignancy are often insidious at the onset, precluding early diagnosis and effective treatment. Dysphagia is the most common symptom. It usually begins with solid foods and then, over a period of weeks to months, progresses to include liquids. Retrosternal pain with swallowing (odynophagia) is the second most common symptom. Constant pain in the midback or midchest may be an ominous symptom of mediastinal invasion. Patients seem to ignore these symptoms and seek medical evaluation only after anorexia or weight loss occurs. Hoarseness may occur with local invasion in upper esophageal or midesophageal cancer. Some patients with cervical or upper thoracic esophageal cancer have acquired tracheoesophageal fistula as a result of erosion of the tumor into the trachea or bronchus. They may also have frequent episodes of pneumonia as a result of recurrent aspiration. Frequently, the disease is so advanced that patients cannot swallow their own saliva.

The presentation of carcinoma of the esophagus ranges from early carcinoma that is limited to the mucosa to more advanced forms that extend through the muscle layers and beyond. It infiltrates locally and involves the adjacent lymph nodes after spreading along the numerous submucosal lymphatics. The absence of a serosal layer allows earlier extension into adjacent structures (e.g., tracheobronchial tree, pericardium, aorta), and 75% of patients have supraclavicular, mediastinal, or celiac nodes at initial presentation.

The presumptive diagnosis of esophageal cancer is made by the typical ragged edge, shelf, or apple core appearance on barium contrast studies of the esophagus (Figure 12-10). An upper gastrointestinal series is often followed by endoscopy and biopsy of the lesion. Few esophageal cancers remain occult after barium and endoscopic studies of the esophagus are completed.

Screening esophagoscopy with Lugol's solution is used with some success to detect abnormal areas that represent malignancy. Lugol's solution contains iodine, which reacts with the high content of glycogen in normal esophageal mucosa, producing a black or green-brown color. Unstained areas are abnormal and are likely malignant.

CT is commonly used to stage esophageal cancer. However, CT is more reliable in detecting extranodal

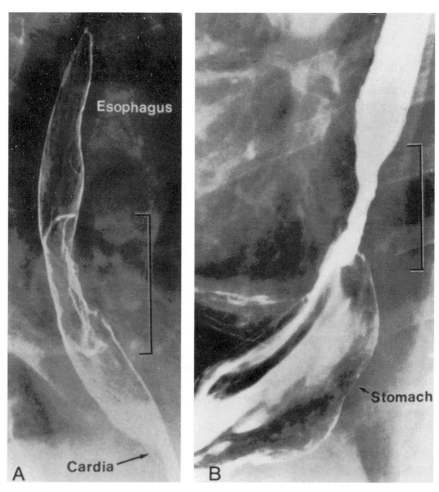

Figure 12-10 A, Contrast radiograph showing the typical "apple core" lesion of carcinoma of the middle one-third of the esophagus. **B,** Ragged edge seen in carcinoma of the distal esophagus.

metastases or recurrent cancer. Endoscopic ultrasound is used with some success in pretreatment staging and posttreatment follow-up. Laparoscopy is the most accurate modality (96%) for detecting intraabdominal metastases, and it allows biopsy confirmation. Despite its accuracy, it is not commonly used in assessing patients with esophageal cancer.

Abrasive brush cytology is of value in detecting early esophageal cancer in high-risk areas in China and South Africa. Brush biopsy is performed by having the patient swallow a brush biopsy capsule that contains the brush attached to a long thread. After 10 minutes, the capsule dissolves, the brush expands and is withdrawn, and the cytologic material is smeared onto a slide, fixed, stained, and examined. The predictive value of the brush cytology screening program in South Africa was 90%.

Treatment

Approximately 7% to 10% of esophageal malignancies arise in the cervical esophagus. When feasible, surgical treatment includes removal of all tumor-containing tissue. This treatment may involve cervical esophagectomy with en bloc laryngectomy and esophageal replacement with stomach, colon, or jejunum. If en bloc bilateral lymph node dissection is included, the jugular veins are spared.

Tumors in the upper and middle thirds of the thoracic esophagus are managed by resection with a transthoracic approach and by reestablishing continuity with esophagogastrostomy. If an adequate amount of stomach is not available, colon and jejunal grafts may be used. For patients with lesions of the distal esophageal and gastric cardia, resection is traditionally carried out with a left thoracoabdominal esophagogastrectomy and either pyloroplasty or pyloromyotomy to prevent delayed gastric emptying.

Transhiatal total esophagectomy without thoracotomy is used, regardless of the level of the tumor. Gastrointestinal continuity is reestablished by bringing up the stomach through the posterior mediastinum and performing an anastomosis between the fundus and the cervical esophagus. Pyloromyotomy and feeding jejunostomy are also performed. This procedure avoids the morbidity associated with making a major thoracic incision and performing a gastrointestinal anastomosis in the chest.

Because patients with squamous cell carcinoma or adenocarcinoma of the esophagus have a poor prognosis, treatment should be directed toward restoring effective swallowing. Treatment of patients with favorable tumors (small, possibly curable lesions and those without evidence of overt lymph node dissemination) should be aggressive and based on tumor location. Radiation therapy is the primary mode of treatment for cancer that arises in the upper esophagus. Surgical treatment at this level usually requires removal of the esophagus en bloc with the larynx, permanent tracheostomy, and restoration of swallowing by a free microsurgically constructed vascular pedicle of jejunum

or colon into the neck. Tumors that involve the middle third of the esophagus are usually treated by a staged procedure with total thoracic esophagectomy and bypass. Reconstructive options include pulling the stomach into the neck and interposing a segment of colon. Cancer involving the lower third of the esophagus or proximal stomach is best treated by esophagogastric resection and an end-to-end anastomosis in the midchest.

Prognosis

Squamous cell carcinomas and adenocarcinomas of the esophagus have a very poor prognosis. The cure rate for very favorable cases seldom exceeds 20% and, in general, the overall cure rate for all esophageal cancer is only 5%. In theory, combined preoperative chemotherapy and radiation therapy may be helpful in some patients. Palliation is available with a number of endoesophageal tubes (Celestin, Souttar, Mousseau-Barbin). The placement of these tubes is often associated with high morbidity and mortality rates, and the average survival is less than 6 months. Expansive metal stents for palliation are being tried, with lower operative morbidity and better palliation. Endoscopic laser provides temporary relief of obstruction, but must be repeated frequently. Photodynamic therapy with laser ablation decreases the overt incidence of adenocarcinoma in some patients with Barrett's esophagus. This approach remains to be proven.

Traumatic Esophageal Disorders

Because of their frequent occurrence and because of the morbidity and mortality associated with their lack of recognition and aggressive management, two traumatic injuries of the esophagus deserve brief mention: disruption or perforation of the esophagus and ingestion of caustic substances.

Esophageal Perforation

Esophageal perforation is usually the result of instrumentation. Causes include endoscopic or biopsy procedures, the passage of blind nasogastric tubes or instruments designed to dilate strictures, and the occasional inflation of devices used to tamponade bleeding varices in the esophagus (e.g., Sengstaken-Blakemore tubes, balloon dilation for achalasia). Spontaneous perforation of the esophagus also occurs, usually after an episode of forceful vomiting or retching that dramatically increases intraesophageal pressure (**Boerhaave's syndrome**). In this condition, the lack of a serosal layer makes perforation more common in the esophagus than at any other location in the alimentary tract. Perforation by external trauma is discussed in Chapter 9.

Clinical Presentation and Evaluation

The symptoms of esophageal perforation may be dramatic or occult, depending on the location of the perforation and its etiology. Perforation by nasogastric

tube may be insidious, and only after several hours will the patient be found in extremis and in profound shock from mediastinal sepsis. At other times, the event is catastrophic from the onset, with severe chest or abdominal pain, hypotension, diaphoresis, nausea, and vomiting to suggest the diagnosis in relation to the events that preceded the collapse.

Treatment

Treatment requires aggressive surgical intervention because the mortality rate is directly related to the interval between occurrence and intervention. Surgical drainage and repair, if possible, are necessary.

Caustic Ingestion

Ingestion of caustic materials, either accidentally (e.g., children) or intentionally (e.g., adult suicide attempt), is a medical emergency. The most ominous is the ingestion of alkaline-containing products (e.g., Drano, Liquid-Plumr). These solutions can destroy the tissue, from the lips well into the small intestine, to varying degrees.

Evaluation

The most important aspect of treatment is the early identification of the etiologic agent (e.g., acid, alkaline, specific toxin) because each agent requires a different approach. Second, careful physical examination of the oropharyngeal cavity is required to estimate the severity of injury. Invasive endoscopic procedures are usually urgently necessary.

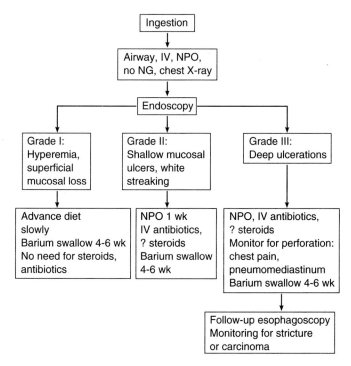

Figure 12-11 Algorithm for caustic ingestion. *IV,* intravenous; *NPO,* nothing by mouth; *NG,* nasogastric tube.

Treatment

Induced vomiting and neutralization of caustic substances are generally not suggested because they are potentially harmful and ineffective. Airway maintenance is the first priority, followed by maintenance of patency of the esophagus. The use of anti-inflammatory agents is generally recommended for alkaline or acid burns if they are seen within the first 24 hours. Steroids should not be used when perforation has occurred. Long-term therapy is directed toward the prevention, by dilation and ultimate surgical management, of stricture formation. The use of antibiotics as adjuvant therapy is controversial. Figure 12-11 shows an algorithm for caustic ingestion.

Summary

In summary, diseases that affect the esophagus are quite common and represent disabling problems for some patients. The diagnosis of virtually all illnesses can be accomplished with a careful barium study of the upper gastrointestinal tract and skilled endoscopic examination and biopsy. CT scans of the chest are useful in examining the esophagus in relation to other anatomic structures in the thorax and in assessing the status of the mediastinum, particularly in esophageal cancer. MRI provides no advantage over CT imaging in esophageal disease. An occasional patient whose disease is not clarified by these studies will require manometric study of the esophagus. Treatment of benign diseases of the esophagus is usually successful, unless distal esophageal inflammation progresses to stricture. The treatment of cancer of the esophagus at the time of clinical presentation is usually for palliation. Most recent efforts to improve cure rates for esophageal cancer focused on modifying risk factors and diagnosing the disease earlier. Traumatic injury of the esophagus requires prompt, aggressive management, with surgical consultation from the onset.

Multiple-Choice Questions

1. Asymptomatic hiatal hernias should be surgically repaired when:
   A. They are of the paraesophageal type
   B. They are seen on an upper gastrointestinal series
   C. Other abdominal surgery is being performed
   D. They are associated with esophagitis
   E. They are documented by two consecutive upper gastrointestinal examinations in 6 months

2. Pharyngoesophageal (Zenker's) diverticula:
   A. Occur just above the cricopharyngeal muscle
   B. Produce aspiration approximately 3 to 7 days after birth
   C. Cause few symptoms
   D. Result from traction on the esophagus
   E. Rarely require surgical therapy

3. Spontaneous perforation of the esophagus:
   A. Results from a peptic ulceration of the esophagus
   B. Is best managed by antibiotics and tube thoracostomy
   C. Is usually associated with Mallory-Weiss syndrome
   D. Is often misdiagnosed as myocardial infarction
   E. Usually occurs in the proximal third of the esophagus

4. Match the following phrase with the best single response. Manometric studies are diagnostic for:
   A. Achalasia
   B. Reflux esophagitis
   C. Both
   D. Neither
   E. Zenker's diverticula

5. The primary diagnosis of a patient who has emesis followed by chest pain and subcutaneous emphysema is:
   A. Acute myocardial infarction
   B. Spontaneous pneumothorax
   C. Ruptured aortic aneurysm
   D. Carcinoma of the esophagus
   E. Rupture of the esophagus

6. After the ingestion of alkaline material:
   A. Vomiting should be induced early
   B. Neutralization with dilute acid is advised
   C. Early endoscopy is necessary
   D. Steroids are not indicated
   E. Antibiotics prevent secondary infection

7. All of the following regarding the lower esophageal sphincter are true EXCEPT:
   A. A high-pressure zone is shown manometrically.
   B. A dense collection of circular smooth muscle is identified.
   C. A shortened intraabdominal esophagus may contribute to the loss of the pressure zone.
   D. Extraesophageal anatomic relations contribute to sphincter function.
   E. It is hormonally responsive.

8. Which of the following statements regarding achalasia is INCORRECT?
   A. Balloon dilation is the most successful means of therapy.
   B. Diverticula are common.
   C. Vomiting is rarely forceful, and may be positional.
   D. Surgical therapy involves myotomy and partial fundoplication.
   E. Calcium channel blockers produce relief in some patients.

9. In Boerhaave's syndrome:
   A. The tear occurs in the proximal part of the esophagus

B. The chest x-ray normally shows a left hydropneumothorax
   C. Only immediate resection of the esophagus is lifesaving
   D. The superficial hemorrhagic defect involves only the proximal gastric mucosa
   E. The diagnosis is generally made by computed tomography scan of the mediastinum

10. Operative intervention for a hiatal hernia is indicated when:
    A. Celestin tube therapy has failed
    B. Lye ingestion contributes to the symptoms of the hernia
    C. There is objective evidence of esophagitis or stenosis in a symptomatic patient
    D. A Schatzki ring is identified radiologically
    E. There is simultaneous peptic ulcer disease

11. Match the following phrase with the single best response. Barrett's esophagus is associated with:
    A. Adenocarcinoma of the esophagus
    B. Squamous carcinoma of the esophagus

12. Which of the items listed below is NOT associated with a high incidence of carcinoma of the esophagus? Select the single best answer.
    A. Low dietary intake of ascorbic acid
    B. Low dietary intake of alpha-tocopherol
    C. High levels of nitrosamines
    D. High intake of alcohol
    E. Low levels of folate

13. A 55-year-old man has dysphagia, midchest pain, blood-tinged sputum, and a 30-lb weight loss over 5 months. What procedure would you perform next?
    A. Computed tomography scan of the chest
    B. Magnetic resonance imaging scan of the chest
    C. Transesophageal ultrasound
    D. Esophagram or upper gastrointestinal series
    E. Esophagoscopy with multiple biopsies and bronchoscopy

14. A 45-year-old man has a long history of smoking and consumption of alcohol equivalent to more than 9.0 g ethanol daily for 20 years. The patient has carcinoma of the midesophagus on biopsy. Transesophageal ultrasound shows an 8-cm lesion with invasion into the pericardium. What are the chances that he will have supraclavicular, mediastinal, or celiac nodes at the time of initial presentation?
    A. 25%
    B. 10%
    C. 35%
    D. 75%
    E. 60%

15. Lugol's solution can be used to identify early neoplastic changes in the esophagus.
    A. True
    B. False

16. A 57-year-old man with a 15-year history of consuming a six-pack of beer daily has a 5- × 2-cm area of mucosa that is unstained with Lugol's solution in the midesophagus. What is the most appropriate next step?
    A. Advise the patient to stop drinking alcohol.
    B. Perform a barium swallow.
    C. Perform multiple biopsies and brush cytology of the unstained areas.
    D. Perform ultrasound of the esophagus.
    E. Perform an acid perfusion test.

17. Palliation for a 75-year-old man with a middle esophageal obstructing cancer can be done with some success with an expansive endoesophageal tube.
    A. True
    B. False

18. A 70-year-old man has a 25-lb weight loss, dysphagia for solid foods, and an obstructing esophageal lesion at the level of the left mainstem bronchus. Chest x-ray shows left lower lobe pneumonic infiltrate. Biopsy of the esophageal lesion shows squamous carcinoma. Alkaline phosphatase is elevated to twice the normal value. What is the most appropriate next step?
    A. Magnetic resonance imaging scan of the chest
    B. Computed tomography scan of the chest and abdomen
    C. Transesophageal ultrasound
    D. Diagnostic laparoscopy
    E. Sputum cytology

19. Primary prevention of esophageal neoplasm in the United States includes all BUT one of the following:
    A. Reduction of cigarette smoking
    B. Decreased consumption of alcohol
    C. Reduction of fat intake
    D. Increase in consumption of an oxidant vitamin
    E. Vigorous control of reflux esophagitis

20. Which of the statements regarding achalasia is INCORRECT?
    A. Balloon dilation is the most successful means of therapy.
    B. A bird's beak deformity on barium swallow is common.
    C. Vomiting is rarely forceful, and may be positional.
    D. Surgical therapy involves myotomy and partial fundoplication.
    E. Calcium channel blockers provide relief in some patients.

Oral Examination Study Questions

CASE 1

A 45-year-old man comes to your office with a history of difficulty in swallowing of 6 months' duration.

OBJECTIVE 1

The student elicits the following history.
  A. Initially, the patient had difficulty swallowing solids, but the condition has progressed, and now he can swallow only pureed food and liquids.
  B. He has been a two-pack-a-day smoker for 25 years and drinks 12 to 16 beers per week, especially on weekends.

OBJECTIVE 2

The student relates the possible findings on physical examination.
  A. Evidence of weight loss
  B. Possible evidence of metastases (e.g., Virchow's node, enlarged liver)

OBJECTIVE 3

The student formulates a differential diagnosis.
  A. Carcinoma of the esophagus
  B. Carcinoma of the stomach
  C. Benign esophageal stricture
  D. Benign esophageal tumor

The student develops an investigational plan for this patient.
  A. Upper gastrointestinal (GI) barium study
  B. Endoscopy with biopsy
  C. Complete blood count
  D. Serum total protein and albumin
  E. Chest x-ray
  F. Urinalysis

The student compares the x-ray findings in carcinoma of the esophagus with those in a benign stricture.
  A. Ragged, space-occupying lesion versus smooth, tapered lesion
  B. Evidence of space-occupying fungating lesion in the fundus of the stomach

The biopsy shows that the lesion is adenocarcinoma of the lower esophagus. The student presents the alternatives in management and expected outcomes for this patient.
  A. Surgery for cure
  B. Surgery with radiation (not indicated)
  C. Chemotherapy (not indicated)
  D. Palliation with a stent, radiation, or laser resection

Minimum Level of Achievement for Passing

The student makes the diagnosis of adenocarcinoma of the lower esophagus and describes the therapy for cure (surgery) or palliation (stent, radiation therapy, or laser resection). The student knows the results of surgery for cure (at best, 20%; in general, 5%).

Honors Level of Achievement

The student describes the therapy for cure of upper, mid-, and lower esophageal tumors and knows the types, origins, and etiologic factors in the development of esophageal malignancy.

CASE 2

A 42-year-old woman comes to your office with a history of heartburn of 1 year's duration that recently increased in severity.

OBJECTIVE 1

The student elicits the following history.

A. The heartburn occurs after eating, particularly after eating spicy foods.

B. The heartburn is precipitated by bending over or lying down, and the patient is awakened at night by it.

C. The patient has not lost weight and is not taking any medication.

D. The symptoms are relieved by taking antacids.

E. The rest of the history and physical examination are unremarkable.

OBJECTIVE 2

The student discusses the differential diagnosis.

A. Reflux esophagitis

B. Scleroderma

C. Diffuse spasm

D. Achalasia

The student sets forth a plan of investigation for the patient, including:

A. Upper GI barium swallow and upper GI series (hiatal hernia)

B. Endoscopy (reflux esophagitis)

C. Esophageal manometry (loss of lower esophageal high-pressure area)

The student sets forth a plan of management to include:

A. Administration of antacids

B. Elevation of the head of the bed

C. Avoidance of foods that precipitate symptoms

D. Weight loss

E. Abstinence from drinking or eating within several hours of sleeping

OBJECTIVE 3

The patient follows this regimen, but continues to have symptoms. She is given cimetidine, which is helpful at first, but later does not reduce her symptoms. She presents 2 years later with severe symptoms. In addition, she notes fluid on her pillow at night and often awakes coughing and choking.

The student sets out the further investigation of this patient to include:

A. Physical examination

B. Chest x-ray

C. Repeat barium swallow with cineradiography or video imaging (reflux esophagitis)

D. Endoscopy

E. Manometry (disordered esophageal contraction)

OBJECTIVE 4

The student discusses the further management of this patient, including operation and the expected outcome of fundoplication (95% relief of symptoms).

Minimum Level of Achievement for Passing

The student diagnoses esophageal reflux and describes the medical and surgical management.

Honors Level of Achievement

The student describes the appropriate manometric findings and knows that medical therapy is fully effective in 50% of patients. The student also knows that of the two-thirds of patients who respond to medical therapy initially, one-half ultimately require surgery.

CASE 3

A 58-year-old woman is seen in the emergency room with a history of dysphagia of 3 months' duration.

OBJECTIVE 1

The student elicits a thorough history. This patient had three pregnancies and had severe heartburn during the last trimester of each pregnancy. She was then symptom-free until 10 years ago, when heartburn developed. The symptoms occurred after eating and were related to changes in posture. She occasionally took antacids, with some relief. Three months ago, she had difficulty swallowing solids. The difficulty progressed, and now she can swallow only liquids. She has lost 10 lb.

OBJECTIVE 2

The student provides a differential diagnosis.

A. Reflux esophagitis with benign stricture

B. Carcinoma of the esophagus

C. Carcinoma of the stomach

D. Benign tumor of the esophagus

The student sets out a plan of investigation for this patient.

A. Barium swallow

B. Endoscopy with biopsy

C. Esophageal manometry

OBJECTIVE 3

The barium swallow shows a hiatal hernia with a smooth stricture of the lower 4 cm of esophagus. Endoscopy shows marked inflammation of the lower esophagus, with a smooth stricture. Biopsies show chronic esophagitis. Manometry shows the absence of the lower esophageal pressure zone.

The student discusses the diagnosis and formulates a plan for the management of this patient, including:

A. Conservative management (unlikely to help because a stricture has formed)

B. Dilation of the stricture (less desirable)

C. Dilatation of the stricture with fundoplication (the best approach)

Minimum Level of Achievement for Passing

The student obtains the appropriate history, physical, and laboratory studies to rule out the differential diag-noses and make the diagnosis of sliding hiatal hernia with stricture.

Honors Level of Achievement

The student describes the mechanism of stricture formation, including reflux acid esophagitis and loss of lower esophageal sphincter or manometry.

SUGGESTED READINGS

Brown LM, Blot WJ, Shuman SH, et al. Environment factors and high risk of esophageal cancer among men in Coastal South Carolina. *J Natl Cancer Inst* 1988;80:1620.

Haddad NG, Fleischer DE. Neoplasms of the esophagus. In: Castell DO, ed. *The Esophagus.* Boston, Mass: Little Brown & Co, 1995:269.

Hiebert CA. Clinical features. In: Pearson FG, ed. *Esophageal Surgery,* 1st ed. New York, NY: Churchill Livingstone, 1995:63–69.

Orringer MB. The esophagus. In: Sabiston DC, ed. *Textbook of Surgery: The Biological Basis of Modern Surgical Practice,* 15th ed. Philadelphia, Pa: WB Saunders, 1997:697.

Richardson JD, Martin LF, Borzotta AP, Polk HC Jr. Unifying concepts in treatment of esophageal leaks. *Am J Surg* 1985:149.

Sabiston DC, Spencer FC, eds. *Surgery of the Chest,* 6th ed. Philadelphia, Pa: WB Saunders, 1995.

Yang CS. Research on esophageal cancer in China: a review. *Cancer Res* 1980;40:2633.

Zuidema GD, ed. *Shackelford's Surgery of the Alimentary tract,* 4th ed. Philadelphia, Pa: WB Saunders, 1996.

13

Stomach and Duodenum

J. Patrick O'Leary, M.D.
Daniel J. Jurusz, M.D.
Glen Steeb, M.D.

OBJECTIVES

1. Compare and contrast the common symptoms and pathogenesis of gastric and duodenal ulcer disease, including patterns of acid secretion.
2. Discuss the significance of the anatomic location of gastric and duodenal ulcers.
3. Discuss the diagnostic value of upper gastrointestinal roentgenograms, endoscopy with biopsy, gastric analysis, serum gastrin levels, and the secretin stimulation test in patients with suspected peptic ulcer disease.
4. Describe in detail the nonoperative management of patients with peptic ulcer disease.
5. Discuss the complications of peptic ulcer disease, including the clinical presentation, diagnostic workup, and appropriate surgical treatment.
6. List the clinical and laboratory features that differentiate Zollinger-Ellison syndrome (gastrinoma) from duodenal ulcer disease.
7. Compare the risk of carcinoma in patients with gastric ulcer disease with the risk in those with duodenal ulcer disease.
8. Describe the common operations performed for duodenal and gastric ulcer disease, and discuss the morbidity rates associated with each procedure.
9. Discuss the commonly recognized side effects associated with surgery for duodenal and gastric ulcer disease.
10. Identify the premalignant conditions, epidemiologic factors, and clinical features in patients with gastric adenocarcinoma.
11. Describe the common types of neoplasms that occur in the stomach, and discuss the appropriate diagnostic procedures, therapeutic modalities, and prognosis for each.
12. List the general principles of curative and palliative surgical procedures for patients with a gastric neoplasm.

Anatomy

The Stomach

The stomach is a pliable, saccular organ that is located in the left hypochondrium and epigastrium. Its major function is to prepare ingested food for digestion and absorption. The stomach is separated from the rest of the gastrointestinal tract by two sphincters. The proximal sphincter, located at the junction of the esophagus and the stomach, is marked histologically by a mucosal change from squamous to columnar epithelium. This area is known as the lower esophageal sphincter, or esophageal distal high-pressure zone. In healthy individuals, this zone prevents reflux of caustic gastric contents into the esophagus. The distal end of the stomach, or antrum, joins with the duodenum. At this point, a definite mucosal change is seen histologically. This region has a well-defined sphincter (pylorus) that is composed of smooth muscle. The restricted lumen of the pylorus, or pyloric channel, is 1 to 3 cm long. The pylorus prevents the reflux of duodenal contents into the stomach and, in association with the antral pump, controls the rate of gastric emptying. After ingestion of a meal, particles larger than 3 to 5 mm are not allowed to leave the stomach until the final "cleansing" wave of peristalsis occurs several hours later.

The arterial blood supply to the stomach includes the right and left gastric arteries, right and left gastroepiploic

Acknowledgments
We thank the following colleagues for their contributions to this chapter: James F. Lind, M.D.; Raymond J. Joehl, M.D.; Edwin C. James, M.D.; Talmadge A. Bowden Jr., M.D.; Mary McCarthy, M.D.; Rudy G. Danzinger, M.D.; Guy Legros, M.D.; Gordon Telford, M.D.; Ajit K. Sachdeva, M.D., F.R.C.S.(C), F.A.C.S.; Thomas A. Miller, M.D., F.A.C.S.; and Steven T. Ruby, M.D.

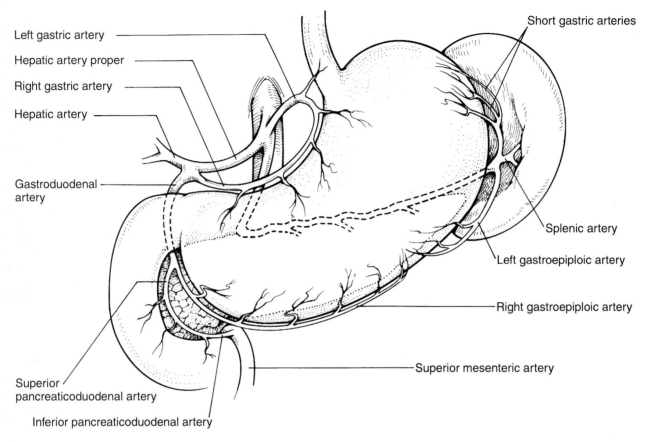

Figure 13-1 The major arteries that supply the stomach. The gastroduodenal artery is located behind the duodenum. Posterior penetrating duodenal ulcers may erode into this artery and cause hemorrhage.

arteries, short gastric arteries, and gastroduodenal arteries (Figure 13-1). Because of its abundant blood supply, it is difficult to devascularize the stomach surgically. Sympathetic innervation parallels arterial flow, and parasympathetic innervation passes through the vagus nerves. As the vagus nerves traverse the mediastinum, the left trunk rotates so that it enters the abdomen anterior to the esophagus (Figure 13-2). The right trunk rotates so that it enters the abdomen posterior to the esophagus. Both nerves innervate the stomach from the lesser curvature. The right vagus gives off a posterior branch to the celiac plexus, from which nerves pass to the midgut (pancreas, small intestine, and proximal colon). Also, the right vagus occasionally gives off a small branch that travels behind the esophagus. This branch is called the criminal nerve of Grassi because when it is not identified and divided, it may cause a recurrent peptic ulcer. The left vagus gives off a hepatic branch that innervates the gallbladder, biliary tract, and liver. The vagus nerves stimulate the **parietal cell** mass to secrete hydrochloric acid and control the motor activity of the stomach.

The wall of the stomach has four layers: the mucosa, submucosa, muscularis, and serosa. The mucosa is separated from the submucosa by the muscularis mucosa.

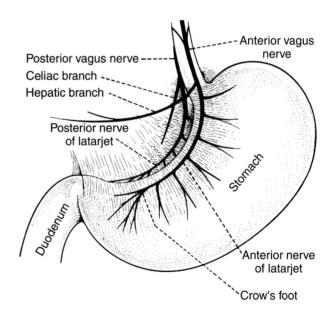

Figure 13-2 Branches of the vagus nerve innervate the stomach, pylorus, and duodenum. If the distal nerve of Latarjet is denervated, the pylorus does not relax in response to normal stimuli.

The submucosa has a rich vascular network that accounts for the abundant blood supply to the mucosa. The mucosa is arranged in a coarse rugal pattern and has a complex glandular structure. Although mucus-secreting cells are found throughout the stomach, parietal cells and chief cells are found only in the fundus. The pace-making area of the stomach is also found in the fundus, on the greater curvature, near the short gastric vessels.

The parietal cells produce both hydrochloric acid and intrinsic factor. Intrinsic factor is required for the absorption of vitamin B_{12} in the terminal ileum. The chief cells are responsible for the production of pepsinogen. Gastrin-producing G cells are found primarily in the antrum of the stomach, but are also found in lesser quantities in the mucosa of the duodenum and the proximal small intestine. The simplest way to differentiate antral tissue from fundic tissue is to demonstrate the absence of the brightly eosin-staining parietal cells that are present in the fundus.

The Duodenum

The duodenum is a metabolically active organ that receives chyme from the stomach and bile and pancreatic secretions through the ampulla of Vater. The duodenum produces a myriad of hormonally active agents. It has four regions: the first part (duodenal bulb), second part (descending duodenum), third part (transverse duodenum), and fourth part (ascending duodenum to ligament of Treitz). The descending duodenum is the site of the pacemaker for the entire small intestine.

The blood supply to the duodenum comes primarily from the gastroduodenal artery, although other smaller vessels are contributors. This vessel is the first branch of the proper hepatic artery. It courses immediately posterior to the duodenal bulb and divides into the pancreaticoduodenal arcades. A **duodenal ulcer** that penetrates through the posterior wall of the duodenal bulb does so in the vicinity of the gastroduodenal artery. If the vessel wall is exposed to the gastric digestive enzymes and acid, massive bleeding may occur.

Physiology

Mechanisms of Hydrochloric Acid Secretion

The human is the only mammal that secretes hydrochloric acid in the fasting state. This finding prompted some investigators to hypothesize that duodenal ulcer disease is an affliction of civilization.

Three general phases of stimulation cause the release of hydrochloric acid from the parietal cell mass: the cephalic phase, which is mediated by the release of acetylcholine by the vagus nerve; the gastric phase, which is mediated by the antral release of **gastrin;** and the intestinal phase, which is mediated by the release of various gastrointestinal peptides and histamine by the small intestine.

Cephalic Phase

Stimulation of the central nervous system by the sight, smell, or thought of food causes efferent activity in the vagus nerve. Acetylcholine is released in the region of the parietal cell. This release is associated with an increase in the metabolic activity of the cell, the consumption of adenosine triphosphate, and the release of hydrochloric acid. This response is suppressed by surgical division of the nerves that supply the parietal cell mass and by anticholinergics.

Gastric Phase

Antral alkalinization, antral distension, and the presence of food in the antrum (particularly amino acids) promote the release of gastrin from the G cells. Gastrin is a true hormone that is released into the venous circulation and exerts its effect on the parietal cell. There are at least three species of gastrin. Basal serum gastrin measured in the fasting state is predominantly "big" gastrin that contains a chain of 34 amino acids. The half-life of this molecule is long, and its potency is low. In the stimulated state, "small" gastrin is released. This molecular species has a 17–amino acid chain, with a short half-life and intense biologic activity. A third variety, "big, big" gastrin is also identified, but its physiologic function is not well understood.

Intestinal Phase

The intestinal phase of gastric acid production occurs when the products of digestion reach the small intestine. This phase is associated with substantial elevations in various serum peptides, some of which stimulate gastric acid output. Other peptides are thought to be inhibitory. Stimulation of the H_2 (histamine) receptor, located on the parietal cell, may play a role in this phase of acid production.

Physiology of Hydrochloric Acid Secretion

The parietal cell membrane has at least three receptors: one each for gastrin, acetylcholine, and histamine (Figure 13-3). Hydrochloric acid is secreted from the cell when any one of these sites is occupied by its appropriate ligand. The effect of any of the ligands is amplified when two receptor sites are occupied simultaneously (synergism). Conversely, when any one of these sites is blocked, the other sites become less responsive to stimulation. Thus, when vagal innervation is interrupted (e.g., with a vagotomy), the parietal cells become less responsive to stimulation by gastrin.

The parietal cell secretes hydrogen ion against a 1,000,000:1 concentration gradient. Hydrogen ion is stored within the cytosol of the parietal cell in packets that are surrounded by a membrane. When stimulated, these membranes fuse with the surface membrane and hydrogen ion is released into the lumen. Secretion is an active process that exchanges hydrogen ion for potassium in a 1:1 ratio. Chloride ion is transported into the lumen in conjunction with this process. As by-products

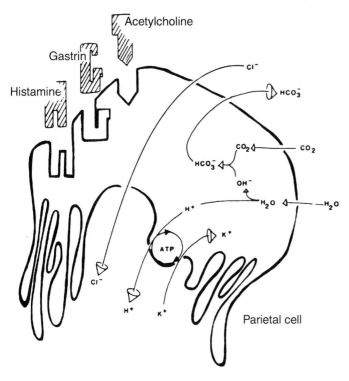

Figure 13-3 The parietal cell in the stomach has three receptors. When stimulated, these receptors elicit the secretion of hydrochloric acid. *ATP* = adenosine triphosphate.

of the reaction, water and bicarbonate passively diffuse into the plasma and extracellular space.

Several mechanisms suppress the production of gastric acid. **Secretin,** which is released from the duodenal wall in response to acidic chyme from the stomach, inhibits gastric acid secretion and gastric emptying. When gastric luminal pH drops to less than 1.5, antral release of gastrin is inhibited by somatostatin. These are the first autoregulation steps in the control of gastric acid release. Additionally, stimulation of the pancreas by secretin causes an increased volume of pancreatic secretion, with an increase in bicarbonate concentration and total protein content.

Duodenal sodium bicarbonate production is up to six times greater than that of the stomach. The transmucosal electrical gradient is responsible for the transport of the bicarbonate ion into the lumen. Sodium bicarbonate can neutralize all of the hydrogen ions that are normally presented to the duodenal bulb. The secretin-stimulated pancreatic bicarbonate contributes only a small amount to neutralization of the total acid load. Bicarbonate is also secreted from the gastric glandular epithelium in exchange for chloride ions. It can neutralize a small portion of the maximum acid output. When this effect is added to the protective effect of secreted mucus, the gastric surface epithelium is generally protected from autodigestion. The goblet cells of the stomach produce a mucopolysaccharide that attaches to the luminal surface of the gastric mucosa. Although the luminal pH may drop to as low as 1.0, the pH within the

mucus, and therefore at the luminal surface of the mucosal cells, rarely falls below 7.0.

In the acid milieu of the stomach, pepsinogen produced by the chief cell is converted to pepsin. Pepsin actively hydrolyzes proteins to peptones and amino acids. The combination of pepsin and hydrochloric acid is potentially damaging to the gastric mucosal cells. Within the mucosa is a sophisticated, highly efficient mechanism (the gastric mucosal barrier) through which back-diffusion of hydrogen ions is rapidly neutralized and cleared. If this mechanism is not functioning adequately, damage to the mucosa occurs.

Pathophysiology

Although they are grouped together for this discussion, ulcers that occur in the duodenum and those that occur in the stomach exhibit many differences in pathophysiology (and clinical presentation, as discussed later). Peptic ulcers of the upper gastrointestinal tract form when the mechanisms for defense are inadequate to deal with the physiologic, but hostile, intraluminal milieu. When this type of imbalance is present, autodigestion of the mucosa ensues. The mechanism that produces **gastric ulcers,** however, is unknown. Suggested etiologies include a defective mucosal barrier, delayed gastric emptying, antecedent **gastritis,** increased hydrogen ion back-diffusion, alkaline reflux, a defective pyloric sphincter mechanism, and the presence of the bacterium *Helicobacter pylori.*

Duodenal Ulcer Disease

Each year, approximately 18 to 20 million patients have acute ulcerations of the duodenum. Although the vast majority of these heal spontaneously, complications sometimes occur.

Ulcers most commonly occur in the first part of the duodenum and are associated with burning epigastric abdominal pain that is accentuated by fasting. A special variant of duodenal ulcer disease is the lesion found in the prepyloric area or the pyloric channel. These ulcers usually occur near the junction between the antral and the duodenal mucosa. The pattern of gastric acid secretion is similar to that found in a duodenal ulcer (as opposed to a gastric ulcer), and the patient is treated as though the lesion were a duodenal ulcer.

Acute Ulcer Disease
Clinical Presentation and Evaluation

In acute peptic ulcer disease, massive upper gastrointestinal hemorrhage may occur if the ulcer erodes into the gastroduodenal artery, producing symptoms of syncope, tachycardia, hypotension, nausea, and hematemesis. An ulcer that perforates through the superior or anterior aspect of the duodenal bulb may spill duodenal contents into the abdominal cavity. In this case, the

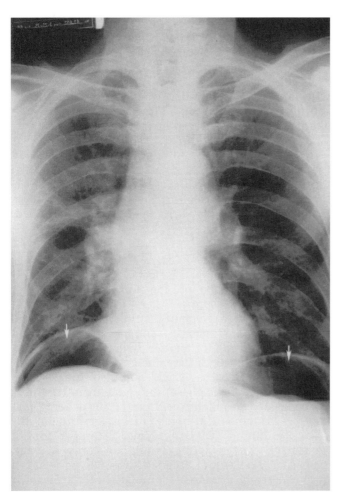

Figure 13-4 An upright posteroanterior chest x-ray often shows subdiaphragmatic air in patients with a perforated ulcer.

patient has the signs and symptoms of an acute abdomen. These include tachycardia, severe abdominal tenderness and pain, guarding, and rigidity. Upright chest x-ray shows free intraperitoneal air outlining the diaphragm or liver **(pneumoperitoneum),** confirming the diagnosis of a perforated viscus (Figure 13-4). Other patients who have repeated bouts of acute ulceration may have a scarred duodenal bulb. As this cicatrix progresses, **gastric outlet obstruction** may occur. These patients have weight loss, persistent vomiting immediately after eating, and chronic gastric dilation. Chronic antral dilation produces sustained release of gastrin, initiating a vicious cycle of exacerbation of ulcer disease.

Treatment

The three complications described earlier (i.e., perforation, hemorrhage, and obstruction) as well as failure of nonoperative management (intractability) are the classic constellation of complications that require surgical intervention.

In patients with free perforation and without other medical diseases that preclude an operation, an exploratory celiotomy (laparotomy) is performed imme-

diately. The combination of abrupt onset of severe abdominal pain, a rigid surgical abdomen, and free air noted under the diaphragm on upright chest x-rays suggests this diagnosis. If the perforation is less than 6 hours old, the ulcer is plicated (oversewn), and an acid-reducing procedure is performed. This procedure may be either a **truncal vagotomy** and pyloroplasty or a **proximal gastric vagotomy,** with buttressing of the perforation with a tag of omentum (Graham patch). If the perforation is greater than 6 hours old, plication alone is performed.

In patients who have upper gastrointestinal hemorrhage, the stomach is decompressed with a nasogastric tube. Gastric lavage and antacid therapy are initiated. At the initial evaluation, coagulation parameters are also assessed. At least two large-bore intravenous lines are inserted, and blood is prepared for administration to the patient. Endoscopy is performed to establish the source of hemorrhage. Although each case is judged on an individual basis, a patient who requires six or more units of blood in the initial 12-hour period to maintain hemodynamic stability is taken to the operating room. Patients who are elderly or hemodynamically unstable are candidates for earlier surgical intervention than younger, stable patients, because hypotension is poorly tolerated in the elderly. The surgical treatment is ligation of the bleeding artery, with the addition of an acid-reducing procedure to prevent further ulcer complications.

In patients with gastric outlet obstruction, the stomach is decompressed with a nasogastric tube for 5 or 6 days, or until it returns to near-normal size. During this time, the patient is allowed nothing by mouth. Nutrition and fluids are administered intravenously. Malnutrition is ameliorated by total parenteral nutrition. Careful monitoring for electrolyte abnormalities is undertaken. The classic metabolic abnormality seen in gastric outlet obstruction is hypochloremic, hypokalemic metabolic alkalosis. An acid-reducing operation as well as a procedure to allow emptying of the stomach is necessary.

This condition is considered intractable if persistent symptoms interfere with the patient's lifestyle despite what is normally adequate medical management. In this situation, surgical intervention may be considered.

Chronic Ulcer Disease

Clinical Presentation and Evaluation

As mentioned earlier, duodenal ulcers are associated with burning epigastric abdominal pain that is accentuated by fasting. The pain often awakens patients from sleep and is relieved by antacids or food. When pain is alleviated by eating, weight gain may be noted. The pain is often characterized as "boring," and may radiate to the back in patients with posterior-penetrating ulcers. A definitive diagnosis of duodenal ulcer disease is established by objective evidence.

Upper Gastrointestinal Series

Classically, the diagnosis of duodenal ulcer disease is made by an upper gastrointestinal barium examination (upper gastrointestinal series) [Figure 13-5]. In this examination, barium and air are swallowed; the esophagus, stomach, and duodenum are observed fluoroscopically; and radiographs are made for permanent documentation. Swallowing and peristaltic and sphincteric function, size, shape, displacement by other organs, flexibility, distensibility, and mucosal pattern are all observed. Ulcers, scars, strictures, cancers, and postoperative changes are shown. Because this test is widely available, inexpensive, and safe, an upper gastrointestinal series is often the first diagnostic study that is used when a duodenal ulcer is suspected, especially when symptoms are vague. However, many acute lesions of the duodenum and almost all superficial lesions of the stomach are undetected by this type of examination. Even if an active ulcer is not visualized, ancillary signs of peptic ulcer disease (e.g., duodenal spasm, deformity, mucosal swelling) usually point to the correct diagnosis.

Endoscopy

To visualize the mucosal surface, upper gastrointestinal endoscopy is even more reliable than an upper gastrointestinal series. This study involves the passage of a gastroscope from the mouth into the esophagus, stomach, and duodenum. The mucosa is examined in detail, and if an ulcer is present, it can usually be seen. Photographs of the lesions may be taken; they can be used for documentation and evaluation of subsequent healing. In patients who are bleeding, the exact site of hem-

orrhage can usually be determined. Endoscopic therapy with a heater probe or bipolar coagulator may be used initially to control the hemorrhage. Because of its diagnostic and therapeutic potential, the endoscope is the most effective tool in the initial management of patients with upper gastrointestinal hemorrhage. Endoscopy can also identify concomitant disease or suggest an alternative diagnosis in certain patients. Analysis for the Gram-negative bacterium *H. pylori* may also be performed endoscopically. Although adenocarcinoma of the duodenum occurs, it is rare. Only if a duodenal ulcer is associated with a mass should a biopsy be performed. In contrast, if a gastric ulcer is present, multiple biopsies are mandatory each time an ulcer is identified.

Gastric Acid Analysis

A gastric analysis provides a substantial amount of meaningful information. The test is performed by placing a nasogastric tube into the stomach and collecting samples of gastric aspirate. After a 1-hour basal period, a secretagogue (e.g., pentagastrin) is usually given intravenously, and gastric samples are collected at 15-minute intervals for another hour. In most patients with duodenal ulcer disease, the gastric analysis classically shows a high basal acid output of greater than 4.0 mEq/hr (cephalic phase), and more than two-thirds have elevated stimulated acid output. In patients who have gastrinoma **(Zollinger-Ellison syndrome)**, the basal acid output may be ten times the upper limit of normal. However, with stimulation, only a small increase in acid output occurs because the parietal cell mass is already maximally stimulated by the elevated basal serum gastrin levels.

Medical Treatment

The fundamental problem in patients with duodenal ulcer disease is an accentuation of the cephalic phase of gastric acid output. Therapy is directed at reducing basal acid secretion. Nonoperative treatment of duodenal ulcer disease is aimed at blocking the stimulation of the parietal cells by the vagus nerve or blocking the response of the parietal cells to stimuli.

Dietary Regimens

Most dietary regimens are ineffective and actually slow gastric emptying. Diet is only a minor component of nonsurgical treatment. Once the diagnosis of duodenal ulcer is confirmed, the medical regimen consists of the avoidance of foods that are secretagogues (e.g., caffeine, alcohol, chocolate), use of intraluminal antacids to neutralize excreted acid, blockade of the H_2 receptor at the parietal cell membrane, inhibition of the Na^+/H^+ pump in the parietal cell, use of surface coating agents and, in certain cases, administration of systemic anticholinergics. With this regimen, most patients are asymptomatic within a 7-day treatment period.

H_2 Blockade

At this time, the most commonly used treatment modality is **H_2 blockade.** The advantages of these

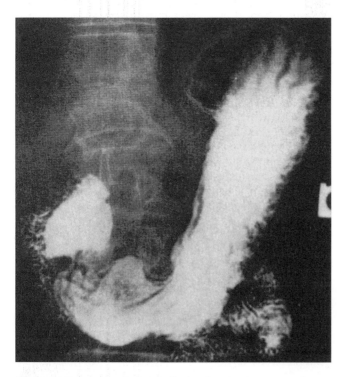

Figure 13-5 An upper gastrointestinal series showing a normal stomach and duodenum. (Reprinted with permission from Robbins LL, ed. *Golden's Diagnostic Radiology.* Baltimore, Md: Williams & Wilkins, 1969:5:187.)

medications include ease of administration, excellent patient compliance, and therapeutic efficacy of more than 90%. In addition, they block acid production rather than neutralizing released hydrogen ions. Antacids are also highly effective if taken appropriately. Antacids that contain aluminum hydroxide often cause constipation, whereas those that contain magnesium salts may cause diarrhea. **Omeprazole**, a Na^+/H^+ pump inhibitor, is a potent antisecretory agent. By directly inhibiting the proton pump of the parietal cell, it greatly decreases hydrochloric acid production. Because the vast majority of patients are rendered achlorhydric with this drug, it is used to treat peptic ulcer disease that is refractory to conventional therapy. Omeprazole is also used to treat Zollinger-Ellison syndrome and intractable gastroesophageal reflux.

H. pylori *Eradication*

Much attention is given to the role of *H. pylori* in the pathogenesis of duodenal and gastric ulcers. *H. pylori* organisms are small, curved, microaerophilic Gram-negative rods with multiple flagella. These bacteria infect the gastroduodenal mucosa, and most infected patients have evidence of chronic gastritis. However, only a small portion of infected people have an ulcer during their lifetime.

The presence of *H. pylori* in the stomach can be diagnosed by serologic tests, breath tests, or endoscopic biopsy of the gastric mucosa. All of these tests are based on the high concentrations of the enzyme urease, which is produced by the *H. pylori* infection. Urease hydrolyzes urea to form ammonia. The presence of *H. pylori* in gastric biopsy specimens is determined by the use of a pH-sensitive dye to detect any increase in pH caused by the production of ammonia (CLO test). Because this test is quick and inexpensive, it can be conducted during routine endoscopy.

Proper treatment of *H. pylori* leads to more rapid healing of duodenal ulcers, resolution of gastritis, and lower recurrence rates for both duodenal and gastric ulcers. *H. pylori* infection is difficult to eradicate. Multiple treatment regimens were proposed, but triple therapy is typically used to eliminate the infection. Triple therapy usually consists of colloidal bismuth, with amoxicillin or tetracycline, and metronidazole for a 2-week period. Increasing the gastric pH increases the effectiveness of the antimicrobial drugs. Bismuth compounds may prevent the adhesion of the bacteria to the gastric epithelium or inhibit their urease and proteolytic activity.

Surgical Treatment

Medical therapy is directed at the underlying disease state that predisposes the patient to the development of a duodenal ulcer. The surgical approach is similarly guided. Because the most salient feature in the patient with duodenal ulcer disease is a pronounced cephalic phase of gastric acid production, the most critical aspect of surgical intervention is interruption of the neural pathway that is responsible for this excess. The vagus nerve is divided in one of three ways: truncal vagotomy, selective vagotomy, or proximal gastric vagotomy (parietal cell vagotomy, or highly selective vagotomy).

Truncal Vagotomy

Truncal vagotomy involves the complete transection of all vagal trunks at or above the esophageal hiatus of the diaphragm. This procedure denervates not only the parietal cell mass, but also the antral pump, pyloric sphincter mechanism, and most of the abdominal viscera. Because the truncal vagotomy disrupts gastric motility, a gastric drainage procedure is required to facilitate gastric emptying. Otherwise, gastric antral dilation occurs and stimulates gastrin release. The most common complementary procedure is pyloroplasty, which is performed by incising the pylorus horizontally and closing it vertically (Figure 13-6). Various modifications of pyloroplasty were proposed, and most are known by eponyms. If pyloroplasty is not possible, gastroenterostomy is an alternative. Many surgeons add distal gastrectomy (**antrectomy**) to the truncal vagotomy (Figure 13-7), performing an anastomosis between the distal end of the stomach and the end of the duodenum (**Billroth I**). Gastrointestinal continuity is reestablished by joining the end of the stomach to a loop of the jejunum (**Billroth II**) [Figure 13-8] or by performing a Roux-en-Y gastroenterostomy (Figure 13-9). Antrectomy augments the effect of vagotomy by removing the bulk of the gastrin-producing cells (G-cells). Therefore, these procedures interrupt both the cephalic phase and the gastric phase of acid stimulation. This combined procedure (vagotomy and antrectomy) is associated with a lower recurrence rate than vagotomy and pyloroplasty (1.5% vs 10%).

Selective Vagotomy

Selective vagotomy provides total denervation of the stomach, from above the crus of the diaphragm, down to and including the pylorus (Figure 13-10). This procedure spares the parasympathetic innervation of the

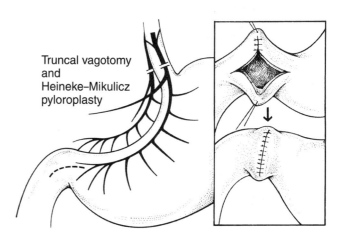

Truncal vagotomy and Heineke–Mikulicz pyloroplasty

Figure 13-6 When the trunk of the vagus nerve is divided, a pyloroplasty is also performed to allow gastric emptying. This pyloroplasty is the most common type performed.

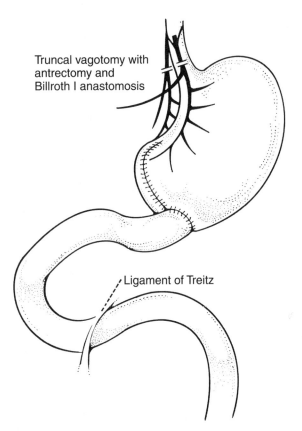

Truncal vagotomy with
antrectomy and
Billroth I anastomosis

Ligament of Treitz

Truncal vagotomy with
antrectomy and
Billroth II anastomosis

Figure 13-7 An antrectomy removes the distal portion of the stomach, where gastrin is produced. In addition, it removes the pylorus, thus allowing gastric emptying after vagotomy. In a Billroth I reconstruction, the duodenum is anastomosed to the stomach in continuity.

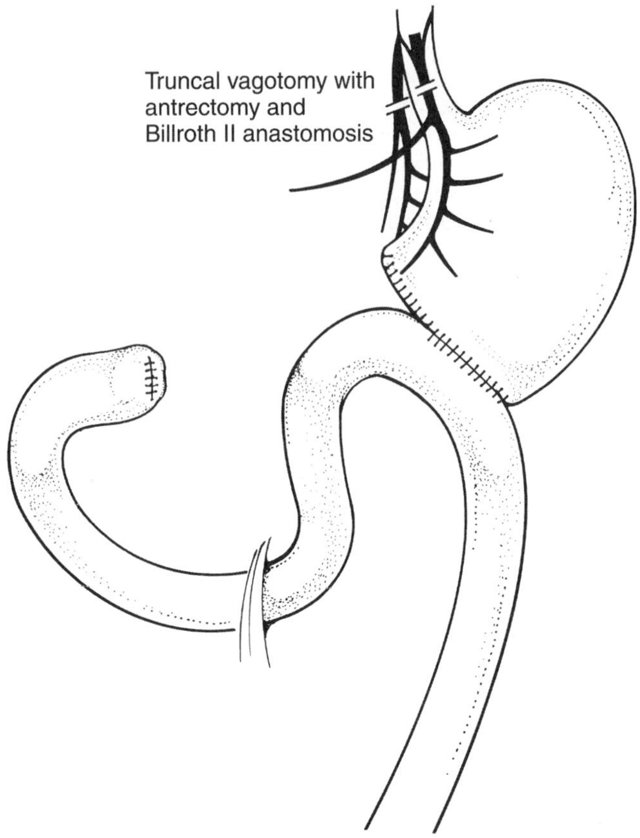

Figure 13-8 In a Billroth II reconstruction, the duodenum is not attached to the stomach; the stomach is anastomosed to a proximal loop of jejunum. This procedure is particularly useful when the duodenum is extensively scarred.

abdominal viscera. However, like truncal vagotomy, it denervates the antral pump and pylorus, necessitating some type of drainage procedure. Most surgeons employ pyloroplasty. Advocates of this type of vagotomy claim that it provides more total gastric denervation than does truncal vagotomy, but does not denervate other abdominal organs (liver, gallbladder, pancreas, small intestine, and proximal colon). The frequency of postgastrectomy syndromes with selective vagotomy is equal to that with truncal vagotomy and pyloroplasty.

Proximal Gastric Vagotomy

The most recent operation to gain popularity is proximal gastric vagotomy (Figure 13-11). In this procedure, the vagus nerve is identified as it courses along the lesser curvature of the stomach, and only the branches that innervate the parietal cell mass are divided. Preservation of the crow's foot allows the antral pump and pyloric sphincter mechanisms to continue to function normally, obviating the need for a drainage procedure. Patients with gastric outlet obstruction as a result of peptic ulcer disease are not candidates for this procedure. This procedure has the lowest incidence of postgastrectomy syndromes. The ulcer recurrence rate is

greater than 10%, but the morbidity and mortality rates are relatively low. Patients with ulcer recurrence after proximal gastric vagotomy are relatively easily managed with newer antacid drugs.

In some patients, especially those with Zollinger-Ellison syndrome (see later), total gastrectomy may be required to control the ulcer diathesis (Figure 13-12). Although this procedure provides absolute protection from recurrent ulcer disease, it is associated with significant aberrations in metabolism (e.g., decreased levels of vitamin B_{12}, absent intrinsic factor, pernicious anemia, malnutrition, weight loss). The operative mortality rate is also significant because of the difficulty involved in performing an esophageal anastomosis.

The decision about which procedure to perform on an individual patient is complicated. It is based on the age of the patient, the likelihood of ulcer recurrence, the severity of symptoms, and the patient's sex and weight. The procedures that have the highest cure rate (i.e., truncal vagotomy and antrectomy) also have the highest incidence of postgastrectomy side effects, such as **dumping syndrome.** Likewise, procedures with the lowest cure rate have the lowest incidence of side effects. Therefore, the surgeon's responsibility is to select the procedure for each patient that is likely to be

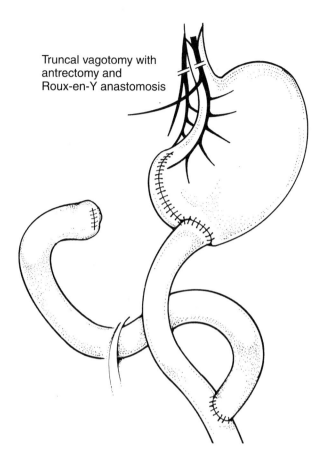

Truncal vagotomy with antrectomy and Roux-en-Y anastomosis

Figure 13-9 A Roux-en-Y anastomosis reduces the reflux of small bowel contents into the stomach. Peristalsis in the small bowel carries food and fluid away from the stomach. This procedure is particularly useful when a patient has a history of alkaline reflux gastritis.

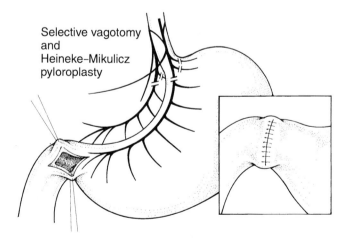

Selective vagotomy and Heineke-Mikulicz pyloroplasty

Figure 13-10 Because a selective vagotomy denervates the pylorus, a pyloroplasty is performed to allow gastric emptying.

effective in treating the ulcer diathesis while minimizing the likelihood of side effects. It is possible to predict which patients are at high risk for postgastrectomy complications; young, thin women are particularly vulnerable. In these patients, it may be advantageous to

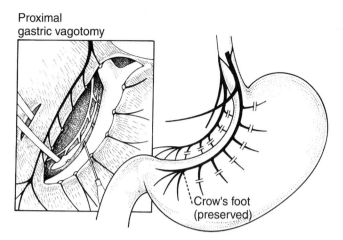

Proximal gastric vagotomy

Crow's foot (preserved)

Figure 13-11 A proximal gastric vagotomy (highly selective vagotomy) denervates the acid-producing parietal cells without interfering with the antral pump or pylorus.

avoid performing truncal vagotomy, especially with the availability of proximal gastric vagotomy, which is an excellent alternative.

Zollinger-Ellison Syndrome

A special variant of duodenal ulcer disease is Zollinger-Ellison syndrome. This syndrome is the direct result of the independent production of gastrin by a tumor (gastrinoma) arising in the pancreas or paraduodenal area. Approximately 60% of these tumors are malignant. Although long-term survivors are not uncommon, approximately 50% of patients with the malignant variant of the disease die within 5 years of the diagnosis. However, because this tumor has a slow growth pattern, many people survive 10 to 15 years.

Clinical Presentation and Evaluation

A high degree of suspicion is necessary to identify patients with Zollinger-Ellison syndrome. Patients at risk are those with refractory peptic ulcer disease or those with an extremely virulent ulcer diathesis. Many of the latter group have multiple ulcers in the duodenum or ulcers in unusual locations (i.e., jejunum, ileum). Zollinger-Ellison syndrome is also suspected in patients who have a family history of peptic ulcer or endocrine disease, those with a personal history of endocrine disease, and those with severe secretory diarrhea. Gastrinomas also occur in patients with familial disease associated with multiple endocrine neoplasia syndrome type 1.

The diagnosis is suspected if fasting serum gastrin levels are high (> 300 pg/mL). In addition, a secretin infusion test, performed by injecting secretin intravenously and measuring serum gastrin levels at 2, 5, 10, 15, 30, 45, and 60 minutes after the infusion, is often confirmatory. Patients with Zollinger-Ellison syndrome often have a profound increase in serum gastrin. In most laboratories, an increase of 200 pg/mL over the baseline level is considered diagnostic. This test is safe and has a high specificity and sensitivity.

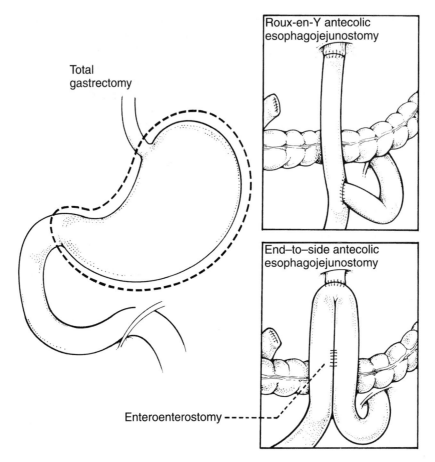

Figure 13-12 A total gastrectomy is performed in selected patients to eliminate ulcer disease. The operation is technically more difficult than other procedures and has a higher incidence of postgastrectomy complications.

Treatment

Therapy for Zollinger-Ellison syndrome is controversial. Pharmacologic doses of H_2 receptor antagonists are advocated and are effective in selected patients, at least in the short term. Omeprazole is also very effective in the treatment of Zollinger-Ellison syndrome. Long-acting synthetic analogues of somatostatin (octreotide) suppress elevated gastrin concentrations. This pharmacologic therapy lowers the production of hydrochloric acid and helps to alleviate the associated hypersecretory diarrhea. Others advocate exploratory laparotomy and biopsy or excision of the tumor, if located, to confirm the diagnosis. In a small subset of patients, this approach is curative. If an isolated tumor is identified, then the tumor is resected and a proximal gastric vagotomy is performed. Even if the tumor cannot be found or totally excised, some recommend proximal gastric vagotomy and long-term treatment with an H_2 blocker or omeprazole. These procedures must be compared with the standard of therapy, total gastrectomy, which removes the end organ, abolishes all acid production, and ablates most symptoms of the disease.

Gastric Ulcer Disease

Gastric ulcers are usually found on the lesser curvature of the stomach, within 1 cm of the transition zone between the antrum and the body of the stomach. As mentioned earlier, the mechanism that produces gastric ulcers is unknown. Suggested etiologies include a defective mucosal barrier, delayed gastric emptying, antecedent gastritis, increased hydrogen ion back-diffusion, alkaline reflux, a defective pyloric sphincter mechanism, and the presence of the bacterium *H. pylori*.

Clinical Presentation and Evaluation

Although both duodenal ulcer disease and gastric ulcer disease commonly cause abdominal pain, the character of the pain is different. Gastric ulcer pain usually occurs in the epigastrium and may radiate through to the back. It is produced by the ingestion of food. In contrast, duodenal ulcer pain is relieved by eating. A lack of appetite, leading to weight loss, is common in patients with gastric ulcers.

Gastric ulcers are classified into three types. Type I gastric ulcers occur along the lesser curvature of the stomach in the transition zone between the acid-secreting mucosa and antral mucosa. Type II gastric ulcers are a combination of a gastric ulcer and a duodenal ulcer. Type III gastric ulcers are pyloric or prepyloric ulcers. Types II and III, in contrast to type I ulcers, are similar to duodenal ulcers and are usually associated with acid hypersecretion. For this reason, they are treated in a similar fashion to duodenal ulcer disease.

Diagnosis

Approximately 80% of patients with gastric ulcers have a pattern of normal or low gastric acid secretion. Some researchers believe that hydrochloric acid is necessary for mucosal damage to occur, but the underlying cause of the ulcer probably is not acid hypersecretion. Because an acidic environment may be necessary for the formation of gastric ulcers, the patient who has achlorhydria has an increased risk of malignancy. Even with normal hydrochloric acid production, a substantial number of gastric erosions are malignancies that mimic gastric ulcer disease. In contrast, duodenal ulcers are seldom malignant.

The diagnosis can be made by upper gastrointestinal series or endoscopy. All patients with gastric ulcers require multiple biopsies to establish the presence or absence of carcinoma. Cytology and brushings are also helpful as an adjunct to biopsy. Despite these procedures, false-negative results are still common because of the small sample size of the biopsy specimens.

Medical Treatment

The treatment regimen proposed for patients with gastric ulcer disease is similar to that for patients with duodenal ulcer disease. However, anticholinergics are usually avoided because they aggravate gastric stasis. Additional options in the treatment of gastric ulcer disease include sucralfate and misoprostol. Sucralfate binds to injured gastric tissue and creates a physical barrier to prevent further mucosal destruction. Misoprostol is a prostaglandin E analogue and functions as a cytoprotective agent. In more than 90% of patients with duodenal ulcer disease, the ulcer heals with a medical regimen. In patients with gastric ulcers, fewer than 50% completely heal. In these patients, all medications that promote ulcer formation or retard mucosal healing (e.g., aspirin, prostaglandin antagonists, steroids, alcohol) are withdrawn. In the nonoperative management of patients with gastric ulcer disease, repeat endoscopy must be performed after 6 weeks of therapy. If the ulcer does not show substantial healing (> 50%), then surgical therapy is considered. If the patient is a poor operative candidate, then the medical regimen is continued, and repeat endoscopy is scheduled. If, after 4 weeks of therapy, the ulcer persists, then it is unlikely that the ulcer will heal without operative intervention. Suspicion that the ulcer harbors a malignancy is heightened. At each endoscopy examination at which a gastric ulcer is iden-

tified, multiple biopsy specimens of the margin of the ulcer are taken. It is only when these biopsy specimens are reviewed histologically that an ulcer can be said to be benign. Despite the efforts of the best pathologists, there is still a substantial false-negative rate. Even with the best of medical care, the nonhealing and recurrence rates of gastric ulcer disease are extremely high.

Surgical Treatment

Indications for surgical intervention in gastric ulcer disease are similar to those for duodenal ulcer disease: hemorrhage, perforation, obstruction, and intractability. An additional relative indication for operation is a high index of suspicion for cancer. The operative approach to benign gastric ulcer disease depends in part on the gastric acid secretory status of the patient. Because most of these patients have low or normal production of hydrochloric acid, antrectomy that includes excision of the ulcer, without truncal vagotomy, is the appropriate therapy. In gastric ulcer disease, the lesion is excised, whereas in duodenal ulcer disease, the lesion is left in situ. Each resected gastric ulcer is evaluated histologically to verify that a gastric carcinoma is not hidden in the depths of the crater. If the patient has gastric acid hypersecretion (types II and III gastric ulcers), then truncal vagotomy is added to the procedure.

The recurrence rate after surgical treatment for a gastric ulcer is extremely low. Although postgastrectomy sequelae may occur, they appear to be less common after this procedure than after procedures for duodenal ulcer disease.

Complications

Postgastrectomy Syndromes

The innervated intact stomach is a careful guardian of the gastrointestinal tract. When the stomach is denervated and especially when the pyloric mechanism is ablated, the exquisite control of gastric emptying is abolished. This change, in association with the anastomotic characteristics of many reconstructions, is the reason for most common postgastrectomy syndromes. Several reconstructions produce a defunctionalized limb of intestine or place the duodenum or jejunum at risk for obstruction or bacterial overgrowth. Others allow easy ingress of bile and duodenal secretions into the gastric pouch. These aberrations in normal anatomy produce the various postgastrectomy syndromes.

In the evaluation of a patient with a complicated postoperative course, an upper gastrointestinal series may be performed. This series is used to document the extent of gastric resection and type of reconstruction, to determine the cause of vomiting (if present), and to assess gastric emptying and motility. Gastric emptying can also be defined more physiologically by administering a radionuclide-labeled meal followed by sequential imaging. Clues to the diagnosis can also be acquired by examination with an endoscope, which allows direct visualization and biopsy.

Early Dumping Syndrome

Early dumping syndrome is characterized by a select set of symptoms that occur after the ingestion of food of high osmolarity. This type of meal may contain a large quantity of simple and complex sugars (e.g., milk products). Approximately 15 minutes after the meal is ingested, the patient has anxiety, weakness, tachycardia, diaphoresis and, frequently, palpitations. The patient may also describe feelings of extreme weakness and a desire to lie down. Crampy abdominal pain may also be present. Often borborygmi are heard, and diarrhea is not uncommon. Gradually, the symptoms clear.

The patient with early dumping has uncontrolled emptying of hypertonic fluid into the small intestine. Fluid moves rapidly from the intravascular space into the intraluminal space, producing acute intravascular volume depletion. As the simple sugars are absorbed and as dilution of the hypertonic solution occurs, symptoms gradually abate. Intravascular volume is replenished as fluid shifts from the intracellular space and is absorbed from the intestinal lumen. Fluid shifts, however, do not explain all of the symptoms associated with early dumping. The release of several hormonal substances, including serotonin, neurotensin, histamine, glucagon, vasoactive intestinal peptide, kinins, and others, is believed to contribute to the symptom complex. The use of a somatostatin analogue to block these hormonal substances may be of benefit to some patients.

This problem is best treated by avoiding hypertonic liquid meals, altering the volume of each meal, and ingesting some fat with each meal to slow gastric emptying. Liquids are ingested either before the meal or at least 30 minutes after the meal. Some authors claim that β-blockers (10–20 mg propranolol hydrochloride) taken 20 minutes before a meal are helpful in approximately 50% of cases. In some patients with recalcitrant symptoms, surgical construction of a Roux-en-Y gastrojejunostomy may be necessary. This procedure works by delaying gastric emptying.

Late Dumping Syndrome

As in early dumping, the patient suddenly has anxiety, diaphoresis, tachycardia, palpitations, weakness, fatigue, and a desire to lie down. In late dumping, the symptoms usually begin within 3 hours after the meal. This variant of dumping is not associated with borborygmi or diarrhea. The physiologic explanation for late dumping involves rapid changes in serum glucose and insulin levels. After the meal, a large bolus of glucose-containing chyme is presented to the mucosa of the small intestine. Glucose is absorbed much more rapidly than when the intact pylorus is present to meter gastric emptying. Extremely high serum glucose levels may occur shortly after the meal and may elicit a profound outpouring of insulin. The insulin response exceeds what is necessary to clear the glucose from the blood, and subsequently, hypoglycemia results. The symptoms in late dumping are the direct result of rapid fluctuations in serum glucose levels.

Nonoperative therapy for this syndrome includes the ingestion of a small snack 2 hours after meals. Crackers and peanut butter make an excellent supplement to abort or ameliorate the symptoms. If symptoms cannot be controlled by nonoperative management, then either conversion of the previous procedure to a Billroth I (if not already present) or construction of a Roux-en-Y gastrojejunostomy is considered. Surgical intervention is considered only in patients who do not respond to aggressive nonoperative therapy.

Postvagotomy Diarrhea

As many as 50% of patients who undergo truncal vagotomy experience a change in bowel habits (i.e., increased frequency, more liquid consistency). In most cases, the symptoms improve or disappear with time. However, a small percentage of patients (< 1%) have severe diarrhea that does not relent with time. These patients may experience diarrhea that is explosive in onset, is not related to meals, and occurs without warning.

The pathophysiology of postvagotomy diarrhea is not entirely known. Gastric hypoacidity and the effects of vagal denervation on intestinal motility are possible etiologies. A diminished bile salt concentration secondary to biliary dysfunction may also be a contributing factor. In most patients with postvagotomy diarrhea, fluid intake is restricted and the intake of foods that are low in fluid content is increased. Antidiarrheal agents, such as codeine, diphenoxylate hydrochloride (Lomotil), or loperamide (Imodium), may be of benefit. Cholestyramine, which binds bile salts, or somatostatin analogues may also be used. If the postvagotomy diarrhea is severe or is refractory to medical management, a reversed 10-cm segment of jejunum is inserted 100 cm distal to the ligament of Treitz. This procedure delays small bowel transit time, but has many inherent problems.

Afferent Loop Obstruction

Afferent loop obstruction occurs only after gastrectomy with a Billroth II reconstruction. It is usually associated with a kink in the afferent limb adjacent to the anastomosis. Pancreatic and biliary secretions are trapped in the afferent limb, where they cause distension. Symptoms usually include severe cramping abdominal pain that occurs immediately after the ingestion of a meal. Patients often characterize the pain as crushing. Within 45 minutes, the patient feels an abdominal rush that is associated with increased pain, followed by nausea and vomiting of a dark brown, bitter-tasting material that has the consistency of motor oil. These symptoms result from the spontaneous, forceful decompression of the obstructed limb. Classically, no food is present. The symptoms resolve with vomiting. These patients often have profound weight loss because they stop eating to prevent the pain. The best treatment is exploration of the abdomen and conversion of the Billroth II anastomosis to either a Roux-en-Y gastrojejunostomy or a Billroth I gastroduodenostomy.

Blind Loop Syndrome

Blind loop syndrome is more common after a Billroth II procedure than after a Roux-en-Y procedure. It also occurs in patients who underwent bypass of the small intestine secondary to radiation injury or morbid obesity. Blind loop syndrome is associated with bacterial overgrowth in the limb of intestine that is excluded from the flow of chyme. This excluded limb of intestine harbors bacteria that proliferate and interfere with folate and vitamin B_{12} metabolism. A deficiency of vitamin B_{12} leads to megaloblastic anemia. The bacterial overgrowth may cause deconjugation of bile salts and lead to steatorrhea. Patients often have diarrhea, weight loss, and weakness, and they are often anemic. A Schilling test is often positive. Treatment consists of orally administered, broad-spectrum antibiotics that cover both aerobic and anaerobic bacteria (e.g., tetracycline). This regimen is often a temporizing step because many patients require conversion to a Billroth I gastroduodenostomy.

Alkaline Reflux Gastritis

Alkaline reflux gastritis is seen in patients in whom duodenal, pancreatic, and biliary contents reflux into the denervated stomach. These patients have weakness, weight loss, persistent nausea, and epigastric abdominal pain that often radiates to the back. In addition, they are often anemic. The diagnosis is made by upper gastrointestinal endoscopy that shows that the gastric mucosa are edematous, bile-stained, atrophic, and erythematous. The visual diagnosis is confirmed by multiple biopsy specimens taken from the gastric mucosa, away from the stoma. The microscopic appearance is often characteristic, showing inflammation and a corkscrew appearance of blood vessels in the submucosa.

Although a variety of medical regimens were proposed to treat alkaline reflux gastritis (e.g., oral ingestion of cholestyramine, antacids, H_2 blockers, or metoclopramide), none is uniformly satisfactory. Surgical correction consists of diverting the duodenal contents away from the stomach with a long-limb Roux-en-Y gastrojejunostomy. The minimum distance between the gastrojejunostomy and the stoma that brings the bile and pancreatic juices into the intestine is 40 cm (18 inches). This procedure is effective in most patients.

Recurrent Ulcer Disease

The most common cause of recurrent ulcer disease is incomplete vagotomy. The vagal branch that is most often missed is the right posterior nerve (criminal nerve of Grassi). Each operation has an accepted recurrence rate. The operation that has the lowest recurrence rate is total gastrectomy, but it is rarely indicated because of its high early and late morbidity rates. The next lowest recurrence rate is seen in patients who undergo truncal vagotomy and antrectomy (1%–2%). The highest recurrence rate appears to be in patients who undergo proximal gastric vagotomy (approximately 12%), although results vary substantially among different centers. Table 13-1 shows the average recurrence rate for each operative procedure and the incidences of various postgastrectomy syndromes.

Gastric Atony

One of the most difficult problems after any operation that denervates the stomach and ablates the pylorus is an aberration in gastric motility. Rapid emptying, especially of liquids, is common and was discussed earlier. Delayed gastric emptying, especially of solids, is a poorly understood phenomenon that may be the single most common problem after gastric resection. More than 50% of patients with a Roux-en-Y gastrojejunostomy have substantial delays in gastric emptying identified by a ^{99m}Tc-labeled egg albumin scan. However, only 50% of these patients have symptoms, and most improve with time. If medication is necessary, urecholine or metoclopramide may prove beneficial.

Table 13-1. Relative Incidence of Recurrence and Operative Mortality Rate Expressed as Percentages[a]

	Recurrence Rate (%)	Operative Mortality Rate (%)	Dumping Early	Dumping Late	Afferent Loop Syndrome	Blind Loop Syndrome	Alkaline Reflux Gastritis	Metabolic Sequelae
Vagotomy/pyloroplasty	5–10	1–2	2+	2+	0	0	1+	1+
Vagotomy/antrectomy Billroth I	1–2	1–4	2+	2+	0	0	1+	1+
Vagotomy/antrectomy Billroth II	1–3	1–4	3+	3+	2+	2+	2+	2+
Selective vagotomy	5–10	1–2	2+	2+	0	0	0	1+
Proximal gastric vagotomy	10–15	1	0	0	0	0	0	0
Total gastrectomy	0	2–5	3+	2+	0			2+

[a]These numbers are averages taken from the larger series published in the literature. The relative incidences of the postgastrectomy syndromes are expressed on a scale of 0 to 4+, with 0 indicating relative absence of symptoms and 4+ indicating frequent profound symptoms.

Nutritional Disturbances

Although a variety of metabolic abnormalities are identified after gastric resection, megaloblastic anemia (vitamin B_{12} or folate deficiency) and microcytic anemia (iron deficiency or blood loss) are the most common. Other patients experience steatorrhea and, in many cases, weight loss. Diarrhea secondary to vagotomy is extremely rare, although changes in stooling pattern are common. As many as 25% of patients have loose, frequent stools postoperatively.

Other Gastric Diseases

Gastritis

Diffuse erythema and disruption of the mucosa of the stomach can occur and may be associated with a myriad of symptoms, including bleeding, nausea, and vomiting. Gastritis is often associated with the intake of caustic agents (e.g., alcohol, aspirin, steroids, prostaglandin antagonists). Treatment consists of withdrawal of the noxious agents, decompression of the stomach, antacids and H_2 blockers, and nutritional repletion.

Stress Gastritis

In the past, bleeding from stress gastritis was a common cause of morbidity and mortality in patients with burn injuries (Curling's ulcer), those with head trauma (Cushing's ulcer), and patients in intensive care units. With the advent of aggressive neutralization of gastric acidity by titrating intraluminal pH to 4.0 or greater, these syndromes were virtually eliminated. In a patient at risk, a nasogastric tube is positioned and the gastric contents aspirated. An antacid is instilled and left for 1 hour. Then gastric aspiration is performed again. If the pH is less than 4.0, the amount of antacid is increased until the pH is greater than 4.0. Other methods of prophylaxis include H_2 blockers (continuous infusion or bolus infusions), sucralfate, misoprostol, or omeprazole. However, monitoring of the gastric pH is still vital to judge the effectiveness of therapy.

If a patient has upper gastrointestinal hemorrhage, the physician aspirates the stomach and performs endoscopy. Gastric lavage with either water or saline is performed before endoscopy is undertaken to aid in evacuating the stomach of blood clots and further decrease the stimulation of acid production caused by antral distension. Isolated sites of bleeding are controlled endoscopically with a bipolar coagulator or heater probe. If the bleeding is caused by stress gastritis and persists despite aggressive, nonoperative management, then a surgical procedure may be needed. Vagotomy and pyloroplasty with oversewing of the bleeding erosions is a quick, conservative procedure that controls bleeding in approximately 50% of patients. If bleeding recurs, total gastrectomy is considered.

Gastric Polyps

Gastric polyps are rare, but greater numbers are being diagnosed as more patients are undergoing upper gastrointestinal endoscopy. The polyps are either hyperplastic or adenomatous. Hyperplastic polyps are more common and have a lower rate of malignant degeneration than adenomatous polyps. If the polyp measures less than 0.5 cm, the risk of malignancy is low. A polyp that is greater than 1.5 cm in diameter has a considerably greater risk. When a gastric polyp is diagnosed, the physician may evaluate the patient for the presence of other polyps. The presence of multiple benign polyps in the small intestine and melanous spots on the lips and buccal mucosa is known as Peutz-Jeghers syndrome. Peutz-Jeghers syndrome is a mendelian dominant trait that has a high degree of penetrance. In these patients, conservative therapy is indicated because the tumors are hamartomas and are infrequently malignant.

Bezoar

The accumulation of a large mass of indigestible fiber within the stomach is known as a **bezoar.** If the material is made up of vegetable fiber, it is called a phytobezoar. If it is predominantly hair, the mass is called a trichobezoar. Trichobezoars are more common in children and among inmates of mental institutions. Although most bezoars may be broken up endoscopically, others must be removed surgically.

Malignant Diseases of the Stomach

Gastric Carcinoma

The incidence of gastric carcinoma in the population varies greatly. In the United States, the frequency has steadily fallen in the past three decades, whereas in Japan, China, Chile, Finland, and Russia, the incidence is considerably higher and has remained essentially unchanged. Immigrants from these countries to the United States seem to have a lower incidence of the disease, suggesting an environmental or dietary factor as a possible etiologic agent.

Conditions in the stomach that are believed to be premalignant and therefore warrant close observation are adenomatous polyps, chronic gastritis, or caustic injury secondary to lye ingestion. Patients with blood group A have a higher risk of gastric carcinoma. Pernicious anemia, which includes gastric achlorhydria and extreme atrophic gastritis, is also considered a premalignant condition (approximately 40% of these patients eventually have gastric cancer). Therefore, patients with pernicious anemia and without other contraindications should undergo yearly endoscopy.

Clinical Presentation and Evaluation

Patients with early gastric cancer are usually asymptomatic. Symptoms usually do not occur until the disease is far advanced. The earliest symptom may be weight loss; however, many patients experience epigastric pain as a prodrome that is so vague that a diagnosis cannot be made. Patients may have dysphagia, hematemesis, or melena. Laboratory studies often show iron deficiency anemia or a positive stool guaiac test.

An upper gastrointestinal series may show a fixed deformity of the stomach, with or without an ulcer. The superficial spreading type of carcinoma, commonly found in Japan, often shows no abnormality on this type of examination. Computed tomography scans and magnetic resonance imaging may yield additional information about invasion of adjacent organs and retroperitoneal structures. However, neither test is reliable in predicting the resectability of gastric carcinoma. Endoscopy with biopsy is the best way to establish the diagnosis.

All gastric carcinomas are adenocarcinomas. The morphologic variants that are most common in the United States are ulcerating, polypoid, and linitis plastica (leather bottle stomach). The prognosis for this disease depends on the extent of involvement. Resected polypoid lesions have a better 5-year survival rate than do ulcerating lesions. Patients with linitis plastica have the poorest prognosis.

Sixty percent of gastric carcinomas originate in the distal half of the stomach. Most of these occur in the pyloric gland area. Metastatic spread occurs to regional lymph nodes, the omentum, the left supraclavicular area (Virchow's node), the ovary, and the peritoneum. Metastases in the pelvis can often be palpated through the rectum or vagina (Blumer's shelf), in the ovary (Krukenberg's tumor), or at the umbilicus **(Sister Mary Joseph's node)**.

Treatment

The only cure for gastric carcinoma is complete surgical resection. However, complete removal of a gastric carcinoma is rarely possible. Because this condition causes few early symptoms, patients often have advanced disease. The best cure rates are reported in Japan, where there is a high percentage of the superficial spreading type. Even with this type of tumor, the 5-year survival rate is less than 50%. In most studies from English-speaking countries, curative resection is associated with a 5-year survival rate of less than 10%. Pathologic staging of the resected specimen is the best predictor of survival (Figure 13-13). The case for early diagnosis is made in studies that evaluated the 5-year survival rate in patients who had an incidental carcinoma found during stomach surgery for supposed benign disease. Some studies report that the 5-year survival rate in this highly selected cohort approaches 75%.

There is considerable debate among surgeons as to the extent of resection that is necessary to control the gastric tumor. Many surgeons favor radical subtotal gastrectomy with extensive lymph node removal. In this procedure, approximately 85% of the stomach is removed, and gastrointestinal continuity is reestablished with a gastrojejunostomy. Extended total gastrectomy may be required for large distal lesions or more proximally located lesions. Splenectomy or pancreatectomy may also need to be included in the operative procedure.

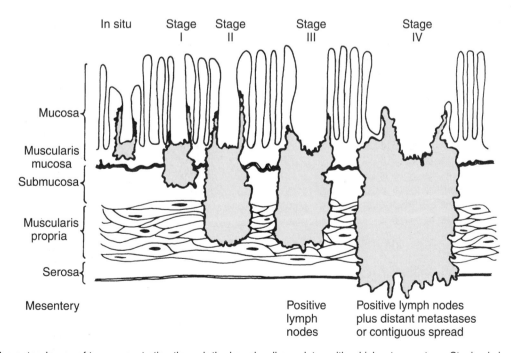

Figure 13-13 A greater degree of tumor penetration through the bowel wall correlates with a higher tumor stage. Staging is important because survival is severely limited with advanced stages.

Prognosis

In the hands of experienced surgeons, these procedures have acceptable operative morbidity and mortality rates. The 5-year survival rate, although improved, is still less than 10%.

Despite these dismal results in the general population, the best palliation is still associated with gastric resection. Surgical resection for palliation is carried out if possible, even if disease is left behind, to reduce bleeding and improve the patient's ability to eat. The resection should include the lesion, with an adequate cephalic margin, and the entire stomach distal to the tumor. Radiation and chemotherapy have no significant value, even for palliation.

Gastric Lymphoma

Gastric lymphoma is clinically similar to and may be mistaken for gastric carcinoma. The diagnostic evaluation is similar, and the treatment of choice is exploratory laparotomy and resection. After the diagnosis is confirmed pathologically, radiation therapy is indicated. The 5-year survival rate for these patients approaches 75% when the lesion is confined to the stomach.

Leiomyoma and Leiomyosarcoma

Both of these entities occur as a submucosal mass. Some observers believe that a leiomyoma may degenerate into a leiomyosarcoma. The most common symptom of these lesions is vague epigastric gastrointestinal pain. Occasionally, massive bleeding occurs. These lesions appear as a submucosal mass on upper gastrointestinal radiography. At endoscopy, the smooth, raised lesion often has a central ulceration. Computed tomography scan is used to evaluate the size of the tumor, its relation to surrounding organs, and the presence of liver metastases. The treatment is surgical resection. The prognosis for the benign lesion is excellent, but the malignant variant may be aggressive.

Multiple-Choice Questions

1. Which of the following arteries does NOT supply blood to the stomach?
   A. Hepatic artery
   B. Splenic artery
   C. Gastroduodenal artery
   D. Superior mesenteric artery
   E. Gastroepiploic artery

2. Regarding the vagus nerves, all of the following are true EXCEPT:
   A. The right vagus nerve innervates the midgut.
   B. The left vagus innervates the gallbladder.
   C. Both innervate the stomach from the lesser curvature.
   D. The vagi provide sympathetic innervation to the stomach.

E. The vagi stimulate the parietal cell mass to secrete hydrochloric acid.

3. Hydrochloric acid is produced by:
   A. G-cells
   B. Delta cells
   C. Parietal cells
   D. Goblet cells
   E. Chief cells

4. Match the following phrase with the best single response.
   Found predominantly in the gastric antrum:
   A. Mucus-secreting cells
   B. Parietal cells
   C. Chief cells
   D. Gastrin-producing G-cells
   E. Calcium-producing C-cells

5. The primary stimulus of secretin release is:
   A. Protein digestion products in the stomach
   B. Fat digestion products in the duodenum
   C. Acid in the duodenum
   D. Distension of the stomach
   E. Carbohydrate in the duodenum

6. The complication that is most often associated with an anterior duodenal ulcer is:
   A. Zollinger-Ellison syndrome
   B. Obstruction
   C. Massive upper gastrointestinal hemorrhage
   D. Carcinomatous change in the ulcer
   E. Perforation

7. Which of the following presentations best describes gastric outlet obstruction that occurs as a result of repeated bouts of acute ulceration?
   A. Progressive weight loss, emesis, and gastric dilation
   B. Severe abdominal pain, guarding, and rigidity
   C. Hematemesis, melena, and hypotension
   D. Persistent symptoms despite aggressive nonoperative management
   E. Epigastric pain associated with weight loss and an abdominal mass

8. The radiologic examination that is generally used to diagnose perforation of a peptic ulcer is:
   A. Upper gastrointestinal series with a water-soluble contrast agent
   B. Flat plate and upright x-rays of the abdomen
   C. Upright chest x-ray
   D. Abdominal ultrasound
   E. Computed tomography scan of abdomen

9. The most effective method to establish the specific source of blood loss in a patient who is hemorrhaging in the upper gastrointestinal tract is:
   A. Upper gastrointestinal barium contrast study
   B. Selective angiography

C. Bleeding scan with labeled red blood cells

D. Computed tomography scan with injected contrast material

E. Fiberoptic endoscopy

10. In the medical treatment of peptic ulcer disease, the component of therapy that seems to be LEAST effective is:

A. H$_2$ blocking agents

B. Dietary manipulations

C. Anticholinergics

D. Avoidance of secretagogues

E. Antacids

11. *H. pylori* infection of the gastroduodenal mucosa:

A. Results in peptic ulceration in most infected individuals

B. Is diagnosed only after a prolonged, relatively expensive workup

C. Presents a picture of chronic gastritis on endoscopic examination

D. Can be eradicated with a single high dose (2 g) of metronidazole

E. Even if properly treated, does not affect recurrence rates for peptic ulcers

12. Truncal vagotomy:

A. Is associated with elevated basal acid output

B. Results in markedly decreased serum gastrin levels

C. Selectively denervates the pyloric sphincter mechanism

D. Alters the cephalic phase of gastric acid production

E. Does not require a gastric emptying procedure

13. Which of the following procedures is associated with the lowest incidence of recurrent duodenal ulcer disease?

A. Selective vagotomy with gastroenterostomy

B. Proximal gastric vagotomy

C. Truncal vagotomy and pyloroplasty

D. Truncal vagotomy and antrectomy

E. Selective gastric vagotomy

14. Zollinger-Ellison syndrome is a gastrin-producing tumor that:

A. Is malignant in approximately 20% of cases

B. Occurs primarily in the large intestine

C. Responds to secretin infusion by increasing circulating levels of serum gastrin

D. Is managed most effectively by antrectomy

E. Is associated in most cases with a normal life span

15. All of the following statements about gastric ulcers are true EXCEPT:

A. Rates of acid secretion are normal or decreased.

B. They commonly develop in the transition area between the body and the antrum of the stomach.

C. They are usually found along the lesser curvature of the stomach.

D. They require surgical management less than 10% of the time.

E. They do not respond to medical management as well as duodenal ulcers.

16. Of the following, which is the most appropriate operation for a prepyloric gastric ulcer?

A. Total gastrectomy

B. Truncal vagotomy and antrectomy

C. 50% distal gastrectomy

D. Excision of the ulcer

E. Truncal vagotomy

17. What is the best diet for a patient who has undergone gastric surgery and has early dumping syndrome?

A. High-carbohydrate, low-fat, low-liquid diet

B. All liquid diet

C. High-protein, high-carbohydrate diet

D. Low-liquid, low-carbohydrate, high-fat diet

E. Low-liquid, low-carbohydrate, low-fat diet

18. Match the following phrase with the best single response.

Associated with persistent nausea and pain:

A. Blind loop syndrome

B. Afferent loop syndrome

C. Early dumping syndrome

D. Late dumping syndrome

E. Alkaline reflux gastritis

19. A 60-year-old man has left upper quadrant pain and had a 20-lb weight loss in the last 6 months. An upper gastrointestinal series showed a 1.5-cm ulcer on the lesser curvature of the stomach. The next step in his management is:

A. Antacids, H$_2$ blocking agents, and repeat evaluation in 6 weeks

B. Upper gastrointestinal endoscopy with biopsy and cytologic examination

C. Gastric acid analysis

D. Testing to obtain fasting serum gastrin levels

E. Resection of the ulcer

20. All of the following statements about gastric carcinoma are correct EXCEPT:

A. It is decreasing in incidence in the United States.

B. It is more common in patients who have pernicious anemia.

C. Prominent radiating rugal folds seen on upper gastrointestinal series are pathognomonic.

D. It usually has a dismal prognosis.

E. It is surgically resected if possible, even in the presence of metastases.

Oral Examination Study Questions

CASE 1

A 36-year-old man comes to your office with mid-epigastric abdominal discomfort. Although the symptoms are intermittent, their intensity has progressively increased over the last 6 months. The pain is most severe when the patient has not eaten, and it frequently wakes him from sleep at approximately 5:00 AM. The pain is relieved by antacids and fasting. Within the past 3 months, he has gained 6 lb.

OBJECTIVE 1

On the basis of this history, the student formulates a differential diagnosis, including:

A. Duodenal ulcer

B. Zollinger-Ellison syndrome

C. Gastric ulcer

D. Gastric malignancy

OBJECTIVE 2

The student understands the pathophysiology of peptic ulcer disease, including:

A. Accentuation of the cephalic phase of gastric acid output and excess acid production in duodenal ulcer

B. Independent production of gastrin by pancreatic or paraduodenal tumor in Zollinger-Ellison syndrome

C. Defective mucosal barrier, antecedent gastritis, increased hydrogen ion back-diffusion, alkaline reflux, or defective pyloric sphincter in gastric ulcer

OBJECTIVE 3

The student outlines the appropriate diagnostic procedures:

A. Upper gastrointestinal series

B. Endoscopy with biopsy or cytology if a gastric ulcer is seen

C. Fasting serum gastrin and secretin tests if the gastrin level is high

D. Gastric analysis, with and without betazole (Histalog) or pentagastrin

OBJECTIVE 4

Assuming that a duodenal ulcer is found, the student outlines the medical management of this patient, including:

A. Avoidance of secretagogues (caffeine, alcohol, chocolate)

B. Intraluminal antacids

C. H_2 receptor blockers

This plan provides relief of symptoms in 90% of patients within 7 days.

OBJECTIVE 5

The student names the indications for surgical intervention in patients with a duodenal ulcer and outlines which surgical procedures may be used, indicating the advantages, risks, and outcomes.

A. Indications
   1. Perforation
   2. Obstruction
   3. Hemorrhage
   4. Intractability

B. Procedures
   1. Truncal vagotomy and drainage
      a. The recurrence rate is 10%.
      b. The procedure denervates other organs.
   2. Truncal vagotomy and antrectomy
      a. The procedure has the lowest recurrence rate (1.5%).
      b. It denervates other organs (postgastrectomy syndrome).
   3. Selective vagotomy and pyloroplasty
      a. The procedure provides more total gastric vagotomy.
      b. It causes postgastrectomy syndromes.
   4. Proximal gastric vagotomy
      a. The procedure allows the antral pump and pyloric sphincter to function normally, obviating the need for a drainage procedure.
      b. It has the lowest incidence of postgastrectomy syndrome.
      c. It has the highest incidence of recurrence.
   5. Total gastrectomy
      a. The procedure has no risk of recurrent ulcer.
      b. Malnutrition, weight loss, and pernicious anemia may occur.
      c. It has the highest operative mortality rate.

Minimum Level of Achievement for Passing

The student identifies a duodenal ulcer and gives a differential diagnosis. The student knows, in general, the pathophysiology of peptic ulcer disease, the diagnostic procedures, the medical therapy, and the indications for surgery.

Honors Level of Achievement

The student provides an in-depth discussion of the pathophysiology and diagnosis of peptic ulcer disease. The student describes the various operations for duodenal ulcer as well as their risks and benefits.

CASE 2

A 36-year-old man comes to your office with a chief complaint of epigastric distress of 10 years' duration. Three years ago, he had a perforated duodenal ulcer that was closed and patched with omentum. He later had persistent ulcer symptoms despite aggressive treatment with antacids and H_2 blockers and avoidance of stimulatory foods and drugs.

OBJECTIVE 1

The student obtains the pertinent history, performs a physical examination, and begins a diagnostic workup.

A. The patient has a history of diarrhea and post-prandial epigastric pain.

B. Physical examination shows an asthenic habitus and a healed incision.

C. Workup
1. Upper gastrointestinal series shows prominent gastric folds and duodenal and proximal jejunal ulcers.
2. Endoscopy shows the same findings as the upper gastrointestinal series.
3. Fasting serum gastrin level is 400 nm/mL (high).
4. Secretin infusion test shows a profound increase in serum gastrin.
5. Gastric analysis shows Histalog or pentagastrin basal output of 30 mEq/hr (high), with a small increase with stimulation.

OBJECTIVE 2

The student describes the therapeutic options for Zollinger-Ellison syndrome, including the outcome:

A. Therapy
1. High-dose H_2 receptor blockers provide relief of symptoms in 50% of patients.
2. Excision of gastrinoma, from either the pancreas or the paraduodenal area, is curative in a small group of patients.
3. Proximal vagotomy and H_2 blockers can also be used.
4. Total gastrectomy causes postgastrectomy syndromes and may not relieve diarrhea.

B. Outcomes
1. 60% of tumors are malignant.
2. 50% of patients with malignant tumor die within 5 years.
3. A substantial number of patients survive 10 to 15 years.

Minimum Level of Achievement for Passing

The student identifies Zollinger-Ellison syndrome with a history and laboratory tests.

Honors Level of Achievement

The student describes the treatment and outcome of patients with Zollinger-Ellison syndrome.

CASE 3

A 54-year-old man comes to your office with a chief complaint of constant epigastric pain.

OBJECTIVE 1

The student obtains a history and physical examination consistent with gastric ulcer disease and its differential diagnosis.

A. History
1. The pain is boring and constant. It is exacerbated by eating and ameliorated by fasting.
2. The patient lost 10 lb in the last 6 months.
3. The patient has no history of the use of ethanol, aspirin, or prostaglandin blockers; smoking; or biliary tract disease.

B. Physical
1. The patient has an asthenic habitus, with depleted temporal fat pads, but no jaundice.
2. The patient has a scaphoid abdomen, with mild midepigastric tenderness, but no masses.
3. No nodes are palpable.

C. Differential diagnosis
1. Duodenal ulcer
2. Gastric cancer
3. Gastric lymphoma
4. Pancreatitis or biliary tract disease
5. Gastritis

OBJECTIVE 2

The student begins a diagnostic workup.

A. Upper gastrointestinal series shows a gastric ulcer.

B. Endoscopy findings are the same as those of upper gastrointestinal series. Results of gastric washings and biopsy are negative.

C. Fasting serum gastrin level is normal.

D. Gastric acid analysis is normal.

E. Biliary tract studies (e.g., ultrasound) are normal.

OBJECTIVE 3

The student makes the diagnosis of gastric ulcer and describes the options for treatment and the expected results.

A. Medical therapy includes H_2 blockers, antacids, and avoidance of acid stimulators (e.g., coffee). Fifty percent of ulcers heal.

B. If, after 4 weeks of medical treatment, the ulcer does not heal, malignancy is suspected. Biopsies of the ulcer are performed, and surgery is considered.

C. The appropriate surgery is 50% gastrectomy, with excision of the ulcer. If the gastric acid level is high, vagotomy is added.
1. The recurrence rate is low.
2. Postgastrectomy syndromes include:
   a. Dumping
   b. Afferent loop obstruction
   c. Blind loop syndrome
   d. Alkaline reflux gastritis
   e. Recurrent ulcer
   f. Gastric atony
   g. Megaloblastic anemia
   h. Steatorrhea

Minimum Level of Achievement for Passing

The student makes the diagnosis of gastric ulcer with the history and physical examination findings. The student performs the appropriate diagnostic workup, institutes medical therapy and knows the expected results, and knows that malignancy is suspected. The student also describes the surgical therapy for gastric ulcer.

Honors Level of Achievement

The student also describes the complications of 50% gastrectomy.

SUGGESTED READINGS

Feldman M. Gastric secretion. In: Sleisenger MH, Fordtran J, eds. *Gastrointestinal Disease: Pathophysiology, Diagnosis, Management,* 4th ed. Philadelphia, Pa: WB Saunders, 1989.

Fink AS, Longmire WT Jr. Carcinoma of the stomach. In Sabiston DC Jr, ed. *Textbook of Surgery.* Philadelphia, Pa: WB Saunders, 1986.

Moody FG, Miller TA. Stomach. In: Schwartz SI, ed. *Principles of Surgery,* 6th ed. New York, NY: McGraw-Hill, 1994.

Richardson CT. Gastric ulcer. In: Sleisenger MH, Fordtran J, eds. *Gastrointestinal Disease: Pathophysiology, Diagnosis, Management,* 4th ed. Philadelphia, Pa: WB Saunders, 1989.

Soll AH. Duodenal ulcer and drug therapy. In: Sleisenger MH, Fordtran J, eds. *Gastrointestinal Disease: Pathophysiology, Diagnosis, Management,* 4th ed. Philadelphia, Pa: WB Saunders, 1989.

Thompson JC. The stomach and duodenum. In: Sabiston DC Jr, ed. *Textbook of Surgery.* Philadelphia, Pa: WB Saunders, 1991.

Zollinger RM, Ellison EH. Primary peptic ulcerations of the jejunum associated with islet cell tumors of the pancreas. *Ann Surg* 1955;142:709.

14 Small Intestine and Appendix

Bruce V. MacFadyen, Jr., M.D.
David W. Mercer, M.D.
John R. Potts, III, M.D.

OBJECTIVES

1. Discuss the signs, symptoms, and differential diagnosis of acute appendicitis, and describe how diseases that mimic it may be differentiated.
2. Outline the diagnostic workup of a patient with suspected appendicitis, and describe the laboratory findings that would confirm the diagnosis.
3. List and discuss the common complications of appendicitis and subsequent appendectomy, and explain how each can be prevented or managed.
4. Describe the presentation and management of appendiceal carcinoid and its significance as an incidental finding.
5. Discuss the location, frequency, size, and various clinical presentations of a patient with a Meckel's diverticulum.
6. Describe the treatment of Meckel's diverticulum that is incidentally found at surgery and the treatment of one that is symptomatic.
7. Describe the various clinical presentations of a patient with Crohn's disease, and explain how they can differ from the presentation of a patient with ulcerative colitis.
8. Outline a diagnostic approach to a patient with Crohn's disease.
9. Discuss the medical and surgical treatment plans for patients with Crohn's disease. Describe the complications associated with the disease process, and explain when surgery is indicated.
10. Discuss the relative frequency of the most common malignant and benign small bowel tumors.
11. Describe the carcinoid syndrome, and list the features of a carcinoid tumor that suggest it may be malignant. List the features that must be present for carcinoid syndrome to occur.
12. Discuss the clinical presentation and diagnostic approach to the following types of small

bowel tumors: adenocarcinoma, carcinoid, and lymphoma.
13. Discuss the role of surgery in the management of patients with small bowel tumors.
14. Describe the common etiologies, signs, and symptoms of small intestinal mechanical obstruction, and contrast them with those of paralytic ileus.
15. Discuss the complications of small intestinal obstruction, including fluid and electrolyte shifts, vascular compromise of the small intestine, and sepsis.
16. Outline the appropriate laboratory tests and x-rays that are used in the diagnostic evaluation of a patient with a suspected small intestinal obstruction.
17. Discuss the clinical appearance of small bowel strangulation and the potential difficulty of making that diagnosis.
18. Compare and contrast mechanical small intestine obstruction with colon obstruction.
19. Outline a treatment plan for a patient with small intestinal obstruction. Discuss the indications for operative therapy.

Appendicitis is one of the most common surgical emergencies in the United States, and the differential diagnosis of right lower quadrant abdominal pain in all ages is extremely important. An accurate differential diagnosis and appropriate therapeutic management allow the physician to provide cost-efficient treatment, an important consideration in this age of managed care. **Crohn's disease,** which affects the small bowel, is also common, and differentiating between it and other inflammatory diseases expedites patient care. Crohn's disease can also cause right lower quadrant pain; differentiating it from acute appendicitis is sometimes a diagnostic dilemma.

Small bowel tumors, although rare, are usually malignant. Accurate diagnosis and management can improve a patient's long-term survival. Small bowel intestinal obstruction is common in postoperative patients, found in approximately 3% of patients who have abdominal surgery. Differentiating between paralytic ileus and small bowel obstruction is necessary to help determine whether conservative or surgical management is necessary.

This chapter explains the anatomy, embryology, and pathophysiology of the small intestine and appendix. Understanding and applying these concepts helps the physician to provide cost-effective medical care.

Anatomy

From a surgical perspective, the small intestine is composed of three anatomic sections: duodenum, jejunum, and ileum. The duodenum begins at the pylorus and ends at the **ligament of Treitz.** The jejunum is the first 40% of small intestine distal to the ligament of Treitz. The remaining 60% is ileum. In contrast to the duodenum, both the jejunum and the ileum are mobile and are tethered to the mesentery, which is attached to the posterior peritoneal wall beginning in the left upper abdomen and extending across the midline to the right lower abdomen. The arterial blood supply originates from the superior mesenteric artery. The major branches are the middle colic artery and the right colic artery. The vascular arcades to the jejunum and ileum terminate in the ileocolic and appendiceal arteries. Venous drainage from the small intestine is into the superior mesenteric vein. This vein forms the portal vein in conjunction with the splenic and inferior mesenteric veins. Lymphatic drainage is through numerous channels that are parallel to the superior mesenteric vein. They empty into the cisterna chyli located in the retroperitoneum between the aorta and vena cava. They eventually drain into the thoracic duct and left subclavian vein.

The **ileocecal valve** is the termination of the small intestine. It regulates the passage of intestinal contents into the large intestine and prevents reflux of the colonic contents into the small bowel. Removal of this valve increases the amount of liquid chyme that enters the colon, decreases colonic transit time, allows reflux of colonic contents into the small intestine, and decreases the absorption of bile salts and nutrients from the ileum. The appendix is located at the tip of the cecum at the junction of the three taenia coli. This landmark is sometimes used by surgeons to find the appendix.

Physiology

The primary function of the small intestine is efficient digestion of a meal and absorption of ingested nutrients into the bloodstream. The alkaline intestinal fluid (succus entericus) is composed of mucus and other digestive enzymes, principally enterokinase and amylase. The volume of succus entericus increases during the first 2 hours after a meal. Absorption is a dynamic process that is carried out by simple diffusion and active transport and requires the expenditure of energy. The jejunum absorbs the greatest magnitude of ingested material. Although the mucosa of the jejunum possesses the necessary transport enzymes, much of the absorptive process occurs through passive transfer of nutrients and water. In contrast, the ileum makes greater use of specific transport mechanisms and contains the necessary receptors for fat-soluble vitamins, vitamin B_{12}, and bile salt absorption. In addition, because the small bowel is responsible for reabsorbing approximately 80% of the fluid that is secreted into the digestive tract (5–10 L/day), small changes in permeability or transport can cause diarrhea.

Intestinal motility is regulated by both sympathetic and parasympathetic stimuli. These nerves follow the blood vessels into the mesentery through the celiac and superior mesenteric ganglia. The parasympathetic nerve supply originates from the vagus nerve, increasing the tone and enhancing the motility of the small intestine. Sympathetic nerves have the opposite effect. However, the small bowel also contains a prominent plexus of neurons called the enteric nervous system. These nerves lie between the circular and longitudinal smooth muscle layers of the bowel and constitute the myenteric nerve plexus. This plexus contains both inhibitory and excitatory enteric neurons that respond to various stimuli. In general, acetylcholine is the excitatory neurotransmitter. Other substances, such as vasoactive intestinal peptide and somatostatin, are the inhibitory neurotransmitters. The enteric nervous system, in conjunction with the parasympathetic and sympathetic nerves, facilitates digestion by propulsion of the ingested nutrients.

During fasting, a cyclic pattern of small bowel electric activity occurs. This activity consists of muscular contractions that migrate from the duodenum to the terminal ileum. These contractions are referred to as the migrating motor complex (MMC). The MMC has four phases: phase 1, quiescence, with no spikes or contractions; phase 2, accelerating, irregular spiking activity; phase 3, activity front, a series of high-amplitude, rapid spikes that correspond to strong, rhythmic gut contractions; and phase 4, subsiding activity. This cycle lasts approximately 90 to 120 minutes and is interrupted after the ingestion of a meal. Although the gut peptide motilin appears to correlate most closely with MMC activity, other gut peptides (e.g., pancreatic polypeptide, somatostatin) also parallel this activity. The function of this interdigestive pattern is not entirely understood.

Diseases of the Appendix

Acute Appendicitis
Significance and Incidence

The first accurate description of acute appendicitis was provided in 1886 by Reginal Fitz. After that time, several physicians recommended that appendectomy be performed before rupture of the appendix. Today, appendectomy is the most common emergent surgical procedure and the most common cause of an acute surgical abdomen, occurring in 4% to 6% of the population. More than 80% of these patients are between 5 and 35 years of age, and they usually present within 1 to 2 days of the onset of symptoms. However, children and the elderly often present atypically. As a result, there may be a delay in diagnosis and treatment. In these patients, there is a higher incidence of perforation, as high as 15% to 25%, before surgery.

Anatomy

The vermiform appendix is located in the right lower quadrant at the apex of the cecum and at the junction of the three taenia coli muscles. It is between 6 and 10 cm long and usually lies in one of four positions in relation to the cecum: inferior, medial, lateral, and retrocecal. Where the inflamed appendix lies determines the presenting location of the pain. The blood supply to the appendix is contained in the mesoappendix and is derived from the appendicular vessels, which originate as branches of the ileocolic vessels. The appendiceal mucosa consists of columnar epithelium and has a high concentration of lymph follicles, often as many as 200. These follicles occur in the greatest number in people who are between the ages of 10 and 20 years, decreasing after the age of 30 years. By the age of 60 years, few lymph follicles are left. These low numbers of lymph follicles in children and the elderly probably account for the low incidence of acute appendicitis in these age groups.

Pathophysiology

Acute appendicitis usually develops as a result of obstruction of the appendiceal lumen. Obstruction may be related to lymphoid hyperplasia, which occurs in more than 60% of patients with acute appendicitis, or it may be caused by the accumulation of fecal material, which occurs in another 35%. Less commonly, a foreign body causes obstruction and appendicitis. Often, in younger patients, lymphoid hyperplasia caused by an acute viral or bacterial illness causes narrowing of the appendiceal lumen. This narrowing leads to secretion of mucus, distension of the distal appendix, and ischemia of the appendiceal wall. Bacterial proliferation and patchy necrosis may occur and may lead eventually to gangrene and perforation. As the appendix distends, the visceral peritoneum stretches and causes ill-defined, poorly localized pain in the periumbilical region. As inflammation progresses, parietal peritoneal irritation develops and the pain becomes more localized at this site. During the inflammatory process, the proliferation of bacteria and the release of exotoxins and endotoxins causes damage to the epithelium, leading to ulceration and ischemia of the mucosa. Perforation may occur if all layers of the appendix are involved. With perforation, an abscess may form that is localized to the right lower quadrant or pelvis, or diffuse peritonitis may develop. If the inflammatory process is not controlled, it potentially can spread through the portal system (pyelophlebitis) to the liver, causing multiple liver abscesses. If the sepsis continues and becomes more generalized, death occurs. In the United States each year, approximately 10,000 deaths are recorded that are attributable to diseases of the appendix. Death is more common in children younger than 2 years of age and in the elderly because, in these patients, the presentation of symptoms is delayed and infection is not sufficiently localized if the appendix perforates.

Clinical Presentation and Evaluation

Often the clinical presentation of acute appendicitis is pain that develops in the upper abdomen or periumbilical region. It may be associated with anorexia, nausea, or vomiting. Often within 4 to 6 hours, as the inflammation progresses, the pain spreads to the right lower quadrant. A fever of as high as 100° F (orally) may occur. It is usually associated with a leukocytosis of 11,000 to 13,000. Initially, the pain is often vague, but as the peritoneal irritation increases, it becomes more specific. There is often rebound tenderness on palpation, and the pain becomes localized to the right lower quadrant. Clinically, this pain is found at **McBurney's point,** which is located between the middle and outer third of a line drawn between the anterior iliac spine and umbilicus. Pain may also be elicited on rectal and pelvic examination if the appendix lies inferior to the cecum. Bowel sounds are usually decreased or absent.

Rovsing's sign is elicited when pressure applied in the left lower quadrant of the abdomen causes pain in the right lower quadrant. A positive **psoas sign** occurs when there is pain on extension of the right hip; it often indicates inflammation of a retrocecal appendix as it lies adjacent to the iliopsoas muscle. A positive **obturator sign** is detected when there is passive rotation of the flexed right thigh when the patient is in the supine position. This sign is caused by inflammation adjacent to the obturator internus muscle.

As inflammation progresses, the appendix may rupture. Abdominal pain becomes more intense and diffuse, and temperature may increase to greater than 102° F. In addition, the white blood cell count increases to greater than 14,000 to 18,000.

In pregnancy, the enlarging uterus pushes the cecum and appendix superiorly causing them to lie at the same level as the fundus of the uterus. The presentation may be that of pain in the right upper quadrant, thus making diagnosis difficult. If the diagnosis of acute appendicitis is not made before perforation, generalized peritonitis may occur, with resulting fetal death in more than 35% of patients. Leukocytosis normally occurs in pregnancy and can range from 15,000 to 17,000, thus adding to the dilemma of diagnosis.

The most important method of diagnosis for acute appendicitis is the history and physical examination. Rebound tenderness in the right lower quadrant is one of the most important and consistent signs. The leukocyte count is important as well; it is often between 11,000 to 13,000, with a left shift. Although a normal leukocyte count may occur in the elderly patient, a left shift indicating infection is usually observed. Urinalysis is also important because it may show a few red or white blood cells. These factors may indicate other possible causes for right lower quadrant pain (e.g., kidney stone, urinary tract infection).

Radiographic studies, such as plain films of the abdomen, are not particularly useful, although they may show a calcified fecalith or foreign body in the right lower quadrant, a nonspecific gas pattern in the small bowel, possible loss of the right psoas margin, or dilation of the cecum. A barium enema is usually not performed except when there is concern about a cecal mass or diverticulitis. When the appendix does not fill with barium, acute appendicitis is suggested. This test may be more helpful in young children and elderly patients. Ultrasonography may also be helpful in identifying a large appendix or abscess or to differentiate diseases in the fallopian tubes and ovaries. A computed tomography (CT) scan of the abdomen may also be useful in establishing the diagnosis of an abscess. However, in most situations, these studies are not necessary, and the patient undergoes surgery expeditiously based on the history, physical examination, and leukocytosis.

Differential Diagnosis

The differential diagnosis of right lower quadrant pain includes gastroenteritis, colitis, pyelitis, salpingitis, tuboovarian abscess, and ruptured ovarian cyst. In younger children, intussusception must be considered as well. Less common diagnoses include Meckel's diverticulum, acute ileitis, obstructing tumors of the ascending colon, sigmoid or cecal diverticulitis, and perforated gastric or duodenal ulcer. In addition, appendicitis must be differentiated from nonoperative conditions (e.g., right lower lobe pneumonia, acute hepatitis, acute pyelonephritis, cystitis, epididymitis, testicular torsion). Therefore, when the patient is seen initially, laboratory tests should include complete blood count (CBC), urinalysis, and chest x-ray. Optional studies might include an abdominal series and ultrasound and CT of the abdomen and pelvis. Barium enema is more effective in helping to make a diagnosis in young children and elderly patients. Because appendiceal perforation is associated with increased morbidity and mortality, diagnosis may be confirmed only by diagnostic laparotomy or laparoscopy. The appendix is normal in 10% to 20% of these cases.

Treatment

The primary treatment for acute appendicitis is appendectomy. Before surgical intervention, fluid and electrolyte replacement should be instituted. Antibiotics, such as a second- or third-generation cephalosporin, are given intravenously to treat aerobic and anaerobic organisms. If the appendix has not ruptured, antibiotics can be discontinued within 24 hours. Other antibiotic combinations include piperacillin and metronidazole. An aminoglycoside, ampicillin, and clindamycin combination may be particularly effective against the colonic flora.

When surgery is considered, it should be undertaken expeditiously. Perforation must be considered if symptoms have been present for more than 24 hours. Surgery can be performed either as an open procedure through a right lower quadrant transverse incision or by laparoscopy. In the open procedure, a transverse incision is made in the right lower quadrant that crosses McBurney's point and splits the external and internal oblique muscles as well as the transversus abdominis muscle in the lines of its fibers. Initial evaluation of the appendix for inflammation is important. If the diagnosis is acute appendicitis, the mesoappendix and the appendicular artery and vein are divided, and the appendix is amputated at the junction with the cecum. If the appendix is not inflamed, careful assessment of the small and large intestine, pelvis, and right upper quadrant organs should be done and the appendix removed to eliminate the appendix as a source of right lower quadrant pain. If an abscess is found, it is drained externally and the appendix removed. If the appendix is not removed, there is a 20% chance of appendicitis recurring within 2 months and as high as a 50% chance in the next 5 years.

Laparoscopy allows for a thorough evaluation of the entire abdomen and easy removal of the appendix. A prospective randomized trial by Frazee et al. compared open and laparoscopic appendectomy and found that patients had an equal length of hospital stay. However, those who underwent laparoscopy had a shorter duration of postoperative pain and returned to work twice as fast as those who underwent the open procedure. However, there is debate about laparoscopic management in patients who have a ruptured appendix because there may be a higher incidence of recurrent abscess. It is suggested that these patients undergo an open operation for effective drainage of the appendiceal abscess and removal of the appendix.

When an appendiceal abscess is identified by CT preoperatively and is localized in the right lower quadrant, nonoperative management may be considered. In these patients, the abscess is drained radiologically, the patient is given antibiotics for 10 to 14 days, and an interval appendectomy is performed 6 to 12 weeks later.

Complications

The most common complication of acute appendicitis is postoperative wound infection. A pelvic or right lower quadrant abscess may develop from inadequate irrigation of the abdomen at surgery or from a leaking appendiceal stump. Bleeding can occur as a result of insufficient ligation of the mesoappendix and, specifically, the appendiceal artery.

Appendicitis in young children is often difficult to diagnose preoperatively, especially in patients who are younger than 1 year of age who have perforation. In addition, the diagnosis of acute appendicitis in pregnancy can be difficult. In these patients, laparoscopy may be particularly useful to make the diagnosis.

However, introduction of the trocars during laparoscopy can injure the uterus, or the uterus may undergo contractions and cause fetal loss, especially in the first and third trimesters.

In elderly patients, appendicitis may also be difficult to diagnose. It may cause only mild elevations of temperature and leukocyte count, even in the presence of acute perforation.

Tumors of the Appendix

The most common tumor of the appendix is a **carcinoid tumor.** It is found in 0.5% of all appendices that are removed, and it accounts for approximately 50% of all carcinoid tumors of the gastrointestinal tract. Only 3% of appendiceal carcinoids are malignant. Patients are often asymptomatic. If the lesion is less than 2 cm in diameter, the treatment of choice is usually appendectomy. If the lesion extends through the serosa or is greater than 2 cm in diameter, the incidence of malignancy is higher and a right hemicolectomy is indicated.

Other tumors of the appendix include adenocarcinoma with or without a mucoid component. These tumors constitute fewer than 1% of all appendiceal diseases. A malignant mucocele of the appendix may occur secondary to luminal obstruction and distension of the appendix. Pathologically, it is often a well-differentiated adenocarcinoma. Patients with appendiceal carcinoma usually have symptoms of perforated acute appendicitis with an appendiceal abscess. The tumor is often mucinous, and a significant number have pseudomyxoma peritonei. A right hemicolectomy is the treatment of choice. The cure rate for adenocarcinoma of the appendix averages 55% at 5 years.

Diseases of the Small Intestine

Meckel's Diverticulum

Significance and Incidence

The most common congenital anomaly of the small intestine is **Meckel's diverticulum,** a remnant of the embryonic vitelline (omphalomesenteric) duct. It was initially described in detail by Johann Meckel in 1809. Its frequency in the general population is approximately 1% to 3%, with a male:female predominance of 2:1 in symptomatic patients. Although previous investigators noted a 25% frequency of symptoms in patients with Meckel's diverticulum, recent studies suggest a much lower rate of 4% to 5% in infants, 1.5% by the age of 40 years, and 0% by the age of 75 years.

Anatomy

Embryologically, Meckel's diverticulum originates from the vitelline duct that is connected to the midgut loop. The vitelline duct remains open until the 8th to 10th week of gestation, at which time it becomes obliterated (Figure 14-1). In patients who have Meckel's diverticulum, at birth, it is located on the antimesenteric bor-

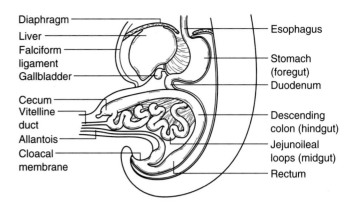

Figure 14-1 Embryologic development of Meckel's diverticulum.

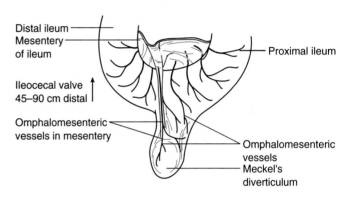

Figure 14-2 Anatomy of Meckel's diverticulum.

der of the ileum, 45 to 90 cm proximal to the ileocecal valve (Figure 14-2). Its blood supply is from the vitelline vessels that remain open and lie in close association with the mesentery of the ileum.

Pathophysiology

Because the cells that line the vitelline duct have the potential to develop into several types of mucosa, it is common to find heterotopic tissue within the diverticulum. The most common type is gastric mucosa (50%). Other types of mucosa include pancreatic cells and, less commonly, colonic mucosa. Benign tumors have been reported in Meckel's diverticulum, including lipoma, **leiomyoma,** neurofibroma, and angioma. A malignant tumor is very uncommon. However, any one of these tumors can be the lead point for intussusception, and all of these findings can potentially lead to complications and symptomatic presentation.

Because of the persistence of the vitelline duct and its connection to the umbilicus, various complications of this duct are reported, including a fistula between the umbilicus and ileum, and an umbilical sinus on the umbilical side of the vitelline duct, which may cause continuous drainage from the umbilicus. In addition, a fibrous cord can remain between the umbilicus and the ileum and can potentially produce small bowel obstruction. Any combination of these entities may also occur.

Clinical Presentation and Evaluation

Most commonly, Meckel's diverticulum is discovered incidentally at the time of an abdominal operation. Overall, only 4% of patients with Meckel's diverticulum become symptomatic during their lifetime. Symptoms can include gastrointestinal hemorrhage, small bowel obstruction, diverticulitis, perforation, and symptoms of an umbilical fistula or tumor (Table 14-1). The most common age for symptoms is younger than 2 years old. In elderly patients, the surgical mortality rate can approach 5% to 6%.

When hemorrhage occurs, it is often bright red rectal bleeding originating from an ulcer in the ileum adjacent to the Meckel's diverticulum that contains gastric mucosa. The bleeding is often painless, occurs in children younger than 2 years of age, and is often diagnosed (90%) with ^{99m}Tc pertechnetate radioisotope scanning (which identifies the gastric mucosa). Angiography may be helpful in making the diagnosis if the rate of bleeding is greater than 0.1 to 0.5 mL/min.

Intestinal obstruction can occur because of **volvulus** of the small bowel around the diverticulum or the fibrous band between the intestine and umbilicus (Figure 14-3). If intussusception of the diverticulum in the small intestine occurs, a currant jelly stool may pass, and there may be a palpable mass in the intestine. A barium enema may be used to reduce the intestinal intussusception, but surgery with resection of the diverticulum and any fibrous band must be performed.

Diverticulitis accounts for approximately 10% to 20% of symptomatic patients. It is indistinguishable from acute appendicitis. In these cases, a diverticulectomy should be done.

Less common complications of Meckel's diverticulum include iron deficiency anemia, malabsorption, foreign body impaction, perforation, and incarceration or strangulation of the diverticulum in a hernia (Littre's hernia). Of these, 50% are inguinal, 20% are femoral, and 20% are umbilical.

The diagnosis of Meckel's diverticulum is difficult and is often based on a combination of symptoms similar to those of acute appendicitis. When there is pain, it is often sudden in onset, and when hemorrhage is present, it can be bright red or currant jelly in color.

Differential Diagnosis

The differential diagnosis often includes acute appendicitis, regional enteritis, and small bowel obstruction, particularly when volvulus around a fibrous band or intussusception occurs. If Meckel's diverticulum is located in an inguinal hernia, a nonreducible tender mass may be palpated in that region. When lower gastrointestinal bleeding from Meckel's diverticulum occurs, it must be differentiated from bleeding from the colon, stomach, or duodenum, which are more frequent sites of gastrointestinal bleeding.

An abdominal series may be useful in the presence of intestinal obstruction. Barium studies of the small and large intestine may also help in the diagnosis.

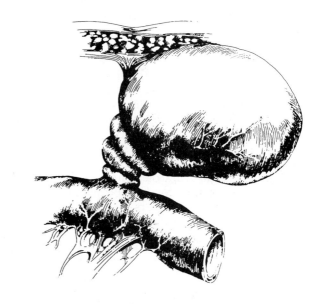

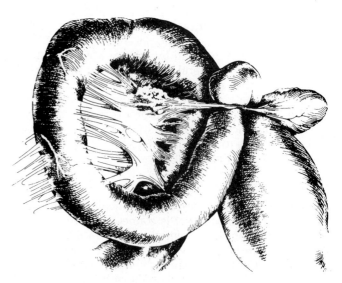

Figure 14-3 Obstruction caused by a mesodiverticular band.

Table 14-1. Clinical Presentation in Meckel's Diverticula[a]

Clinical Presentation	Frequency (%)
Hemorrhage	23
Ileus	31
Intussusception	14
Diverticulitis	14
Perforation	10
Miscellaneous (e.g., fistula, tumor)	8

[a]Occurrence in 1044 cases of Meckel's diverticula compiled from previously published reports.
Adapted with permission from Scharli AF. In: Freeman NV, Burge DM, Griffiths DM, Malone PSJ, eds. *Surgery of the Newborn.* Edinburgh, Scotland: Churchill Livingstone, 1994.

Treatment

In the past, the management of Meckel's diverticulum found incidentally at laparotomy was controversial. The indications for removal included a diverticulum 2 inches long in a patient younger than 40 years of age, palpable heterotopic tissue, inflammation, or a mesodiverticular band. However, because resection is associated with a low operative morbidity rate (2%), most authors now agree that the diverticulum should be resected when found incidentally.

Symptomatic Meckel's diverticulum should be resected, even though the mortality rate in elderly patients can be as high as 5% to 10%. The increased morbidity and mortality rate is related to the presenting problem (e.g., bowel obstruction, diverticulitis, bleeding). With a broad-based diverticulum, segmental bowel resection may be necessary to remove all of the associated heterotopic gastric, pancreatic, or colonic mucosa that may be present. With newer laparoscopic techniques, Meckel's diverticulum can be resected safely with a complication rate equivalent to that of the open procedure.

Crohn's Disease of the Small Intestine

Significance and Incidence

Crohn's disease of the small intestine was described in 1932 by Crohn, Ginsburg, and Oppenheimer. Its worldwide prevalence is estimated as 10 to 70 cases per 100,000 population, and its incidence in 1 year varies from 0.5 to 6 cases per 100,000 population. Interestingly, demographic surveys showed an increase in its frequency in the 1950s, with subsequent stabilization in the 1970s. The disease process predominantly affects young individuals who live in industrialized nations, suggesting that environmental factors play an important role in its pathogenesis. Although genetic and familial factors may also play a role, there is no direct evidence of simple Mendelian transmission or human leukocyte antigen (HLA) typing.

There are two peak periods during which Crohn's disease occurs. The first peak occurs in the late teens and early twenties. Most patients have disease involving the small intestine and terminal ileum. The second peak is in the sixth and seventh decades of life. Most patients have colonic involvement. Because the disease runs a chronic course with intermittent exacerbations, is not curable, and involves a potentially economically productive patient population, the disease has a major impact on society.

Pathophysiology

Crohn's disease is a chronic, transmural inflammatory condition that may involve any segment of the alimentary tract. The precise etiology of Crohn's disease is elusive, but the common extraintestinal manifestations suggest that it is a systemic disorder rather than a localized intestinal disease. In addition, the presence of noncaseating granulomas in the inflammatory tissue lends credence to an infectious cause. However, the infectious agent that causes this inflammatory reaction (if one exists) is not known. Nonetheless, after infection, it is hypothesized that the immune system responds appropriately to the infection to initiate an inflammatory response. In contrast, others hypothesize that the immune system reacts inappropriately to an antigenic challenge independent of any infectious process. Although numerous alterations in systemic and mucosal immunity are reported in Crohn's disease, no specific defect has been identified. Further, a unifying mechanism linking all of the aberrations in the intestinal mucosal immune system is lacking. As a result, further research in epidemiology, bacteriology, and immunology is necessary to better define the exact mechanisms that contribute to the pathogenesis of this inflammatory bowel disease.

The disease may occur anywhere from the mouth to the anus and characteristically has "skip lesions," as opposed to the contiguous disease pattern observed in **ulcerative colitis** (Table 14-2). Aphthous mucosal ulcerations, lymphoid aggregates, and noncaseating granulomas characterize the acute, or active, phase. Later, transmural chronic inflammation develops and is accompanied by the formation of fissures and fistulas. The quiescent, or healing, phase is exemplified by chronic ulcerations, fibrosis, and resultant stricture formation.

On gross examination of the bowel, the serosa appears beefy red and is often covered with a gray exudate. Mesenteric fat is characteristically observed to be "creeping" over the antimesenteric bowel wall in the areas of greatest inflammation. The mesentery is thickened and foreshortened and often contains enlarged mesenteric lymph nodes. Additionally, the inflammatory process is not necessarily confined to the intestine

Table 14-2. Characteristics of Crohn's Disease and Ulcerative Colitis

Crohn's Disease	Ulcerative Colitis
Transmural involvement	Mucosal disease
Segmental involvement	Diffuse involvement of the entire colon
Rectum uninvolved with disease	Rectum involved with disease
Thickened bowel wall with creeping fat	Normal thickness of bowel wall
Pseudopolyps (occasionally)	Pseudopolyps common
Small bowel may be involved	Small bowel not involved (except as backwash ileitis)
Fistulas common	Fistulas rare
Anal complications common	Anal complications rare
Toxic megacolon uncommon	Toxic megacolon common
Bleeding rare	Bleeding uncommon
Surgery relatively effective	Surgery curative
Cobblestoning	Pseudopolyps
Narrow, deeply penetrating ulcers	Shallow, wide ulcers
Granulomas common	Granulomas rare
Mucus secretion increased	Mucus secretion decreased

and may extend into adjacent structures, with resultant fistula or abscess formation. Fistula formation between diseased bowel and nearly any organ or structure is one of the pathognomonic features of Crohn's disease. Often, the development of intraabdominal abscesses accompanies the formation of a fistula. These abscesses are classified as interloop, intramesenteric, retroperitoneal, ileopsoal, and enteroperitoneal (bounded by parietal peritoneum and abdominal viscera). Perianal complications (e.g., ulcers, fissures, perirectal fistulas, abscesses) also occur in 30% to 60% of patients with colonic disease and 8% to 30% of patients with small bowel disease. Last, the inflammation and fibrosis that characterize this disease often result in distortion of normal anatomic relations. This distortion can lead to deviation of ureters or bowel obstruction of involved or uninvolved segments.

Microscopically, the inflammatory process originates in the submucosa and spreads transmurally. These changes begin with the accumulation of inflammatory cells adjacent to a crypt, which is followed by the formation of an aphthoid ulceration, fissure-like ulcers, and crypt abscesses that can later develop into fistulas or sinus tracts. Although epithelial cell injury with necrosis and apoptosis occurs, it is not the initial inciting event, which again originates in the submucosa. Not uncommonly, the submucosal compartment has prominent edema and infiltration by inflammatory cells, and the overlying mucosa is only minimally involved. In contrast, in ulcerative colitis, the mucosa is always involved. Although not all patients with Crohn's disease have noncaseating granulomas, more than 60% have this microscopic finding that consists of epithelioid histiocytes surrounded by lymphocytes and giant cells.

Clinical Presentation

In general, the clinical presentation depends on the anatomic location of the disease within the digestive tract. Three major categories of the disease process exist and determine not only the clinical features, but also the types of complications that arise. Ileocolic involvement occurs in roughly 50% of patients, followed by small intestinal involvement only in 30% to 40% of patients. In contrast, isolated involvement of the colon is present in roughly 20% of patients. Although certain clinical features are more commonly associated with specific locations, most patients have the triad of abdominal pain, diarrhea, and weight loss. These signs and symptoms are usually gradual in onset and are typified by a progressive, but waxing and waning, course that varies from patient to patient.

Abdominal pain is the most common presenting symptom. It may be intermittent or constant. Intermittent or colicky abdominal pain occurs as a result of partial or complete bowel obstruction. More constant pain is induced by irritation of the parietal peritoneum. Diarrhea is also a common symptom that results from a variety of causes. However, the diarrhea associated with Crohn's disease rarely contains blood. In contrast, in ulcerative colitis, bloody diarrhea commonly occurs.

Other nonspecific signs and symptoms include fever, anorexia, nausea, and vomiting.

Another common manifestation of Crohn's disease is perianal involvement, with the development of abscesses, fistulas, and fissures. Perianal disease may develop at any time, but is present at initial presentation in approximately one-third of patients. Perianal disease is most common in patients with ileocolic involvement. In this group, as many as 50% of patients have perianal involvement. In addition, 40% of patients with isolated colonic involvement have perianal complications. However, only approximately 25% of patients with ileitis ever have perianal disease.

Extraintestinal manifestations are commonly associated with Crohn's disease. They primarily involve the skin, eyes, joints, and liver. Their prevalence is higher with colonic involvement than with small bowel disease. Extraintestinal involvement of the skin may include pyoderma gangrenosum, erythema nodosum multiforme, vasculitis, and aphthous stomatitis. Conjunctivitis, iritis, iridocyclitis, episcleritis, uveitis, and vasculitis can occur in the eyes. Joint involvement is characterized by arthritis, ankylosing spondylitis, or hypertrophic osteoarthropathy. Less commonly, the liver is involved, with changes such as sclerosing cholangitis, pericholangitis, or granulomatous hepatitis. In general, these extraintestinal manifestations resolve when the disease is in remission or as a result of medical or surgical therapy.

Patients with Crohn's disease often appear chronically ill. In 65% of patients, a 10% to 20% loss of body weight is apparent at initial presentation. Hypoproteinemia (decreased serum albumin), edema, muscle weakness, increased basal metabolic rate, and deficiencies of vitamins A, D, E, and K are often seen. Protein secretion into the gut may be increased up to 15 times the normal level of 24 mg albumin/kg body weight/day. In addition, 40% to 50% of patients may have malabsorption of carbohydrate, protein, fat, and vitamin B_{12}. These consequences are especially deleterious in children, resulting in growth retardation and delayed maturation in 10% to 40%. Despite their severity, these nutritional deficits can be reversed or significantly attenuated by aggressive nutritional therapy, which effectively decreases morbidity and mortality rates.

Crohn's disease may be rapidly progressive or run an indolent, chronic course characterized by intermittent exacerbations. More than 90% of patients have intermittent, but progressive abdominal pain and diarrhea. In these patients, the disease is characterized by a waxing and waning of symptoms. Usually, the presenting symptoms are primarily related to the complications of the disease (e.g., bowel obstruction, abscess, fistula, perianal disease). Nevertheless, the presenting symptom complex in 10% of patients is similar to that of acute appendicitis, with fever and pain in the midabdomen or right lower quadrant that may or may not be associated with a mass. Differentiating acute Crohn's disease from appendicitis is difficult, and surgery is often necessary to determine the correct diagnosis.

The signs and symptoms of Crohn's disease are nonspecific and resemble a variety of other conditions that involve the gastrointestinal tract. Thus, establishing the diagnosis can be challenging. Nonetheless, after a careful history and physical examination, routine laboratory studies are generally obtained. Unfortunately, there is no specific laboratory test to diagnose Crohn's disease. Consequently, the diagnosis depends on obtaining radiologic studies and performing endoscopic examinations. Radiology is useful for determining not only the diagnosis, but also the extent and severity of the disease. Radiologic examination is used for patients with progressive disease in whom surgical therapy is being considered or for patients who require a major change in their medical management. Radiologic investigation is also warranted for the patient who has recurrent symptoms after surgical resection.

Clinical presentation dictates which radiologic studies are necessary. When surgery is contemplated, an expeditious and proper sequence of studies should be planned so that one study does not interfere with another or delay intervention. Radiologic consultation for planning can greatly increase the diagnostic yield and minimize radiation and expense. In general, barium expulsion is slow and interferes with nuclear scans, ultrasonography, plain films, and intravenous contrast studies. As a result, barium studies should be done last and in the following order: barium enema, upper gastrointestinal series, small bowel series, and enteroclysis.

Water-soluble contrast agents also interfere with the interpretation of ultrasound and plain films; hence, the latter should be done first.

The first radiologic studies should be plain films of the abdomen to search for biliary and urinary calculi, skeletal manifestations, and intestinal complications. If biliary calculi or intestinal complications are suspected, ultrasonography should follow. This study may also show the thickened walls and narrowed lumens of involved bowel segments and may detect surrounding abscesses or masses. CT scan may show abscess or phlegmon formation in even greater detail. However, cost and radiation dose, especially to the female pelvis, must be considered. Excretory urography, if needed, should be done before CT. If extraintestinal (enterocutaneous, enterovesical, or enterovaginal) fistulas are suspected, they should be investigated next with fluoroscopically and endoscopically guided catheter placement and a water-soluble contrast agent. Nuclear scans are less helpful because they cannot distinguish inflammation in the bowel from that surrounding it.

Thereafter, double-contrast barium enema, double-contrast esophagram, an upper gastrointestinal series, and a small bowel series should be done (Figure 14-4). If all of the segments of the small bowel are not exceptionally well shown, enteroclysis (small bowel enema) should be used to show skip lesions as well as enteroenteric and

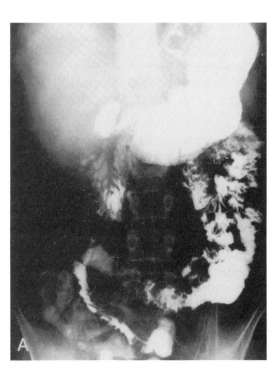
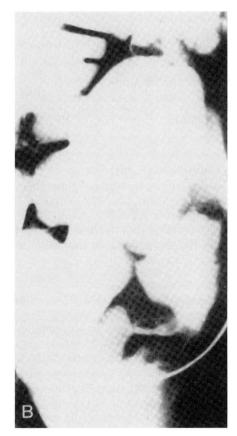

Figure 14-4 A, Small bowel study showing a narrowed segment of distal small bowel and a similar change in the antrum of the stomach. The mucosal pattern of the bowel is altered by pseudopolyps, and the valvulae conniventes are absent. The upper small bowel suggests skip areas of Crohn's involvement, whereas the distal bowel is narrowed and contiguously involved with Crohn's disease. **B,** Small bowel study showing the "string sign" in the terminal ileum adjacent to the cecum, with proximal dilation of the ileum.

other fistulous connections. Enteroclysis involves passing a tube under fluoroscopic guidance through the nose and gastrointestinal tract into the proximal small bowel and rapidly injecting a large quantity of barium to fully distend the bowel loops while multiple radiographs are made.

Radiographic interpretation depends on finding the earliest and the most advanced Crohn's lesions. The earliest mucosal lesion is an aphthous ulcer, which appears on a double-contrast barium study as a white fleck (ulcer) on a dark doughnut (edema) in an otherwise normal-appearing mucosa. As the disease progresses, the mucosa thickens and becomes nodular. The mucosal folds become unrecognizable, cracks (representing linear ulcers) appear between the nodules, and the lumen narrows as the bowel wall thickens. Mesenteric involvement adds to the thickening, and the final result is a narrowed string-like lumen, fixed in position and size, and separated by mass effect from the next adjacent loop. Although spasm, a common fluoroscopic finding, and edema account for some of the lumen narrowing, irreversible stricturing and partial obstruction eventually occur. In general, these strictures are smooth, without the shouldering seen in neoplasms.

After a radiologic overview of the gastrointestinal tract, endoscopic confirmation and biopsy of Crohn's lesions is needed. Proctocolonoscopy and biopsy are extremely important in differentiating the type of inflammatory bowel disease in the colon. Even though Crohn's disease less commonly involves the rectum, full-thickness rectal biopsy must be performed, even when the mucosa appears normal, to differentiate Crohn's disease from ulcerative colitis (see Table 14-2). Esophagogastroduodenoscopy is necessary to document the rare involvement of the foregut structures by Crohn's disease. If sclerosing cholangitis is a concern, endoscopic retrograde cholangiography can be performed.

Differential Diagnosis

Often, this disease causes right lower quadrant pain and fever. Sometimes it cannot be differentiated from acute appendicitis, tuberculosis of the cecum, or inflammation of the fallopian tubes and ovaries. In addition, it may be difficult to differentiate it from ulcerative colitis when it is examined microscopically.

Treatment

Medical Therapy

Crohn's disease cannot be cured by any medical or surgical therapy. For this reason, it presents a major therapeutic challenge. Because disease-specific treatment does not exist, the goals of therapy are to alleviate symptoms, provide nutritional support, and suppress the inflammatory process. Further, any planned therapeutic regimen must take into account the natural history of Crohn's disease, with its acute exacerbations and prolonged remissions, especially when assessing the efficacy of drug therapy.

Control of abdominal pain with opiates and other analgesics must be done with great caution. Use of these agents obscures the abdominal examination and results in decreased bowel motility that might potentiate the risk of ileus and obstruction. Diarrhea can be managed with diphenoxylate, codeine, or loperamide. These agents are most effective when the diarrhea is a result of long-standing disease or intestinal resection. These agents must also be given cautiously because they are associated with a slight risk of toxic megacolon. However, central nervous system depression is the principal side effect observed with these antidiarrheal agents. For this reason, loperamide is sometimes better tolerated because of its incomplete penetration of the blood–brain barrier. Finally, cholestyramine is often effective in patients with bile-salt induced diarrhea from ileal resection or as a result of Crohn's disease involving the ileum.

As previously indicated, these patients are often chronically ill, malnourished, and have a 10% to 20% loss of body weight at presentation. As a result, intensive parenteral or enteral nutritional therapy is necessary to correct these deficiencies and increase visceral protein status and nitrogen balance. Further, bowel rest accompanied by total parenteral nutrition or enterally fed elemental diets has been used to treat acute disease, both as supportive and primary therapy. Elemental diets are constructed so that they are absorbed primarily in the proximal gut, which effectively puts the distal small bowel and large bowel at rest. Although prospective, controlled, randomized trials comparing total parenteral nutrition with elemental enteral diets have not been performed, total parenteral nutrition in combination with bowel rest as primary therapy is reported to heal fistulas in as many as 50% to 75% of patients. Despite its obvious benefits, a program of total parenteral nutrition in preparing a patient for surgical intervention remains controversial. Nevertheless, most studies suggest that patients with the most severe disease or nutritional deficits should receive or be considered for preoperative total parenteral nutrition.

Several options are available to suppress the inflammatory process associated with Crohn's disease. These include the use of corticosteroids, aspirin derivatives, antibiotics, and other immunosuppressant agents. Corticosteroids have been used to treat Crohn's disease since the 1940s. Although the exact mechanism of action is not entirely understood, several studies show their efficacy in the treatment of acute exacerbations. Approximately 60% of patients achieve and maintain a remission for the duration of therapy versus 30% of patients receiving placebo. However, patients with quiescent disease or those in remission did not benefit from long-term continued corticosteroid treatment.

Sulfasalazine, which contains a sulfonamide moiety that is linked to the aspirin analogue 5-aminosalicylate (5-ASA), is given orally. After it passes into the distal ileum and colon, it is cleaved by bacteria. As a result, the sulfonamide portion is absorbed. The 5-ASA moiety, in turn, is available to the intestinal mucosa, where it acts locally and is excreted intact. Its mechanism of action is likely the inhibition of the cyclooxygenase pathway and possibly the lipoxygenase pathway. Inhibition of these pathways prevents the formation of inflammatory arachidonic acid metabolites (e.g., prostaglandins, leukotrienes). Like corticosteroids, sulfasalazine is more effective than placebo in achieving remission of the acute exacerbations of the disease. Interestingly, patients with predominantly colonic disease receive the most benefit. This drug is not as effective as steroids in treating patients with small bowel disease. In addition, patients who are asymptomatic do not seem to benefit from prophylactic treatment. Recently, several similar agents became available (e.g., Pentasa); like sulfasalazine, they have a similar mechanism of action.

Broad-spectrum antibiotics and immunosuppressants are also used to treat Crohn's disease. Usually, antibiotics are prescribed to treat the septic complications associated with this disease. Metronidazole is often used to treat the perianal complications. Interestingly, the cooperative Crohn's disease study in Sweden found that metronidazole was as effective as sulfasalazine in the treatment of symptomatic patients. On the other hand, the immunosuppressant agents azathioprine, 6-mercaptopurine, methotrexate, and cyclosporine have been used at one time or another to treat Crohn's disease. Although they are effective, they have numerous side effects that are primarily dose-dependent. Future trials are necessary to determine the role of these agents, especially cyclosporine.

Surgical Therapy

Surgical therapy can cure ulcerative colitis, but for Crohn's disease, it is only palliative. Surgical intervention is undertaken when complications develop, or when medical management fails and the patient's lifestyle, well-being, and socioeconomic status are significantly impaired because of intractable symptoms or the side effects of medical therapy. If possible, the patient is prepared preoperatively with mechanical bowel preparation (including cathartics, oral antibiotics, and lavage solutions). If this preparation is not possible, gentle cleansing enemas and a clear liquid diet will suffice. As a rule, prophylactic parenteral antibiotics are given preoperatively, but their continued use is reserved for cases of obvious sepsis.

After preoperative preparation, an abdominal exploration is performed. Acute terminal ileitis precipitated by *Yersinia* bacteria can produce an inflammatory response in the terminal ileum in 20% of patients with Crohn's disease. Although this problem resolves spontaneously in 90% of cases, the appendix should be removed if the cecum is normal. This intervention eliminates the possibility of appendicitis in the differential diagnosis if the patient has more attacks of right lower quadrant abdominal pain. However, for the other varieties of Crohn's disease involving the gastrointestinal tract, it is imperative to assess the extent of disease intraoperatively, rule out any skip lesions, and note the length of uninvolved small intestine. If a bowel resection is required, the proposed sites of transsection are chosen conservatively. In general, these sites should be adjacent to clinically obvious gross involvement of Crohn's disease, extending only a few centimeters proximal and distal to the site of macroscopic or visible evidence of disease (i.e., narrowing of the intestinal lumen, bowel wall thickening, serositis, mesenteric fat creeping, mesentery thickening, tortuosity of serosal vessels). Microscopic confirmation of the absence of Crohn's disease at the resection margins does not determine future recurrence and is not necessary for a safe anastomosis. Consequently, frozen-section examination of the resection margins is not indicated.

Complications

Various complications can develop during medical and surgical therapy. Small bowel obstruction can occur as a result of a strictured intestinal lumen. Nutritional deficiencies may also occur, including protein-calorie malnutrition and vitamin, electrolyte, and mineral deficiencies.

Gastrointestinal fistulas and abscesses are a particularly complicated treatment problem. After a fistula is diagnosed, its tract and its communication with other abdominal structures must be determined. Surgical intervention is best performed when the active inflammatory process is under control, nutritional status is optimized, and adequate bowel preparation is obtained. Some gastrointestinal fistulas are more severe than others. If the fistula is of low output and does not compromise the patient's overall status, it may be observed. However, once a fistula becomes clinically symptomatic, surgical intervention is necessary. For enterocutaneous fistulas, patients are prepared preoperatively (previously described), and their nutritional status optimized with either parenteral or enteral nutritional support. At exploration, the diseased segment of intestine from which the fistulous tract arises is resected. At the abdominal wall, the tract is debrided and excised at the skin level. For communications to other intraabdominal viscera that are not actively involved with Crohn's disease, the diseased segment of intestine is resected and the fistula is excised. The intraabdominal organ with which the fistulous tract communicates is excised in a wedge fashion and then closed primarily. If a fistula or Crohn's disease is associated with an intraabdominal abscess, percutaneous drainage of the abscess under CT guidance may not be prudent because loops of matted bowel (diseased and nondiseased) may have to be transgressed. In this case, open surgical drainage with bowel resection is safer and better tolerated.

Management of perianal complications of Crohn's disease also requires a conservative surgical approach. An abscess requires standard incision and drainage, whereas chronic anal fistulas may be safely observed if they are not debilitating. For patients with severe perianal disease associated with active rectal disease, a proctectomy may be needed. Alternatively, a diverting proximal colostomy may provide symptomatic relief, but does not result in healing of the lesions.

Because recurrence of Crohn's disease is the rule rather than the exception, it is likely that these patients will be reoperated on in the course of their disease. Resection of multiple segments of small bowel may result in the short-bowel syndrome. Consequently, when managing strictures of the small bowel, stricturoplasty is an excellent alternative to resection. Stricturoplasty is especially helpful for patients with multiple strictures. Short strictures may be widened in the manner of a Heineke-Mikulicz pyloroplasty (see Chapter 13). Longer strictures may need to be opened and closed in a Finney pyloroplasty fashion. Moreover, resection and stricturoplasty can be combined and are complementary techniques that are useful in the surgical management of Crohn's disease.

If given enough time, recurrence is inevitable. The incidence of recurrence is particularly high in patients who have this disease during their youth. Recurrences can be either early or late. Early recurrence is an exacerbation of symptoms that develops within the first 2 years after surgery. A late recurrence develops after 2 years, usually between 5 and 10 years. Overall, early and late recurrences are greater in patients with small bowel involvement than in patients with colonic involvement. Postoperatively, recurrences are seen clinically in almost 40% of all patients within 5 years; 60% appear within 10 years, and 75% within 15 years. These recurrences are usually found proximal to the anastomosis after resection. For example, in patients with ileitis or ileocolitis, the most common site of recurrence is the neoterminal ileum. However, not all patients with a recurrence require reoperation because the indications for surgical intervention are the same. Nevertheless, after operation for recurrent Crohn's disease, the rate of recurrence is similar to that for primary resections.

In light of the high rate of recurrence, several trials assessed the efficacy of prophylactic pharmacotherapy after bowel resection in preventing recurrence. Unfortunately, these trials do not show convincingly that these agents are of any benefit, whether given alone or in combination, at preventing recurrence, compared with placebo. Thus, although Crohn's disease is benign, it produces significant morbidity to the young, economically productive patient population that is predominantly affected. Fortunately, only approximately 10% of affected patients die as a direct or indirect result of their disease. Nonetheless, optimal treatment requires the highest level of both medical and surgical judgment.

Small Bowel Tumors

A wide variety of tumors arise from the epithelial and mesenchymal components of the small intestine. Tumors occur 50 times more frequently in the colon and rectum than in the small intestine, despite its much greater length and mucosal surface area. The diagnosis of small bowel tumor is usually made with contrast studies. Particularly useful is enteroclysis, which is analogous to an air-contrast barium enema. Upper endoscopy and extended colonoscopy identify tumors at the extreme ends of the bowel. Small intestinal enteroscopy is being used with increasing frequency to visualize the jejunoileum.

Benign Tumors

Benign tumors are much more common than malignancies in the small bowel. Men and women appear equally affected. Although the average age at presentation is in the sixth decade, there is a wide range. More than half of the benign tumors of the small intestine are completely asymptomatic and discovered incidentally at operation or autopsy. Symptomatic tumors can cause luminal obstruction, bleeding, or intussusception.

Leiomyomas

Leiomyomas are the most common benign tumor of the small intestine. They are most commonly found in the jejunal region. These tumors are of smooth muscle origin and tend to have extraluminal growth. Ulceration of the overlying mucosa can lead to bleeding and, less commonly, obstruction. Most gastrointestinal lipomas occur in the small bowel. They are more often found in the ileum and duodenum than in the jejunum. Unlike most other benign small bowel tumors, they occur more commonly in men. Lipomas rarely become symptomatic.

Adenomas

Three types of **adenomas** are found in the small bowel. Simple tubular and Brunner's gland adenomas are usually incidental findings and require treatment only if they are symptomatic. Because approximately 30% of villous adenomas harbor malignancies, they should be excised. Villous adenomas have a distinct propensity for the periampullary region and other duodenal sites (Figure 14-5). They may cause occult bleeding or, much more likely, intussusception.

Hemangiomas

Hemangiomas constitute 5% of benign small bowel tumors. They can cause either occult or active bleeding and are often multiple. In Osler-Weber-Rendu disease, they can involve the entire small intestine. Symptomatic hemangiomas should be removed.

Hamartomas

Hamartomas are usually isolated, except in Peutz-Jeghers syndrome, in which mucocutaneous melanotic pigmentation is seen in association with multiple gastrointestinal hamartomas. The syndrome is an autosomal dominant trait with a very high penetrance. Hamartomas usually cause intussusception and are resected only if they are symptomatic. Fibromas, lymphangiomas, neurogenic tumors, and myxomas also occur in the small bowel.

Malignant Tumors

Unlike other areas of the gut, the small intestine is host to a variety of malignant tumors that occur with similar frequency. Only 2% of all gastrointestinal malignancies occur in the small intestine, bringing the

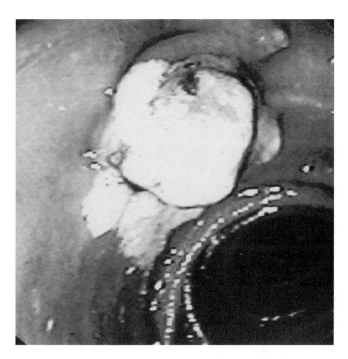

Figure 14-5 Ampullary villous adenoma. Reconstruction of the biliary and pancreatic ducts was necessary after local excision of the tumor.

incidence to approximately 1 per 100,000 population. The average age at presentation is in the sixth decade, and there is a slight male preponderance.

Adenocarcinomas

Adenocarcinomas account for approximately half of all small bowel malignancies. They are most common in the duodenum and least common in the ileum. Obstruction is the most common finding, and it is often associated with weight loss. Occult bleeding can occur in the presence of mucosal ulceration, but massive bleeding is rare. Periampullary adenocarcinomas can cause jaundice. Nearly half of small intestinal adenocarcinomas are diagnosed at operation.

Treatment consists of wide resection to include the associated mesentery, which contains the lymphatic drainage of the involved segment. Chemotherapy has little established role in treatment, and the 5-year survival rate is 10% to 30%, depending on the stage at diagnosis. This poor prognosis is the result of the relatively early spread of the disease and its relatively late diagnosis.

Carcinoid Tumors

Carcinoid tumors originate in the Kulchitsky cells within the crypts of Lieberkühn. These cells are a part of the amine precursor uptake and decarboxylation (APUD) system. Carcinoid tumors are considered malignant lesions. Metastasis occurs in only 2% of patients with primary tumors that are smaller than 1 cm, but in 90% of patients in whom the primary tumor is greater than 2 cm in diameter. The average age at

presentation is in the sixth decade, although there is a wide range. Men are more commonly affected. Some 40% to 50% of all gastrointestinal carcinoids are found in the appendix. The small intestine is the second most common gastrointestinal site for carcinoids. In the small intestine, they occur most frequently in the ileum and least frequently in the duodenum. As many as 30% of patients have multicentric primary tumors. Obstruction is the most common presentation, but the obstruction is often not caused by the relatively small primary mass itself. Rather, the obstruction occurs as a result of an intense desmoplastic reaction in the adjacent mesentery, which leads to kinking of the bowel lumen. Bleeding from overlying mucosal ulceration and intussusception are less common. Patients may also have nonspecific symptoms of anorexia, weight loss, and fatigue. With appendiceal carcinoids, the appropriate treatment depends on the size of the primary. With primary tumors smaller than 2 cm, simple appendectomy is appropriate. When the primary tumor is greater than 2 cm, right colectomy is necessary to achieve an adequate lymphadenectomy. Carcinoids in the small intestine should be resected with free margins of bowel along with mesentery draining the segment. For those located in the terminal ileum, appropriate mesenteric resection may require right colectomy. Because of the high incidence of multicentricity, a thorough search should be made for a second primary. If liver metastases are noted at the time of operation, they should be resected if feasible.

The **carcinoid syndrome** is a fascinating complex of signs and symptoms that can occur in association with carcinoid tumors. Episodic attacks of cutaneous flushing (mostly about the head and trunk), hyperperistalsis with watery diarrhea, bronchospasm and wheezing, pellagra-like skin lesions, and vasomotor instability are seen as well as valvular disorders in the right side of the heart (Figure 14-6). These attacks can occur spontaneously or may be induced by excitement, physical activity, certain foods, alcohol ingestion, anesthesia, or manipulation of the tumor. Carcinoid tumors are responsible for increased elaboration of serotonin (5-hydroxytryptamine), which is degraded in the liver to 5-hydroxyindole acetic acid as well as many other peptides, including 5-hydroxytryptophan, kallikrein, histamine, and adrenocorticotropic hormone (ACTH), all of which are eventually degraded by the liver. Which of these peptides is responsible for each of the multiple manifestations of the syndrome is not known. Many, if not all, of the manifestations are the result of two or more peptides acting in concert. Therefore, for the syndrome to occur, the tumor (primary or metastatic) must be located in a site that is not drained by the portal vein. The liver is one such site, and carcinoids that originate in the appendix or small bowel can be responsible for the syndrome only if they have metastasized to that organ. Primary carcinoids in the rectum, bronchus, ovary, or testes can ignite the syndrome. In the presence of the clinical manifestations, the diagnosis of carcinoid syndrome is best confirmed by an elevated urinary level of 5-hydroxyindole acetic acid. Treatment consists of

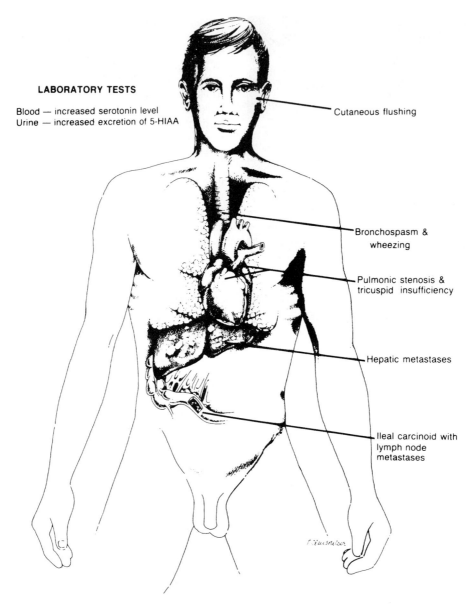

LABORATORY TESTS

Blood — increased serotonin level
Urine — increased excretion of 5-HIAA

Cutaneous flushing

Bronchospasm &
wheezing

Pulmonic stenosis &
tricuspid insufficiency

Hepatic metastases

Ileal carcinoid with
lymph node
metastases

Figure 14-6 Clinical manifestations of malignant carcinoid syndrome.

excising the tumor or symptomatic therapy if resection is not feasible.

Lymphoma

Lymphoma accounts for 10% to 15% of all small bowel malignancies. The small intestine can be one involved site in systemic **lymphoma** or the site of primary disease. It is the most common extranodal primary site for lymphoma, but such disease accounts for only approximately 5% of all cases of lymphoma. The age at presentation is usually the fifth or sixth decade and, as with other small bowel malignancies, there is a predilection for males. Because it is the site of the greatest concentration of lymphoid follicles in the small bowel, the ileum is more commonly the site of primary lymphoma than the jejunum or duodenum. The presen-

tation of primary small bowel lymphoma is usually nonspecific, including weight loss, fatigue, malaise, and vague abdominal pain. However, one-fourth of patients have an abdominal emergency (e.g., perforation, obstruction, bleeding, intussusception). The diagnosis can be suspected if small bowel contrast studies show submucosal nodules or mucosal ulcerations. On CT scan, a thickening or mass in the wall of the bowel, along with bulky lymphadenopathy, may be seen. Surgical resection is indicated for most patients with small bowel lymphoma. At operation, the diagnosis can be confirmed, staging can be performed, and any complications can be treated. Chemoradiation is usually administered once the diagnosis is confirmed. The prognosis depends on the stage of disease at diagnosis, but the overall 5-year survival rate is 20% to 40%.

Leiomyosarcoma

The incidence of **leiomyosarcoma** is similar to that of lymphoma in the small bowel. Although the peak age for small bowel leiomyosarcoma is in the sixth decade, it can occur at any age. These tumors occur with equal frequency in each region of the small intestine. They tend to grow as bulky, extraluminal masses, so obstruction is a late manifestation. Ulceration and bleeding occur in two-thirds of patients, and bleeding can be massive. Approximately 10% of patients have perforation. At operation, wide en bloc resection is performed because of the risk of complications, but these tumors have usually metastasized widely at the time of diagnosis.

Small Bowel Obstruction

Significance and Incidence

The most common indication for operation on the small intestine is obstruction, and worldwide, the most common cause of intestinal obstruction is hernia. Most hernias that cause small bowel obstruction are located in the abdominal wall, either in the groin or through an old incision site. Occasionally, internal hernias are responsible for bowel obstruction. These hernias can be congenital or postoperative and consist of a mesenteric defect through which the small intestine protrudes and becomes trapped. In the United States and other industrialized nations, the most common cause of small bowel obstruction is postoperative **adhesions.** More than two-thirds of patients who have had any form of open abdominal operations have adhesions. Adhesions are present in more than 90% of patients who have had two or more open abdominal operations. As a result, more than 5% of all individuals who have undergone open abdominal operations will have small bowel obstruction at some time. Occasionally, adhesions are responsible for small bowel obstruction in individuals who have not had an operation. Presumably, these adhesions have formed in response to an inflammatory condition (i.e., appendicitis, diverticulitis, cholecystitis, pelvic inflammatory disease) that did not require operation. Small bowel obstruction can also develop during the acute phase of such inflammatory conditions.

Volvulus is another cause of small bowel obstruction. In this condition, a length of small bowel becomes twisted on itself and causes a closed-loop obstruction. Intussusception is a condition in which a more proximal portion of the intestine telescopes itself through the lumen of the adjacent distal bowel. It is much more common in children, where it can occur spontaneously. In adults, the leading edge is almost always a neoplastic or inflammatory mass. Intestinal tumors, whether primary or metastatic and whether intrinsic or extrinsic to the bowel lumen, can also cause obstruction. **Gallstone ileus** is an unusual cause of small bowel obstruction that is notable because of the high associated mortality rate. In this condition, a large (usually > 2.5 cm) stone passes from the gallbladder or common duct through a fistula to the gastrointestinal tract, usually in the duodenum. The stone then passes through the intestine to a point where it becomes lodged, usually in the terminal ileum. The classic abdominal series shows a distal small bowel obstruction along with air in the biliary tree. The associated high mortality rate is caused by the usually advanced age of the patient and the delay in presentation. Inflammatory bowel disease can also cause small bowel obstruction.

Pathophysiology

One of the most critical issues in dealing with small bowel obstruction is the recognition and repair of the accrued and ongoing volume and electrolyte losses. Intraluminal volume losses occur as a result of decreased absorption, increased secretion (hormonally stimulated by luminal distension), and vomiting. Additional volume losses occur as a result of bowel wall edema and transudation into the peritoneal cavity. The electrolyte losses are essentially isotonic early in the process. Later, they vary with the site of obstruction and cannot be easily predicted.

In addition to volume and electrolyte losses, a major risk in small bowel obstruction is strangulation. A segment of bowel can be rendered ischemic by occlusion of its mesenteric blood supply as a result of kinking or external compression by edematous tissues. Strangulation is much more likely to occur in the presence of a closed-loop obstruction in which both ends of the involved bowel segment are occluded. Perforation may occur as a result of strangulation. Local or systemic sepsis can develop as a further consequence of strangulation, with or without perforation. It is more common in association with closed-loop obstruction.

It is important to distinguish partial from complete small bowel obstruction. Complications other than volume and electrolyte deficits are rarely seen with partial obstruction. For this reason, and because partial obstruction often resolves with more conservative measures, operation is often unnecessary. However, it is almost always indicated for complete obstruction. Again, because of the greater incidence of complications in strangulated obstruction, it is important to distinguish this entity from simple obstruction. Tachycardia, fever, focal abdominal tenderness, and leukocytosis are seen with strangulation. If one of these signs is present, the risk of strangulation is approximately 7%. If all four signs are present, the risk approaches 67%.

Clinical Presentation and Evaluation

History

A thorough history should elicit any previous abdominal operations and episodes of abdominal pain. The pain associated with small bowel obstruction is perceived in the periumbilical region and is crampy. The waves of pain are usually separated by a few minutes and may be transiently relieved by vomiting. In uncomplicated obstruction, the cramps may dissipate in favor of a steady, dull pain after several hours as the bowel becomes exhausted and unable to generate peristaltic waves.

Abdominal distension is more pronounced with more distal obstructions. It is usually perceived by the patient shortly after the onset of pain followed by nausea and vomiting. It is important to obtain a history of the passage of gas or stool per rectum because stooling and flatus stop entirely in complete obstruction, but may persist (even with diarrhea) in partial obstruction.

Examination

On examination, the patient's general appearance may range from relative comfort to profound distress. Tachycardia and dry mucous membranes are often noted, and hypotension shows a profound fluid deficit. The abdomen may or may not appear distended, depending on body habitus and the level of obstruction. On rare occasions, visible peristaltic waves are seen. Old surgical scars should be noted, especially because less invasive surgical approaches are commonly performed and scars may be difficult to visualize. Auscultation classically shows infrequent bowel sounds that are often high-pitched, with occasional rushes. Palpation usually shows a taut abdominal wall that is mildly, but diffusely tender. Surgical incisions, the groins, and less common sites of abdominal wall hernias should be thoroughly palpated for hernias. Percussion may show tympany, and any evidence of peritonitis on percussion is a sign of a poor prognosis and an indication for emergent operation.

Radiographs

The most important x-ray is an abdominal series that includes supine and upright views of the abdomen as well as an anterior–posterior view of the chest. One of the primary aims in obtaining these films is to rule out other diseases and complications. They should be carefully viewed for evidence of pneumonia, free air under the diaphragm, pneumobilia (gas in the biliary tree), pneumatosis intestinalis (gas in the bowel wall), and renal, biliary, and intestinal calculi. Typically, the gut proximal to the point of obstruction is dilated, with visible air–fluid levels. The presence of differential air–fluid levels in the same loop of bowel is helpful in diagnosing obstruction (Figure 14-7). The gut distal to the point of obstruction should be collapsed and therefore not apparent on x-ray films. In partial bowel obstruction, residual gas is seen in the colon and rectum. Rarely, no gas is seen in the abdomen when the gut lumen is totally filled by fluid. Serial abdominal films taken at least several minutes apart are useful in determining the presence of a gut loop that is fixed in location and may represent a closed loop. In addition, a loop that is persistently dilated after proximal decompression by nasogastric suction may represent a closed loop. When there is massive distension of the gut by air, it is difficult to distinguish small bowel from colon. In this situation, or when either the location of the obstruction is unclear or the diagnosis of obstruction is uncertain, a contrast enema can be obtained. Likewise, to distinguish among ileus, partial obstruction, and complete obstruction, it may be necessary to obtain a contrast study of the small bowel. The contrast enema should

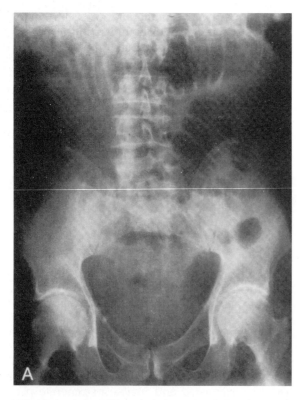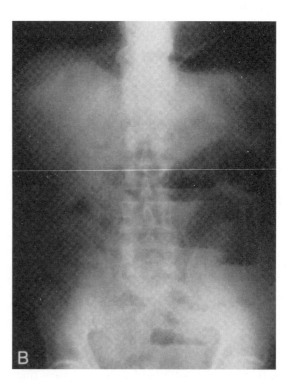

Figure 14-7 Mechanical small intestinal obstruction. **A,** Decubitus abdominal x-ray. There are many centrally located loops of air-filled small intestine and no gas at the periphery of the abdomen. Valvulae conniventes are shown. **B,** Upright abdominal x-ray. Multiple air-filled levels are seen.

always be obtained before the small bowel series because residual contrast in the small bowel may render a contrast enema impossible to obtain. Contrast agent in the colon must always be cleared to allow other studies.

Laboratory Data

Laboratory data cannot confirm the diagnosis of bowel obstruction. However, these studies are useful to rule out other problems that could confound the diagnosis and to evaluate possible complications. A complete blood count, an electrolyte panel, and a urinalysis should be obtained. An elevated white blood cell count may be seen with dehydration and sepsis. Elevated blood urea nitrogen (BUN), creatinine, urine specific gravity, or hemoglobin concentration also indicates dehydration. The serum electrolytes may be entirely normal, particularly early in the process and before any vomiting. Hypovolemic, hypokalemic metabolic alkalosis may accrue over time.

Differential Diagnosis

Paralytic Ileus

Perhaps the primary consideration in the differential diagnosis is paralytic ileus. In this condition, peristalsis is absent or ineffective, but there is no physical obstruction to the passage of the luminal contents of the bowel. A number of problems encountered by the general surgeon can cause ileus. Sepsis, whether within, adjacent to, or remote from the peritoneal cavity, can give rise to ileus. Many medications are associated with ileus, including opiates, anesthetic agents, and certain psychotropics. Other causes include retroperitoneal hematoma, electrolyte abnormalities (Na, K, Ca, Mg, P), and inactivity in institutionalized individuals. Paralytic ileus may be associated with low-grade, diffuse, and continuous pain, and with the inability to pass stool or flatus per rectum. On examination, the abdomen is distended, bowel sounds are infrequent or absent, and there may be mild diffuse tenderness. Abdominal radiographs show generalized distension of the bowel, often including the colon (Figure 14-8). It is occasionally necessary to obtain a contrast study of the small bowel to differentiate ileus from obstruction (Table 14-3).

Colonic Obstruction

Colonic obstruction is also considered in the differential diagnosis of small bowel obstruction. When colonic obstruction is present, nausea and vomiting usually occur much later after the onset of pain than is seen in small bowel obstruction. Typically, on abdominal radiographs, the colon is distended proximal to the site of the obstruction, but the small bowel is spared (Figure 14-9). However, if a patient with colonic obstruction has an incompetent ileocecal valve, the radiographs may show markedly dilated loops of small bowel that are impossible to distinguish from the colonic component. A contrast enema may be necessary to differentiate colonic from small bowel obstruction.

Treatment

The first priority in proven or suspected small bowel obstruction is the correction of fluid and electrolyte abnormalities. Often large volumes of fluid must be infused. The patient must be given sufficient fluid not only for maintenance requirements, but also to correct losses from vomiting and nasogastric output. Finally, the volume lost before presentation through vomiting and extraluminal third-space loss should be estimated and replaced. Half of that volume should be given in the first 8 hours and the second half over the ensuing

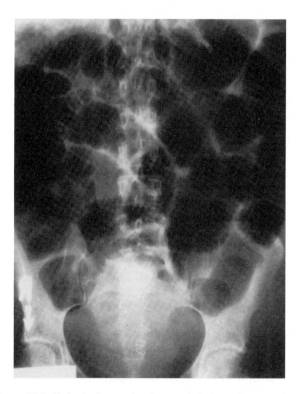

Figure 14-8 Abdominal x-ray showing paralytic ileus of the small bowel. This condition is differentiated from mechanical small bowel obstruction and colonic obstruction by air in the distal sigmoid colon and rectum.

Table 14-3. Characteristics of Paralytic Ileus and Small Intestinal Obstruction

Paralytic Ileus	Small Intestinal Obstruction
Minimal abdominal pain	Crampy abdominal pain
Nausea and vomiting	Nausea and vomiting
Obstipation and failure to pass flatus	Obstipation and failure to pass flatus
Abdominal distension	Abdominal distension
Decreased or absent bowel sounds	Normal or increased bowel sounds
Gas in the small intestine and colon on x-ray	Gas in the small intestine only on x-ray

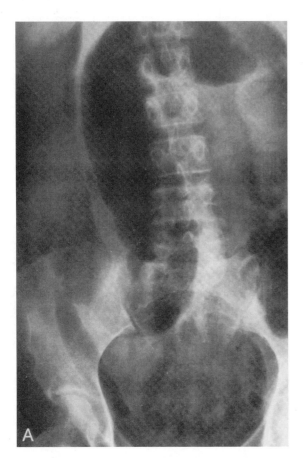 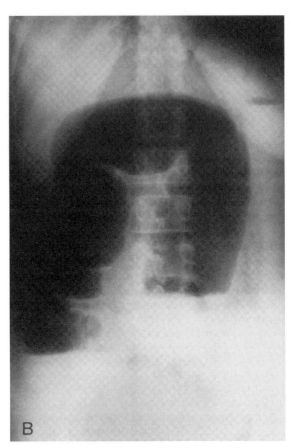

Figure 14-9 Large bowel obstruction. **A,** Decubitus abdominal x-ray. **B,** Upright abdominal x-ray. The presence of dilated air-filled loops of colon at the periphery of the abdomen and centrally located air-filled loops of small intestine with no rectal gas suggests that this patient has a sigmoid obstruction. The patient has carcinoma of the colon.

16 hours. The resuscitation should begin with an iso-tonic solution (normal saline or lactated Ringer's solu-tion) and, when renal function is assured by adequate urine output, potassium should be added. Unless other-wise indicated by the serum electrolytes, the patient should be given 20 to 40 mEq potassium chloride/L fluid. The adequacy of volume replacement is most conveniently and accurately monitored by measuring urine output with a Foley catheter. Output should equal at least 0.5 mL/kg/hr. The patient should take nothing by mouth, and a nasogastric tube should be inserted and attached to low intermittent suction.

If the patient has a partial small bowel obstruction, no detectable hernia, and a history of operation, resolu-tion may occur with the measures discussed, and oper-ation may be unnecessary. The urine output should be closely monitored for the adequacy of hydration, and the white blood cell count, temperature, heart rate, and level of abdominal tenderness should be monitored to rule out the presence of a complication. The patient should begin to show improvement within 12 to 24 hours and continue to improve steadily thereafter. Fail-ure to improve clinically or as shown by an abdominal series may indicate the need for surgery. If the patient has no apparent etiology for obstruction (i.e., no previ-ous operation and no hernia), an etiology should be

determined aggressively by upper gastrointestinal and small bowel series. Partial obstructions that are treated nonoperatively may be at risk for future recurrence. Fre-quent recurrences may lead to surgery during an episode of obstruction so that the point of obstruction can be ascertained and treated.

A patient with a complete small bowel obstruction should undergo operation at the earliest opportunity, once the fluid and electrolyte repair is sufficient to estab-lish adequate urine output. Complete obstruction is unlikely to resolve without surgery, and the risk of com-plications increases with time. Preoperatively, prophy-lactic antibiotics that adequately cover both aerobic and anaerobic organisms (which can proliferate in the small bowel in the presence of obstruction) should be admin-istered. The primary aim of the operation is to relieve the obstruction and remove the cause. Adhesions should be divided, and any hernia that is found should be closed. Resection and primary anastomosis of the bowel should be performed if there is nonviable bowel or if a tumor is present. Intussusceptions should be excised in adults because of the high likelihood that a tumor is the lead point. Unresectable tumors should be bypassed.

Complications

Before surgery, bowel strangulation can occur and result in gangrene of the intestinal segment. This complication is more likely to occur in a closed-loop obstruction or when there has been significant delay in relief of the obstruction. The most common complication after surgery for small bowel obstruction is wound infection, which is most likely to develop if the bowel lumen is entered. With any breach of bowel integrity, peritonitis and intraabdominal abscesses can also develop.

The risk of mortality with simple bowel obstruction is less than 1%, but the risk of death increases to greater than 25% in patients with strangulated bowel obstruction. Thus, the need for a thorough and aggressive approach to bowel obstruction is emphasized. Operation for small bowel obstruction, like other abdominal operations, can result in adhesion formation. Thus, even though the obstruction has been completely relieved, the patient retains at least the same risk for future obstruction as any other patient who has had an abdominal operation.

Small intestinal and appendiceal diseases are common and often require surgical treatment. A working knowledge of these problems is important to provide efficient and cost-effective medical care.

Multiple-Choice Questions

1. The most common age for acute appendicitis is:
   A. 0 to 2 years
   B. 5 to 10 years
   C. 10 to 40 years
   D. 60 to 70 years
   E. 70 to 80 years

2. The most common cause of acute appendicitis is:
   A. Foreign body of the appendix
   B. Fecalith
   C. Lymphoid follicle swelling in the appendix
   D. Adhesive bands in the abdomen
   E. Tumor of the appendix

3. The preferred treatment for acute appendicitis is:
   A. Observation and bowel rest
   B. Antibiotics and observation
   C. Antibiotics and appendectomy
   D. Antibiotics, intravenous hydration, and appendectomy
   E. Antibiotics and delayed appendectomy 3 months later

4. The most common tumor of the appendix is:
   A. Adenocarcinoma
   B. Carcinoid
   C. Mucocele
   D. Lymphoma
   E. Leiomyosarcoma

5. Meckel's diverticulum originates from the:
   A. Foregut
   B. Midgut
   C. Hindgut
   D. Stomach
   E. Colon

6. The most common complication of Meckel's diverticulum is:
   A. Gastrointestinal bleeding
   B. Small bowel obstruction
   C. Perforation
   D. Diverticulitis
   E. Fistula formation

7. The types of ectopic mucosa that are found in Meckel's diverticulum include all of the following EXCEPT:
   A. Colonic mucosa
   B. Gastric mucosa
   C. Pancreatic mucosa
   D. Esophageal mucosa
   E. Duodenal mucosa

8. All of the following are characteristic pathologic features of Crohn's disease EXCEPT:
   A. Disease anywhere from the mouth to the anus
   B. Mesenteric fat creeping
   C. Fistula formation
   D. Transmural inflammation
   E. Absence of "skip lesions"

9. All of the following are true in patients who have Crohn's disease EXCEPT:
   A. The clinical presentation depends on the anatomic location of disease within the digestive tract.
   B. Isolated colonic involvement is the most frequent site of disease.
   C. Abdominal pain is the most frequent presenting symptom.
   D. Perianal disease is common.
   E. Patients often have nutritional deficits.

10. Which of the following treatments can cure Crohn's disease?
    A. Bowel rest and total parenteral nutrition
    B. High-dose steroids
    C. Removal of all segments of the bowel that are involved with microscopic disease
    D. Broad-spectrum antibiotics in combination with immunosuppressants
    E. None of the above

11. All of the following are goals of therapy in patients with Crohn's disease EXCEPT:
    A. Alleviate symptoms
    B. Provide nutritional support
    C. Suppress the inflammatory process
    D. Maintain patients in remission with continued corticosteroid treatment
    E. Use broad-spectrum antibiotics for the septic complications associated with the disease

12. All of the following are true regarding surgical therapy for Crohn's disease EXCEPT:
    A. Surgical therapy for Crohn's disease is palliative.
    B. Surgical intervention is undertaken for the complications of the disease or for failure of medical therapy.
    C. For patients with acute terminal ileitis at the time of abdominal exploration, the appendix should be left in place.
    D. In patients who require bowel resection, the proposed sites of transection should be adjacent to areas of clinically obvious gross involvement of Crohn's disease.
    E. Microscopic confirmation of the absence of disease at the resection margins does not determine future recurrence.

13. The most common site of recurrent Crohn's disease in patients who underwent previous bowel resection is:
    A. Stomach
    B. Perianal involvement
    C. Distal to the resection margin
    D. Proximal to the resection margin
    E. Recurrences occur equally throughout the digestive tract

14. What is the most common cause of small bowel obstruction worldwide?
    A. Postoperative adhesions
    B. Volvulus
    C. Gallstone ileus
    D. Hernia
    E. Tumor

15. The amount of intravenous fluid received by a patient with small bowel obstruction should equal the:
    A. Calculated maintenance fluid rate
    B. Calculated maintenance fluid rate plus an estimated replacement of vomitus before presentation
    C. Estimated replacement of vomitus before presentation plus volume-for-volume replacement of ongoing nasogastric tube output
    D. Calculated maintenance fluid rate plus volume replacement of ongoing nasogastric tube output
    E. Estimated replacement of vomitus and third-space losses before presentation plus calculated maintenance therapy plus volume-for-volume replacement of ongoing nasogastric tube output

16. Volume replacement in a patient with small bowel obstruction is probably adequate when:
    A. Urine output is established
    B. The blood urea nitrogen and creatinine values are within the normal range
    C. The urinary sodium concentration exceeds 40 mEq/L
    D. Urinary output exceeds 0.5 mL/kg body weight/hr
    E. The serum electrolytes are normal

17. Gallstone ileus is:
    A. The most common cause of small bowel obstruction in patients older than 70 years of age
    B. Commonly seen in elderly patients who have acute calculous cholecystitis
    C. Best treated by laparoscopic rather than open cholecystectomy because of the age and comorbid conditions in the typical patient
    D. Caused by repeated passage of small stones through the ampulla of Vater and their constant presence in the small intestine
    E. Pathognomonic for the presence of a cholecystenteric or choledochoenteric fistula

18. Malignant tumors of the small intestine:
    A. Are best treated surgically by wide resection with en bloc resection of the mesentery draining the involved segment
    B. Are much more common than their benign counterparts in the small intestine
    C. Are usually asymptomatic and found incidentally at operation or autopsy
    D. Are unusual and affected patients have a much better 5-year survival rate than those with malignancies in the colon
    E. Always arise from the epithelial layer

19. The carcinoid syndrome is:
    A. Usually seen in patients with primary carcinoid tumors in the midgut
    B. Caused by increased circulating levels of serotonin and its metabolites
    C. Seen only when a carcinoid tumor is drained by tributaries of the portal vein
    D. Seen only when the carcinoid tumor is in the liver
    E. Seen only when the carcinoid tumor is not drained by tributaries of the portal vein

20. Which small bowel tumor has the greatest malignant potential?
    A. Villous adenoma
    B. Brunner's gland adenoma
    C. Fibroadenoma
    D. Leiomyoma
    E. Hamartoma

21. Which of the following small bowel neoplasms is associated with the highest incidence of bleeding?
    A. Carcinoid
    B. Leiomyosarcoma
    C. Adenocarcinoma
    D. Villous adenoma
    E. Brunner's gland adenoma

Oral Examination Study Questions

CASE 1

You are a surgeon in a 300-bed community hospital. You are called to see a 42-year-old patient in the emergency room. He has a 24-hour history of nausea and vomiting, obstipation, crampy abdominal pain, and gradually increasing abdominal distension. Initial vital signs are blood pressure of 120/80 mm Hg, pulse rate of 100/min, respiratory rate of 16/min, and temperature of 99.2° F (37.3° C).

OBJECTIVE 1

The student elicits the following history and physical examination findings.

A. The patient had an appendectomy 5 years ago.

B. He has passed no flatus in 24 hours, and the crampy abdominal pain is intermittent.

C. Abdominal examination shows distension, increased bowel sounds, diffuse mild tenderness, and voluntary guarding. The psoas and obturator signs are negative.

D. There is no stool in the rectum on rectal examination.

OBJECTIVE 2

The student makes the probable diagnosis of small intestinal obstruction and asks for the following tests.

A. Plain and upright x-rays of the abdomen show multiple loops of air-filled small intestine, with air-fluid levels and no colon gas. There is no evidence of closed or fixed loops or of ischemic mucosa to indicate strangulated bowel.

B. Electrolytes are normal. Blood urea nitrogen is 25 mg/dL, and creatinine is 1.0 mg/dL.

C. Complete blood count shows a white blood cell count of 11,200/mm^3, with a left shift. Hematocrit is 42%, and hemoglobin is 14.5 g/dL.

D. Chest x-ray is normal.

E. Urinalysis is normal, except for a specific gravity of 1.030.

OBJECTIVE 3

The student plans appropriate therapy on the basis of the diagnosis.

A. Insert a nasogastric tube and obtain 700 mL bile-stained fluid.

B. Insert a Foley catheter and obtain 50 mL urine.

C. Start the administration of 5% glucose and normal saline or Ringer's lactate at 200 to 300 mL/hr IV.

D. Reevaluate the patient for adequacy of resuscitation 1 hour later. The patient has only 30 mL urine output and should have a bolus of fluids (500–1000 mL). Then his urine output increases to adequate levels.

OBJECTIVE 4

The student prepares the patient for early operation.

A. Administer antibiotics. Many choices are appropriate (i.e., clindamycin, gentamicin).

B. Cross-match for blood.

C. Repeat serum electrolyte tests. The results are normal.

OBJECTIVE 5

The student gives the most likely diagnosis that will be found at operation.

A. The diagnosis is small intestinal obstruction secondary to adhesions (the differential diagnosis may include hernia, neoplasm, regional enteritis, and intussusception).

B. Colonic obstruction and paralytic ileus should not be choices because the x-ray has made them unlikely.

C. The student realizes that strangulation obstruction is possible, even with no fever, no signs of gross peritonitis, and no radiologic signs.

D. The student knows the radiologic signs of strangulation (fixed loop, mucosal edema, and intramural gas).

OBJECTIVE 6

The student discusses why early operation is necessary.

Strangulation obstruction cannot be distinguished from simple obstruction because the signs and symptoms can be the same.

OBJECTIVE 7

The student discusses which operation should be performed if the following are found at the time of surgery.

A. A simple adhesive peritoneal band across the intestine (lyse the band).

B. A short segment of Crohn's ileitis of the terminal ileum (resection and primary anastomosis).

C. An incarcerated femoral hernia with viable intestine (reduce and repair the hernia).

D. A nonviable loop of small intestine that was entrapped under an adhesive band (resect the bowel and perform primary anastomosis).

E. Extensive metastatic carcinoma with an unresectable segment of small intestine that is obstructed (bypass the segment with a side-to-side technique).

Minimum Level of Achievement for Passing

The student recognizes the signs and symptoms of small intestinal obstruction and orders the appropriate tests (plain and upright abdominal x-rays, complete blood count, electrolytes, blood urea nitrogen and creatinine, and urinalysis). Appropriate therapy is instituted, including a nasogastric tube, a Foley catheter, and fluid resuscitation. The student recognizes the necessity of operating early because strangulated obstruction cannot be distinguished from simple obstruction in the early stages.

Honors Level of Achievement

The student discusses the operative therapy of most lesions that can be found at surgery.

CASE 2

You are a surgeon in a 200-bed community hospital and are called to the emergency room to see a 20-year-old woman with a 3-week history of nausea, malaise, crampy abdominal pain, watery diarrhea six times per day, and weight loss of 10 lb in the past 3 weeks. Vital signs are blood pressure of 110/70 mm Hg, pulse rate of 110/min, respiration rate of 16/min, and oral temperature of 100.5° F.

OBJECTIVE 1

The student elicits the following history and physical examination findings.

  A. The patient had two previous episodes of perirectal abscesses. They were treated with incision and drainage.

  B. She was told that she has an irritable intestine.

  C. She had occasional pain in her knees over the past 3 weeks.

  D. Abdominal examination shows the abdomen to be scaphoid. The bowel sounds are hyperactive, and there is deep and rebound tenderness, particularly in the right lower quadrant. There is a vague mass in the right lower quadrant.

  E. Rectal examination shows perirectal tenderness, with swelling and erythema at the 6 o'clock position.

OBJECTIVE 2

The student makes the diagnosis of suspected Crohn's disease and a perirectal abscess and orders the following tests.

  A. Plain and upright x-rays of the abdomen show gas in the small and large intestines, with no obstruction.

  B. Serum electrolytes are normal. Blood sugar is 100 mg/dL, and creatinine is 0.7 mg/dL.

  C. Complete blood count shows hemoglobin of 15 g/dL, hematocrit of 43%, and a white blood count of 15,500/mm³, with a left shift.

  D. Urinalysis is normal, except for a specific gravity of 1.025.

OBJECTIVE 3

Based on this information, the appropriate therapy includes:

  A. Administering antibiotics (many choices are acceptable, i.e., aminoglycoside, clindamycin)

  B. Starting the administration of 5% glucose and 0.45% saline at 125 to 150 mL/hr IV

OBJECTIVE 4

The findings at surgery confirm the perirectal abscess, which was incised and drained. Sigmoidoscopy shows minimal erythema of the rectal wall. After the patient recovers from the incision and drainage, the following diagnostic procedures are appropriate.

  A. Upper gastrointestinal and small bowel series show a "string sign" in the terminal ileum and several areas in the jejunum and ileum with thickened intestinal wall and decreased luminal size.

  B. Enteroclysis and (after the perirectal area is healed) barium enema with air contrast are normal, with no other skip lesions found.

  C. Colonoscopy is normal.

OBJECTIVE 5

At this point, the patient's temperature returns to normal, but she still has abdominal pain, malaise, and diarrhea. The appropriate therapy is as follows:

  A. Begin oral sulfasalazine (Azulfidine) 4 g/day.

  B. Begin oral steroids (40–60 mg prednisone/day).

  C. Start a low-residue, low-roughage oral diet.

  D. Consider the options of total bowel rest and total parenteral nutrition if prednisone and Azulfidine are not effective.

OBJECTIVE 6

The student gives the indication for surgical intervention for Crohn's disease.

  A. Abscess formation

  B. Persistently draining internal or external fistula

  C. Intractable disease

  D. Perforation

  E. The possibility of carcinoma

OBJECTIVE 7

The student relates the arthritis symptoms to the Crohn's disease.

  A. Extracolonic manifestations are more common with ulcerative colitis than with Crohn's disease.

  B. Symptoms may respond to surgical therapy.

  C. The student lists the extracolonic manifestations.

Minimum Level of Achievement for Passing

The student recognizes the signs and symptoms of Crohn's disease and associated perirectal fistula. The student recognizes the appropriate initial and early therapy of incision, drainage, and sigmoidoscopy. The student thoroughly evaluates the patient with appropriate radiologic tests, including barium and radionuclide studies, computed tomography scan and ultrasonography, and colonoscopy. The student also institutes therapy with sulfasalazine and prednisone and recognizes the indications for surgical intervention.

The student knows the extraintestinal manifestations of Crohn's disease. The student also knows the timing and duration of medical therapy, the appropriate radiologic workup, and the appropriate surgical therapy when confronted with a fistula, persistent disease (in singular and multiple sites), or an abscess, and when carcinoma is present.

CASE 3

You are a surgeon in a community hospital and are called to see a 23-year-old woman with lower abdominal pain of 12 hours' duration. The pain is more severe on the right side and is associated with anorexia, but no vomiting. The initial vital signs are blood pressure 110/70 mm Hg, temperature 99.5° F, pulse 90/min, and respiration 14/min.

OBJECTIVE 1

The student elicits the following history and physical examination findings:

A. The patient had no previous episodes of abdominal pain.

B. Pain is not associated with menses (period 1 week ago).

C. The pain shifted from the periumbilical area to the right lower quadrant and is more definitely localized.

D. Deep tenderness and definite referred rebound tenderness of the right lower quadrant are observed.

E. There is pain on extension of the psoas muscle.

F. The student recognizes that appendicitis is usually a progressive disease that can lead to serious complications if it is not treated in a timely fashion.

G. Pelvic and rectal examination shows right lower quadrant tenderness, no cervical tenderness, and no masses. The stool is heme-negative.

OBJECTIVE 2

The student differentiates possible appendicitis from the following conditions.

A. Acute cholecystitis: location, radiation, food intolerance, predisposing age, parity, and weight

B. Tubal pregnancy: bleeding or anemia, irregular or absent menses, palpable tender mass in the pelvis

C. Acute salpingitis: cervical discharge, exquisite tenderness of the cervix, previous history of this disease or multiple opportunities for exposure to infection

D. Miscellaneous diverticulitis of the sigmoid and cecum and Meckel's diverticulitis

E. Ileitis secondary to Crohn's disease.

F. Gastroenteritis: diarrhea and active bowel sounds

OBJECTIVE 3

The student makes the diagnosis of acute appendicitis and requests the following studies.

A. Complete blood count, which shows hemoglobin of 12.5 g/dL; hematocrit of 36%; and white blood count of 11,000/mm^3, with 78% polymorphonuclear leukocytes, 4% bands, 12% lymphocytes, 5% monocytes, and 1% eosinophils

B. Plain and upright abdominal x-rays to look for renal stones, bowel obstruction, and fecalith ($\leq 10\%$)

C. Serum electrolytes, blood urea nitrogen, and blood sugar, which are normal (the value of these tests has little direct diagnostic bearing on appendicitis)

D. Pregnancy test, which is negative

OBJECTIVE 4

The student prepares the patient for surgery.

A. Immediate operation is essential.

B. Observation for 4 to 6 hours, with repeat temperatures, white blood cell counts, and physical examination, may be considered, but is not preferred.

C. Broad-spectrum antibiotics to cover aerobes should be administered because perforation is unlikely.

D. Insertion of a nasogastric tube is appropriate, but not required unless the patient is vomiting.

E. The patient is given intravenous fluid, and a Foley catheter is inserted to monitor urine output.

OBJECTIVE 5

The student discusses the operative management after the following findings are established.

A. Inflamed, swollen appendix with patchy necrosis: appendectomy

B. A 6-cm abscess secondary to a ruptured appendix with adhesions
   1. Drain the abscess, insert an external drain, and leave the skin open.
   2. Appendectomy is performed only if it is easily accomplished.

C. Normal appendix, but inflamed Meckel's diverticulum: resection of Meckel's diverticulum

D. Acute ileitis, with normal appendix: appendectomy if the cecum is normal

E. Normal appendix with no other findings: appendectomy

F. Mucoid cyst (3 cm) of the appendix: appendectomy

Minimum Level of Achievement for Passing

The student recognizes the presenting symptoms of acute appendicitis and its progressive nature. The student differentiates this condition from other acute conditions of the abdomen by history and physical examination.

Honors Level of Achievement

The student differentiates acute appendicitis from all other common inflammatory diseases of the abdomen and knows the variations in treatment based on operative findings. The student also discusses the pathogenesis of acute appendicitis, the progression of the disease, and the potential complications of abscess and generalized peritonitis. The student describes the appropriate roentgen workup for complicated appendicitis.

SUGGESTED READINGS

Small Intestine and Appendix

Frazee RC, Roberts JW, Symmonds RE, et al. A prospective randomized trial comparing open versus laparoscopic appendectomy. *Ann Surg* 1994;219:725–731.

Gomez A, Wood M. Acute appendicitis during pregnancy. *Am J Surg* 1979;137:180–183.

Nitecki SS, Wolff BG, Schlinkert R, Sarr MG. The natural history of surgically treated primary adenocarcinoma of the appendix. *Ann Surg* 1994;219:51–57.

Hoffman J, Lindhard A, Jensen HE. Appendix mass: conservative management without interval appendectomy. *Am J Surg* 1984;148:379–382.

Knishern JH, Eskin EM, Fletcher HS. Increasing accuracy in the diagnosis of acute appendicitis with modern diagnostic techniques. *Ann Surg* 1986;52:222–225.

Meckel's Diverticulum

Mackey W, Dineen P. A fifty-year experience with Meckel's diverticulum. *Surg Obstet Gynecol* 1983;156:56–64.

Cullen JJ, Kelly KA, Moir CR, et al. Surgical management of Meckel's diverticulum. *Ann Surg* 1994;220:564–569.

Crohn's Disease of the Small Intestine

Peppercorn M. Advance in drug therapy for inflammatory bowel disease. *Ann Intern Med* 1990;112:50–60.

Pennington L, Hamilton SR, Bayless TM, Cameron JL. Surgical management of Crohn's disease: influence of disease at margin or resection. *Ann Surg* 1980;192:311–318.

Rutgeerts P, Geboes K, Vantrappen G, et al. Natural history of recurrent Crohn's disease at the ileocolic anastomosis after curative surgery. *Gut* 1984;25:665–672.

Tumors

Godwin JD II. Carcinoid tumors: an analysis of 2,837 cases. *Cancer* 1975;36:560–569.

Levine BA, Kaplan BJ. Polyps and polypoid lesions of the jejunum and ileum: clinical aspects. *Surg Oncol Clin North Am* 1996;5:609–619.

Ashley SW, Wells SA Jr. Tumors of the small intestine. *Semin Oncol* 1988;15:116–128.

Morgan BK, Compton C, Talbert M, et al. Benign smooth muscle tumors of the gastrointestinal tract: a 24-year experience. *Ann Surg* 1990;211:63–66.

Haber DA, Mayer RJ. Primary gastrointestinal lymphoma. *Semin Oncol* 1988;15:154–169.

Small Bowel Obstruction

Reisner RM, Cohen JR. Gallstone ileus: a review of 1001 reported cases. *Am Surg* 1994;60:441–446.

Seror D, Feigin E, Szold A, et al. How conservatively can postoperative small bowel obstruction be treated? *Am J Surg* 1993;165:121–125.

Eskelinen M, Ikonen J, Liponen P. Contributions of history taking, physical examination, and computer assistance to diagnose small bowel obstruction: a prospective study of 1333 patients with acute abdominal pain. *Scand J Gastroenterol* 1994;29:715–721.

Brolin RE, Krasna MJ, Mast BA. Use of tubes and radiographs in the management of small bowel obstruction. *Ann Surg* 1987;206:126–133.

15

Colon, Rectum, and Anus

Merril T. Dayton, M.D.
Judith L. Trudel, M.D.

OBJECTIVES

Diverticular Disease

1. Describe the clinical findings of diverticular disease of the colon.
2. Discuss five complications of diverticular disease and their appropriate surgical management.
3. List the differential diagnosis, initial management, diagnostic studies, and indications for medical versus surgical treatment in a patient with left lower quadrant pain.

Polyps and Carcinoma of the Colon, Rectum, and Anus

1. Identify the common symptoms and signs of carcinoma of the colon, rectum, and anus.
2. Discuss the appropriate laboratory, endoscopic, and x-ray studies for the diagnosis of carcinoma of the colon, rectum, and anus.
3. Using the TNM and Dukes' classification systems, discuss the staging and 5-year survival rate of patients with carcinoma of the colon and rectum.

Ulcerative Colitis and Crohn's Disease of the Colon

1. Differentiate ulcerative colitis from Crohn's disease of the colon in terms of history, pathology, x-ray findings, treatment, and risk of cancer.
2. Discuss the role of surgery in the treatment of patients with ulcerative colitis and Crohn's colitis.

Colonic Obstruction and Volvulus

1. List the signs, symptoms, and diagnostic aids for evaluating presumed large bowel obstruction.
2. Discuss at least four causes of colonic obstruction in adults, including the frequency of each cause.

3. Outline a plan for diagnostic studies, preoperative management, and treatment of volvulus, intussusception, impaction, and obstructing colon cancer.
4. Given a patient with mechanical large or small bowel obstruction, discuss the potential complications if the treatment is inadequate.

Hemorrhoids

1. Discuss the anatomy of hemorrhoids, including the four grades encountered clinically, and differentiate internal from external hemorrhoids.
2. Describe the symptoms and signs of patients with external and internal hemorrhoids.
3. Outline the principles of management of patients with symptomatic external and internal hemorrhoids, including the roles of nonoperative and operative management.

Perianal Infections

1. Outline the symptoms and physical findings of patients with perianal infections.
2. Outline the principles of management of patients with perianal infections, including the role of antibiotics, incision and drainage, and primary fistulectomy.

Anal Fissures

1. Describe the symptoms and physical findings of patients with anal fissures.
2. Outline the principles of management of patients with anal fissures.

Anal Malignancy

1. Name the two most common cancers of the anal canal and describe their clinical presentation.
2. Describe the recent changes in the approach to the treatment of anal canal cancers.

The colon and rectum are the terminal portion of the alimentary tract. Although the colon and rectum are biologically nonessential, it is important to understand their physiology, anatomy, and pathophysiology because of the high incidence of disease originating in them. Conditions such as diverticulosis coli, colonic polyps, adenocarcinoma of the colon and rectum, and ulcerative colitis affect a large number of patients in the United States, and the economic, social, and personal costs are enormous. Paradoxically, although the colon is much less vital for nutrition, fluid maintenance, and overall homeostasis then the small intestine, disease is far more common in the colon and rectum.

The anus, anal canal, and sphincters play a critical role in continence, a function that is important for comfortable social interaction. Benign conditions (e.g., hemorrhoids, anal fissures) are common and result in frequent visits to the physician as well as a large expenditure for nonprescription medications.

Anatomy

The large intestine may be divided into several parts (Figure 15-1). The cecum is the largest part and is the site where the small bowel enters the colon. There is no distinct division between the cecum and the ascending colon, which is fixed posteriorly in the right gutter of the posterior abdominal cavity and is therefore a retroperitoneal structure. The hepatic flexure is the bend in the ascending colon where it becomes the transverse colon, which is suspended freely in the peritoneal cavity by the transverse mesocolon. The transverse colon bends again at the spleen (splenic flexure) and again becomes retroperitoneal. The descending colon remains retroperitoneal up to the sigmoid colon, which is a loop of redundant colon in the left lower quadrant. The distal sigmoid colon, which is intraperitoneal, becomes the rectum at the sacrum and becomes partially retroperitoneal. The rectum continues to the sphincters that form the short (3 cm) anal canal.

The rectum is 12 to 15 cm long. Its origin is marked by anatomic change from the colon. The teniae coli disperse at approximately the level of the sacral promontory. As a result, the longitudinal muscle layer becomes a continuous, homogeneous layer. In addition, the proximal rectum is covered by peritoneum anteriorly, but not posteriorly, down to approximately 8 to 9 cm above the anal verge, where the rectum becomes an extraperitoneal structure. Rectal biopsy higher than 8 to 9 cm above the anal verge is more hazardous on the anterior wall because of the risk of perforation into the peritoneal cavity.

The anal canal is approximately 3 to 4 cm long and extends from the anorectal junction (dentate, or pectinate, line) to the anal verge (Figure 15-2). The **dentate line** marks the junction between the columnar rectal epithelium, which is insensate, and the squamous anal epithelium, which is richly innervated by somatic sensory nerves. For this reason, pathologic conditions that arise below the level of the dentate line cause severe pain. Immediately proximal to the dentate line are longitudinal folds called the columns of Morgagni (rectal columns). Perianal glands normally discharge their secretions at the base of these columns, at the level of the anal crypts. Perirectal abscesses usually originate in this area (discussed later).

The blood supply to the colon (see Figure 15-1) is more complex than that to the small bowel. Like the small intestine, the ascending colon and proximal half of the transverse colon are supplied by branches of the superior mesenteric arteries, whereas the distal half of the transverse colon, descending colon, sigmoid colon, and upper half of the rectum are supplied by branches of the inferior mesenteric artery. The distal rectum and anus are supplied by branches of the internal iliac artery (middle and inferior hemorrhoidal arteries). The importance of understanding this complex arterial blood supply is that in certain areas of the colon (e.g., splenic flexure) that are at the junction of two separate blood vessel systems, the blood supply may be relatively poor. For this reason, anastomoses in this region would carry a higher risk of ischemic complications. The venous drainage of the large bowel is less complex because most branches accompany the arteries and eventually drain into the portal system.

The arterial supply to the rectum is derived from a branch of the inferior mesenteric artery (superior hemorrhoidal artery) for the upper rectum, and from branches of the internal iliac arteries (middle hemorrhoidal arteries) and the internal pudendal arteries (inferior hemorrhoidal arteries) for the middle and lower rectum. Veins from the upper rectum drain into the portal system through the inferior mesenteric vein. The middle and inferior rectal veins drain into the systemic circulation through the internal iliac and pudendal veins. Hemorrhoids are physiologic vascular cushions that connect the two systems. They may become distended or thrombose, leading to symptoms of hemorrhoid disease.

Lymphatic drainage of the large intestine parallels the arterial blood supply, with several levels of lymph nodes as one moves toward the aorta. In general, tumor metastases move from one level to another in an orderly progression, with the paracolic lymph nodes involved

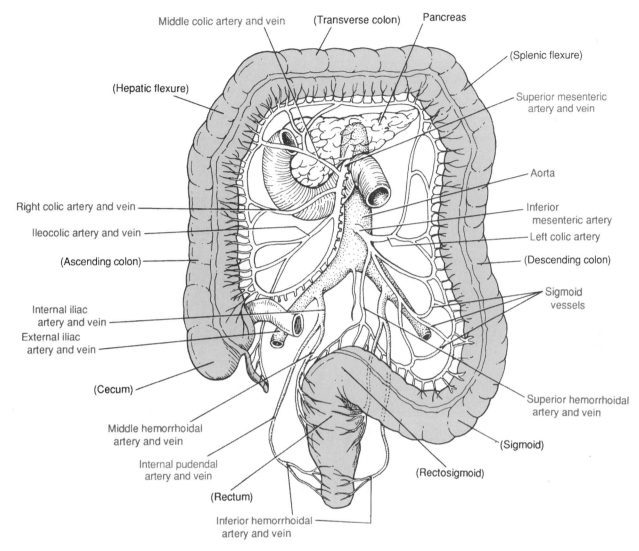

Middle colic artery and vein
(Transverse colon)
Pancreas
(Splenic flexure)
(Hepatic flexure)
Superior mesenteric
artery and vein
Right colic artery and vein
Ileocolic artery and vein
(Ascending colon)
Aorta
Inferior
mesenteric artery
Left colic artery
(Descending colon)
Sigmoid
vessels
Internal iliac
artery and vein
External iliac
artery and vein
(Cecum)
Middle hemorrhoidal
artery and vein
Internal pudendal
artery and vein
(Rectum)
Inferior hemorrhoidal
artery and vein
Superior hemorrhoidal
artery and vein
(Sigmoid)
(Rectosigmoid)

Figure 15-1 Normal anatomy and blood supply of the colon and rectum.

first, followed by the middle tier of lymph nodes, and last by the periaortic lymph nodes.

The bowel wall of the colon has the same layers as the small intestine: mucosa, submucosa, muscularis, and serosa (Figure 15-3). The major difference is that the colon has no villi (i.e., the mucosal crypts of Lieberkühn form a more uniform surface with less absorptive area). Another major difference is that the outer longitudinal smooth muscle layer is separated into three bands (teniae coli) that cause outpouchings of bowel between the teniae (haustra).

The anal sphincter mechanism resembles a tube enclosed in a funnel. The tube is the internal sphincter, which is a continuation of the circular muscular layer of the rectum. This involuntary sphincter is made of smooth muscle. The funnel is the external sphincter, which is a striated voluntary muscle. The external sphincter has three parts: the subcutaneous, superficial, and deep portions. The deep portion is in continuity with the levator ani muscles, which form the base of the

pelvic floor. The anatomy of the sphincters must be kept in mind in the diagnosis and treatment of perirectal pathology (discussed later).

Innervation of the colon is primarily from the autonomic nervous system. Sympathetic nerves pass from the spinal cord through the sympathetic chains and sympathetic ganglia to postganglia that end in Meissner's and Auerbach's plexuses in the bowel wall. Sympathetic stimulation causes inhibition of colonic muscular activity. Parasympathetic innervation comes through the vagus nerve for the first half of the colon. The second half (distal transverse and beyond) is innervated by branches from the second through the fourth sacral cord segments. Parasympathetic activity results in stimulation of colon muscle activity. However, the most important control of colon activity appears to be mediated by regional reflex activity that occurs in the submucosal plexuses (patients with spinal cord transection continue to have relatively normal bowel function).

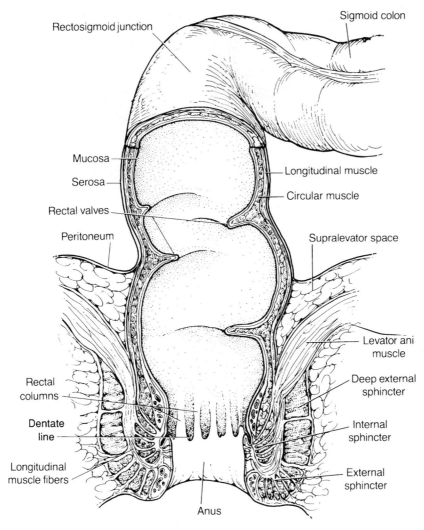

Figure 15-2 Normal anatomy of the anorectal canal.

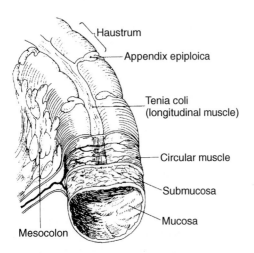

Figure 15-3 Oblique cross-section showing the layers of the colon wall. (Reprinted with permission from Hardy JD. *Hardy's Textbook of Surgery*, 2nd ed. Philadelphia, Pa: Lippincott-Raven, 1983.)

Physiology

The colon and rectum have two primary functions: (1) absorption of water and electrolytes from liquid stool and (2) storage of feces. Some 600 to 700 mL of chyme enters the cecum each day. Most of the stool water is absorbed in the right portion of the colon, leaving 200 mL of stool evacuated as solids daily. This amount is a small fraction of the total water absorbed in the intestinal tract. The left portion of the colon and the rectum store solid fecal material, and the anorectal apparatus regulates the evacuation of solids, permitting defecation at a socially acceptable time and place. Because little digestion and absorption of nutrients occurs in the colon, the organ is not essential to life. The composition of colonic gas varies among individuals and is influenced substantially by diet. Some 800 to 900 mL/day is passed as flatus, 70% of which is nitrogen (N_2) derived from swallowing air. Other gases include oxygen, carbon dioxide, hydrogen, methane, indole, and skatole. Indole and skatole give colonic gas its characteristic odor.

Colonic motility is unique among organs of the alimentary canal because of the multiple types of contraction patterns, including segmentation and **mass contractions.** These contractions are unique to the colon and are characterized by the contraction of long segments of colon, resulting in mass movement of stool. Movement of residue through the colon occurs at a slower rate (18–48 hours) than through the small bowel (4 hours). Colonic transit is accelerated by emotional states, diet, disease, infection, and bleeding.

The physiology of anal continence is the result of complex interactions between sensory and involuntary and voluntary motor functions. When stool distends the proximal rectum, the internal sphincter relaxes, allowing sensory sampling of the rectal contents. This very sensitive mechanism allows, among other things, the passage of gas without incontinence to stool. Defecation involves a complex interplay among the pelvic floor muscles, rectum, and distal colon.

The normal frequency of defecation is approximately every 24 hours, but it may vary from 8 to 72 hours. Any patient who has a significant change in bowel habits should be evaluated for the possibility of serious disease. Severe constipation (ability to pass flatus, but not stool) and obstipation (inability to pass stool or flatus) are examples of changes that should be evaluated.

The colon harbors a greater number and variety of bacteria than any other organ in the body. Most of these organisms are anaerobes; *Bacteroides fragilis* is the most common. The most common aerobes are *Escherichia coli* and enterococci. Although the bacteria perform a number of important functions for the host (e.g., degradation of bile pigments, production of vitamin K), their high number and variety increase the risk of infection during colon surgery. Some studies show postoperative infection rates as high as 25% to 30% after surgery on colon that was "prepared" (cleaned out) before operating.

Colon and Rectum

Diagnostic Evaluation

Patients who have signs or symptoms that are referable to the colon or rectum may be evaluated by several modalities. The digital examination is an important means of detecting many disease processes, including tumors or polyps, abscesses, ulcers, hemorrhoids, and colorectal bleeding. The tendency to defer the digital rectal examination because of patient discomfort or physician inconvenience is a serious error.

Although rigid sigmoidoscopy was the standard method of visualizing the distal colon and rectum for many years, it has largely been replaced by fiberoptic flexible sigmoidoscopy. This method provides a higher diagnostic yield and is much less uncomfortable for the patient. This examination allows visualization of the last 30 to 65 cm of the colorectal complex and results in detection of 60% of colorectal neoplasms. In addition to detecting polyps and neoplasms, it can aid in detecting sites of hemorrhage, ascertaining the etiology of obstruction, evacuating excessive colonic gas, and removing foreign bodies from the rectum. Because of the frequency of colorectal disease, this examination should be an integral part of the routine examination of patients who are older than 50 years of age. In the absence of other symptoms, flexible sigmoidoscopy should be performed every 3 to 5 years.

An abdominal series (flat plate and upright x-ray) should be obtained on any patient who has significant abdominal pain. This series is helpful in detecting pneumoperitoneum, large bowel obstruction (e.g., volvulus, tumor), paralytic ileus, appendicolith, and less common diseases. Both of these x-rays should be obtained, not simply an abdominal flat plate.

Barium enema remains an important diagnostic modality in detecting disease in this region. After the colon and rectum are prepared, contrast medium is introduced under mild pressure to fill the entire organ. Air insufflation, with some intraluminal barium remaining, allows particularly sensitive detection of polyps and small lesions (Figure 15-4). Barium enema is particularly helpful in diagnosing tumors, diverticulosis, volvulus, and sites of obstruction.

The most accurate diagnostic tool is fiberoptic **colonoscopy.** This instrument allows visualization of the entire colon and rectum and the last few centimeters of terminal ileum. It also provides diagnostic and therapeutic options that were not previously available without surgery (e.g., polyp removal, colonic decompression, stricture dilation, hemorrhage control, foreign body removal). After the patient undergoes thorough bowel preparation and mild sedation, the device is inserted into the anus and advanced with a steering mechanism located on the handle (Figure 15-5). Although this instrument was initially used primarily to evaluate ambiguous findings on barium enema studies, more physicians are using it for diagnostic purposes and postoperative follow-up. Colonoscopy is now a primary diagnostic modality to evaluate lower gastrointestinal bleeding of unknown etiology, inflammatory bowel disease, stricture, equivocal barium enema findings, posttumor removal, pseudo-obstruction, and polyps (Figure 15-6).

Angiography is useful in detecting the source of moderate or rapid colonic bleeding. It is not helpful in patients with slow, chronic blood loss.

Terminology

Understanding the treatment of colonic diseases requires familiarity with terms that are unique to this organ. **Colostomy** is the surgical procedure in which the colon is divided and the proximal end is brought through a surgically created defect in the abdominal wall (Figure 15-7). Its purpose is nearly always to divert stool from a diseased segment distally in the colon or rectum or to protect a distal anastomosis. The distal segment is either oversewn and placed in the peritoneal cavity as a blind limb **(Hartmann's procedure)** or brought

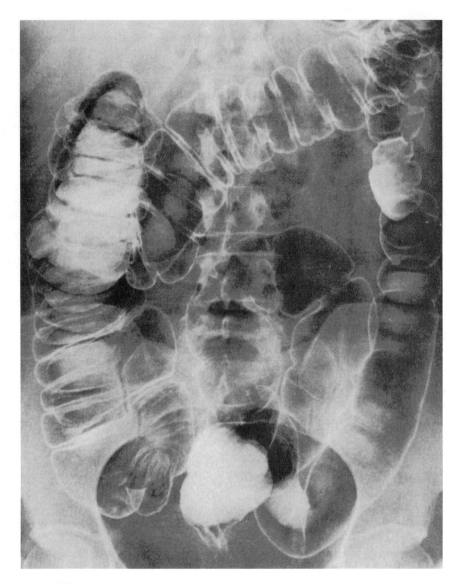

Figure 15-4 Normal air-contrast barium enema.

out inferiorly to the colostomy through the abdominal wall (mucous fistula). A loop colostomy is created by bringing a loop of colon through a defect in the abdominal wall, placing a rod underneath, and making a small hole in the loop to allow stool to exit into a colostomy bag. Ileostomy is a similar procedure in which ileum is brought through the abdominal wall to divert its contents from distal disease or, in proctocolectomy, to serve as a permanent stoma.

Other terms that often confuse medical students include **proctocolectomy, abdominoperineal resection,** and **low anterior resection.** Proctum is a synonym for rectum. Proctocolectomy is operative removal of the entire colon and rectum (e.g., for ulcerative colitis or polyposis syndromes). Abdominoperineal resection, which is used in the surgical treatment of low rectal cancers, is the operative removal of the lower sigmoid colon and the entire rectum and anus, leaving a permanent proximal sigmoid colostomy (e.g., for low rectal cancer). Low anterior resection, which is used to surgically treat

cancers in the middle and upper sections of the rectum, is removal of the distal sigmoid colon and approximately one-half of the rectum, with primary anastomosis of the proximal sigmoid to the distal rectum.

Diverticular Disease

Diverticular disease develops at different rates in different countries with widely varying dietary habits, suggesting the probable influence of diet on the development of this condition. The incidence of diverticular disease is progressive from the fifth to the eighth decade of life, and 70% of elderly patients may have asymptomatic diverticula. Clearly, there is some influence of the aging process on the incidence, but whether it is related to general relaxation of the colonic tissue or to lifelong dietary habits is not clear. Dietary influences have been implicated based on comparative geographic epidemiology; these studies implicate the lower fiber diet found in

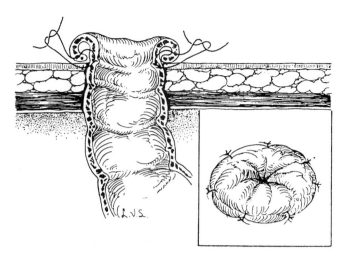

Figure 15-7 Lateral and anterior appearance of an end colostomy. (Reprinted with permission from Way L. *Current Surgical Diagnosis,* 7th ed. Stamford, Conn: Appleton & Lange, 1985.)

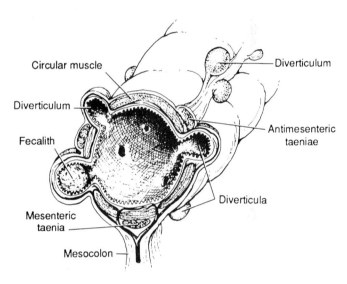

Figure 15-8 Mucosal herniation characteristic of diverticulosis. Most herniations occur at a site where the blood vessel penetrates the bowel wall.

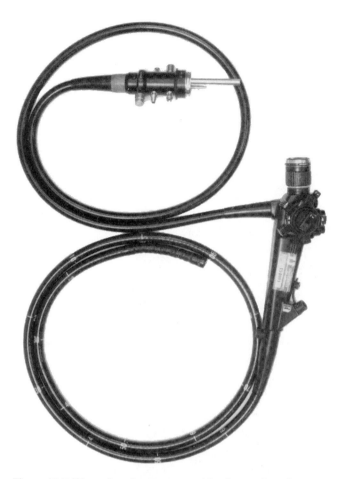

Figure 15-5 Fiberoptic colonoscope used for diagnostic and therapeutic maneuvers in the colon.

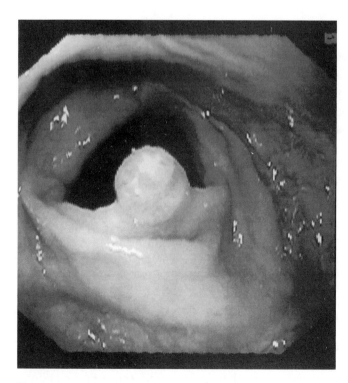

Figure 15-6 A polyp detected during colonoscopy.

Western Europe and the United States. Some postulate that lower stool bulk results in higher generated luminal pressures for propulsion. The resultant increased work causes hypertrophy that leads to diverticulosis.

Two types of diverticula are found in the colon. **Congenital,** solitary, **"true" diverticula** (full-wall thickness in the diverticular sac) are uncommon, but when present, are found in the cecum and ascending colon. **Acquired (false) diverticula** are very common in Western countries, and 95% of patients with the condition have involvement of the sigmoid colon. These diverticula are mucosal herniations through the muscular wall. The muscles of the colon have an inner circular smooth muscle layer and a thinner outer layer, which includes three longitudinal bands, the teniae. The most favorable area for herniation occurs where branches of the marginal artery penetrate the wall of the colon (Figure 15-8).

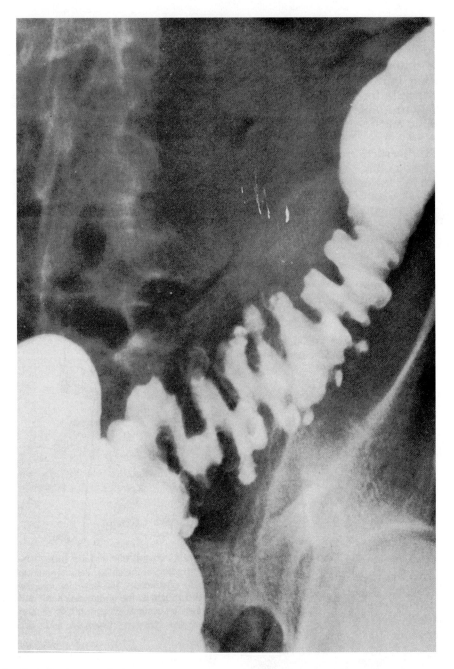

Figure 15-9 Sigmoid diverticulosis shown on barium enema.

The etiology of herniation is probably related to the colon's exaggerated adaptation for fecal propulsion. One theory suggests that diverticular disease results from higher than normal segmental contractions of the sigmoid colon that lead to high intraluminal pressure. These high intraluminal pressures are confined to the segments that have diverticula. Specifically, the sigmoid colon has localized pressure increases because of segmentation between contraction rings. Contraction of the wall generates high-pressure zones within the segment. As a result, herniation occurs at the weakest point, near the vascular penetration of the bowel wall.

Diverticulosis

General use of the term diverticulosis is reserved for the presence of multiple false diverticula in the colon. This condition is most often an asymptomatic (80%) radiographic finding when a barium enema is performed for some other diagnostic purpose (Figure 15-9). Nevertheless, certain symptoms are attributed to diverticula in the absence of either inflammation or bleeding.

Clinical Presentation and Evaluation

Symptoms include recurrent abdominal pain, often localized to the left lower quadrant, and functional changes in bowel habits, including bleeding, constipation, diarrhea, or alternating constipation and diarrhea. The physical examination is most often unremarkable, or it shows mild tenderness in the left lower quadrant. By definition, fever and leukocytosis are absent. Additional roentgenographic findings may include segmental spasm and luminal narrowing. Endoscopic evaluation of the lumen generally does not show anything except the openings of the diverticula.

Treatment

Management of asymptomatic patients with diverticular disease is controversial. Although certain public health organizations recommend a diet with increased fiber content, no specific definition of fiber dietary content has been given for the normal adult. Patients are encouraged to consume fresh fruits and vegetables, whole-grain breads, cereals, and bran products. Pharmacologic preparations of fiber (e.g., psyllium seed products) are more expensive, but are more likely to be taken by patients.

Diverticulitis

Diverticulitis describes a limited infection of one or more diverticula, including extension into adjacent tissue. The condition is initiated by obstruction of the neck of the diverticulum by a fecalith. The obstruction leads to microperforation that results in swelling in the colon wall or macroperforation that involves the pericolic tissues.

Clinical Presentation and Evaluation

The clinical presentation depends on the progression of infection after the perforation. If the perforation is small, it may spontaneously regress. If it is large, it may be confined to pericolic tissues and abate after treatment with antibiotics. The process may enlarge to form an extensive abscess in the mesenteric fat that remains contained, eventually requiring surgical drainage. It may burrow into adjacent hollow organs, resulting in fistula formation. Occasionally, the diverticulum freely ruptures into the peritoneal cavity, causing peritonitis and requiring urgent exploration.

Approximately one-sixth of patients with diverticulosis have signs and symptoms of diverticulitis. The hallmark symptoms of diverticulitis are left lower quadrant abdominal pain (subacute onset), alteration in bowel habits (constipation or diarrhea), occasionally a palpable mass, and fever. Occasionally, free perforation with generalized peritonitis occurs, but the most common picture is one of localized disease. The disease is often called left lower quadrant appendicitis. When cicatricial obstruction develops secondary to repeated bouts of inflammation, the patient will have distension, high-pitched bowel sounds, and severe constipation or obstipation. Fistula formation may be associated with diarrhea, stool per vagina (colovaginal fistula), pneumaturia and recurrent urinary tract infections (colovesical fistula; most commonly associated with diverticular disease), or skin erythema and a furuncle that ruptures

and is associated with stool drainage (colocutaneous fistula). The clinical spectrum is a function of the complications of the diverticular perforation, including abscess formation, fistula development, and partial or total obstruction. Of all life-threatening complications that arise from diverticulitis, 44% involve perforation or abscess, 8% involve fistula, and 4% involve obstruction.

Diagnostic evaluation of diverticulitis or its complications is directed by the clinical presentation. If acute diverticulitis is suspected, abdominal x-rays are obtained; a barium enema is contraindicated in the acute phase. Barium enema may be obtained 2 to 3 weeks after the episode to confirm the clinical impression. If the patient has obstructive symptoms or evidence of a fistula (e.g., pneumaturia), a contrast enema is indicated. If free perforation has occurred, upright abdominal x-rays show pneumoperitoneum.

Colovesical fistula is the most common type of fistula encountered in diverticulitis, with a complication occurring in approximately 4% of cases. The differential diagnosis includes carcinoma of the colon, cancer of other organs (e.g., bladder), Crohn's disease, radiation injury, and trauma as a result of foreign bodies. Some patients are symptom-free or mildly symptomatic. However, others have refractory urinary tract infections, fecaluria, and pneumaturia. The most common physical finding is a palpable mass, and leukocytosis secondary to urinary tract infection is frequently found. The diagnostic triad includes barium enema, cystography, and intravenous pyelogram. However, in a patient with no demonstrable lesion, a dye marker (e.g., methylene blue) can be instilled into the bladder or rectum.

Treatment

Treatment of the complications of diverticular disease is directed at the specific complication (Table 15-1). Treatment of acute diverticulitis is initially medical in 85% of cases. It consists of admitting the patient to the hospital, instituting intravenous hydration, giving the patient nothing by mouth, and administering intravenous antibiotics (usually an aminoglycoside and coverage for *B. fragilis*) for 5 to 7 days. Most patients respond to nonoperative treatment and do not require further therapy. However, a subsegment of this group have repeated bouts of acute diverticulitis, requiring hospitalization. The natural history of diverticulitis in those who have repeated bouts is gradual progression to one of the serious complications. For this reason, most surgeons believe that any patient who has had two severe bouts of diverticulitis requiring hospitalization

Table 15-1. Indications for Surgery of Diverticular Disease

Perforation

Obstruction

Intractability

Bleeding

Fistula

should be scheduled for elective sigmoid colectomy (the site of the problem in 95% of cases). In the case of perforation, obstruction, or abscess, immediate surgical resection of the diseased sigmoid colon is indicated, with a temporary diverting colostomy and a Hartmann procedure (Figure 15-10). No attempt at a primary reanastomosis should be made in this setting of unprepared bowel because of the high risk of infection and bowel leak. If the disease is refractory or a fistula is present, the patient may undergo bowel preparation and formal sigmoid colectomy with primary anastomosis.

The treatment for colovesical fistula is surgery. Primary closure of the bladder and resection of the sigmoid colon with primary anastomosis is the usual treatment. However, in the presence of severe infection, the colon anastomosis may be delayed and a temporary colostomy performed. Generally, the operation is successful, and recurrence is rare.

Diverticular Bleeding

Diverticulosis is occasionally associated with gastrointestinal hemorrhage. Bleeding is the primary symptom in 5% to 10% of all patients with diverticular disease. Bleeding from diverticula is occasionally massive (diverticulosis is the most common cause of massive lower gastrointestinal bleeding) and may be lethal. Massive bleeding is defined as bleeding that is sufficient to warrant transfusion of more than four units of blood in 24 hours to maintain normal hemodynamics. Of all patients with bleeding distal to the ligament of Treitz, approximately 70% have diverticulosis as the source of the bleeding. Approximately 25% of the time, the bleeding is massive.

Clinical Presentation and Evaluation

The patient generally has profuse bright or dark red rectal bleeding and hypotension. Unfortunately, the age, sex, and symptoms of patients with bleeding diverticular disease are the same as those with cancer and other lesions. Patients with cancer are unlikely to bleed as severely as patients with diverticulosis, but carcinomas bleed more frequently.

After the history, physical examination, and resuscitation with volume expanders and blood transfusions, the diagnostic approach to the patient with lower gastrointestinal hemorrhage includes insertion of a nasogastric tube with aspiration (to rule out an upper gastrointestinal source) and rectal examination to rule out severe hemorrhoidal bleeding (e.g., portal hypertension) or ulcer. The next diagnostic procedure is flexible sigmoidoscopy to rule out other causes of bleeding. If massive bleeding continues, angiography is the next diagnostic procedure of choice. If the bleeding is intermittent or angiography is indeterminate, colonoscopy after rapid colonic lavage is the preferred modality. In addition to diverticulosis, the differential diagnosis includes angiodysplasia, solitary ulcers, varices, cancer and, rarely, inflammatory bowel disease.

Treatment

If the bleeding does not cease spontaneously, surgical resection of the involved segment is indicated.

Polyps and Carcinoma of the Colon and Rectum

Colorectal Polyps

Polyp is a morphologic term that is used to describe small mucosal excrescences that grow into the lumen of the colon and rectum. A variety of polyp types have been described, all with different biologic behaviors (Table 15-2). Approximately 5% of all barium enema studies show polyps. Approximately 50% occur in the rectosigmoid region, and 50% are multiple.

Distinguishing among polyp types is important because some types are clearly associated with carcinoma of the colon. Inflammatory polyps (pseudopolyps) are common in inflammatory bowel disease and have no malignant potential. Hamartomas (juvenile polyps and polyps associated with Peutz-Jeghers syndrome) similarly have very low malignant potential and often spontaneously regress or autoamputate. They may be safely observed. However, polyps that fall into the general category of "adenoma" are clearly premalignant, and appropriate vigilance is indicated. Three subdivisions of adenomas are described: (1) tubular (Figure 15-11), (2) tubulovillous, and (3) **villous adenoma**. Most polyps are either **sessile** (flat and intimately attached to the mucosa) or **pedunculated** (rounded and attached to the mucosa by a long, thin neck; Figure 15-12). Tubular and tubulovillous adenomas are more commonly pedunculated, whereas villous

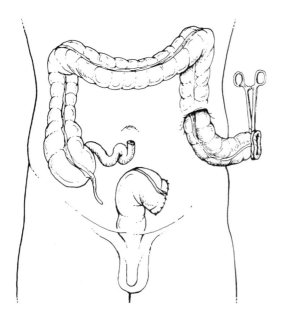

Figure 15-10 Operative therapy for diverticular disease usually involves resection of the sigmoid portion of the colon. If the operation is done for acute perforation or obstruction, the segment may be resected, a diverting colostomy brought to the abdominal wall, and the distal rectal stump oversewn (Hartmann procedure). A second stage of the operation involves colostomy take-down and anastomosis to the rectal stump.

Table 15-2. Comparison of Colonic Polyps

Type	Frequency	Location	Malignant Potential	Treatment
Tubular	Common: 10% of adults	Rectosigmoid in 20%	7% malignant	Endoscopic excision
Villous	Fairly common, especially in the elderly	Rectosigmoid in 80%	33% malignant	Surgical removal
Hamartoma	Uncommon	Small bowel	Low; uncommon	Excise for bleeding or obstruction
Inflammatory	Uncommon, except in IBD	Colon and rectum	None	Observation
Hyperplastic	Fairly common	Stomach, colon, and rectum	None	Observation

IBD, irritable bowel disease.

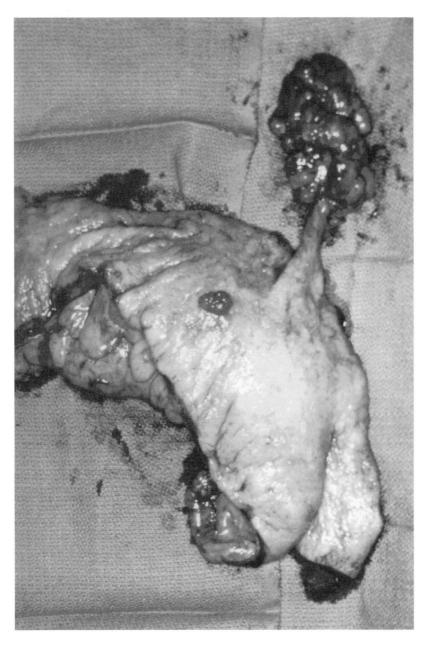

Figure 15-11 Large tubular adenoma in the sigmoid colon.

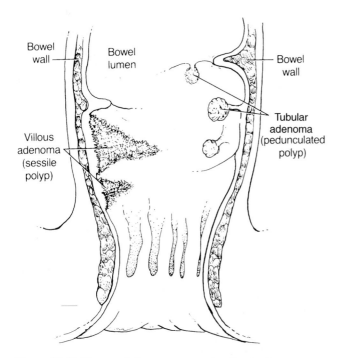

Figure 15-12 Characteristic appearance of a villous adenoma (sessile polyp) compared with a tubular adenoma (pedunculated polyp). Sessile polyps tend to be more difficult to manage because they are difficult to remove endoscopically and because their malignant potential is greater.

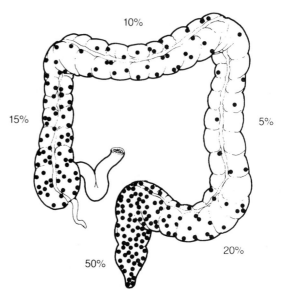

Figure 15-13 Frequency distribution of adenocarcinoma of the colon and rectum.

adenomas are more commonly sessile. Evidence for malignant potential includes: (1) the high incidence of cancer associated with the polyps in familial polyposis syndrome or Gardner's syndrome, (2) simultaneous occurrence of cancers and polyps in the same specimen, (3) carcinogens that experimentally produce both adenomas and cancers in the same model, and (4) lower cancer risks associated with those who have polyps removed. Approximately 7% of tubular, 20% of tubulovillous, and 33% of villous adenomas become malignant. Villous adenomas greater than 3 cm in diameter have a greater probability of malignancy.

Clinical Presentation and Evaluation

Polyps are usually asymptomatic, but occasionally bleed enough to cause the patient to seek medical evaluation. They are most commonly detected during routine endoscopic surveillance. Occasionally, a family history of polyps causes the patient to seek endoscopic screening.

Treatment

Treatment of adenomatous polyps involves colonoscopic polypectomy of pedunculated polyps where possible. If some cannot be safely removed colonoscopically, biopsy should be performed and a segmental resection of the colon done if the lesion is a villous adenoma or is large, ulcerated, or indurated. For disease conditions that are characterized by extensive polyposis (familial polyposis syndrome or Gardner's syndrome),

the treatment most commonly performed is total abdominal colectomy, mucosal proctectomy, and ileoanal pull-through.

Carcinoma of the Colon and Rectum

Cancer of the colon and rectum is a major cause of death in the United States. The American Cancer Society estimates that approximately 60,000 to 63,000 people die of this disease annually. Approximately 140,000 to 145,000 new cases are identified each year. Although a large number of factors are associated with the development of this disease, theories about its etiology center around the impact of intraluminal chemical carcinogenesis. There are various theories as to whether these carcinogens are ingested or are the result of biochemical processes that occur intraluminally from existing substances that are found normally in the fecal stream. Geographic epidemiologic studies show that certain populations have a very low incidence of cancer of the colon and rectum, apparently as a result of identifiable dietary factors (e.g., high fiber, low fat), although social customs and a lack of environmental carcinogens cannot be excluded. Certain health agencies promote a low-fat, high-fiber diet as protective against cancer of the colon and rectum. Chemoprevention by ingestion of such agents as carotenoids and other antioxidants has been suggested, but the efficacy of this measure is unproven.

Most large bowel cancers occur in the lower left side of the colon, near the rectum (Figure 15-13), although recent studies suggest a slow shifting to right-side lesions. Synchronous (simultaneously occurring) tumors develop in 5% of patients, whereas 3% to 5% of patients have metachronous tumors (a second tumor developing after resection of the first).

Familial polyposis syndrome, Gardner's syndrome, and the cancer family syndrome (Lynch syndrome) clearly show that certain patient subsets are genetically predisposed to cancer of the colon. Other predisposing diseases include ulcerative colitis, Crohn's colitis, lymphogranuloma venereum, and certain polyps (described previously).

The peak incidence of colon cancers occurs at approximately 70 years of age, but the incidence begins to increase in the fourth decade of life. Rectal cancer is more common in men, and colon cancer appears to be more common in women.

Clinical Presentation and Evaluation

The clinical signs and symptoms of colorectal cancer are determined largely by the anatomic location. Cancers of the right colon are usually exophytic lesions associated with occult blood loss, resulting in iron deficiency anemia (Table 15-3). At advanced stages of the disease, patients may have a palpable right lower abdominal mass. Recent retrospective studies indicated that the incidence of right colon cancers is increasing at a greater rate than that of left colon cancers. Right-sided lesions may account for as many as one-third of all new cases seen, with most diagnosed at a late stage. Cancers that arise primarily in the left and sigmoid colon are more frequently annular and invasive, resulting in obstruction and macroscopic rectal bleeding (see Table 15-3). Cancers of the rectum (the terminal 12–14 cm of large bowel) also cause a symptom complex of rectal bleeding, obstruction and, occasionally, alternating diarrhea and constipation. Tenesmus occurs with far advanced disease.

Any patient with a change in bowel habits, iron deficiency anemia, or rectal bleeding should undergo the following studies: (1) a digital rectal examination with testing to rule out occult blood, (2) flexible sigmoidoscopy, and (3) a barium enema study (Figure 15-14). If rectal bleeding occurs, workup for a possible malignancy should be initiated, even if the apparent source is a benign lesion (e.g., hemorrhoid).

If the results of all of these are inconclusive, a total colon survey by flexible colonoscopy should be considered. Bright red rectal bleeding should always be evaluated by an examination of the perianal region, digital rectal examination, and flexible sigmoidoscopy. The value of preoperative total colonoscopy lies in its ability to detect the 3% to 5% of patients with synchronous colon cancers, allowing better planning of surgical therapy. Liver scans and computed tomography of the abdomen are not routinely indicated before surgery. Preoperative blood tests should evaluate the patient's overall nutritional status and should include liver function tests and a carcinoembryonic antigen study. Results of the antigen study are elevated in many gastrointestinal malignancies and, although it is not specific for colorectal cancer, it may be useful in following patients after resection to detect recurrence.

Diagnostic studies often show an obstructing lesion in the sigmoid colon that occurs in the presence of diverticula, but is suspicious for malignancy. Because both conditions may coexist and it is occasionally impossible to

Table 15-3. Symptoms of Colon and Rectal Cancers

Symptom	Site of Cancer		
	Right Colon	Left Colon	Rectum
Weight loss	+	+/0	0
Mass	+	0	0
Rectal bleeding	0	+	+
Tympany	0	0	+
Virchow's node	+	0	0
Blumer's shelf	+	+	0
Anemia	+	0	0
Obstruction	0	+	+

distinguish between the two, the surgeon should proceed with a "cancer operation," which includes a wide lymph node resection, whenever there is any question. Diverticular stricture, polyps, benign tumors, ischemic structure, and Crohn's colitis are included in the differential diagnosis.

Treatment

The surgical treatment used by most surgeons includes adequate local excision of the tumor, with a length of normal bowel on either side, and resection of the potentially involved lymph node draining basin found in the mesentery that is determined by the vascular supply. Removal of the lymphatics that drain the tumor region should be part of the operation because nodal involvement is present in more than 50% of specimens. A certain subset of patients with carcinoma of the colon and rectum and lymph node metastasis at a site that is fairly distant from the primary lesion, but is included in the resected specimen, may be rendered disease-free by the surgical resection. Colorectal cancer may also spread hematogenously, intraluminally, or by direct extension or peritoneal seeding (Blumer's shelf on rectal examination). The most common organ involved in distant colorectal metastases is the liver.

Patients whose tumors are no longer confined to the bowel and are adherent to extraperitoneal structures in the pelvis, upper abdomen, or other area should have en bloc resections (which include resection of the tumor and any other invaded structure) whenever possible, with the area being subsequently marked with metal clips to identify it as a site of potential recurrence. When the small bowel is involved, it should be included en bloc in the resection. Studies indicate that small bowel involvement does not change the stage-for-stage prognosis. Similarly, a partial cystectomy or total hysterectomy should be performed with the resection if the tumor is adherent to these organs. Bilateral oophorectomy is recommended by some in menopausal or post-menopausal women to remove occult ovarian metastasis and improve staging.

Tumors of the cecum and ascending colon are treated with right hemicolectomy that includes resection of the

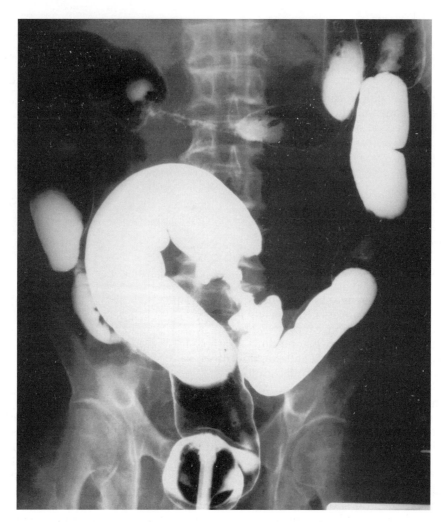

Figure 15-14 Carcinoma of the sigmoid colon causing high-grade obstruction and showing a classic "apple core" lesion.

distal portion of the ileum and the colon to the mid-transverse colon with an ileomidtransverse colon anastomosis (Figure 15-15). Hepatic flexure lesions are best treated by an extended right colectomy that includes resection to or beyond the level of midtransverse colon. Lesions in the transverse colon require a transverse colectomy with complete mobilization and anastomosis of ascending to descending colon. Splenic flexure and left-sided lesions are treated with a left hemicolectomy that includes resection from the level of the midtransverse colon to the sigmoid. Sigmoid colon lesions are treated with sigmoid resection. However, obstructing sigmoid lesions may require left hemicolectomy and sigmoid colectomy. Obstructive or perforating tumors that prevent bowel preparation and primary anastomosis should be treated with resection, diverting colostomy, and Hartmann's pouch or mucous fistula.

Tumors in the upper and middle one-third of the rectum are treated with low anterior resection with primary anastomosis. Tumors in the lower one-third of the rectum require specialized procedures (e.g., abdominoperineal resection with permanent end-sigmoid colostomy; Figure 15-16). When the expertise and

equipment are available, selected high-risk patients with rectal lesions that are smaller than 2 cm, exophytic, mobile, and well differentiated may be treated with transanal full-thickness resection of the lesion or local laser ablation.

Recent developments in minimally invasive surgery involving the use of the laparoscope raise the question of possible laparoscopic resection of colon cancers. A number of studies show that the operation can be done technically with resection of an acceptable number of lymph nodes in the lymphadenectomy specimen. The procedure is usually done with a small transverse incision to facilitate removal of the tumor and to assist in the anastomosis. However, most laparoscopic resections are now being done in protocol because of a disturbing finding of tumor recurrences in the port sites of the laparoscopic procedure. Further experience is needed to determine whether laparoscopy can be safely used for resection of colorectal tumors.

The use of adjuvant therapies in the treatment of colon and rectal carcinoma generated considerable research in the last several decades. The main outcome from the randomized trials with 5-fluorouracil (5-FU) as

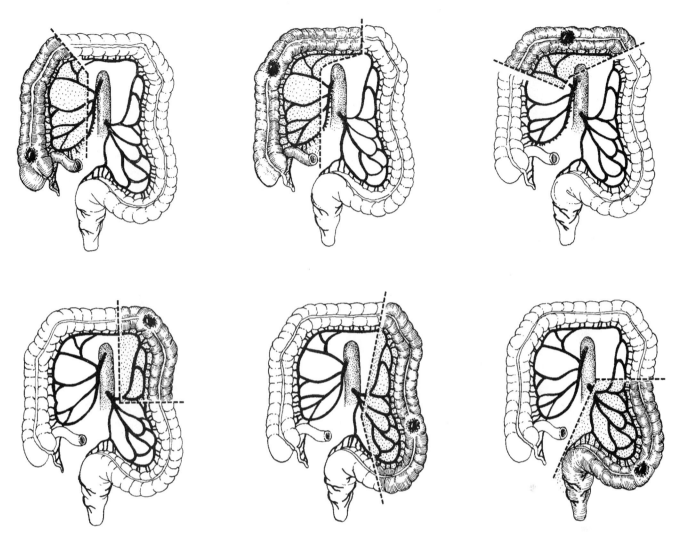

Figure 15-15 Indicated operative resection for colon cancer in different sites. The boundaries of the resection are dictated by lymphatic drainage patterns that parallel the blood supply.

a single agent in an adjuvant setting was that no improvement occurred in the disease-free interval, nor was there an increase in cure rate compared with surgery alone. However, recent studies show conclusively that 5-FU used in combination with levamisole or leucovorin lowers the mortality rate in patients with Dukes' stage C tumors.

Because of their significant rate of recurrence (30%) despite the most radical surgical procedure, rectal tumors that have completely penetrated the rectal wall, with or without lymph node metastases, are treated additionally by radiation combined with 5-FU. The question of whether to use preoperative or postoperative radiation seems to be strictly a matter of choice. However, postoperative radiation seems more widely applicable because it permits a selection based on the final pathologic staging and prevents treating patients who are not at risk for local recurrence. It also eliminates those who are not candidates because of distant disease. The usual tumoricidal doses of approximately

50 to 60 cGy can be tolerated in the postoperative period if the surgeon and the radiation oncologist plan the adjuvant radiation therapy before surgery, even if it is to be given postoperatively. Well-conducted trials indicate that postoperative radiation therapy prevents recurrence, increasing disease-free intervals and survival rates.

Prognosis

Because a clinical staging system does not exist for colon cancer, final pathologic staging is used. A system of staging large bowel cancer was first proposed by **Dukes** more than 50 years ago. There have been subsequent modifications, particularly those by Astler and Coller (Table 15-4). The TNM (tumor, node, metastasis) system was developed by the American Joint Committee on Cancer (Table 15-5). There have been other attempts to look at clusters of prognostic factors (e.g., tumor markers, size of the lesion) and elements that are not included in Dukes' original classification, which

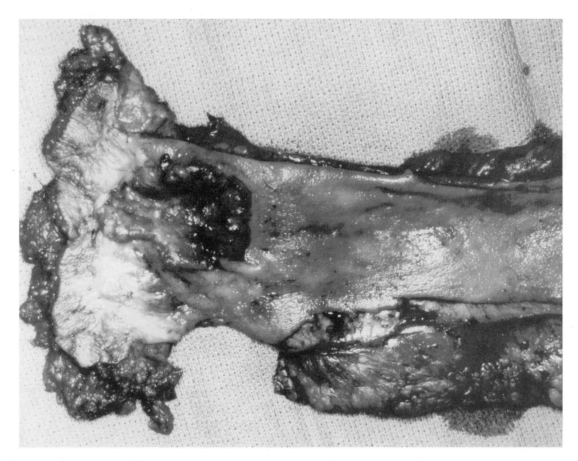

Figure 15-16 Adenocarcinoma of the low rectum invading the anal canal and requiring abdominoperineal resection.

Table 15-4. Dukes-Astler-Coller System

Stage	Description	5-Year Survival Rate (%)
A	Confined to the mucosa	85–90
B1	Negative nodes; extension into, but not through, the muscularis propria	70–75
B2	Negative nodes; extension through the muscularis propria	60–65
C1	Same level of penetration as B2, but with positive nodes	30–35
C2	Same level of penetration as B2, but with positive nodes	25
D	Distant metastases	< 5

was based on the depth of invasion. The most important prognostic variable is lymph node involvement.

For patients who have had curative resection and for whom no adjuvant therapy is appropriate, the question of follow-up surveillance is of maximal importance. Certain large centers recommend monthly physical examination, bimonthly measurement of carcinoembryonic levels, and either endoscopy or barium enema study every 6 months for the first 2 years of follow-up because most recurrences occur in the first 18 to 24 months. The use of **carcinoembryonic antigen** is well established, with recurrence suggested not by the absolute level of this antigen, but rather by a progressive rise. A progressive rise mandates a complete evaluation of the patient, including computed tomography or magnetic resonance imaging, and possible second-look surgical procedure. Although the number of patients who benefit from this thorough survey is not large, a sufficient number benefit to make it worthwhile. The prognosis of colon and rectal carcinoma depends on the classification detailed in Table 15-4. For patients who have recurrences, the effective management of liver metastases, pelvic and anastomotic recurrences, and solitary pulmonary metastases has been demonstrated.

Ulcerative Colitis and Crohn's Disease of the Colon

Ulcerative colitis is an idiopathic inflammatory bowel disorder that involves the mucosa and submucosa of the large bowel and rectum. It has a bimodal distribution with regard to age. The first, and largest, peak (two-thirds of all cases) includes ages 15 to 30, whereas the second, smaller peak (one-third of all cases) occurs at approximately age 55. The disease is slightly more common in Western countries, and its annual incidence is 10 per 100,000 population. A family history of ulcera-

Table 15-5. TNM Staging System

Primary Tumor (T)

TX	Primary tumor cannot be assessed
TO	No evidence of primary tumor
Tis	Carcinoma in situ; intraepithelial tumor or invasion of the lamina propria
T1	Tumor invading the submucosa
T2	Tumor invading the muscularis propria
T3	Tumor invading through the muscularis propria into the subserosa, or into nonperitonealized pericolic or perirectal tissues
T4	Tumor directly invading other organs or structures or perforating the visceral peritoneum

Regional Lymph Nodes (N)

NX	Regional lymph nodes cannot be assessed
NO	No regional lymph node metastasis
N1	Metastasis in 1–3 pericolic or perirectal lymph nodes
N2	Metastasis in ≥4 pericolic or perirectal lymph nodes
N3	Metastasis in any lymph node along the course of a named vascular trunk or metastasis to ≥ 1 apical node (when marked by the surgeon)

Distant Metastasis (M)

MX	Presence of distant metastasis cannot be assessed
M0	No distant metastasis
M1	Distant metastasis

tive colitis is positive in 20% of patients, suggesting a genetic predisposition.

Crohn's disease is a transmural disease that can involve any portion of the alimentary canal. In a minority of patients, disease is limited to the colorectal region. Like ulcerative colitis, it occurs in a bimodal distribution. Although it more commonly occurs in the region of the terminal ileum, when it occurs exclusively in the colorectum, it is often confused with ulcerative colitis. Gross differences that may be used to distinguish it from ulcerative colitis include rectal sparing, skip lesions (in which diseased segments alternate with normal segments), aphthous sores, and linear ulcers. Crohn's disease is discussed in greater detail elsewhere. This section focuses on ulcerative colitis.

The exact etiology of ulcerative colitis is unknown. Infectious, immunologic, genetic, and environmental factors are implicated, but none is proven. The female:male occurrence ratio among patients with ulcerative colitis is 5:4. There is an increased incidence of the disease among Jews, but it is uncommon among blacks and Native Americans.

Pathologic findings include invariable involvement of the rectum (< 90%) with variable proximal extension. Occasionally, the rectum alone is involved (ulcerative proctitis). In contrast to Crohn's disease, skip areas of normal bowel between diseased segments are not seen. The mucosa is initially involved, with lymphocyte and leukocyte infiltration that then involves the submucosa with microabscess formation. The crypts of Lieberkühn are commonly affected (crypt abscesses), but muscle

layers are rarely involved. The coalescing of these abscesses and erosion of the mucosa lead to **pseudopolyp** formation, which is identified readily on endoscopic examination. Approximately one-third of the patients affected with ulcerative colitis have pancolitis, in which the entire colon is severely involved.

In addition to the material contained here, the student should refer to Chapter 14 for a discussion of ulcerative colitis and Crohn's disease.

Clinical Presentation and Evaluation

The clinical presentation of ulcerative colitis is variable. The disease may have a sudden onset, with a fulminant, life-threatening course, or it may be mild and insidious. Patients often have watery diarrhea that contains blood, pus, and mucus, accompanied by cramping, abdominal pain, tenesmus, and urgency. To varying degrees, patients have weight loss, dehydration, pain, and fever. Fever is usually indicative of multiple microabscesses or endotoxemia secondary to transmural bacteremia. Approximately 55% of patients have a mild, indolent course; 30% have a moderately severe course that requires large doses of prednisone or sulfasalazine (Azulfidine); and 15% have a fulminant, life-threatening course. The fulminant presentation is often associated with massive colonic dilation secondary to transmural progression of the disease and destruction of the myenteric plexus (toxic megacolon). Patients have severe constitutional symptoms related to sepsis, malnutrition, anemia, acid–base disturbances, and electrolyte abnormalities.

Extraintestinal manifestations occur in a small percentage of patients, including ankylosing spondylitis, peripheral arthritis, uveitis, pyoderma gangrenosum, sclerosing cholangitis, pericholangitis, and pericarditis. The amount of information obtained on physical examination depends on the acuteness and severity of the disease process at the time of examination. If the patient is seen in a quiescent phase, there may be few or no findings; if the patient is seen in an acute phase, there may be a finding of an acute abdomen.

The mainstay of diagnosis is endoscopy with biopsy. Typical endoscopic findings include friable, reddish mucosa with no normal intervening areas, mucosal exudates, and pseudopolyposis (Figure 15-17A and B). A secondary diagnostic study is barium enema, in which mucosal irregularity may be seen. Frequently, shortening of the colon, loss of normal haustral markings, and a "lead-pipe" appearance may be seen (Figure 15-18). No specific laboratory tests are diagnostic for ulcerative colitis; however, leukocytosis and anemia may be present.

The differential diagnosis includes other inflammatory or infectious disorders, including Crohn's disease, bacterial colitis, and pseudomembranous colitis. The disease that is most commonly confused with ulcerative colitis is Crohn's disease of the colon. In approximately 10% of cases, there is an overlap of features; this type of colitis is called indeterminate colitis. Its clinical behavior appears to be more like ulcerative colitis than

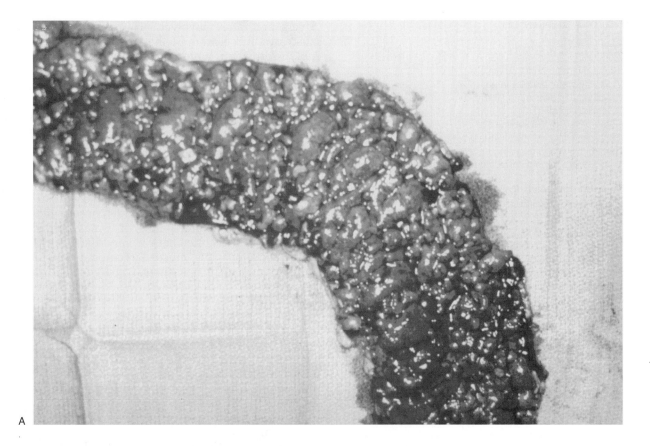

A

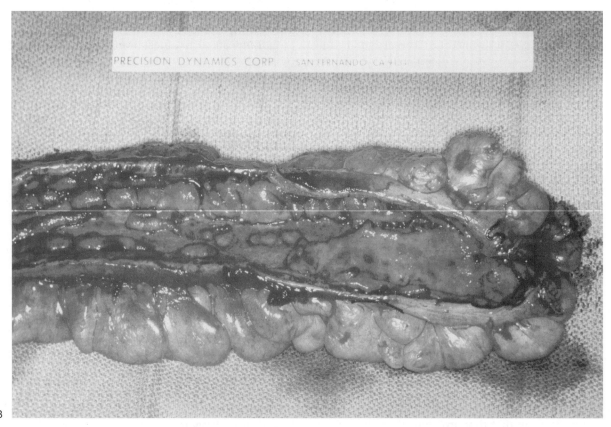

B

Figure 15-17 A, Severe ulcerative colitis showing pseudopolyps, deep ulceration, and friability. **B,** Severe Crohn's colitis showing linear ulcers and "cobblestoning."

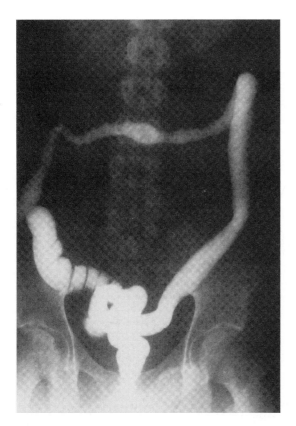

Figure 15-18 Barium enema showing the characteristic changes associated with chronic ulcerative colitis. Shown are loss of the haustral pattern, ulcerations, and foreshortening. Because of these changes, the colon is said to resemble a "lead pipe."

Crohn's disease, however. Table 15-6 shows distinguishing characteristics of both disease processes.

Treatment

Medical therapy is usually the initial treatment. It is successful in approximately 80% of cases. In mild disease, the treatment is primarily symptomatic, with the use of antidiarrheal agents that slow gut transit (e.g., loperamide) and bulking agents (psyllium seed products) that result in semiformed, less watery stools. In more severe disease, sulfasalazine, which is the anti-inflammatory agent of choice, should be tried because it induces remission in approximately half of all patients initially. Steroids are a mainstay of therapy, and most patients respond dramatically to steroid administration. Unfortunately, because of severe side effects, the dose is tapered and minimized whenever possible. Elimination of milk from the diet is occasionally helpful. Supportive therapy, including physical and emotional support, is important.

Major complications are toxic megacolon, colonic perforation, massive hemorrhage, serious anorectal complications, and carcinoma development after years of disease. Initial therapy for toxic megacolon is aggressive medical care, including gastric decompression, antibiotics, intravenous administration of fluids, hyperalimentation, and elimination of all other medications, specifically anticholinergics.

Surgical therapy is indicated when medical therapy fails or surgically treatable complications ensue (e.g., hemorrhage, perforation, obstruction, carcinoma). Because of

Table 15-6. Comparison of Ulcerative Colitis and Crohn's Colitis

	Ulcerative Colitis	Crohn's Colitis
Symptoms and signs		
Diarrhea	Severe, bloody	Less severe, bleeding infrequent
Perianal fistulas	Rare	Common
Strictures or obstruction	Uncommon	Common
Perforation	Free, uncommon	Localized, common
Pattern of development		
Rectum	Virtually always involved	Often normal
Terminal ileum	Normal	Diseased in majority of patients
Distribution	Continuous	Segmented, skip lesions
Megacolon	Frequent	Less common
Appearance		
Gross	Friable, bleeding granular exudates, pseudopolyps, isolated ulcers	Linear ulcers, transverse fissures, cobblestoning, thickening, strictures
Microscopic	Inflamed submucosa and mucosa, crypt abscesses; fibrosis uncommon	Transmural inflammation, granulomas, fibrosis
Radiologic	Lead-pipe, foreshortening, continuous, concentric	String sign in small bowel; segmental, asymmetric internal fistulae
Couse		
Natural history	Exacerbations, remissions, dramatic flare-ups	Exacerbations, remissions, chronic, indolent
Medical treatment	Initial response high (> 80%)	Response less predictable
Surgical treatment	Curative	Palliative
Recurrence	No	Common

the increased risk of carcinoma, long-standing ulcerative colitis is also an indication for surgical intervention. The risk increases 1% to 2% per year after the initial 10 years of disease. In the past, the definitive operative procedure for ulcerative colitis was total proctocolectomy with permanent ileostomy. Recently, procedures were devised to maintain fecal continence, including an operation that involves constructing a reservoir with a continence-producing nipple valve out of the small intestine (Kock's continent ileostomy). This operation has met with limited success. Subtotal colectomy with ileoproctostomy is attempted in some patients who have less severe rectal involvement and absolutely no perianal problems. Unfortunately, this operation does not cure the disease and subjects the patient to the risks of recurrent disease or the development of a malignancy in the remaining remnant. Total colectomy with mucosal proctectomy and **ileoanal pull-through** (Figure 15-19*A–D*) is now the operation of choice. The procedure is performed with a surgically constructed ileal reservoir, thereby sparing the patient a permanent abdominal ileostomy. A recent variation of this procedure removes the colon and all but 2 cm of the rectum. The remaining rectal stump receives a stapled anastomosis. There is, however, significant concern that this operation does not represent a cure because diseased mucosa is left behind, raising the possibility of subsequent development of cancer in the retained rectal stump. The advantage of the stapled operation is that very often it can be done without a diverting ileostomy. Because patients with toxic megacolon, perforation, or other complications have much higher morbidity and mortality rates, early surgery may be indicated.

Colonic Obstruction and Volvulus

Obstruction of the Large Intestine

Only 10% to 15% of intestinal obstruction in adults is the result of obstruction of the large bowel. The most common anatomic site of colonic obstruction is the sigmoid colon. The three most common causes are adenocarcinoma (65%), scarring associated with diverticulitis (20%), and volvulus (5%). Inflammatory disorders, benign tumors, foreign bodies, fecal impaction, and other miscellaneous problems account for the remainder. Obstructive adhesive bands, which are often seen in the small bowel, are extremely uncommon in the colon.

Clinical Presentation and Evaluation

Signs and symptoms include abdominal distension; cramping abdominal pain, usually in the hypogastrium; nausea and vomiting; and obstipation. Radiologic findings show distended proximal colon, air–fluid levels, and no distal rectal air (Figure 15-20).

Physical examination usually shows abdominal distension, tympany, high-pitched metallic rushes, and gurgles. On palpation, a localized, tender, palpable mass may indicate a strangulated closed loop or an area of inflamed diverticular disease.

An important element that affects the clinical expression of large bowel obstruction is whether the ileocecal

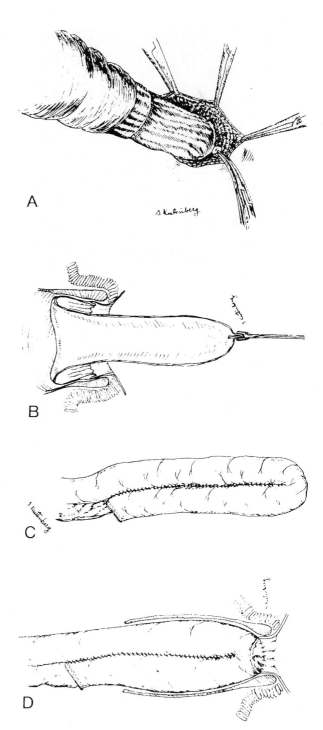

Figure 15-19 Ileoanal pull-through is the operation of choice for definitive treatment of ulcerative colitis and familial polyposis syndrome. **A,** After removal of the entire colon, the mucosa is stripped away from the muscular layers of the rectum. **B,** This dissection is continued down to the dentate line, and the mucosa is everted out through the anus and resected. **C,** A small reservoir is constructed from the terminal ileum using a J-shaped configuration. **D,** This J-shaped pouch is then pulled through the muscular cuff and anastomosed to the dentate line to create a neorectum.

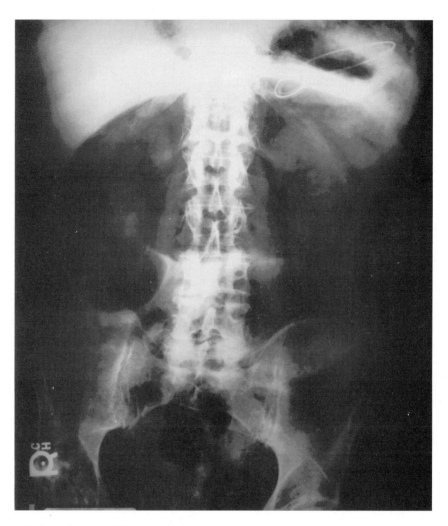

Figure 15-20 Massive colonic distension caused by a cecal volvulus.

valve is competent. If it is incompetent, the signs and symptoms produced are indistinguishable from those of routine small bowel obstruction. If the ileocecal valve is competent, as is the case in approximately 75% of patients, a "closed loop" obstruction occurs between the ileocecal valve and the obstructing point distally. Massive colonic distension results, and the cecum may reach a diameter of 12 cm, increasing the possibility of perforation, with or without gangrene. It is critically important for the clinician to distinguish between complete large bowel obstruction and partial large bowel obstruction. Patients with complete large bowel obstruction have obstipation that includes a history of no flatus or stool passage for 8 to 12 hours. On the other hand, patients with partial large bowel obstruction describe the passage of some gas or stool. Distinguishing between the two is important because a patient with complete bowel obstruction should undergo emergent operation. Those with partial large bowel obstruction may often be treated by nasogastric decompression and intravenous fluids with resolution of the acute obstruction. This distinction has important surgical ramifications because patients with partial large bowel obstruc-

tion can then be prepared for surgery by cleaning out the large intestine, thus avoiding a colostomy.

The appropriate diagnostic techniques include plain films of the abdomen. In patients in whom the cecum measures more than 12 cm and a definitive lesion cannot be delineated, laparotomy is undertaken. The use of barium enema confirms the diagnosis of colonic obstruction and identifies the exact location. If the obstruction is shown on plain abdominal films, barium enema is not necessary. Barium should never be given orally in the presence of suspected colonic obstruction because it may accumulate proximal to the obstruction and cause a barium impaction. Colonoscopic examination plays a major role in Ogilvie's syndrome (localized paralytic ileus of the colon without mechanical obstruction); otherwise, it is reserved for the occasional case of volvulus for decompression.

Treatment

All patients with large bowel obstruction should be treated with intravenous fluids, nasogastric suction, and continuous observation until the diagnosis is established and definitive therapy is undertaken. Potentially lethal complications of large bowel obstruction are perforation and abdominal peritonitis and sepsis. The major causes of severe colonic obstruction leading to these complications include carcinoma of the colon, with or without perforation; diverticulitis; sigmoid volvulus; and cecal volvulus.

Emergency laparotomy is undertaken for acute large bowel obstruction with cecal distension beyond 12 cm, severe tenderness, evidence of peritonitis, or generalized sepsis. Perforation caused by volvulus, obstructing cancers, or diverticular strictures usually requires laparotomy with the appropriate surgical procedures, usually resection and diverting colostomy.

For the occasional case of Ogilvie's syndrome in which there is enormous dilation of the right side of the colon without mechanical obstruction (pseudo-obstruction), the current therapy is fiberoptic colonoscopy, with decompression and placement of a long rectal decompression tube. Cecostomy may be necessary in cases of recurrence.

The various conditions that lead to large bowel obstruction result in differing prognoses, most of which depend on the patient's age and the comorbidity of existing diseases, particularly cardiovascular disease. Unfortunately, the overall death rate of patients who have a cecal perforation approaches 30%. Thus, prompt laparotomy is the mainstay of treatment.

Volvulus of the Large Intestine

Volvulus is rotation of a segment of the intestine on the axis formed by the mesentery (Figure 15-21). The most common sites of occurrence in the large bowel are the sigmoid (70%) and cecum (30%). Volvulus accounts for 5% to 10% of cases of large bowel obstruction and is the second most common cause of complete colonic obstruction. Stretching and elongation of the sigmoid with age is a predisposing factor. The first occurrence of volvulus in more than 50% of cases is in patients 65 years of age or older. For unknown reasons, patients who are confined to mental institutions or nursing homes have an increased risk of this disease. Volvulus also occurs in patients who have a hypermobile cecum because of incomplete fixation of the ascending colon at the time of intrauterine development. This condition allows the cecum to twist about the mesentery, forming a closed-loop obstruction at the entry and exit points, with major pressure at the sites of the twist. The vessels are partially occluded, and circulatory impairment leads to prompt gangrene and perforation.

Clinical Presentation and Evaluation

The patient has abdominal distension, which is often massive; vomiting; abdominal pain; obstipation; and tachypnea. Physical examination shows distension, tympany, high-pitched tinkling sounds, and rushes. Diagnostic studies include abdominal x-ray films and barium enemas. Abdominal x-rays show a massively dilated cecum or sigmoid without haustra that often assumes a kidney bean appearance. Barium enema study shows the exact site of obstruction, with a charac-

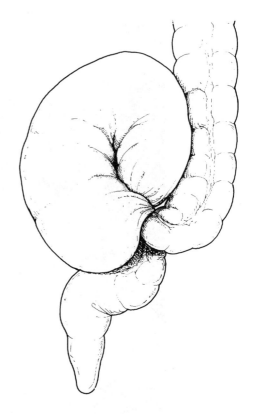

Figure 15-21 Volvulus of the sigmoid colon.

teristic funnel-like narrowing that often resembles a bird's beak or an ace of spades.

Treatment

Sigmoidoscopy with rectal tube insertion to decompress sigmoid volvulus is the recommended initial treatment for that location. Emergency operation is performed promptly if strangulation or perforation is suspected or if attempts to decompress the bowel are unsuccessful. Surgical therapy involves resection without anastomosis and the construction of a temporary colostomy. Most patients with sigmoid volvulus are easily decompressed and subsequently require elective resection, except for very high-risk elderly patients. Cecal volvulus is always treated surgically, either with cecopexy (suturing the cecum to the parietal peritoneum) or with right hemicolectomy with ileotransverse colostomy if the cecum is gangrenous.

Anus and Rectum

Diagnostic Evaluation

The anus and rectum are the site of many conditions that cause pain, protrusion, bleeding, discharge, or a combination of these. Most people complain generally about their "hemorrhoid problem"; it is up to the physician to distinguish between various pathologies that may present similarly.

Examination of the perianal and rectal area is an integral part of every physical examination. The importance of gentleness and empathy cannot be overemphasized. A complete history must be obtained before the examination; this information alone suggests the diagnosis in more than 80% of the cases. Gentle parting of the buttocks allows inspection that may show fissures, skin tags, hemorrhoids, fistulae, tumors, and dermatologic or infectious conditions. Gentle digital examination may show tumors, polyps, fluctuation, and sphincter weakness.

Anoscopic examination is mandatory because many visible lesions are not palpable. It may be deferred, however, in the presence of acute pain. The anoscope is a beveled instrument devised to examine the anal canal. It allows detection of more subtle lesions (e.g., ulcers, villous adenomas, infectious disorders) than the rigid or flexible proctosigmoidoscope. The proctosigmoidoscope, however, is the instrument of choice for a proper evaluation of the rectum because is the only instrument that allows exact localization of rectal lesions.

Hemorrhoids

Hemorrhoids are vascular cushions located in the anal canal. Hemorrhoidal disease, which most often causes hemorrhoidal protrusion or bleeding, is usually precipitated by constipation and straining at stool. Pregnancy, increased pelvic pressure (ascites, tumors), portal hypertension, and excessive diarrhea may influence the development of hemorrhoidal symptoms.

Hemorrhoids are usually found in three constant positions: left lateral, right anterior, and right posterior. It is preferable to refer to the actual anatomic position of the anorectal processes because the old "o'clock" system referred to the findings when the examination was performed in the lithotomy position. In the modern ambulatory setting, most patients are examined either in the left lateral (Simm's) or the knee-chest position, which change the terms of reference by 90° to 180°.

Hemorrhoids are classified as either internal or external. **Internal hemorrhoids** originate above the dentate line; external hemorrhoids are located below the level of the dentate line. Because the rectal mucosa above the dentate line is insensate, bleeding from internal hemorrhoids is usually painless. Conversely, external hemorrhoids are covered by richly innervated anoderm and usually cause pain when thrombosis occurs.

Clinical Presentation and Evaluation

A patient with hemorrhoids has symptoms of hemorrhoidal protrusion or bleeding. In cases of protrusion, the hemorrhoids are graded according to the level of prolapse. First-degree internal hemorrhoids do not prolapse; the anoscope must be used to visualize them. Second-degree internal hemorrhoids prolapse with defecation and return spontaneously to their anatomic position. Third-degree internal hemorrhoids prolapse

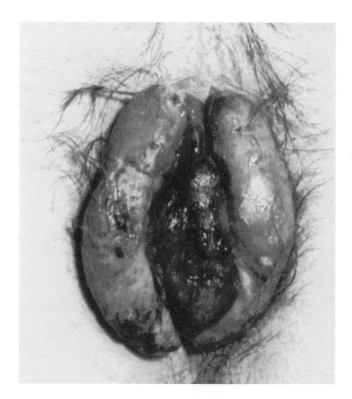

Figure 15-22 Fourth-degree hemorrhoids associated with thrombosis.

with defecation and require manual reduction. Fourth-degree hemorrhoids are not reducible (Figure 15-22). There is no classification for external hemorrhoids; they are either present or absent. Mixed hemorrhoids are a combination of internal and external hemorrhoids.

Bleeding may be minimal, appearing only on toilet paper, or it may occasionally be severe enough to cause anemia. It is usually bright red, coats the stool (rather than being mixed with it), and is painless, unless there is thrombosis, ulceration, or gangrene.

Treatment

Treatment is based on the presence of symptoms and the degree of disease (Table 15-7). Asymptomatic hemorrhoids are best left alone; cosmetic treatment is not indicated. Bulk-forming agents (e.g., psyllium derivatives) and avoidance of constipation are recommended. First-degree internal hemorrhoids are treated similarly; rubber-band ligation (banding) or infrared coagulation may be indicated, depending on the size of the hemorrhoids on anoscopic examination. Historically, sclerotherapy and cryosurgery were used in these cases, but these modalities have been abandoned by most colorectal surgeons. Second-degree internal hemorrhoids and some third-degree hemorrhoids are treated with banding. Formal surgical hemorrhoidectomy is used for fourth-degree hemorrhoids, for mixed third-degree hemorrhoids with a large external component, and in some emergency situations (e.g., gangrene, severe ulceration).

External hemorrhoids usually cause few problems. Contrary to popular belief, hemorrhoids do not itch or

Table 15-7. Internal Hemorrhoids: Classification and Treatment

Degree	Definition	Treatment
First	Bulge in the anal canal lumen; does not protrude outside the lumen	*Asymptomatic:* take bulking agents; avoid constipation; increase water intake *Symptomatic:* same treatment as asymptomatic; rubber-band ligation; infrared coagulation
Second	Protrudes with defecation Reduces spontaneously	Rubber-band ligation
Third	Protrudes with defecation Must be reduced manually	*Selected cases:* rubber-band ligation *Mixed:* surgical hemorrhoidectomy
Fourth	Protrudes permanently Incarcerated	Surgical hemorrhoidectomy

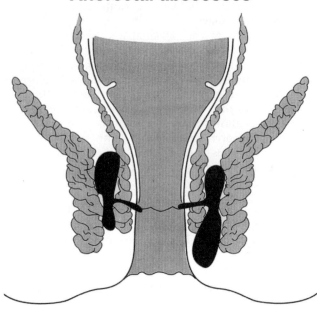

Anorectal abscesses

Intersphincteric   **Perianal**

Figure 15-23 Progression of intersphincteric abscess to perianal abscess.

burn; it is the perianal skin that is the site of pruritus ani. However, large external hemorrhoids may interfere with perianal hygiene and thus be indirectly associated with pruritus. In these cases, excision may be indicated. It is usually done under local anesthesia.

Some patients may have severe perianal pain and a lump close to the anus after a bout of constipation or prolonged sitting. Examination shows an obvious thrombosed external hemorrhoid. This condition is self-limited and resolves progressively over 7 to 10 days; creams, suppositories, and topical adjuncts are useless. If the patient is seen early in the course of the disease (the first 24–48 hours), treatment consists of excision of the thrombosed hemorrhoid under local anesthesia. If the patient is seen later in the course of the disease, spontaneous resolution is usually underway and conservative treatment is indicated. Sitz baths and a mild nonnarcotic analgesic are recommended.

Perianal Infections: Abscess and Fistula-in-Ano

Abscess

Most anorectal abscesses are believed to start with obstruction of the perianal glands that are located between the internal and external sphincters (intersphincteric space). These glands normally discharge their secretions at the level of the anal crypts that are located at the base of the columns of Morgagni. The term "of cryptoglandular origin" describes the origin of perirectal abscesses. As the early intersphincteric abscess (Figure 15-23, *left*) increases in size, it tends to spread along the planes of lesser resistance and to manifest fully as a perianal abscess (Figure 15-23, *right*) or as an ischiorectal abscess in the ischiorectal fossa, located

outside the external sphincter mechanism and below the level of the levatores ani muscles (Figure 15-24, *left*). If the infection spreads above the levators (Figure 15-24, *right*), the supralevator abscess may be very difficult to diagnose clinically. Perianal and ischiorectal abscesses are the most common. They account for as many as 70% of perirectal abscesses.

Clinical Presentation and Evaluation

Except for early intersphincteric abscesses and supralevator abscesses, perianal pain and swelling are readily apparent in perirectal abscesses. Spontaneous drainage of pus may occur. The cardinal signs of infection (pain, fever, redness, swelling, and loss of function) are usually present.

Treatment

The treatment is drainage of the abscess. Antibiotics alone have no role in their primary treatment. However, antibiotics may be used in conjunction with surgical incision and drainage in patients who are immunocompromised; those who have diabetes, leukemia, or acquired immune deficiency syndrome; or those who are undergoing chemotherapy.

Fistula-in-Ano

After drainage of a perirectal abscess, the patient has a 50% chance of having a chronic **fistula-in-ano.** An anorectal fistula is an abnormal communication between the anus at the level of the dentate line and the perirectal skin, through the bed of the previous abscess.

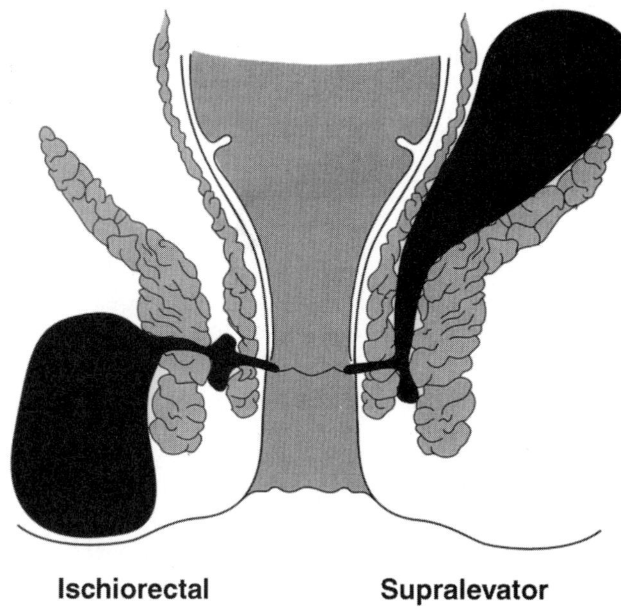

Anorectal abscesses

Ischiorectal **Supralevator**

Figure 15-24 Simple intersphincteric abscesses may progress to more complex ischiorectal and supralevator abscesses.

Table 15-8. Perianal Infections

Abscess: acute phase
  Intersphincteric
  Perianal
  Ischiorectal
  Supralevator
Fistula: chronic phase
  Intersphincteric
  Transsphincteric
  Suprasphincteric
  Extrasphincteric

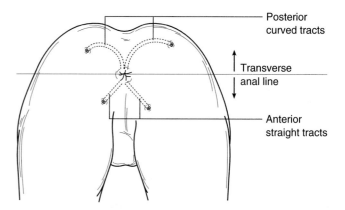

Figure 15-25 Goodsall's rule. (Reprinted with permission from Schwartz SI, et al. *Principles of Surgery*, 6th ed. New York, NY: McGraw-Hill, 1994. Reproduced with permission of The McGraw-Hill Companies.)

Fistulae are named in relation to the sphincter mechanism (Table 15-8). Intersphincteric fistulae are the result of perianal abscesses; transsphincteric fistulae are the result of ischiorectal abscesses; suprasphincteric fistulae are the result of supralevator abscesses. Extrasphincteric fistulae bypass the anal canal and the sphincter mechanism and open high up in the rectum.

Clinical Presentation and Evaluation

Fistulae manifest as chronic drainage of pus and sometimes stool from the skin opening. They never heal spontaneously, and surgical correction is indicated to eliminate the symptoms.

Goodsall's rule helps the examiner to predict the trajectory of the fistulous tract and the probable location of the internal anal opening (Figure 15-25). With the patient in the lithotomy or the knee-chest position, an imaginary line is drawn at the level of the anus, parallel to the floor. For external openings located anterior to this line, the fistula tract usually goes radially straight into the anal crypt. For external openings located posterior to this imaginary line, the fistula tract generally curves around, and the internal opening is in a frank midline position. However, the greater the distance between the anus and the external opening, the less reliable and helpful Goodsall's rule becomes. The trajectory of complex anal fistulae is unpredictable.

Treatment

Fistulotomy consists of unroofing the fistula tract, allowing the fistula to heal slowly by secondary intention. Judgment must be exercised to avoid cutting a large portion of the sphincter muscle, which may precipitate incontinence.

Preliminary identification of the fistula tract by gentle insertion of a probe into the external skin opening, through the tract, until the internal anal opening is found, allows intraoperative evaluation of the structures that need division. Staged fistulotomy with a Seton stitch permits immediate division of all nonsphincteric structures. Then the sphincter muscle is progressively divided to avoid incontinence.

Anal Fissures

Anal fissures are painful linear tears in the lining of the anal canal, below the level of the dentate line. They are most often located posteriorly in both sexes, but women also have anterior anal fissures. They occur in the posteroanterior plane because pelvic muscular support is weakest along this axis. Ectopic lateral fissures suggest an unusual diagnosis (e.g., Crohn's disease, leukemia, sexually transmitted disease, malignancy).

Clinical Presentation and Evaluation

Fissures are secondary to local trauma, either from constipation or excessive diarrhea. Pain typically starts with defecation and may persist from minutes to hours. It is disproportionate to the size of the lesion. If bleeding is present, it is usually minimal and bright red.

If the history suggests an anal fissure, gentle retraction of the buttocks will reveal the tear. In cases of chronic recurrent anal fissures, the classic triad of an external skin tag, a fissure exposing the internal sphincter fibers, and a hypertrophied anal papilla at the level of the dentate line is pathognomonic.

Treatment

Treatment is based on the duration and severity of the symptoms. Acute anal fissures usually respond to conservative treatment, avoidance of diarrhea or constipation, bulk laxatives to keep bowel movements atraumatic, and a mild nonnarcotic analgesic. Sitz baths are helpful for comfort. If conservative treatment fails, or if the fissure is chronic, surgery is recommended. Several surgical options are available. In uncomplicated cases, the operation of choice is a lateral internal sphincterotomy. A small portion of the internal sphincter is cut, which releases the sphincter spasm, relieves pain, and allows the fissure to heal. The operation carries a small risk of minor incontinence.

Anal Malignancy

Perianal and anal canal malignancies are rare, accounting for only 3% to 4% of all anorectal carcinomas. There are essentially two types of anal cancers: epidermoid carcinoma (a generic type that includes squamous cell, basaloid, cloacogenic, mucoepidermoid, and transitional carcinomas) and malignant melanoma. The anus is the third most common site for malignant melanoma, after the skin and the eyes.

Clinical Presentation and Evaluation

Either type of malignancy may cause pain, bleeding, or a lump. Delay in diagnosis is often a consequence of both patient and physician neglect. In cases of malignant melanoma, lymph node involvement and widespread metastasis are common at presentation. The diagnosis is often delayed because of the lack of pigmentation of these lesions (amelanotic melanoma). Examination should include palpation of the inguinal lymph nodes, a site of potential metastasis.

Treatment

In the past, abdominoperineal resection and permanent colostomy were the mainstay of treatment. This approach has been almost completely abandoned in favor of combined modality chemotherapy and radiation therapy, using a protocol of pelvic radiation with infusion of 5-FU and mitomycin C. With this treatment, 5-year survival rates range from 82% to 87%. Surgery is indicated in cases in which residual tumor is present after radiation and chemotherapy. Abdominoperineal resection is indicated in this setting.

Prophylactic inguinal node dissection is not recommended unless clinically palpable nodes are present because of the high morbidity associated with this procedure. Synchronous inguinal node metastasis is an ominous sign, and survival rates are poor. Conversely, metachronous inguinal node involvement has a better prognosis. Inclusion of the groins in the radiated fields decreases the incidence of metachronous lymph node involvement without adding much morbidity.

For malignant melanoma, the prognosis is dismal, regardless of the treatment. For good-risk patients, abdominoperineal resection is a reasonable option to maximize survival.

Anorectal Sexually Transmitted Diseases

More than 20 sexually transmitted diseases can be present in the anorectal area. Therefore, it is important to inquire about a complete sexual history in patients with anorectal symptoms.

Anal Condylomas

Anal condylomas are caused by human papilloma virus. They are the most common anorectal infection affecting homosexual men, but may also be seen in heterosexual men and women and even children. Transmission at birth and by close contact with infected patients has been reported.

Anal warts are more common in homosexual men who practice anal-receptive intercourse. The lesions are found perianally, intraanally, on the penis, and in the urethra. In women, the lesions may be found in the vagina, vulva, cervix, or urethra. Condylomas acuminata are pink or white papillary lesions. They vary in size from less than 1 mm to large cauliflower-like lesions. They bleed easily, and difficulty in maintaining perianal hygiene leads to pruritus ani. Discomfort and pain are often present.

Various topical caustic agents (bichloracetic acid, podophyllin) and local destructive therapies (electrocoagulation, cryotherapy, laser excision) have been tried with mitigated success. Regardless of the technique, the recurrence rate is high (10%–50%). Persistent causative sexual behavior obviously increases the recurrence rate.

Chlamydia and Lymphogranuloma Venereum

Chlamydial infections are among the most common sexually transmitted diseases. Chlamydial proctitis is increasing in both men and women who practice anal-receptive sex. The disease usually begins as vesicles and progresses to an ulcer. Inguinal adenopathy is a prominent sign. The rectal symptoms are tenesmus and pain. Patients who have lymphogranuloma venereum usually have hematochezia. Sigmoidoscopy may show a friable, ulcerating, erythematous mucosa. Biopsy findings are not definitive. The microimmunofluorescent antibody titer is the test of choice; however, the complement fixation test is still used. Most patients are successfully treated with tetracycline or doxycycline. Erythromycin is reserved for those who are insensitive to tetracyclines.

Gonorrhea

Neisseria gonorrhoeae infections of the rectum account for as many as 50% of the cases of gonorrhea in homosexual men. Evaluation and follow-up of patients with rectal gonorrhea require cultures of the urethra, rectum, and pharynx. Most patients have nonspecific complaints, including pruritus, tenesmus, and hematochezia. Sigmoidoscopy shows a thick, yellow mucopurulent discharge. The rectal mucosa ranges from normal to erythematous and edematous. Culture and Gram stain are used for organism identification. Treatment is aqueous procaine penicillin G 4.8 million units intramuscularly with probenecid 1 g orally.

Herpes Simplex Virus

Herpes simplex virus type 2 causes herpetic proctitis. The infection is acquired by direct inoculation. Approximately 15% of homosexual men with rectal symptoms have only this virus identified by rectal culture. The symptoms begin 4 to 28 days after inoculation. The majority of patients have pain and burning worsened by bowel movements. Some patients have a syndrome that is characterized by lumbosacral radiculopathy associated with sacral paresthesias. Symptoms include impotence; lower abdominal, buttock, and thigh pain; and urinary dysfunction. Lesions include vesicles with red areolae, ruptured vesicles, and aphthous ulcers. The usual locations include the perianal skin, anal canal, and lower rectum. Patients who are seen in the relapsing stage may report a history of crusting lesions followed by healing. Scrapings for cytologic examination show intranuclear inclusion bodies and giant cells. Treatment is aimed at relieving symptoms: sitz baths, topical anesthetics, and analgesics. Acyclovir has benefit in the acute and relapse phases. Continuous suppressive therapy is warranted only in the most severe cases.

Multiple-Choice Questions

1. What is the most common cause of massive lower gastrointestinal bleeding?
   A. Colon cancer
   B. Ulcerative colitis
   C. Familial polyposis syndrome
   D. Diverticulosis
   E. Colonic varices

2. Diverticulosis of the colon is associated with all of the following complications EXCEPT:
   A. Perforation
   B. Fistula
   C. Obstruction
   D. Hemorrhage
   E. Carcinoma

3. The polyps associated with the following conditions are all premalignant lesions EXCEPT:
   A. Gardner's syndrome
   B. Peutz-Jeghers syndrome
   C. Familial polyposis syndrome
   D. Villous adenoma
   E. Tubular adenomas (adenomatous polyps)

4. What is the most common cause of large bowel obstruction?
   A. Volvulus
   B. Fecal impaction
   C. Diverticular disease
   D. Carcinoma
   E. Adhesions

5. A cachectic 72-year-old white woman is admitted with a history of lethargy, weakness, 10-lb weight loss, and anemia. The most probable location of a colon tumor is in the:
   A. Sigmoid colon
   B. Rectum
   C. Transverse colon
   D. Splenic flexure
   E. Cecum

6. The proper operative management of a perforated diverticulum with fecal soilage is:
   A. Transverse loop colostomy
   B. Sigmoid colon resection with primary anastomosis
   C. Sigmoid colon resection, diverting colostomy, and Hartmann's pouch
   D. Nasogastric suction, laparotomy, and drainage
   E. Intravenous antibiotics and hydration

7. A 29-year-old man has a fever, exquisite perianal tenderness, edema, erythema, and fluctuance. Appropriate management is:
   A. Fissurectomy
   B. Incision and drainage
   C. Hemorrhoidectomy
   D. Diverting colostomy
   E. Antibiotics and warm soaks

8. The most common cause of chronic anorectal pain is:
   A. Hemorrhoids
   B. Anal fissure
   C. Anal fistula
   D. Low rectal cancer
   E. Crohn's proctitis

9. The appropriate management of prolapsing internal hemorrhoids that spontaneously reduce is:
   A. Observation only
   B. Hemorrhoidectomy
   C. Incision and drainage
   D. Suppositories and stool softeners
   E. Aspiration

10. The operation of choice for most patients with ulcerative colitis is:
    A. Subtotal colectomy with ileoproctostomy
    B. Colectomy, mucosal proctectomy, and ileoanal pull-through
    C. Proctocolectomy with ileostomy
    D. Proctocolectomy with Kock's continent ileostomy
    E. Abdominoperineal resection

11. The initial therapy for a sigmoid volvulus is:
    A. Nasogastric suction and intravenous hydration
    B. Immediate laparotomy with loop colostomy
    C. Placement of a Cantor tube and intravenous hydration
    D. Subtotal colectomy
    E. Sigmoidoscopic decompression

12. A 61-year-old man has guaiac-positive stools. Barium enema evaluation shows an "apple core" lesion in the cecum. On laparotomy, the patient has a large cecal mass as well as metastatic tumors in both lobes of the liver. You should now:
    A. Close the abdomen and do nothing further
    B. Perform a biopsy on the primary lesion only
    C. Perform a biopsy on the liver lesions only
    D. Perform a biopsy on both the primary and the liver lesions
    E. Remove the primary lesion and perform a biopsy on the liver section

13. Of the following veins that drain the colorectal region, which one does NOT eventually enter the portal venous system?
    A. Right colic vein
    B. Middle colic vein
    C. Superior hemorrhoidal vein
    D. Inferior hemorrhoidal vein
    E. Left colic vein

14. What is the 5-year survival rate after the diagnosis of a Dukes' stage B2 adenocarcinoma of the colon?
    A. 85%
    B. 65%
    C. 45%
    D. 25%
    E. 5%

15. The radiologic "bird's beak" on barium enema is associated with:
    A. Ulcerative colitis
    B. Crohn's disease
    C. Diverticular disease
    D. Carcinoma
    E. Volvulus

16. A "string sign" on enteroclysis is associated with:
    A. Ulcerative colitis
    B. Crohn's disease
    C. Diverticular disease
    D. Carcinoma
    E. Volvulus

17. Match the following phrase with the best single response. Lateral subcutaneous sphincterotomy:
    A. Fistula-en-ano
    B. Anal fissure
    C. Perirectal abscess
    D. Hemorrhoids
    E. Anal cancer

18. A diagnosis of ulcerative colitis is confirmed by:
    A. Digital examination of the rectum
    B. A bowel obstruction pattern on x-ray film
    C. Endoscopy (sigmoidoscopy or colonoscopy) with biopsy
    D. The finding of an anorectal abscess
    E. The presence of microcytic anemia

19. The most common symptom or sign of carcinoma in the descending colon is:
    A. High-volume, high-frequency diarrhea
    B. Anemia, with bloody, mucus-containing stool
    C. A palpable left lower quadrant mass
    D. Abdominal pain on defecation
    E. Crampy abdominal pain, with a change in bowel habits

20. The prognosis in colon carcinoma is best related to the:
    A. Blood supply of the involved segment
    B. Age of the patient
    C. Amount of hematochezia
    D. Depth of penetration of the primary lesion
    E. Size of the primary lesion

Oral Examination Study Questions

CASE 1

You are a general surgeon on staff at a large private medical center. A gastroenterologist asks you to see a 64-year-old white woman who was admitted with a 10-day history of worsening severe abdominal pain and a fever of 38.8° C.

OBJECTIVE 1

The student obtains a thorough history, pointing out pertinent negative findings.
   A. The pain is located in the left lower quadrant. It is unrelieved by passing flatus. The patient has no history of similar pain. The pain does not radiate, and it is worsened by coughing or sneezing.
   B. The onset of fever was 2 days before admission. The patient had chills yesterday.
   C. Pertinent negative findings include no melena, constipation, obstipation, weight loss, diarrhea, or previous abdominal disease. The patient is anorexic.
   D. The patient has no history of abdominal disease. She underwent appendectomy 20 years ago.
   E. The review of systems is noncontributory.

OBJECTIVE 2

The student elicits the pertinent physical findings and discusses their significance.
   A. The patient's temperature is 38.8° C, blood pressure is 130/75 mm Hg, and pulse is 108/min.

B. Abdominal examination shows left lower quadrant tenderness with rebound locally; a mass is palpable in the same area.

C. Rectal examination shows guaiac-negative stool, with no tenderness.

D. Bimanual examination shows a left lower quadrant mass that is palpable with the abdominal hand.

OBJECTIVE 3

The student outlines the initial diagnostic and treatment plans. The student also suggests a differential diagnosis.

A. The complete blood count is 15,000/mm^3, with a shift to the left. Hematocrit is 43%, amylase is 81 IU/L, and urinalysis shows 1 to 2 white blood cells/high-power field.

B. Abdominal x-ray series shows nonspecific findings.

C. Barium enema is contraindicated if diverticulitis is included in the differential diagnosis.

D. Colonoscopy is nondiagnostic in diverticulitis.

E. Intravenous fluid administration and intravenous antibiotics (aminoglycoside and metronidazole) are initiated.

F. The patient is given nothing by mouth.

G. The differential diagnosis includes gastroenteritis, appendicitis, kidney stones, ovarian torsion, foreign body perforation, diverticulitis, and perforated colon cancer.

OBJECTIVE 4

The student describes the natural history of this disease and an algorithm for disease that does not improve or recurs.

A. Most patients whose initial attack of diverticulitis results in hospitalization are successfully treated with intravenous hydration, antibiotics, and gut rest. If the disease resolves with conservative measures only, no further treatment is recommended, except for eating a high-fiber diet.

B. If the patient does not improve (decreased white blood count and fever, resolution of abdominal pain and mass) with intravenous antibiotics and gut rest, operative therapy is indicated. The operative procedure of choice is sigmoid colectomy with diverting colostomy and Hartmann's procedure.

C. If patient has a second bout that results in hospitalization (i.e., leukocytosis, fever, rebound pain), conservative measures are used to resolve the acute event, and the patient is electively scheduled for a sigmoid colectomy with primary anastomosis.

OBJECTIVE 5

The student describes the indications for operative therapy in diverticular disease (i.e., complications).

A. Hemorrhage

B. Obstruction

C. Fistula

D. Perforation

E. Abscess

F. Intractability

OBJECTIVE 1

Minimum Level of Achievement for Passing

A. The student obtains an accurate history and points out the pertinent negative findings.
   1. The student describes the characteristics of the pain, including location, radiation, duration, nature, aggravating factors, and previous occurrence.
   2. In contrast to appendicitis, which is a 48-hour disease, diverticulitis often smolders for a number of days before it achieves full expression.
   3. There is usually no melena, constipation, weight loss, or obstipation in diverticulitis.

B. The student describes the age group in which this disease commonly occurs (older than 55 years of age).

Honors Level of Achievement

The student describes the incidence of diverticulosis in the general population (60% of patients older than 60 years of age).

OBJECTIVE 2

Minimum Level of Achievement for Passing

A. The student consolidates the clinical findings and makes a presumptive diagnosis of diverticulitis (left lower quadrant pain and mass in an older person).

B. The student describes the most common location for diverticular complications in the colon (sigmoid colon).

Honors Level of Achievement

The student explains why cancer in the sigmoid colon is rarely associated with a mass, whereas a palpable mass is common in diverticular disease (a large phlegmon develops in diverticulitis; sigmoid cancers are usually relatively small).

OBJECTIVE 3

Minimum Level of Achievement for Passing

A. The student explains that the diagnosis of diverticulitis is usually made clinically, with treatment started before absolute confirmation of the diagnosis.

B. The student knows that leukocytosis and a fever usually accompany acute diverticulitis.

C. The student realizes that a barium enema is not obtained during the acute phase of the disease (because of the risk of barium extravasation), but it may be obtained later.

D. The student describes the appropriate management of an initial attack (i.e., surgery is not immediately indicated), including the use of antibiotics.

E. The student generates a relatively inclusive differential diagnosis.

Honors Level of Achievement

The student understands and can explain the choice of antibiotics (aminoglycoside for *Escherichia coli* coverage, metronidazole for *Bacteroides fragilis*).

OBJECTIVE 4

Minimum Level of Achievement for Passing

A. The student describes the natural history of most cases of diverticulitis (resolution with conservative treatment).

B. The student recommends alternative treatment if the patient does not improve with conservative measures alone (sigmoid colectomy, Hartmann's procedure).

C. The student describes the recommended treatment if the patient has a second severe attack of diverticulitis (conservative measures until the disease is quiescent, then elective sigmoid colectomy with primary anastomosis).

Honors Level of Achievement

A. The student knows the difference between a sigmoid colectomy and a low anterior resection and between Hartmann's pouch and a mucous fistula.

B. The student explains why complications of diverticular disease do not occur in the rectum.

OBJECTIVE 5

Minimum Level of Achievement for Passing

A. The student names five of the six indications for surgery in diverticular disease.

B. The student describes the correct management of a perforated diverticulum with fecal contamination.

Honors Level of Achievement

A. The student describes the most common fistula that occurs as a complication of diverticular disease (colovesical).

B. The student describes the amount of colon that is resected when a sigmoid diverticulum becomes inflamed and causes obstruction in the colon, with many diverticula throughout its length. The sigmoid colon is the only portion removed, even in pandiverticulosis.

CASE 2

You are a general surgeon practicing in a small town of 10,000. A family practitioner calls you to consult on a 72-year-old man with a 36-hour history of obstipation, moderate abdominal distension, and vomiting.

OBJECTIVE 1

The student obtains an accurate history.

A. The patient's last bowel movement was 36 hours ago. He has had severe constipation for 2 months.

B. The patient's stools are pencil-thin.

C. The patient lost 10 lb in the last 4 months.

D. The patient is having minimal abdominal pain now.

E. The patient has had nausea and vomiting for the last 14 hours.

F. Pertinent negative findings include no diarrhea, no history of previous operation, no history of hernia, and no blood noted in the stool.

G. The patient's history and review of systems are unremarkable in this previously healthy man. He has no recent history of antibiotic use.

OBJECTIVE 2

A careful physical examination is performed and initial diagnostic studies recommended.

A. This thin, distressed elderly man has a moderately distended abdomen with obvious tympani to percussion.

B. Auscultation shows high-pitched, tinkling bowel sounds. Palpation shows mild tenderness to palpation throughout the abdomen.

C. Rectal examination shows guaiac-positive stool; otherwise, it is unremarkable.

D. An abdominal x-ray series shows a tremendously dilated colon from the splenic flexure proximally. Air-fluid levels are seen in the small intestine.

E. Barium enema shows an apple core lesion of the splenic flexure, with virtual obliteration of the lumen.

F. Colonoscopy shows a ragged, friable lesion in the splenic flexure. A biopsy is performed.

OBJECTIVE 3

The student forms a differential diagnosis, including a discussion of the most common causes of large bowel obstruction.

A. The differential diagnosis includes the three most common causes of large bowel obstruction (in order): (1) carcinoma, (2) diverticular disease, and (3) volvulus. Other diseases in the differential diagnosis include fecal impaction, stricture, internal hernia, foreign body and, rarely, adhesions.

B. In contrast to small bowel obstruction, adhesions from previous operative procedures are rarely the cause of large bowel obstruction.

OBJECTIVE 4

The student describes the appropriate treatment for this patient, including preoperative preparations.

A. Preoperative preparations include giving the patient nothing by mouth, performing naso-gastric suction, providing preoperative hydration, and correcting the most likely acid–base abnormality, metabolic alkalosis, with normal saline.

B. Bowel preparation, although usually performed before colon surgery, cannot be safely done in a patient with colonic obstruction.

C. The patient is given preoperative antibiotics.

D. The operative procedure of choice is left hemi-colectomy with diverting colostomy and mucous fistula. Primary anastomosis should not be done in unprepared bowel. The operative procedure should resect all lymph node–bearing tissue that drains the area of the tumor.

OBJECTIVE 5

The student describes the modified Dukes system that is used to predict prognosis based on the depth of invasion in patients with colon cancer.

A. Dukes' stage A: involvement of the mucosa only, with an 85% to 90% 5-year survival rate

B. Dukes' stage B: involvement of the muscularis, but not the serosa, with a 70% 5-year survival rate

C. Dukes' stage B2: invasion of the serosa, with a 60% 5-year survival rate

D. Dukes' stage C: lymph node involvement, with a 25% 5-year survival rate

E. Dukes' stage D: distant metastasis, with a 5% 5-year survival rate

OBJECTIVE 1

Minimum Level of Achievement for Passing

A. The student obtains enough information from the history to suggest a diagnosis of bowel obstruction (i.e., obstipation, distension, nausea, and vomiting).

B. The student distinguishes obstipation from constipation.

C. The student provides a differential diagnosis for (1) small bowel obstruction and (2) large bowel obstruction. The student lists the three most common causes of large bowel obstruction in order of incidence.

Honors Level of Achievement

The student describes how the presentation of right colon cancer differs from that of left colon cancer (right colon: palpable mass, anemia, weight loss, guaiac-positive stool; left colon: constipation, gross blood in the stool, thin stools, mass that usually is not palpable).

OBJECTIVE 2

Minimum Level of Achievement for Passing

A. The student contrasts the physical findings in mechanical bowel obstruction with those in para-lytic ileus.

1. Mechanical obstruction causes high-pitched, tinkling sounds, rushes associated with waves of pain (colic), and distension.

2. Paralytic ileus causes hypoactive or absent bowel sounds, colic (much less common), and distension.

B. The student describes the x-ray findings in an abdominal series that suggest large bowel obstruction instead of small bowel obstruction.

1. In large bowel obstruction, haustra are present, but do not completely cross the width of the bowel; there is a greater diameter of distended colon, especially in the cecum; and the ascending and descending colon are placed laterally. In incompetent ileocecal valve, the entire small bowel is dilated.

2. In small bowel obstruction, plicae circulares are present that completely cross the bowel width, the diameter of the distended bowel is less than that of the colon, and no colonic air is seen.

C. The student describes the two most commonly used diagnostic tests that confirm the diagnosis as well as their advantages and disadvantages.

1. Barium enema is noninvasive and quick, has a lower incidence of complications, and is technically easier. However, it does not permit biopsy.

2. Colonoscopy allows the lesion to be visualized and permits actual biopsy. However, it requires increased technical skill and poses a higher risk to the patient.

Honors Level of Achievement

The student explains why the workup of bowel obstruction always begins with an evaluation of the lower gastrointestinal system (to minimize the risk of barium impaction proximal to an obstructing colon lesion, something that does not occur in small bowel obstruction).

OBJECTIVE 3

Minimum Level of Achievement for Passing

A. The student gives the three most common causes of large bowel obstruction, preferably in order.

B. The student knows that adhesions rarely cause large bowel obstruction.

Honors Level of Achievement

A. The student describes volvulus and its most common site (sigmoid colon).

B. The student describes the initial management of sigmoid volvulus (including sigmoidoscopic decompression).

OBJECTIVE 4

Minimum Level of Achievement for Passing

A. The student describes the preoperative management of a patient with a diagnosed large bowel obstruction.

B. The student explains why primary anastomosis is not possible in this case (high risk of infection: 25%).

C. The student describes the rationale for removing the entire left colon, even though the lesion is a 2.5-cm isolated lesion at the splenic flexure (splenic flexure has a relatively poor blood supply because there is no dominant artery).

Honors Level of Achievement

A. The student explains the difference between a mucous fistula and Hartmann's pouch.

B. The student defines left hemicolectomy, proctocolectomy, low anterior resection, and abdominoperineal resection.

OBJECTIVE 5

Minimum Level of Achievement for Passing

The student describes the modified Dukes system, which predicts 5-year survival rates for patients with colon cancer. This system is based on the depth of invasion.

Honors Level of Achievement

A. The student explains when surgery is indicated in hepatic metastasis from colorectal cancer (single lesion, on one side of the liver only, no metastatic disease elsewhere).

B. The student describes how a patient is followed clinically after resection of a Dukes' stage B2 colon cancer (complete blood count, carcinoembryonic antigen, and liver function test every 3 months for the first year and every 4 months for the second year; colonoscopy yearly for 5 years).

CASE 3

You are a board-certified general surgeon practicing in a large town with a 25-bed hospital. A 27-year-old woman comes to your office with intractable diarrhea, abdominal discomfort, and lethargy.

OBJECTIVE 1

The student obtains a thorough history.

A. The onset of the diarrhea was 6 weeks ago.

B. The diarrhea is usually watery, with blood mixed in occasionally.

C. Associated symptoms include cramping, tenesmus, and loss of appetite.

D. Weight loss was 5 lb in 6 weeks.

E. The patient has not traveled outside the United States.

F. The patient has had no new, unrefrigerated, or unusual foods.

G. The patient has no previous history of diarrhea or abdominal disease.

OBJECTIVE 2

The student requests the results of a careful physical examination.

A. Abdominal examination shows mild, diffuse tenderness to deep palpation throughout, with hyperactive bowel sounds.

B. Rectal examination shows normal results, except for guaiac-positive stools.

C. Skin examination shows questionable scleral icterus.

OBJECTIVE 3

The student describes the appropriate workup.

A. Stool that was sent for ova, parasites, and routine cultures has negative results.

B. Stool that was sent for microscopic evaluation shows sheets of white blood cells.

C. Complete blood count shows a white blood cell count of 11,700/mm³ (normal, 5000–10,000/mm³) and hematocrit of 30% (low). Differential count shows 75 polymorphonuclear leukocytes, 5 bands, and 10 lymphocytes (shift to the left).

Liver function tests show total bilirubin of 2.4 mg/dL, direct bilirubin of 1.8 mg/dL, alkaline phosphatase of 295 U/L, serum glutamic pyruvic transaminase of 141 IU/L, serum glutamic oxaloacetic transaminase of 170 U/L, and LDH of 240 mg/dL (all abnormally high).

D. Flexible sigmoidoscopy shows granular mucosa, a foreshortened rectum with contact friability, and mucosal exudates.

E. Colonoscopy shows these characteristics extending to 55 cm from the anal verge. Biopsy shows lymphocyte infiltration of the mucosa with crypt abscesses present. This test is not indicated in the acute, severe phase of the disease.

F. Barium enema is not indicated during the acute, severe phase of the disease. When it is done 2 weeks later, it is essentially normal.

G. Enteroclysis is done primarily to rule out Crohn's disease; it is normal.

OBJECTIVE 4

The student compiles a differential diagnosis and suggests the correct treatment of the disease at this stage.

A. The differential diagnosis includes bacterial diarrhea, diarrhea secondary to Giardia or amebae, gastroenteritis, ulcerative colitis, Crohn's colitis, and spastic colitis.

B. The endoscopic appearance and biopsy findings suggest ulcerative colitis. Management at this point is conservative, with rest; oral sulfasalazine (Azulfidine), prednisone, or both; and avoidance of foods that aggravate the patient's symptoms (e.g., milk products).

C. If the symptoms are more severe (i.e., fever, abdominal pain, frequent bloody bowel movements, tenesmus), gut rest and total parenteral nutrition may be indicated, along with high doses of intravenous steroids.

OBJECTIVE 5

The student explains when surgery is indicated in ulcerative colitis and describes the surgical options.

A. Indications for surgery include hemorrhage, toxic megacolon, intractable disease (no improvement with medications), inability to tolerate medications, cancer prophylaxis after 10 years, and severe interference with lifestyle.

B. Surgical options
   1. Proctocolectomy
   2. Total colectomy, mucosal proctectomy, and ileoanal pull-through

OBJECTIVE 6

The student names the extraintestinal complications associated with ulcerative colitis.

A. Hepatic: sclerosing cholangitis, pericholangitis

B. Joint: peripheral arthritis, ankylosing spondylitis

C. Skin: pyoderma gangrenosum, acanthosis nigricans

D. Other: uveitis, conjunctivitis

OBJECTIVE 1

Minimum Level of Achievement for Passing

A. The student obtains a thorough history regarding the diarrhea, including the time of onset, appearance, frequency, travel history, bowel habits, associated symptoms, and dietary review.

B. The student distinguishes the diarrhea associated with ulcerative colitis from that associated with Crohn's disease (ulcerative colitis: bloody with associated pus and mucus; Crohn's disease: watery diarrhea, often associated with obstructive symptoms).

Honors Level of Achievement

The student describes the epidemiology of ulcerative colitis with regard to age, race, and genetics.

A. Age distribution is bimodal, with one peak at 20 to 35 years of age and a second peak at 55 to 65 years of age.

B. This condition is uncommon in blacks and American Indians, and common in certain Jewish populations.

C. Approximately 20% of patients have an affected family member.

OBJECTIVE 2

Minimum Level of Achievement for Passing

A. The student realizes that the physical examination is usually not remarkable, except in toxic megacolon (toxic, septic presentation with abdominal distension) or hemorrhage (anemia).

B. The student realizes that hepatic disease is often associated with ulcerative colitis and can explain why this patient might be jaundiced.

Honors Level of Achievement

The student describes the most common hepatic lesion associated with ulcerative colitis (pericholangitis: 40%).

OBJECTIVE 3

Minimum Level of Achievement for Passing

A. The student describes the appropriate workup in a patient with chronic diarrhea (stool for culture, ova, and parasites, and microscopic examination; routine laboratory tests, including complete blood count with differential and liver function tests; stool for clostridia toxin when indicated by history). Flexible sigmoidoscopy is indicated if the test results are negative.

B. The student understands that the diagnosis is usually made by endoscopy and the clinical pattern of involvement.

C. The student knows what "enteroclysis" is and how it is used to distinguish ulcerative colitis from Crohn's disease (contrast study in which barium is placed directly into the jejunum; it is helpful in detecting strictures of the terminal ileum).

Honors Level of Achievement

The student describes how the endoscopic appearance of ulcerative colitis differs from that of Crohn's disease. Ulcerative colitis virtually always involves the rectum and extends proximally in a continuous fashion, it has pseudopolyps and discrete ulcers, and mucosal exudates are common. Crohn's disease more commonly involves the right colon and terminal ileum. It is associated with skip lesions and may not involve the rectum; it also has "cobblestoning," linear ulcers, and aphthous ulcers.

OBJECTIVE 4

Minimum Level of Achievement for Passing

A. The student formulates a differential diagnosis for chronic diarrhea.

B. The student suggests six ways in which Crohn's disease is different from ulcerative colitis.

C. The student defines toxic megacolon and describes its clinical appearance.

D. The student describes the conservative management of ulcerative colitis.

	Crohn's Disease	Ulcerative Colitis
Depth of involvement	Transmural	Mucosal
Pattern of involvement	Right colon, terminal ileum	Rectum, left colon
Presence of bleeding	Uncommon	Common
Cancer risk	Increased somewhat	High
Risk of obstruction	High	Low
Organs affected	Entire gastrointestinal tract	Colon and rectum only

Honors Level of Achievement

The student states what percentages of patients have mild (50%), moderate (30%), and fulminant (15%) colitis.

OBJECTIVE 5

Minimum Level of Achievement for Passing

A. The student describes the indications for surgery in ulcerative colitis.

B. The student describes the two operations commonly used to treat ulcerative colitis and discusses their advantages and disadvantages.
   1. Proctocolectomy is curative and relatively quick. It results in permanent ileostomy and requires one operation.
   2. Ileoanal pull-through is curative. It results in preservation of sphincter control, with no ileostomy required. It is a long operation that requires two procedures.

Honors Level of Achievement

The student describes the risk of colon cancer in a patient with ulcerative colitis over a period of 20 years (risk increases 2% per year each year after 10 years).

OBJECTIVE 6

Minimum Level of Achievement for Passing

A. The student names six extraintestinal complications associated with ulcerative colitis.

B. The student realizes that all extraintestinal complications of ulcerative colitis may be seen in Crohn's disease.

Honors Level of Achievement

The student realizes that sclerosing cholangitis is the most dreaded extraintestinal complication of ulcerative colitis, and explains why.

SUGGESTED READINGS

American Society of Colon and Rectal Surgeons Standards Task Force. Practice parameters for the management of anal fissure. American Society of Colon and Rectal Surgeons, 1993.

American Society of Colon and Rectal Surgeons Standards Task Force. Practice parameters for the treatment of hemorrhoids. *Dis Colon Rectum* 1993;36:1118.

August L, Wise L. Surgical management of perforated diverticulitis. *Am J Surg* 1981;141:122.

Evans JT, Vena J, Aronoff BL, et al. Management and survival of carcinoma of the colon: results of a national survey by the American College of Surgeons. *Ann Surg* 1978;188:716.

Lavery IC, Jagelman DG. Cancer in the excluded rectum following surgery for inflammatory bowel disease. *Dis Colon Rectum* 1982;25:52.

Ovaska J, Heikki J, Kujarii H, et al. Follow-up of patients operated on for colorectal carcinoma. *Am J Surg* 1990;159:593.

Quan SHQ. Malignant melanoma of the anorectum. *Semin Colon Rectal Surg* 1995;6(3):166.

Riddell RH, et al. Dysplasia in inflammatory bowel disease: standardized classification and the provisional clinical applications. *Hum Pathol* 1983;14:931.

Sanfey H, Bayless TM, Cameron JL. Crohn's disease of the colon: is there a role for limited resection? *Am J Surg* 1984;147:38.

Wexner SD. Managing common anorectal sexually transmitted disease. *Infect Surg* 1990;9:9.

16

Biliary Tract

Ajit K. Sachdeva, M.D.
Harvey H. Sigman, M.D.
Rudy G. Danzinger, M.D.

OBJECTIVES

1. Discuss the factors that contribute to the formation of the three most common types of gallstones.
2. Describe the epidemiology of gallstone disease as it relates to patient evaluation and management.
3. Discuss the most useful laboratory tests and radiologic studies to evaluate patients with diseases of the biliary tract.
4. Describe the management of asymptomatic gallstones found incidentally on radiologic studies or at celiotomy.
5. Compare and contrast the: (1) clinical presentation, (2) laboratory and radiologic findings, and (3) management of a patient with chronic cholecystitis (biliary colic) and a patient with acute cholecystitis.
6. List the differences in the clinical presentation and evaluation of a jaundiced patient with choledocholithiasis and a jaundiced patient with biliary obstruction secondary to malignancy.
7. Describe the clinical presentation, evaluation, and management of a patient with: (1) acute cholangitis and (2) acute suppurative cholangitis. Highlight the differences between the two conditions.
8. Discuss the clinical presentation, evaluation, and management of a patient with acute biliary (gallstone) pancreatitis.
9. Outline the clinical presentation, evaluation, and management of a patient with gallstone ileus. Contrast these with the corresponding features of other types of small bowel obstruction.
10. Discuss the epidemiology, clinical presentation, evaluation, and management of carcinoma of the gallbladder.
11. Outline the clinical presentation, evaluation, and management of carcinoma of the extrahepatic biliary ducts.
12. List the common causes of benign strictures of the common bile duct, and describe the clinical features of patients who have such strictures.
13. Discuss the various options available to treat stones in the gallbladder and the extrahepatic biliary ducts.
14. Outline the indications for laparoscopic cholecystectomy. Discuss the advantages of this approach over open cholecystectomy.
15. Compare and contrast the complications associated with laparoscopic cholecystectomy with those associated with open cholecystectomy.
16. Describe the postoperative management of a patient after: (1) cholecystectomy and (2) common bile duct exploration.

Diseases of the gallbladder and bile ducts are common in the adult population of North America. Approximately 10% of adults have gallstones, and more than 600,000 cholecystectomies are performed annually in the United States, accounting for more than $5 billion in health care costs. In Canada, approximately 50,000 cholecystectomies are performed each year. Accurate clinical assessment, including pertinent history and accurate physical examination, yields valuable information about the diagnosis of common diseases of the biliary tract. Laboratory tests are helpful in distinguishing among various causes of jaundice, and radiologic studies play a pivotal role in confirming the diagnosis of biliary tract disease. To minimize the risk of iatrogenic injury, the surgeon must possess the skills to recognize common variations in the anatomy of the biliary tract and to perform careful dissection of the vital structures during surgery. This dictum was reemphasized in recent years with the meteoric rise in the popularity of **laparoscopic cholecystectomy,** which has replaced open cholecystectomy as the preferred operation for many patients with gallstone disease.

Anatomy

The anatomy of the extrahepatic biliary system varies considerably from individual to individual, and many anomalies are reported. To prevent inadvertent injury to the extrahepatic bile ducts and related structures during cholecystectomy, anticipation of anomalous anatomy and careful, bloodless dissection are vitally important.

The gallbladder is a thin-walled, contractile storage bag attached to the undersurface of the liver at the anatomic division of the right and left lobes. It is usually tubular, approximately 10 cm long, and 5 cm in diameter. Most commonly, 75% of the gallbladder is covered by peritoneum, and the remainder is intimately attached to the liver. In some patients, the gallbladder is completely covered by peritoneum and is suspended by a mesentery. In others, it is almost completely embedded in the liver. In general, the less the gallbladder is attached to the liver, the easier is its surgical removal. The gallbladder consists of the fundus, body, neck, and cystic duct, which is lined by the spiral valves of Heister.

The cystic duct joins the common hepatic duct (formed by the confluence of the left and right hepatic ducts) to form the common bile duct. The hepatocystic triangle **(triangle of Calot)** is the anatomic area that is bounded by the inferior margin of the liver superiorly, the common hepatic duct medially, and the cystic duct laterally. A number of important normal (i.e., right hepatic artery) and anomalous structures traverse this triangle. The common bile duct passes through the head of the pancreas, usually joins the pancreatic duct within 1 cm of the wall of the duodenum, and then empties into the second portion of the duodenum, through the ampulla of Vater. Bile flow into the duodenum is regulated in part by the sphincter of Oddi, which encircles the distal bile duct. The most common anatomic configuration of this region is shown in Figure 16-1, which demonstrates the usual relations of the important ductal and arterial structures.

Physiology

The liver secretes 500 to 1000 mL bile/day under physiologic conditions. The volume of bile secretion is highest during gastric emptying and lowest during prolonged fasting. When the sphincter of Oddi is closed, most hepatic bile is diverted into the gallbladder for storage and concentration. The gallbladder concentrates the bile by absorbing Na$^+$, Cl$^-$, and water. Throughout gastric emptying, cholecystokinin and autonomic neural activity cause oscillating contractions of the gallbladder along with relaxation of the sphincter of Oddi. The result is a slow, sustained emptying of most of the gallbladder bile into the duodenum. Simultaneously, mainly through the activity of secretin on bile ductular cells, hepatic bile flow is increased because of the addition of water and bicarbonate.

The electrolyte composition of hepatic bile is similar to that of plasma. Bile also contains cholesterol, bile

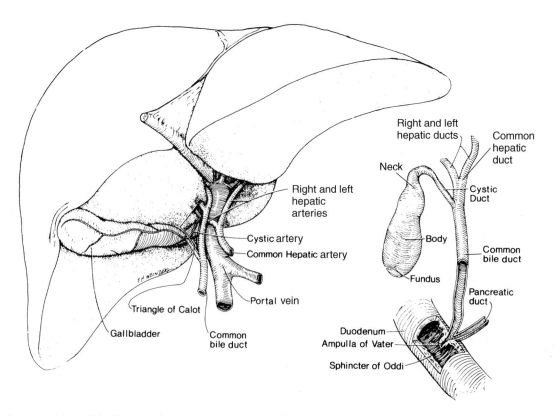

Figure 16-1 Anatomy of the gallbladder, porta hepatis, and extrahepatic bile ducts.

acids, phospholipid (primarily lecithin), and protein. Additionally, the bile pigment bilirubin, a breakdown product of heme, is excreted in the bile. Primary bile acids are synthesized from cholesterol in the liver and are conjugated with glycine or taurine before they are excreted in the bile. Conjugated bile acids and lecithin form vesicles and micelles that help to maintain the cholesterol soluble in the bile. The relative concentrations of cholesterol, bile salts, and lecithin must be maintained within a fairly limited range to maintain the cholesterol in solution. A change in their relative concentrations may favor the formation and precipitation of cholesterol crystals (Figure 16-2). Cholesterol is most soluble in a mixture that contains at least 50% bile salts and smaller amounts of lecithin. Once in the duodenum, bile acids traverse the small intestine; most are returned to the liver through the portal blood. Small amounts of bile acids are reabsorbed passively throughout the small intestine, but most of the reabsorption occurs actively at the level of the terminal ileum. Thus, there is an effective mechanism for enterohepatic circulation of bile acids. Depending on the duration of gastric emptying (e.g., quantity of the meal, fat content), the same bile acid molecules may recirculate two or three times after a meal. Normally, approximately 5% of bile acids escape reabsorption in the ileum. They are deconjugated or dehydroxylated by intestinal bacteria, rendering them less water soluble, or are adsorbed to intraluminal particulate matter. To keep the bile acid pool relatively constant, the lost bile acids are replaced by hepatic synthesis of new bile acids through a feedback mechanism. The liver can compensate for a loss of as much as 20% of the bile acid pool by the synthesis of new bile acids. Greater losses lead to a diminished bile acid pool, making the bile lithogenic and prone to stone formation. Bilirubin is actively excreted by hepatocytes into bile as a conjugated water-soluble diglucuronide (direct bilirubin). This mechanism is responsible for the green-brown color of bile and the brown color of stool. Extrahepatic obstruction to the flow of bile by benign or malignant diseases leads to the accumulation of predominantly conjugated (direct) bilirubin, which is water soluble and is excreted in the urine, making it dark. In contrast, hemolytic diseases, which cause excessive breakdown of heme, and hepatocellular diseases, which preclude adequate conjugation of bilirubin, lead to the accumulation of predominantly unconjugated (indirect) bilirubin, which is fat soluble and is not excreted in the urine.

Bile in the duodenum is important for alkalinizing acid gastric chyme, making luminal contents iso-osmolar, and digesting and absorbing fats and the fat-soluble vitamins (A, D, E, and K). Hence, obstructive jaundice or external bile diversion may cause problems with fat assimilation (steatorrhea) and blood coagulation (prolonged prothrombin time secondary to vitamin K malabsorption), along with light-colored stools.

Gallstone Disease

Pathogenesis of Gallstones

The most common types of gallstones in the Western population are of the mixed variety, which contain a high proportion of cholesterol. These stones account for approximately 75% of all types of gallstones. Precipitation of cholesterol as crystals tends to occur if the bile is lithogenic and supersaturated with cholesterol. These crystals, in the presence of enucleating factors (an imbalance between nucleation-inhibiting and nucleation-promoting proteins), may agglomerate to form gallstones and entrap other components of bile (e.g., bilirubin, mucus, Ca^{++}) in the process. Most mixed stones do not contain enough calcium to render them radiopaque; thus, they are usually not seen on plain x-rays. Occasionally, a single large stone forms and is composed almost entirely of cholesterol (cholesterol solitaire). Incomplete emptying of the gallbladder (a normal phenomenon) affords ideal conditions for agglomeration; for this reason, most stones form in the gallbladder.

Pigment stones are of two types, black and brown. Black pigment stones account for approximately 20% of all biliary stones and are generally found in the gallbladder. They typically form in sterile gallbladder bile and are commonly associated with hemolytic diseases and cirrhosis. In chronic hemolysis, there is hypersecretion of bilirubin conjugates in the bile and greater secretion of monoglucuronides compared with diglucuronides, which favors the precipitation of pigment

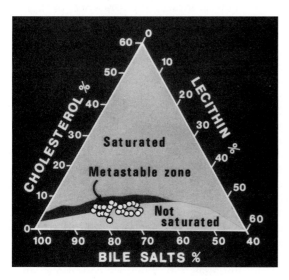

Figure 16-2 The molar percentages of cholesterol, lecithin, and bile salts in bile plotted on triangular coordinates. A relative change in the concentrations of these components can lead to supersaturation of the bile with cholesterol, increasing the likelihood of gallstone formation. In the metastable zone, there is supersaturation of cholesterol, but its precipitation occurs extremely slowly. (Used with permission. Copyright, American Gastroenterological Association, Bethesda, Maryland.)

stones. In contrast, brown stones are associated with infected bile. They are found primarily in the bile ducts and are soft. Pigment stones often contain enough calcium to render them radiopaque.

Gallbladder sludge is amorphous material that contains mucoprotein, cholesterol crystals, and calcium bilirubinate. It is often associated with prolonged total parenteral nutrition, starvation, or rapid weight loss. Gallbladder sludge may be a precursor of gallstones.

The source of most stones found in the biliary ducts (**choledocholithiasis**) is the gallbladder. However, bile stasis and infection involving the bile ducts predispose to the formation of primary bile duct calculi within the ducts.

Epidemiology of Gallstones

Both genetics and the environment appear to influence the incidence of gallstones. The incidence increases with age, and women are affected approximately three times as often as men are. The prevalence of gallstone disease among white women who are younger than 50 years of age is 5% to 15%; in older women, it is approximately 25%. Among white men who are younger than 50 years of age, the prevalence is 4% to 10%; in older men, it is 10% to 15%. Gallstone disease also tends to cluster in families. Native Americans have an extremely high prevalence of gallstones; more than 50% of men and 80% of women have mixed stones by the age of 60 years. Obesity (excessive cholesterol biosynthesis), multiparity (altered steroid metabolism, lithogenic bile, gallbladder hypomotility), high-dose estrogen oral contraceptives, and some cholesterol-lowering agents (alteration of cholesterol and bile acid biosynthesis), rapid weight loss (reduction in bile acid secretion and gallbladder stasis), and prolonged total parenteral nutrition (hyperconcentration of bile and gallbladder stasis) all predispose to the formation of stones. Diseases that diminish the bile acid pool (e.g., Crohn's disease, involving the terminal ileum, resection of the terminal ileum) increase the incidence of stones. Patients with hemolytic disorders and alcoholic cirrhosis tend to form pigment stones.

Theoretically, the following manipulations may help to decrease the risk of gallstone formation: avoiding obesity (see above); following a high-fiber, high-calcium diet (to diminish the enterohepatic circulation of dehydroxylated bile acids); eating meals at regular intervals (to diminish gallbladder storage time); and eating foods with low levels of saturated fatty acids (to diminish the nucleation of lithogenic bile).

Diagnostic Evaluation

History and Physical Examination

In patients who have symptoms that suggest biliary tract disease, the differential diagnosis can be narrowed by obtaining the pertinent history and performing an accurate physical examination. The history may provide valuable clues that point to either an acute or a chronic condition. If the patient is jaundiced, the history can suggest either obstructive or hepatocellular disease and may indicate an underlying malignancy. Specific physical findings may also yield useful information that can help with the differential diagnosis.

The hallmark of chronic gallstone disease is pain, described as **biliary colic.** The pain is usually steady, fairly severe, and located in the epigastrium or the right upper quadrant of the abdomen. The pain is visceral, poorly localized, and may last from 1 to 4 hours. The cause of the pain is transient obstruction of the cystic duct by a gallstone. The pain is secondary to increased pressure in the gallbladder that results from contraction against a stone that is impacted in the cystic duct (ball-valve effect). Typical biliary colic is caused by obstruction and is not associated with acute inflammation or infection. The pain tends to occur postprandially, but it may have no relation to meals, and may awaken the patient at night. The pain can occur after any meal, but larger meals and those that contain fat are most likely to cause pain. Biliary pain is seldom relieved by anything but time or potent analgesics. Nausea and vomiting may accompany this episodic pain. The patient is well before the onset of pain and then again within minutes to a few hours after the pain subsides.

Acute inflammation or infection involving the gallbladder causes sharp, steady, well-localized pain in the right upper quadrant of the abdomen or in the epigastrium. The pain lasts longer than 3 to 4 hours and may continue for several days. It is mediated by somatic sensory nerves, with cortical localization. It is often accompanied by nausea and vomiting.

In patients with jaundice, the presence of light-colored stools and dark, tea-colored urine indicates extrahepatic biliary obstruction. If this combination is present, severe or sharp pain suggests a benign etiology for the jaundice (e.g., calculous disease of the biliary tract). In contrast, patients with malignancies (e.g., carcinoma of the pancreas) generally have dull, vague, or insignificant upper abdominal pain. A history of marked weight loss is often present in patients with malignant conditions. Pruritus is believed to be caused by high tissue concentrations of reabsorbed conjugated bile acids and is often present in patients with obstructive jaundice.

On examination, a patient with biliary colic appears doubled-up or restless, whereas a patient who has pain associated with inflammation tends to be still because the pain is aggravated by movement. The pulse rate may be high secondary to pain, inflammation, or infection. Fever often accompanies inflammatory conditions, and high fever may be present if complications (e.g., gangrene of the gallbladder, abscess) are present or if the patient has infection involving the bile ducts. Low blood pressure signifies severe dehydration or septic shock. The abdomen of patients with biliary colic is soft, but often some tenderness is found in the right upper quadrant. Once the pain subsides, the abdomen is nontender between episodes of colic. In **acute cholecystitis,** examination of the abdomen may show a positive **Murphy's sign** (sharp pain on deep inspiration during palpation in the right upper quadrant) when the visceral peritoneum overlying the gallbladder is inflamed, but the inflammation has not spread to the adjacent parietal peritoneum. Once the inflammation spreads, abdominal examination shows localized guarding and rebound tenderness. A tender mass may also be palpable in the right upper quadrant of the abdomen in acute cholecystitis. The presence of a nontender, palpable gallbladder with jaundice suggests underlying malignant disease, such as carcinoma of the pancreas (Courvoisier's law). In such conditions, the gallbladder is passively distended as a result of back pressure caused by the distal malignant obstruction. If a stone is the cause of the distal ductal obstruction, the site of origin of the stone is generally a diseased thick-walled gallbladder, which is incapable of passive distension. An irregular abdominal mass may be present in a patient with advanced malignancy.

Laboratory Tests

A number of laboratory tests aid in the diagnosis and management of biliary tract disease. The hemoglobin or hematocrit may be elevated if the patient is dehydrated, and leukocytosis with a shift to the left suggests acute inflammation and infection. Serum amylase may be elevated in both acute cholecystitis and acute cholangitis, but marked elevations of serum amylase suggest acute pancreatitis. Liver function tests are helpful in detecting hyperbilirubinemia and providing information about the underlying disease process. The serum level of unconjugated or indirect bilirubin increases in hemolytic disorders, whereas the direct, conjugated fraction is elevated with extrahepatic biliary obstruction or cholestasis. Alkaline phosphatase is synthesized by hepatocytes and the biliary tract epithelium. Serum alkaline phosphatase levels increase as a result of overproduction in conditions that cause extrahepatic biliary obstruction or, less commonly, from cholestasis resulting from a drug reaction or primary biliary cirrhosis. The serum level of this enzyme is moderately elevated in hepatitis, and it may also be elevated as a result of bone disease. Alkaline phosphatase of hepatobiliary origin may be differentiated from that originating from bone by confirming its heat stability. The concomitant elevation of 5'-nucleotidase or ϒ-glutamyltranspeptidase also indicates that the source of the elevated alkaline phosphatase is the biliary tract. Aspartate aminotransferase (AST) and alanine aminotransferase (ALT) are released from hepatocytes, and serum levels of both enzymes are increased significantly in various types of hepatitis. AST and ALT are also often elevated with biliary obstruction, particularly when it is acute. As a rule, however, the increase in alkaline phosphatase is greater than the increase in the levels of AST and ALT in biliary obstruction, and the converse is true in hepatitis. If the biliary ductal system is partially obstructed (e.g., by a primary or metastatic neoplasm), alkaline phosphatase is released into the serum from the obstructed ducts, but the serum bilirubin may be normal. Prothrombin time is often prolonged in patients with obstructive jaundice as a result of the malabsorption of vitamin K. In obstructive jaundice, the water-soluble conjugated (direct) bilirubin is excreted in the urine. On the other hand, urobilinogen is produced in the intestine as a result of bacterial metabolism of bilirubin. Then it is reabsorbed from the intestine and secreted in the urine. Bile duct obstruction leads to the disappearance of urobilinogen from the urine because the excretion of bilirubin into the intestine is blocked.

Imaging Studies

Imaging studies are very helpful in establishing the definitive diagnosis in patients who have clinical features that suggest biliary disease. They are also useful in a variety of therapeutic interventions. Table 16-1 lists commonly used imaging studies and their diagnostic and therapeutic potential.

Approximately 10% to 15% of gallstones contain sufficient calcium to render them radiopaque. These stones are visible on plain x-rays of the abdomen (Figure 16-3). Air in the biliary system may be seen as a result of communication between the biliary and gastrointestinal tracts secondary to a pathologic fistula or a previous surgical procedure. Also, air in the lumen or wall of the gallbladder may be seen in acute emphysematous cholecystitis.

Ultrasonography is the initial study of choice in most patients with suspected biliary tract disease. For gallstones, both the sensitivity and the specificity of this study are approximately 95%. Ultrasonography can successfully detect stones as small as 3 mm in diameter, and sometimes even smaller stones may be seen (Figure 16-4). However, the study is not helpful for visualizing stones in the bile ducts. Ultrasonography is highly sensitive for detecting dilation of the bile ducts and may provide information on whether the site of biliary obstruction is intrahepatic or extrahepatic. If the gallbladder is distended and the ducts are dilated, the site of obstruction is likely to be distal to the junction of the cystic duct and the common hepatic duct. The finding of a thickened gallbladder wall or a pericholecystic collection of fluid supports the diagnosis of acute cholecystitis. Additionally, ultrasonography provides information about the liver and pancreas. The study is noninvasive, quick, and relatively inexpensive, and does not entail the use of radiation.

The oral cholecystogram has been replaced by ultrasonography for routine workup of patients with biliary colic. However, in situations where gallstones are suspected on clinical grounds but are not visualized on ultrasonography, oral cholecystogram may be performed as a backup study. The study is also indicated if dissolution therapy or lithotripsy is being considered. The night before an oral cholecystogram, the patient takes an oral contrast agent (Telepaque or Bilopaque). This agent is absorbed through the intestine. It enters the liver and is excreted into the bile and then concentrated in the gallbladder. X-rays of the right upper quadrant are obtained the next day (Figure 16-5). These x-rays may show an opacified gallbladder (with stones, if present) or may not show the gallbladder at all. In the

Table 16-1. Imaging Studies Commonly Used in the Diagnosis and Management of Biliary Disease

Imaging Procedure	Diagnostic or Therapeutic Potential
Plain abdominal x-ray	Calcified gallstone Air in the biliary tree Air in the gallbaldder wall or lumen
Ultrasonography	Stones in the gallbaldder Thickened gallbladder wall Dilation of intrahepatic and extrahepatic ducts Liver lesion Pancreatic mass
Radionuclide scan (HIDA scan)	Filling of gallbladder Filling of bile ducts Passage of bile into the duodenum
Computed tomography	Pancreatic mass Dilation of intrahepatic and extrahepatic ducts Liver lesion Stones in the gallbladder
Transhepatic cholangiogram	Detecting bile duct obstruction Draining obstructed bile duct Bypassing bile duct obstruction with stent Obtaining cytology specimen Detecting bile leak from ducts Extracting bile duct calculus

Endoscopic retrograde
   cholangiopancreatography
	Detecting bile duct obstruction
	Draining obstructed bile duct
	Inserting stent to bypass
	   obstruction or control bile leak
	Detecting pancreatic duct
	   obstruction
	Obtaining cytology specimen
	Detecting bile leak from ducts
	Extracting bile duct calculus
	Obtaining biopsy of a neoplasm
	Performing sphincterotomy

Oral cholecystography	Stones in gallbladder Filling of gallbladder

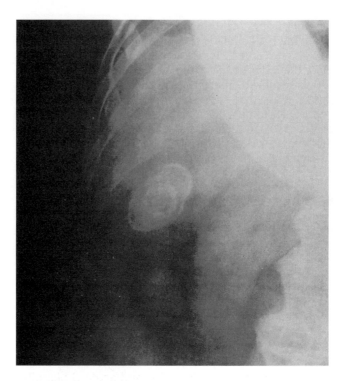

Figure 16-3 Plain x-ray of the abdomen showing gallstones.

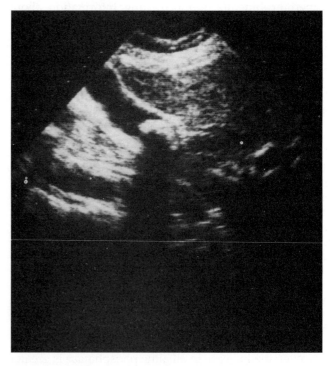

Figure 16-4 Ultrasound of the gallbladder showing gallstones.

latter situation, another dose of the contrast agent is administered and, again, x-rays are obtained the next day. If the gallbladder is still not visualized despite the double dose of contrast agent, there is a 95% chance that the gallbladder is diseased. However, nonvisualization of the gallbladder may also occur in patients with vomiting, intestinal malabsorption, or serum bilirubin levels greater than 2.5 mg/dL.

Radionuclide biliary scanning (HIDA scan) involves the intravenous injection of a ^{99m}technetium-labeled derivative of iminodiacetic acid. The radionuclide is excreted by the liver into the bile in high concentrations. Then it enters the gallbladder (if the cystic duct is patent) and duodenum. The normal gallbladder begins to fill within 30 minutes. Visualization of the common bile duct and duodenum without filling of the gallbladder after 4 hours indicates cystic duct obstruction and supports the diagnosis of acute cholecystitis

(Figure 16-6). The sensitivity and specificity of the HIDA scan for diagnosing acute cholecystitis are 95% to 97% and 90% to 97%, respectively. False-positive results may occur in patients who are receiving total parenteral nutrition or those who have hepatitis. The scan is also of value in identifying a suspected bile leak after surgery.

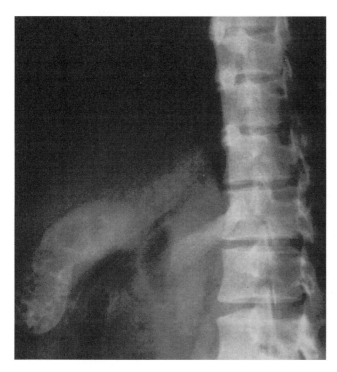

Figure 16-5 Oral cholecystogram showing gallstones.

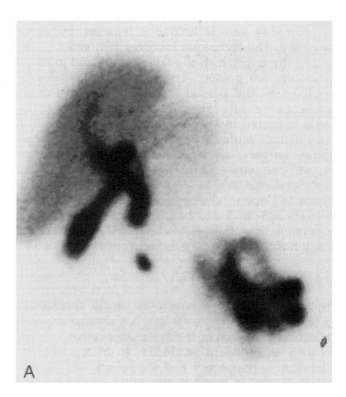

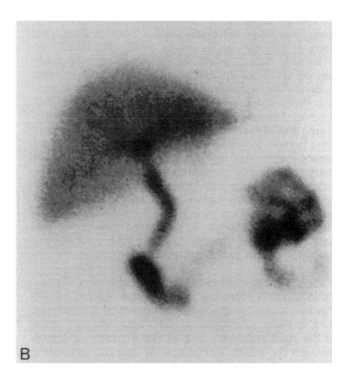

Figure 16-6 Radionuclide biliary (HIDA) scans, **A,** with and **B,** without visualization of the gallbladder.

However, the HIDA scan is not useful for showing stones in either the gallbladder or the common bile duct. The study can be successfully performed even when the serum bilirubin level is elevated.

In patients with jaundice, particularly with dilated ducts and evidence of extrahepatic obstruction on ultrasonography, detailed radiographic visualization of the biliary ductal anatomy may be helpful in confirming the diagnosis and planning therapy. Direct injection of contrast agent into the ducts is necessary in these cases. This may be achieved by performing a **percutaneous transhepatic cholangiogram (PTC)** or an **endoscopic retrograde cholangiopancreatogram (ERCP).** PTC involves inserting a thin needle through the skin and body wall, into the liver parenchyma, and injecting contrast medium directly into the intrahepatic bile ducts. Dilated bile ducts facilitate this procedure, yielding a success rate of more than 95%. If the ducts are of normal caliber, the test is successful only 70% to 80% of the time. PTC is particularly valuable for visualizing the proximal ductal system. It is also used to obtain a cytologic diagnosis, extract stones, and aid in the placement of a biliary drainage catheter into the obstructed bile ducts. ERCP requires a skilled endoscopist, who cannulates the sphincter of Oddi and injects contrast medium to obtain a picture of the biliary and pancreatic ductal anatomy. This study is particularly valuable in patients who have bile ducts of normal size and in those with suspected ampullary lesions, because a diagnostic biopsy specimen can also be obtained in the latter situation. Further, endoscopic brushing of an obstructed site may provide a cytologic diagnosis. In addition to imaging the bile duct and facilitating a biopsy, ERCP is used to perform a sphincterotomy. This procedure includes cutting the sphincter of Oddi with an electrosurgical current through a wire attached to the ERCP catheter. It is used to extract biliary calculi and place a stent through an area of bile duct obstruction. If coagulopathy is present, it must be corrected before either PTC or ERCP.

Computed tomography (CT) scan is especially helpful in identifying the level and cause of the biliary obstruction and in managing neoplasms. Specific anatomic definition of their size, position, and spread by the CT scan greatly assists in planning curative or palliative therapy. Also, percutaneous needle aspiration (cytology) or small-core needle biopsy (histology) performed with the aid of a CT scan can help in establishing a definitive diagnosis. CT scan is not the preferred test for the diagnosis of cholelithiasis because of its lower sensitivity in detecting gallstones, its higher cost compared with ultrasonography, and its use of radiation.

Magnetic resonance cholangiography is a new imaging technique that may prove helpful in diagnosing cal-

culi in the common bile duct. The obvious advantages of this diagnostic procedure are that it is noninvasive and does not involve the use of x-rays.

Intravenous cholangiography (IVC) consists of intravenous injection of an iodine-containing contrast material that is excreted through the liver into the bile ducts. It allows imaging of the common bile duct and gallbladder soon after injection because concentration of the contrast in the gallbladder is not necessary. The study indicates whether the cystic duct is patent (similar to an HIDA scan) and may also show stones in the bile duct. However, IVC has certain disadvantages. Some patients are allergic to the contrast material, and serious anaphylactic reactions have been reported. Also, the contrast agent is not excreted in the presence of jaundice. Because of these disadvantages, HIDA scanning has superceded IVC for the diagnosis of acute cholecystitis.

Figure 16-7 shows an algorithm for the evaluation of a jaundiced patient.

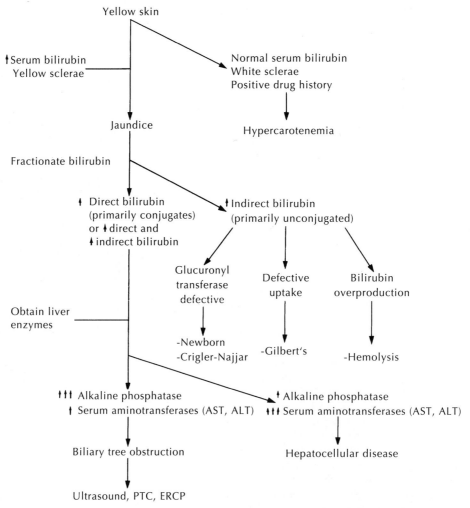

Figure 16-7 Algorithm for the evaluation of a jaundiced patient. *PTC* = percutaneous transhepatic cholangiogram; *ERCP* = endoscopic retrograde cholangiopancreatogram.

Clinical Presentation and Treatment of Gallstone Disease

Asymptomatic Gallstones

Many individuals have asymptomatic gallstones that remain silent throughout life. Of these individuals, approximately 1% to 2% per year will develop symptoms or complications of gallstone disease. Thus, two-thirds of these people remain free of symptoms or complications after 20 years. Also, the likelihood of complications decreases as the length of time the gallstones remain silent increases. Although complications secondary to gallstones may occur at any time, most patients experience symptoms for some time before a complication develops. Thus, in adults, prophylactic cholecystectomy is not routinely indicated for asymptomatic gallstones. However, after patients have even mild symptoms of biliary colic, they are at considerable risk for complications and should undergo elective cholecystectomy. Because the risk of septic complications in diabetic patients with gallstone disease may be higher than in the nondiabetic population, prophylactic cholecystectomy was recommended in the past for diabetic patients with asymptomatic gallstones. However, because of existing comorbid conditions, patients with diabetes mellitus are at increased risk for complications even after elective cholecystectomy. For this reason, prophylactic cholecystectomy is not routinely recommended for patients with diabetes mellitus and asymptomatic gallstones. The risk of gallbladder carcinoma in patients with gallstones is too low to justify cholecystectomy for asymptomatic gallstones. An exception to the conservative approach is made in the patient with a calcified ("porcelain") gallbladder because the incidence of gallbladder cancers is significantly higher in these cases.

Management of asymptomatic gallstones that are found at celiotomy for an unrelated intraabdominal problem requires special consideration. More than 50% of these patients become symptomatic postoperatively, and as many as 70% have symptoms within 6 months of the laparotomy. Acute cholecystitis is more likely to occur during the postoperative period as a result of a number of factors (e.g., prolonged fasting, dehydration, hypoxia, hypotension), and emergency cholecystectomy may be needed for the ensuing complications. In many elective operations, the addition of cholecystectomy to other abdominal procedures does not significantly alter the risk of morbidity and mortality. For this reason, when gallstones are found incidentally, cholecystectomy is indicated if it can be performed without technical difficulty. However, this approach is contraindicated in unstable patients, poor-risk individuals, and those with cirrhosis and portal hypertension. Also, because of the possibility of increased risk of graft infection, there is no consensus about the advisability of adding cholecystectomy to an aortic reconstruction procedure if asymptomatic gallstones are found at the time of the operation.

Chronic Cholecystitis

Biliary colic is the classic symptom associated with chronic calculous cholecystitis. Characteristic features of biliary colic were described earlier. Nausea and vomiting may accompany this pain. Other associated symptoms include intolerance to fatty foods, flatulence, belching, and indigestion. These symptoms are encompassed by the collective term dyspepsia. However, the symptoms of dyspepsia are nonspecific and may be secondary to other diseases. Because the condition is not associated with acute infection, fever and chills are absent. In contrast to patients who have acute inflammatory conditions, patients with biliary colic are typically not still and are often doubled-up or writhing during the episode of pain. Palpation of the abdomen during the episode of biliary colic may elicit tenderness in the right upper quadrant or the epigastrium, but there are no clinical signs of peritoneal irritation. The abdomen is generally soft, and bowel sounds are active. Between episodes of biliary colic, the abdomen shows no specific abnormality. The differential diagnosis includes angina pectoris, peptic ulcer disease, gastroesophageal reflux, ureteral obstruction, and irritable bowel syndrome.

Because biliary colic is not associated with acute inflammation, the total and differential leukocyte counts are within the normal range. In addition, liver function tests may be entirely normal. Typically, biliary colic is distinguished from acute cholecystitis by the presence of the characteristic clinical features described previously and by the absence of leukocytosis or a shift to the left. Ultrasonography is the preferred study for evaluation of the biliary tract in these patients. If the results of ultrasonography are equivocal, an oral cholecystogram is performed. ERCP with collection of bile for examination of microlithiasis is recommended for the occasional patient who presents with a clinical picture of biliary colic, but has negative findings on both ultrasonography and oral cholecystogram.

Management of the episode of biliary colic includes administration of parenteral analgesics for severe pain and observation. After cholelithiasis is confirmed, the optimum treatment is elective cholecystectomy. In most cases, the laparoscopic approach is used. An intraoperative **cholangiogram** may be added to evaluate the biliary ducts for stones (if these are suspected) or to delineate the ductal anatomy (which can facilitate the performance of the procedure). If the operative cholangiogram performed during the laparoscopic cholecystectomy shows common duct calculi, the duct should be explored laparoscopically, or the patient may be referred subsequently for ERCP and sphincterotomy to extract the stones. Both laparoscopic cholecystectomy and open cholecystectomy are highly effective in managing chronic calculous cholecystitis, and they are associated with very low rates of morbidity and mortality. Elective cholecystectomy is associated with an operative mortality rate of less than 0.5%, except in older or high-risk individuals, regardless of whether the laparoscopic or open approach is used. The risk of injury to the bile duct with laparoscopic cholecystectomy is 0.3% to 0.5%, slightly higher than the risk with open cholecystectomy. However, these injuries usually occur during the steep portion of the learning curve of the surgeon, and the risk diminishes as a surgeon gains experience.

In patients with comorbid conditions that preclude the performance of safe cholecystectomy and in those who refuse surgery, oral dissolution therapy may be considered. Bile acids have been used for this purpose, and ursodeoxycholic acid is the most desirable agent. However, the stones should be small and composed of cholesterol (floating, radiolucent stones), within a functioning gallbladder. Oral dissolution therapy, which may take 6 to 12 months to dissolve the stones, yields a dissolution rate of 90% for stones smaller than 5 mm and a dissolution rate of 60% for calculi smaller than 10 mm. However, in approximately 50% of these patients, the gallstones recur within 5 years of discontinuing the therapy. **Extracorporeal shock wave lithotripsy (ESWL) is** used to manage gallstone disease in selected patients, but support for this procedure has waned with the rise in popularity of laparoscopic cholecystectomy.

Acute Cholecystitis

The underlying pathology in acute cholecystitis is similar to that of biliary colic associated with chronic cholecystitis, except that there is sustained obstruction of the cystic duct in this condition. Thus, the gallbladder becomes progressively more distended and inflamed. As the disease progresses, inflammation extends from the visceral peritoneum overlying the gallbladder to involve the parietal peritoneum. Complications of empyema, gangrene, or perforation of the gallbladder may result from progression of the disease process and bacterial involvement. Most patients with acute cholecystitis have a history of biliary colic or dyspepsia. The pain of acute cholecystitis is constant. It is located in the right upper quadrant of the abdomen or the epigastrium and occasionally radiates to the back. Nausea and vomiting are common. The patient is usually febrile, but the fever rarely exceeds 38.3° C (101° F) unless a complication has supervened. On examination, the patient has tenderness in the right upper quadrant and a positive Murphy's sign. Once inflammation progresses to involve the parietal peritoneum, the patient has rebound tenderness and guarding. A tender mass is palpable in the right upper quadrant in approximately 20% of cases, and generalized peritonitis with rebound tenderness involving all quadrants may be present if the disease has progressed to free perforation. Free uncontained perforation with spillage of the gallbladder contents into the peritoneal cavity occurs in fewer than 1% to 2% of patients with acute cholecystitis.

The differential diagnosis includes acute pancreatitis, penetrating peptic ulcer (erosion into the pancreas), perforated peptic ulcer, and acute appendicitis. Laboratory studies show leukocytosis with a total leukocyte count of approximately 12,000 to 15,000/mL, and a shift to the left. Many patients with acute cholecystitis have mild

hyperbilirubinemia (total bilirubin level < 3–4 mg/mL). If the patient has higher levels of serum bilirubin, stones in the common bile duct should be suspected; however, perforation of the gallbladder also leads to high serum bilirubin levels. Mild increases in serum AST, ALT, and alkaline phosphatase are usually present, and the serum amylase level may also be moderately elevated.

Radiologic studies should include plain x-rays of the chest and abdomen. Upright views are necessary to exclude pneumoperitoneum from another underlying cause of the acute abdomen. Plain x-rays may also show gallstones if they are radiopaque. However, the finding of stones does not in itself establish the diagnosis of acute cholecystitis. Ultrasonography is very helpful in making a definitive diagnosis. In addition to detecting gallstones with a high degree of accuracy, the study often shows specific characteristic findings of acute cholecystitis, such as a distended gallbladder, thickened gallbladder wall (> 3–4 mm), pericholecystic fluid collection, and ultrasonographic Murphy's sign. This sign is elicited by demonstrating the presence of the most tender spot directly over the sonographically localized gallbladder with the ultrasound probe. This sign is present in 98% of patients with acute cholecystitis. HIDA scan is very useful in confirming the diagnosis of acute cholecystitis in cases in which ultrasonography shows gallstones, but there is no other ultrasonographic evidence to support the diagnosis. Nonvisualization of the gallbladder after 4 hours of the study indicates cystic duct obstruction and is interpreted as positive for acute cholecystitis. However, certain patients (e.g., individuals receiving total parenteral nutrition, those who have fasted for a long time), may demonstrate nonvisualization of the gallbladder on HIDA scan, yielding a false-positive result. Therefore, ultrasonography is preferred over HIDA scanning as the initial definitive radiologic study to confirm acute cholecystitis. It can also provide additional information about the liver, intrahepatic bile ducts, common bile duct, and pancreas, and it can be conveniently performed over a shorter period.

The initial management of acute cholecystitis includes a regimen of giving the patient nothing by mouth, administering intravenous fluids, and starting antibiotic therapy. The bacteria commonly associated with acute cholecystitis are *Escherichia coli*, *Klebsiella pneumoniae*, *Streptococcus faecalis*, and *Clostridium welchii* or *Clostridium perfringens*. Severe cases require broad antibiotic coverage, sometimes with multiple agents, to cover a wide spectrum of Gram-negative aerobes and enterococcus. Parenteral analgesics may be administered judiciously after the diagnosis is confirmed and further plans for therapy are made. A nasogastric tube is inserted if the patient has abdominal distension (with paralytic ileus) or is vomiting.

The optimum approach to treatment includes early cholecystectomy within 3 days of the onset of symptoms. This approach prevents complications (e.g., perforation, gangrene) and makes the surgical procedure easier than if it were performed later in the course of the disease, when the inflammatory reaction and edema are more severe. However, the timing of the operation must be based on other factors as well. It should be delayed if major medical problems must be addressed and performed earlier if perforation or abscess is suspected. The cholecystectomy may be performed laparoscopically, but this approach should be converted to an open one if bleeding or poor definition of the anatomy leads to technical difficulty. Overall, operations for acute cholecystitis are associated with higher mortality and morbidity rates compared with those for chronic cholecystitis, often as a result of underlying cardiovascular, pulmonary, or metabolic disease.

Patients with acute cholecystitis who are too ill to undergo cholecystectomy may require cholecystostomy performed under local anesthesia. This procedure involves the removal of the gallbladder contents and drainage of the gallbladder. Percutaneous cholecystostomy under radiologic guidance is another option.

Acute gangrenous cholecystitis is associated with a morbidity rate of 16% to 25% and a mortality rate of 20% to 25%. Patients with this condition tend to be older and generally have more serious comorbid conditions than patients with nongangrenous cholecystitis. Laboratory findings include leukocytosis with a shift to the left. HIDA scan may show pericholecystitic hepatic uptake along with nonvisualization of the gallbladder. Treatment includes stabilization of the medical condition, administration of broad-spectrum antibiotics, and performance of emergency cholecystectomy.

Acute emphysematous cholecystitis results from gas-forming bacteria and is associated with a higher risk of gangrene and perforation compared with nonemphysematous cholecystitis. It generally affects older individuals, and diabetes mellitus is present in 20% to 50% of these patients. The classic findings on plain x-rays include air within the wall or lumen of the gallbladder, air–fluid level within the lumen of the gallbladder, or air in the pericholecystic tissues. Air in the bile ducts may also be seen. Patients with acute emphysematous cholecystitis should receive broad-spectrum antibiotics, including coverage for anaerobes. In addition, they should undergo emergency cholecystectomy.

Although most patients with acute cholecystitis have associated calculi, acute cholecystitis can occur without calculi. **Acute acalculous cholecystitis** may complicate the course of a patient who is being treated for other conditions in a medical or surgical intensive care unit. Many patients are receiving total parenteral nutrition and mechanical ventilatory support and have received blood transfusions. Establishing the diagnosis of acute acalculous cholecystitis can present significant difficulty. The clinical features resemble those of acute calculous cholecystitis; however, the patient often cannot give a coherent history, and the associated conditions result in complex physical findings that are less revealing and more difficult to interpret. Ultrasonography is helpful in establishing the diagnosis. CT scan can also be useful. Ultrasonography may show gallbladder distension, thickened gallbladder wall, pericholecystic fluid, and a sonographic Murphy's sign. HIDA scan

may help to establish the diagnosis, but it often yields a false-positive result and is associated with a specificity of only 38% in such cases. After the diagnosis is established, the management is similar to that of patients with acute calculous cholecystitis. However, patients with acute acalculous cholecystitis are more likely to be candidates for operative or percutaneous cholecystostomy (instead of cholecystectomy) in view of their associated medical problems and higher risk for perioperative complications.

Choledocholithiasis and Acute Cholangitis

In approximately 15% of patients with gallstones, the stones pass through the cystic duct and enter the common bile duct, resulting in choledocholithiasis. Although the smaller stones that enter the common bile duct can progress further into the duodenum, choledocholithiasis may lead to sequelae associated with significant morbidity and mortality (e.g., cholangitis, pancreatitis).

Patients with choledocholithiasis often have a history of previous episodes of biliary colic. The characteristic feature in the clinical presentation is jaundice accompanied by light-colored stools and dark, tea-colored urine. The jaundice associated with choledocholithiasis typically fluctuates in intensity compared with the progressive jaundice caused by malignant disease. If infection supervenes, **acute cholangitis** will develop. It is characterized by jaundice, right upper quadrant abdominal pain, and fever associated with chills **(Charcot's triad)**. The condition can become further complicated with the presence of pus in the biliary ducts, resulting in **acute suppurative cholangitis.** In this condition, the patient may also have hypotension and mental confusion in addition to Charcot's triad. These five features together constitute **Reynold's pentad.**

On examination, a patient with choledocholithiasis appears deeply jaundiced if a stone is obstructing the duct. Fever is characteristically associated with acute cholangitis and acute suppurative cholangitis; however, septic and debilitated patients may have hypothermia. Examination of the abdomen may be unremarkable in a patient with choledocholithiasis or may reveal tenderness (without a palpable mass) in the right upper quadrant if cholangitis is present. Rebound tenderness is not usually found, even in the presence of acute cholangitis. Bowel sounds are generally audible and may even be normal.

The differential diagnosis in patients with obstructive jaundice or cholangitis includes choledocholithiasis, malignancy (e.g., carcinoma of the pancreas, bile ducts, or gallbladder), and stricture.

The diagnostic workup of jaundice associated with probable choledocholithiasis starts with laboratory studies described previously. In patients with cholangitis, the leukocyte count is elevated, with a shift to the left. Bile duct obstruction leads to elevation in total bilirubin, with a predominance of the direct fraction, marked elevation of serum alkaline phosphatase, and mild elevations of AST and ALT. Serum amylase may also be moderately elevated. Ultrasonography is the best initial imaging study in patients with choledocholithiasis and cholangitis. It often shows dilated intrahepatic and extrahepatic ducts along with the presence of gallstones, suggesting that stones are the likely cause of the common duct obstruction. As stated previously, stones in the common bile duct are not usually seen on ultrasonography. PTC and ERCP are the best studies to define the specific site and determine the source of the bile duct obstruction. Figure 16-8 shows a PTC demonstrating the typical meniscus sign in the distal common bile duct, indicating that the obstruction is secondary to stones. ERCP may be very useful for extracting stones from the common bile duct. Oral cholecystography, IVC, and HIDA scan are not helpful in the evaluation of a patient with common bile duct obstruction.

The management of patients with choledocholithiasis varies with the clinical situation. A patient with choledocholithiasis without evidence of cholangitis should undergo elective cholecystectomy and extraction of stones from the common duct. Extraction may be achieved operatively or endoscopically (through ERCP and sphincterotomy). The management of acute cholan-

gitis, especially acute suppurative cholangitis, requires urgent intervention, and septic shock (if present) necessitates prompt resuscitation. A patient with cholangitis is started on a regimen of nothing by mouth, administration of intravenous fluids, and antibiotic therapy after blood cultures are obtained. The broad spectrum of aerobic and anaerobic bacteria listed in the section on acute cholecystitis as well as *Enterobacter* and *Pseudomonas* species must be considered in selecting the appropriate antibiotic coverage. Any clotting abnormalities should be corrected by giving vitamin K or administering fresh frozen plasma before an invasive procedure. Vomiting or abdominal distension resulting from paralytic ileus necessitates the insertion of a nasogastric tube. More than 70% of patients with cholangitis respond to this regimen, thus allowing for completion of the workup and adequate planning for the definitive treatment, which includes cholecystectomy and extraction of stones from the common bile duct. If a patient does not respond to this therapy, urgent decompression of the bile duct through open surgery, PTC, or ERCP can be lifesaving. Patients with acute suppurative cholangitis require urgent decompression of the common bile duct after the initial resuscitation and administration of broad-spectrum antibiotics.

Stones detected in the bile duct by any type of cholangiography before cholecystectomy may be managed by performing an open procedure, which includes cholecystectomy and bile duct exploration. Alternatively, bile duct calculi can be removed through ERCP and sphincterotomy, and the patient can then undergo laparoscopic cholecystectomy. The success rate with ERCP and sphincterotomy in these cases is greater than 90%, with a complication rate of approximately 10%. If the surgeon is experienced in advanced laparoscopic biliary surgery, laparoscopic cholecystectomy and extraction of the bile duct calculi through the cystic duct or choledochotomy is also an option. If the gallbladder was previously removed, the bile duct calculi should be removed endoscopically with ERCP and sphincterotomy. Lithotripsy can be used to break large stones. The fragments can then pass spontaneously or be removed with ERCP and sphincterotomy or PTC. If the stones cannot be removed by these methods, an open procedure is necessary.

Acute Biliary (Gallstone) Pancreatitis

Approximately 60% of nonalcoholic patients with acute pancreatitis have associated gallstones. Although the occurrence of **acute biliary (gallstone) pancreatitis** is usually attributed to transient or persistent obstruction of the ampulla of Vater by a large stone, passage of small stones and biliary sludge rather than the impaction of a large stone is often the cause of the pancreatitis. Patients with acute biliary pancreatitis have the classic clinical picture of pancreatitis; however, the serum amylase levels are characteristically very high compared with patients with alcoholic pancreatitis, who may have less functioning pancreatic tissue because of chronic alcohol consumption.

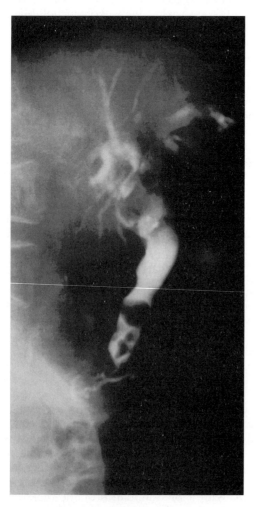

Figure 16-8 Percutaneous transhepatic cholangiogram showing common bile duct obstruction secondary to gallstones.

Management of patients with acute biliary pancreatitis includes initial resuscitation and supportive care, with correction of any existing fluid deficits and treatment of respiratory insufficiency, if present. Antibiotics are added for severe pancreatitis and for the management of septic complications. Parenteral analgesics may be administered once the diagnosis is made and treatment is initiated. Determination of the severity of the disease and prognostication of outcomes are carried out with the same criteria as for alcoholic pancreatitis. After the initial conservative management, a definitive operation should be performed after the patient improves clinically, during the same hospitalization. This procedure includes cholecystectomy, cholangiography, and extraction of stones from the common bile duct if any are detected on the cholangiogram. Acute pancreatitis recurs in 25% to 60% of patients if a definitive operation is not performed at this time. However, the operation should be delayed in patients with very severe pancreatitis unless infected pancreatic necrosis or cholangitis is present, both of which occur infrequently in patients with acute biliary pancreatitis. Progression of the disease despite conservative management may necessitate urgent ERCP and sphincterotomy.

Gallstone Ileus

Although **gallstone ileus** accounts for only 1% to 3% of all cases of intestinal obstruction, the condition is the cause of nonstrangulated small intestinal obstruction in approximately 25% of patients older than 70 years of age. It occurs more commonly in women than in men (3.5:1 ratio). Gallstone ileus results from the erosion of a large stone through the gallbladder directly into the small intestine through an internal fistula between the gallbladder and the intestinal tract, usually at the level of duodenum. Passage of the stone along the length of the small intestine may cause episodes of partial small bowel obstruction until the stone becomes impacted in a narrow portion of the intestine, usually in the distal ileum just proximal to the ileocecal valve. A history of biliary colic or gallstone disease suggests the diagnosis. Patients present with the clinical picture of small intestinal obstruction; however, the intermittent nature of the obstruction in the early stages (before impaction of the stone) often results in delay in the diagnosis.

Plain x-rays of the abdomen show findings of small intestinal obstruction and may show air in the biliary tree. Ultrasonography is useful in detecting gallstones and may even reveal the offending stone, although it may be difficult to visualize because of the overlying gas-containing loops of intestine. Barium study of the small intestine may demonstrate the biliary-enteric fistula and confirm the distal small intestinal obstruction. However, even with the availability of imaging studies, the correct diagnosis of gallstone ileus as the cause of small intestinal obstruction is made preoperatively in fewer than one-half of patients.

Appropriate management of gallstone ileus includes celiotomy and enterolithotomy (extraction of the stone from the small intestine to relieve the obstruction). In selected patients who are otherwise healthy, cholecystectomy and definitive correction of the internal fistula may also be performed. Because many patients with gallstone ileus are elderly and have other comorbid conditions, cholecystectomy and correction of the fistula are often deferred, sometimes being performed during a second operation. The mortality rate remains high because of the frequent coexistence of medical problems (e.g., cardiac disease, diabetes mellitus, obesity). There is also a high risk of postoperative wound infection.

Gallbladder Cancer

Gallbladder cancer is uncommon and accounts for less than 2% of all malignant tumors. It generally occurs in the elderly and is more common in women than in men. Nearly 80% of patients have gallstones. Gallbladder cancer tends to spread early through direct invasion of the liver and porta hepatis, and by metastasizing to the regional lymph nodes and liver. Histologically, most such cancers are adenocarcinomas.

Presenting symptoms include vague right upper quadrant abdominal pain, weight loss, and malaise. Jaundice is present in approximately 50% of cases. Physical examination may show a mass in the right upper quadrant of the abdomen. Gallbladder cancer is seldom detected early and is often not diagnosed preoperatively. The disease may be discovered unexpectedly during cholecystectomy for chronic calculous cholecystitis.

If the disease is found to be localized during elective cholecystectomy, wedge resection of the gallbladder fossa and liver bed and regional lymphadenectomy should be performed. The 5-year survival rate is still poor (< 5% at 5 years) unless the cancer is detected incidentally as a small focus within the gallbladder wall during pathologic examination of the gallbladder specimen.

Extrahepatic Bile Duct Malignancies

Cancer of the extrahepatic bile ducts is uncommon, with an autopsy incidence of 0.01% to 0.5%. It occurs with equal frequency in both sexes and is most common in individuals between 50 and 70 years of age. The risk of bile duct malignancy is significantly higher in patients with ulcerative colitis and sclerosing cholangitis. Other risk factors include choledochal cysts and parasitic disease. Approximately one-third of patients with bile duct carcinoma have associated gallstones. The bile duct tumors are usually well circumscribed, and two-thirds of these carcinomas are located above the junction of the cystic duct with the common hepatic duct. Histologically, the lesions are usually mucin-producing adenocarcinomas. In general, these are slow-growing, locally invasive tumors that rarely metastasize to distant sites. However, because of the intimate anatomic relation of the extrahepatic bile ducts to the liver, portal vein, and common hepatic artery, curative resection of these lesions is the exception rather than the rule.

Common symptoms include jaundice, weight loss, abdominal pain, and pruritus; fever is less common. In contrast to the fluctuating jaundice that is often seen in patients with common duct calculi, the jaundice associated with bile duct cancers is progressive. On physical examination, hepatomegaly may be found. A palpable, nontender gallbladder indicates that the site of the obstructing tumor is distal to the junction of the cystic duct with the common duct.

Laboratory studies show a typical picture of obstructive jaundice. As with other patients who have jaundice, ultrasonography is a good initial study. It may show dilated intrahepatic ducts; however, the absence of intrahepatic ductal dilation does not rule out obstruction. The ducts may not be dilated because of incomplete obstruction, tumor encasement, or sclerosing cholangitis. Both ultrasonography and CT scanning are helpful in determining the extrabiliary extent of the tumors and providing information about their resectability. PTC and ERCP are very helpful in demonstrating the lesion, determining the intraductal tumor extent, and obtaining cytologic specimens. PTC is particularly useful for evaluation of the proximal lesions.

Tumors in the proximal one-third of the ductal system may require resection of both the left and right hepatic ducts with a Roux-en-Y hepaticojejunostomy. If resection is not possible, the tumor may be dilated and a stent passed through it to relieve the biliary obstruction. Resection of bile duct cancers offers the best chance of survival, although the prognosis after resection of these proximal lesions remains poor: the 5-year survival rate is only 0% to 5%. Middle-third tumors are also best treated by resection and a Roux-en-Y hepaticojejunostomy. The 5-year survival rate after resection of middle-third lesions is approximately 10%. Like proximal regions, unresectable lesions may be bypassed with a stent. The operation of choice for distal common duct tumors is a Whipple procedure, which involves resecting the distal stomach, distal common duct (with the tumor), pancreatic head, and entire duodenum. Three anastomoses (i.e., pancreaticojejunostomy, choledochojejunostomy, and gastrojejunostomy) must be performed after the resection. The 5-year survival rate after a Whipple procedure for a lesion in the distal third of the common duct is approximately 30%. If resection is not possible, palliation can be achieved through internal surgical bypass (Roux-en-Y choledochojejunostomy) or stent insertion. Surgical bypass is preferable in good-risk patients because the anastomosis will probably be associated with longer patency and improved quality of life. Stents may become obstructed and are often complicated by cholangitis.

Bile Duct Injury and Stricture

Because bile ducts have a low elastin content, little redundancy, and a poor blood supply, injury can be potentially disastrous. More than 90% of bile duct strictures result from iatrogenic injury during an operative procedure. Most severe injuries involve the common hepatic duct or the confluence of the right and left hepatic ducts. Approximately 75% of injuries occur during simple cholecystectomy, underscoring the importance of recognizing the anatomic variations of the biliary tree correctly and proceeding in a cautious, systematic fashion, even during routine cholecystectomy. The incidence of bile duct injuries associated with laparoscopic cholecystectomy is higher than that associated with open cholecystectomy, but should decrease with the surgeon's experience. Unfortunately, many iatrogenic injuries go unrecognized until they cause complications from delayed stricture formation.

When bile duct injury is suspected at the time of the initial operation, intraoperative cholangiography should be performed. If a duct smaller than 3 mm is found to be injured, it should simply be ligated. If the injured duct is 4 mm or larger, immediate operative repair should be carried out. Primary repair of a simple ductal injury may be performed over a T-tube stent, which is brought out through another location in the common duct. A choledochoenteric anastomosis should be performed if there is significant loss of length of the common duct. In the early postoperative period, bile duct injury may cause unexpected abdominal pain, jaundice, drainage of bile (from a drain or through the wound), signs of acute abdomen, and sepsis. HIDA scan is useful in confirming the presence of bile extravasation. Ultrasonography or CT scan may be obtained to detect or exclude an intraabdominal collection. Definition of the exact location of the ductal injury requires either PTC or ERCP. A minor leak from an accessory hepatic duct is likely to heal spontaneously and merely requires placement of a percutaneous catheter under CT or ultrasonic guidance. Leakage from a cystic duct stump requires placement of a stent with the aid of ERCP. If major ductal injury is detected postoperatively, repair should be undertaken after the initial management, which includes control of the bile leak and treatment of sepsis.

Late development of stricture leads to obstructive jaundice and recurrent cholangitis, and long-standing strictures may result in biliary cirrhosis and portal hypertension. The diagnosis of stricture is confirmed by PTC or ERCP. Cholangitis should be managed with antibiotics and the stricture treated by anastomosing the dilated proximal bile duct to a Roux-en-Y loop of jejunum. A stent is passed through the anastomosis and left in place long enough to prevent restricturing. In the hands of experienced surgeons, excellent outcome from the operative repair is achieved in 70% to 90% of patients. For poor-risk patients, balloon dilation and stenting may be an option.

Table 16-2 summarizes the common clinical syndromes and complications that result from cholelithiasis.

Table 16-2. Summary of the Common Clinical Syndromes that Result from Cholelithiasis and the Complications of Cholelithiasis

Syndrome	Etiology	Findings
Biliary colic	Transient cystic duct obstruction	Episodes of upper abdominal pain Nonspecific physical findings Ultrasound: cholelithiasis
Acute cholecystitis	Sustained cystic duct obstruction Acute inflammation of gallbladder	Constant, severe right upper quadrant pain Elevated temperature Murphy's sign Rebound tenderness Leucocytosis Mild hyperbilirubinemia Ultrasound: cholelithiasis, with or without other signs of gallbladder inflammation HIDA: nonvisualization of gallbladder
Choledocholithiasis	Stone in the common bile duct (can cause intermittent obstruction, "ball-valve" effect) Infected bile; septicemia	History of abdominal pain, jaundice, light stool, dark urine Laboratory findings: obstructive jaundice picture Ultrasound: cholelithiasis with dilated ducts
Acute cholangitis	Stone impacted in the common bile duct Stricture of the common bile duct (previous biliary surgery); tumor Tumor obstructing the common bile duct (especially after an invasive diagnostic procedure which might have seeded the bile with bacteria)	History same as choledocholithiasis but acutely ill patient with abdominal pain, jaundice, fever, chills; may also have hypotension and change in mentation (in acute suppurative cholangitis) Laboratory findings: same as choledocholithiasis, plus elevated white blood cell count Ultrasound: same as choledocholithiasis, but gallbladder may have been removed previously if the etiology is a stricture
Biliary (gallstone) pancreatitis	Passage of small stones or sludge through the sphincter of Oddi Acute pancreatitis	Acutely ill, severe constant epigastric pain, with or without radiation through to the back With or without history of biliary colic Tenderness, guarding in upper abdomen Markedly elevated serum amylase Ultrasound and CT scan: cholelithiasis, with or without inflammatory mass in pancreas

HIDA, radionuclide biliary scan.
CT, computed tomography.

Brief Description of Selected Procedures

Open Cholecystectomy and Common Bile Duct Exploration

Open cholecystectomy is generally performed through a right subcostal incision. After the abdomen is entered, the gallbladder is exposed by packing off the adjacent viscera. The gallbladder is held with a clamp, and the triangle of Calot is exposed by applying appropriate traction. Dissection is carried out to isolate the cystic artery and cystic duct. Both of these structures are divided and ligated or clipped. The gallbladder is dissected free from the liver and removed. A drain is not routinely placed after elective cholecystectomy. An intraoperative cholangiogram may be performed through the cystic duct to define the biliary anatomy and confirm or exclude suspected choledocholithiasis.

There are absolute and relative indications for common bile duct exploration during open cholecystec-

tomy. Absolute indications include a palpable common duct calculus and common duct calculi visualized on preoperative or intraoperative cholangiography. Relative indications include jaundice, acute biliary pancreatitis, ductal dilation, small gallbladder stones (smaller than the cystic duct), and a single-faceted gallbladder stone (facets on a gallstone require the presence of at least two stones, suggesting that a second stone may have passed through into the common duct). Operative cholangiography is performed to confirm or exclude the stones in the bile duct when only relative indications for bile duct exploration are present.

The procedure for common bile duct exploration involves mobilizing the duodenum (Kocher maneuver) and making a small vertical incision in the common duct. Then the lumen is irrigated with saline using flexible catheters to help flush out stones and debris from the duct. Inflatable balloon catheters are passed in both proximal and distal directions in an attempt to extract stones. A small endoscope (choledochoscope) is advanced through the opening, and the duct is carefully visualized both proximally and distally. A variety of instruments, including stone forceps and collapsible wire "baskets," are available to remove stones that remain impacted and resist removal by flushing and balloon catheters. All stones, mucus, and debris are removed, and the duct is irrigated with saline. A T-tube is then placed in the lumen of the duct, and the opening in the duct is closed around the T-tube. A completion cholangiogram is obtained to ensure that no other stones remain in the duct before the abdomen is closed. A closed drainage catheter is often left in the subhepatic space. When there are multiple stones and the surgeon believes that stones may have been left in the bile duct, it is prudent to perform a choledochoduodenostomy, sphincteroplasty, or choledochojejunostomy so that residual stones can pass easily from the duct into the intestine.

The peritoneal drain is usually removed within 24 to 48 hours postoperatively if the drainage is minimal, but it should be left in place longer if it is draining significant amounts of blood or bile. These complications must be addressed further. A T-tube is placed to gravity drainage for 1 week. Then a T-tube cholangiogram is obtained. In the absence of residual filling defects, the T-tube is clamped for 24 hours, and if the patient remains asymptomatic, the tube is removed. The tract should drain for 1 to 3 days and then close spontaneously. If there is any concern about the interpretation of the cholangiogram, the T-tube is left in place for a longer period.

Occasionally, despite thorough duct exploration, a filling defect is noted in the postoperative T-tube cholangiogram, indicating a missed or retained stone. In approximately 20% of patients, these stones pass spontaneously, especially if they are small. The T-tube is left in place for 4 to 6 weeks. Then the retained stone or stones may be extracted with one of two approaches. The usual approach is to remove the T-tube and advance a basket through the T-tube tract into the duct under fluoroscopy to retrieve the stones (Figure 16-9). This approach is successful in as many as 95% of cases in the hands of skilled operators. A flexible choledochoscope may also be advanced through the tract to assist with stone retrieval under direct vision, using the basket. The other approach involves ERCP and sphincterotomy. Stones may pass spontaneously after the sphincterotomy or may be extracted with balloon catheters or baskets. Lithotripsy may be used to fragment larger stones in the common duct to facilitate extraction. If none of these methods is successful, operative reexploration of the duct is necessary. Dissolution of cholesterol stones with solvents has been described by some investigators, but this approach requires prolonged treatment, has a significant failure rate, and is not frequently used because of the high likelihood of success with the techniques described earlier.

Laparoscopic Cholecystectomy

Laparoscopic cholecystectomy has replaced open cholecystectomy as the preferred approach to the management of gallstone disease in most elective and many emergency situations. The procedure begins with inflation of the peritoneal cavity with carbon dioxide gas to a pressure of 15 mm Hg or less and insertion of a 10-mm

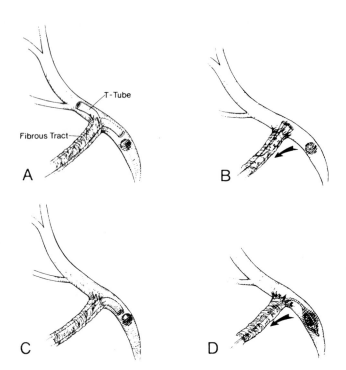

Figure 16-9 Extraction of a retained common bile duct stone through the T-tube tract using a basket.

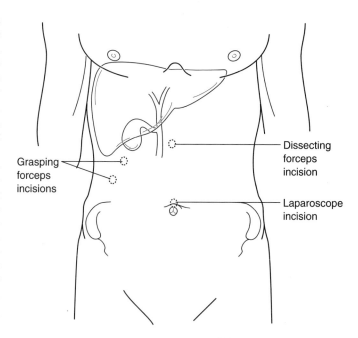

Figure 16-10 Sites for ports used in laparoscopic cholecystectomy.

sheath into the peritoneal cavity through an umbilical port. This port may also be inserted with the open technique. The laparoscope, with an attached video camera and light source, is inserted through the sheath into the peritoneal cavity. The image is viewed on a television monitor, and a 10-mm sheath is inserted under direct vision into the upper abdomen to the right of the midline (Figure 16-10). Two 5-mm sheaths are inserted into the right abdomen, again under direct vision. The fun-

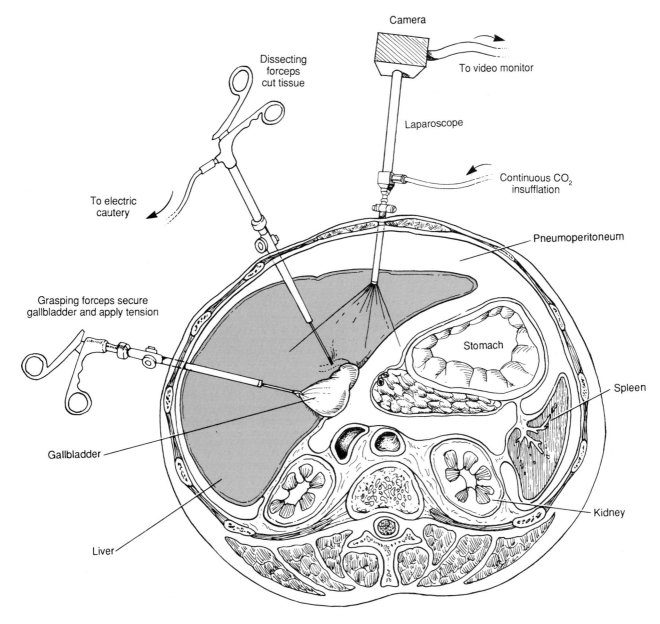

Figure 16-11 Cross-section of a laparoscopic cholecystectomy.

dus of the gallbladder is grasped with a forceps, and the gallbladder and liver are pushed cephalad (Figure 16-11). The triangle of Calot is exposed by applying appropriate traction, and the cystic artery and duct are dissected, clipped, and divided. The gallbladder is then dissected free from the liver bed. The gallbladder and its contents are extracted from the peritoneal cavity, usually through the umbilical port. The advantages of the laparoscopic approach are minimal postoperative pain, minimal wound and pulmonary complications, the possibility of ambulatory surgery or a short hospitalization, and rapid recovery, with early return to normal activity. The main risk associated with the laparoscopic approach is injury to the bile ducts, intestine, and major vessels (almost always resulting from blind trocar insertion). However, with greater experience of the operating

surgeon, the risk of complications should diminish significantly. If anatomy is obscured because of the pathologic process or technical difficulty is encountered with the laparoscopic approach, it is prudent to convert it to an open procedure. There is some controversy as to whether cholangiography should be performed routinely or selectively at the time of laparoscopic cholecystectomy. If stones are found in the common bile duct on cholangiography, they may be removed laparoscopically (if the operator is skilled) or with ERCP and sphincterotomy postoperatively. The procedure can also be converted to an open one to extract the stones.

Extracorporeal Shock Wave Lithotripsy

ESWL is used to fragment kidney stones so that they can pass through the urinary tract. Some believe that the same principle could be applied to the treatment of gall-stones. The gallstones are imaged by ultrasonography, and a shock wave is delivered to the stones with special equipment. The criteria for patient selection include the history of at least one recent episode of biliary colic, cholelithiasis confirmed by ultrasonography, a function-ing gallbladder (as seen by oral cholecystography), the absence of acute gallbladder inflammation, the presence of one to three radiolucent stones, and a total stone bur-den that does not exceed 30 mm. ESWL is most effective in patients who have a single stone 20 mm in diameter or smaller. Contraindications to ESWL include acute cholecystitis, cholangitis, pancreatitis, choledocholithia-sis, liver disease, coagulopathy, pregnancy, and a pace-maker. The procedure is generally safe, but patients fre-quently have colic after the procedure. The fragments and sand that result from lithotripsy must be dissolved with a bile acid (e.g., ursodeoxycholic acid) that is taken for at least 1 year. ESWL may need to be repeated if the fragments are large. Between 20% and 30% of treated patients will have gallstones again 5 years after the com-pletion of ESWL and dissolution therapy. ESWL has not gained wide acceptance because of limited patient eligi-bility, a high failure rate, a high recurrence rate, the need for long-term use of an expensive solvent (e.g., ursodeoxycholic acid), and the need for expensive equipment.

Multiple-Choice Questions

1. The most common types of gallstones in western society are caused by the supersaturation of the fol-lowing substance in bile:
   A. Bilirubin
   B. Bile salts
   C. Cholesterol
   D. Lecithin
   E. Calcium

2. Each of the following is associated with an increased incidence of gallstones EXCEPT:
   A. Regional enteritis
   B. Essential hypertension
   C. Native American race
   D. Total parenteral nutrition
   E. Sickle cell anemia

3. Biliary colic is caused by:
   A. A stone obstructing the cystic duct
   B. Passage of a stone through the ampulla of Vater
   C. Acute infection within the bile ducts
   D. Inflammation of the pancreas
   E. Inflammation of the gallbladder

4. A 45-year-old obese woman has a 6-hour history of constant pain in the upper abdomen. It is most pro-nounced in the epigastrium and right upper quadrant. On examination, she has a temperature of 37.8° C (100° F), and there is tenderness and guarding in the

right upper quadrant of the abdomen. The total leuko-cyte count is 12,000/mm³, with a shift to the left. The total serum bilirubin level is 1.5 mg/dL, with mild elevations of serum aspartate aminotransferase (AST), alanine aminotransferase (ALT), alkaline phos-phatase, and amylase.
   The most likely diagnosis is:
   A. Acute hepatitis
   B. Acute cholangitis
   C. Acute pancreatitis
   D. Acute duodenal ulcer
   E. Acute cholecystitis

5. A 50-year-old obese man has a history of episodic postprandial upper abdominal pain, located mainly in the right upper quadrant. The pain lasts for 1 to 4 hours each time and is associated with nausea. The patient has a history of excessive flatulence. The ini-tial diagnostic study of choice is:
   A. Ultrasonography
   B. Barium upper gastrointestinal series
   C. Oral cholecystography
   D. Radionuclide biliary (HIDA) scan
   E. Computed tomography (CT) scan

6. A 48-year-old woman is found to have gallstones on ultrasonography performed to evaluate the right kid-ney. She has no symptoms attributable to the gall-stones and was previously in good health. The appro-priate management of the gallstones includes:
   A. Laparoscopic cholecystectomy
   B. Open cholecystectomy
   C. Observation
   D. Extracorporeal shock wave lithotripsy (ESWL)
   E. Dissolution therapy

7. A 60-year-old man has a 2-week history of jaundice, dark urine, and pruritus. On examination, he is icteric, afebrile, and has a palpable, nontender glob-ular mass in the right upper quadrant of the abdomen.
   The most likely diagnosis is:
   A. Choledocholithiasis
   B. Acute cholecystitis
   C. Acute hepatitis
   D. Carcinoma of the head of the pancreas
   E. Acute cholangitis

8. The following statement about gallbladder cancer is true:
   A. Gallstones are present in approximately 80% of cases.
   B. The usual symptoms include episodic abdominal pain, fever, and jaundice.
   C. Abdominal examination often shows a tender mass in the right upper quadrant.
   D. Cholecystectomy is adequate treatment.
   E. The overall 5-year survival rate is approximately 45%.

9. A 69-year-old woman is brought to the emergency room with a history of upper abdominal pain, vomiting, jaundice, and fever. On examination, her temperature is 38.9° C (102° F), pulse rate is 110/min, and blood pressure is 120/80 mm Hg. She is in moderate distress, but is alert and oriented. The abdomen is distended, with tenderness in the right upper quadrant. Laboratory studies include the following: total leukocyte count, 15,000/mm³, with a shift to the left; total serum bilirubin, 12 mg/dL; conjugated bilirubin, 8 mg/dL; serum alkaline phosphatase, 680 U/L (normal 35–125 U/L); aspartate aminotransferase (AST), 112 U/L (normal 15–35 U/L); alanine aminotransferase (ALT), 170 U/L (normal 10–50 U/L); prothrombin time, 30 seconds (control, 12–14 seconds). Initial management includes all of the following EXCEPT:
   A. Intravenous fluids
   B. Intravenous antibiotics
   C. Nasogastric intubation
   D. Administration of vitamin K
   E. Emergency celiotomy

10. Which of the following statements about extrahepatic bile duct malignancies is true?
   A. Extrahepatic bile duct malignancies occur more commonly in women than in men.
   B. Neoplasms most frequently involve the distal one-third of the common bile duct.
   C. Neoplasms metastasize early to distant sites.
   D. The 5-year survival rate after resection of malignancies in the distal one-third of the common bile duct is approximately 30%.
   E. Neoplasms in the proximal one-third of the common bile duct are best treated by radiation therapy.

11. Antibiotic treatment for acute cholecystitis should include coverage of all of the following microorganisms EXCEPT:
   A. *Escherichia coli*
   B. *Klebsiella pneumoniae*
   C. *Streptococcus faecalis*
   D. *Helicobacter pylori*
   E. *Clostridium welchii*

12. The following statement about gallstone ileus is true:
   A. The patients are usually 40 to 50 years old.
   B. An internal fistula is present.
   C. Jaundice and fever are common.
   D. Abdominal x-rays show a picture consistent with paralytic ileus.
   E. Nonoperative therapy usually results in resolution of the problem.

13. All of the following statements about bile duct injury are true EXCEPT:
   A. Approximately 75% of bile duct injuries occur during simple cholecystectomy.
   B. The incidence of injuries associated with laparoscopic cholecystectomy is higher than that associated with open cholecystectomy.

C. Most injuries are not recognized at the time of occurrence.
   D. Delay in recognition and repair of the injury often results in stricture formation.
   E. Repair of bile duct structures yields good results in only 10% to 20% of cases.

14. Advantages of laparoscopic cholecystectomy over open cholecystectomy include all of the following EXCEPT:
   A. Minimal postoperative pain
   B. Shorter hospitalization
   C. Minimal wound complications
   D. Lower risk of bile duct injury
   E. Earlier return to normal activity

15. Optimum management of acute cholecystitis includes all of the following EXCEPT:
   A. Giving nothing by mouth
   B. Administering intravenous antibiotics
   C. Administering a parenteral analgesic
   D. Selective nasogastric intubation
   E. Delayed operation, after the condition resolves clinically

16. The following statement about acute biliary (gallstone) pancreatitis is true:
   A. The usual underlying cause is a large stone impacted at the ampulla of Vater.
   B. Abdominal pain is less severe than with alcoholic pancreatitis.
   C. After clinical improvement, definitive operation should be performed during the same hospitalization.
   D. The serum amylase level is generally lower than in alcoholic pancreatitis.
   E. Endoscopic retrograde cholangiopancreatogram (ERCP) and sphincterotomy should be performed as soon as possible after the diagnosis is made.

17. Radionuclide biliary (HIDA) scan is most helpful in diagnosing:
   A. Acute cholecystitis
   B. Acute cholangitis
   C. Chronic calculous cholecystitis
   D. Acute pancreatitis
   E. Choledocholithiasis

Questions 18–20
   A. Endoscopic retrograde cholangiopancreatogram (ERCP)
   B. Percutaneous transhepatic cholangiogram (PTC)
   C. Both
   D. Neither

18. Higher success rate if ultrasonography shows dilated intrahepatic ducts

19. May be used to obtain a specimen for cytologic diagnosis

20. May be used to extract biliary calculi

Oral Examination Study Questions

CASE 1

A 52-year-old obese woman comes to your office with episodic severe pain in the epigastrium and right upper quadrant of the abdomen for the past 8 months. The patient has a history of accompanying nausea and one episode of vomiting.

OBJECTIVE 1

The student obtains the relevant history.

A. The pain is episodic, steady, and severe. It generally lasts 1 to 3 hours each time, and then subsides.

B. The pain is poorly localized. It is located mainly in the epigastrium and right upper quadrant of the abdomen.

C. The patient has two to three episodes of pain each month. On occasion, it awakens the patient at night.

D. The pain is often triggered by meals. The patient achieves some relief of pain if she is doubled-up in bed. She obtains no relief with antacids.

E. The patient also has nausea. She had a single episode of vomiting. She also has occasional heartburn after large meals, and excessive flatulence.

F. The patient has no jaundice, no fever, no change in the color of urine or stool, no melena, and no weight loss. She has diet-controlled diabetes mellitus. She had no previous surgery.

OBJECTIVE 2

The student requests pertinent information about the physical examination.

A. The student observes an obese patient who is in no distress.

B. The skin shows no icterus.

C. The eyes show no scleral icterus.

D. The pulse rate is 80 beats/min, blood pressure is 120/85 mm Hg, respiratory rate is 20/min, and temperature is 37.1° C (98.8° F).

E. The abdomen is soft and nontender, with no palpable mass.

OBJECTIVE 3

The student discusses the differential diagnosis and explains reasons in support of the most likely diagnosis.

A. The differential diagnosis includes biliary colic secondary to chronic calculous cholecystitis, peptic ulcer disease, reflux esophagitis, and angina pectoris.

B. Factors that justify the most likely diagnosis include the patient's age, obesity, and sex. The characteristics of the pain, the associated complaints, the absence of fever, the absence of jaundice, and the negative findings on abdominal examination all support the diagnosis of biliary colic secondary to chronic calculous cholecystitis.

OBJECTIVE 4

The student requests the appropriate laboratory tests.

A. Complete blood count shows hemoglobin of 12.5 gm/dL, hematocrit of 38%, and total leukocyte count of 6500/mm^3, with no shift to the left.

B. Urinalysis shows normal results and is negative for bile.

C. Liver function studies show total bilirubin of 0.9 mg/dL; alkaline phosphatase of 85 U/L (normal, 35–125 U/L); aspartate aminotransferase (AST) of 18 U/L (normal, 15–35 U/L); and alanine aminotransferase (ALT) of 15 U/L (normal, 10–50 U/L).

D. Blood glucose level is 135 mg/dL.

OBJECTIVE 5

The student requests the appropriate imaging studies to establish the definitive diagnosis.

A. Plain x-ray of the abdomen is normal.

B. Ultrasonography shows that the gallbladder contains multiple stones. The gallbladder wall is not thickened, and the common bile duct is normal in size.

C. An upper gastrointestinal series is normal.

OBJECTIVE 6

The student discusses the management of this patient.

A. Laparoscopic cholecystectomy is the optimum approach (preferred approach for removal of the gallbladder). The student discusses the principles of applied anatomy (significance of the triangle of Calot), the advantages of laparoscopic cholecystectomy over open cholecystectomy, and the complications associated with laparoscopic cholecystectomy.

B. The student discusses the selection of patients for extracorporeal shock wave lithotripsy (ESWL) and the limitations of ESWL.

C. The student describes dissolution therapy for gallstones, including patient selection and limitations of the therapy.

ADDITIONAL QUESTION

The student discusses the appropriate management of asymptomatic gallstones (incidentally found on ultrasonography done for unrelated reasons).

A. Risk that symptoms will develop and complications will occur

B. Role of continued observation

C. Special considerations for asymptomatic gall-stones: "porcelain" gallbladder, associated diabetes mellitus, gallstones found during celiotomy for an unrelated condition

OBJECTIVE 1

Minimum Level of Achievement for Passing

A–D. The student asks for information about the nature, location, and frequency of the pain, and exacerbating and alleviating factors.

E. The student asks about the patient's history of associated nausea, vomiting, and dyspepsia.

F. The student asks about the patient's history of jaundice, fever, change in the color of urine or stool, weight loss, and previous surgery.

Honors Level of Achievement

A–D. The student obtains complete information about the nature, location, and frequency of the pain, and exacerbating and alleviating factors without prompting by the examiner. The student discusses the differences in the characteristics of biliary colic secondary to chronic calculous cholecystitis and those of pain associated with acute cholecystitis. The student explains the reasons for these differences and compares the characteristics of biliary colic with those of pain secondary to peptic ulcer disease, reflux esophagitis, and coronary artery disease.

E. The student obtains a complete history of the associated complaints without prompting by the examiner. The student discusses the importance of each complaint in supporting the diagnosis of biliary colic.

F. The student obtains other relevant history without prompting by the examiner. The student explains the relevance of the presence or absence of jaundice, fever, change in the color of urine and stool, and weight loss in the context of this patient's clinical presentation.

OBJECTIVE 2

Minimum Level of Achievement for Passing

A–E. The student requests pertinent information about the patient's general appearance, skin, eyes, vital signs, and abdominal findings.

Honors Level of Achievement

A–E. The student requests the pertinent information without prompting by the examiner. The student explains the relevance of the presence or absence of jaundice, fever, and abdominal tenderness in the context of this patient's presentation.

OBJECTIVE 3

Minimum Level of Achievement for Passing

A. The student lists the differential diagnoses.

B. The student identifies items from the history and physical examination that support the diagnosis of biliary colic.

Honors Level of Achievement

A. The student discusses the possible diagnoses and prioritizes them without prompting by the examiner.

B. The student explains the reasons for the prioritization and discusses the features that support or refute each diagnosis.

OBJECTIVE 4

Minimum Level of Achievement for Passing

A–D. The student requests the appropriate laboratory tests.

Honors Level of Achievement

A–D. The student requests the appropriate laboratory tests without prompting by the examiner. The student explains the relevance of each test in the evaluation and management of this patient. The student does not request irrelevant tests that would merely increase the expense of evaluating and managing the patient.

OBJECTIVE 5

Minimum Level of Achievement for Passing

A–C. The student requests ultrasonography. The student should not order invasive studies that are not indicated.

Honors Level of Achievement

A–C. The student requests the relevant imaging studies without prompting by the examiner and explains the relevance of each study in the evaluation and management of this patient. The student describes the ultrasonographic findings in a patient with gallstones and discusses other studies that may help to establish the diagnosis of gallstones if the clinical picture is suggestive of the problem, but the ultrasonography is questionable.

OBJECTIVE 6

Minimum Level of Achievement for Passing

A. The student describes the management of the patient, including the need for cholecystectomy; outlines the relevant anatomy; and discusses the advantages of laparoscopic cholecystectomy over open cholecystectomy.

B–C. The student recognizes the limited role of ESWL and dissolution therapy in managing gallstones.

Honors Level of Achievement

A. The student discusses the complications associated with laparoscopic cholecystectomy.

B. The student outlines the selection of patients for ESWL and discusses the limitations of ESWL.

C. The student outlines the selection of patients for dissolution therapy and discusses the limitations of this therapy.

ADDITIONAL QUESTION

Minimum Level of Achievement for Passing

A. The student recognizes the low incidence of symptoms in patients with asymptomatic gallstones.

B. The student discusses the appropriate management of patients with asymptomatic gallstones (with continued observation).

C. The student recognizes the need for cholecystectomy in patients with a "porcelain" gallbladder because of the significant risk of carcinoma.

Honors Level of Achievement

A. The student discusses the specific risks that symptoms and complications will develop in patients with asymptomatic gallstones, quoting the relevant statistics.

B. The student explains the need for elective cholecystectomy once symptoms develop, and the need for more urgent intervention if complications occur.

C. The student outlines the appropriate management of a diabetic patient with asymptomatic gallstones and discusses the appropriate management of asymptomatic gallstones found incidentally at celiotomy.

CASE 2

A 45-year-old man comes to the emergency room with a 10-hour history of severe pain in the upper abdomen. The patient is nauseous and had two episodes of vomiting.

OBJECTIVE 1

The student elicits the relevant history from the patient.

A. The pain is severe and constant, and became progressively worse. The patient had no previous episode of similar pain.

B. The pain is located in the epigastrium and right upper quadrant of the abdomen. It radiates to the right flank.

C. The pain is worse when the patient moves or coughs.

D. The patient has a history of accompanying nausea, vomiting, fever (no chills), and anorexia. He had no weight loss and no change in the color of urine or stools.

E. The patient has a history of alcohol abuse. He has no history of diabetes mellitus, no history of ulcer disease, and underwent no previous surgery.

OBJECTIVE 2

The student requests information about the pertinent physical findings.

A. The patient is lying still. He appears to be in distress, especially when he moves.

B. The skin is normal.

C. On examination of the eyes, the sclerae are not icteric.

D. The pulse rate is 100 beats/min, blood pressure is 110/70 mm Hg, respiratory rate is 20/min, and temperature is 38.3° C (101° F).

E. The abdomen is slightly distended. There is marked guarding and tenderness in the right upper quadrant, extending to the epigastrium. There is rebound tenderness in the right upper quadrant, and bowel sounds are hypoactive.

OBJECTIVE 3

The student discusses the differential diagnosis and explains the reasons that support or refute each diagnosis.

A. The differential diagnosis includes acute cholecystitis, acute pancreatitis, peptic ulcer (penetrating or perforated), and acute appendicitis.

B. The history and physical examination findings are consistent with acute cholecystitis. The history of alcohol abuse and other items in the history and physical examination are consistent with acute pancreatitis. The findings are also consistent with a penetrating or locally perforated and walled-off peptic ulcer. (A free, uncontained ulcer perforation would cause signs of generalized peritonitis.) In addition the history and physical examination findings could result from inflammation of a high-lying, retrocecal appendix.

OBJECTIVE 4

The student orders the appropriate laboratory tests.

A. Complete blood count and differential count show hemoglobin of 13 g/dL, hematocrit of 40%, and total leukocyte count of 15,000/mm³, with a shift to the left.

B. Urinalysis results are normal, with no bile.

C. Liver function tests show total bilirubin of 2 mg/dL; alkaline phosphatase of 130 U/L (normal, 35–125 U/L); aspartate aminotransferase (AST) of 50 U/L (normal, 15–35 U/L); and alanine aminotransferase (ALT) of 75 U/L (normal, 10–50 U/L).

D. Serum amylase is 195 U/L (normal, 30–110 U/L).

OBJECTIVE 5

The student orders the appropriate imaging studies to establish the diagnosis.

A. Upright x-rays of the abdomen and chest show mild paralytic ileus, with no pneumoperitoneum.

B. Ultrasonography shows gallstones but no dilatation of the common bile duct. The pancreas is not well visualized.

C. Radionuclide biliary (HIDA) scan shows nonvisualization of the gallbladder after 4 hours.

Radionuclide fills the bile ducts and enters the duodenum.

OBJECTIVE 6

The student outlines an appropriate management plan. The plan includes:

A. Nothing by mouth

B. Nasogastric intubation

C. Intravenous fluids

D. Intravenous antibiotics

E. Parenteral analgesic

F. Type and crossmatch of blood

G. Cholecystectomy, with possible intraoperative cholangiogram, within 3 days

ADDITIONAL QUESTIONS

1. The student discusses the special items that must be considered in the diagnosis and management of acute gangrenous cholecystitis.

   A. Fever; leukocytosis, with a shift to the left; pericholecystic hepatic uptake and nonvisualization of the gallbladder on radionuclide (HIDA) scan

   B. Stabilization of comorbid conditions, intravenous broad-spectrum antibiotics, and emergency cholecystectomy

2. The student discusses the special items that must be considered in the diagnosis and management of acute emphysematous cholecystitis.

   A. Association with diabetes mellitus; high risk of gangrene and perforation; high fever; leukocytosis, with shift to the left; air within the wall or lumen of the gallbladder or air in the bile ducts on plain x-rays

   B. Stabilization of comorbid conditions (diabetes mellitus), intravenous broad-spectrum antibiotics (with special consideration of anaerobic coverage), and emergency cholecystectomy

3. The student describes the special items that must be considered in the diagnosis and management of acute acalculous cholecystitis

   A. Treatment for other medical problems (e.g., total parenteral nutrition, mechanical ventilatory support)

   B. Ultrasonography shows a thickened gallbladder wall, gallbladder distension, pericholecystic fluid, and a positive sonographic Murphy's sign.

   C. Radionuclide (HIDA) scan has a specificity of 38%.

   D. Management is similar to that of acute calculous cholecystitis; cholecystostomy may be needed.

OBJECTIVE 1

Minimum Level of Achievement for Passing

A–C. The student obtains the relevant history regarding the characteristics and location of the pain and information about the exacerbating and alleviating factors.

D. The student asks about the patient's history of nausea, vomiting, fever, anorexia, weight loss, and change in the color of urine or stool.

E. The student asks for the patient's history of diabetes mellitus, alcohol abuse, ulcer disease, and previous surgery.

Honors Level of Achievement

A–C. The student obtains the relevant history without prompting by the examiner. The student compares and contrasts the characteristics of this pain with the biliary pain associated with chronic calculous cholecystitis (biliary colic).

D. The student obtains the relevant history without prompting by the examiner. The student explains the significance of change in the color of urine or stool in the context of this patient's clinical presentation.

E. The student obtains the relevant history without prompting by the examiner. The student explains the relevance of the positive history of alcohol abuse in the differential diagnosis and describes the significance of diabetes mellitus as a comorbid condition.

OBJECTIVE 2

Minimum Level of Achievement for Passing

A–D. The student requests the relevant information about the general appearance, examination of the skin and eyes, and vital signs.

E. The student requests the relevant information about the abdominal examination.

Honors Level of Achievement

A–D. The student requests the relevant information without prompting by the examiner. The student explains the relevance of the patient's distress on movement (local peritonitis secondary to acute cholecystitis) and compares the physical examination findings with those associated with biliary colic secondary to chronic calculous cholecystitis.

E. The student requests the pertinent information without prompting by the examiner. The student discusses the significance of rebound tenderness and explains the progression of the disease process from the presence of a positive Murphy's sign to the presence of rebound tenderness. The student recognizes the paralytic ileus associated with acute cholecystitis.

OBJECTIVE 3

Minimum Level of Achievement for Passing

A–B. The student lists the differential diagnosis and identifies items from the history and physical examination that support the most likely diagnoses (acute cholecystitis and acute pancreatitis).

Honors Level of Achievement

A. The student discusses the possible diagnoses and prioritizes the diagnoses without prompting by the examiner.

B. The student explains the reasons for the prioritization of the possible diagnoses and discusses the features that support or refute each diagnosis.

OBJECTIVE 4

Minimum Level of Achievement for Passing

A–D. The student requests the appropriate laboratory tests.

Honors Level of Performance

A–D. The student requests the appropriate laboratory tests without prompting by the examiner, justifies each test, and explains the relevance of each abnormal result. The student does not request irrelevant tests that would merely add to the expense of evaluating and managing this patient. The student explains the reasons for the differences between the results of specific laboratory tests in acute cholecystitis versus acute cholangitis.

OBJECTIVE 5

Minimum Level of Achievement for Passing

A–C. The student requests the relevant imaging studies, recognizes the significance of the absence of pneumoperitoneum, and diagnoses acute cholecystitis based on the results of the studies. The student does not request invasive studies that are not indicated in this case.

Honors Level of Achievement

The student orders the relevant imaging studies without prompting by the examiner.

A. The student compares and contrasts the radiologic findings of paralytic ileus with those of mechanical small intestinal obstruction and describes the techniques available to visualize free intraperitoneal air if the patient cannot be placed in an upright position.

B. The student explains the relevance of the findings on ultrasonography in this patient and describes other ultrasonographic findings that suggest acute cholecystitis (not found here). The student discusses the significance of the finding of a common bile duct of normal size.

C. The student explains the reasons for ordering the radionuclide scan in this patient. The student discusses the significance of nonvisualization of the gallbladder on the scan and lists other reasons for nonvisualization of the gallbladder.

OBJECTIVE 6

Minimum Level of Achievement for Passing

A–D. The student outlines an appropriate management plan, including the items covered in these sections.

E. The student recognizes the need to order parenteral analgesic after the diagnosis is made.

F. The student recognizes the need to have blood available before surgery because of the higher risk of bleeding in patients with acute cholecystitis.

G. The student recognizes the optimum approach of performing cholecystectomy within 3 days of the onset of the disease and not routinely waiting for acute cholecystitis to resolve with antibiotic treatment.

Honors Level of Achievement

A–C. The student explains the reasons for each intervention and discusses the choice of intravenous fluids.

D. The student discusses the selection of antibiotics based on the anticipated bacteriology and justifies the specific choice.

E. The student recognizes the need to use analgesics judiciously.

F–G. The student describes the preoperative preparation of the patient and discusses the selection of the procedure. The student recognizes the choice between laparoscopic and open cholecystectomy and the higher conversion rate from the laparoscopic to the open procedure in acute cholecystitis compared with chronic calculous cholecystitis. The student discusses the therapeutic options available if calculi are found on intraoperative cholangiogram.

ADDITIONAL QUESTIONS

Minimum Level of Achievement for Passing

A–B. The student recognizes the special features of acute gangrenous cholecystitis and the need for emergency cholecystectomy.

Honors Level of Achievement

A–B. The student discusses the special findings on radionuclide (HIDA) scan that suggest acute gangrenous cholecystitis, describes in detail the management, justifies the choice of antibiotics, and explains the reasons for emergency cholecystectomy.

Minimum Level of Achievement for Passing

A–B. The student recognizes the high risk of gangrene and perforation, the association with diabetes mellitus, and the significance of air in the gallbladder or biliary ducts. The student outlines the management of these patients and recognizes the need for emergency cholecystectomy.

Honors Level of Achievement

A. The student discusses the differential diagnosis of pneumobilia found on plain x-rays of the abdomen.

B. The student discusses in detail the management of these patients, justifies the choice of specific antibiotics, and explains the reasons for emergency cholecystectomy.

Minimum Level of Achievement for Passing

A. The student recognizes the comorbid conditions associated with acute acalculous cholecystitis.

B–C. The student discusses the imaging studies available to confirm the diagnosis.

D. The student outlines the management of these patients.

Honors Level of Achievement

A. The student recognizes the difficulty in making a clinical diagnosis of acute acalculous cholecystitis.

B–C. The student compares the findings on ultrasonography and radionuclide (HIDA) scan in patients with acute calculous cholecystitis versus acute acalculous cholecystitis. The student recognizes the lower specificity of the radionuclide (HIDA) scan in the latter condition.

D. The student discusses various aspects of the management of patients with acute acalculous cholecystitis and recognizes other options (e.g., open or percutaneous cholecystostomy) available for very sick patients.

CASE 3

A 70-year-old woman is brought to the emergency room with a history of jaundice that was noticed by her daughter 4 days ago. The patient had upper abdominal pain for the same duration, and was febrile for 2 days.

OBJECTIVE 1

The student obtains the relevant history.

A. The abdominal pain is steady and progressively worsening. The patient has no history of similar pain.

B. The pain is located in the epigastrium and right upper quadrant of the abdomen.

C. Nothing seems to help the pain.

D. The patient's daughter noticed that the patient's skin became progressively more yellow over the past 4 days. The patient has pruritus.

E. The patient was febrile for the past 2 days. Her temperature on the day before presentation was 38.6° C (101.5° F). She had chills just before arriving in the emergency room.

F. The patient has a history of nausea, three episodes of vomiting, and anorexia. She had light-colored stool 2 days ago, and no bowel movement since then.

G. The patient's urinary output is decreased. The urine is dark and tea-colored.

H. The patient has no history of malignancy, no travel history, no history of blood transfusion, no history of weight loss, no diabetes mellitus, and no previous abdominal surgery.

OBJECTIVE 2

The student requests pertinent information about the physical examination.

A. The patient appears to be in some distress because of the abdominal pain. She is alert and oriented.

B. The eyes have deep yellow sclerae.

C. The skin is yellow, and both forearms and legs appear scaly.

D. The pulse rate is 110 beats/min, blood pressure is 110/70 mm Hg, respiratory rate is 22 breaths/min, and temperature is 38.9° C (102° F).

E. Abdominal examination shows mild distension; tenderness in the right upper quadrant, extending to the epigastrium; no rebound tenderness; and no mass. Bowel sounds are present, but hypoactive.

F. Rectal examination shows a small amount of pasty, gray stool.

OBJECTIVE 3

The student discusses the differential diagnoses and lists items that support or refute each possible diagnosis.

A. The differential diagnosis includes acute cholangitis secondary to choledocholithiasis, stricture, or neoplasm.

B. The clinical features of obstructive jaundice and Charcot's triad strongly suggest acute cholangitis. The most likely underlying cause is choledocholithiasis. Stricture is unlikely (no previous history of surgery). Neoplasm is possible, but less likely (no weight loss, no palpable gallbladder, no invasive diagnostic intervention that might have seeded the bile with bacteria).

OBJECTIVE 4

The student requests the appropriate laboratory tests.

A. Complete blood count with differential count shows hemoglobin of 13 g/dL; hematocrit of 43%; and total leukocyte count of 17,500/mm^3, with a shift to the left.

B. Serum electrolytes are sodium, 143 mEq/L; potassium, 3.7 mEq/L; chloride, 101 mEq/L; and CO_2, 29 mEq/L.

C. Blood glucose is 125 mg/dL.

D. Blood urea nitrogen is 20 mg/dL, and serum creatinine is 1.1 mg/dL.

E. Liver function tests are total bilirubin, 14.0 mg/dL; conjugated bilirubin, 10.5 mg/dL;

alkaline phosphatase, 850 U/L (normal, 35–125 U/L); aspartate aminotransferase (AST), 175 U/L (normal, 15–35 U/L); and alanine aminotransferase (ALT), 195 U/L (normal, 10–50 U/L).

F. Serum amylase is 200 U/L (normal, 30–110 U/L).

G. Urinalysis shows no urobilinogen. Bile is 3+.

H. Prothrombin time is 16 seconds (control, 12–14 seconds).

I. Blood cultures were sent.

OBJECTIVE 5

The student requests the appropriate imaging studies to establish the diagnosis.

A. Plain supine and upright x-rays of the abdomen are ordered. Upright x-ray of the chest shows a gas pattern consistent with paralytic ileus, no pneumoperitoneum, and no air in the biliary tract.

B. Ultrasonography shows multiple gallstones. The gallbladder is not distended, there is marked dilation of the intrahepatic and extrahepatic bile ducts, and the pancreas is not well visualized.

C. Percutaneous transhepatic cholangiogram (PTC) shows dilated intrahepatic ducts, a dilated common hepatic duct, a dilated common bile duct, and obstruction in the distal common bile duct (consistent with a stone), with no flow into the duodenum.

OBJECTIVE 6

The student should discusses the management of this patient.

A. Nothing by mouth

B. Intravenous fluids

C. Intravenous broad-spectrum antibiotics

D. Nasogastric intubation

E. Parenteral analgesic

F. Parenteral Vitamin K

G. Cholecystectomy and extraction of the stone or stones from the common bile duct after response to this therapy; if the response is not adequate, urgent drainage of the common bile duct with PTC or ERCP

ADDITIONAL QUESTION

The patient has a change in mentation and hypotension in addition to the abdominal pain, fever and chills, and jaundice.

1. The student recognizes the significance of Reynold's pentad.

2. The student makes the diagnosis of acute suppurative cholangitis.

3. The student discusses the immediate steps to combat septic shock (adequate resuscitation, antibiotics).

4. The student recognizes the need for urgent ductal drainage.

OBJECTIVE 1

Minimum Level of Achievement for Passing

A–C. The student elicits the pertinent information about the characteristics and location of the abdominal pain as well as exacerbating and alleviating factors.

D. The student elicits the information about the change in the color of the skin and pruritus.

E. The student elicits the information about fever and chills.

F. The student elicits the information about the associated gastrointestinal symptoms (nausea, vomiting, anorexia, and light-colored stool).

G. The student elicits the information about the urinary symptoms, including dark-colored urine.

H. The student obtains the history of malignancy, travel, blood transfusion, weight loss, and abdominal surgery.

Honors Level of Achievement

A–C. The student obtains the history without prompting by the examiner. The student distinguishes the pain associated with acute cholangitis from that associated with obstructive jaundice secondary to malignancy with no accompanying cholangitis. Pain in the latter condition is usually dull and less severe, or jaundice may be present without pain.

D. The student obtains the history without prompting by the examiner. The student explains the cause of pruritus in patients with obstructive jaundice.

E. The student obtains the history without prompting by the examiner. The student explains the significance of fever and chills in the diagnosis of acute cholangitis.

F–G. The student obtains the history without prompting by the examiner. The student recognizes the significance of light-colored stool and dark-colored urine in supporting the diagnosis of obstructive jaundice and explains the reasons for their occurrence. The student explains the differences in the color of urine in obstructive jaundice versus hemolytic disease.

H. The student obtains the history without prompting by the examiner. The student discusses the significance of the history of weight loss in suggesting a diagnosis of malignancy and describes various types of malignancies (primary and metastatic) that can cause extrahepatic biliary obstruction. The student recognizes the significance of various items in the context of evaluating patients for possible hepatitis.

OBJECTIVE 2

Minimum Level of Achievement for Passing

A–D. The student obtains the relevant information about the patient's general appearance, scleral discoloration, skin changes, and vital signs.

E. The student obtains the relevant information about the abdominal examination.

F. The student obtains the information about the appearance of stool in the rectum.

Honors Level of Achievement

A–D. The student requests the relevant information about the physical examination without prompting by the examiner. The student explains the significance of the high fever in this jaundiced patient.

E. The student requests the relevant information about the physical examination without prompting by the examiner. The student compares and contrasts the abdominal findings in acute cholangitis with those in acute cholecystitis.

F. The student requests the relevant information about the physical examination without prompting by the examiner. The student recognizes the significance of heme-positive stool (if present) and its association with periampullary carcinoma (if it is the cause of the obstructive jaundice).

OBJECTIVE 3

Minimum Level of Achievement for Passing

A–B. The student lists the differential diagnoses for this patient and identifies items from the history and physical examination that support the most likely diagnosis.

Honors Level of Achievement

A. The student discusses the possible diagnoses and prioritizes them without prompting by the examiner.

B. The student discusses various items in the history and examination that support or refute each possible diagnosis. The student explains the significance of Charcot's triad.

OBJECTIVE 4

Minimum Level of Achievement for Passing

A–H. The student requests the laboratory tests listed, identifies the abnormalities found, and recognizes that the results support the diagnosis of obstructive jaundice with acute infection.

I. The student requests blood cultures before antibiotic therapy is initiated.

Honors Level of Achievement

The student requests the appropriate tests without prompting by the examiner and does not request irrelevant tests that would merely add to the expense of evaluating and managing this patient.

A. The student recognizes the differences in the level of leukocytosis in acute cholangitis verses acute cholecystitis.

B–D. The student explains the reasons for requesting these tests.

E. The student explains the differences in the liver function test abnormalities found in this patient versus those in a patient with hepatitis.

F. The student discusses the significance of hyperamylasemia.

G. The student discusses the reasons for the absence of urobilinogen and the presence of bile in the urine.

H. The student explains the reason for the prolonged prothrombin time.

OBJECTIVE 5

Minimum Level of Achievement for Passing

The student orders the relevant imaging studies and does not request invasive studies that are not indicated in this patient.

A. The student requests plain x-rays of the abdomen and chest.

B. The student requests ultrasonography and recognizes that the findings described are consistent with the diagnosis of obstructive jaundice secondary to choledocholithiasis.

C. The student corrects the coagulopathy before the PTC and discusses the relevance of the findings.

Honors Level of Achievement

The student orders the relevant imaging studies without prompting by the examiner.

A. The student discusses the techniques available to rule out pneumoperitoneum if the patient cannot be placed upright. The student explains the significance of air in the biliary tract (if present).

B. The student compares and contrasts the ultrasonographic findings in this patient with those in a patient with acute cholecystitis. The student recognizes the infrequent visualization of common bile duct calculi on ultrasonography.

C. The student compares and contrasts the use of PTC and ERCP in the evaluation and management of patients with obstructive jaundice secondary to stone disease and malignancy.

OBJECTIVE 6

Minimum Level of Achievement for Passing

A–F. The student discusses the management plan, including the items listed, and orders the parenteral analgesic after the diagnosis is made.

G. The student recognizes that 70% of patients with acute cholangitis respond to the therapy listed in items A through F. Then they need to undergo the definitive operation, including cholecystectomy and extraction of the common bile duct calculi. The student also recognizes the need for urgent ductal decompression if there is no response to the initial therapy.

Honors Level of Achievement

A. The student discusses the reasons for continuing to give the patient nothing by mouth.

B. The student explains the choice of intravenous fluids.

C. The student justifies the choice of antibiotics based on the underlying bacteriology.

D. The student discusses the reasons for nasogastric intubation.

E. The student recognizes the need to use the analgesic judiciously.

F. The student explains the reasons for vitamin K administration and describes the approach to correct the coagulopathy if an invasive procedure is to be performed urgently (give fresh frozen plasma).

G. The student discusses the various approaches available for extraction of common bile duct calculi, including the timing of such interventions.

ADDITIONAL QUESTION

Minimum Level of Achievement for Passing

The student recognizes the components of Reynold's pentad, clinically distinguishes between acute cholangitis and acute suppurative cholangitis, outlines the resuscitation for patients in shock, and recognizes the need for urgent ductal decompression in acute suppurative cholangitis.

Honors Level of Achievement

The student justifies the choice of intravenous fluids in combating shock, explains in detail the steps taken to monitor the efficacy of resuscitation, justifies the choice of antibiotics, and discusses the options available for urgent decompression of the common bile duct.

SUGGESTED READINGS

Carey MC. Pathogenesis of gallstones. *Am J Surg* 1993;165:410–419.

Diehl AK. Epidemiology and natural history of gallstone disease. *Gastroenterol Clin North Am* 1991;20(1):1–19.

Friedman GD. Natural history of asymptomatic and symptomatic gallstones. *Am J Surg* 1993;165:399–404.

Kadakia SC. Biliary tract emergencies: acute cholecystitis, acute cholangitis, and acute pancreatitis. *Med Clin North Am* 1993;77(5):1015–1034.

Lipsett PA, Pitt HA. Acute cholangitis. *Surg Clin North Am* 1990;70(6):1297–1312.

NIH Consensus Development Panel on Gallstones and Laparoscopic Cholecystectomy. Gallstones and laparoscopic cholecystectomy. *JAMA* 1993;269(8):1018–1024.

Oría A, Alvarez J, Chiappetta L, et al. Choledocholithiasis in acute gallstone pancreatitis. *Arch Surg* 1991;126:566–568.

Phillips EH. Controversies in the management of common duct calculi. *Surg Clin North Am* 1994;74(4):931–948.

Pitt HA, Dooley WC, Yeo CJ, Cameron JL. Malignancies of the biliary tree. *Curr Probl Surg* 1995;32:1–90.

Reisner RM, Cohen JR. Gallstone ileus: a review of 1001 reported cases. *Am Surg* 1994;60:441–446.

Sharp KW. Acute cholecystitis. *Surg Clin North Am* 1988;68(2):269–279.

Wanebo HJ, Vezeridis MP. Carcinoma of the gallbladder. *J Surg Oncol Suppl* 1993;3:134–139.

17

Pancreas

Kenneth W. Sharp, M.D.
Walter E. Pofahl, M.D.

OBJECTIVES

1. Classify pancreatitis on the basis of the severity of injury to the organ.
2. List four etiologies of pancreatitis.
3. Describe the clinical presentation of a patient with acute pancreatitis, including indications for surgical intervention.
4. Discuss at least five potential early complications of acute pancreatitis.
5. Discuss the criteria that are used to predict the prognosis for acute pancreatitis.
6. Discuss four potential adverse outcomes of chronic pancreatitis as well as the surgical diagnostic approach, treatment options, and management.
7. Discuss the mechanism of pseudocyst formation with respect to the role of the duct, and list five symptoms and physical signs of pseudocysts.
8. Describe the diagnostic approach to a patient with a suspected pseudocyst, including the indications for and the sequence of tests.
9. Discuss the natural history of an untreated pancreatic pseudocyst as well as the medical and surgical treatment.
10. List four pancreatic neoplasms, and describe the pathology of each with reference to cell type and function.
11. Describe the symptoms, physical signs, laboratory findings, and diagnostic workup of a pancreatic mass on the basis of the location of the tumor.
12. Describe the surgical treatment of pancreatic neoplasms.
13. Discuss the long-term prognosis for pancreatic cancers on the basis of pathology and cell type.

Diseases of the pancreas are common and often require surgical intervention. The pancreas is subject to congenital, inflammatory, infectious, posttraumatic, and neoplastic diseases. Its exocrine role in digestion was not known until the 1800s, and its ability to modulate glucose metabolism was demonstrated in 1921 by Banting and Best. Inflammatory diseases of the pancreas were described in the late 1800s by Fitz, and surgery for pancreatic neoplasms was popularized by the work of Whipple et al. in the 1930s. As a result of our greater understanding of pancreatic anatomy, physiology, and pathophysiology, we can now identify patients with pancreatic disease who will benefit from surgical intervention.

Anatomy

The pancreas is a gland that lies in a transverse orientation in the retroperitoneum at the level of the second lumbar vertebra. It is usually between 12 and 18 cm long, and it weighs between 70 and 110 g. The gland is divided into four distinct parts: head, neck, body, and tail (Figure 17-1). The head of the pancreas accounts for approximately 30% of the gland. It is surrounded by the "C-loop" of the duodenum. The head is the part of the gland that extends to the right of the superior mesenteric veins. Anteriorly, this section is marked by the gastroduodenal artery. The uncinate process is considered a portion of the head. The neck of the gland is the portion overlying the superior mesenteric vein and artery. The body extends from the left of the superior mesenteric vessels toward the splenic hilum. The tail is the most distal portion of the gland. The anatomic boundary between the body and the tail is vague and has little effect on the management of pancreatic disease. The anterior surface of the gland is in contact with the transverse mesocolon as well as the posterior wall of the stomach. Its posterior surface is devoid of peritoneum and is bounded by the common bile duct, superior mesenteric vessels, inferior vena cava, and aorta.

Ductal Anatomy

An understanding of pancreatic ductal anatomy necessitates familiarization with the embryology of pancreatic development. The pancreas begins as dorsal

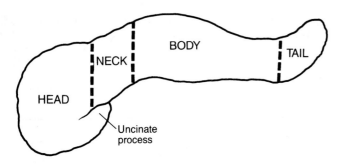

Figure 17-1 Regional anatomy of the pancreas.

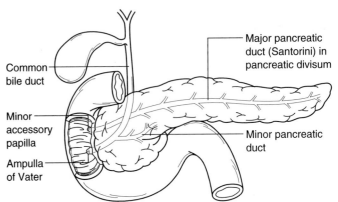

Figure 17-2 Anatomy of the pancreatic ductal system showing the ducts of Wirsung (main duct) and Santorini (accessory duct) and their relation to the common bile duct.

and ventral buds that arise from the duodenal tube. Because of differential growth and gut rotation, the ventral bud passes posteriorly to the duodenal tube and fuses with the larger dorsal bud. Fusion of the ducts of the ventral and dorsal buds forms the main pancreatic duct (Figure 17-2). The caliber of the pancreatic duct ranges from 3 to 4 mm in the head to 1.5 to 2 mm in the tail. In approximately 90% of cases, the main pancreatic duct **(duct of Wirsung)** drains through the major papilla (ampulla of Vater) into the second portion of the duodenum. The common bile duct often forms a common channel with the main pancreatic duct before it enters the ampulla. In confusing terminology, the major ampulla (Vater) always drains the common bile duct and the minor pancreatic duct. The major pancreatic duct may empty through an accessory (minor) papilla that is located more proximally in the duodenum.

Two important anomalies can occur during embryologic development of the pancreas. **Pancreas divisum** occurs when the ventral and dorsal ducts do not fuse. This condition, which is seen in 5% to 10% of the population, results in the drainage of most of the pancreatic secretions through the minor papilla. The drainage from the head and uncinate process is through the major papilla. This condition is a proposed etiology of idiopathic recurrent pancreatitis. The other anomaly, **annular pancreas**, is less common. Its exact etiology is unknown, but presumably it is caused by incomplete rotation of the ventral pancreatic bud, leading to a ring of pancreatic tissue around the second portion of the duodenum. Annular pancreas is one of the causes of duodenal obstruction in infants and children.

Arterial Blood Supply

The pancreatic head shares a blood supply with the duodenum, necessitating resection of both structures when the pancreatic head must be resected (e.g., cancer of the pancreatic head). The gastroduodenal artery arises from the common hepatic artery, marking the beginning of the proper hepatic artery, and passes posteriorly to the duodenal bulb. It divides to form the anterior and posterior superior pancreaticoduodenal arteries. These vessels anastomose with the anterior and posterior inferior pancreaticoduodenal arteries that arise directly from the superior mesenteric artery.

The dorsal pancreatic artery is present in 90% of people, but has a variable origin. In most cases, it arises from the proximal splenic artery, but may be a branch of the celiac axis or superior mesenteric artery. It divides into a right branch, which passes along the upper margin of the uncinate process and joins the anterior arcade, and a left branch, which becomes the inferior pancreatic artery and supplies the pancreatic body and tail. The splenic artery is the source of multiple superior pancreatic branches that supply the body of the pancreas. The largest is the **pancreatic magna** (great pancreatic artery).

Venous Drainage

The venous drainage of the pancreas and duodenum corresponds to the arterial supply. The veins are immediately superficial to the arteries. The anterior venous arcade drains into the superior mesenteric vein. The posterior venous arcade usually drains into the portal vein (Figure 17-3).

An important point in the surgical anatomy is the fact that venous tributaries enter the portal and superior mesenteric veins along their lateral borders. The anterior vascular plane allows dissection behind the neck of the pancreas, anterior to the portal mesenteric veins. The venous drainage of the body and tail is through tributaries that enter the splenic vein and the inferior pancreatic vein, which enters either the inferior or superior mesenteric vein.

Innervation

Inflammatory and neoplastic diseases of the pancreas often cause pain that is mediated through the abundant supply of afferent sensory nerve fibers. The pancreas is also innervated by fibers of both the sympathetic (greater splanchnic nerve) and parasympathetic (vagus nerve) autonomic nervous systems. All fibers pass through the celiac or superior mesenteric plexus. Pain fibers accompany the sympathetic fibers and follow the blood vessels to the gland.

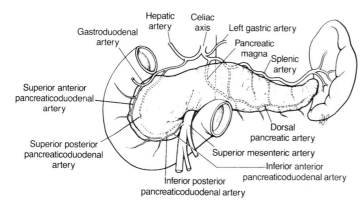

Figure 17-3 Blood supply of the pancreas.

Physiology

Exocrine

The exocrine pancreas secretes 1000 to 2000 mL/day of isotonic, alkaline fluid that contains electrolytes and digestive enzymes. Although the sodium and potassium concentrations are similar to those in plasma, the bicarbonate concentration is elevated, accounting for the alkaline pH (approximately 8.0). Many of the 20 different digestive enzymes that are synthesized by the pancreas are secreted as inactive precursors (e.g., trypsin and chymotrypsin are secreted as trypsinogen and chymotrypsinogen) and are activated by contact with the duodenal contents.

Two hormones play a central role in regulating pancreatic exocrine secretion: secretin and cholecystokinin (CCK). Duodenal acidification stimulates the release of secretin, which stimulates the secretion of pancreatic juice that is rich in bicarbonate. The intraluminal products of digestion, especially peptides, amino acids, and free fatty acids, stimulate the release of CCK, which stimulates the secretion of pancreatic digestive enzymes. In addition, CCK potentiates the action of secretin and causes gallbladder contraction so that bile is mixed with pancreatic secretions to digest fat, protein, and carbohydrate.

Endocrine

The islets of Langerhans make up 1.5% of the pancreas by weight. They are responsible for the endocrine functions of the gland. The islets measure 75 to 150 μm and are more abundant in the tail of the gland. Their major function is the control of glucose homeostasis. In response to a low serum glucose, alpha cells secrete glucagon, a peptide that is composed of 20 amino acids. The resulting glycogenolysis releases glucose into the bloodstream. Beta cells, which constitute 60% of the islets, secrete insulin in response to increases in serum glucose. Insulin promotes the transfer of glucose across cell membranes. Delta cells, which constitute a small proportion of islet cells (5%–10%), secrete somatostatin,

the most potent known inhibitor of pancreatic exocrine secretion.

Pathophysiology

Acute Pancreatitis

Acute pancreatitis is a diffuse inflammation of the pancreas that is often associated with complications that occasionally lead to death. Several well-known factors are associated with acute pancreatitis, although the precise etiology is not well understood. The two most common causes, alcohol ingestion and biliary calculi, account for 85% of cases.

Acute pancreatitis is characterized by enzymatic destruction of the pancreatic substance by the release and activation of pancreatic enzymes into the glandular parenchyma. The microscopic (histologic) changes range from interstitial edema and inflammation in mild cases to hemorrhage and necrosis in severe cases.

Etiology

All causes of acute pancreatitis can be categorized into the following groups: metabolic, mechanical, and vascular. The most common etiology within the metabolic group is alcohol, which accounts for as many as 40% of all cases of pancreatitis. Generally, the first episode is preceded by 6 to 8 years of significant alcohol ingestion and is often followed by recurring acute attacks. After multiple attacks of acute pancreatitis, the pancreas is permanently damaged, and the clinical syndrome of **chronic pancreatitis** develops. Exactly how alcohol causes pancreatitis is not known. A common theory is that alcohol induces changes in the secretory response of the pancreas and that these changes result in a higher protein content in the secretions. This higher content leads to the precipitation of protein and the blockage of small pancreatic ductules. Other metabolic causes of pancreatitis include hyperlipidemia and hyperparathyroidism. Drugs associated with acute pancreatitis include corticosteroids, thiazide diuretics, furosemide, estrogens, azathioprine, and dideoxyinosine.

The most common mechanical etiology of acute pancreatitis is gallstones. It is estimated that as many as 60% of nonalcoholic patients with pancreatitis have gallstones. Like the etiology of alcohol-induced pancreatitis, the etiology of gallstone-induced pancreatitis is not completely understood. In 1901, Opie proposed the common channel theory based on his observation of a common channel within the ampullae made up of the common bile duct and the pancreatic duct. He proposed that a gallstone could block the pancreatic duct within the ampulla, leading to a reflux of bile into the pancreatic duct and resulting in acute pancreatitis. This theory is disputed by some who have shown experimentally that bile in the pancreatic duct at physiologic pressures does not cause pancreatitis. It has been suggested that transient obstruction of a common channel might lead to reflux of pancreatic juice into the common bile duct.

The mixing of bile and pancreatic juice may lead to the formation of a substance that is highly toxic to the pancreas. Other mechanical causes of pancreatitis include blunt and penetrating trauma to the pancreas and malignant obstruction of the pancreatic duct by tumors of the distal common duct, pancreas, ampulla of Vater, and duodenum.

Ischemic injuries to the pancreas, secondary to hypotension or devascularization during upper abdominal surgery, may initiate pancreatitis or may play a role in the progression of pancreatic edema to pancreatic necrosis. Postoperative pancreatitis is seen after gastric surgery in as many as 15% of cases and after biliary surgery in 10% of cases. Acute pancreatitis is a complication in 1% of patients who undergo endoscopic retrograde cholangiopancreatography (ERCP). This complication is believed to be caused by an acute increase in intraductal pressure. Approximately 8% to 10% of cases of pancreatitis have no recognizable etiology (idiopathic pancreatitis).

Clinical Presentation and Evaluation

Patients with acute pancreatitis have noncrampy, epigastric abdominal pain. The character of the pain is variable, and it frequently radiates to the left or right upper quadrant or the back. The pain may be relieved by sitting or standing. It is associated with nausea and often a significant amount of vomiting. Physical examination is characterized by fever, tachycardia, and upper abdominal tenderness with guarding. Bowel sounds are generally absent because of the presence of an adynamic ileus. Generalized abdominal and rebound tenderness may also occur in severe pancreatitis. Laboratory evaluation shows leukocytosis and elevated serum amylase and lipase. In severe cases of pancreatitis, there may also be abnormal liver chemistries, hyperglycemia, hypocalcemia, elevated blood urea nitrogen (BUN) and creatinine levels, and hypoxemia. The differential diagnosis of acute pancreatitis includes acute cholecystitis, perforated peptic ulcer, mesenteric ischemia, esophageal perforation, and myocardial infarction. Patients with suspected acute pancreatitis should be evaluated radiologically with (1) a chest x-ray to show possible left pleural effusion, plate atelectasis, or hemidiaphragm elevation, and to exclude free air; (2) plain and upright abdominal x-rays to show possible calcifications indicating chronic pancreatitis, gallstones, or local adynamic ileus; and (3) ultrasonography to show gallstones, pancreatic enlargement, and pseudocysts. If complicated acute pancreatitis is suspected, computed tomography (CT) is preferred over ultrasound because of its greater sensitivity. CT scans are useful in cases of unclear clinical diagnosis or severe pancreatitis, and to detect local complications (e.g., pancreatic necrosis, abscess, pseudocyst).

Prognosis

Outcome after acute pancreatitis is directly proportional to the severity of the attack. One of the first systems for grading severity was developed by Ranson.

This system **(Ranson's criteria)** uses readily measured laboratory and clinical variables (Table 17-1). Five variables are measured at admission, and six additional variables are measured over the ensuing 48 hours. The presence of three or more criteria indicates severe pancreatitis and is associated with an increased incidence of local and systemic complications.

The other main prognostic index is the Acute Physiology and Chronic Health Evaluation II (APACHE II) score. Although it was first used to stratify intensive care unit patients, this scoring system was adapted to assess patients with acute pancreatitis. Although it is not as simple and straightforward as Ranson's criteria, the APACHE II system also uses readily obtainable variables (Table 17-2). Numeric scores are assigned to

Table 17-1. Prognostic Factors: Risk of Major Complications or Death (Ranson's Criteria)

At admission
  Age > 55
  WBC > 16,000
  Glucose > 200 mg/100 mL
  LDH > 350
  AST > 250
During 48 hr after admission
  HCT > 10-point decrease
  BUN > 5 mg/100 mL increase
  Ca++ < 8.0
  pO_2 < 60 mm Hg on room air
  Base excess > 4 mEq/L
  Estimated fluid sequestration > 6000 mL

WBC, white blood cell count.
LDH, lactic dehydrogenase.
AST, aspartate aminotransferase.
HCT, hematocrit.
BUN, blood urea nitrogen.

Table 17-2. Variables Scored in the APACHE II Severity of Disease Classification System

Physiologic Variables	Age Ranges	Chronic Health Problems and Variables
Temperature	≤ 44	Liver
Mean arterial pressure	45–44	Cardiovascular
Heart rate	55–64	Respiratory
Respiratory rate	65–74	Renal
Oxygenation	≥ 75	Immunocompromised
Arterial pH		
Serum sodium		
Serum potassium		
Serum creatinine		
Hematocrit		
White blood cell count		
Glasgow Coma Score		

The actual physiologic ranges and points assigned are not indicated in this table; only the variables considered are listed.
APACHE, Acute Physiology and Chronic Health Evaluation.

physiologic measurements, age, and preexisting organ insufficiencies to provide a score that reflects the severity of the disease. The main advantage of the APACHE II system is that a score can be derived at any time during the patient's hospital course. With Ranson's criteria, the variables that indicate severity are prognostic only during the first 48 hours after admission. Patients with APACHE II scores of 8 or greater are considered to have severe acute pancreatitis.

Finally, CT scans can yield prognostic information. The severity and complications of the attack are correlated to the amount of pancreatic necrosis and the size and location of peripancreatic and extrapancreatic fluid collections seen on abdominal contrast CT scans.

Treatment

Medical

The medical therapy of acute pancreatitis can be divided into general supportive therapy and specific treatment of pancreatic inflammation. In patients with pancreatitis, it is important to maintain adequate tissue perfusion by monitoring cardiovascular parameters and also to maintain adequate intravascular volume. A massive amount of fluid can be sequestered in the retroperitoneal tissues because of the presence of activated enzymes and inflammation. Pancreatitis is often compared with a retroperitoneal "burn" because of the magnitude of fluid extravasation and third-space fluid loss that it causes. In severe cases, administration of several liters of isotonic solution may be required. Fluid management is aided by the use of a central venous line or pulmonary artery catheter to monitor cardiac function and a Foley catheter to evaluate urine output. Electrolytes and blood glucose are carefully monitored.

Respiratory function is monitored carefully because severe hypocalcemia and respiratory failure can cause early death in severe pancreatitis. Oxygenation is monitored with pulse oximetry or arterial blood gas measurements if necessary. Patients with severe pancreatitis can also have respiratory distress syndrome that requires intubation and aggressive ventilatory support.

Specific inhibition of pancreatic secretions in an effort to decrease peripancreatic inflammation has been attempted with the use of nasogastric suction. Studies in patients with mild alcoholic pancreatitis do not show a benefit with this mode of therapy. However, nasogastric suction may be useful in patients with more severe forms of pancreatitis with ileus and vomiting. Anticholinergics, somatostatin, specific enzyme inhibitors (e.g., aprotinin, snake antivenom), and antacids have been used in an attempt to decrease the degree of pancreatic inflammation, but none has any significant benefit. Similarly, antibiotics do not decrease morbidity or mortality in patients with mild pancreatitis; however, they are used quite liberally in the treatment of **gallstone pancreatitis** because of concern that this condition might be confused with cholangitis. Patients with severe pancreatitis (more than three positive Ranson's criteria) are often treated with prophylactic antibiotics, but there is not common support for this approach.

Surgical

The surgical management of patients with pancreatitis is controversial. When the diagnosis is not clear, diagnostic laparotomy is recommended, not only to establish the diagnosis of pancreatitis but also to rule out other nonpancreatic lesions that may mimic pancreatitis (e.g., perforated ulcer, gangrenous cholecystitis, mesenteric infarction).

In some cases, patients with severe gallstone pancreatitis may be treated with early removal of an impacted stone at the ampulla of Vater. This procedure is considered only in severe cases and in cases with suspected cholangitis complicating the diagnosis. Removal is accomplished endoscopically by a skilled endoscopist using a side-viewing duodenoscope and a wire-cautery sphincterotome. Patients with mild to moderate gallstone pancreatitis should be allowed to recover from their pancreatitis. Cholecystectomy may be performed during the same hospital admission to reduce the length of convalescence or the probability of another episode of gallstone pancreatitis and to avoid another hospitalization.

Complications

Acute pancreatitis has many major and minor complications. Metabolic complications include hyperglycemia, hypocalcemia, and renal failure. Varying degrees of respiratory insufficiency and hypoxemia may also be present. They develop secondary to a combination of factors that include diaphragmatic elevation resulting in decreased ventilation, fluid overload during resuscitation, pulmonary thromboemboli, and the release of an antisurfactant factor. Severe cases may require mechanical ventilation with positive end-expiratory pressure. Coagulopathy and hemorrhage may also occur as a result of the depletion of coagulation factors or erosion into a major vessel. The most common local complications are paralytic ileus and sterile peripancreatic fluid collections. Patients may have obstruction of the biliary tree or duodenum because of edema as well as thrombosis of the nearby splenic vein, which can lead to esophageal varices.

Necrosis of the gland is a common finding in patients with severe episodes. This finding is determined by contrast-enhanced dynamic CT scan. In general, necrosis of less than 30% usually resolves without further sequelae. Patients with greater degrees of necrosis are at increased risk of tissue infection and organ dysfunction. The management of sterile necrosis is controversial. Several authors advocate early operative intervention and debridement of the necrotic tissue to prevent infection and interrupt development of the systemic inflammatory response syndrome, with its associated organ dysfunction. Other groups advocate operative intervention only in cases of organ dysfunction or infection. Regardless of the decision regarding operative therapy in these patients, the mainstay of treatment is aggressive support to optimize oxygen delivery.

Local infectious complications of acute pancreatitis markedly increase the mortality associated with a given attack. Infected pancreatic necrosis is associated with the highest mortality rate (> 40%). The risk of infection is directly proportional to the extent of necrosis. Typically, necrosis becomes manifest 2 to 3 weeks into the patient's illness. Frequently, patients have worsening of organ dysfunction. The diagnosis is made by CT-guided needle aspiration of necrotic pancreatic tissue, with demonstration of organisms by Gram's stain. Therapy for infected pancreatic necrosis is operative debridement with blunt dissection. Multiple operations are needed to remove the infected debris without damaging adjacent structures. Percutaneous drainage usually fails because the large pieces of infected necrotic material cannot drain through small catheters.

A pancreatic abscess is a collection of pus adjacent to the pancreas, without underlying necrosis. Typically, an abscess is an infected acute fluid collection, or pseudocyst. Treatment is the same as for any intraabdominal abscess: external drainage. Drainage can be accomplished by open operation or, in some cases, by nonoperative percutaneous drainage. The mortality risk for pancreatic abscess is less than that for infected necrosis.

Chronic Pancreatitis

Etiology

Inflammation of the pancreas progresses to a chronic state for a variety of reasons. If the initial inflammatory insult is severe enough to cause permanent ductal damage, recurring pancreatitis can develop, usually because of ductal obstruction or stasis (Table 17-3). The causes of such a significant injury include trauma and cholelithiasis. The most important cause of **chronic pancreatitis** is persistent alcohol ingestion.

Congenital causes include cystic fibrosis, familial pancreatitis, and pancreatic divisum. The last entity occurs when the dorsal and ventral segments of the fetal pancreas do not meet and fuse. As a result, most of the pancreas is drained by the smaller **duct of Santorini**, with consequent stasis and increased likelihood of inflammation.

Repeated episodes of pancreatitis result in interruption and obstruction of large and small pancreatic ducts, with subsequent autodigestion. As a result of the edema and tissue destruction, the pancreas undergoes scarring and fibrosis, with loss of functional substance. The result of this process is pancreatic insufficiency, which manifests as exocrine and endocrine failure. Loss of exocrine function leads to malabsorption. When pancreatic secretion of enzymes decreases to 10% of normal, protein and fat cannot be adequately absorbed. The resulting steatorrhea is quantitated by measuring stool fat in a patient who is receiving a prescribed fat diet. Pancreatic endocrine dysfunction causes diabetes. Generally, these patients respond to insulin treatment and do not seem to be as vulnerable to small vessel disease as other diabetic patients. Nonetheless, insulin administration is difficult in this population because most continue their heavy alcohol intake.

Clinical Presentation and Evaluation

Pain is the most common symptom of chronic pancreatitis. The pain is usually intermittent, but with the development of subsequent attacks of pancreatitis and more scarring and fibrosis, the pain may become inexorable and unrelenting. Eating may be impossible because of the resulting pain. Patients often resort to increased alcohol intake and the use of painkilling drugs to obtain relief. Drug dependency, malnutrition, and vitamin B_{12} deficiency are common. Malabsorption as a result of exocrine insufficiency may cause steatorrhea and fat-soluble vitamin deficiency.

Patients with suspected chronic pancreatitis and those with known chronic pancreatitis who have new symptoms should be assessed by CT scan to search for surgically correctable causes or complications. CT has the greatest sensitivity for showing gland enlargement or atrophy, duct enlargement, calcifications, masses, pseudocysts, inflammation, and extensions beyond the pancreas (Figure 17-4). The liver, gallbladder, and bile ducts are also visualized. Ultrasonography is less expensive than CT, but it is also less successful in show-

Table 17-3. Marseilles Classification of Pancreatitis

Category	Characteristics
I	Acute pancreatitis: a single episode of pancreatitis in a previously normal gland
II	Acute relapsing pancreatitis: recurrent attacks that do not lead to permanent functional damage; clinical and biologic normalcy in the interval between attacks
III	Chronic relapsing pancreatitis: progressive functional damage persisting between attacks; frequent pain-free intervals
IV	Chronic pancreatitis: inexorable and irreversible destruction of pancreatic function; constant pain

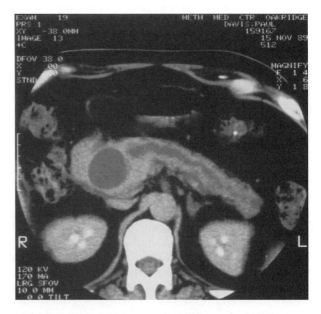

Figure 17-4 Computed tomography scan showing the pancreas of a patient with chronic pancreatitis. A pseudocyst is seen in the head of the pancreas, and a dilated pancreatic duct is seen distally.

ing the pancreas, especially in obese patients and those with gas-filled intestines. However, ultrasonography is the preferred diagnostic study for following changes in pseudocysts if they are clearly visualized. It is also the preferred method for the initial study of jaundiced patients, even if the jaundice has a pancreatic cause.

Treatment

Patients with chronic pancreatitis are managed conservatively, with the intention of reducing trauma to the pancreas. When necessary, surgery is considered for appropriate complications, such as pseudocysts. Because alcoholism is the leading cause of pancreatitis, abstinence is strongly advised. If other specific causes are identified, they are corrected to minimize further injury. Medical treatment of chronic pancreatitis is a low-fat diet (to minimize steatorrhea), enzyme replacement, and insulin for hyperglycemia. Medical treatment rarely resolves the pain of chronic pancreatitis.

Surgery is indicated in patients with chronic pancreatitis who have incapacitating pain that is resistant to medical therapy and in patients with anatomic abnormalities that cause recurrent bouts of acute pancreatitis. Preoperative delineation of pancreatic ductal anatomy by ERCP is necessary. In this procedure, endoscopy and fluoroscopy are used in combination to facilitate cannulation and opacification of the pancreatic and biliary ducts with contrast agent. Radiographs are made during the filling and emptying phases to map the ductal anatomy and to delineate obstructions, strictures, calculi, duct ectasia, and pseudocysts. ERCP is invasive and carries a small, but definite, risk of exacerbating pancreatitis, biliary or pancreatic sepsis, or pseudocyst infection. ERCP is very useful in identifying dilated pancreatic ducts, strictures, fistulas, and common bile duct obstructions.

The surgical options for treating chronic pancreatitis are ductal decompression and pancreatic resection. Patients with segmental ductal obstruction or alternating areas of stricture and dilation ("chain of lakes") are best treated by decompression of the duct into a loop of jejunum (pancreaticojejunostomy, or Puestow procedure). The long-term results of this procedure are good, with approximately 70% of patients achieving lasting relief of pain. Pancreatic resection is reserved for patients without pancreatic duct dilation who have disease limited to a segment of the gland. Results are similar to those obtained with ductal decompression. These procedures have no effect on the progression of exocrine and endocrine insufficiency. A significant number of patients will have progression to exocrine insufficiency and diabetes after these procedures. Near-total and total pancreatectomy is rarely indicated because these operations leave the patient with no exocrine or endocrine function.

Surgical intervention is also indicated to treat several complications of chronic pancreatitis. Patients with biliary strictures and associated liver enzyme abnormalities benefit from biliary enteric decompression. Pseudocysts are common in patients with chronic pancreatitis; however, unlike acute fluid collections associated with acute pancreatitis, these are less likely to resolve. Operative drainage should be undertaken in patients with symptoms or a pseudocyst that is larger than 5 cm.

Pseudocysts

The most common complication of pancreatitis is the development of an acute fluid collection in the peripancreatic area or, in more severe cases, at distant locations in the retroperitoneum. This complication is caused by ductal disruption and gland autolysis. Enzymatic fluid collects in and around the pancreas and is walled off by surrounding viscera. Most of these acute fluid collections resolve. Those that persist become **pseudocysts.** Over the course of 4 to 6 weeks after the initial attack, the wall of these persistent fluid collections matures into a fibrotic rind. By definition, a pseudocyst is lined by nonepithelial tissue.

Clinical Presentation and Evaluation

The most common symptoms of pseudocysts are related to the causative inflammation. Epigastric pain is the most common symptom, but nausea and vomiting may also occur. On occasion, pseudocysts can create mechanical obstruction of either the stomach or duodenum, but this is uncommon. Jaundice secondary to biliary obstruction can occur as a result of pseudocyst formation, but this is also unusual.

A thorough history and a complete physical examination are essential in the evaluation of a pseudocyst. Obviously, obtaining a history of alcoholism and previous pancreatitis is important. Fever, weight loss, and a history of jaundice are other salient clinical features. Clinical features that lead to suspicion of a pseudocyst include persistent abdominal pain for longer than 1 week after an episode of pancreatitis, persistent elevations of serum amylase or lipase, and the development of a palpable abdominal mass.

Sonography and CT scans are the first-line noninvasive studies to assess an abdominal mass. Sonography is a useful technical advance because it is relatively inexpensive and is quite accurate in distinguishing solid from cystic masses. Further delineation of the mass and surrounding tissue structures is obtained with a CT scan (Figure 17-5). Not only can the mass and its relation to surrounding structures be clearly outlined, but serial examinations can also show growth or shrinkage of the mass over time. Further, CT and sonography can be used in more invasive techniques that permit direct needle or catheter aspiration or drainage of the fluid collection. Thus, these tools may aid in the diagnosis or may serve in the primary treatment. More and more literature supports radiologically directed biopsies, aspirations, or drainage procedures. This modality clearly has a major impact on the diagnosis and treatment of many lesions. A pseudocyst that lies adjacent to the abdominal wall is easily accessible to catheter drainage under local anesthesia. Moreover, a septic patient who has a pseudocyst that is the possible origin of the infection can undergo aspiration to determine whether the pseudocyst contains pus.

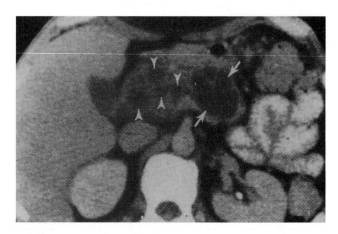

Figure 17-5 Computed tomography scan showing multiple pseudocysts (*arrows*) in a patient with chronic pancreatitis.

Treatment
Medical

Approximately 30% of pseudocysts resolve spontaneously with conservative medical management. The conservative approach consists of allowing the pancreas to rest by maintaining the patient on total parenteral nutrition and avoiding oral intake that would stimulate pancreatic secretion. During observation of the patient over a period of weeks, progressive decrease in size is seen if the pseudocyst will resolve. Simple palpation on daily examination shows reduced tenderness and diminished size. Ultrasound and, if necessary, CT can document the disappearance of the pseudocyst very accurately.

Medical management continues until the cyst resolves or a mature cyst wall forms. Maturation of the cyst wall, during which the cyst wall develops enough fibrosis to support suturing to the stomach or jejunum for internal drainage, generally requires more than 4 weeks.

Clearly, pseudocysts that occur suddenly in patients with acute pancreatitis are much more likely to resolve than long-standing masses in patients with a history of chronic pancreatitis. Complications from pseudocysts (e.g., infection, hemorrhage) can be catastrophic. A patient who has a pseudocyst and sudden onset of fever may have an infected pseudocyst that requires drainage. Hemorrhage from a pseudocyst is rare, but can be life-threatening. Pseudocysts may abut large peripancreatic vessels (splenic, inferior and superior pancreaticoduodenal), and the digestive enzymes in the pseudocyst fluid may affect the vessel wall. Erosion into an artery can occur, with rapid onset of hypotension and severe abdominal pain. A patient with known pancreatitis who has sudden, severe abdominal pain (from sudden expansion of a pseudocyst with blood) or hypotension should undergo volume resuscitation and prompt to angiography to search for a bleeding pseudoaneurysm. Embolization should also be performed if possible.

Surgical

If the cyst does not resolve within 4 to 6 weeks and the patient is still symptomatic, drainage is performed. If the pseudocyst is approachable by CT-directed drainage, aspiration may be attempted, but recurrence rates are high. This decision is best made jointly by the radiologist and surgeon. Two basic techniques are used to drain pseudocysts surgically. Internal drainage is accomplished by anastomosis of the lumen of the pseudocyst to the lumen of a limb of the jejunum in a Roux-en-Y cyst-jejunostomy. If the cyst is fixed to the stomach by inflammation, a cyst-gastrostomy is performed. Internal drainage is preferred, but if it cannot be done because of technical problems, an immature cyst wall, or infection, then external drainage is used. Internal drainage is acceptable in more than 90% of cases. External drainage often requires a second operation because of pancreatic fistula. Biopsy of the cyst wall is recommended at the time of surgical drainage to confirm that the process is benign. Rarely, cystadenocarcinoma of the pancreas mimics a pseudocyst.

Pancreatic Neoplasms
General Considerations

Pancreatic adenocarcinoma is the fourth most common cause of cancer deaths in the United States, accounting for more than 27,000 deaths per year. The male:female ratio in most series is approximately 2:1, and the annual incidence is between 9 and 10 cases per 100,000 population. The principal risk factors for pancreatic carcinoma appear to be increasing age and cigarette smoking. Although controversy exists over the etiologic role of diabetes and alcohol, cigarette smoking appears to double the risk of pancreatic carcinoma. The most common location for pancreatic carcinoma is in the head of the gland, accounting for approximately two-thirds of all cases. The most common malignancy of the pancreas is an adenocarcinoma originating from the ductal epithelium. Several studies show a high incidence of multicentricity. The rest of the neoplasms that arise in the pancreas are islet cell tumors and cystadenocarcinomas, which account for fewer than 10% of pancreatic malignancies.

Clinical Presentation and Evaluation

The signs and symptoms of pancreatic carcinoma are related to the anatomy of the region. Tumors that originate in the periampullary region may present relatively early with asymptomatic jaundice. However, most patients have a combination of weight loss, jaundice, and pain as a result of infiltration of the tumor in the peripancreatic region. Pain tends to be in the posterior epigastric region, with radiation to the back. The pain of pancreatic disease is constant, posterior, and radiating. In contrast, intermittent colic is usually associated with biliary tract disease. A palpable nontender gallbladder in a jaundiced patient is more commonly associated with malignancy than with cholelithiasis (**Courvoisier's sign**). This unusual sign is explained by the distensibility of a nonfibrotic gallbladder wall in a patient without gallstones as opposed to a chronically scarred and inflamed gallbladder in a patient with chronic cholelithiasis.

The evaluation of patients with jaundice should begin with ultrasonography, which accurately shows biliary dilation, liver lesions, and (to a lesser degree) pancreatic lesions. In patients who have a history and physical findings that suggest pancreatic carcinoma, CT can be used as the initial diagnostic test. CT provides better detail of the periampullary region without sacrificing accuracy in detecting biliary dilation. It is also helpful in detecting liver metastases and assessing local tumor invasion. In many centers, a high-quality, contrast-enhanced CT scan is accurate for making the determination of tumor resectability. In Figure 17-6, a large pancreatic head mass is seen on CT scan. Radiographic features that deem these lesions unresectable include liver metastases, ascites, and vascular invasion (portal or superior mesenteric vein, superior mesenteric artery, vena cava, or aorta). ERCP (or, less commonly, percutaneous transhepatic cholangiography) also delineates the biliary and pancreatic ductal anatomy. Biliary drainage can also be achieved by either of these methods. Angiography is also used selectively to define the regional vascular anatomy that is prone to anomalies and to elucidate vascular invasion. However, this test has been supplanted by high-resolution CT scans in many cases. Except in cases of unresectable malignancy or in patients who are not candidates for operation, preoperative tissue sampling is not indicated.

Treatment

Patients with obstructive jaundice who are undergoing major surgical procedures should have correction of vitamin K–related coagulopathies that may be present because of biliary obstruction and liver injury. Baseline studies are recommended to evaluate hepatic function and nutritional status, including albumin, transferrin, and prothrombin time. Prolonged parenteral nutritional support and preoperative biliary tract decompression remain controversial. However, they may lower operative morbidity and mortality rates in selected patients.

The operative approach to pancreatic cancer involves assessment for regional and local spread. Patients without preoperative evidence of systemic or regional dissemination (which makes the tumor unresectable) undergo exploration with curative intent. For lesions in the head of the pancreas and the periampullary region, a **pancreaticoduodenectomy (Whipple procedure)** is performed. Lesions of the body and tail are treated with a distal pancreatectomy. With the advent of laparoscopic technology, many surgeons begin the procedure laparoscopically to avoid a laparotomy in patients whose lesion is found at exploration to be unresectable. At laparoscopy or laparotomy, incurable disease is defined by liver metastases or peritoneal seeding of tumor, both of which may be missed by CT scan. Invasion of the mesenteric root, celiac axis, or mesenteric vessels also constitutes unresectability. In patients with

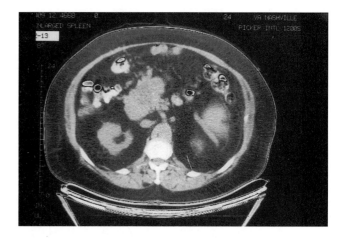

Figure 17-6 Computed tomography scan showing a large pancreatic head mass.

unresectable disease, palliation can be achieved with minimally invasive techniques. Biliary drainage is accomplished by endoscopic stenting in most cases. Patients with gastric outlet obstruction can be managed with gastrojejunostomy.

Pancreaticoduodenectomy involves resection of the distal common bile duct, duodenum, and head of the pancreas. Classically, an antrectomy has been performed; however, many surgeons currently perform a pylorus-preserving procedure. After resection, continuity is restored with choledochojejunostomy, pancreaticojejunostomy, and gastrojejunostomy (Figures 17-7, 17-8, and 17-9).

Given the magnitude of the procedure, complications are common. However, most complications are managed without operation, and the mortality rate of the procedure is less than 5% in modern series. A frequent complication is leakage of the pancreaticojejunostomy. This leakage may manifest as amylase-rich drainage from drains placed intraoperatively or abscess formation with overwhelming sepsis. The incidence of this complication is approximately 20% in most series. Management includes assurance of adequate drainage of pancreatic secretions, provision of nutrition (often including total parenteral nutrition), and control of fistula output. Most of these leaks close with nonoperative therapy.

Prognosis

Despite the removal of all gross disease, a significant number of patients die of recurrent disease. Factors associated with a poor prognosis include lymph node metastasis, tumor size greater than 3 cm, and perineural invasion. Patients who undergo resection for cure have a median survival of approximately 12 months, whereas patients with unresectable disease have a median survival of 6 months. Patients without lymph node metastases have a 5-year survival rate of approximately 25% to 30%. Although surgical therapy is the only curative modality, further advances in the treatment of pancreatic

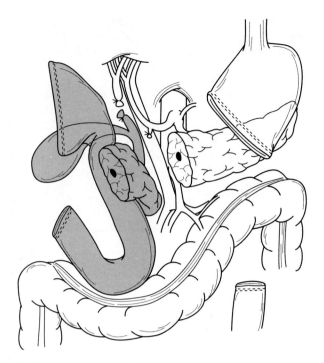

Figure 17-7 Details of Whipple resection (pancreaticojejunostomy) showing antrectomy, duodenectomy, cholecystectomy, distal common bile duct resection, and partial pancreatectomy. A vagotomy is also performed.

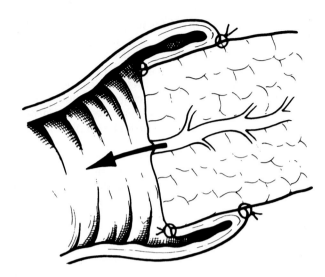

Figure 17-9 Detailed view of pancreaticojejunostomy. The pancreas inverts into the jejunum.

cancer will require the development of effective chemotherapeutic regimens and radiation protocols. Adjuvant radiation and chemotherapy after curative resection are common, but little data support their efficacy.

Cystadenoma and Cystadenocarcinoma

Cystadenomas and cystadenocarcinoma of the pancreas typically occur in middle-aged women. They are associated with malignancy in the mucosal lining approximately 60% of the time. Because these tumors usually arise in the body and tail of the pancreas, a distal pancreatectomy is usually adequate treatment. Cystadenocarcinoma of the pancreas is uncommon (1%–2%). These lesions originate in the body or tail of the gland and present as cystic lesions lined by epithelial cells. They are distinct from pseudocysts, which have no true epithelial lining. The prognosis for cystadenocarcinoma of the pancreas is much better than for the more common ductal (noncystic) adenocarcinomas. Cystadenocarcinoma is usually diagnosed incidentally on a CT scan or sonogram performed for another indication. Aggressive treatment of cystic lesions in the body and tail of the pancreas is recommended because of the favorable prognosis associated with resection. Biopsy should be performed for all cystic lesions of the pancreas to look for epithelial cells in the cyst wall. All epithelial-lined cysts of the pancreas should be excised, not drained internally.

Islet Cell Tumor of the Pancreas

The two most common islet cell neoplasms of the pancreas arise from the beta cells (insulinoma) and the delta cells (gastrinoma). Other islet cell neoplasms of the pancreas secrete glucagon and somatostatin, but they are extremely rare.

The classic symptoms of insulin-producing neoplasms are attacks (palpitations, tremulousness, and

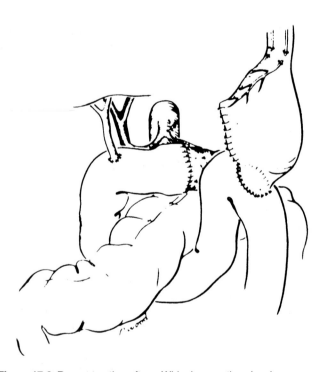

Figure 17-8 Reconstruction after a Whipple resection showing pancreaticojejunostomy, choledochojejunostomy, and gastroenterostomy.

tachycardia) precipitated by Whipple's triad: fasting, fasting blood sugar levels less than 50 mg/100 mL, and relief of symptoms after eating. Simultaneous measurement of serum insulin and blood glucose levels is diagnostic in showing an inappropriately high serum insulin level relative to blood glucose. Patients classically have been treated for psychiatric illness because of abnormal behavior associated with prolonged, recurrent hypoglycemia.

Localization of the tumor is the goal of the preoperative evaluation. The majority of insulinomas are solitary and benign. Angiography shows hypervascular lesions in approximately one-half of patients. Percutaneous transhepatic sampling of portal and splenic vein blood for measurement of insulin levels may also be helpful in the detection of insulinoma. CT scans of the abdomen show the lesion less than 50% of the time. The most successful means to identify a tumor is careful exposure of the pancreas surgically for careful palpation. Intraoperative ultrasound is used to confirm the findings and establish the anatomic relation to the pancreatic duct.

Surgical resection is the preferred management for patients with insulinoma. Delay in treatment is associated with neurologic damage as a result of recurrent episodes of hypoglycemia. The surgical treatment is resection of the tumor if it can be found. Usually, the tumor is simply enucleated without major pancreatic resection. Medical treatment is reserved for patients with unresectable malignant lesions. Streptozotocin and diazoxide are used with limited success.

Zollinger-Ellison Syndrome

Zollinger-Ellison syndrome is severe peptic ulcer disease caused by a gastrin-secreting islet cell tumor. These tumors are most commonly found in the gastrinoma triangle of the cystic duct: the junction of the second and third portion of the duodenum and the superior mesenteric artery as it crosses under the pancreatic neck.

The diagnosis of Zollinger-Ellison syndrome should be considered in patients with ulcers in unusual locations (distal duodenum or jejunum), recurrent duodenal ulcers, profuse watery diarrhea, or large gastric rugal folds seen on endoscopy. Elevations of the fasting serum gastrin greater than 750 pg/dL are common, but not diagnostic. The most common false-positive elevation of serum gastrin is found in patients with atrophic gastritis. These patients have no peptic ulcers on endoscopy and have a neutral gastric pH while they are not taking H_2 blockers or proton pump inhibitors. Patients with suspected gastrinomas and low levels of fasting serum gastrin should have a secretin-stimulation test to confirm the diagnosis before they undergo further imaging studies or an operation. A fasting gastrin level is obtained, followed by rapid intravenous administration of 2 units/kg secretin. Serum gastrin levels are obtained at 1, 3, 5, 7, 10, and 15 minutes. A positive test result is indicated by a doubling of the fasting level or an absolute increase of 200 pg/dL over the fasting level.

CT scan and ultrasound of the abdomen are used to attempt preoperative localization of gastrinomas, but they fail in as many as 50% of cases. Selective angiography to look for vascular blush may detect gastrinomas in as many as 75% of cases. Patients with gastrinomas as part of multiple endocrine neoplasia (MEN) syndrome are much more likely to have multicentric lesions than patients with sporadic gastrinomas; these lesions are difficult to localize. Octreotide-labeled nuclear medicine scans are highly sensitive and specific in detecting gastrinomas and metastatic disease, but precise correlation to the exact anatomic locations is difficult.

Surgical removal of gastrinomas should be attempted in good-risk surgical patients, especially if the lesion can be localized preoperatively and is not multicentric. Intraoperative ultrasound can be extremely useful in determining the location of tumors and the relation of the tumor to the bile duct, pancreatic duct, or major vessels. Many of these tumors can be removed with simple enucleation, but some require major pancreatic resection.

Currently, blind distal subtotal pancreatic resection is rarely used for gastrinomas. Instead, the detection and removal of these tiny lesions located in the duodenal wall is accomplished by intraoperative duodenal transillumination provided by intraoperative endoscopy. In the past, total gastrectomy to prevent intractable complications of peptic ulcers was done for undetectable or metastatic gastrinomas but, with the availability of potent acid secretion inhibitors (e.g., proton pump inhibitors), it is rarely used today.

Most gastrinomas are malignant, although histologic differentiation between benign and malignant tumors is extremely difficult. Clinical differentiation is based on the detection of metastatic disease with imaging studies or surgical exploration.

Multiple-Choice Questions

1. What is the most important component of the initial management of patients with acute pancreatitis?
   A. Adequate intravenous fluids
   B. Intravenous antibiotics
   C. Morphine
   D. Cimetidine
   E. Urgent celiotomy

2. Each of the following indicates a poor prognosis in patients with acute pancreatitis EXCEPT:
   A. White blood cell count greater than 16,000/mm^3
   B. Blood glucose greater than 200 mg/dL
   C. Serum calcium less than 8 mg/dL
   D. Serum amylase greater than 450 units/dL
   E. Aspartate aminotransferase (AST) greater than 250 sigma Frankel units/dL

3. What is the most common indication for operative intervention in patients with chronic pancreatitis?
   A. Exocrine deficiency
   B. Persistent abdominal pain

C. Endocrine deficiency
D. Weight loss
E. Risk of development of carcinoma

4. Pancreatic carcinoma is:
   A. Most common in younger individuals
   B. More common in female than in male patients
   C. Decreasing in incidence in the United States
   D. Associated with heavy cigarette smoking
   E. Not associated with diabetes mellitus

5. Secretin:
   A. Increases the secretion of gastrin
   B. Increases pancreatic secretion of water and bicarbonate
   C. Increases gastrointestinal motility
   D. Decreases bile flow from the liver
   E. Is released from the duodenum in response to luminal carbohydrate

6. The two most common predisposing factors for the development of acute pancreatitis are:
   A. Trauma and type I and V hyperlipidemia
   B. Alcoholism and hypercalcemia
   C. Cholelithiasis and alcoholism
   D. Hypercalcemia and peptic ulcer
   E. Multiple endocrine neoplasia and trauma

7. What is the best surgical treatment of a pancreatic pseudocyst?
   A. Cholecystojejunostomy
   B. Cyst enterostomy or cyst gastrostomy
   C. Duodenotomy and sphincteroplasty of the sphincter of Oddi
   D. Sump tube drainage through a separate stab wound
   E. Resection of the pancreatic pseudocyst

8. The most common pancreatic neoplasm arises from which of the following:
   A. Islet delta cells
   B. Acinar cells
   C. Islet alpha cells
   D. Muscularis layer of the pancreatic ducts
   E. Ductal epithelium

9. The most frequent and characteristic symptom of acute pancreatitis is:
   A. Ascites with bulging flanks
   B. Abdominal pain that radiates to the back and is relieved by sitting or bending forward
   C. Substernal or epigastric pain with radiation to the left shoulder and arm
   D. Waking up in the middle of the night with nausea and vomiting
   E. Loose, watery diarrhea six to ten times a day

10. A 64-year-old man with painless jaundice of 3 weeks' duration suggests a diagnosis of:
    A. Carcinoma of the pancreas
    B. Hydrops of the gallbladder

C. Acute pancreatitis
D. Common duct stones
E. Sclerosing cholangitis

11. Beta cell pancreatic islet tumors are characterized by:
    A. Recurrent peptic ulcer disease
    B. Intermittent diarrhea
    C. Metastases
    D. Hypoglycemia
    E. Excessive thirst

12. The most common location of carcinoma of the pancreas is the:
    A. Head region
    B. Isthmus
    C. Body
    D. Tail
    E. Distal main pancreatic duct

13. In carcinoma of the pancreas, the highest cure rates are encountered when the primary lesion is:
    A. In the body of the pancreas
    B. In the tail of the pancreas
    C. In the periampullary region
    D. Not found, but pulmonary metastasis exists
    E. Diffuse, with a weight loss of less than 10%

14. When considering screening tests for carcinoma of the pancreas, which of the following statements is correct?
    A. There are no useful screening tests.
    B. The carcinoembryonic antigen level is directly related to the presence of hepatic metastasis.
    C. The CA 19/9 test is the most specific.
    D. The galactosyl transferase II test is the most sensitive.
    E. Screening is performed only on patients who have a history of alcohol abuse.

15. The most useful test for the preoperative staging of carcinoma of the pancreas is:
    A. Celiac axis arteriogram
    B. Endoscopic retrograde cholangiopancreatography
    C. Upper gastrointestinal x-ray with oral contrast
    D. Computed tomography scan of the abdomen
    E. Ultrasound of the liver

16. The primary stimulus of cholecystokinin release is:
    A. Protein digestion products in the stomach
    B. Fat digestion products in the duodenum
    C. Carbohydrate in the duodenum
    D. Acid in the duodenum
    E. Distension of the stomach

17. Gastrinoma should be suspected in which of the following cases:
    A. A 25-year-old patient with a single duodenal ulcer that causes pain
    B. A 55-year-old patient with distal gastric and duodenal ulcers

C. A 45-year-old patient who requires an operation for a bleeding ulcer

D. A 35-year-old patient whose father had peptic ulcer disease

E. A 55-year-old patient who has recurrent ulcers after vagotomy and antrectomy

18. Steatorrhea occurs when:
   A. Chronic pancreatitis causes biliary stricture
   B. There is a pseudocyst
   C. Pancreatic enzyme secretion drops to less than 50% of normal
   D. Pancreatic enzyme secretion drops to less than 10% of normal
   E. Pancreatic duct stricture impairs pancreatic bicarbonate secretion

19. Which of the following statements regarding pancreatic pseudocysts is true?
   A. The lining of the pseudocyst cavity is columnar epithelium.
   B. The majority of acute fluid collections associated with acute pancreatitis require operation.
   C. Hemorrhage into a pseudocyst is a common complication.
   D. Pseudocysts that persist for longer than 4 to 6 weeks usually require drainage.
   E. Drainage of the pseudocyst into the biliary tree is the preferred operation.

20. The pancreas receives portions of its arterial blood supply from all of the following EXCEPT the:
   A. Proper hepatic artery
   B. Splenic artery
   C. Gastroduodenal artery
   D. Superior mesenteric artery
   E. Anterior pancreaticoduodenal arcade

Oral Examination Study Questions

CASE 1

A 45-year-old man has a 2-day history of severe, constant pain in the epigastrium and right upper quadrant of the abdomen.

OBJECTIVE 1

The student obtains the relevant history.
   A. The patient has noncrampy, penetrating upper abdominal pain radiating to the flank and back. The patient has some relief of pain on bending forward.
   B. The patient has nausea and vomiting.
   C. The patient has a history of alcohol intake.
   D. The patient had one previous episode of similar pain 6 months ago.

OBJECTIVE 2

The student elicits the following physical findings.
   A. The patient is a thin man who is bending forward and is in moderate distress.
   B. The temperature is 100.6° F, pulse is 110/min, blood pressure is 100/60 mm Hg, and respiratory rate is 20/min.
   C. The patient has mild scleral icterus.
   D. The abdomen is slightly distended. There is tenderness in the epigastrium and right upper quadrant, with rigidity and positive rebound. The lower quadrants are soft and nontender. Tenderness and rebound may be generalized in severe pancreatitis. Bowel sounds are hypoactive. Rectal examination shows guaiac-positive stool.

OBJECTIVE 3

The student discusses the differential diagnosis.
   A. Acute cholecystitis
   B. Perforated peptic ulcer
   C. Mesenteric ischemia
   D. Ruptured esophagus
   E. Myocardial infarction
   F. Pancreatitis

OBJECTIVE 4

The student orders appropriate laboratory and radiologic studies.
   A. Complete blood count shows hemoglobin of 12.5 g/dL and hematocrit of 36%. Hemoglobin and hematocrit may be low in hemorrhagic pancreatitis. White blood cell count is 14,000/mm^3, with a left shift.
   B. Serum amylase is 525 IU/L (normal, 50–200 IU/L).
   C. Serum lipase is 3.5 IU/L (normal, 0–1.5 IU/L).
   D. Total serum bilirubin is 3 mg/dL.
   E. Blood glucose is 290 mg/dL.
   F. Serum calcium is 10.1 mg/dL.
   G. Aspartate aminotransferase (AST) is 70 IU/L (normal, 3–35 IU/L).
   H. Lactic dehydrogenase (LDH) is 170 IU/L (normal, 50–140 IU/L).
   I. Upright x-rays of the chest and abdomen show no free intraperitoneal air, plate-like atelectasis in the left lobe of the lung, a sentinel loop of small bowel in the upper midabdomen, and a plain abdomen.
   J. Ultrasonography or computed tomography (CT) shows a normal gallbladder and biliary tree, with pancreatic enlargement.

OBJECTIVE 5

The student plans appropriate initial management.

A. The patient is given nothing by mouth.

B. A nasogastric tube is inserted.

C. Intravenous fluids are administered (with careful monitoring of output).

D. The abdomen is reexamined at frequent intervals.

The student should know the indications for the use of H_2 blockers (associated ulcer disease, gastritis).

OBJECTIVE 6

The student knows the indications for early surgical intervention.

A. Uncertain diagnosis

B. Associated calculus disease of the biliary tract

C. Pancreatic abscess

OBJECTIVE 7

The student discusses the complications of acute pancreatitis.

A. Hypovolemia

B. Renal failure

C. Respiratory failure

D. Hemorrhage

E. Coagulopathy

F. Sepsis

G. Pseudocyst

H. Abscess

I. Necrosis

J. Paralytic ileus

Minimum Level of Achievement for Passing

The student obtains the relevant history, elicits the pertinent physical findings, discusses the differential diagnosis, orders the appropriate tests, and plans the initial management. The student also names the complications.

Honors Level of Achievement

The student discusses in detail the management of complications of acute pancreatitis. The student is also familiar with the poor prognostic indicators and their significance.

ADDITIONAL INFORMATION

A. Etiology of acute pancreatitis
   1. Alcoholism
   2. Biliary tract disease
   3. Trauma
   4. Hyperparathyroidism
   5. Hyperlipidemia
   6. Medications (chlorothiazide, corticosteroids)
   7. Idiopathic causes

B. Poor prognostic indicators in acute pancreatitis
At admission:
   1. Age > 55 years
   2. White blood cell count > 16,000/mm³
   3. Blood glucose > 200 mg/dL
   4. Serum LDH > 350 IU/L
   5. AST > 250 sigma Frankel units/dL
During the initial 48 hours:
   6. Hematocrit decrease > 10%
   7. Blood urea nitrogen increase > 5 mg/dL
   8. Serum calcium < 8 mg/dL
   9. Arterial PO_2 < 60 mm Hg
   10. Base deficit > 4 mEq/L
   11. Estimated fluid sequestration > 6 L

If three or more of these signs are present, the risk of mortality is significant.

CASE 2

A 38-year-old man has a long-standing history of persistent upper abdominal pain and a history of significant alcohol consumption.

OBJECTIVE 1

The student obtains the pertinent history.

A. The patient has persistent pain in the epigastrium, radiating to the back, of 1.5 years' duration. For the past 6 months, the patient has received narcotics for pain relief.

B. The patient has significant weight loss.

C. The patient has steatorrhea.

D. The patient stopped drinking alcohol 1.5 years ago.

OBJECTIVE 2

The student elicits the pertinent physical findings.

A. The patient is a thin man in some distress.

B. Temperature is 98.6° F, pulse is 80/min, blood pressure is 100/60 mm Hg, and respiratory rate is 18/min.

C. The patient has no scleral icterus (some patients may be mildly jaundiced).

D. The abdomen is scaphoid, with no tenderness and no mass. The abdomen is soft in all quadrants, and bowel sounds are normal.

OBJECTIVE 3

The student orders the appropriate laboratory and radiologic studies.

A. Complete blood count is normal.

B. Blood glucose is 350 mg/dL.

C. Serum amylase is 85 IU/L (normal, 50–200 IU/L).

D. Total serum bilirubin is 0.8 mg/dL (normal, < 1.4 mg/dL).

E. Stool shows increased fat excretion.

F. The chest x-ray is normal, but the abdominal film shows pancreatic calcification.

G. Ultrasonography shows no cholelithiasis. A small pancreas is seen, but no cyst is visualized.

H. Endoscopic retrograde cholangiopancreatography (ERCP) shows a significantly dilated pancreatic duct, with areas of obstruction and stenosis ("chain of lakes" appearance).

The student should be familiar with the appropriate use of ERCP (as a preoperative study to determine the configuration of the pancreatic ductal system).

OBJECTIVE 4

The student discusses the medical management of this patient.

A. Low-fat diet

B. Pancreatic enzyme replacement

C. Insulin to control diabetes

D. Abstinence from alcohol

E. Treatment of narcotic addiction

The student should be aware of the poor response to medical therapy in most patients.

OBJECTIVE 5

The student discusses the indications for surgery.

A. Chronic, persistent abdominal pain

B. Correction of associated biliary tract disease

C. Associated pseudocyst

Minimum Level of Achievement for Passing

The student knows the clinical manifestations of chronic pancreatitis and the principles of medical and surgical therapy.

Honors Level of Achievement

The student discusses in detail the sequelae of chronic pancreatitis. These include endocrine and exocrine deficiencies, malabsorption, vitamin B_{12} deficiency (as a result of the binding of vitamin B_{12} to nonintrinsic factor proteins), persistent abdominal pain, and jaundice. The student is familiar with the social problems associated with the treatment of the patient (e.g., alcoholism, drug addiction). The student has a superior understanding of the surgical procedures carried out on these patients.

ADDITIONAL INFORMATION

A. If present, associated calculus disease of the biliary tract is eradicated (by cholecystectomy and possibly common bile duct exploration).

B. Successful pain relief is obtained in 70% to 80% of patients after surgical intervention.

C. If ERCP shows a dilated pancreatic duct with a "chain of lakes," a drainage procedure (pancreaticojejunostomy) is preferred (to preserve the pancreas). If the duct is narrow, a previous drainage procedure failed, or there is segmental involvement, resection of the pancreas is indicated, especially in patients who are diabetic.

CASE 3

A 62-year-old man has a history of vague upper abdominal pain, weight loss, and jaundice.

OBJECTIVE 1

The student obtains the pertinent history.

A. The patient has vague epigastric pain, radiating to the back, of 4 months' duration.

B. The patient had a weight loss of 15 lb over the past 6 weeks.

C. The patient noticed jaundice 3 days ago.

D. There is a history of dark urine and clay-colored stools.

E. The patient has a history of smoking one pack of cigarettes per day for 30 years.

F. The patient has a history of pruritus.

G. There is no history of diabetes.

H. The patient has no history that suggests migratory phlebitis.

I. The patient is not having fever or chills.

OBJECTIVE 2

The student elicits the pertinent physical findings.

A. The patient is a thin man who is in no distress.

B. The patient is afebrile. Pulse, blood pressure, and respiratory rate are normal.

C. There is deep scleral icterus.

D. The abdomen is flat and nontender. The liver is palpable 2 cm below the costal margin. A globular, nontender mass is palpable in the right upper quadrant. It moves with respiration. (What is Courvoisier's sign?) Bowel sounds are normal. The stool is positive for occult blood.

OBJECTIVE 3

The student orders the appropriate laboratory and radiologic studies.

A. Complete blood count is normal.

B. Urinalysis is positive for bilirubin and shows a decrease in urobilinogen.

C. Serum bilirubin is 9.8 mg/dL [total, 6.2 mg/dL (direct)].

D. Alkaline phosphatase is 850 IU/L (normal, 35–125 IU/L).

E. AST is 150 IU/L (normal, 3–40 IU/L).

F. AST is 180 IU/L (normal, 3–40 IU/L).

G. Prothrombin time and partial thromboplastin time are normal.

H. Total protein is 6.5 g/dL, and albumin is 3.6 g/dL.

I. Ultrasonography shows a mass in the head of the pancreas, an enlarged gallbladder without calculi, a dilated common bile duct, and dilated intrahepatic ducts.

J. CT to assess peripancreatic tissue, extrapancreatic extension, and metastases shows a moderate-sized mass in the pancreatic head, with associated bile duct enlargement.

K. Arteriography to assess the resectability of the pancreatic carcinoma is normal.

OBJECTIVE 4

The student discusses the differential diagnosis of obstructive jaundice (neoplasm vs calculus). The student develops an algorithm for the evaluation of jaundice.

ADDITIONAL QUESTIONS

1. What is the role of percutaneous transhepatic cholangiography or ERCP in the workup of a patient with obstructive jaundice? [delineation of the proximal extent of disease, internal biliary drainage, and external biliary decompression (of controversial worth)]

2. What is the 5-year survival rate for patients with pancreatic carcinoma? Is the rate different for periampullary carcinoma? (carcinoma of the pancreas: 10%–20%; periampullary carcinoma: 25%–45%)

3. What are the palliative procedures for unresectable carcinoma of the head of the pancreas?

4. What is the average survival after these palliative procedures? (6 months)

Minimum Level of Achievement for Passing

The student is aware of the low cure rate for pancreatic cancer, even with surgery. The student is familiar with the clinical features of carcinoma of the head of the pancreas and discusses the workup of patients with obstructive jaundice. The student knows that coagulopathy results from vitamin K malabsorption in patients with obstructive jaundice.

Honors Level of Achievement

The student discusses the role of ERCP and percutaneous transhepatic cholangiography in the workup of these patients. The student is also familiar with newer diagnostic techniques (e.g., fine-needle aspiration cytology). The student knows the criteria for unresectability (hepatic involvement, peritoneal metastasis, nodal involvement, superior mesenteric artery involvement, portal vein involvement, vena cava involvement).

SUGGESTED READINGS

Delcore R, Friesen SR. Gastrointestinal neuroendocrine tumors. *J Am Coll Surg* 1994;178:187–211.

Hodgkinson DJ, ReMine WH, Weiland LH: Pancreatic cystadenoma: a clinicopathologic study of 45 cases. *Arch Surg* 1978;113:512–519.

Lillemoe KD. Current management of pancreatic carcinoma. *Ann Surg* 1995;221:133–148.

Modlin IM, Brennan MF. The diagnosis of and management of gastrinoma. *Surg Gynecol Obstet* 1984;158:97–104.

Ranson JHC, Rifkind KM, Roses DF, et al. Prognostic signs and the role of operative management in acute pancreatitis. *Surg Gynecol Obstet* 1974;139:69.

Soper NJ, Brunt LM, Caller MP, et al. Role of laparoscopic cholecystectomy in the management of acute gallstone pancreatitis. *Am J Surg* 1994;167:42–51.

Steer ML, Waxman I, Freedman S. Chronic pancreatitis. *N Engl J Med* 1995;332:1482–1490.

Steinberg W, Tenner S. Acute pancreatitis. *N Engl J Med* 1994; 330:1198–1210.

Tann HP, Smith J, Garberoglic CA. Pancreatic carcinoma: an update. *J Am Coll Surg* 1996;183:164–184.

Warshaw AL, Richter JM. A practical guide to pancreatitis. In: Current Problems in Surgery, Vol 21. Chicago, Ill: Year Book Medical Publishers, 1984.

18

Liver

John R. Potts, III, M.D.
William C. Chapman, M.D.

OBJECTIVES

1. List at least three common benign tumors of the liver, and describe their appropriate treatment.
2. List four factors that favorably influence the prognosis after resection of hepatic metastasis from colorectal cancer.
3. List the two most common primary hepatobiliary malignancies and their relative frequency.
4. List the steps involved in diagnosing a hepatic mass.
5. Compare and contrast the clinical and pathologic features and the treatment of hepatic adenoma and focal nodular hyperplasia.
6. List the three major complications of portal hypertension.
7. List four forms of specific therapy for acute variceal hemorrhage in the order in which they are typically applied.
8. List at least three sites of portosystemic collateral formation in patients with portal hypertension.
9. List at least four causes of portal hypertension in addition to cirrhosis.
10. List three complications associated with ascites formation in the patient with portal hypertension.
11. List four common indications for liver transplantation.
12. List three common causes of fulminant hepatic failure.
13. Describe the settings in which opportunistic bacterial, fungal, and viral infections occur after liver transplantation.

In the liver, mass lesions (tumors, cysts, and abscesses), complications of **portal hypertension,** organ failure, and trauma constitute the vast majority of hepatic diseases for which surgical intervention is warranted.

Anatomy

The liver is the largest single gland in the body. In the average adult, it weighs approximately 1500 g. It is located below the diaphragm, with its greatest mass to the right of the midline. It is covered by the tough, fibrous Glisson's capsule, which extends into its parenchyma along penetrating vessels. Except for the bare area over its posterior surface near the vena cava, the liver is invested in peritoneum. Reflections of the peritoneum (falciform, coronary, and triangular "ligaments") attach the liver to the diaphragm and abdominal wall. Another reflection of the peritoneum, the gastrohepatic ligament, attaches the liver to other abdominal viscera.

A plane passing from the left side of the gallbladder and through the left side of the vena cava divides the left and right lobes of the liver. Each lobe has four segments described by vertical passage of the major hepatic veins and horizontal passage of the major portal venous and hepatic arterial branches. This surgically important segmental anatomy is not visible on the surface of the liver (Figures 18-1 and 18-2).

The liver enjoys a dual blood supply. In most individuals, the hepatic artery arises from the celiac axis. Occasionally, it comes from the superior mesenteric artery (i.e., replaced hepatic artery). The portal vein represents the confluence of drainage from the bowel and spleen. The portal vein supplies 70% of the blood flow to the liver. The right, middle, and left hepatic veins drain directly into the inferior vena cava.

Physiology

The functional unit of the liver is the lobule. On the periphery of each lobule lie hepatic arterial and portal venous branches. Centrally lies a draining vein. Blood from these vessels converges in the hepatic sinusoids with which each hepatocyte has intimate contact.

The liver performs more than 2000 metabolic functions, including bile production and the metabolism of protein, carbohydrates, fats, vitamins, drugs, and toxins. The hepatocyte, which is the principal cell of the liver, accounts for the majority of metabolic activity.

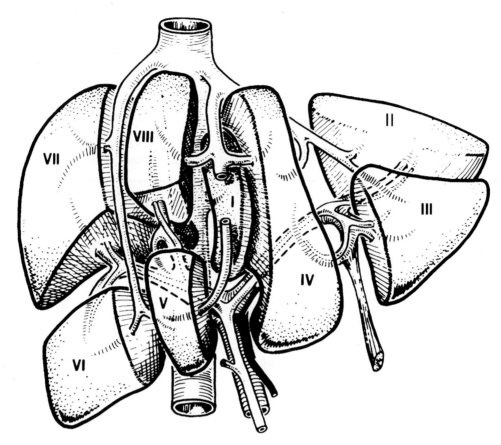

Figure 18-1 The functional division of the liver and liver segments according to Couinaud's nomenclature (segments *I–VIII*). (Reprinted with permission from Blumgart LH, ed. *Surgery of the Liver and Biliary Tract*. New York, NY: Churchill Livingstone, 1994:5.)

These cells continually divide and can potentially reproduce the entire cell mass of the liver every 50 days. The cells are aligned in a single layer along the hepatic sinusoids, and they transport essential substrates and hormones intracellularly. The hepatocytes then transport metabolic products either back into the plasma or into the bile canaliculus, which is positioned on the opposite side of this single layer of cells. In this way, the hepatocyte monitors and regulates plasma levels of proteins and assures that metabolic requirements are met.

The liver also performs many important immunologic functions. **Kupffer cells** line the vascular endothelium and are in close proximity to hepatocytes. These macrophages represent 80% to 90% of the fixed macrophages of the body and are subject to frequent turnover. Their unique position within the liver allows them to interface directly with damaging agents (e.g., endotoxin) from the portal circulation. These cells secrete a variety of effectors on hepatocytes and other cells within the body, including tumor necrosis factor (TNF-α), interleukin-1 (IL-1), interleukin-6 (IL-6), and other important cytokines.

Hepatic Tumors, Cysts, and Abscesses

With the increased availability and use of abdominal imaging techniques, including computed tomography (CT) scanning, symptomatic and incidental liver abnormalities are discovered with greater frequency. An important role of the physician who is treating a patient with a newly discovered hepatic abnormality is to determine both the likely etiology of the abnormality and whether further diagnostic or therapeutic measures are needed. Careful patient assessment is needed because incidental benign liver tumors and cysts are common and usually require no specific therapy. On the other hand, some benign liver tumors are resected, if feasible, even in the asymptomatic patient. An important principle is to avoid liver biopsy early in the workup of a newly discovered liver mass in an otherwise asymptomatic patient. Needle biopsy is usually not necessary to determine the most likely diagnosis. It is subject to sampling error and may introduce additional risks of bleeding or tumor seeding in a patient who might undergo tumor resection regardless of the biopsy result.

Benign Tumors

Hemangioma

Cavernous hemangioma of the liver is the most common benign liver tumor and occurs in as many as 8% of patients. These are probably congenital lesions and are embryologic hamartomas (benign tumors with two distinct cell types). They may enlarge over

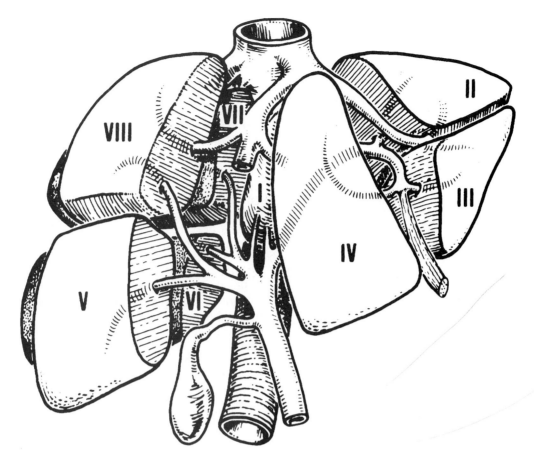

Figure 18-2 The biliary anatomy of the segments of the liver. The caudate lobe (segment *I*) drains into both the right and left ductal systems. (Reprinted with permission from Blumgart LH, ed. *Surgery of the Liver and Biliary Tract*. New York, NY: Churchill Livingstone, 1994:11.)

the lifetime of a patient. Some reports suggest hormonal responsiveness, including enlargement during pregnancy. Cavernous hemangiomas that are larger than 4 cm are defined as giant hemangiomas. These lesions are often incidental findings and require no specific therapy. Ultrasonography is usually diagnostic, showing focal hyperechoic abnormalities that are characteristic of these lesions. Contrasted CT imaging usually shows a progressive peripheral-to-central prominent enhancement and a central hypodense region.

Most patients are asymptomatic at presentation and remain so in follow-up. Spontaneous rupture is extremely rare. Longitudinal studies assessing long-term (> 10 years) follow-up in patients with giant cavernous hemangiomas confirm the absence of spontaneous rupture. Occasionally, patients with very large hemangiomas have pain, and surgical resection may be considered. Microscopic evaluation shows endothelial vascular spaces separated by fibrous septa. Nonresectional strategies used in the past (e.g., radiation, high-dose steroid administration, hepatic artery ligation, embolization) did not show efficacy. These lesions may undergo spontaneous thrombosis, which causes transient pain, elevation in hepatic transaminases, and involution on imaging studies.

Hepatic Adenoma

A **hepatic adenoma** is a benign tumor that usually occurs in young women between 30 and 50 years of age. Most patients have a history of estrogen exposure, usually in the form of long-standing use of oral contraceptives and occasionally from estrogen replacement therapy. These tumors grossly appear as solitary, unencapsulated masses. Their cut surfaces have a smooth, soft appearance. Microscopically, they appear as sheets of hepatocytes without portal triads or bile ducts.

The usual treatment of hepatic adenoma is surgical resection, if it can be safely performed, because of the risk of subsequent growth and possible rupture. In approximately 20% to 35% of cases, patients have pain or shock as a result of spontaneous rupture of the tumor. Hepatocellular carcinoma occasionally develops within these tumors. This risk appears to be increased for larger lesions (> 5 cm).

The clinical presentation is often highly suggestive of hepatic adenoma, but definite preoperative diagnosis may not be possible. CT scanning usually shows a solid hypodense lesion, sometimes with evidence of adjacent hemorrhage. ^{99m}Tc sulfa colloid scanning usually shows a corresponding filling defect because these tumors do not contain Kupffer cells and do not take up this tracer.

Needle biopsy may help to establish the diagnosis, but sampling errors can make it difficult to distinguish hepatic adenoma from focal nodular hyperplasia or hepatocellular carcinoma on the basis of needle biopsy alone.

The treatment of choice for these tumors is hepatic resection whenever possible. Occasionally, patients note tumor regression on withdrawal of hormonal therapy, but this situation is uncommon, and this treatment should not be used as primary therapy for an otherwise resectable tumor in a healthy patient. Intraoperative ultrasonography is performed in these patients, as in any patient with a hepatic neoplasm, to search for unsuspected additional tumors and to define the relation of the tumor to adjacent portal venous and hepatic arterial structures. Women with a history of hepatic adenoma should use alternative methods of contraception and avoid subsequent use of oral contraceptives. Avoidance of subsequent pregnancy is optimal, but if a patient becomes pregnant, she should undergo periodic surveillance ultrasound assessment of the liver.

Focal Nodular Hyperplasia

Focal nodular hyperplasia (FNH) is a well-circumscribed benign lesion. It usually has a central scar with fibrous septa and nodular hyperplasia. Unlike in hepatic adenoma, bile ducts are scattered throughout. These tumors do not have premalignant potential, and rupture or hemorrhage is extremely rare. These tumors are usually found incidentally when ultrasound or CT scanning is performed for some other cause.

The major difficulty in managing FNH lies in establishing a diagnosis. CT scanning does not differentiate this lesion from other solid liver masses, nor does ultrasonography provide assistance with the differential diagnosis. Arteriography may show a characteristic spoke-wheel pattern, but even needle biopsy may not distinguish this tumor from hepatic adenoma. For these reasons, FNH is often excised in the good-risk medical candidate who has a symptomatic tumor, but may be observed in the patient who is a poor operative candidate and in whom the diagnosis is strongly suspected based on imaging studies.

Malignant Tumors

Hepatocellular Carcinoma

Hepatocellular carcinoma (HCC), or hepatoma, accounts for more than 90% of all primary liver malignancies. This tumor usually occurs in patients with underlying liver disease (70%–80%). It occurs at high rates in areas where hepatitis B is endemic. Although cirrhosis from any cause appears to be associated with the development of HCC, it is also found at increased rates in noncirrhotic chronic carriers of hepatitis B and C.

HCC is suspected in any patient with known cirrhosis and sudden clinical decompensation, including worsening jaundice, encephalopathy, or increasing ascites. HCC is also part of the differential diagnosis for any solid liver tumor. Alpha-fetoprotein (AFP) is an

α_1-globulin serum marker that is elevated in 60% to 80% of patients with HCC. This tumor marker may also be elevated to 200 to 400 mg/dL in patients with cirrhosis who do not have a hepatoma. Elevations greater than 500 to 1000 mg/dL are almost always associated with HCC.

When HCC is suspected, ultrasound, CT, or magnetic resonance scanning may show the tumor mass. HCC has a propensity for vascular invasion, particularly into portal venous tributaries, and the likelihood of vascular invasion increases with increasing tumor size. This property accounts for the common finding of satellitosis (multifocal tumors within a similar segmental distribution in the liver) seen with HCC.

The best treatment for HCC is resection with clear surgical margins, whenever possible, in a patient with no evidence of extrahepatic disease. Unfortunately, surgical resection is often impossible because of the underlying cirrhosis that is so common in patients with HCC. Although it is possible to remove as much as 70% of the normal hepatic parenchyma at liver resection, the presence of cirrhosis limits the regenerative capacity of the liver. No specific studies conclusively determine the extent of hepatic parenchyma that can be safely resected in a cirrhotic patient, and most surgeons attempt only small peripheral wedge or segmental resections in this setting. When patients with HCC and cirrhosis undergo successful tumor resection, the remaining liver is the most common site of future recurrence ($\geq$ 50% of patients), probably because similar etiologic factors are present in the remaining liver (e.g., hepatitis with the formation of second primary lesions) and also from satellite lesions that were not detected at initial resection. Other sites of tumor metastasis include lung and bone. Brain and intraperitoneal metastases are less common.

Liver transplantation has theoretical appeal for patients with HCC because it not only removes the malignant tumor, but also eliminates possible sites of recurrence in the remaining diseased liver. It also provides hepatic replacement in patients who usually have severely limited hepatic reserve in addition to their tumor. Major limitations to the use of liver transplantation in the treatment of patients with hepatoma include the limited number of donor livers for transplantation and the high cost of this treatment modality. Additionally, the results are poor when extrahepatic tumor is present. This tumor may undergo accelerated growth under the influence of the immunosuppression that is required to prevent rejection of the transplanted liver. Recent strategies used preoperative chemoembolization followed by posttransplant adjuvant chemotherapy in carefully selected patients. Chemoembolization involves the infusion of chemotherapy [usually doxorubicin (Adriamycin)] combined with gelatin foam particles. This process induces tumor ischemia while prolonging chemotherapy dwell times at the site of hepatic tumors. This procedure is possible for hepatic tumors because of the dual blood supply present for the liver. Further, because most hepatomas derive 85% or more of their blood supply from a hepatic arterial source, this treatment modality induces a much greater effect than on the surrounding nontumor hepatic parenchyma, where at least 50% of the oxygen and nutrient supply is derived from a portal venous source. In many centers, liver transplantation in combination with pretransplantation chemoembolization is the treatment of choice for patients with advanced cirrhosis and small (< 5 cm), but unresectable HCC.

The fibrolamellar variant of HCC occurs more often in younger patients and often is not associated with underlying cirrhosis. Patients with this tumor usually do not have elevated AFP levels and have a better long-term prognosis after resection than patients with standard HCC. It is unclear whether this improved prognosis is related to the less aggressive nature of the tumor or to the absence of underlying liver disease and a greater resectability rate.

Cholangiocarcinoma

Cholangiocarcinoma (see Chapter 16) usually causes obstructive jaundice and a bile duct stricture on endoscopic retrograde cholangiopancreatography. There is often no visible tumor mass on CT scanning. Occasionally, primary tumors of bile duct origin present as a solid tumor within the substance of the liver. These tumors are treated with liver resection. Other rare primary tumors of the liver include angiosarcoma and epithelioid hemangioendothelioma.

Metastatic Tumors

The most common malignant tumors found in the liver represent metastatic carcinoma, most commonly from a gastrointestinal source (probably because the hepatic sinusoids are the first capillary bed encountered for blood from a gastrointestinal source). In patients who die of malignant disease, 30% to 40% have hepatic metastases at autopsy. Although hepatic metastases usually are indicative of widespread metastatic carcinoma, in selected cases, hepatic metastases may be the only residual disease and therefore can be treated with hepatic-only directed therapy. This approach is clearly established for colorectal carcinoma, where successful resection of metastatic foci can result in 5-year survival rates of 30% to 40% in properly selected patients.

Requirements for successful hepatic resection of colorectal metastases include the absence of extrahepatic disease and the ability to safely resect all hepatic disease. Patients who have hepatic metastasis more than 1 year after colon resection and those without regional lymph node involvement at the time of colon resection fare better than those with synchronous colon and metastatic liver lesions and those with mesenteric lymph node involvement. Patients with three or fewer liver lesions resected appear to fare better than those with more lesions. However, long-term survival is reported with resection of as many as five metastatic foci. Patients with multilobar metastases resected appear to do as well as those in whom all metastatic foci are confined to a single lobe.

Although resection of hepatic metastases may afford long-term survival, most of these patients (60%–70%) have recurrence of colorectal carcinoma, and the residual liver is the most common site of recurrence. For this reason, resected patients require careful selection and close follow-up. It is unclear whether patients who undergo successful hepatic resection of colorectal metastases benefit from adjuvant systemic or regional chemotherapy after liver resection. Current clinical trials that address this question may provide results within the next several years.

Hepatic Cysts

Simple Cysts and Polycystic Liver Disease

Cystic disease of the liver is a common finding, particularly with the increased use of CT to investigate many abdominal conditions. Simple cysts occur in as many as 10% of patients. They are usually small and asymptomatic. They usually contain clear serous fluid and do not communicate with the biliary tree. Although they may appear in multiples, they usually number fewer than three to four and are scattered throughout the liver.

Simple cysts are most often asymptomatic, but occasionally may become quite large and may be associated with pain or early satiety because of the mass effect. Needle aspiration provides temporary relief, but the cysts almost always recur. For this reason, standard treatment includes unroofing or fenestrating the cyst wall and allowing the cyst fluid to drain into and be resorbed by the peritoneal cavity. Surgical resection of simple cysts is not usually required and may be dangerous because large portal and hepatic venous branches may be compressed in the cyst–parenchyma interface and because there is usually no clear plane for resection of the cyst wall.

Polycystic liver disease (Figures 18-3 and 18-4) is an autosomal dominant disorder that causes multiple cysts that are microscopically similar to simple cysts. Unlike simple cysts, however, these cysts are innumerable, and progressive enlargement is the norm. Additionally, patients with polycystic liver disease often have polycystic kidney disease that may progress to end-stage renal disease. The hepatic cysts in this condition may be treated with resection of the dominant area of cystic involvement, but simple cyst unroofing alone is rarely effective because of the extensive involvement. Some patients have extensive involvement of the entire liver, but even in this situation, it is rare for hepatic synthetic function to be significantly altered.

Cystic Neoplasms

Although most patients with liver cysts have non-neoplastic simple cysts that require treatment only if they are symptomatic, some cystic lesions are cystadenoma or cystadenocarcinoma. A clue to the neoplastic nature of these cysts is the presence of thick walls with multiple septations within the cyst. Unlike simple cysts or polycystic liver disease, which occur with similar

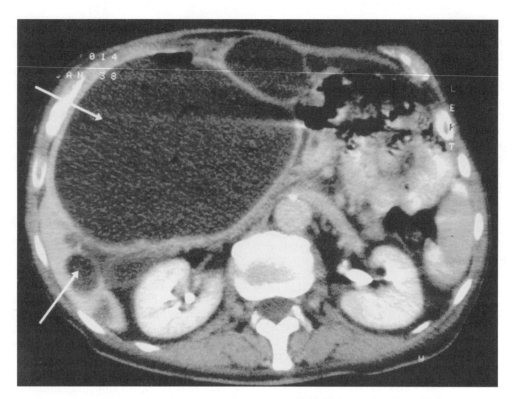

Figure 18-3 Computed tomography scan showing multiple large and small cysts within the liver *(arrows)* in a patient with polycystic liver disease.

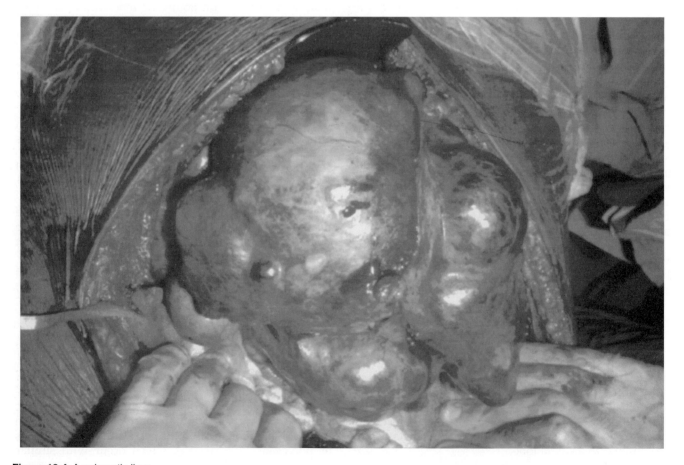

Figure 18-4 A polycystic liver.

frequency in men and women, cystadenoma occurs with a much higher frequency in women, usually in middle age. Calcifications in the cyst wall may also be noted and are more common in cystadenocarcinoma than in the benign variety. Because of the malignant potential of these lesions, the preferred treatment is surgical excision. Nonresectional procedures, including marsupialization (creation of a pouch), drainage into the peritoneal cavity, and drainage into the gastrointestinal tract, are associated with a high rate of cyst recurrence and the development of infected cysts. Therefore, they are not indicated.

Hydatid Cysts

Hydatid cystic disease occurs when humans become infected with echinococcal organisms and act as an accidental host. The normal life cycle of this parasite involves sheep and carnivores (wolves or dogs). Humans are infected by contact with dog feces. The most common infecting organism is *Echinococcus granulosis,* which forms unilocular cysts within the hepatic parenchyma that may grow as large as 10 to 20 cm. Within the larger cysts are multiple daughter cysts that contain innumerable protoscolices.

The diagnosis of hydatid cyst disease is suspected in any patient who has lived in an endemic region (Alaska, regions of the southwest United States, and many foreign countries) and who has cystic hepatic lesions that contain characteristic daughter cysts. Calcifications may also be present and are sometimes indicative of long-standing indolent infection. The diagnosis is confirmed with serologic testing. If the diagnosis is suspected, needle aspiration or biopsy must not be performed because it may produce disastrous results from seeding of protoscolices throughout the abdominal cavity and may also induce profound anaphylaxis. After the diagnosis is established, antiparasitic therapy with mebendazole is initiated. Open exploration is performed, and the area of cystic involvement is walled off with a scolicidal agent (e.g., hypertonic saline). The cyst contents are then carefully removed, with care taken to dissect out the inner cyst lining, which may contain infective parasites. Extreme caution is used to avoid spillage of any of the cyst contents into the peritoneal cavity because spillage can lead to intraperitoneal recurrence of hydatid cyst disease.

Hepatic Abscesses

Pyogenic Abscess

Patients with bacterial liver abscess usually have right upper quadrant pain, fever, and leukocytosis. The alkaline phosphatase level is elevated in most patients, and CT and ultrasound imaging show a hypoechoic abnormality that sometimes is associated with a hyperechoic or hypervascular wall. Although hepatic abscess may develop as a consequence of hematogenous seeding from any site, this complication usually occurs from a gastrointestinal (i.e., diverticulitis) or biliary tract source.

Percutaneous aspiration and drain placement aid in the diagnosis and facilitate resolution of the infectious process. Antimicrobial therapy is directed by the results of blood and abscess cultures. Biliary stenting may be required if biliary obstruction contributed to the abscess formation. As part of the hepatic abscess workup, a source is sought and treated if indicated.

Amebic Abscess

Although rare in the United States, amebic hepatic abscess is relatively common in regions endemic for amebiasis, including Central and South America. For this reason, it should be considered in immigrants from these regions. Liver abscess occurs in as many as 10% of patients with amebiasis and is one of the most common sites of extraintestinal infection. Percutaneous aspiration shows a sterile fluid that has a characteristic "anchovy paste" appearance. These abscesses respond dramatically to metronidazole. Unlike pyogenic abscesses, they do not require percutaneous drainage.

Portal Hypertension and Its Complications

Portal hypertension is simply abnormally high pressure in the portal vein or its tributaries. Figure 18-5 shows the normal portal circulation. One uncommon, but relatively straightforward form of portal hypertension is sinistral, or left-sided, portal hypertension. In this disorder, thrombosis of the splenic vein (usually caused by pancreatitis or pancreatic tumor) leads to increased pressure in the spleen, which causes splenomegaly and secondary hypersplenism. Another consequence of this disorder is the development of gastric varices because of the return of splenic blood flow to the portal vein through the short gastrics, the submucosal veins of the stomach, and the coronary vein. Splenectomy cures this compartmentalized form of portal hypertension.

Much more common is generalized portal hypertension, in which the portal vein and all of its tributaries are under high pressure. Cirrhosis causes approximately 90% of all portal hypertension in the United States. Approximately 70% of cases of cirrhosis are caused by chronic ethanol ingestion. Portal hypertension can also result from portal vein thrombosis (which accounts for 50% of portal hypertension in children, often related to umbilical vein catheter placement in infancy) and schistosomiasis (which, worldwide, is the most common cause of presinusoidal portal hypertension). In addition, portal hypertension occasionally results from excessive inflow (e.g., a large arteriovenous fistula to a portal vein tributary). Obstruction of hepatic

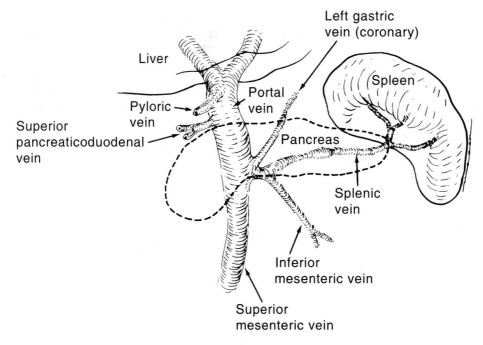

Figure 18-5 Anatomy of the portal circulation. (Reprinted with permission from Rikkers LF. Portal hypertension. In: Goldsmith HS, ed. *Practice of Surgery: General Surgery.* Vol. 3, Chap. 4. Philadelphia, Pa: Harper & Row, 1981.)

venous outflow can transmit high pressure to the portal vein. The best known example of this phenomenon is the Budd-Chiari syndrome of hepatic venous occlusion, which can result from various thrombotic states or from the formation of vascular webs in the vena cava. Rarely, congestive heart failure causes portal hypertension in adults. Regardless of the etiology, the increased pressure in the portal vein is compensated for in part by dilation of the portal venous tributaries and in part by the development of collateral channels to the systemic venous system. **Portosystemic collateral routes** form where portal and systemic veins normally meet (Figure 18-6). These sites include the submucosal veins of the esophagus, which communicate with the azygous system cephalad; the hemorrhoidal veins, which communicate with the iliac system caudad; the umbilical vein, which communicates with veins of the anterior abdominal wall; and the retroperitoneum, which communicates with the vena cava. Adhesions to the abdominal wall can also carry large portosystemic collateral channels. With the development of portal hypertension, the patient may have three complications: ascites, **hepatic encephalopathy,** and variceal bleeding.

Ascites

Ascites is the accumulation of serous fluid in the peritoneal cavity. In portal hypertension, ascites forms as a result of increased hydrostatic pressure and decreased colloid oncotic pressure caused by deficient protein production. This situation favors transudation of fluid out of the vascular space, into the parenchyma, and ultimately into the peritoneal cavity. Clinically significant volumes of ascites are usually detected on

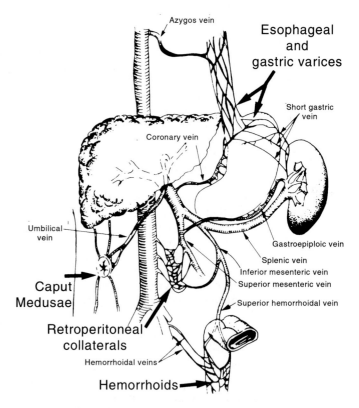

Figure 18-6 Sites of portal-systemic collateralization. (Reprinted with permission from Rikkers LF. Portal hypertension. In: Goldsmith HS, ed. *Practice of Surgery: General Surgery.* Vol. 3, Chap. 4. Philadelphia, Pa: Harper & Row, 1981.)

physical examination by dependent dullness to percussion and by eliciting a fluid wave. Smaller amounts are detected by ultrasound or CT scan. A number of conditions other than portal hypertension can result in ascites accumulation, including hypoproteinemic states (nephrotic syndrome, protein-losing enteropathy, malnutrition); carcinomatosis; pancreatic, chylous, or bile ascites; and end-stage renal disease. The differential diagnosis emphasizes the need for diagnostic paracentesis in the patient with newly diagnosed ascites. Studies on the fluid should include cytology, cell count and differential, amylase, triglyceride and protein levels, pH, and bacterial cultures.

In patients with portal hypertension related to cirrhosis and without complicating features, the cell count and differential of ascitic fluid usually shows a predominance of monocytes with a total neutrophil cell count of fewer than 250 cells/mL. The cytology shows nonneoplastic cells. The amylase level is less than or equal to the serum amylase level, as is the triglyceride level. Bacterial cultures are negative. The pH is usually 7.3 or greater in noninfected ascites, and the protein content is usually less than 2.5 g.

Ascites in portal hypertension can lead to substantial morbidity. Umbilical, groin, and other abdominal wall hernias can enlarge dramatically with the added pressure of ascites. The skin overlying hernias can become thinned and ulcerated. Rupture of the hernias can occur and is associated with a high mortality rate. Spontaneous bacterial peritonitis occurs in approximately 10% of cirrhotic patients with ascites. It is usually associated with an ascitic fluid white blood cell count of more than 500 cells/mL and a predominance of neutrophils. The mechanism of inoculation is speculative, but most infections are monomicrobial with enteric organisms. This disorder is associated with an exceedingly high mortality rate and requires aggressive antibiotic therapy.

The decreased circulating volume in the patient with significant ascites leads to decreased renal blood flow, aldosterone secretion, and redistribution of renal blood flow. As a result, urinary volume and urinary sodium concentration are decreased. Ultimately, renal failure can occur. This unfortunate, but common sequence is called hepatorenal syndrome, but there is no clear evidence to show that it represents anything other than profound prerenal azotemia secondary to intravascular volume depletion. Acute renal failure against a background of ascites rarely occurs spontaneously but, sadly, is usually precipitated by overzealous use of diuretics.

Treatment

Medical management effectively controls ascites in more than 90% of patients. Fluid intake is moderately restricted, and sodium intake is limited to less than 40 mEq/day. Diuresis begins with spironolactone, an aldosterone antagonist, which promotes sodium excretion. The dose is gradually increased until urinary excretion of sodium exceeds that of potassium. If further diuresis is necessary, loop or thiazide diuretics are cautiously added. When the ascitic volume severely limits respiration, or mobility and rapid decompression are desired, therapeutic paracentesis is performed, particularly in patients who have peripheral edema in addition to ascites. Large volumes (8–10 L) can safely be removed in one sitting. At paracentesis, it is probably prudent to administer salt-poor albumin intravenously to replace the estimated protein content of ascites that is withdrawn.

Rarely, when medical management and paracentesis fail, more invasive treatment is required. One option is the placement of a peritoneal venous shunt. This device is a tube approximately the diameter of intravenous tubing that originates in the peritoneal cavity and runs subcutaneously to its insertion in the internal jugular vein. The peritoneal end has multiple side-hole perforations, and the tubing contains a one-way valve that precludes the reflux of blood into the tubing. When properly functioning, these devices restore circulating volume and enhance urinary output. Placement is technically simple, but they are associated with a number of complications (e.g., infection, occlusion of the tubing by proteinaceous debris, congestive heart failure). Variceal bleeding can also occur as a result of the increased venous pressure associated with increased circulating volume.

Portosystemic shunts (Figure 18-7) are another means of controlling ascites by reducing portal pressure. At one time, surgical portacaval shunts were used for this purpose, but this effort was largely abandoned. Not only did the operative morbidity exceed the benefit of ascites reduction, but a number of survivors had portosystemic

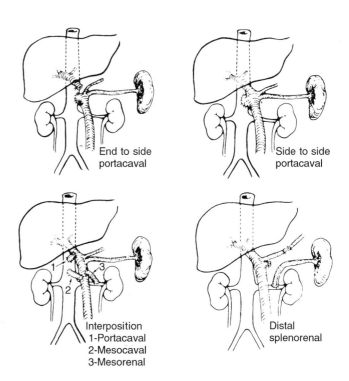

Figure 18-7 Surgical portal–systemic shunts.

encephalopathy. Thus, one complication of portal hypertension was merely traded for another. Recently, there was some enthusiasm for radiologically placed portosystemic shunts in the treatment of ascites. These **transjugular intrahepatic portacaval shunts (TIPS),** although associated with less procedure-related morbidity than surgical shunts, are not uniformly successful. Like surgical shunts, they often merely trade ascites for encephalopathy. Both TIPS and surgically constructed central shunts (nonselective) allow portal blood to bypass the metabolic actions of the liver. As a result, amino acid imbalances may occur and are believed to play an important role in hepatic encephalopathy (discussed below).

Hepatic Encephalopathy

Hepatic encephalopathy is a poorly understood neuropsychiatric disorder that can develop in patients with severe liver disease. Clinical features include confusion, obtundation, tremor, asterixis, and fetor hepaticus (sweet, slightly feculent smell of the breath noted in advanced liver disease). The pathogenesis of encephalopathy is not understood. A number of theories were advanced, including increased circulating levels of toxins (e.g., ammonia), the presence of false neurotransmitters (e.g., aromatic amino acids), and the concerted effect of two or more metabolic abnormalities (e.g., alkalosis, hypoxia, infection, electrolyte imbalance). Certain factors can precipitate encephalopathy. Among these are infection, gastrointestinal bleeding, constipation, dehydration, and metabolic disorders. In some cases, the ingestion of even modest amounts of dietary protein induces encephalopathy.

The diagnosis of hepatic encephalopathy is made clinically. The serum ammonia level is often elevated in encephalopathic patients, but this test lacks sufficient specificity to be diagnostic. Certain electroencephalographic patterns are seen in encephalopathy, but again, they are not diagnostic. It is important to exclude other causes of altered mental status (e.g., acute intoxication, organic brain syndrome and infection, injury or tumor in the central nervous system).

Treatment

In patients with hepatic encephalopathy, protein intake is moderately restricted. In patients who have gastrointestinal bleeding or constipation, the gut is purged. One particularly useful substance is lactulose, which can be administered by mouth, nasogastric tube, or enema. Lactulose not only acts as a cathartic but also alters the pH in the colon and inhibits bacterial production of ammonia. Intraluminal antibiotics (e.g., neomycin) decrease ammonia production by decreasing bacterial flora.

Variceal Bleeding

Although ascites and encephalopathy cause substantial morbidity in the portal hypertensive population, the complication that is clearly associated with the greatest mortality is bleeding from esophageal varices. The percentage of patients with cirrhosis who have esophageal varices is not known, but only approximately 30% of patients who have varices bleed from them. Esophageal varices are submucosal veins that become dilated and fragile in the presence of portal hypertension. As noted earlier, esophageal varices are collateral routes that drain the short gastric and coronary (left gastric) veins from the portal system into the azygous vein in the systemic venous circulation. The higher the pressure in these veins, the greater the risk of rupture. However, what causes rupture of a given vein at a given time is unclear. Theories include spontaneous rupture, erosion by esophagitis, and disruption by passing food. Two aspects of therapy for variceal bleeding must be considered: cessation of the acute bleeding and prevention of recurrent bleeding.

Cessation of Acute Bleeding

The mortality rate per admission for variceal bleeding is between 25% and 50%. This staggering figure speaks to the need for rapid, aggressive management. The initial goal of treatment is volume resuscitation through large-bore intravenous lines to maintain tissue perfusion. As with other causes of massive hemorrhage, the volume that is lost is blood. Thus, replacement consists predominantly of blood components, particularly in variceal bleeding, because the salt and water in crystalloid solutions may later contribute to ascites formation. Although it is important to restore adequate circulating volume, it may be equally important to refrain from excessive volume replacement. Variceal pressure varies directly with central venous pressure. Thus, excessive volume replacement may lead to further bleeding. Urinary output is the best clinical indicator of circulatory perfusion. For this reason, a urinary catheter is placed early in the resuscitation effort. The hemoglobin and coagulation factors are monitored frequently to determine the adequacy of blood component therapy. Oxygen is also administered, and the hemoglobin–oxygen saturation closely monitored.

It is critical to establish the diagnosis of variceal bleeding early in the course of the disease so that therapy can be properly directed. The diagnoses of cirrhosis and portal hypertension can often be made from the history and physical examination (e.g., temporal muscle wasting, spider angiomata over the chest, ascites, splenomegaly). However, numerous studies show that as many as 50% of acute upper gastrointestinal bleeds in cirrhotic patients originate not from esophageal varices, but from such sources as peptic ulcer disease and Mallory-Weiss tears (mucosal tears at the gastroesophageal junction). Endoscopy is necessary to determine the source of bleeding. It is performed as soon as possible because the passage of even a few hours may not only prevent identification of the source of bleeding, but may also delay appropriate therapy. Gastric lavage before endoscopy is beneficial both in achieving a thorough examination and in purging blood from the gut and abating the subsequent development of encephalopathy from the extra protein load. Lavage is not performed with cold solutions because they can cause rapid loss of body temperature which, among other things, can induce coagulopathy. During endoscopy, the diagnosis is made by visualizing the bleeding varix or by documenting the presence of varices and the absence of other bleeding sources.

Pharmacologic Therapy

Pharmacologic therapy for variceal hemorrhage is usually well tolerated and has no adverse effect, even if there is a nonvariceal cause of bleeding. For this reason, it is initiated before the diagnosis of variceal bleeding is confirmed. Intravenous **somatostatin** acts promptly to decrease variceal bleeding by splanchnic vasoconstriction and decrease of portal venous flow. It decreases or halts variceal bleeding in more than 50% of patients and has few clinically significant side effects. Intravenous vasopressin also acts by splanchnic vasoconstriction, but in prospective randomized trials, was not as effective as somatostatin in controlling variceal hemorrhage. The vasoconstrictive effect of vasopressin is not limited to the splanchnic circulation. If given to patients with atherosclerotic disease, the coronary and peripheral vasoconstriction can cause serious complications (e.g., myocardial infarction, limb ischemia). The simultaneous infusion of nitroglycerin with vasopressin ameliorates these complications and may help to stop variceal bleeding.

Endoscopic Therapy

Endoscopic therapy is effective in approximately 80% of patients with acute variceal hemorrhage. One form of endoscopic therapy is sclerotherapy, in which small amounts of caustic solutions are injected either into or adjacent to varices to induce edema and scarring and obliterate the variceal lumen. A number of complications can occur, including additional bleeding from tearing a delicate varix, ulceration of the epithelium over the varix, perforation of the esophagus, and dissemination of the sclerosing agent to the pulmonary or systemic circulation.

To accomplish the same effect of luminal obliteration of the varix without many of the complications of sclerotherapy, banding of varices recently gained popularity. This treatment is similar to the banding of internal hemorrhoids, which has been successfully used for years. A hollow extension of the endoscope is placed in contact with the epithelium surrounding a varix, and suction is applied to elevate both the epithelium and the underlying varix. A very small rubber band is then used to encircle and tightly gather the varix, thus obliterating its lumen. Banding is at least as effective as sclerotherapy in the cessation of acute variceal hemorrhage, and has few of its undesirable side effects.

One limitation on both forms of endoscopic therapy is that the varices must be clearly seen for accurate and safe application. Thus, if the patient has massive active bleeding that fills the lumen of the esophagus, it may not be possible to proceed with endoscopic therapy.

Another limitation of both sclerotherapy and banding is that they are much more difficult to apply safely to gastric varices (which may be difficult to visualize in the fundus) than to esophageal varices.

Luminal Tamponade

When both pharmacologic and endoscopic treatments do not control variceal hemorrhage, luminal tamponade can be applied. The **Sengstaken-Blakemore tube** (Figure 18-8) is one specific device available for luminal tamponade, but a number of other tubes with various modifications are available. All of these devices have a distal port to suction the luminal contents of the stomach, a large round balloon that places traction on the gastric fundus and tamponades the submucosal veins that approach the esophagus and, above that, a cylindrical balloon to directly tamponade the esophageal varices. If the available device does not have a port proximal to the esophageal balloon to suction swallowed saliva, then a second tube is placed for this purpose. When properly applied, variceal tamponade effectively controls variceal bleeding in approximately 90% of cases. However, a number of serious complications (e.g., aspiration, asphyxiation, esophageal rupture) can occur. Thus, placement and maintenance of these tubes follows a very strict protocol. One other limitation of variceal tamponade is that it can be applied

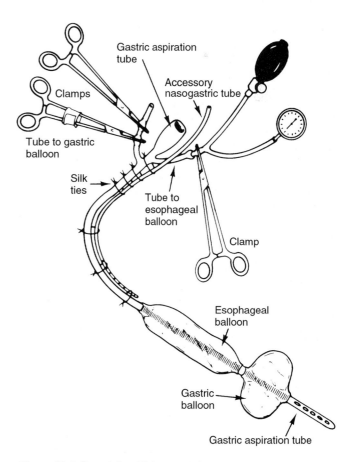

Figure 18-8 Sengstaken-Blakemore tube.

only for a relatively short period (24–36 hours) because of the risk of necrosing underlying tissue. Thus, a plan must be devised for further treatment when the tamponade is released.

TIPS

If all other available forms of therapy fail, TIPS can be attempted to control acute variceal hemorrhage. This procedure consists of cannulating the jugular vein, directing a semirigid wire into a large hepatic vein, and puncturing the hepatic vein wall, the intervening hepatic parenchyma, and the wall of a large portal vein branch nearby. An expandable stent is then used to dilate and maintain a channel between the portal and hepatic vein branches. This procedure is truly a portacaval shunt that is created within the liver. The diameter of the lumen of the channel is adjusted until the reduction in portal pressure is sufficient to halt the variceal bleeding. TIPS is technically accomplished in approximately 95% of patients. Except in profoundly coagulopathic patients, it is highly successful in controlling acute variceal hemorrhage.

After the acute variceal hemorrhage is controlled, attention is turned to correcting ascites, encephalopathy, and any other problems (e.g., sepsis, malnutrition). At the same time, plans are made to prevent recurrent variceal hemorrhage.

Prevention of Recurrent Variceal Hemorrhage

As noted earlier, in most patients, varices do not bleed. However, once variceal bleeding occurs, the chance of repeated bleeding approaches 70%. Most recurrent bleeding occurs within a few weeks of the index bleed. A number of options are available to prevent recurrent bleeding. The choice of options for a given patient depends on a number of factors. During the initial hospital stay, the patient is thoroughly evaluated to arrive at a thoughtful plan for preventing recurrent hemorrhage. A hepatitis profile is obtained as well as a history of ingestion of alcohol or exposure to other hepatotoxins (e.g., acetaminophen, nonsteroidal anti-inflammatory drugs). A reliable social history is also important because the long-term success of some forms of therapy depends heavily on patient accessibility and reliability. One of the most important factors in determining future therapy is an estimation of the functional reserve of the liver. **Child's classification** (Table 18-1) uses readily available clinical information to make this estimation. The portal venous anatomy of the patient is also important because it may strongly influence the choice of definitive therapy. This anatomy is best shown by angiography (Figure 18-9), with selective injection of the superior mesenteric and splenic arteries. At the same time that these studies are done, images are obtained of the left renal vein and inferior vena cava, which may serve as outflow tracts for shunt procedures. At the time of angiography, a hepatic vein tributary is cannulated to obtain the free and wedged hepatic vein pressures. Subtracting the former from the latter provides an estimate of the sinusoidal pressure within the

Table 18-1. Child's Classification

Criteria	Good Risk (A)	Moderate Risk (B)	Poor Risk (C)
Serum bilirubin (mg/100 mL)	<2.0	2.0–3.0	>3.0
Serum albumin (mg/100 mL)	>3.5	3.0–3.5	<3.0
Ascites	None	Easily controlled	Not easily controlled
Encephalopathy	None	Minimal	Advanced
Nutrition	Excellent	Good	Poor

liver, which is a reflection of the portal venous pressure. Angiography may also provide diagnostic information if portal or hepatic vein occlusion is identified.

In a stable Child's A or B patient, treatment options include endoscopic therapy and surgical shunting. If the patient lives near the endoscopist and is expected to be reliable in pursuing followup evaluations, it is reasonable to pursue endoscopic therapy as the initial treatment. Because regular, longterm sessions are necessary to limit rebleeding with endoscopic therapy, it is probably advisable for the unreliable patient or one who lives far away to have either a distal splenorenal shunt or a small-bore portacaval shunt. These procedures maintain prograde hepatic portal perfusion and have lower rates of associated encephalopathy than nonselective or total shunts. TIPS should not be used in Child's A and B patients, except under unusual circumstances.

Child's C patients are candidates for either TIPS or endoscopic therapy, although complete variceal obliteration may be difficult to achieve endoscopically in these patients. Regardless of the therapy that is initially chosen, Child's C patients should undergo evaluation for liver transplantation.

Endoscopic Therapy

The same forms of endoscopic therapy that are available for acute bleeding (sclerotherapy and banding) can also be used on a long-term basis to prevent recurrent bleeding. The aim is to systematically eradicate all visible esophageal varices through a series of endoscopic sessions over the first few weeks and then to periodically identify and treat newly developed variceal channels. One problem with endoscopic therapy is that eradication of esophageal varices often leads to the development of gastric varices, which are much less successfully treated endoscopically.

Surgical Therapy

Three forms of surgical therapy are used to prevent recurrent variceal hemorrhage: portosystemic shunts, **selective shunts,** and nonshunt operations. In portosystemic shunts, large-caliber connections are made between some point in the portal circulation and a point in the systemic circulation. The portal vein can be sewn

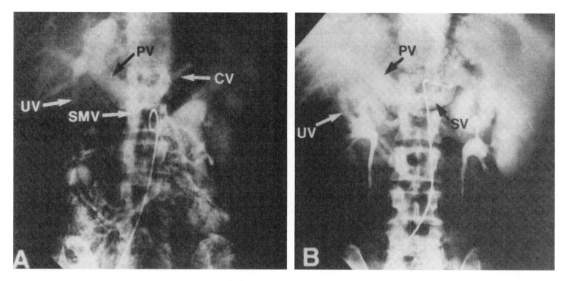

Figure 18-9 A and **B,** Venous phase of an angiogram showing the superior mesenteric vein *(SMV)*, portal vein *(PV)*, splenic vein *(SV)*, common vein *(CV)*, and umbilical vein *(UV)*.

directly to the inferior vena cava in an end-to-side or a side-to-side fashion. Alternatively, the interposition of prosthetic graft material can be used for a side-to-side portacaval shunt. A variety of other options (see Figure 18-7) are hemodynamically equivalent. Prosthetic grafts often make the shunt easier to construct, but are associated with a relatively high incidence of thrombosis in long-term follow-up. Portosystemic shunts very effectively lower variceal pressure and prevent bleeding. In addition, they effectively control ascites. However, they divert portal flow to such a great degree that deterioration of hepatic function and hepatic encephalopathy frequently occur. Selective shunts were developed to decompress varices and prevent variceal bleeding while preserving portal blood flow to the liver. They do so by isolating the gastrosplenic compartment from the remainder of the portal circulation and decompressing only that compartment into the systemic circulation. The distal splenorenal shunt is the most commonly performed selective shunt procedure in the United States. It is as effective as portosystemic shunts at preventing variceal hemorrhage, but produces much lower rates of encephalopathy. Because no prosthetic material is used in its construction, the distal splenorenal shunt has excellent long-term patency. The coronary–caval shunt is another option for selective shunting and achieves the same desired effect. The small-bore portacaval shunt was designed to achieve the same goals as selective shunts, but is much more easily performed. In this operation, a small-diameter (8–10 mm), short (2–3 cm), and straight piece of polytetrafluoroethylene (PTFE) [Teflon] graft is sewn between the portal vein and the inferior vena cava. The small diameter of the shunt limits the amount of portal blood stolen from the liver while lowering portal pressure sufficiently to prevent bleeding. The short, straight PTFE graft also appears to substantially reduce the rate of thrombosis seen with longer, curved pieces of Dacron grafts.

Nonshunt operations are designed to control bleeding by interrupting blood flow to the varices. One operation is division and reanastomosis of the esophagus, which is usually done with an end-to-end stapling device. The other operation is devascularization of the stomach and lower esophagus, usually with splenectomy, to halt flow through the varices. Although nonshunt operations are successful in other parts of the world for certain disease conditions, they do not enjoy great success in the United States.

TIPS

TIPS, described earlier in association with acute variceal bleeding, is also used to prevent variceal bleeding. Although these devices are initially successful in decreasing portal pressure, they have two recurrent problems. The first is the high rate of encephalopathy ($\leq 30\%$) that accompanies a patent TIPS. Because these procedures are radiographically constructed portacaval shunts, it is not surprising that they share this complication with their surgically created equivalents. The other problem with TIPS is a potentially high rate of thrombosis when not carefully followed. The result is a substantial incidence of recurrent variceal hemorrhage.

TIPS is also associated with the development of intimal hyperplasia along the intrahepatic course of the shunt. Because this hyperplasia can lead to shunt occlusion, close follow-up is required, with Doppler ultrasound examination of the shunt at 3- to 4-month intervals. If progressive myointimal hyperplasia is shown, balloon dilation with revision of the TIPS often maintains the patency of the shunt. Most centers consider TIPS a shorter-term solution for portal hypertension and use it only in patients who need this decompression for a period of 5 years or less.

Prognosis

The most important indicator of long-term survival in patients who have bled from varices (regardless of the therapy chosen) is the functional reserve of the liver. Because cirrhosis, both with continued alcohol abuse and with viral hepatitis, tends to progress relentlessly, only 50% of patients who have had variceal bleeding survive for 5 years.

End-Stage Liver Disease and Liver Transplantation

End-stage liver disease has many recognized complications, some of which are life-threatening. Liver transplantation is now considered standard treatment for many causes of acute and chronic liver failure. However, significant risks are associated with the transplant procedure, and it is costly. Additionally, there is limited organ availability, and the procedure commits the transplant recipient to lifelong immunosuppressive therapy, with its inherent risks. Thus, physicians must exercise careful judgment to determine which patients can be treated with medical measures or less complicated surgical procedures and which ones are likely to require transplantation because of disease progression.

Indications for Transplantation

Patients who are under consideration for liver transplantation usually have irreversible hepatic failure for which there is no suitable alternative therapy. Thus, for most patients, medical measures are tried initially to treat specific complications associated with cirrhosis and liver failure. Transplantation is considered only when these measures are not effective. Three common severe complications seen in association with end-stage liver disease are hepatic encephalopathy, intractable ascites (which may be associated with spontaneous bacterial peritonitis), and variceal hemorrhage. When these occur as isolated complicating factors in patients with otherwise well-preserved hepatic synthetic function, then attention can be directed toward correcting the isolated problem (e.g., performing a portal–systemic or peritoneal–venous shunt procedure). However, when complications occur in the patient with advanced liver disease, they serve as markers of declining hepatic functional reserve, and consideration is usually given to liver transplantation.

Liver transplantation in adults is generally performed for two major indications: chronic, progressive advanced liver disease and **fulminant hepatic failure.** Other indications (in < 10% of patients) include unresectable malignancies and inborn errors of metabolism in patients who may not have underlying cirrhosis. Table 18-2 lists contraindications to liver transplantation.

Chronic liver disease usually results from either hepatocellular injury (e.g., viral hepatitis, alcohol-induced injury) or cholestatic liver disease (e.g., primary biliary cirrhosis, sclerosing cholangitis) [discussed later]. Because of the risks and expense associated with transplantation, patients are usually considered for this procedure when their 1- to 2-year survival rate is estimated at 50% or less. Although it is sometimes difficult

Table 18-2. Absolute Contraindications to Liver Transplantation

Uncontrolled sepsis
Human immunodeficiency virus–positive status
Extrahepatic malignancy
Active alcohol or substance abuse
Advanced cardiac or pulmonary disease

to predict expected survival in patients with advanced liver disease, certain markers assist in this prediction. For example, in patients with chronic liver disease, clinical factors that indicate advanced liver disease include nutritional impairment and muscle wasting, hepatic encephalopathy, difficult-to-control ascites, variceal hemorrhage, and renal insufficiency.

Laboratory parameters may be altered depending on the etiology of liver failure. When cirrhosis has a hepatocellular cause, the prothrombin time is prolonged beyond 18 to 20 seconds (INR ≥ 2.0). A serum albumin level of less than 2.5 to 3.0 g/L is associated with diminished hepatic synthetic reserve. Patients whose cirrhosis has a cholestatic etiology may have near-normal prothrombin times and serum albumin values of 3 g/L or greater. However, elevation of the serum bilirubin above 10 mg/dL suggests advanced liver disease in this group. Laboratory parameters are only guides to hepatic functional reserve and must be considered in the context of the clinical condition of the individual patient. When patients have complications of liver disease (e.g., difficult-to-manage ascites, variceal hemorrhage, marginally controlled encephalopathy), the decision to proceed with transplantation rather than to continue observation of the patient is likely to be made.

Chronic and Progressive Advanced Liver Disease
Chronic Hepatitis C

Chronic hepatitis C infection is one of the most common indications for liver transplantation today. Hepatitis C was previously categorized under the heading non-A, non-B hepatitis, but molecular techniques allowed identification of this single-stranded RNA virus in 1989. Although it was a common cause of transfusion-associated hepatitis in the past, this risk is now less than 0.05% per unit of blood product transfused with current testing of banked blood. Many patients with chronic hepatitis C have such identifiable risk factors as previous drug use, previous transfusions, and multiple sexual partners, but approximately 50% have no definable risk factors. Its course is usually slowly progressive, and most patients have chronic infection for 10 to 20 years before complications of liver disease occur or a liver transplant is needed. Only approximately 20% of patients clear the hepatitis C virus in response to acute infection.

After liver transplantation for chronic hepatitis C, reinfection of the transplanted liver is nearly universal, but fortunately, the course of hepatocellular injury is indolent in most patients. New strategies, including antiviral therapies, are under investigation, but no effective measures to prevent allograft infection have been established. Although the short-term results of liver transplantation for hepatitis C are satisfactory in most cases, it is not known how often patients require retransplantation in long-term follow-up.

Chronic Hepatitis B

Chronic hepatitis B infection, unlike hepatitis C infection, shows a marked propensity to cause significant hepatocellular injury in the transplanted allograft, with a high incidence of early graft loss and death of the transplant recipient. Although at one time hepatitis B infection was an absolute contraindication to liver transplantation, many centers now use hepatitis B immunoglobulin to suppress viral expression in the posttransplant recipient. Although there is short-term success with this approach, the long-term outcome is not known.

Alcoholic Liver Disease

Transplantation for alcoholic liver disease is one of the most controversial indications for liver transplantation. With intensive pretransplant screening, including completion of an alcohol rehabilitation program and a period of supervised abstinence (usually ≥ 6 months), the risk of recidivism is less than 10% to 15%. Of those who consume alcohol after transplantation, continued alcohol use to the point of causing liver disease in the allograft is extremely rare. For reasons that are not well understood, as many as one-third of patients with a history of alcohol abuse also have serologic markers for hepatitis C infection without other known risk factors.

Autoimmune Hepatitis

Autoimmune hepatitis can usually be distinguished from other causes of chronic liver disease on the basis of immunologic and serologic testing. These patients usually have positive antinuclear or other self-directed antibodies. Initial treatment is usually with immunosuppressive medication, including corticosteroids and azathioprine. Patients in whom this treatment fails are usually good candidates for liver transplantation. Recurrent disease does not usually occur in the transplanted liver.

Hemochromatosis

Hemochromatosis is an autosomal recessive disease that causes iron overload as a result of excessive absorption from the intestinal tract. Multiple organs are affected by iron deposition, including the liver, heart, pancreas, spleen, adrenal glands, pituitary, and joints. The peak incidence of liver disease is between 40 and 60 years of age. Men show clinical manifestations and cirrhosis earlier than women, who may be protected by iron loss during menstruation and childbirth. Treatment in recognized patients is with serial phlebotomy. Withdrawal of 500 mL blood/wk is often required until the excessive iron stores are depleted. Effective treatment

may reverse many of the damaging effects of iron deposition. Hemochromatosis is associated with a significant risk of hepatocellular carcinoma, up to 200 times that of other patients with cirrhosis. This risk is not fully diminished by phlebotomy. Liver transplantation is effective for patients with hemochromatosis and end-stage cirrhosis, but may be complicated by the preexisting cardiomyopathy and diabetes often found in these patients. The increased absorption of iron continues after liver transplantation, necessitating careful surveillance, even in patients who undergo successful transplantation.

Wilson's Disease

Wilson's disease is a rare autosomal recessive disorder of copper metabolism. Patients have increased deposition of copper in the liver, corneas (Kayser-Fleischer rings), kidneys, brain, and other locations. Patients with Wilson's disease have decreased circulating levels of ceruloplasmin and increased urinary excretion of copper. In normal individuals, excess copper is excreted into bile, but patients with Wilson's disease appear to have diminished biliary excretion. Some patients with Wilson's disease may have acute hepatitis and fulminant hepatic failure, whereas others have chronic progressive liver disease. Patients who have chronic liver disease are initially treated with D-penicillamine, which chelates copper and increases urinary excretion. Liver transplantation is effective in patients with fulminant failure and those in whom initial medical therapy fails. After transplantation, the metabolic defect is corrected, and no further damage from excessive copper occurs.

Alpha$_1$-antitrypsin Deficiency

Alpha$_1$-antitrypsin deficiency is an autosomal dominant disorder that causes varying degrees of lung and liver damage over a patient's lifetime. The diagnosis is established by the determination of low levels of serum alpha$_1$-antitrypsin levels and confirmed with phenotypic studies. Most patients with liver disease have relatively mild pulmonary involvement, but more advanced pulmonary disease can complicate attempts at liver transplantation. There is no effective medical treatment, except for supportive measures. After liver transplantation, alpha$_1$-antitrypsin levels return to normal as the recipient takes on the phenotype of the transplanted liver.

Primary Biliary Cirrhosis

Primary biliary cirrhosis, which primarily affects middle-aged women, causes progressive bile duct destruction, probably from cytotoxic T cells. Patients often have pruritus without jaundice and usually have a positive anti-mitochondrial antibody finding (≥ 1/40). The course of the disease may be indolent, with patients living 10 years or longer from presentation. Elevation of the serum bilirubin level is associated with disease progression and usually prompts consideration of liver transplantation.

Primary Sclerosing Cholangitis

Primary sclerosing cholangitis is an idiopathic disease that causes chronic fibrotic strictures that can involve any portion of the intrahepatic or extrahepatic biliary tree. One-half to two-thirds of patients also have inflammatory bowel disease, usually ulcerative colitis. The risk of cholangiocarcinoma is increased in patients with primary sclerosing cholangitis, and rapid progression of disease should prompt a search for malignant strictures within the biliary tree. Disease progression in patients with primary sclerosing cholangitis is more variable than in patients with primary biliary cirrhosis. When patients become jaundiced and do not have a correctable biliary stricture (usually with stenting, but occasionally with surgical bypass), then transplantation is considered. After transplantation, patients who have primary sclerosing cholangitis and ulcerative colitis require close colonic surveillance because of the increased risk of colon carcinoma.

Fulminant Hepatic Failure

Fulminant hepatic failure occurs when massive hepatocyte necrosis or severe impairment of liver function occurs. These patients do not have evidence of chronic liver disease. Liver dysfunction occurs within 8 to 12 weeks of the onset of symptoms. In these patients, hepatic encephalopathy develops and can progress to coma, brain stem herniation, and death without liver replacement. The prothrombin time is usually significantly prolonged, and reversible renal insufficiency (hepatorenal syndrome) may develop. Because these patients do not have chronic liver disease, muscle wasting and portal hypertension usually are not present. For this reason, liver transplantation is technically easier to perform than in the setting of chronic liver disease. However, because of the rapidly advancing nature of liver dysfunction in this setting, most patients die within 1 to 2 weeks of presentation without liver transplantation.

At most centers, fulminant hepatic failure is the indication for approximately 5% to 10% of liver transplantations. Common causes of fulminant hepatic failure include viral infection and hepatotoxic drugs (e.g., anesthetic drugs, acetaminophen, isoniazid). Mushroom poisoning occurs in certain areas of the United States (Pacific Northwest) and Europe, where wild mushrooms are gathered and eaten by unsuspecting individuals.

Because of the rapid progression of fulminant hepatic failure, patients require an aggressive and accelerated workup in addition to aggressive supportive measures. Patients in hepatic coma usually undergo placement of an intracerebral pressure monitor so that adequate cerebral perfusion pressures can be maintained and increases in cerebral pressures minimized. To be successful, liver transplantation must be performed before irreversible brain injury occurs. Some patients with milder forms recover without liver transplantation, but the period of observation cannot extend for too long, or it may not be possible to obtain a suitable donor liver in time to perform a successful transplant. Thus, the decision to proceed with liver transplantation requires careful judgment by the treating physicians, who must weigh the risks of death without a transplant against the potential commitment to lifelong immunosuppression in a patient who might otherwise recover without this procedure. Clinical trials with extracorporeal liver support systems are underway. These systems may prevent cerebral injury while the injured liver recovers or until a suitable donor liver is located. In the future, these systems may successfully assist patients during this critical period.

Technical Aspects of Liver Transplantation

After brain death is declared in a prospective donor and consent for organ donation is given by the next of kin, organ procurement representatives assess the donor's suitability for organ transplantation. Consideration is usually given for heart, lung, liver, pancreas, and kidney donation, depending on individual donor factors. Rapid assessment for evidence of underlying liver disease is carried out based on the medical history, social history, and results of physical examination, serologic testing (hepatitis B and C, human immunodeficiency virus), and laboratory studies. In general, liver transplantation is considered in donors younger than 60 years of age, but older donors are sometimes acceptable.

After a suitable donor is identified, a member of the organ procurement team maintains the donor in a hemodynamically stable condition until members of the various transplant teams travel to the donor hospital for the procurement procedure. This procedure usually begins within 12 to 24 hours of the time of the initial assessment for donation. As in any major operative procedure, the donor procurement procedure is performed in the operating room with standard sterile techniques. The specific techniques vary depending on the organ that is being procured, but the general approach is similar. The surgeon performs enough dissection to identify the important structures (including anomalies) and prevent inadvertent injury during organ removal. Perfusion catheters are placed to flush the organs with cold preservation solution at the time of procurement. The liver, kidneys, and pancreas are flushed with University of Wisconsin solution, then removed and placed in cold storage until the time of reimplantation into the recipient. Liver preservation times with this approach allow for a cold ischemic time of 12 to 18 hours. In this way, the same team can perform the donor and recipient operations.

After anesthesia is induced and monitoring catheters are placed, the recipient operation is initiated with a bilateral subcostal incision and a midline extension to the xiphoid process. The attachments of the liver to the diaphragm and retroperitoneum are divided, and portal structures are carefully dissected and identified. The vena cava is encircled and dissected free infrahepatically and suprahepatically.

After the initial dissection is completed, the anhepatic phase is begun by removal of the diseased liver. Depending on the hemodynamic stability of the recipient, venovenous bypass may be used during the anhepatic phase to direct blood from the temporarily occluded infrahepatic vena cava and superior mesenteric venous system. This bypass is performed by placing cannulas into the femoral and portal veins, with a return circuit to the superior vena cava. The donor liver is then placed into the recipient, and anastomoses are serially completed to the suprahepatic vena cava, infrahepatic vena cava, portal vein, hepatic artery, and bile duct. After the operation is completed, the patient is carefully monitored in the intensive care unit for signs of satisfactory graft function.

Immunosuppression is usually started just before the transplant procedure or intraoperatively. It usually consists of corticosteroids, azathioprine, and either cyclosporin A or tacrolimus (FK-506), or some combination of the two, depending on patient circumstances and transplant center preference.

Complications of Liver Transplantation

In addition to the complications that may accompany any major operative procedure (e.g., postoperative bleeding, wound infection, deep venous thrombosis), liver transplantation has unique complications. These may result from liver allograft dysfunction or may be related to immunosuppressive drug therapy.

Liver Allograft Dysfunction

Liver allograft dysfunction can have diverse etiologies, but certain etiologies are more likely to occur at certain time points. Severe dysfunction in the first week after transplantation most likely results from either a preservation injury or hepatic artery thrombosis. A preservation injury may be reversible, depending on the degree of insult to the allograft. Hepatic artery thrombosis, which occurs in 5% of transplants, usually requires retransplantation. Unlike renal transplantation, in which hyperacute rejection may be seen in the face of a positive crossmatch, hyperacute rejection is rare in liver transplantation, and usually involves an ABO blood group mismatch.

Acute cellular rejection usually occurs from day 5 to day 30 posttransplant. It is seen in as many as 40% to 70% of transplant recipients. The major targets in the immune response are the biliary ductal epithelial cells and the endothelium of the hepatic vessels. Acute rejection is usually suspected based on rising serum transaminase levels (aspartate transaminase and alanine transaminase) and confirmed by liver biopsy. In most patients, this condition resolves with bolus corticosteroid therapy. Usually, nonresponders are satisfactorily treated with the monoclonal antibody OKT3.

Biliary tract complications can occur at any time after transplantation. Early complications usually involve bile duct leaks. Late complications include anastomotic strictures and leaks at the T-tube entry site at the time of T-tube removal. These problems are usually satisfactorily treated with radiologic or endoscopic stenting, sometimes with percutaneous drain placement for bile collection.

As noted earlier, recurrent viral hepatitis can occur at any time after transplantation. Hepatitis B and C have a high rate of recurrence after transplantation, but hepatitis B appears to have a much more aggressive course, with progression to liver disease and cirrhosis 1 year or less after transplantation. The administration of high-dose hepatitis B immunoglobulin decreases the risk of recurrent hepatitis B, but will likely be required for life and is expensive, costing approximately $25,000 to $30,000 per year of treatment. Hepatitis C usually has a less aggressive course in the posttransplant setting. However, there is no satisfactory treatment, and the long-term outlook is unclear.

Complications of Immunosuppressive Drug Therapy

Numerous complications occur as a result of immunosuppressive medication. Infectious complications are common and vary with the time elapsed since transplantation. Infections that occur within 2 to 4 weeks of transplantation are more commonly bacterial, particularly Gram-negative organisms. Patients who require prolonged hospitalization before transplantation are at increased risk of posttransplant fungal infections. Opportunistic infections, particularly cytomegalovirus, occur 1 to 6 months posttransplant.

Many side effects of immunosuppressive medication require close attention. Cyclosporine and tacrolimus both cause nephrotoxicity, with a decrease in the glomerular filtration rate in most patients. They can also cause hypertension, tremor, and headaches. Corticosteroid therapy can lead to weight gain, hyperglycemia, and cortical bone loss. The primary side effect of azathioprine is myelosuppression, but it can also cause hepatotoxicity in the early posttransplant period.

Multiple-Choice Questions

1. Hepatic adenoma:
   A. Is the most common benign tumor in the liver
   B. Is left untreated once the benign nature is certain
   C. Cannot transform into hepatocellular carcinoma
   D. Is associated with the use of oral contraceptives
   E. Has a central stellate pattern on radiographic studies

2. Hepatocellular carcinoma:
   A. Accounts for more than 90% of all primary liver malignancies
   B. Accounts for more than 90% of all liver malignancies
   C. Occurs with equal frequency in patients with and without cirrhosis
   D. Can be safely removed in most patients with modern operative techniques, including venovenous bypass
   E. Rarely recurs in the liver after resection

3. Colorectal carcinoma that metastasizes to the liver:
   A. Cannot be resected for cure
   B. Is often suspected on the basis of an elevated alpha-fetoprotein level

C. Is usually found in the periphery of the liver
D. Can be resected with curative intent, even if multiple lesions are present
E. Responds better to chemotherapy than to surgery

4. Choose the correct statement.
A. Polycystic liver disease is an autosomal dominant disorder that is often found in association with polycystic kidney disease.
B. Simple cysts of the liver usually become symptomatic and are therefore resected when found.
C. Polycystic liver disease usually causes progressive deterioration of synthetic function and is an indication for liver transplantation.
D. Simple cysts of the liver are usually first diagnosed incidentally during surgery for another disease.
E. Simple cysts of the liver have thick walls and multiple septations.

5. Choose the correct statement.
A. Cystadenocarcinoma often develops in patients with polycystic liver disease.
B. Calcification in the walls of a hepatic cystic lesion suggests a benign condition.
C. Cystadenomas are simply drained into the peritoneal cavity after benignancy is established.
D. Thick walls and septations in cystic hepatic lesions are indications of neoplasia.
E. Simple hepatic cysts are more common in women than in men.

6. Choose the correct statement.
A. Amebic abscesses usually require surgical drainage.
B. Needle aspiration for culture is the preferred method to diagnose echinococcal cysts.
C. The preferred treatment of echinococcal cysts is metronidazole.
D. Humans are accidental hosts for the organisms that cause amebic abscesses in the liver, and carnivores are the vector.
E. Daughter cysts and cyst wall calcifications on imaging studies should prompt serologic testing for echinococcal cysts.

7. Pyogenic abscesses of the liver:
A. Have thin walls and are therefore surgically drained
B. Are treated with metronidazole after a diagnosis is made
C. Are almost always associated with an identifiable primary source of infection
D. Are best diagnosed serologically
E. Often show septations and calcifications on computed tomography (CT) scan

8. The most common cause of portal hypertension in children is:
A. Cirrhosis
B. Portal vein occlusion
C. Schistosomiasis

D. Budd-Chiari syndrome
E. Hepatitis

9. The best way to diagnose hepatic encephalopathy is:
A. Determination of the serum ammonia level
B. Clinical evaluation
C. Electroencephalography
D. Psychomotor testing
E. Analysis of the ratio of aromatic and branch chain amino acids in the peripheral blood

10. Transjugular intrahepatic portacaval shunting (TIPS):
A. Is the treatment of choice to prevent ascites
B. Is associated with a lower incidence of hepatic encephalopathy than distal splenorenal shunting
C. Is technically possible in a limited number of patients
D. Is the treatment of choice to prevent recurrent variceal bleeding in Child's B patients
E. May act as a bridge to transplantation in patients with advanced liver disease (Child's C) and variceal bleeding

11. The distal splenorenal shunt is:
A. Associated with a high incidence of thrombosis and recurrent variceal hemorrhage
B. The best operation to control ascites
C. Easier to construct than a small-bore portacaval shunt
D. An operation that requires splenectomy
E. Associated with a low incidence of rebleeding and a lower incidence of encephalopathy than portacaval shunting

12. In the patient with suspected variceal bleeding, endoscopy:
A. Is not performed because of the risk of tearing varices
B. Is performed before somatostatin is administered
C. Is performed as soon as possible to enhance the accuracy of the diagnosis
D. Cannot be performed if the patient has encephalopathy
E. Is performed only if pharmacologic therapy does not abate the bleeding

13. The Sengstaken-Blakemore tube:
A. Is the first line of therapy in the patient with proven variceal hemorrhage
B. Can cause mild or pronounced hepatic encephalopathy
C. Is the first line of therapy in the patient with suspected variceal hemorrhage
D. Is dangerous if not used according to a strict protocol
E. Prevent the need for further therapy

14. Choose the correct statement.
A. All patients with cirrhosis have clinically significant esophageal varices, but some do not bleed from them.

B. Esophageal varices develop in only approximately 30% of patients with cirrhosis.

C. Each admission for variceal bleeding is associated with a 25% to 50% mortality rate.

D. Lactulose decreases portal pressure by constricting the mesenteric vasculature.

E. Approximately three-fourths of all patients with varices experience variceal bleeding at some point in their lives.

15. Choose the correct statement.

A. Initial resuscitation of the patient with variceal bleeding includes placement of two large-bore intravenous lines and administration of lactated Ringer's solution at a calculated maintenance rate.

B. Patients with cirrhosis rarely have massive upper gastrointestinal bleeding from sources other than esophageal varices.

C. Lactulose acts by decreasing colonic flora.

D. Somatostatin is slightly more effective than vasopressin in stopping acute variceal hemorrhage.

E. The operation of choice in a stable Child's C patient is a distal splenorenal shunt.

16. Transplantation:

A. In the patient with chronic hepatitis B rarely results in hepatocellular injury in the transplanted allograft

B. Is contraindicated in patients with chronic hepatitis C

C. In the patient with chronic hepatitis C rarely results in reinfection of the transplanted liver

D. In the patient with chronic hepatitis C almost uniformly results in reinfection of the transplanted liver, but these infections are wholly indolent and well tolerated

E. In the patient with chronic hepatitis B rarely results in early loss of the graft and death of the patient

17. Absolute contraindications to liver transplantation include:

A. Variceal bleeding, chronic hepatitis B, and age younger than 12 years

B. Extrahepatic malignancy, human immunodeficiency virus (HIV)–positive status, and uncontrolled sepsis

C. Uncontrolled sepsis, encephalopathy, and alcoholic liver disease

D. Active alcohol use, massive ascites, and chronic hepatitis C

E. HIV-positive status, advanced pulmonary disease, and obesity

18. Causes of liver failure that may be completely corrected with liver transplantation include:

A. Ethanol abuse, hemochromatosis, and Wilson's disease

B. Autoimmune hepatitis, chronic hepatitis C, and variceal bleeding

C. Alpha$_1$-antitrypsin deficiency, massive ascites, and hepatitis B

D. Substance abuse, encephalopathy, and autoimmune hepatitis

E. Autoimmune hepatitis, Wilson's disease, and alpha$_1$-antitrypsin deficiency

19. Acute rejection after liver transplantation:

A. Occurs in fewer than 25% of cases

B. Is first manifested by a rising serum bilirubin level approximately 90 days after transplantation and is usually diagnosed on clinical grounds

C. Is treated by retransplantation if the patient is to survive

D. Usually occurs 5 to 30 days after transplantation and is first manifested by rising serum transaminase levels

E. Is best treated with cyclosporine

20. Choose the correct statement.

A. Liver donors may be hepatitis B–positive if the recipient is hepatitis B–positive.

B. Liver dysfunction from technical complications at transplantation is usually apparent 14 to 28 days postoperatively.

C. Hepatorenal syndrome established in the recipient before liver transplant is rarely correctable after transplantation.

D. Immunosuppression of the patient undergoing liver transplant begins after the transplant to decrease the risk of complications.

E. The allowable cold ischemia time for the liver is 12 to 18 hours.

Oral Examination Study Questions

CASE 1

You are a senior resident on call in the emergency room. A 55-year-old white man comes to the emergency room complaining of "vomiting up a pint of red blood." A quick appraisal of his vital signs shows a pulse of 130/min, blood pressure of 95/65 mm Hg, and a respiratory rate of 24/min.

OBJECTIVE 1

The student rapidly obtains the patient's pertinent history and forms a differential diagnosis.

A. Prior history
   1. No history of bleeding
   2. No history of ulcer disease
   3. No history of varices
B. Recent history
   1. The patient had mild epigastric discomfort 3 to 4 days ago, but nothing severe.
   2. This morning after breakfast, he felt nauseous and light-headed, and he vomited.

C. Drug history
1. The patient has been a moderately heavy drinker for the last 35 years. His wife volunteered that he has been on a drinking "binge" lately.
2. The patient denies the use of aspirin or nonsteroidal anti-inflammatory drugs.

D. The patient has had normal bowel movements, but describes one since his vomiting started as being "tarry" and foul-smelling.

E. The patient was slightly jaundiced 2 weeks ago, but the condition resolved.

F. Differential diagnosis
1. Peptic ulcer disease
2. Varices
3. Erosive gastritis
4. Mallory-Weiss syndrome

OBJECTIVE 2

The student obtains the pertinent physical findings and requests the pertinent negative findings about the stigmata of portal hypertension.

A. Physical findings
1. The patient has a mildly distended abdomen, with a few collateral veins apparent. A fluid wave is noted on percussion.
2. The patient has no pain to deep palpation.
3. Mild jaundice is noted in the sclerae.

B. Pertinent negative findings. The patient has none of the following:
1. Spider angiomas
2. Palmar erythema
3. Muscle wasting
4. Encephalopathy
5. Hepatosplenomegaly

OBJECTIVE 3

The student describes the appropriate initial resuscitative efforts in this patient with upper gastrointestinal bleeding.

A. A nasogastric tube is placed to confirm an upper gastrointestinal source of bleeding. It shows blood clots.

B. Two large-bore intravenous lines (16 gauge or larger) are placed.

C. Intravenous infusion of a volume expander (lactated Ringer's solution, normal saline, etc.) is initiated.

D. Blood is drawn for a complete blood count, prothrombin time (PT), and partial thromboplastin time (PTT). The platelet count and clot are sent for typing and crossmatch for six units of blood.

E. A Foley catheter is placed to monitor fluid administration.

F. Intensive care unit monitoring is begun.

G. Laboratory results show hematocrit of 24%, hemoglobin of 8 g/dL, platelet count of 85,000/mm^3, PT of 16 seconds, and PTT of 45 seconds.

OBJECTIVE 4

The student describes the appropriate diagnostic workup.

A. Urgent upper gastrointestinal endoscopy (the most appropriate immediate diagnostic test) shows multiple tortuous varices, with active bleeding apparent in the distal esophagus.

B. Barium upper gastrointestinal study is performed. (It is suboptimal to order this study as the initial diagnostic test because it is less accurate than endoscopy and it takes a barely stabilized patient out of the intensive care unit.) No ulcers are seen, but distal esophageal opacities consistent with varices are shown.

C. Further blood studies
1. Total bilirubin is 2.5 mg/dL.
2. Direct bilirubin is 1.6 mg/dL.
3. Alanine transaminase is 150 IU/L.
4. Alkaline phosphatase is 186 IU/L.
5. Lactic acid dehydrogenase (LDH) is 290 IU/L.
6. Amylase is 93 IU/L.
7. Albumin is 3.1 g/dL.
8. Blood urea nitrogen is 52 mg/dL.
9. Electrolytes are normal.

D. Arteriography is not indicated during the emergency workup.

OBJECTIVE 5

The student suggests appropriate short-term management now that the diagnosis is made.

A. Restore the blood volume.

B. Stop the variceal bleeding as soon as possible.
1. A Sengstaken-Blakemore tube is placed. Complications include perforation, ischemic necrosis, aspiration, and asphyxiation. In addition, 20% to 50% of patients bleed after deflation.
2. Systemic vasopressin administration is initiated. Vasopressin controls variceal bleeding in 50% of patients, but it is avoided in patients with coronary artery disease.
3. Endoscopic sclerotherapy is performed. This therapy results in temporary control in 85% to 95% of patients, but rebleeding occurs in as many as one-half to two-thirds.

C. Prevent hepatic encephalopathy.
1. Nasogastric aspiration of intraluminal blood
2. Administration of cathartics
3. Administration of neomycin orally and through enemas

D. Support the failing liver.
1. Administration of hypertonic glucose with minimal Na$^+$ intravenously.
2. Administration of vitamins.
3. Provision of adequate nutritional intake.

E. Correct clotting abnormalities.

OBJECTIVE 6

The student makes a recommendation for the long-term management of this problem and discusses the available surgical options and their complications.

A. This patient will almost certainly rebleed. Some form of definitive therapy is necessary.

B. Possible operations include:
1. Portacaval shunt, both side-to-side and end-to-side
2. Distal splenorenal shunt
3. Mesocaval shunt
4. Endoscopic sclerotherapy
5. Nonshunting operations

C. Postoperative complications
1. Hepatic failure (jaundice, coagulopathy, ascites)
2. Stress erosions (high stress in this group)
3. Renal failure (acute tubular necrosis, hepatorenal syndrome)
4. Infections, especially pulmonary and urinary
5. Delirium tremens
6. Inadequate nutrition
7. Rebleeding (slightly higher incidence with distal splenorenal shunts; lower incidence with portacaval shunts)
8. Encephalopathy (higher incidence with portacaval shunts; much lower incidence with distal splenorenal shunts)
9. Recurrent ascites (worse with end-to-side portacaval shunts)
10. Surgical mortality rate of 0% to 5% in Child's class A, 5% to 15% in Child's class B, and 20% to 50% in Child's class C

OBJECTIVE 1

Minimum Level of Achievement for Passing

A. The student formulates a differential diagnosis.

B. The student distinguishes the clinical signs that establish the level of bleeding.

C. The student asks the appropriate questions to obtain enough information to establish the likely diagnosis.

Honors Level of Achievement

A. The student provides a reasonably complete differential diagnosis for upper gastrointestinal bleeding.

B. The student recognizes that 25% of patients with varices have nonvariceal lesions as the source of bleeding.

OBJECTIVE 2

Minimum Level of Achievement for Passing

A. The student knows the stigmata of portal hypertension.

B. The student explains the significance of a fluid wave.

OBJECTIVE 3

Minimum Level of Achievement for Passing

A. The student describes the appropriate precautions for resuscitation for gastrointestinal bleeding.

B. The student knows the value of volume expanders in resuscitation.

Honors Level of Achievement

A. The student describes the use of O-negative and type-specific, uncrossmatched blood in emergency situations.

B. The student understands how to monitor fluid administration through a central venous pressure line and through a Swan-Ganz catheter, and understands the differences between the two methods.

OBJECTIVE 4

Minimum Level of Achievement for Passing

A. The student knows that endoscopy is the diagnostic procedure of choice for upper gastrointestinal bleeding.

B. The student knows what tests are used to assess liver function.

OBJECTIVE 5

Minimum Level of Achievement for Passing

A. The student identifies two methods to stop variceal bleeding.

B. The student knows why these patients have clotting abnormalities.

Honors Level of Achievement

A. The student states that systemic vasopressin administration is as effective as selective administration in stopping variceal bleeding.

B. The student describes how clotting abnormalities are corrected (e.g., fresh frozen plasma, vitamin K).

OBJECTIVE 6

Minimum Level of Achievement for Passing

A. The student realizes that first-time variceal bleeding has a high likelihood of recurrence.

B. The student names two types of operations to decompress the portal system.

Honors Level of Achievement

A. The student explains the differences between the types of portal decompression operations.

B. The student knows the relative operative risks as determined by Child's classification.

CASE 2

You are a general surgeon working in a large university hospital. A gastroenterologist asks you to see a

60-year-old woman whom he has been unable to diagnose. The patient's only complaints are weakness and malaise.

OBJECTIVE 1

The student obtains an accurate history (even though it was done before) and performs a careful review of systems.

A. The patient felt well until 2 months ago, when she started to feel tired, weak, and devoid of energy.

B. The patient has a mild dull, aching sensation in the right upper quadrant, for which she takes Tylenol. The pain is recurrent and is not relieved or worsened by food. It is occasionally worsened by physical activity.

C. The patient lost 15 lb over the last 2-1/2 months.

D. Her appetite is decreased, but she denies nausea, vomiting, change in bowel habits, exposure to hepatitis, jaundice, or chills. She has occasional low-grade fever at night.

E. She is taking no drugs, but has a history of heavy alcohol consumption.

F. She denies hematemesis, melena, prior blood transfusions, or jaundice.

OBJECTIVE 2

The student requests the pertinent physical findings and initiates an appropriate diagnostic workup.

A. Physical examination shows a slightly emaciated white woman with normal physical findings, with the exception of hepatomegaly without splenomegaly.

B. Complete blood count shows hematocrit of 29% and white blood cell count of 5600/mm^3.

C. Total bilirubin is 1.6 mg/dL, alanine transaminase is 74 IU/L, alkaline phosphatase is 140 IU/L, LDH is 275 IU/L, and albumin is 2.9 g/dL (normal).

D. PT and PTT are 14/12 seconds and 50/35 seconds, respectively (abnormal).

E. Plain and upright abdominal x-rays are normal.

F. Ultrasound shows a normal gallbladder and common bile duct without stones or evidence of dilation. The right hepatic lobe is enlarged, with an inhomogeneous area noted inferiorly. Ultrasound is useful as a screening test because it is noninvasive and less expensive than other screening modalities.

G. Computed tomography (CT) shows a large right hepatic mass measuring 7 × 9 cm that does not appear to cross the midline of the liver. The lesion is solid.

H. Radionuclide scan shows an area of decreased uptake in the right hepatic lobe, consistent with a solid neoplasm. This test has a higher incidence of false-positive findings than CT scan or ultrasound.

I. Arteriography shows a normal celiac axis and normal common hepatic artery and branches. There is a rounded effacement of the peripheral vessels near a hypervascular area in the right lobe. Some contrast blush is noted in the hypervascular region. No other lesions are seen.

J. Alpha-fetoprotein is 10,000 μg/L. It is positive in 50% to 80% of patients with malignant hepatoma.

K. Oral cholecystogram is normal.

OBJECTIVE 3

The student recommends appropriate treatment for this lesion and describes the risk factors that predispose to its development.

A. Although there is no definitive diagnosis, this patient almost certainly has a malignant hepatoma. Exploration is warranted to confirm this suspicion.

B. Surgical resection is the only hope of curing this lesion. Chemotherapy and radiation therapy are essentially ineffective.

C. If the lesion is confined to one lobe of the liver and does not cross the anatomic midline (demarcated by the gallbladder), surgical resection may be attempted. In younger patients, 70% to 80% of the liver may be resected without loss of hepatic function.

D. Resection is not attempted in patients with significant cirrhosis or marginal liver function.

E. Predisposing factors:
1. Hepatitis B infection
2. Hemochromatosis
3. Alpha$_1$-antitrypsin deficiency
4. Aflatoxin ingestion
5. Cirrhosis
6. Chronic active hepatitis
7. Chronic hepatitis C

OBJECTIVE 4

The student describes possible postoperative complications after a major hepatic resection. The student also describes the prognosis.

A. Postoperative complications
1. Bleeding from the resected liver surface secondary to marginal clotting status
2. Bile leak from unligated ductules (usually taken care of by drains)
3. Subphrenic abscess
4. Bile peritonitis
5. Hepatic failure manifested by elevated liver function test results, elevated bilirubin, and encephalopathy
6. Profound hypoglycemia (loss of glycogen stores in the resected lobe, liver failure)
7. Recurrent carcinoma
8. Pneumothorax, empyema, or pleural effusion (if chest tubes are used)
9. Renal failure
10. Atelectasis

B. Prognosis
1. Without hepatic resection, the 5-year survival rate is 0%.
2. With hepatic resection, the 5-year survival rate is 10%–40%.

OBJECTIVE 1

Minimum Level of Achievement for Passing

A. The student obtains a good gastrointestinal review of systems.

B. With this patient's history of right upper quadrant pain, the hepatobiliary systems review is emphasized.

OBJECTIVE 2

Minimum Level of Achievement for Passing

A. The student recognizes laboratory evidence of mild hepatic dysfunction (abnormal liver function test results, PT, and PTT).

B. The student initiates a diagnostic workup by ordering the appropriate tests to evaluate hepatobiliary disorder (especially ultrasound and CT).

C. The student gives a reasonable differential diagnosis for a solid hepatic mass (metastatic carcinoma, malignant hepatoma, adenoma, focal nodular hyperplasia, hemangioma, sarcoma).

Honors Level of Achievement

A. The student orders an alpha-fetoprotein level and interprets the results.

B. The student explains the importance of arteriography before laparotomy (to delineate the blood supply to each hepatic lobe and prepare the surgeon for anomalies).

OBJECTIVE 3

Minimum Level of Achievement for Passing

A. The student knows that surgery is the treatment of choice for malignant hepatoma.

B. The student is aware of the extent of resection possible in removing a hepatoma (≤ 75% of the liver may be removed).

Honors Level of Achievement

A. The student knows that the gallbladder demarcates the anatomic midpoint of the liver.

B. The student lists three to four factors that predispose the patient to the development of malignant hepatoma.

OBJECTIVE 4

Minimum Level of Achievement for Passing

A. The student lists five postoperative complications of major liver surgery.

B. The student gives 5-year survival data for patients with hepatoma who undergo resection (approximately 10%–40%).

Honors Level of Achievement

The student describes hepatic failure and postoperative hypoglycemia and their pathophysiology.

CASE 3

You are a newly board-certified general surgeon practicing in a large Midwestern city hospital. As your partner leaves for vacation, he mentions that he has a 62-year-old patient with a history of alcohol abuse who was admitted because of a distended abdomen. He asks you to evaluate the patient and initiate treatment in his absence.

OBJECTIVE 1

The student obtains an accurate history to suggest the possible source of this man's problem.

A. Although the patient minimizes it, the family describes a long history of severe alcohol abuse (a fifth of hard liquor every other day).

B. The patient denies abdominal pain, but states that his distended abdomen is "uncomfortable because of the pressure."

C. He denies nausea, vomiting, hematemesis, melena, constipation, obstipation, change in stool habits, or weight loss.

D. The patient states that he had two previous episodes of abdominal distension that spontaneously disappeared.

E. He denies a history of peptic ulcer disease, pancreatitis, blood transfusions, or gallbladder disease.

F. The patient describes the recent development of a yellow hue to his skin (jaundice).

OBJECTIVE 2

The student elicits the pertinent physical findings to confirm the diagnosis. The student also knows the stigmata of portal hypertension.

A. Physical examination shows a thin, jaundiced man with a massively protuberant abdomen.

B. The patient has no abdominal tenderness. Patients with ascites usually have no abdominal pain.

C. Multiple spider angiomata and caput medusae are noted. He also has gynecomastia and palmar erythema (both stigmata of portal hypertension).

D. The abdomen is tense to palpation, and a fluid wave is noted on percussion. There is no tympany to percussion.

E. No masses are palpated.

F. Mild asterixis and disorientation are noted on neurologic examination.

OBJECTIVE 3

The student obtains the appropriate laboratory values to establish a baseline in this patient with ascites.

Only 5% of patients with cirrhosis and ascites have intractable ascites.

A. Complete blood count shows hematocrit of 43%, white blood cell count of 8500/mm³, and platelet count of 90,000/mm³.

B. Electrolytes show Na^+ of 129 mEq/L, K^+ of 3.9 mEq/L, Cl^- of 105 mEq/L, and CO_2 of 25 mEq/L.

C. Creatinine 1.3 mg/dL, and blood urea nitrogen is 38 mg/dL.

D. Urinalysis is normal, and creatinine clearance is less than 25 mL/min.

E. Total bilirubin is 3.5 mg/dL, alanine transaminase is 250 IU/L, alkaline phosphatase is 225 IU/L, LDH is 380 IU/L, albumin is 2.8 g/dL, and total protein is 5.8 g/dL.

F. PT and PTT are 18 seconds and 60 seconds, respectively.

G. Plain and upright abdominal x-rays are normal, except for a ground-glass appearance that suggests ascites.

OBJECTIVE 4

The student associates these findings with the severity of liver disease.

A. Child described the following five criteria that establish the level of severity in alcoholic cirrhosis and portal hypertension.
1. Jaundice
2. Ascites
3. Nutritional state
4. Encephalopathy
5. Albumin

B. These five criteria were further analyzed, stratified, and considered together to create the classifications A (best prognosis), B (intermediate prognosis), and C (worst prognosis).

C. This patient is classified as Child's C because he has jaundice, low albumin, ascites, malnutrition, and encephalopathy.

D. The operative risk approaches 50% mortality in the patient's current condition.

OBJECTIVE 5

The student identifies the appropriate management, describes it, and knows how often it is successful (95%).

A. Conservative therapy is always initiated and attempted before surgical options are considered.

B. Conservative therapy reduces ascites in most patients.

C. Conservative management includes the following:
1. Abstinence from alcohol
2. Adequate nutritional intake (carbohydrate-rich diet)
3. Salt restriction
4. Mild fluid restriction
5. Use of diuretics
6. Use of antialdosterone drugs
7. Bed rest
8. Vitamin and K^+ supplements

D. Abdominal paracentesis is occasionally done for diagnostic purposes and to offer transient relief. Repeated taps are not performed because of the risk of infection and the loss of substantial amounts of protein in the ascites fluid.

OBJECTIVE 6

The student defines intractable ascites, states its approximate incidence, and describes the available treatment options and their complications.

A. Intractable ascites is ascites that does not respond to vigorous attempts at conservative management.

B. Fewer than 6% of patients with cirrhosis and ascites have intractable ascites.

C. Surgical options include:
1. Side-to-side portacaval shunt is probably the best portal decompressive operation for intractable ascites. Complications include the following:
   a. Sepsis
   b. Poor wound healing and dehiscence
   c. Mortality rate of 30% to 50% (in this patient)
   d. Encephalopathy
   e. Hepatic failure
2. Peritoneovenous shunts have lower morbidity and mortality rates in patients with advanced cirrhosis. Complications include the following:
   a. Coagulopathy
   b. Hypokalemia
   c. Shunt failure
   d. Infection
   e. Congestive heart failure
   f. Air embolus

OBJECTIVE 1

Minimum Level of Achievement for Passing

A. The student identifies questions that distinguish distended abdomen caused by bowel obstruction from that caused by ascites.

B. The student obtains a thorough gastrointestinal review of systems.

Honors Level of Achievement

The student correlates alcohol abuse, jaundice, and distended abdomen and makes a tentative diagnosis of ascites.

OBJECTIVE 2

Minimum Level of Achievement for Passing

A. The student knows the stigmata of portal hypertension.

B. The student explains the significance of a fluid wave.

Honors Level of Achievement

The student defines asterixis and explains how it is elicited.

OBJECTIVE 3

Minimum Level of Achievement for Passing

A. The student orders the appropriate baseline laboratory studies (electrolytes, liver function tests, clotting studies).

B. The student knows the significance of a ground-glass appearance on abdominal radiographs.

OBJECTIVE 4

Minimum Level of Achievement for Passing

The student understands that the presence of Child's criteria worsens the prognosis.

Honors Level of Achievement

The student defines Child's criteria and describes the surgical risk associated with the A, B, and C classifications.

OBJECTIVE 5

Minimum Level of Achievement for Passing

A. The student defines intractable ascites.

B. The student describes the conservative management of ascites.

Honors Level of Achievement

The student states how often conservative management is successful (95% of cases).

OBJECTIVE 6

Minimum Level of Achievement for Passing

A. The student describes two surgical options for intractable ascites.

B. The student describes the complications of the surgical options.

Honors Level of Achievement

A. The student states what type of obstruction most commonly leads to ascites: prehepatic, intrahepatic, or posthepatic; and presinusoidal or postsinusoidal (intrahepatic, postsinusoidal).

B. The student names a syndrome that is associated with posthepatic obstruction (Budd-Chiari syndrome).

SUGGESTED READINGS

Bismuth H, Azoilay D, Dennison A. Recent developments in liver transplantation. *Transplant Proc* 1993;25:2191–2194.

Bismuth H, Chiche L, Adam R, et al. Liver resection versus transplantation for hepatocellular carcinoma in cirrhotic patients. *Ann Surg* 1993;218:145–151.

Coldwell DM, Ring EJ, Rees CR, et al. Multicenter investigation of the role of transjugular intrahepatic portosystemic shunt in the management of portal hypertension. *Radiology* 1995;196:335–340.

Conn HO. Portal-systemic shunting and portal-systemic encephalopathy: a predictable relationship. *Hepatology* 1995;22:365–367.

Gournay J, Lake JR. Management of common problems after liver transplantation. *Adv Gastroenterol Hepatol Clin Nutr* 1996;1(2):59–72.

Henderson JM. Role of distal splenorenal shunt for long-term management of variceal bleeding. *World J Surg* 1994;18:205–210.

Hillarie S, Labianca M, Borgonovo G, Smadja C, Grange D, Franco D. Peritoneovenous shunting of intractable ascites in patients with cirrhosis: improving results and predictive factors of failure. *Surgery* 1993;113:373–379.

Hughes KS. Resection of the liver for colorectal carcinoma metastases: a multi-institutional study of indications for resection. *Surgery* 1998;103:278–288.

Imperiale TF, Teran C, McCullough AJ. A meta-analysis of somatostatin versus vasopressin in the management of acute esophageal variceal hemorrhage. *Gastroenterology* 1995;109:1289–1294.

Infante-Rivard C, Esnaola S, Villeneuve JP. Role of endoscopic variceal sclerotherapy in the long-term management of variceal bleeding: a meta-analysis. *Gastroenterology* 1989;96:1087–1092.

Lake JR, ed. Advances in liver transplantation. *Gastroenterol Clin North Am* 1993;22(2).

Maddrey WC, Sorrell MF, eds. *Transplantation of the Liver,* 2nd ed. Norwalk, Conn: Appleton & Lange, 1995.

Nagorney DM. Benign hepatic tumors: focal nodular hyperplasia and hepatocellular adenoma. *World J Surg* 1995;19:13–18.

Rikkers LF, Burnett DA, Volentine GD, Buchi KN, Cormier RA. Shunt surgery versus endoscopic sclerotherapy for long-term treatment of variceal bleeding: early results of a randomized trial. *Ann Surg* 1987;206:261–271.

Sarfeh IJ, Rypins EB. Partial versus total portacaval shunt in alcoholic cirrhosis: results of a prospective, randomized clinical trial. *Ann Surg* 1994;219:353–361.

Sherlock S. *Diseases of the Liver and Biliary System,* 8th ed. London: Blackwell, 1991.

Spina GP, Henderson JM, Rikkers LF, et al. Distal splenorenal shunt versus endoscopic sclerotherapy in the prevention of variceal bleeding: a meta-analysis of four randomized clinical trials. *J Hepatol* 1992;16:338–345.

Stiegmann GV, Goff JS, Michaletz-Onody PA, et al. Endoscopic sclerotherapy as compared to endoscopic ligation for bleeding esophageal varices. *N Engl J Med* 1992;326:1527–1532.

19 Breast

Gary L. Dunnington, M.D.
Dorothy A. Andriole, M.D.
Susan Kaiser, M.D., Ph.D.

OBJECTIVES

1. Categorize the risk factors for breast cancer into major and minor factors.
2. Provide the guidelines for routine screening mammography.
3. Describe the diagnostic workup and management for common benign breast conditions, including breast pain, cysts, fibroadenoma, nipple discharge, and breast abscess.
4. List the diagnostic modalities and describe their sequence in the workup of a patient with a breast mass or nipple discharge.
5. Describe the preoperative evaluation for a patient with breast cancer.
6. Provide the differential diagnosis of a breast lump in a woman in her 20s and in a woman in her 60s.
7. Describe how ductal cancer in situ differs from invasive breast cancer. Describe its role as a risk factor for invasive cancer.
8. Explain the rationale for breast conservation treatment as the preferred therapeutic option for most stage I and stage II breast cancers.
9. Describe the rationale for adjuvant therapy, radiation therapy, and hormonal therapy in the treatment of breast cancer.
10. Describe the expected survival and local recurrence rates after treatment for early breast cancer.

Familiarity with evaluation of the breast and an understanding of breast disease are critically important for primary care physicians and surgeons. This chapter focuses on the evaluation of the patient who is undergoing routine screening as well as the patient who has a breast complaint. Breast cancer is the second most common cancer in women, only recently surpassed by lung cancer. It is the leading cause of death in women 40 to 55 years of age. In 1995, approximately 180,000 women were diagnosed with breast cancer, and 45,000 died of the disease.

Anatomy

The breast is a heterogeneous structure composed of glandular, ductal, connective, and adipose tissue. It is located on the anterior chest wall, superficial to the pectoralis major muscle. The breast may extend from the clavicle superiorly to the sixth rib inferiorly, and from the midsternal line medially into the axilla laterally (Figure 19-1). The mammary gland has approximately 15 to 20 lobes that are embedded in fibrous and adipose tissue. These lobes radiate from the central nipple area. Each lobe has an excretory duct that drains into the lactiferous sinus beneath the nipple. Cooper's ligaments are connective tissue structures that are derived from the superficial fascia of the skin that suspend the breast on the chest wall. Skin dimpling, produced by retraction of Cooper's ligaments, may be associated with underlying malignancy. The breast is a well-vascularized organ that receives its blood supply predominantly from the perforating branches of the paired internal mammary arteries and from branches of the lateral thoracic artery. The axillary, subclavian, and intercostal veins receive venous drainage from the breast. The long thoracic, thoracodorsal, and intercostobrachial nerves are intimately associated anatomically with the breast and the axillary space. The long thoracic nerve courses vertically along the superficial surface of the serratus anterior muscle in the region of the axilla. It provides motor innervation to the serratus anterior muscle, which abducts and laterally rotates the scapula and holds it against the chest wall. The thoracodorsal nerve, which is located posteriorly in the axillary space, innervates the latissimus dorsi muscle, which adducts, extends, and medially rotates the arm. The medial pectoral nerve most commonly pierces the pectoralis minor en route to the pectoralis major while innervating both. In 15% to 20% of patients, the nerve passes lateral to the pectoralis minor en route to the pectoralis major. For this reason, it is vulnerable to injury during axillary dissection. The intercostobrachial nerves, which are the lateral cutaneous branches of the first and second intercostal nerve, course across the axillary space to provide cutaneous innervation to the inner aspect of the upper arm and the axilla. The axillary lymph nodes provide the main route for lymphatic drainage of the breast (Figure 19-2). Two other routes of lymphatic drainage that may be significant in

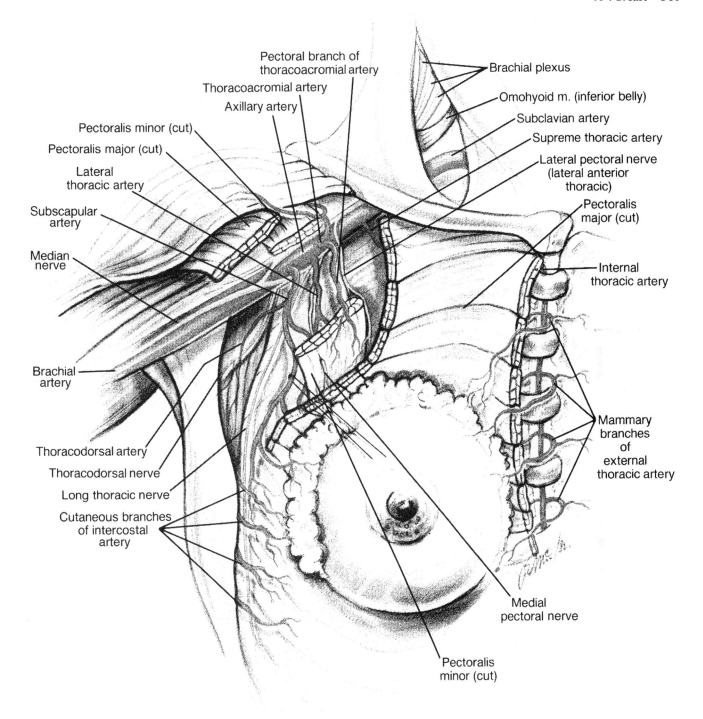

Figure 19-1 Normal breast anatomy showing vascular and neural origins.

women with breast cancer include the interpectoral (Rotter's) nodes and internal mammary nodes (which receive lymphatic drainage predominantly from the medial half of the breast).

Physiology

The female breast is a modified apocrine gland that undergoes considerable structural changes during a woman's lifetime. Increased hormonal production by the ovary at puberty causes ductal budding and the initial formation of acini, which are proliferations of the terminal ducts lined with secretory cells for milk production. With each menstrual cycle, preovulatory estrogen production stimulates proliferation of the breast ductal system. After ovulation, decreased estrogen and progesterone levels cause a decrease in ductal proliferation. In pregnancy, when estrogen and progesterone

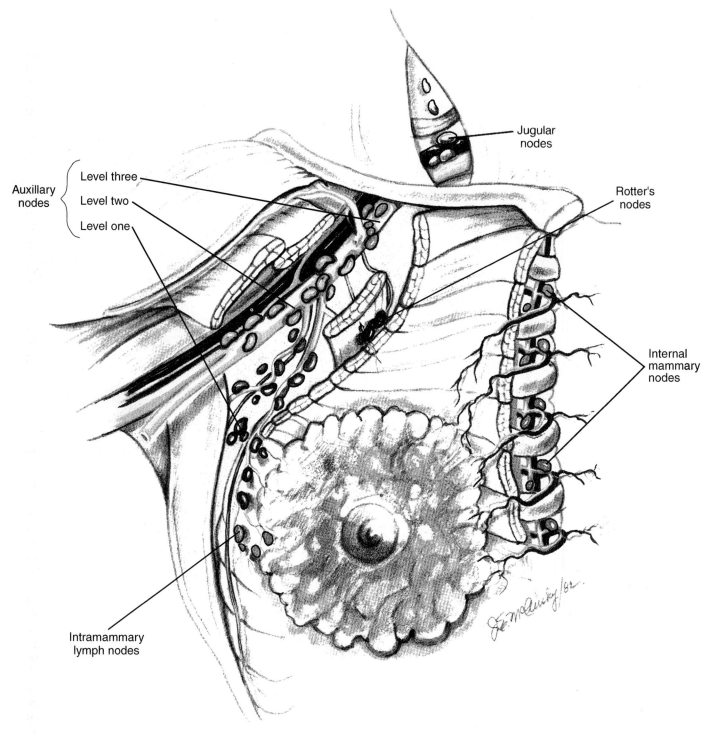

Figure 19-2 Lymphatic drainage of the breast.

levels remain relatively high, there is continued hypertrophy and budding of the ductal system, with associated acinar development. The sudden decrease in hormone levels in the postpartum period, associated with prolactin secretion from the pituitary gland, precipitates the onset of lactation. Postmenopausally, in the absence of the hormonal stimulus for cyclic proliferation of the breast ductal system, breast parenchyma is progressively lost and replaced by adipose tissue. The male breast is anatomically composed of the same heterogeneous tissue as the female breast, but it does not undergo cyclic hormonally related changes.

Clinical Presentation and Evaluation: Assessment of Breast Cancer Risk

A complete medical history should be obtained from any patient who has symptomatic breast disease. Table 19-1 summarizes the key aspects of the history. A careful history allows assessment of the patient's risk of breast cancer. Although breast cancer can occur in younger women, a breast mass in a young patient is more likely to be a fibroadenoma or a breast cyst. A breast mass in a woman who is older than 50 years of age, however, should be considered breast cancer until proven otherwise. The history allows elucidation of the four major risk factors for the development of breast cancer (i.e., factors that increase the relative risk by greater than fourfold). The first major risk factor is family history. The patient should be asked about the number of first-degree relatives who had breast cancer, whether the cancer occurred premenopausally or postmenopausally, and whether it was unilateral or bilateral. A strong family history in association with a young age at diagnosis raises the possibility of the presence of **BRCA-1** (breast cancer gene 1, also associated with ovarian cancer) or BRCA-2 (breast cancer gene 2). Whenever possible, pathology reports of previous benign or malignant breast lesions should be reviewed. Although fibrocystic condition does not significantly increase the risk of breast cancer, a biopsy showing **atypical hyperplasia** is the second major risk factor,

increasing the relative risk of breast cancer by threefold to fourfold, similar to the increased risk of having a mother with breast cancer. The third major risk factor is a personal history of breast cancer. In a woman with unilateral breast cancer, the risk that contralateral breast cancer will develop is 0.5% to 1% per year over the next 15 years. The fourth major risk factor is a previous diagnosis of lobular cancer in situ (LCIS) or ductal cancer in situ (DCIS) on breast biopsy. These diagnoses are associated with an increased relative risk of tenfold to twelvefold. Lobular carcinoma in situ is a risk factor that requires no treatment because subsequent cancer develops in the contralateral breast with equal frequency as it does in the breast where the LCIS was diagnosed. DCIS, however, is treated when identified (discussed later). The rest of the elements in the history elucidate the risk factors that increase relative risk in the range of onefold to twofold. These factors include early menarche, a long interval between menarche and first live birth, nulliparity, a history of ovarian or endometrial cancer, and the use of **estrogen replacement therapy** after menopause. The last risk factor is a common source of concern to patients and physicians because estrogen replacement therapy is often prescribed after surgical or natural menopause. Generally, studies show that although estrogen replacement therapy may slightly increase the risk of breast cancer, this increased risk is likely to be clinically insignificant. In most cases, the benefits of estrogen replacement therapy (e.g., decreased postmenopausal symptoms, decreased osteoporosis, decreased cardiac disease) outweigh this slight increase in risk.

Table 19-1. Patient Evaluation: Key Elements in the History

Family history of breast cancer: number of first-degree relatives affected

Personal history of breast cancer: specific information on diagnosis and treatment

Pathologic results of any previous breast biopsy

History of benign breast disease

Age (breast cancer is predominantly a disease of older women—after the first four decades of life)

Presence of a mass and any noted changes in size (cyclic changes or progressive increase)

Pain in the breast: unilateral or bilateral, cyclic or noncyclic

Medications: oral contraceptive use, exogenous hormone replacement

Family history of ovarian or colon cancer

Age at onset of menses and (surgical or natural) menopause

Age at first full-term pregnancy; number of pregnancies

Lactational history

History of mammograms; results of mammograms

History of nipple discharge: spontaneous or elicited, unilateral or bilateral, bloody or nonbloody

Personal history of endometrial cancer

History of weight loss, pain, or other systemic complaints that suggest metastatic disease

Physical Examination of the Breasts

A systematic approach to the physical examination of the breasts includes both inspection and palpation. The examination begins with the patient in the sitting position. The breasts are inspected first with the arms at the patient's side, second with the arms elevated toward the ceiling, third with the patient pressing tightly at her waist to contract the pectoralis muscles, and finally with the patient leaning forward. These maneuvers are complementary in aiding the detection of dimpling of the skin, a sign of malignancy. Inspection also allows for assessment of breast symmetry, the presence of any discoloration (e.g., redness, ecchymosis), and the presence of edema. The nipples are inspected to be certain that they are everted and without rash or ulceration. With the patient still in the sitting position, both axillae are examined, with the patient's arm resting over the forearm of the examiner to relax the shoulder musculature, allowing for full assessment of axillary contents. Lymph nodes are best detected as the examiner pushes superiorly in the axilla, then moves the fingertips inferiorly against the chest wall, trapping lymph nodes between the finger and the chest wall. A careful lymph node examination also involves palpation in the supraclavicular fossae. Examination of the breasts in the sitting

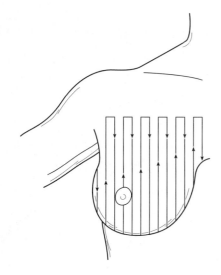

Figure 19-3 The strip method of breast examination.

position is discouraged because it often yields false-positive findings for the examiner (as well as for the patient during self-examination). The breasts should be examined with the patient supine and the arm resting comfortably above the head. This position spreads breast tissue out over the chest wall, allowing more accurate detection of abnormalities. Although several methods for examining the breasts are used, such as larger and larger circles and the "spokes of a wheel" approach, the most consistent and reliable findings are obtained with the strip method (Figure 19-3). With this method, the breast is examined using the touch pads of the index, middle, and ring fingers in vertical strips, covering the breasts from the sternum to the axilla and from the clavicle to near the costal margin. The location of any breast mass is described (e.g., at one o'clock 4 cm from the areolar margin). In addition, the precise size of the mass should be described with the use of a measuring instrument. In addition, the examiner should note whether the mass is tender or nontender, its mobility, and its texture. It is not necessary to squeeze the nipples during a breast examination because unilateral elicited discharge is almost always normal, particularly in younger women. With a history of **spontaneous nipple discharge,** the source of the discharge should be localized with systematic palpation from the outer breast to the nipple circumferentially around the areola. If discharge is identified, it should be heme tested to determine whether it is bloody or nonbloody. A bloody discharge indicates an increased likelihood of cancer.

Diagnostic Evaluation

Mammography

Standard mammography involves one craniocaudal and one mediolateral view of each breast (Figure 19-4). With these two views, a mammographic abnormality can be localized to one of four quadrants in the breast. Mammograms may be obtained for either screening or diagnostic purposes. Screening mammography is mam-

mography obtained in asymptomatic patients. There is substantial evidence that screening mammography can detect clinically occult breast cancers and, as a result, can reduce breast cancer mortality. Table 19-2 summarizes the current American Cancer Society recommendations for the detection of breast cancer in asymptomatic women. These recommendations are general guidelines only. Appropriate screening protocols may vary for women who are at high risk for the development of breast cancer because of the presence of premalignant disease, family history, or other risk factors. A diagnostic mammogram study generally includes the same two-view studies of each breast as the screening mammogram. The initial two-view mammogram is reviewed by a radiologist when it is performed. Then, based on clinical and initial mammographic findings, additional views, such as oblique, **magnified,** or **compression,** are obtained to clarify any questionable abnormalities. Mammography has a 5% to 10% false-negative rate (90%–95% sensitivity). Therefore, a normal, or nondiagnostic, mammogram should never deter the clinician from performing a full evaluation, with tissue diagnosis as indicated, for clinical manifestations in women with breast disease, particularly if they are suspicious for malignancy.

The most common abnormal mammogram findings are dominant masses and microcalcifications. Dominant masses are characterized by their size and the regularity of their margins. A spiculated lesion is probably a malignancy, whereas a round, smooth, dominant mass may be a cyst or a fibroadenoma.

Further workup of a dominant mass may require additional mammographic views, with or without compression of the breast, ultrasound, or directed biopsy. Microcalcifications on mammography are characterized by the number of microcalcifications and their morphology. A few (< 5) smooth, round microcalcifications are considered benign and do not require routine mammography for follow-up. A cluster of several irregular microcalcifications with a branching pattern warrants biopsy for definitive diagnosis.

Ultrasound

Ultrasound provides a noninvasive evaluation tool for mammographically detected breast abnormalities and palpable breast masses. It is not associated with significant radiation exposure, so it is particularly useful in pregnant women. It is often the most useful study in younger women (< 35 years) who have a breast mass because mammography is often limited by the density of the premenopausal breast. Ultrasound delineates the solid versus cystic nature of a mass and can be used to direct needle aspiration or biopsy of nonpalpable or poorly localized abnormalities. Its utility as a screening device for breast cancer is not established. Like mammographic evaluation, however, ultrasound evaluation does not replace clinical judgment.

Biopsy Techniques

Biopsy techniques for the evaluation of breast abnormalities are summarized in Table 19-3. The appropriate

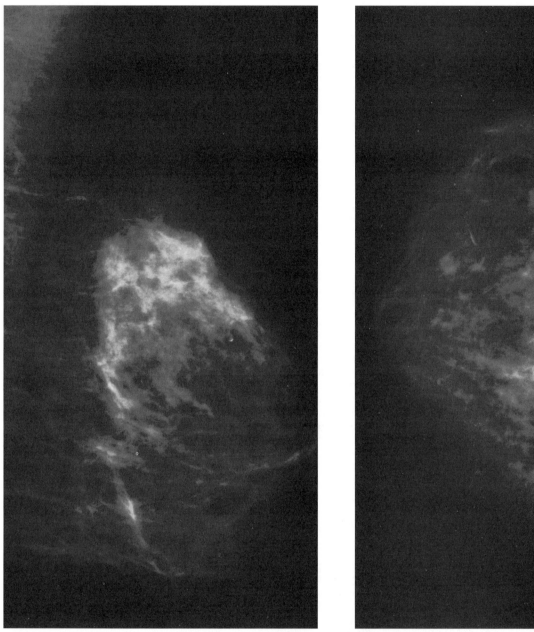

A

B

Figure 19-4 Standard two-view bilateral mammogram. A normal study in a 50-year-old woman. **A,** The mediolateral view of the left breast shows the breast "on profile." The breast is compressed mediolaterally with the patient's arm raised above her head. The functional breast parenchyma is normally most dense in the upper outer quadrant of the breast, and the symmetric appearance of the more dense parenchyma on the upper aspect of the breast is well visualized on these mediolateral films. **B,** The craniocaudal view of the left breast shows the breast compressed in a craniocaudal direction. In this view, the "cc" (craniocaudal) designation is placed on the lateral aspect of the film (a standard labeling convention for mammograms). On these views, the prominent area of density bilaterally is localized to the lateral half of the breast and again represents the normal breast parenchyma.

diagnostic evaluation and biopsy techniques are determined on an individual basis. An algorithm for the evaluation of a palpable mass in a woman who is at least 30 years of age is outlined in Figure 19-5. The preferred method for diagnosis of a palpable solid mass is **fine-needle aspiration cytology** or **core biopsy.** This method usually provides definitive diagnosis in the office and allows only a single trip to the operating room if a

malignancy is detected. For women who are younger than 30 years of age, this algorithm is not necessarily applicable. In this age group, palpable masses are rarely malignant, and not all masses require excision. Mammography is indicated only if cancer is suspected on the basis of physical findings, the patient has a history of premalignant disease, or there is a significant family history of breast cancer. Factors to consider in the selec-

Table 19-2. American Cancer Society Recommendations for Breast Cancer Detection in Asymptomatic Women

Age Group	Examination	Frequency
20–40	Breast self-examination	Every month
	Clinical breast examination	Every 3 years
40–49	Breast self-examination	Every month
	Mammography	Every 1–2 years
	Clinical breast examination	Every year
50 and older	Breast self-examination	Every month
	Mammography	Every year
	Clinical breast examination	Every year

Reprinted with permission from Mettlin C, Smart CR. Breast cancer detection guidelines for women ages 40–49 years: rationale for the American Cancer Society reaffirmation of recommendations. *CA Cancer J. Clin* 1994; 44: 248–255.

tion of biopsy technique include the index of suspicion for malignancy based on clinical findings, patient age, and the presence of any coexisting conditions (e.g., pregnancy, bleeding disorder).

Studies to Evaluate Metastatic Breast Disease

The initial evaluation of the patient with known or suspected breast cancer must include a complete detailed history and physical examination so that clinical staging can be performed accurately. For women with early-stage breast cancer (stage 0, I, or II), posteroanterior and lateral chest x-rays, blood count, and liver function studies are routinely performed. Further diagnostic studies, such as bone scan or computerized tomography (CT) scan of the abdomen, chest, or head, are performed only for specific indications, based on

Table 19-3. Biopsy Techniques: Palpable and Nonpalpable Masses

Technique	Indications	Advantages	Disadvantages
Palpable mass Fine-needle aspiration (FNA)	Establish cytologic diagnosis.	Minimally invasive office procedure that is well tolerated by the patient. Often allows for a single trip to operating room. Specimen can be processed and interpreted rapidly.	False (+) rate for cancer varies from 0%–1% on an institutional basis. Significant false (-) rate (> 20%) for cancer because of small sampling size.
Core-needle biopsy (CNB)	Establish histologic diagnosis.	Minimally invasive, low-morbidity office procedure False (+) rate for cancer is 0.	Rare complications of hematoma and pneumothorax. Significant false (-) rate (> 20%) for cancer because of small sampling size.
Incisional biopsy	Establish histologic diagnosis for a large mass(> 3 cm) when FNA and CNB are nondiagnostic.	Performed under local anesthesia. False (+) rate for cancer is 0. False (-) rate for cancer is close to 0.	Substantially higher cost than FNA or CNB. Open surgical procedure with associated risks of bleeding and wound infection.
Excisional biopsy	Establish definitive histologic diagnosis for a small (< 3 cm) mass when FNA and CNB are nondiagnostic.	Can be therapeutic as well as diagnostic for benign mass and for malignant mass excised with negative microscopic margins. False (+) and false (-) rates for cancer are 0. Performed under local anesthesia.	Open surgical procedure with associated risks of bleeding and wound infection. Substantially higher cost than other biopsy procedures.
Nonpalpable mass CNB (stereotactic or ultrasound-guided)	Establish histologic diagnosis for a nonpalpable mammographically visualized abnormality.	Avoids open biopsy procedure, with associated risks and costs. Well tolerated by patient. False (+) rate for cancer is 0.	False (-) rate for cancer is approximately 1%.
FNA cytology (stereotactic or ultrasound-guided)	Establish cytologic diagnosis for a nonpalpable mass.	Minimally invasive, well tolerated by the patient. Specimen can be processed and interpreted rapidly.	False (+) rate for cancer varies from 0%–1% on an institutional basis. Significant false (-) rate (> 20%) for cancer because of small sampling size.
Needle localization breast biopsy	Establish definitive histologic diagnosis for a nonpalpable mammographically visualized abnormality.	Therapeutic as well as diagnostic for benign masses and for malignant masses excised with negative margins. False (+) rate for cancer is 0. False (–) rate is 0 if mammographic abnormality is completely excised.	Open procedure that requires radiologic localization before surgical excision. Occasional (1%) failure to excise abnormality. May require relocalization and reoperation. Cosmetic deformity may result.

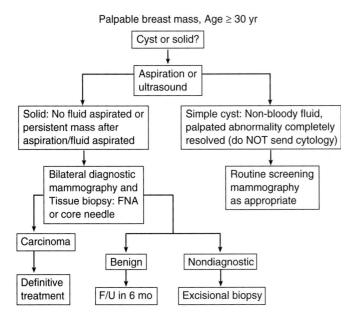

Palpable breast mass, Age ≥ 30 yr

Cyst or solid?

Aspiration or ultrasound

Solid: No fluid aspirated or persistent mass after aspiration/fluid aspirated

Simple cyst: Non-bloody fluid, palpated abnormality completely resolved (do NOT send cytology)

Bilateral diagnostic mammography and Tissue biopsy: FNA or core needle

Routine screening mammography as appropriate

Carcinoma

Benign

Nondiagnostic

Definitive treatment

F/U in 6 mo

Excisional biopsy

Figure 19-5 Algorithm for the evaluation of a palpable mass in a woman at least 30 years of age. *FNA* = fine-needle aspiration; *F/U* = follow-up.

symptoms or physical signs that suggest metastatic disease or based on abnormalities in the initial screening chest x-ray and blood work. For patients with stage III (locally advanced) breast cancer, a metastatic workup, including a bone scan and CT scan of the abdomen and chest, is usually performed because of the high likelihood (up to 50%) of detecting clinically occult metastatic disease that could significantly alter treatment recommendations.

Benign Conditions of the Breast

Nipple Discharge

Spontaneous nipple discharge requires complete evaluation, although elicited discharge is rarely of concern. The incidence of malignancy increases when there is bloody nipple discharge, although an intraductal papilloma is the most common cause of spontaneous, bloody, unilateral discharge. An intraductal papilloma is a benign local proliferation of ductal epithelial cells. It typically occurs in women in the fourth or fifth decade of life. In approximately 40% of patients, unilateral bloody discharge is associated with a palpable mass. When no mass is palpable, the location of the bleeding duct can be determined by gentle palpation in a systematic manner around the nipple–areolar complex. In approximately 10% to 15% of patients, unilateral bloody discharge is caused by an underlying malignancy. Therefore, mammography is an important step in the preoperative workup of a patient with bloody nipple discharge. In the absence of clinical or radiographic evidence of an associated malignancy, ductal excision is the recommended treatment if the unilateral spontaneous

discharge can be localized to a single duct. An intraductal papilloma is usually easily visible in the opened surgical specimen as a pedunculated mass. However, the definitive diagnosis can only be made on the basis of microscopic pathologic inspection of the entire resected specimen to rule out underlying malignancy. Other common causes of spontaneous nipple discharge include cysts and duct ectasia.

Fibroadenoma

Fibroadenoma is a very common benign tumor of the breast. It usually occurs in young women (late teens to early 30s), although it may develop at any age. Typically, the fibroadenoma is 1 to 3 cm in size and presents as a freely movable, discrete, firm, spherical mass in the breast. Often, fine-needle aspiration is performed to establish a presumptive cytologic diagnosis of fibroadenoma. For young women with a typical clinical presentation and cytologic diagnosis of fibroadenoma, excision is no longer uniformly required if the fibroadenoma is small (< 3 cm). In this group, approximately 50% of fibroadenomas resolve within 5 years. In some patients, periodic follow-up and reexamination, with excision if the mass increases in size, is an appropriate alternative to surgical excision after the diagnosis is confirmed with fine-needle aspiration. Giant fibroadenoma is an uncommon benign tumor in adolescent girls. Occasionally, an incisional biopsy is performed before excision because of the rare occurrence of **phyllodes tumor,** a large, usually benign tumor (90%) requiring wide margins of resection to prevent local recurrence.

Breast Cyst

A gross cyst is the most common cause of a breast mass in women in their fourth and fifth decades of life. In this setting, cysts are most likely caused by a relative excess in estrogen stimulation of the breast. Gross cysts may also be present in postmenopausal women who are taking oral hormone replacement therapy. The cyst, which may be solitary or multiple, is a mobile, slightly tender mass on palpation, often with less well-defined margins than fibroadenomas. Unlike fibroadenomas, the size and degree of tenderness of a gross cyst typically fluctuates with the menstrual cycle. Needle aspiration can be both diagnostic and therapeutic. However, aspiration is not necessary for all palpable cysts. If ultrasound examination confirms the presence of a simple cyst (no internal projections) and the patient is asymptomatic, the cyst can be followed. If aspiration is performed, several milliliters of straw-colored or green-tinged fluid are usually found. The breast is reexamined immediately after aspiration to confirm the complete disappearance of the palpable abnormality. Aspiration of bloody fluid or persistence of a palpable mass after cyst aspiration warrants further evaluation, including diagnostic mammography and biopsy. Ultrasound is occasionally useful to further evaluate a cystic mass in the breast, and ultrasound-directed cyst aspiration facilitates the management of ill-defined, poorly localized cysts or cysts located deep in the breast. With the more widespread use of screening mammography, small cysts are detected with increasing frequency. Ultrasound can be used to confirm the cystic nature of these mammographically visualized, nonpalpable masses, although aspiration is not routinely required.

Fibrocystic Breast Condition

Fibrocystic breast condition is a common, progressive condition, and not a true disease. It is a manifestation of normal physiologic changes in the breast related to menstrual hormonal cycles. Most women are likely to have manifestations of fibrocystic breast changes at some point in their lives. Fibrocystic changes in the breast may be associated with the development of microscopic cysts embedded in dense fibrous tissue, giving the characteristic physical examination finding of "lumpy" breasts without a discrete mass. The extent of the dense breast tissue and the degree of tenderness elicited on palpation generally fluctuate with the menstrual cycle. Symptomatic fibrocystic changes typically occur in women between 30 and 50 years of age. Symptoms are typically worst in the several days preceding menses and improve after the onset of menses. It is uncommon for postmenopausal women to have symptomatic fibrocystic changes unless they are receiving oral hormone replacement therapy. Often, reexamination of the woman with symptomatic fibrocystic changes at a different point in her menstrual cycle is very helpful in documenting the fluctuating nature of the symptoms and physical findings. Women with these findings should be reassured that the condition is normal and does not increase their risk of malignancy.

Breast Abscess

Breast abscesses usually develop in lactating women. The patient with a breast abscess typically has a painful, erythematous mass that is exquisitely tender on palpation. It may be fluctuant, depending on its location within the breast. Although mammography is generally not performed, ultrasound may be useful to localize an abscess. Aspiration yields purulent fluid for Gram stain and culture. Gram-positive cocci (staphylococci or streptococci) are the most common infecting organisms. Appropriate systemic antibiotic therapy is indicated for the woman with a breast abscess. This therapy should be accompanied by drainage of the abscess, which is readily accomplished by incision directly over the abscess and evacuation of the contents of the multiloculated cavity. Occasionally, repeated aspiration, rather than open drainage, is sufficient for the management of a small abscess. With appropriate antibiotic therapy and drainage, these infections resolve rapidly, with minimal residual cosmetic defect. Development of a breast abscess in a nonlactating woman, or failure of an abscess to resolve completely with appropriate antibiotic management and drainage, should alert the clinician to the possibility of an atypical infection (microbacterial or fungal) or an underlying malignancy. Inflammatory cancer occasionally mimics breast abscess. In these circum-

stances, careful palpation of the abscess cavity, with biopsy of the abscess wall, is indicated at the time of abscess drainage.

Breast Pain

Slight bilateral breast tenderness is a fairly common physical finding in women and tends to develop on a cyclic (monthly) basis before menses. In postmenopausal women, it may occur in association with estrogen replacement therapy. Women with persistent breast pain or severe breast tenderness in the absence of any other symptoms, physical findings, or mammographic abnormalities can be challenging to manage. Numerous etiologies are proposed for breast pain, but the most likely is either a decrease in the level of progesterone or a sustained increase in the level of prolactin. No single intervention had established efficacy in a large, prospective randomized trial. Thorough clinical evaluation and appropriate diagnostic workup should be performed for any woman who has breast pain, particularly if it is unilateral, to rule out an underlying malignancy or chest wall problem. Once this workup is done, reassurance is often all that is necessary. However, for patients with more severe symptoms, elimination of caffeine and administration of vitamin E supplements, oil of evening primrose capsules, oral contraceptive agents, and bromocriptine appear to provide symptomatic relief. Danazol, an androgen analogue, is effective in relieving breast pain and tenderness, but it should be used only after failure of the previous measures, because its side effects include deepening of the voice and hirsutism.

Breast Cancer

It is estimated that one of every eight women will have breast cancer in her lifetime. Most women with a diagnosis of breast cancer (75%) have no known risk factors. Major public health efforts are being directed toward screening and early diagnosis. The incidence of breast cancer has been rising since 1982, possibly due entirely or in part to screening. Over the last 25 years, there has been a highly significant change in stage at diagnosis, with gradually more in situ cancers and cancers confined to the breast, fewer with spread to axillary lymph nodes, fewer with distant metastases, and smaller tumors at diagnosis. A much higher proportion of cancers are initially found by screening mammogram.

The cause of breast cancer is unknown in the vast majority of cases. Environmental and dietary factors are probably involved. For example, work continues to investigate the possible link between breast cancer and magnetic fields, polyvinyl chlorides, and other environmental factors. Increasing evidence indicates a high-fat diet as a possible factor in breast cancer development and regular exercise over several years as a possible factor in decreasing the incidence of breast cancer. There is increasing understanding of the major role of hormonal factors, particularly estrogen, in the etiology of breast cancer. Knowledge about the genetic basis of breast cancer is progressing rapidly, but still, as far as we know, fewer than 3% of cases of breast cancer are caused by "breast cancer genes." Approximately 1% of breast cancers occur in men. Most of the same diagnostic and treatment modalities are used.

Histologic Types of Breast Cancer

Ductal Carcinoma in Situ

DCIS, also called intraductal, or noninvasive, carcinoma, is characterized by abnormal cells that remain within the confines of the duct, without crossing the basement membrane (Figure 19-6). A mass is rarely seen on physical examination or mammography; it may appear only as **mammographic microcalcifications** in otherwise normal-appearing tissue. The process may be localized by a small cluster of irregular calcifications or microcalcifications spread throughout an entire quadrant of the breast. DCIS progresses to invasive cancer in 30% to 50% of patients. The cribriform type is characterized by punched-out areas, or holes, in the sheets of abnormal cells that fill the ducts. In the micropapillary type, abnormal cells appear in papillary formation within the ducts. In the comedo type, there is central necrosis in the sheets of abnormal cells that fill the ducts. This necrosis suggests rapid growth and has an unfavorable prognostic significance. When DCIS is found, a careful search of the histology must be made for any invasive component; if found, it changes both the treatment and the prognosis.

Infiltrating Ductal Carcinoma

Infiltrating ductal carcinoma constitutes approximately 90% of invasive breast cancers. It produces the characteristic firm, irregular mass on physical examination. These masses are characteristically more well-defined mammographically and histologically than infiltrating lobular cancers.

Tubular carcinoma, a very well-differentiated form of ductal carcinoma, constitutes approximately 1% to 2% of breast cancers. It is so named because it forms small tubules, randomly arranged, with each lined by a single uniform row of cells. This subtype tends to occur in women who are slightly younger than the average patient with breast cancer. The prognosis is better than with other infiltrating ductal carcinomas.

Medullary carcinoma, which is characterized by extensive tumor invasion by small lymphocytes and is slightly less well differentiated than tubular carcinoma, constitutes approximately 5% of breast carcinomas. At diagnosis, it tends to be rapidly growing and large, and it is often associated with DCIS. It less commonly metastasizes to regional lymph nodes and has a better prognosis than the typical infiltrating ductal carcinoma.

Colloid or mucinous carcinoma, which accounts for approximately 2% to 3% of breast carcinomas, is characterized histologically by clumps and strands of epithelial cells in pools of mucoid material. It grows slowly and occurs more often in older women. The pure type has a relatively good prognosis.

True papillary carcinoma accounts for approximately 1% of breast carcinomas. These tumors can be difficult to distinguish histologically from intraductal papilloma, a benign lesion. They tend to be quite small, and even when they metastasize to regional nodes, they have a better prognosis than ductal carcinomas because of their slower rate of growth.

Paget's Disease of the Nipple

Cutaneous nipple abnormalities, which may be moist and exudative, dry and scaly, erosive, or just a thickened area, are symptomatic of Paget's disease of the nipple. The patient may note itching, burning, or sticking pain in the nipple. As time passes, the lesion spreads out from the duct orifice. Histologically, the dermis is infiltrated by Paget's cells, which are of ductal origin, large and pale, with large nuclei, prominent nucleoli, and abundant cytoplasm. Paget's disease of the nipple is seen in approximately 3% of breast cancers and is usually, but not always, associated with an underlying malignancy, which is palpable in half of cases. It may originate in DCIS or in an invasive cancer.

Paget's disease of the nipple is often misdiagnosed as a simple dermatologic eruption and treated with ointments and creams for prolonged periods, during which time the cancer progresses. If a lesion is clinically suspicious for Paget's disease, a biopsy should be done.

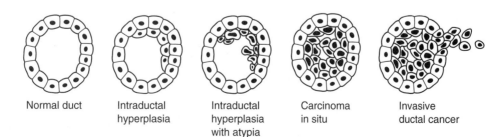

Normal duct Intraductal hyperplasia Intraductal hyperplasia with atypia Carcinoma in situ Invasive ductal cancer

Figure 19-6 The evolution from normal duct to invasive cancer. (Adapted with permission from Love SM. *Dr. Susan Love's Breast Book.* Reading, Mass: Addison-Wesley Longman, 1990;192. Copyright 1990, 1991 by Susan M. Love, MD. Reprinted by permission of Addison-Wesley Longman Inc.)

Lobular Carcinoma

Lobular carcinoma is characterized by small cells with scanty cytoplasm and oval or round nuclei. The cells are arranged linearly ("Indian file") or concentrically ("bull's-eye"). Distribution within the breast tissue may be diffuse and may produce thickening of the tissue rather than a well-defined mass. This characteristic may also make mammographic detection more difficult. Lobular carcinoma constitutes approximately 10% of invasive breast cancers. The percentage varies greatly from one study to another according to the histologic criteria used. A large percentage are estrogen- and progesterone-receptor–positive. It has a slight propensity toward synchronous bilaterality (2%–5%).

Inflammatory Carcinoma

Inflammatory carcinoma often resembles localized or generalized inflammation of the breast, with skin edema (peau d'orange), erythema, warmth, pain, and tenderness. This presentation is caused not by infection, but by invasion of dermal lymphatics with breast cancer cells, predominantly from ductal carcinoma. It accounts for approximately 2% of breast cancers. Diagnosis is established by biopsy of the involved skin. Inflammatory breast carcinoma has a very poor prognosis, with approximately 25% of patients alive 5 years after diagnosis.

Other Breast Malignancies

Malignancies that rarely appear in the breast include various types of sarcomas as well as Hodgkin's and non-Hodgkin's lymphomas, leukemia, and the malignant form of phyllodes tumor.

Histologic types of breast cancer may be mixed. Prognosis and treatment decisions are usually based on the least favorable type (Table 19-4).

Clinical Staging

Patients are staged at the time of diagnosis on the basis of clinical findings (clinical stage) and again after surgery on the basis of microscopic examination of the excised breast tissue and lymph nodes (pathologic stage).

The most commonly used clinical staging system is the TNM system, which is based on tumor size, lymph node involvement, and metastases (Figure 19-7) as defined by the American Joint Committee on Cancer (AJCC; 1992). Tumors are categorized, by maximum diameter, as less than or equal to 2 cm (T1), greater than 2 cm to less than or equal to 5 cm (T2), or greater than 5 cm (T3). These are subcategorized as not fixed (a) or fixed (b) to the underlying pectoralis fascia or muscle. Tumors that cannot be found (e.g., metastatic lymph nodes without a primary) are categorized as T0, and tumors whose size is unknown are categorized as TX. T4 tumors are fixed to the bones or to deep muscles of the chest wall (a); involve the skin, with peau d'orange, edema, or ipsilateral skin nodules (b); involve both the chest wall and skin (c); or show inflammatory carcinoma (d). Lymph nodes are categorized according to

Table 19-4. Histopathologic Classification of Breast Cancer (AJCC)

Ductal carcinoma
  DCIS
    Micropapillary type
    Cribriform type
    Comedo type
  Predominantly DCIS, with an invasive component
  Invasive ductal carcinoma
  Medullary
  Mucinous (colloid)
  Papillary
  Scirrhous
  Tubular
  Mixed types
Lobular carcinoma
  LCIS (not actually a cancer, but rather a marker)
  Invasive lobular carcinoma
Paget's disease of the nipple
  With no other cancer found
  With DCIS
  With invasive ductal carcinoma
Inflammatory carcinoma
Undifferentiated carcinoma

Some of the categories overlap (e.g., DCIS with Paget's disease of the nipple).
AJCC, American Joint Committee on Cancer.
DCIS, ductal carcinoma in situ.
LCIS, lobular carcinoma in situ.

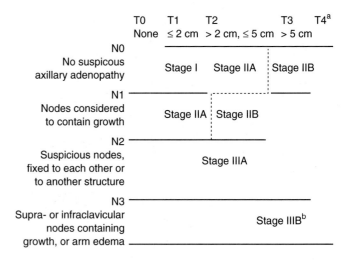

[a]T4 is defined as: (1) fixed to the bones or deep muscles of the chest wall; (2) involving the skin, with peau d'orange, edema, or ipsilateral skin nodules; (3) involving both chest wall and skin, (1), and (2); or (4) showing inflammatory carcinoma.

[b]The presence of any distant metastases automatically defines breast cancer as stage IV, regardless of any factors related to tumor or lymph nodes.

Figure 19-7 The staging of breast cancer.

the extent of involvement, whether no nodes are involved (N0), the involved ipsilateral nodes are mobile (N1), the involved ipsilateral nodes form a matted mass or are fixed to other structures (N2), or the ipsilateral internal mammary nodes are involved (N3). NX denotes unknown nodal status. The absence of distant metastases is denoted as M0, and their presence is denoted as M1. MX denotes unknown metastatic status.

In addition to the status of tumor margins and lymph nodes, pathologic staging involves additional studies that allow more accurate assessment of prognosis and assist in planning **adjuvant therapy.** The most important of these studies is determining the presence of estrogen and progesterone receptors. A positive result on an estrogen and progesterone receptor test indicates that the tumor is responsive to these hormones and allows the likely successful use of tamoxifen, an estrogen receptor (ER) blocker, to prevent recurrence. Overall, ER-positive tumors have a better survival rate than ER-negative tumors. Other prognostic indicators assess the growth rate of the tumor. For example, ploidy, measured by flow cytometry, determines the DNA content per tumor cell; a diploid tumor has a better prognosis than an **aneuploid** tumor. The **S-phase** fraction describes the number of tumor cells that are in the growth phase of the cell cycle; higher S-phase fractions are noted in more aggressive tumors. Cathepsin D, an enzyme produced by tumor cells, is produced in greater quantities by the more aggressive types of breast cancer. **Her-2-neu,** an oncogene produced by some tumors, predicts a poorer prognosis, particularly for node-positive patients.

Treatment of Breast Cancer

Breast cancer treatment is a team effort by mammographers, sonographers, breast and plastic surgeons, medical and radiation oncologists, pathologists, gynecologists, social workers, nurses, and physiatrists. The treatment of breast cancer is divided into local treatment (e.g., surgery, radiation treatment) and adjuvant treatment (e.g., chemotherapy, hormone therapy) designed to decrease systemic recurrence.

Surgery

Definitions of Surgical Procedures

Wide excision, lumpectomy, and segmental resection refer to the excision of a malignancy with at least a 1-cm margin of microscopically normal tissue on all sides (see Chapter 26). Simple, or total, mastectomy removes the entire breast with the pectoralis major fascia. Axillary dissection removes the axillary fat pad and the level I and II lymph nodes, including the nodes in the axillary fat pad (level I), behind the pectoralis major muscle, and between the pectoralis major and pectoralis minor muscles [level II (see Figure 19-2)]. Level III nodes (above the pectoralis minor muscle) are removed if they are grossly involved, a rare finding in early breast cancer. Modified radical mastectomy is simple mastectomy with axillary dissection (see Chapter 26). Radical mastectomy, which involves removal of the breast, both pectoralis muscles down to the chest wall, the axillary contents, and the overlying skin, was developed by Halstead to treat locally advanced breast cancer at a time when no other treatments were available. This procedure is disfiguring, causes significant upper extremity dysfunction, and is no longer performed except in unusual circumstances (e.g., invasion of the pectoral muscles).

After mastectomy, the breast can be reconstructed with a subpectoral prosthesis or with autologous tissue (musculocutaneous flaps on vascular pedicles, taken from the abdomen or back). Reconstruction, which can be done at mastectomy or later, depending on patient preference, should be offered to all patients.

Choosing a Surgical Option

DCIS is treated with lumpectomy followed by radiation to the breast. If it is diffuse, simple mastectomy is chosen. Radiation added to lumpectomy decreases the rate of recurrence of both DCIS and invasive cancer at the site of lumpectomy. Axillary dissection is not indicated because DCIS, confined within the ducts and without access to lymphatics and blood vessels, cannot metastasize.

For small invasive tumors of all types, especially those less than 4 cm in greatest diameter, the patient is offered a choice between two procedures. They are modified radical mastectomy and wide excision with axillary dissection followed by 6 weeks of radiation to the breast. Dermal or lymphatic involvement, a large tumor, multiple tumors, diffuse tumor involvement in the breast, unwillingness or inability to undergo radiation therapy, and the expectation of a cosmetically unacceptable result are all contraindications to lumpectomy. Lumpectomy is usually cosmetically superior to mastectomy. Most important, the patient should understand that there is no statistically significant difference in cure (survival) or chance of recurrence between the two options. Recurrence after mastectomy usually occurs in the skin over the chest wall, whereas recurrence after lumpectomy usually occurs at the lumpectomy site.

Paget's disease is treated with local excision of the nipple–areola complex and any associated mass. Further treatment is chosen according to the underlying lesion. For example, if only DCIS is present, it is treated with wide excision and radiation. If there is underlying invasive cancer, it is treated with wide excision, axillary dissection, and radiation, or with mastectomy.

Prophylactic (simple) mastectomy is being increasingly considered as an option for patients at very high risk for breast cancer. This group includes those with a combination of high-risk lesions on biopsy (atypical hyperplasia, LCIS) and a strong family history. Patients who carry one of the breast cancer genes (BRCA-1, BRCA-2) are also offered the option of prophylactic mastectomy, with or without reconstruction. This procedure significantly decreases, but does not eliminate, the possibility of a future breast cancer.

Adjuvant Treatment

Indications for adjuvant therapy include large tumor size, involved lymph nodes, negative ER status, lymphatic invasion, aneuploidy, elevated S-phase, poor histologic grade, elevated cathepsin D levels, and the expression of her-2-neu oncogene. Other prognostic indicators are investigational. Evidence suggests that premenopausal patients do better if treated with chemotherapy, regardless of cancer stage. The only exception is the patient with a small tumor (< 1 cm), negative lymph nodes, positive ER status, and good prognostic factors. In contemplating adjuvant treatment, consideration should always be given to comorbidities and to the patient's life expectancy. For example, chemotherapy for stage IIa breast cancer is unlikely to be of value to a patient whose life expectancy is only a few years because of advanced age or another disease.

Large tumors and inflammatory cancers are usually treated first with chemotherapy. Surgery is performed after maximal response. There are two reasons for this approach. First, because large tumors are more likely to have spread to distant sites, it is desirable to provide systemic treatment as early as possible. Second, surgery may become much easier if the tumor is reduced in size. Sometimes the response to chemotherapy is complete, and the mass disappears entirely. Radiation therapy usually follows chemotherapy or surgery. Chemotherapy is the primary modality for the treatment of stage IV breast cancer, with biopsy to establish the diagnosis as the only surgical procedure.

Chemotherapy

Both combination chemotherapy and tamoxifen reduce the chance of recurrence, and trials continue to define their optimal role in both premenopausal and postmenopausal women (Table 19-5). The most common chemotherapeutic combination of cyclophosphamide, methotrexate or Adriamycin, and 5-fluorouracil is given over a course of 6 months. Patients who have more than 10 positive axillary lymph nodes may be treated in a clinical investigation with high-dose chemotherapy followed by rescue with **autologous bone marrow transplant.**

Hormonal Therapy

Tamoxifen is used to treat ER-positive tumors, particularly in postmenopausal women, and it may have some benefit for ER-negative tumors in postmenopausal women. Its role in premenopausal women is less well established, but it is often used in this setting after chemotherapy. In addition to decreasing recurrence, tamoxifen decreases the incidence of contralateral breast cancer by approximately 40%. No benefit is shown for continuing tamoxifen longer than 5 years.

Treatment for Recurrent and Metastatic Breast Cancer

Local tumor recurrence in the breast after breast conservation (lumpectomy, axillary dissection, and radiation) is treated with mastectomy. If radiation was never

Table 19-5. Recommendations for Adjuvant Therapy in Early Breast Cancer

Tumor Size	Lymph Nodes	Estrogen Receptors	Adjuvant Therapy
Premenopausal			
< 1 cm	Negative	Positive	None
≥ 1 cm	Negative	Positive	Chemotherapy, tamoxifen
≥ 1 cm	Positive	Positive	Chemotherapy, tamoxifen
≥ 1 cm	Positive	Negative	Chemotherapy
≥ 1 cm	Negative	Negative	Chemotherapy
Postmenopausal			
< 1 cm	Negative	Positive	None
≥ 1 cm	Negative	Positive	Tamoxifen
≥ 1 cm	Positive	Positive	Tamoxifen± chemotherapy
≥ 1 cm	Positive	Negative	Chemotherapy
≥ 1 cm	Negative	Negative	Chemotherapy

given, a small recurrence is treated with lumpectomy and radiation. Local recurrence after mastectomy is treated with surgical excision, if possible, and radiation to the chest wall. Early recurrences are treated with systemic chemotherapy. Local recurrence has a good prognosis in the absence of concomitant systemic recurrence.

Metastatic disease is treated with chemotherapy. Brain metastases, which are often multiple, are treated with radiation. Bony metastases are treated with radiation and surgical fixation if there is a high risk of fracture. For pain reduction, biphosphonates and ^{89}Sr are undergoing trials. Bone marrow transplantation is an experimental treatment for metastatic disease.

Complications of Breast Cancer Treatment

Complications of Surgery

The most common immediate complications of surgery are bleeding and infection, as with any operation, and flap necrosis secondary to inadequate blood supply. Disfigurement can result from poorly planned lumpectomy or mastectomy incisions as well as from excision of too great a proportion of the breast tissue (e.g., a large tumor in a small breast). Seromas and lymphoceles in the axilla or under mastectomy flaps are not uncommon and can usually be treated successfully with intermittent percutaneous needle aspiration. Postoperative bleeding may occur, but it is rarely sufficient to require transfusion or a return to the operating room. Infection is treated in the standard fashion, with antibiotics for cellulitis, wound opening if pus is suspected or present, and debridement of devitalized tissue. Large areas of granulation can be grafted after infection is resolved, but this procedure is rarely necessary.

Longer-term complications are related to the axillary dissection. Skeletonizing or otherwise compromising the axillary vein, which is the superior margin of the axillary dissection, can cause venous thrombosis and intractable **lymphedema** of the arm. Division of the long thoracic nerve denervates the serratus anterior muscle and causes a "winged scapula." Division of the thoracodorsal nerve denervates the latissimus dorsi muscle, but causes minimal functional deficit. Division of the medial pectoral nerve can cause significant denervation of the pectoralis major and minor muscles and result in arm and shoulder weakness and atrophy of the chest wall musculature. Intercostobrachial nerve damage or division often occurs during axillary dissection because the nerve exits the lateral chest wall and passes through the center of the axillary fat pad. The result is abnormality or loss of sensation to the inner upper arm. Although this problem has no functional significance, it is an annoyance to the patient. Restriction of shoulder motion after axillary dissection may require physical therapy, but full range of motion is generally recovered within a month.

In the long term, intractable arm edema may result from compromise to lymphatic return that is caused by axillary dissection. From the moment of surgery, the patient must never allow blood to be drawn, an intravenous line to be placed, or a tourniquet to be used on that arm. Prevention of this complication is crucial because edema may be massive and, once it becomes established, may be impossible to reverse. Over the course of time, permanent fibrotic changes occur.

Complications of Chemotherapy

Nausea, vomiting, leukopenia, thrombocytopenia, amenorrhea, weight gain, and alopecia are so common after chemotherapy that is seems more reasonable to call them secondary or undesirable effects rather than complications. The development of effective drugs to combat nausea has facilitated patient compliance. In the past, many patients discontinued treatment because of their inability to tolerate this almost universal effect.

Much less common adverse effects of chemotherapy include sepsis, hemorrhagic cystitis, thrombophlebitis in the veins that are used to infuse the drugs, mucositis, and cardiotoxicity from Adriamycin. The development of recombinant erythropoietin and **granulocyte colony-stimulating factor** made it possible to maintain hematocrit and neutrophil counts at acceptable levels, decreasing the likelihood of nadir sepsis and allowing more aggressive treatment.

Complications of Treatment with Tamoxifen

Common side effects of tamoxifen include vaginitis, hot flashes, fluid retention, weight gain, nausea, and thrombocytopenia. Less common side effects are increased incidence of vascular thrombosis, pulmonary embolism, and endometrial carcinoma.

Complications of Radiation Therapy

Radiation treatment initially causes the breast to become edematous and inflamed, with altered skin sensation. Over time, the chronic changes evolve to fibrosis, with skin thickening and hyperpigmentation.

Table 19-6. Five-Year Relative Survival Rates for Patients with Treated Breast Cancer by Stage

Stage	Survival Rate (%)
I	96%
II	82%
III	53%
IV	18%

Rates adjusted for deaths from other causes.

More serious, but extremely rare, complications of radiation treatment include pneumonitis and bone necrosis that result from the inclusion of other tissues in the radiation field. The radiation oncologist uses tangential fields to minimize the radiation dose to all but breast tissue.

Prognosis

The prognosis of breast cancer is affected by many factors. The most important predictor is whether the tumor is in situ or invasive. Although tumor size is directly related to lymph node involvement, tumor size and lymph node status are independent predictors of survival. In order, from the most predictive prognostic factor to the least, are tumor size, lymph node status, ER status, and other prognostic factors such as ploidy, S-phase, cathepsin D, her-2-neu oncogene expression and p-53 expression (Table 19-6). After successful treatment of breast cancer, the risk of a second primary tumor is approximately 0.5% to 1% per year for the next 15 years. The risk of recurrence or distant metastases, on the other hand, decreases over time.

Stage for stage, the 5-year survival rate is worse for African-American women than for white women. Some investigators believe that this difference is related to socioeconomic status, and not to race, possibly because women of lower socioeconomic status have less access to health care and tend to receive less aggressive treatment. However, African-American women may also tend to have histologically less favorable tumors.

Multiple-Choice Questions

1. A 64-year-old woman who underwent a left modified radical mastectomy 3 weeks ago has numbness in the upper inner left arm. What is the cause of this complication?
   A. Injury to the thoracodorsal nerve
   B. Injury to the long thoracic nerve
   C. Injury to the intercostal brachial nerve
   D. Thrombosis of the axillary vein
   E. Injury to the medial pectoral nerve

2. A 52-year-old woman has a history of spontaneous bloody nipple discharge every 2 to 3 days for the last

month. She had a mammogram that was read as normal. What is the most important step in her evaluation?
A. Breast ultrasound
B. Ductography
C. Localization of the region of discharge on physical examination
D. Cytology of the discharge
E. Additional mammographic views with the focus on the retroareolar region

3. In which of the following patients would you increase the frequency for mammography and clinical breast examination over the usual recommendations appropriate for the patient's age?
A. A 36-year-old woman with a recent biopsy showing atypical hyperplasia
B. A 60-year-old woman with a family history of breast cancer
C. A 34-year-old woman with a 10-year history of fibrocystic condition
D. A 29-year-old woman with a recent excision of a fibroadenoma
E. A 42-year-old woman with a history of early menarche

4. A 56-year-old woman is diagnosed with ductal cancer in situ after a stereotactic biopsy of a 2-cm cluster of suspicious microcalcification. What is the appropriate management for this patient?
A. Modified radical mastectomy
B. Wide excision only
C. Wide excision and radiation treatment
D. Radiation treatment only
E. Wide excision followed by chemotherapy administration

5. A 46-year-old woman has bloody nipple discharge occurring 5 times over the last 2 weeks. What is the most likely diagnosis?
A. Breast cancer
B. Duct ectasia
C. Fibrocystic changes
D. Intraductal papilloma
E. Cyst

6. Which of the following indicates the worst prognosis in a patient with breast cancer?
A. A 1.5-cm palpable axillary node
B. A 4-cm tumor
C. Cancer presenting as bloody nipple discharge
D. An involved supraclavicular node
E. An enlarged internal mammary node on computed tomography scan

7. Which of the following is true regarding the management of breast cysts?
A. Asymptomatic cysts may be observed without intervention.

B. All cysts must be excised because of the increased risk of the development of cancer.
C. Mammography is the best diagnostic study for cysts.
D. Symptomatic cysts should be treated with oral contraceptives.
E. All cyst fluid should be sent for cytology when aspirated.

8. A 24-year-old woman has a 1.5-cm, smooth, nontender mobile mass in the upper outer quadrant of her right breast. She has no family history of breast cancer and no significant risk factors. Ultrasonography confirms a 1.5-cm solid lesion with regular borders. She is eager to avoid surgery if possible. What is the appropriate next step in her management?
A. No treatment at this time; repeat clinical breast examination in 6 months
B. Mammography to rule out cancer
C. Fine-needle aspiration cytology to confirm the diagnosis
D. Excisional biopsy
E. Stereotactic-guided core biopsy

9. Which of the following would be considered major risk factors for the development of breast cancer (increased relative risk greater than 4 times)?
A. Menarche at age 10
B. Diagnosis of lobular cancer in situ at the time of excisional biopsy for a fibroadenoma
C. Mild hyperplasia diagnosed on a recent biopsy for a breast mass
D. A 10-year history of hormone replacement therapy
E. A history of ovarian cancer

10. A 26-year-old woman has a 3-month history of bilateral breast pain that occurs before menses. Her mother was diagnosed with breast cancer at 58 years of age. Breast examination shows bilateral breast tenderness with no masses present. What is the best plan for her management?
A. Baseline mammography
B. Reassurance that the pain rarely represents cancer; no treatment at this time if the patient can live with the discomfort
C. Danazol
D. Bilateral breast ultrasound
E. Oral contraceptives

11. A 46-year-old woman has a palpable, mobile, 1.5-cm breast cancer in the upper outer quadrant of the right breast. She also has a 1.3-cm, mobile, nontender axillary node on the right side. Her mother had postmenopausal breast cancer. The patient wants to preserve her breast if possible without compromise of cure. What is the best management option?
A. Lumpectomy, axillary dissection, and radiation therapy
B. Modified radical mastectomy

C. Modified radical mastectomy and immediate reconstruction

D. Wide excision of the breast mass and radiation

E. Lumpectomy and axillary dissection with radiation if the palpable lymph node is positive

12. A 42-year-old premenopausal woman is diagnosed with a 1.8-cm infiltrating ductal cancer. She elects modified radical mastectomy and immediate reconstruction. On axillary dissection, 3 of 18 nodes are positive for cancer. The tumor is estrogen receptor–positive. What is the best recommendation for adjuvant therapy?

A. Radiation of the chest wall and axilla

B. Combination chemotherapy

C. Hormonal therapy

D. Bilateral oophorectomy

E. Bone marrow transplantation

13. A 42-year-old woman is considering lumpectomy, axillary dissection, and radiation therapy for a 3-cm infiltrating ductal cancer in the upper outer quadrant of her left breast. Which of the following is a common complication of radiation therapy that she should be aware of as she considers breast preservation?

A. Lung cancer

B. Erythema and exfoliation of the breast skin

C. Hodgkin's lymphoma

D. Anorexia

E. Hair loss

14. A 63-year-old woman underwent modified radical mastectomy for a 3-cm infiltrating ductal cancer with one positive node. The tumor was estrogen receptor–positive. The patient's oncologist recommends tamoxifen. What is the most common side effect that she should be made aware of secondary to tamoxifen treatment?

A. Endometrial cancer

B. Hot flashes

C. Osteoporosis

D. Thrombocytopenia

E. Breast tenderness

15. Which of the following patients would likely have the worst prognosis?

A. A 46-year-old woman with a 2-cm infiltrating ductal cancer, with 1 of 22 nodes positive

B. A 46-year-old woman with a 2.5-cm infiltrating lobular cancer, with 1 of 22 nodes positive

C. A 52-year-old woman with a 5.5-cm infiltrating ductal cancer, with 0 of 20 nodes positive

D. A 51-year-old woman with a 3-cm inflammatory breast cancer, with 2 of 16 nodes positive

E. A 58-year-old woman with a 2-cm medullary cancer, with 1 of 19 nodes positive

16. A 48-year-old woman has a palpable, 2-cm, firm, mobile mass in the upper outer quadrant of her left breast. Mammography confirms the presence of a dominant mass. What is the next step to confirm the diagnosis?

A. Excisional biopsy

B. Incisional biopsy

C. Fine-needle aspiration cytology

D. Stereotactic biopsy

E. Frozen section in the operating room, with plans for definitive treatment if cancer is diagnosed

17. Which of the following patients should undergo a metastatic survey (bone scan and computed tomography scan of the chest and abdomen) before the initiation of treatment?

A. A patient with a 2-cm infiltrating ductal cancer, with two palpable axillary nodes

B. A patient with a 5.5-cm tumor, with a clinically negative axillary examination

C. A patient who has a 4-cm tumor and whose mother and maternal grandmother had breast cancer

D. A patient with a 3-cm lobular cancer, with no visualization of the tumor on mammography

E. All patients with the diagnosis of invasive breast cancer

18. Which of the following is true regarding hormonally induced changes in the breast?

A. With each menstrual cycle, the production of progesterone before ovulation stimulates ductal proliferation.

B. In pregnancy, high levels of estrogen and progesterone stimulate ductal proliferation and acinar development.

C. A sudden postpartum increase in estrogen and prolactin precipitates lactation.

D. Postmenopausally, the lack of hormonal stimulation results in the conversion of ductal tissue to fibrosis.

19. Which of the following is the strongest predictor of systemic recurrence of disease after breast cancer treatment?

A. Age < 40 years

B. S-phase

C. Tumor size

D. Estrogen receptor status

E. Her-2-neu oncogene status

20. Which of the following provides the most significant advantage for a patient who chooses modified radical mastectomy over lumpectomy with axillary dissection and radiation treatment?

A. Improved 5-year survival with modified radical mastectomy

B. Decreased chance of local recurrence

C. Avoidance of radiation treatment

D. Decreased likelihood of the need for combination chemotherapy

E. Decreased likelihood of the need for tamoxifen

Oral Examination Study Questions

CASE 1

A 43-year-old premenopausal woman has a 3-cm palpable mass in the upper outer quadrant of her left breast.

OBJECTIVE 1

The student elicits the following history.

A. The mass is nontender and has been present for 4 weeks.

B. The patient has no history of breast problems or biopsy.

C. She has no family history of breast cancer.

D. She experienced menarche at age 12, and her last menstrual period was 1 week ago.

E. She had three pregnancies and three live births, the first at age 21.

F. She has never used oral contraceptives.

OBJECTIVE 2

The student elicits the following physical examination findings.

A. The mass is irregular, firm, nontender, and mobile.

B. The patient also has a 1-cm, mobile, nontender lymph node in the left axilla.

OBJECTIVE 3

The student formulates a differential diagnosis.

A. Breast cancer

B. Breast cyst

C. Fibroadenoma

D. Fibrocystic changes

The student develops a plan for diagnostic workup.

A. Fine-needle aspiration cytology shows infiltrating ductal cancer.

B. Bilateral mammograms show a spiculated 3-cm mass in the upper outer quadrant of the left breast.

OBJECTIVE 4

The student provides the options for management.

A. Lumpectomy, axillary dissection, and radiation treatment

B. Modified radical mastectomy, with or without immediate or delayed reconstruction

The final pathology shows a 3.5-cm infiltrating ductal cancer with clear margins. The tumor is estrogen receptor–positive. There are 2 positive lymph nodes among 18 removed. The student recommends appropriate adjuvant therapy.

A. Chemotherapy

B. Consideration for tamoxifen

Minimum Level of Achievement for Passing

The student takes an appropriate history and elicits the physical examination findings. The student presents the two options for management of breast cancer.

Honors Level of Achievement

The student identifies both fine-needle aspiration cytology and mammography as critical components of the diagnostic workup. The student also identifies chemotherapy as appropriate adjuvant therapy and suggests the consideration of tamoxifen.

CASE 2

A 54-year-old woman has a 1.5-cm cluster of pleomorphic microcalcifications in the upper inner quadrant of her left breast on mammography.

OBJECTIVE 1

The student elicits the results of breast examination, which are entirely normal. The student also provides a differential diagnosis.

A. Fibrocystic changes

B. Ductal cancer in situ

C. Invasive cancer

OBJECTIVE 2

The student suggests a plan for further evaluation.

A. Needle-directed breast biopsy

B. Stereotactically guided core biopsy

If a needle-directed breast biopsy is done, the diagnosis is ductal cancer in situ with clear surgical margins. If a stereotactically guided biopsy is done, the diagnosis is ductal cancer in situ.

OBJECTIVE 3

The student explains the definitive treatment for this condition. If needle-directed biopsy was done, the definitive treatment includes 6 weeks of radiation therapy to decrease local recurrence. If stereotactically guided core biopsy was done, the definitive treatment includes wide excision followed by 6 weeks of radiation therapy. The student explains why axillary dissection is unnecessary in this case. Ductal cancer in situ involves cancer cells that have not invaded the basement membrane; therefore, lymphatic and hematogenous spread is not possible.

Minimum Level of Achievement for Passing

The student develops a differential diagnosis that includes ductal cancer in situ. The student suggests one of the two appropriate diagnostic studies.

A. Needle-directed breast biopsy

B. Stereotactically guided core biopsy

Honors Level of Achievement

The student includes fibrocystic changes in the differential diagnosis. The student also describes the definitive therapy and explains why axillary dissection is unnecessary.

CASE 3

A 40-year-old premenopausal woman has a 10-day history of intermittent bloody nipple discharge from the left breast.

OBJECTIVE 1

The student elicits the patient's history.

A. The discharge is spontaneous and is noted on the patient's clothing at the end of the day.

B. She has no history of a similar discharge and no previous breast problems.

C. The family history is negative for breast cancer.

D. The patient experienced menarche at age 13, and her last menstrual period was 2 weeks ago.

E. The patient has had no pregnancies and has used oral contraceptives for the last 5 years.

The student elicits the findings of breast examination.

A. No skin changes and no palpable masses are found in either breast.

B. Findings of axillary and supraclavicular examination are negative.

The student elicits the following physical examination finding:

The discharge is localized to be coming from the 2 o'clock area of the breast.

OBJECTIVE 2

The student recommends appropriate further evaluation. Bilateral mammography shows no abnormality in either breast. The student suggests a differential diagnosis.

A. Intraductal papilloma (most common)

B. Duct ectasia

C. Fibrocystic changes

D. Breast cyst

OBJECTIVE 3

The student suggests appropriate treatment. The patient undergoes duct excision, which shows a 5-mm benign intraductal papilloma. The student suggests a plan for follow-up that includes resumption of normal screening appropriate for a 40-year-old patient. This plan includes clinical breast examination and mammography every year.

Minimum Level of Achievement for Passing

The student elicits an appropriate history and physical examination. The student identifies the need to localize the area of discharge on breast examination. The student identifies intraductal papilloma as the most likely diagnosis.

Honors Level of Achievement

The student describes at least one possible diagnosis other than intraductal papilloma. The student identifies duct excision as the appropriate surgical management. The student describes the appropriate ongoing follow-up after treatment.

SUGGESTED READINGS

Balch CM, Singletary SE, Bland KI. Clinical decision-making in early breast cancer. *Ann Surg* 1993;217:207–225.

Bland KI, Copeland EM III, eds. *The Breast: Comprehensive Management of Benign and Malignant Diseases*, 4th ed. Philadelphia, Pa: WB Saunders, 1991.

Dupont WD, Page DL. Risk factors for breast cancer in women with proliferative breast disease. *N Engl J Med* 1985;312:146–157.

Goldhirsch A, Wood WC, Senn H, Glick JH, Gelber RD. Meeting highlights: international consensus panel on the treatment of primary breast cancer. *J Natl Cancer Inst* 1995;87:1441–1445.

Mettlin C, Smart CR. Breast cancer detection guidelines for women ages 40–49 years: rationale for the American Cancer Society reaffirmation of recommendations. *Ca Cancer J Clin* 1994;44:248–255.

20

Surgical Endocrinology

Thyroid Gland

Nicholas P. W. Coe, M.D.
Glenn H. Lytle, M.D.
Anne T. Mancino, M.D.

Parathyroid Glands

Chris Jamieson, M.D.
Glenn H. Lytle, M.D.

Adrenal Glands

Michael K. McLeod, M.D.
Anne T. Mancino, M.D.

Multiple Endocrine Neoplasia Syndromes

Jeffrey A. Norton, M.D.

OBJECTIVES

Thyroid Gland

1. Discuss the evaluation and differential diagnosis of a patient with a thyroid nodule.
2. List the different types of carcinoma of the thyroid gland and their cell type of origin; discuss the appropriate therapeutic strategy for each.
3. Understand the major risk factors for carcinoma of the thyroid gland and the prognostic variables that dictate therapy.
4. Describe the symptoms of a patient with hyperthyroidism; discuss the differential diagnosis and treatment options.

Parathyroid Glands

1. Understand the role of the parathyroid glands in the physiology of calcium homeostasis.
2. List the causes, symptoms, and signs of hypercalcemia.
3. Know the difference between primary, secondary, and tertiary hyperparathyroidism.

4. Discuss the evaluation and differential diagnosis of a patient with hypercalcemia.
5. Understand the management of acute and severe hypercalcemia.
6. Describe the indications for surgery for hyperparathyroidism.
7. Describe the complications of parathyroid surgery.

Adrenal Glands

1. Describe the clinical features of Cushing's syndrome and discuss how lesions in the pituitary, adrenal cortex, and extraadrenal sites are distinguished diagnostically.
2. Discuss the medical and surgical management of Cushing's syndrome in patients with an adrenal adenoma, with a pituitary adenoma causing adrenal hyperplasia, and with an adrenocorticotropic hormone (ACTH)-producing neoplasm.
3. Describe the pathology, clinical features, laboratory findings, workup, and management of a patient with primary aldosteronism.
4. Discuss pheochromocytoma, including its associated signs and symptoms, appropriate diagnostic workup, and treatment.
5. Discuss adrenal cortical carcinoma, including its presentation, signs and symptoms, diagnostic workup, and management.
6. Discuss the management and evaluation of an incidentally discovered adrenal mass.
7. Discuss the causes of adrenal insufficiency in the surgical setting as well as the associated clinical and laboratory findings.

Multiple Endocrine Neoplasia Syndromes

1. Describe the multiple endocrine neoplasia syndromes and their surgical treatment.

Thyroid Gland

Anatomy

The thyroid gland forms two lobes in the neck, anterior to the larynx. The lobes are connected by the thyroid isthmus at approximately the second tracheal ring (Figure 20-1). It is the first endocrine gland to appear during embryonic development, at approximately 24 days after conception. It begins as a thickening on the floor of the pharynx at the site of the foramen cecum on the adult tongue. This endodermal thickening grows caudally, as the thyroglossal duct, into the neck, passing ventral to the embryonal hyoid bone and thyroid cartilage. The duct disappears by the fiftieth day of gestation, but may persist anywhere along its migratory pathway as the pyramidal lobe of the thyroid (in 50% of adults) or as a thyroglossal duct cyst. In addition, the ultimobranchial body that stems from the fourth pharyngeal pouch epithelium contributes to the thyroid. This body is the origin of the C cells.

The adult thyroid gland weighs 15 to 25 g and is supplied by the superior (the first branch of the external carotid artery) and inferior (a branch of the thyrocervical trunk that arises from the subclavian artery) thyroid arteries (Figure 20-2). Venous drainage occurs through the superior, middle, and inferior thyroid veins. The thyroid gland lies anterior to the trachea. It is covered anteriorly by the skin and platysma muscle and anterolaterally by the sternocleidomastoid, sternohyoid, and sternothyroid muscles. The parathyroid glands (discussed later) are posterior to the thyroid gland.

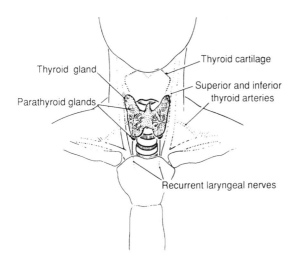

Figure 20-1 The thyroid gland.

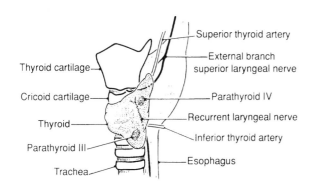

Figure 20-2 The adult thyroid gland.

Physiology

The thyroid gland has two distinct groups of hormone-producing cells. **Follicular cells** produce, store, and release **thyroxine (T_4)** and **triiodothyronine (T_3)**, major regulators of the basal metabolic rate. **Parafollicular cells,** or C cells, secrete calcitonin, a hormone that has a minor role in maintaining calcium homeostasis.

Follicular cells efficiently capture iodide from the circulation, which appears to be the rate-limiting step in thyroid hormone synthesis. Thyroid cells concentrate **iodine** to levels thirty times that found in normal tissues. The iodide (I^-) is then oxidized to I^+ or to iodine (I^0). This reaction is catalyzed by the membrane-bound enzyme thyroid peroxidase (TPO). This reaction, called organification, occurs on the apical membranes of the follicular cells, which form the boundary of an extracellular storage space called the **follicle.** Thyroglobulin is a large [molecular weight (MW) = 660 kDa] glycoprotein that is synthesized by the follicular cells and then secreted into the follicle. The tyrosine residues of thyroglobulin are iodinated by the I^0 or I^+ species, forming monoiodotyrosine (MIT) and diiodotyrosine (DIT), which then couple to form the iodothyronines T_3 (MIT + DIT) and T_4 (DIT + DIT). This iodinated thyroglobulin is the storage form of the thyroid hormones that are kept in the follicle (Figure 20-3). When **thyroid-stimulating hormone** (TSH, or thyrotropin) stimulates the thyroid gland to release active hormone, the iodinated thyroglobulin from the follicle is taken into the follicular cell by endocytosis. There, it is hydrolyzed to T_3 and T_4, which are then released into the circulation. The thyroglobulin itself is not released except under pathologic conditions. T_3 and T_4 are the active forms of circulating hormone. Most (80%) of the circulating hormone is T_4, but T_3, which is generated by the peripheral conversion of T_4 to T_3, is the most active form of thyroid hormone. This reaction can also produce reverse T_3 (rT_3), an inactive form of the hormone.

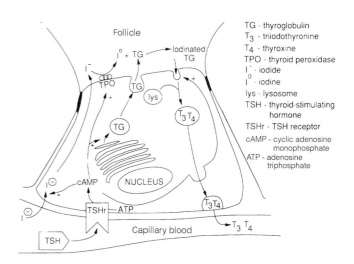

Figure 20-3 Iodinated thyroglobulin stored as thyroid hormones in the follicle.

Follicular cell function is controlled by the anterior pituitary–derived TSH, which stimulates the thyroid to release T_3 and T_4. TSH also stimulates the cell to increase the means of producing thyroid hormones, which includes increasing both thyroglobulin synthesis and iodide transport efficiency. TSH production, in turn, is controlled by two mechanisms. Thyrotropin-releasing hormone (TRH), which is secreted by the hypothalamus into the hypothalamic–pituitary portal venous system, increases TSH release. If excessive concentrations of T_3 and T_4 are present, however, a negative feedback system shuts off the secretion of TSH and probably TRH (Figure 20-4).

The other hormone-producing cells in the thyroid, the parafollicular cells, or C cells, are derived from the neural crest cells of the ultimobranchial body. When these cells are stimulated by high serum calcium levels, they secrete the hormone calcitonin, which inhibits osteoclast activity, thus decreasing the calcium level. Calcitonin secretion, which is also affected by serum estrogen and vitamin D levels, does not normally play a major role in regulating serum calcium levels. Its function probably is to protect the skeleton from excessive scavenging during times of high calcium demand (e.g., growth, pregnancy, lactation). The absence of calcitonin production (e.g., after total thyroidectomy) appears to have no demonstrable negative physiologic effect.

Pathophysiology

Hyperthyroidism

Hyperthyroidism is a syndrome that is caused by excessive secretion of thyroid hormone. The most common cause is **Graves' disease,** or diffuse toxic **goiter.** Less commonly, hyperthyroidism is caused by one **(toxic adenoma)** or more **(toxic multinodular goiter)** hyperfunctioning nodules. Less common causes include thyrotoxicosis factitia, a condition that is caused by the ingestion of excessive amounts of exogenous thyroid hormone, and struma (synonymous with goiter) ovarii, a condition in which the hyperactive thyroid tissue is found in an ovarian teratoma or dermoid.

The lifetime risk of hyperthyroidism is approximately 5% for women and 1% for men. Graves' disease occurs predominantly in young women (8:1 ratio). The yearly rate of occurrence for women 20 to 30 years of age is 59:100,000. For women older than 60 years of age, it is 38:100,000. The incidence of toxic adenoma is lower and less well defined. However, between 10% and 30% of patients with hyperthyroidism may have toxic adenomas, and approximately 75% of these have a single toxic adenoma.

Graves' Disease
Clinical Presentation and Evaluation

Graves' disease (Robert J. Graves, Irish physician, 1797–1853) is a syndrome of diffuse goiter with hyperthyroidism (the most common component), exophthalmos, tachycardia, and tremor. Heat intolerance and weight loss are also common.

The signs and symptoms (Table 20-1) are those of a hypermetabolic state resulting from excessive production of thyroid hormone. The ophthalmologic effects of Graves' disease cover a continuum from a stare with lid lag, to proptosis, to deformity of the periorbital tissues with optic nerve involvement and complete loss of vision.

Serum TSH levels in thyrotoxicosis can determine whether the hyperthyroidism is pituitary-dependent or independent. In thyroid causes of hyperthyroidism, serum TSH levels are decreased, whereas in pituitary causes, they are increased. Total T_3 and T_4 levels are measured, along with the amount of thyroxine-binding globulin (TBG), because elevated T_4 levels may reflect increased serum TBG (e.g., in pregnancy). Alternatively, free T_3 and T_4 estimations are not affected by altered TBG levels. A low level of TSH in the presence of high thyroid hormone levels establishes thyroid-dependent hyperthyroidism, the most common situation.

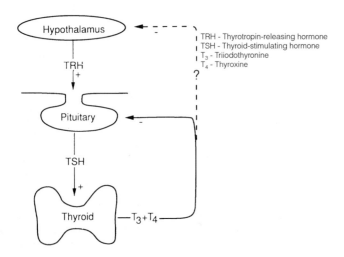

Figure 20-4 The hypothalamus-pituitary-thyroid axis.

TRH - Thyrotropin-releasing hormone
TSH - Thyroid-stimulating hormone
T_3 - Triiodothyronine
T_4 - Thyroxine

Table 20-1. Symptoms and Signs of Hyperthyroidism

Central Nervous System	Cardiovascular and Respiratory Systems	Other Systems
Nervousness	Tachycardia	Lid lag
Restlessness	Palpitations	Proptosis or exophthalmos
Emotional lability	Arrhythmias	Ophthalmopathy
Fast speech	Dyspnea	Increased sweating
Fine tremor		Fatigue
		Weakness
		Hair loss
		Leg swelling
		Pretibial myxedema

The hyperthyroidism associated with Graves' disease is caused by a circulating immunoglobulin G (IgG) immunoglobulin [thyroid-stimulating antibody (TSAb)] that is directed against the TSH receptors on the follicular cells of the thyroid. This antibody stimulates the thyroid to generate and secrete thyroid hormone, but the sensitivity to the negative feedback system that controls normal thyroid function is lost. Thus, TSAb causes excessive production of T_3 and T_4 and progressive hyperthyroidism. The pathogenesis of the exophthalmos and pretibial myxedema of Graves' disease is not well understood.

Treatment

The three possible treatments for Graves' hyperthyroidism are: (1) medical blockade of the hormone and its effects, (2) radioiodine ablation of active thyroid tissue, and (3) surgical resection. Iodide, administered as potassium iodide or as Lugol's solution (5% iodine plus potassium iodide), temporarily inhibits the release of thyroid hormone from the gland. The reason for this counterintuitive effect (the Wolff-Chaikoff effect) is not fully understood. As plasma iodide levels rise, increasing amounts are organified until a critical point is reached. After the critical point, the binding of iodide to tyrosine residues decreases dramatically. The synthesis of an unknown inhibitory iodine-containing compound within the thyroid during exposure to excess iodine has been postulated. The effect is short-lived (1–2 weeks).

Propranolol and other β-blockers ameliorate some of the peripheral effects of excess thyroid hormone. These drugs decrease the peripheral conversion of T_4 to T_3 rather than block β activity. Both iodide and propranolol may have a role in the short-term management or preoperative preparation of patients with hyperthyroidism, but do not provide definitive therapy.

Thionamides [e.g., propylthiouracil (PTU), methimazole (Tapazole)] interfere with the synthesis of thyroid hormones in the gland by inhibiting iodide organification and iodotyrosine coupling. They also reduce the rate of peripheral conversion of T_4 to T_3. Approximately one-third of patients who tolerate thionamide therapy remain in remission after 6 to 12 months of treatment with PTU; however, a significant percentage (5%–10%) have adverse reactions to the drug (Table 20-2).

The other two-thirds of patients need more definitive treatment with either surgery or radioiodine. The isotope of choice for the radioablation of hyperactive thyroid tissue is ^{131}I. A dose of 80 μCi/g estimated thyroid tissue is effective for most patients and has a low incidence of inducing early hypothyroidism. A second and even a third dose may be necessary if the patient has hyperthyroidism after 6 months (see Table 20-2). Over a period of 5 to 10 years, however, hypothyroidism occurs in 50% to 70% of these patients. Radioiodine ablation is safe and effective, and long-term follow-up of these patients suggests that radiation exposure does not appear to cause secondary thyroid cancer. This result probably occurs because the **radioactive iodine** is taken up so avidly by thyroid cells that the cellular radiation

Table 20-2. Complications of Treatment in Graves' Hyperthyroidism

Treatment	Complication	Frequency (%)
Subtotal thyroidectomy	Hypothyroidism	20
	Recurrent hyperthyroidism	< 5
Total or subtotal thyroidectomy	Superior laryngeal nerve injury	< 1
	Recurrent laryngeal nerve injury	< 1
	Hypoparathyroidism	< 2
Radioiodine ablation	Hypothyroidism	
	Early	20
	Late	50
	Delayed control requiring:	
	Second radioiodine treatment	15–20
	Third radioiodine treatment	5
Thionamides	Recurrent/persistent hyperthyroidism	60–70
	Intolerance of medication including:	5–10
	Cholestasis	
	Arthralgia	
	Headache	
	Neuritis	
	Dependent edema	
	Reversible granulocytopenia	0.02

dose completely destroys the cells rather than simply altering their DNA. Subsequent neck exploration in these patients shows minimal, if any, residual thyroid tissue. Therapy with radioactive iodine does not appear to cause injury to the parathyroids, agranulocytosis, or any other radiation-induced phenomena. External beam radiotherapy plays no role in the treatment of hyperthyroidism.

Subtotal (Figure 20-5) or total **thyroidectomy** (see Figure 20-8) can also be used to treat Graves' hyperthyroidism. These procedures provide rapid control of the disease and eliminate exposure to radioactivity. Some studies show total thyroidectomy to be superior to subtotal thyroidectomy because it avoids the possibility of recurrent thyrotoxicosis. Although earlier reports suggested a higher incidence of injury to the nerves or parathyroids with total thyroidectomy, recent data document the safety of the procedure in experienced hands. Surgery may be chosen as the definitive therapy for patients who are pregnant or wish to become pregnant within a year of therapy, cannot comply with antithyroid medications or follow-up because of mental or emotional incapacity, are allergic to iodine, or refuse antithyroid drugs or radioiodine ablation. However, most clinicians favor radioiodine ablation over surgery.

None of the antithyroid therapies significantly affect the exophthalmos or pretibial myxedema that is associated with Graves' disease. These manifestations may respond to local or systemic cortisol treatment, and

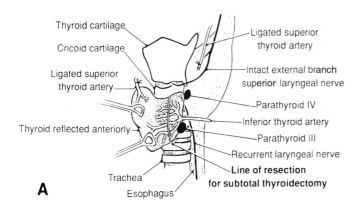

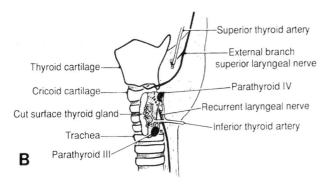

Figure 20-5 A, Anteromedial reflection of the thyroid gland. **B,** Anatomy after bilateral subtotal thyroid lobectomy for Graves' disease.

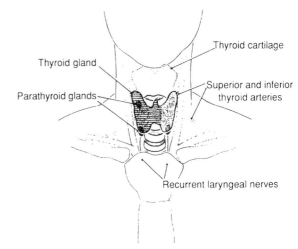

Figure 20-6 Thyroid lobectomy and isthmectomy.

external beam radiation therapy is occasionally used for severe ophthalmopathy. However, stabilization and regression of these signs and symptoms are reported most consistently after total thyroidectomy. This effect is thought to occur by lessening the generalized autoimmune response by removing all thyroid tissue.

Toxic Adenoma

Toxic adenoma is a solitary tumor of the thyroid gland that produces excessive amounts of thyroid hormone and causes clinically overt hyperthyroidism. Malignancy in a toxic nodule is rare. The hyperthyroidism is similar to that seen in Graves' disease. However, patients do not have associated ophthalmopathy or pretibial myxedema because toxic adenoma is not an autoimmune phenomenon such as Graves' disease.

Clinical Presentation and Evaluation

Serum thyroid hormone levels show high T_3 and T_4 and suppressed TSH, consistent with an autonomous thyroid source for the excessive thyroid hormone production. The differentiation between hyperthyroidism caused by Graves' disease and that caused by toxic adenoma depends on the characteristics of the thyroid on physical examination and scan. In patients with Graves' disease, the thyroid is diffusely enlarged. In patients with toxic adenoma, it is normal or small, with a palpable nodule that is "hot," or functional, on thyroid scan.

Treatment

The initial treatment is similar to that for Graves' disease, but definitive treatment depends more on surgery because resolution after treatment with PTU or methimazole is rare. After preoperative preparation, usually with propranolol or one of the thionamides, the lobe with the "hot" nodule is excised by thyroid lobectomy and isthmectomy (Figure 20-6). Surgery is also considered optimal therapy for a toxic multinodular goiter **(Plummer's disease).** Total or subtotal thyroidectomy is indicated, especially if the goiter is large and associated with symptoms such as compression. In general, radioactive iodine ablation is not considered appropriate therapy for toxic adenoma or Plummer's disease. Although the overactive thyroid elements can be ablated, recurrence is more common than with Graves' disease because of the intrinsic autonomy of the thyroid tissue.

Thyroid Carcinoma

The annual incidence of **thyroid carcinoma** is 36 to 60 cases per one million people. The death rate is approximately nine people per million. It is twice as common in women as in men, occurring primarily in those 25 to 65 years of age. Thyroid cancers can arise from any of the cells that make up the gland. Follicular cells give rise to well-differentiated thyroid cancers (papillary and follicular varieties). Parafollicular cells give rise to medullary carcinoma, and lymphoid cells give rise to lymphoma. Hürthle cell or oxyphil cell tumors are a variant of follicular neoplasms and arise from follicular cells. When analyzed by electron microscopy and immunohistochemistry, anaplastic tumors appear to arise from follicular cells, although they have dedifferentiated to the point that they are no longer recognizable as such by light microscopy.

General Principles of Treatment

Surgery is the therapy of choice for localized thyroid cancer, unless the tumor is an anaplastic carcinoma or a

Table 20-3. Common Problems at Presentation of Thyroid Malignancy and Their Management

Diagnosis	Incidence (%)	Age (yr)	Size	Extrathyroidal Invasion	Lymph Nodes	Surgical Therapy[a,b]
Well-differentiated Papillary	70–80	< 45	< 2 cm	None	±	Thyroid lobectomy and isthmusectomy or total thyroidectomy; removes only abnormal nodes
		> 45	> 1 cm	Often	±	Total thyroidectomy
Follicular	10–20	Any	Any	–	–	Total thyroidectomy
		Any	Any	+	–	Total thyroidectomy
Medullary	7%	Any	Any	±	±	Total thyroidectomy and median lymph node dissection
Anaplastic	3%	Any	Any	±	±	Nonsurgical therapy

[a]Thyroid replacement (thyroid-stimulating hormone) is recommended for patients with well-differentiated thyroid cancer after surgery.
[b]Radioactive iodine ([131]) is recommended for all patients with well-differentiated thyroid cancer and extrathyroidal disease that demonstrate uptake on a postsurgical [131] scan.

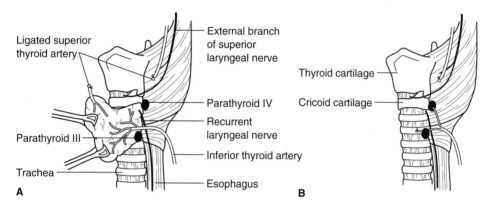

Figure 20-7 A Anteromedial reflection of the thyroid gland. **B,** Anatomy after total thyroidectomy.

lymphoma (see below). The type of surgical resection used for more favorable forms of thyroid cancer, papillary or follicular lesions, is dictated by the extent of disease and the aggressiveness of the tumor (Table 20-3; see Figures 20-6 and 20-7). The prognosis for papillary and follicular tumors is generally good, and the disease seldom shortens life expectancy. The survival benefit demonstrated by some studies and the ease of long-term follow-up when no thyroid tissue remains in the neck justify the risk of complications (e.g., recurrent laryngeal nerve injury, hypoparathyroidism) posed by total thyroidectomy. These risks are minimal if the surgeon is experienced.

Papillary Carcinoma

Papillary carcinoma is the most common thyroid malignancy in the United States, occurring in approximately 70% to 80% of cases.

Clinical Presentation and Evaluation

Tumors with a mix of papillary and follicular features are classified with the papillary cancers because they have similar biologic behavior. Papillary carcinomas are characterized by concentric layers of calcium (psammoma bodies) found in the stalk formations that give this cancer its name. Because papillary cancers grow slowly, most patients with these tumors have an excellent prognosis. Poor prognosis is associated with male sex, age older than 50 years, a primary tumor larger than 4 cm, less well differentiated cells, and locally invasive or distant metastatic disease. Metastases are primarily to regional lymph nodes, although this finding is not associated with a significantly worse prognosis, particularly in young women.

Treatment

Lesions in patients with a good prognosis are treated by thyroid lobectomy and isthmectomy (see Figure 20-6) or total thyroidectomy (see Figure 20-7A, B). All patients with lesions that show evidence of a poor prognosis should undergo total thyroidectomy.

The extent of surgery, either lobectomy or total thyroidectomy, has been hotly debated in the endocrine literature. Several risk stratification systems assess *age, metastatic* disease, *extent* of disease, and tumor *size* (AMES; Lahey Clinic) or *age*, histologic *grade*, *extent* of disease, and tumor *size* (AGES; Mayo Clinic) as prognostic factors. Other classifications of risk assess similar factors. Previously, patients who had lesions smaller than 3 cm were considered to have a good prognosis. Current data suggest, however, that optimal therapy should include total thyroidectomy and postoperative radioiodine ablation of residual or metastatic disease for any lesion larger than 1 cm. On the basis of these data, virtually all patients should undergo total thyroidectomy; stratification into risk groups is necessary only for prognostic calculations, not to dictate the choice of operation. Removal of obviously involved lymph nodes is generally advocated, but random sampling plays little role in planning therapy and has no place in the treatment of thyroid cancer. Although all of these patients will receive thyroid hormone replacement, because thyroid cancer cells are to some degree TSH-dependent, TSH should be suppressed to minimal levels by adjusting the hormone replacement dosage to avoid the potential trophic effect of this hormone on cancer cells.

Distant metastases are usually to the lungs and bones. Excision of all thyroid tissue in the neck facilitates scanning for metastases and treatment of those lesions with radioiodine if they are identified. Scanning and radioactive iodine therapy are not possible if thyroid tissue remains in the neck because the isotope is preferentially taken up by this tissue. Although thyroid cancers are often thought of as "cold," this designation is in reference to normal thyroid tissue. Well-differentiated thyroid cancer metastases often take up radioiodine and can be imaged in areas, such as lung, that do not. Pulmonary metastases more commonly take up iodine and may be cured with aggressive treatment with radioiodine, but bony metastases may need additional treatment with external beam radiation therapy. Although small trials of doxorubicin and cisplatin have been undertaken, there is no well-documented, effective chemotherapy for well-differentiated thyroid cancer.

Follicular Carcinoma

Follicular carcinoma occurs less commonly than papillary carcinoma, accounting for 10% to 20% of cases, except in iodine-deficient areas of the world.

Clinical Presentation and Evaluation

Follicular carcinomas have a monotonous, relatively uniform appearance of microfollicles, without the more complex papillations seen in papillary carcinoma. They closely resemble follicular adenomas on cytologic and frozen-section examination. On permanent section, they are distinguished from adenomas by the presence of capsular and vascular invasion. Follicular cancers also grow slowly, and the prognosis is good for patients with small, minimally invasive tumors. Larger or more invasive tumors have a poorer prognosis. Poor prognostic indicators include age greater than 45 years, local invasion to contiguous neck structures, and distant metastases.

Treatment

Papillary and follicular carcinomas are considered well-differentiated cancers. Treatment for both is similar

(including operative options). Metastases are usually hematogenously disseminated to lung and bone. These lesions may concentrate iodine and be amenable to radioiodine therapy after the thyroid gland is removed.

Medullary Carcinoma

Medullary thyroid carcinoma (MTC) constitutes approximately 7% of all thyroid cancers. Of patients with this cell type, 20% have a genetically transmitted, autosomal dominant inheritance pattern associated with either familial medullary carcinoma or multiple endocrine neoplasia (MEN) type 2A or 2B (discussed later).

Clinical Presentation and Evaluation

In patients with familial medullary cancer or MEN-2, the tumor is always present in both thyroid lobes. The sporadic variant of MTC usually occurs unilaterally. Patients with MTC have a worse prognosis than patients with well-differentiated papillary or follicular carcinoma; only 50% of patients survive 10 years. Medullary cancer is demonstrated by plasma screening that shows elevated calcitonin levels or by screening with a calcium and pentagastrin infusion test that shows elevated calcitonin.

Treatment

Medullary cancer without obvious lymph node metastases requires total thyroidectomy and central lymph node dissection [removal of the cervical lymph nodes medial to both recurrent laryngeal nerves and carotid arteries (Figure 20-8)]. Its tendency to have early lymph channel and bloodborne metastasis and its worse overall prognosis warrant an aggressive approach. Modified radical lymph node dissection is performed if there is lymph node involvement.

Anaplastic Carcinoma

Anaplastic carcinoma of the thyroid gland is an extremely aggressive neoplasm. It arises from the follicular cells, but is nearly totally dedifferentiated. Surgical resection does not appear to improve the outcome because it provides only palliative airway relief. The prognosis is dismal. Chemotherapy and external beam

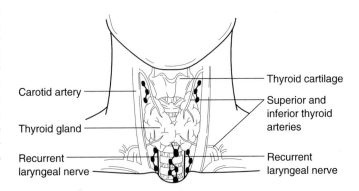

Figure 20-8 Removal of the cervical lymph nodes medial to both carotid arteries to treat medullary cancer, which requires a total thyroidectomy and central lymph node dissection.

radiation therapy are equally ineffective. Patients are considered to have Stage IV disease at presentation, and few survive longer than 2 years.

Lymphoma

Lymphoma can present as a thyroid mass lesion and is treated similarly to lymphomas that present in other sites. To distinguish a lymphoma from florid **Hashimoto's thyroiditis,** a core-needle or open biopsy may be necessary.

Thyroid Nodule

Palpable thyroid nodules occur in 4% of the population of the United States: half are solitary and half are multinodular. The frequency of undetected nodules is unknown, but autopsy studies suggest that the true incidence is much higher. At autopsy, 50% of thyroid glands contain one or more nodules, and 12% have a solitary nodule. Thyroid nodules are a common presentation of a potentially curable cancer.

Clinical Presentation and Evaluation

In evaluating a patient with a thyroid nodule, a thorough history and physical examination should be performed. Although thyroid cancer is more common in women, a solitary lesion in a man is significantly more likely to be malignant than a comparable nodule in a woman. Although the initial evaluation is the same, a heightened index of suspicion should be maintained in a man with a thyroid nodule. Certain factors, such as the duration of the presence of a nodule, and local symptoms, such as pain, pressure, or hoarseness, may suggest local invasiveness, and should be assessed. The patient should be asked about symptoms of toxicity because toxic adenomas can present as a solitary palpable thyroid nodule. A family history of MEN syndrome should be investigated.

A history of childhood radiation is significant because radiation exposure increases the risk of thyroid cancer, which is often multicentric. Beginning at a dose of as low as 200 rad, the risk rises as the dose increases to 2000 rad. A dose of radiation greater than 2000 rad usually causes actual destruction of the thyroid tissue. Patients may have radiation exposure as the result of treatment of an enlarged thymus in infancy or treatment for ringworm, acne, tubercular lymphadenopathy (therapies popular between 1930 and 1955), capillary hemangioma, or keloid scars (still used occasionally today). Patients who lived in the Ukraine or the Gomel region of Belorussia at the time of the Chernobyl incident (1986) are also at significant risk.

Although the primary concern in patients with a thyroid nodule is to confirm or exclude carcinoma, many patients have symptoms from benign disease. Multinodular goiters, especially those that extend retrosternally, and occasionally thyroids associated with Hashimoto's thyroiditis, may grow to great size and cause symptoms of compression with a feeling of choking and difficulty breathing or swallowing. These patients may present for thyroidectomy to relieve their symptoms.

The physical examination should include careful palpation of the remainder of the thyroid gland and regional lymph nodes. Symptoms of compression may be confirmed by a Pemberton's test, especially in patients whose goiter is retrosternal. Raising the arms above the head, as while brushing the hair, may cause venous compression at the thoracic inlet, with engorgement of the head and neck and a feeling of strangulation. Indirect laryngoscopy is indicated when there is hoarseness or when the signs and symptoms suggest malignancy. The simplest baseline laboratory study is a TSH test. A low level suggests thyrotoxicosis, and a high level suggests underactivity (e.g., associated with Hashimoto's thyroiditis). Thyroid function is measured whenever the TSH is abnormal. Serum calcium levels are measured in patients who have a history of radiation exposure (which may also cause parathyroid adenoma) or a family history of MEN syndrome. Patients who are related to someone who has MEN-2A syndrome should also have urinary catecholamines and catecholamine metabolites screened for functional **pheochromocytoma.** Medullary carcinoma is the only thyroid cancer that reliably expresses a tumor marker that is measurable in the serum (calcitonin). Serum thyroglobulin levels may be elevated in follicular or papillary carcinomas, but not reliably so. Thyroglobulin levels may also be elevated in benign diseases.

Fine-needle aspiration cytology (FNA) is extremely accurate and is the single most important study in evaluating a thyroid mass. Only 3% of patients with a benign diagnosis on FNA have thyroid cancer, and 85% of nodules identified as malignant on FNA are cancers at resection. FNA has decreased unnecessary operative procedures in patients with benign nodules and increased the probability that surgery will be performed only on patients with malignant nodules. The major difficulty remains in patients whose FNA diagnosis is indeterminate, usually those with follicular neoplasms. Follicular adenomas are often difficult to distinguish from follicular carcinomas because the distinction rests on architectural characteristics, such as capsular and vascular invasion, which are not detectable by cytology. In these cases, surgical resection is necessary to obtain a diagnosis.

Ultrasound examination of the neck may be used to supplement physical examination to determine whether a nodule is cystic or solid, whether additional nodules or nodes exist, and the exact size of the nodule (Figure 20-9). Multiple nodules, usually benign, are difficult to evaluate with percutaneous FNA and may require surgical resection for diagnosis. If a solitary thyroid nodule is cystic, it is aspirated with a fine needle. If the fluid obtained is cytologically benign and the mass disappears, the nodule is considered resolved, and no further evaluation or treatment is necessary. Recurrent cystic nodules are reaspirated and reevaluated cytologically as necessary. Most cystic masses resolve after a single needle aspiration. The presence of a residual mass after complete aspiration of a thyroid cyst may warrant surgical resection, particularly if the cytologic findings are suspicious. A thyroid nodule that is solid on ultrasound also requires aspiration or biopsy for diagnosis.

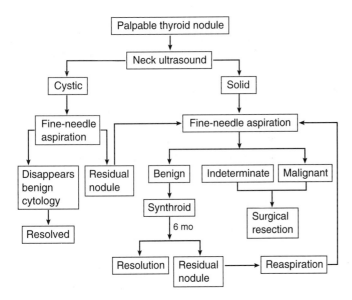

Figure 20-9 Ultrasound examination of the neck can determine whether a nodule is cystic or solid, whether additional nodules or nodes exist, and the exact size of the nodule. Follicular neoplasms are commonly intermediate on aspiration.

Treatment

Patients with solid nodules that are diagnosed as benign on FNA should be followed for a period of 3 to 6 months and treated with oral thyroid hormone to suppress TSH stimulation of tumor growth. The decrease in TSH should be carefully monitored to ensure the adequacy of suppression. If the nodule remains the same size, it is reaspirated. If it shrinks, suppression therapy is continued. If it enlarges on suppressive therapy (undetectable serum TSH levels), it has a higher risk of being a cancer and must be excised.

Surgical exploration in a patient with a thyroid nodule is undertaken with a working diagnosis of cancer. The initial procedure is thyroid lobectomy and isthmectomy to remove the ipsilateral lobe of the thyroid gland as well as the isthmus (see Figure 20-6). Simple nodulectomy incompletely removes the tumor and should not be performed. Lobectomy allows the pathologist to assess the relation between the nodule and its surrounding thyroid tissue to determine whether it is malignant. If the pathologist cannot provide a definitive diagnosis on frozen-section analysis, especially in the case of follicular neoplasms, no further surgery is undertaken at that time. Definitive therapy is dictated by the permanent pathologic analysis and may require completion thyroidectomy in a few days. If frozen-section analysis of the specimen shows cancer, further resection (total thyroidectomy) is performed if it is indicated according to the criteria in Table 20-3. In patients with symptomatic thyroid enlargement, the extent of thyroidectomy is dictated by the disease. Lobectomy may be sufficient, or subtotal or total thyroidectomy may be necessary to remove all diseased tissue. Surgical resection should be definitive if possible because reoperation poses much greater risk to the nerves and parathyroids.

In performing lobectomy or total thyroidectomy, great care is taken to preserve the parathyroid glands and their blood supply. Occasionally, autografting of a parathyroid into the sternocleidomastoid muscle is necessary if the glandular blood supply is injured during the procedure. Preservation of the recurrent laryngeal nerve and the external branch of the superior laryngeal nerve is also essential. Injury to the recurrent laryngeal nerve causes paralysis of the ipsilateral vocal cord, which is immobile in the paramedian position. The other cord may not be opposable, leaving the patient with a weak, breathy voice. Bilateral injury causes total loss of speech and airway control, and requires tracheostomy. Injury to the external branch of the superior nerve results in loss of voice quality. Transient hypoparathyroidism or neurapraxia of the nerves is more common than permanent injury, and it usually resolves without sequelae. Hemorrhage, always a risk with any surgical procedure, is uncommon.

Parathyroid Glands

Anatomy

The **parathyroid glands** are paired organs, normally with two on the posterior surface of each thyroid lobe. Their embryologic development is from the dorsal portions of the third and fourth pharyngeal pouches. The inferior parathyroid gland and thymus gland develop from the third pharyngeal pouch and migrate downward together. The superior parathyroid gland develops from the fourth pharyngeal pouch, as do the ultimobranchial bodies, which eventually fuse with the thyroid gland to form the parafollicular cells.

In the adult, the parathyroid glands are yellow-brown, ovoid, and lobulated. They vary from 30 to 50 mg each. The main blood supply is from branches of the inferior thyroid arteries. The usual location of each parathyroid gland is on the dorsal thyroid capsule, with the superior gland posterior and lateral to the recurrent laryngeal nerve and superior to the inferior thyroid artery (see Figure 20-2), and the inferior parathyroid glands anterior and medial to the recurrent laryngeal nerve and inferior to the inferior thyroid artery. Although the superior parathyroid glands are more consistent in their location, any of the parathyroid glands can be ectopically positioned along the path of their descent from the pharynx, within the thyroid gland, posterior in the neck, or even in the mediastinum.

Physiology

The parathyroid glands synthesize and secrete **parathyroid hormone,** or parathormone. This hormone, along with vitamin D, maintains calcium homeostasis. The active metabolites of vitamin D regulate the overall amount of calcium in the body through control of intestinal calcium absorption. The production of parathyroid hormone is stimulated by low serum calcium concentration. The feedback loop is rapid, so the level of parathyroid hormone is quickly influenced by changes in serum calcium in the normal patient.

Parathyroid hormone controls the minute-to-minute serum calcium concentration by increasing the rate of dissolution of bone minerals, stimulating the resorption of calcium in the distal tubules of the kidney, and inhibiting the renal tubular resorption of phosphate.

Pathophysiology

Primary hyperparathyroidism, the most common cause of hypercalcemia, is usually a chronic disorder. It is often discovered while patients are relatively asymptomatic. It may cause irreversible skeletal damage through the depletion of calcium and kidney damage through hypercalciuria and the formation of renal stones. Malignancy is the second most common cause of hypercalcemia, either because of ectopic parathormone production or because of extensive lytic metastases. Less common causes of hypercalcemia include vitamin D or A intoxication, sarcoidosis, multiple myeloma, hyperthyroidism, thiazide or lithium therapy, familial hypercalcemic hypocalciuria, and milk-alkali syndrome.

Primary hyperparathyroidism is distinguished by an elevated serum calcium level in a patient with a higher than expected parathyroid hormone level and normal renal function. Three distinct conditions cause primary hyperparathyroidism: parathyroid adenoma (83%), parathyroid hyperplasia (15%), and parathyroid carcinoma (1%–2%).

A **parathyroid adenoma** is a benign functional tumor of the parathyroid gland. It is usually single, up to 1 to 2 cm in size, and rarely palpable. In **parathyroid hyperplasia,** each of the parathyroid glands is enlarged (< 2 cm). The condition may occur in a sporadic or familial setting. Enlargement of more than a single gland suggests hyperplasia because adenoma usually involves only one gland.

Secondary hyperparathyroidism is a response of the parathyroid glands to clinically low plasma levels of ionized calcium, usually because of chronic renal failure. In these patients, an impaired glomerular filtration rate (GFR) leads to phosphate retention and decreased serum calcium levels. These changes cause increased secretion of parathyroid hormone by the parathyroid gland, which in turn leads to the normalization of serum calcium and phosphate levels. This cycle is repeated with gradual development of parathyroid hyperplasia and subsequent secondary hyperparathyroidism. The increase in serum levels of parathyroid hormone decreases renal tubular phosphate resorption, thus compensating for the lower GFR. When the GFR falls below 30 mL/min, calcium–phosphate homeostasis is no longer maintained. Serum phosphate and parathyroid hormone levels increase, and serum calcium levels decrease. This sequence may be exacerbated by decreased renal production of vitamin D, leading to decreased intestinal absorption of calcium. The conse-

quences of secondary hyperparathyroidism may be abnormal calcification in some tissues, spontaneous bone fractures, or tendon ruptures.

In **tertiary hyperparathyroidism,** the chronically stimulated, hyperplastic glands of a patient with secondary hyperparathyroidism become autonomous producers of parathyroid hormone. Correction of serum levels of phosphate and calcium does not decrease levels of parathyroid hormone, and continued secretion of parathyroid hormone may cause hypercalcemia, severe bone disease as a result of resorption, dangerous elevation of calcium levels, and soft tissue calcification.

Clinical Presentation

Patients with hyperparathyroidism have been characterized as presenting with "stones (renal calculi), bones (painful resorption of bone), moans (fatigue, depression, or confusion), and abdominal groans (peptic ulcer and pancreatitis)." Patients with mild hyperparathyroidism, sometimes found only after routine serum calcium analysis, may have few, if any, symptoms.

Diagnosis

In hyperparathyroidism, serum calcium (total or ionized levels) and parathyroid hormone levels (determined by immunoassay) are elevated. The levels of calcium and parathyroid hormone do not help to distinguish parathyroid adenoma from hyperplasia. The distinction is usually made only at surgery. The use of preoperative localization studies (i.e., ultrasound, isotope scanning, computed tomography (CT), magnetic resonance imaging) to localize an adenoma is controversial because many experienced surgeons rely on the operative findings. Imaging studies are useful for patients who are undergoing reoperation after previous surgery did not identify the adenoma.

Treatment
Medical Treatment

Acute, severe hypercalcemia is treated by correcting dehydration with intravenous saline, enhancing renal excretion of calcium with diuretics, pharmacologically inhibiting accelerated bone resorption, and treating the underlying disorder.

In secondary hyperparathyroidism, abnormalities of calcium and phosphate metabolism secondary to renal failure usually can be managed medically, with dialysis on a high-calcium bath, supplemental vitamin D, and oral phosphate binders. These measures lower the serum phosphate and parathyroid hormone levels, raise the serum calcium levels, and decrease subsequent bone resorption.

Surgical Treatment and Complications

Primary hyperparathyroidism is treated surgically, with identification and excision of the adenoma. Resection of an adenoma usually is curative.

If parathyroid hyperplasia is found, the treatment is either removal of three complete glands and much of the fourth (leaving some viable parathyroid tissue) or removal of all four parathyroid glands (with or without autotransplantation of some parathyroid tissue into muscle of the forearm).

Parathyroid surgery may be indicated for tertiary, but not secondary, hyperparathyroidism. In patients with renal failure, renal transplantation corrects defects in renal phosphate excretion as well as vitamin D metabolism. Secondary hyperparathyroidism is thus corrected by the normalization of serum calcium and phosphate levels. Tertiary hyperparathyroidism is also usually corrected by a successful transplant. Indications for surgery in patients with tertiary hyperparathyroidism include persistent, significant hypercalcemia; severe bone disease; and extensive soft tissue calcification.

Complications of surgery for primary hyperparathyroidism are:

1. Persistent hypercalcemia because the adenoma was not found and removed
2. Hypoparathyroidism if all glands are damaged or removed
3. Recurrent laryngeal nerve injury

The risk of complication is greater with reoperation.

Adrenal Glands

Anatomy

The adrenal glands are located superiorly and medially to the upper pole of each kidney. The anatomic relations of each adrenal are different. The right adrenal is posterior to the liver, in close proximity to the inferior vena cava. The left adrenal abuts the aorta close to the pancreas and spleen. The arterial supply to the adrenals is from multiple small arteries that arise from the phrenic artery, the renal artery, and a small branch of the aorta. The venous drainage is more consistent. The right adrenal drains directly into the vena cava through a short, but relatively large, vein. The left adrenal vein empties into the left renal vein (Figure 20-10).

The adrenal gland has two types of tissue: the cortex, which is derived from the mesoderm, and the medulla, which is derived from neural crest ectoderm. The cortex has three layers: the outer zona glomerulosa, the middle zona fasciculata, and the inner zona reticularis.

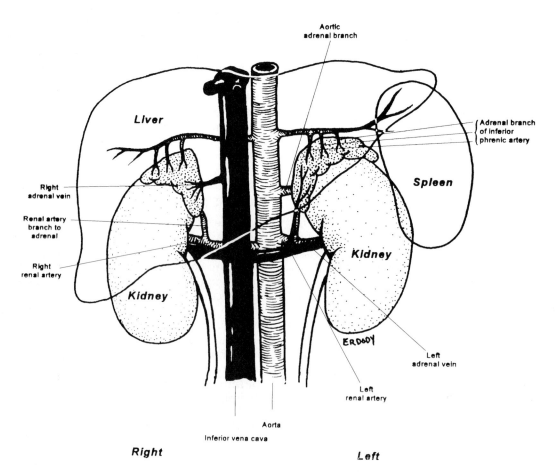

Figure 20-10 Anatomy of the adrenal glands showing their relations to adjacent structures and their blood supply.

Physiology

The adrenal cortex produces many hormones. They are divided into three major categories according to their function:

1. Glucocorticoids (cortisone and hydrocortisone). These are secreted in the zona fasciculata and involved in protein and carbohydrate metabolism. They are essential for survival.
2. Mineralocorticoid (aldosterone). This hormone is secreted in the zona glomerulosa. It exerts predominant action on electrolyte metabolism.
3. Progesterone, androgens, and estrogen. These hormones are secreted in the zona reticularis. Adrenal progesterone is not secreted into the bloodstream, but acts as a precursor for androgens and estrogen, both of which circulate in the blood.

The adrenal medulla primarily produces the catecholamines epinephrine and norepinephrine. Although chromaffin cells of the sympathetic nervous system also produce norepinephrine, only the adrenal medulla contains the enzyme phenylethanolamine n-methyltransferase (POMT), which converts norepinephrine to epinephrine.

Dysfunction in the adrenal gland may be primary or may be secondary to abnormal function in other endocrine organs, especially the pituitary gland. Each hormonal disturbance causes a disease state with specific characteristics (Table 20-4).

Pathophysiology

Cushing's Syndrome and Cushing's Disease

Cushing's syndrome is a constellation of clinical findings that results from excessive circulating glucocorticoids. The term **Cushing's disease,** first defined in 1932, refers to Cushing's syndrome that occurs secondary to excess ACTH production by an adenoma of the pituitary gland. The most common cause of true, or organic, Cushing's syndrome is the presence of an anterior pituitary basophilic adenoma (Cushing's disease) that secretes excess ACTH, which leads to diffuse adrenal cortical hyperplasia. Cushing's disease is the cause of Cushing's syndrome in 60% of cases. Unilateral benign adenomas and carcinomas of the adrenal gland are seen in 15% of cases. Occasionally, excess glucocorticoid secretion is secondary to a malignant tumor (e.g., lung cancer) that produces ectopic ACTH (5%–10%).

Clinical Presentation

Cushing's syndrome is usually seen in patients who are between 30 and 40 years of age. It affects women four times as often as men. Clinical features include the following: fatigue and weakness; moon facies, a "buffalo hump," and truncal obesity (all caused by rapidly developing adiposity of the face, neck, and trunk); dusky complexion with purple skin markings (striae); glucose intolerance; hypertension; amenorrhea or menstrual irregularity; easy bruising; muscular wasting; nervousness, irritability, and psychological changes;

Table 20-4. Correlation of Adrenal Zones with Disease Syndromes and Abnormal Adrenal Function

Adrenal Zone	Hormone Produced	Normal Function	Hypersecretory Syndrome	Symptoms	Pearls
Zona glomerulosa	Aldosterone	Electrolyte metabolism	Conn's syndrome	Hypokalemia Hypertension Muscle weakness	Unsuppressible hyperaldosteronism and suppressed plasma renin
Zona fasciculata	Cortisone Hydrocortisone	Protein and carbohydrate metabolism	Cushing's syndrome or disease	Buffalo hump Violaceous striae Moon facies Truncal obesity Hypertension	Exclude exogenous intake of glucocorticoids
Zona reticularis	Progesterone Androgen Estrogen	Sexual differentiation	Adrenogenital syndrome	Virilism/feminization Hyponatremia Hypertension	Presents in early childhood
Medulla	Epinephrine Norepinephrine	Sympathetic response	Pheochromocytoma	Episodic hypertension Headache Sweating Palpitations	10% are: Malignant Bilateral Familial Extraadrenal

back and bone pain; osteoporosis; hirsutism; headache; ankle and hand edema; diminished libido; impotence; and feminization in men. A single patient seldom displays all of these features simultaneously.

The most common signs and symptoms of Cushing's syndrome occur in patients who do not have true Cushing's syndrome (i.e., factitious disease). Factitious Cushing's syndrome is caused either by the exogenous intake of glucocorticoids or by another disease that interferes with normal steroid metabolism.

Diagnosis

The physical findings may be prominent or subtle. A tumor is rarely palpated on physical examination. When Cushing's syndrome is suspected clinically, initial screening should involve the measurement of glucocorticoid hormones or their breakdown products. The 24-hour urinary excretion of free cortisol and 17-hydroxycorticosteroid is elevated, and plasma cortisol is generally elevated. The diurnal variation in glucocorticoid secretion and the ability of the adrenal gland to increase cortisol secretion in response to ACTH stimulation are either lost or blunted. ACTH can be accurately measured with an immunoradiometric assay. Other biochemical changes in Cushing's syndrome include mild hyperglycemia, glycosuria, low serum potassium, and elevated carbon dioxide content. However, serum glucose, potassium, and carbon dioxide content may be normal in patients with Cushing's syndrome and therefore cannot be used by themselves to exclude or establish a diagnosis.

The **dexamethasone suppression test** is used to confirm the presence of Cushing's syndrome and to discriminate between Cushing's syndrome and Cushing's disease. Dexamethasone in low doses (1–2 mg) suppresses cortisol secretion in normal subjects. In Cushing's syndrome, cortisol secretion is not suppressed by this dose of dexamethasone. In Cushing's disease, dexamethasone in large doses (8 mg) suppresses plasma cortisol levels by more than 50% and is associated with normal or mildly elevated ACTH. When Cushing's syndrome is caused by ectopic ACTH production, cortisol levels are not suppressed by large doses of dexamethasone, and plasma ACTH is very high. When Cushing's syndrome is caused by an autonomously functioning adrenal tumor, cortisol levels are not suppressed by large doses of dexamethasone. The secretion of ACTH by the pituitary is suppressed by the elevated levels of cortisol. Consequently, plasma ACTH is low (Figure 20-11).

Radiologic examinations may be helpful in identifying adrenal lesions. The initial study is abdominal axial CT with thin cuts through the adrenal glands. An autonomous adenoma appears as a unilateral mass 2 cm or larger. The contralateral gland is normal or atrophic. A unilateral mass larger than 4 to 6 cm should raise suspicion of carcinoma. Bilateral adrenal enlargement suggests hyperplasia. Except for very specific circumstances, the CT scan has replaced the use of invasive techniques (e.g., intravenous pyelogram with nephrotomography, selective arteriography, selective retrograde

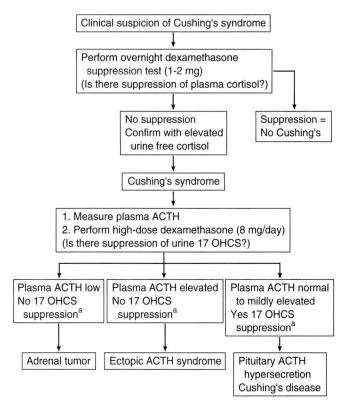

17 OHCS = 17-hydroxycorticosteroids. ª Refers to whether dexamethasone suppresses 17-hydroxycorticosteroid levels in the urine.

Figure 20-11 Algorithm for the management of a patient whose symptoms suggest Cushing's syndrome. *ACTH* = adrenocorticotropic hormone.

adrenal venography). Adrenal photoscanning or scintigraphy with radiolabeled cholesterol (^{59}NP scan) is helpful in differentiating ACTH-dependent disease (bilateral uptake) from ACTH-independent disease (unilateral uptake associated with an ipsilateral adrenal mass). It is also helpful in localizing ectopic adrenal tissue and in identifying a destructive lesion of the adrenal gland (unilateral uptake associated with a contralateral adrenal mass), as in metastases, hemorrhage, or infection (e.g., tuberculosis).

Treatment

The treatment of choice for Cushing's disease is transsphenoidal microadenomectomy, which has an initial cure rate that approaches 95%. When persistent or recurrent disease prompts a second exploration of the pituitary with this method, the cure rate is approximately 50%. Nonsurgical treatment includes pituitary irradiation and medications that inhibit steroid biosynthesis (i.e., metapyrone, ketoconazole, and aminoglutethimide). Bilateral total adrenalectomy is indicated when pituitary therapy is unsuccessful. In 90% of cases, adrenal gland exploration discloses pathologic changes in one or both glands. Exploration of both glands is indicated because of the possibility of multiple adenomas, nodular hyperplasia, or diffuse hyperplasia of both adrenals. This procedure is performed either transabdominally or with a combined bilateral posterior approach. After bilateral adrenalectomy, **Nelson's syndrome** may occur because of the progression of neoplastic growth of an ACTH-secreting pituitary adenoma. Enlargement of the pituitary tumor can cause visual field loss, headaches, and hyperpigmentation.

The treatment of primary adrenal causes of Cushing's syndrome depends on the etiology. Total adrenalectomy on the involved side is the treatment of choice for solitary adenomas and carcinomas of the adrenal. For bilateral adrenal cortical hyperplasia, total (bilateral) adrenalectomy is the procedure of choice to prevent recurrence.

Perioperative cortisone therapy is used when adrenalectomy is planned. After unilateral adrenalectomy, the adrenocortical function of the remaining normal adrenal is suppressed in cases of Cushing's syndrome with a primary adrenal cause. This suppression is caused by the associated suppression of ACTH that results from negative feedback inhibition of ACTH by cortisol. Therefore, after adrenalectomy, daily maintenance doses of hydrocortisone (25–37.5 mg) are continued until adequate adrenal reserve or an intact hypothalamic-pituitary-adrenal axis is shown by the **ACTH stimulation test.** When total adrenalectomy is performed, daily maintenance hydrocortisone is necessary for the life of the patient.

Primary Aldosteronism

Primary aldosteronism (Conn's syndrome) was first described by Jerome Conn in a patient who was treated at the University of Michigan in 1955. Although Conn originally described the syndrome as primary hyperaldosteronism, primary aldosteronism is the current term. Patients with primary aldosteronism produce excess aldosterone from a solitary adenoma, diffuse hyperplasia, or nodular (adenomatous) hyperplasia of the adrenal cortex. On rare occasions, hyperaldosteronism arises from a functional adenocarcinoma of the adrenal cortex that secretes excess aldosterone.

Clinical Presentation

The clinical characteristics of primary aldosteronism include hypokalemia, hypertension, and metabolic alkalosis, but can include hypomagnesemia, tetany, and periodic paralysis. The classic biochemical findings include persistently elevated plasma and urinary aldosterone secretion and decreased plasma renin activity that cannot be stimulated to rise. Aldosterone is normally secreted in response to a reduced effective blood volume, sodium depletion or restriction, and potassium loading. Aldosterone stimulates the reabsorption of sodium (chloride) at the distal convoluted and cortical collecting tubules. Under the influence of aldosterone, sodium is reabsorbed at the expense of potassium and hydrogen ions. Thus, excess aldosterone causes hypokalemia and a metabolic alkalosis.

Diagnosis

First, it is necessary to distinguish primary from secondary aldosteronism. This distinction is made biochemically, primarily based on the status of plasma renin activity. Primary aldosteronism is associated with elevated aldosterone secretion and suppressed plasma renin activity. In contrast, secondary aldosteronism, which is a normal homeostatic response to volume or salt depletion, is associated with elevated plasma renin activity and elevated or high normal aldosterone levels. Clinical settings in which secondary hyperaldosteronism can occur include cirrhosis, nephrotic syndrome, and congestive heart failure. To establish the diagnosis, after the discontinuation of antihypertensive sympathetic inhibitors such as clonidine and a-methyldopa (1 week), diuretics (4 weeks), and spironolactone (6 weeks), the patient is given 200 mEq/day sodium for 3 to 4 days **(sodium loading).** Plasma and 24-hour urine collections are measured for aldosterone, potassium, and plasma renin activity. Primary aldosteronism is confirmed if plasma and urinary aldosterone levels are increased in the presence of suppressed plasma renin activity.

Second, once primary aldosteronism is established, the cause of the hyperaldosteronism must be determined. The two most common causes are an aldosterone-producing adenoma (aldosteronoma) and bilateral nodular hyperplasia of the adrenal cortex. Both conditions cause autonomous secretion of excess aldosterone. Adrenocortical adenocarcinoma is a rare cause of hyperaldosteronism. Primary aldosteronism caused by diffuse nodular hyperplasia is referred to as idiopathic aldosteronism. It is important to differentiate primary aldosteronism caused by an aldosteronoma from that caused by idiopathic aldosteronism, because the treatment of each is different. The measurement of plasma aldosterone concentration after 4 hours of upright posture may be helpful in distinguishing aldosteronomas from bilateral adrenal hyperplasia. In patients with an aldosteronoma, the renin–angiotensin system is completely suppressed. As a result, postural stimulation, which normally activates the renin–angiotensin system, does not increase plasma aldosterone. Most patients who have an aldosteronoma respond to postural stimulation with no change or with a decrease in plasma aldosterone. Patients who have bilateral adrenal hyperplasia respond with an increase in plasma aldosterone. This response is theoretically caused by the increased sensitivity of diffusely hyperplastic adrenocortical tissue to small increases in angiotensin II that are induced by upright posture.

Finally, localization of the adrenal gland that contains the anatomic abnormality (tumor or dominant nodule) in the setting of primary aldosteronism is the next important step in management. The imaging studies of choice include CT and iodocholesterol **adrenal scintigraphy** (^{59}NP scan), when it is available, under dexamethasone suppression. The role of ultrasonography in identifying solitary adrenal adenomas remains unclear. The use of arteriography and adrenal venography has declined significantly. Adrenal vein sampling to lateralize the source of excess aldosterone secretion by measuring concomitant cortisol and aldosterone levels in adrenal venous effluent is useful in certain cases. Adrenal vein sampling is useful to establish unilateral and functionally dominant disease (i.e., one adrenal secretes at least three times more aldosterone than the contralateral gland in a patient with primary aldosteronism). In some cases, this finding alone justifies unilateral adrenalectomy on the side with dominant aldosterone secretion.

Treatment

Unilateral adrenalectomy is the treatment of choice for patients with primary aldosteronism secondary to an aldosterone-secreting adrenal adenoma. Patients with hyperaldosteronism that cannot be localized to one adrenal gland (idiopathic aldosteronism) are managed with spironolactone and symptomatic treatment. In most of these patients, bilateral adrenal hyperplasia (diffuse disease) causes hyperaldosteronism, and bilateral adrenalectomy is not recommended.

Pheochromocytoma

Pheochromocytoma has an incidence among hypertensive patients of 0.1% to 2%. These tumors arise from chromaffin tissue and secrete excess catecholamines. As a result, vasoconstriction (alpha-adrenergic stimulation), increased cardiac output (beta-adrenergic stimulation), and hypertension occur. Approximately 85% to 90% of these tumors arise from the adrenal medulla, but they may arise from extraadrenal sites (**paraganglionoma**) of chromaffin tissue in the peripheral autonomic nervous system, anywhere from the base of the skull to the pelvis, usually in a paraaortic position. Approximately 10% of pheochromocytomas are malignant, 10% are bilateral, 10% are found in children, 10% are familial, and 10% are extraadrenal.

Clinical Presentation

The signs and symptoms of pheochromocytomas are a direct result of the effects of sustained or paroxysmal (in either case, uncontrolled) secretion of norepinephrine or epinephrine. The hallmark manifestation of these tumors is hypertension, which usually occurs in one of three patterns: episodic, sustained, or widely fluctuating superimposed on sustained hypertension. Other clinical symptoms include paroxysmal attacks manifested by palpitations, headaches, pallor, flushing, and sweating. Patients may experience a sense of impending doom and significant anxiety. Most attacks are short-lived, lasting 15 minutes or less, and can be precipitated by trauma, physical activity, exertion, changes in position, alcohol intake, micturition, or smoking.

Pheochromocytomas may occur as a sporadic tumor, as a dominant neoplasm in several members of a family (familial pheochromocytoma), or as one of several endocrine tumors found in the MEN syndrome complex. MEN-2A disease is associated with medullary thyroid cancer, pheochromocytomas, and primary hyperparathyroidism. MEN-2B disease is associated with a specific phenotype or distinct physical features, ganglioneuromatosis, medullary thyroid cancer, pheochromocytomas, and a much rarer incidence of hyperparathyroidism. The MEN syndrome is discussed in greater detail elsewhere in this chapter.

Pheochromocytomas are associated with four related familial disorders that involve abnormalities of the central nervous system and skin. **Von Recklinghausen's disease** is one of the most common of these neuroectodermal dysplasias. It is manifested by multiple neurofibromas of the peripheral nerves that present as subcutaneous or intradermal nodules of varying size. These may be associated with central nervous system involvement in the form of vascular malformations of the brain, meningiomas, and gliomas. **Von Hippel–Lindau** disease is associated with cystic cerebellar hemangioblastomas and angiomatous malformation of the retina. **Sturge-Weber syndrome** is manifested by a port wine stain (facial hemangioma) that occupies the cutaneous distribution of the trigeminal nerve and by angiomatous malformations of the brain and meninges. Finally, tuberous sclerosis is associated with the triad of mental deficiency, seizures, and facial nevi. In all of these familial disorders, pheochromocytomas occur more frequently than in the general population.

Diagnosis

The diagnosis of a pheochromocytoma or functional paraganglionoma is made by demonstrating elevated levels of urinary catecholamines and their metabolites [metanephrine, normetanephrine, and vanillylmandelic acid (VMA)]. The measurement of serum epinephrine and norepinephrine has a sensitivity of only 75%, but may lead to the diagnosis in rare cases in which only transient rises in plasma catecholamines during paroxysmal attacks are the sole significant finding. Free plasma metanephrines are elevated in pheochromocytomas. However, with a more standard approach, when pheochromocytoma is suspected or must be excluded (e.g., an incidentally discovered adrenal mass), a 12- or 24-hour urine collection should be obtained and measured for epinephrine, norepinephrine, metanephrine, normetanephrine, and VMA. Certain medications interfere with the measurement of catecholamines and metabolites. Medications that elevate measured levels of catecholamines and metabolites include tricyclic antidepressants, benzodiazepines, amphetamines, labetalol, L-dopa, methyldopa, clonidine, and alcohol. Medications that decrease these measured values include metyrosine and methylglucamine (a component of iodinated contrast media). Therefore, it is important to assure that the patient is not taking any medication that is known to affect catecholamine secretion or the measurement of catecholamines and metabolites before sampling begins.

Once endogenous catecholamine excess is identified, the responsible tumor must be localized. Because the enzyme necessary to convert norepinephrine to epinephrine (POMT) is present only in the adrenal medulla, the rare tumor that secretes predominantly excess epinephrine is likely to be located in the adrenal gland until proven otherwise. However, excess norepinephrine secretion from anywhere can increase epinephrine production in the adrenal medulla of an active normal gland.

In 98% of cases, pheochromocytomas are located in the abdominal cavity; however, they can be located anywhere that chromaffin tissue is found normally. Chromaffin tissue is found anywhere from the base of the skull to the pelvis in a periaortic or paravertebral position. Special locations for chromaffin tissue that can give rise to occult pheochromocytomas include the bladder and a region of chromaffin tissue that is inferior to the take-off of the inferior mesenteric artery and anterior to the aorta. This latter region is referred to as the organ of Zuckerkandl. Technically, any tumor of chromaffin tissue outside of the adrenal medulla is called a paraganglionoma. All extraadrenal pheochromocytomas are paraganglionomas by definition.

CT scan is the first-line imaging study used to screen for and locate a possible pheochromocytoma in either the adrenal or a known site of distribution of chromaffin tissue. Magnetic resonance imaging (MRI) is also useful in distinguishing pheochromocytomas from benign adrenocortical adenomas. With MRI, pheochromocytomas can usually be distinguished based on their increased T2-weighted image. Further, the use of ^{123}I-metaiodobenzylguanidine (MIBG) scintigraphy has helped to locate occult pheochromocytomas or paraganglionomas. Chromaffin tissue takes up the radiolabeled MIBG in a way that directly correlates with its active biosynthesis and secretion of catecholamines.

Treatment

Once a pheochromocytoma is identified and localized, the patient is prepared for surgical excision by administration of alpha-adrenergic blockers, usually with phenoxybenzamine in a daily dose that is sufficient to cause nasal stuffiness or borderline postural hypotension (usually 40–160 mg/day in divided doses). Beta-adrenergic blockade with propranolol is added whenever the patient shows cardiac arrhythmia or tachycardia that suggests excess beta-adrenergic stimulation of the heart. Beta blockade should never be administered to a patient who was not pretreated with adequate alpha-adrenergic blockade to obviate the adverse effects of uncompensated alpha-adrenergic stimulation. In addition to adrenergic blockade, volume replacement to ensure adequate effective circulating volume is an important step in preoperative management.

The adverse effects of uncompensated alpha-adrenergic stimulation are better understood in the following context. The excessive alpha-adrenergic stimulation that is caused by the secretion of excess catecholamines by a pheochromocytoma leads to severe peripheral vasoconstriction. Peripheral vasoconstriction leads to increased systemic vascular resistance and increased cardiac afterload. The body compensates by increasing tonic sympathetic outflow from vasomotor centers in the brain and reflex increases in heart rate, cardiac output, and blood pressure through beta-adrenergic stimulation of the heart. When the pheochromocytoma arises from the adrenal gland, there is usually excess epinephrine secreted with the excess catecholamines elaborated by the tumor. The excess epinephrine associated with excess beta-adrenergic stimulation of the heart and the peripheral alpha-adrenergic stimulation of the heart are crucial aspects of the cardiac compensatory mechanisms for these patients. The patient overcomes increased peripheral vasoconstriction and cardiac afterload by increasing stroke volume, heart rate, and cardiac output (cardiac effects of increased beta-adrenergic stimulation). If cardiac compensation of the increased peripheral vasoconstriction is blocked by beta-adrenergic blockers before alpha-adrenergic blockers are administered, then the patient is at risk for cardiovascular collapse and the inability to perfuse peripheral tissues adequately.

After the achievement of adequate preoperative adrenergic blockade and volume replacement, surgical excision is the treatment of choice. Bilateral adrenal exploration and exploration of the paraaortic and paracaval retroperitoneum from diaphragm to pelvis (to examine the areas in which chromaffin tissue is normally distributed), through either a midline or a transverse abdominal incision, is the standard approach. Adrenalectomy may also be performed laparoscopically, with either a flank, retroperitoneal (posterior), or transabdominal (anterior) approach. Laparoscopic adrenalectomy is associated with a shorter hospital stay and lower postoperative morbidity rate. However, the surgeon must be entirely confident of his or her ability to exclude the presence of tumors in other locations that are known to give rise to pheochromocytomas. MIBG scintigraphy plays a role in screening patients with catecholamine-secreting neoplasms before laparoscopic adrenalectomy, paraganglionectomy, or tumor excision.

Adrenal Cortical Carcinoma

The incidence of adrenocortical carcinoma (ACC) is estimated at 1 case per 1.7 million people. ACC is bilateral in approximately 5% of cases. It can occur at any age, but shows a peak incidence in the fourth and fifth decades. It also shows a slight left-sided and female preponderance. Functioning tumors are present in 50% of cases and are more often seen in younger patients and women. ACC has a poor prognosis; the 5-year survival rate rarely exceeds 30%.

Most ACCs are large (often > 6 cm or 1000 g), encapsulated, and friable, with extensive central necrosis and hemorrhage. It is often impossible to differentiate large benign adrenal neoplasms from malignant lesions purely on the basis of cellular characteristics. Venous or capsular invasion and distant metastases are the most reliable signs of malignancy. However, tumor necrosis, intratumoral hemorrhage, marked nuclear and cellular pleomorphism, and the presence of many mitotic figures per high-power field all strongly support the diagnosis of ACC.

Clinical Presentation

Patients with ACC may have flank or abdominal pain, a palpable mass, symptoms that result from metastases (e.g., weight loss, weakness, fever, bone pain), or autonomous production of adrenocortical hormones (Cushing's syndrome). The most common hormone produced to excess by an ACC is cortisol. For this reason, Cushing's syndrome is the most common presentation of a functional ACC. In children, however, virilization because of excess androgen production is the more common presentation. Women with virilizing tumors (excess androgen production by their adrenal carcinoma) have hirsutism, temporal balding, increased muscle mass, and amenorrhea. Boys have precocious puberty. A man who has gynecomastia, testicular atrophy, impotence or decreased libido, and an adrenal mass is considered to have an ACC until proven otherwise.

Diagnosis

The diagnosis may not be firmly established until surgical exploration. However, clues to the diagnosis are often present on CT scan or another imaging study used to identify the mass.

ACCs are often large enough to show anatomic distortions or abnormalities on a plain abdominal radiograph, an excretory urogram (intravenous pyelogram), or an adrenal ultrasound. However, CT scan is the imaging modality of choice for adrenal lesions. Features on abdominal CT that suggest that an adrenal mass is a carcinoma include irregular margins or borders, heterogeneity (homogenous lesions are usually benign), evidence of central necrosis, stippled calcifications (seen in 15%–30% of cases), regional adenopathy, invasion of adjacent structures, and the presence of liver or other visceral metastases.

ACCs have a predilection for extension through the adrenal vein into either the renal vein (left-sided neoplasms) or the inferior vena cava (right-sided neoplasms). MRI scans may be helpful in identifying this extension. ACCs have increased T2-weighted images on MRI, as do pheochromocytomas and metastases to the adrenal. However, the clinical presentation and associated findings almost always allow differentiation between these very different adrenal neoplasms. In the current era of CT and MRI, the need to perform adrenal angiography or venography is increasingly rare in the routine workup of a patient with a suspected ACC.

Treatment

Surgical excision with gross total tumor removal whenever possible is the treatment of choice. When gross total tumor removal is not possible, then debulking the tumor to the greatest extent possible is appropriate. In most cases of early disease, treatment requires adrenalectomy and excision of involved regional lymph nodes. In the presence of local invasion or visceral metastases, it may be necessary to include ipsilateral nephrectomy and resection of contiguous structures or hepatic metastases. After adrenalectomy, corticosteroid replacement is usually necessary because of atrophy of the contralateral adrenal gland secondary to the suppression of ACTH secretion caused by the overproduction of cortisol by the ACC.

Adjuvant chemotherapy is indicated in patients who have metastatic and unresectable ACCs. **Mitotane** (o,p'-DDD, which is pronounced ortho-para-DDD) is the most common adrenolytic agent. Other chemotherapeutic agents include cisplatin, suramin (polysulfonated napthylurea), etoposide (VP-16), and gossypol (spermatotoxin). Also, combinations of any of these chemotherapeutic drugs, with and without 5-fluorouracil and doxorubicin, have been tried in an effort to maximize the therapeutic effect. A recent phase II trial of mitotane and cisplatin showed efficacy in patients with metastatic or residual disease in whom complete resection was not possible. However, the combination caused significant toxicity.

Although ACC is relatively resistant to radiation therapy, it is used to treat the adrenal bed postoperatively and for unresectable recurrences and bony metastases. Its role in the management of these neoplasms is controversial.

The overall aggressive nature of ACC leads to a generally poor prognosis, with a median survival of approximately 8 months. The 5-year survival rate for ACC is 19% to 30%, and the 10-year survival rate is less than 10%. Because approximately 98% of ACCs are larger than 4 cm by the time they are diagnosed, this poor prognostic picture may change with the diagnosis of smaller lesions and earlier disease. This change is expected to result from improved imaging technologies and patient access.

Incidentally Discovered Adrenal Mass

An incidentally discovered adrenal mass **(adrenal incidentaloma)** is found in approximately 0.35% to 5% of patients who undergo abdominal CT. When an adrenal mass is recognized in the absence of any symptoms, the question is whether the lesion represents disease. Is the adrenal mass associated with occult or asymptomatic excess adrenocortical hormonal or catecholamine secretion? Is it an early ACC? Is it a benign adrenocortical adenoma or nodule? Does it represent the metastasis of an extraadrenal primary cancer, a normal anatomic variant, or a benign endogenous process?

Among reported cases of incidentally discovered adrenal masses, approximately 38% are benign cortical adenomas, 22% are metastases to the adrenal gland, 3% are adrenal cysts, 2.6% are myelolipomas (benign tumors composed of mature fat and bone marrow elements) or lipomas, 1.7% are ACCs, and 1% or fewer are pheochromocytomas (functional and nonfunctional). Approximately 2.3% are pseudotumors, which are not really tumors of the adrenal gland, but an anatomic abnormality (e.g., pancreatic cyst) masquerading as an adrenal tumor. The rest of these adrenal masses are neuroblastomas, ganglioneuromas, or lymphomas. In approximately 25% to 30% of cases, they are other or unknown entities. Of incidentally discovered adrenal adenomas, 5% to 14% may produce "occult" excess cortisol or have autonomous function that leads to a subclinical or pre-Cushing's syndrome.

Diagnosis

The evaluation of a patient who is incidentally found to have an adrenal mass should be directed by a careful history, physical examination, and review of the abdominal CT scan. If the patient has a history of an extraadrenal primary cancer that is known to metastasize to the adrenal gland (e.g., lung, breast, colon), then it is important to establish whether the adrenal lesion represents metastatic disease. This is probably the most common setting in which FNA biopsy (FNAB) is performed to evaluate a solid mass of the adrenal gland. FNAB is performed after excess glucocorticoid or catecholamine excretion into the urine is excluded, as outlined previously. This approach is recommended because performing an FNAB on a functional pheochromocytoma may precipitate a catecholamine crisis and death. FNAB of an ACC may seed the peritoneal cavity with carcinoma or may yield a falsely negative cytologic specimen as a result of sampling error. The setting in which FNAB may be most useful without untoward risks, other than to exclude metastatic disease, is in evaluating a purely cystic adrenal lesion. If the lesion is identified as a simple cyst on ultrasound and CT, and the aspirate is clear (nonbloody), then the lesion is benign and can be followed. However, if the cyst aspirate is bloody or the lesion is a mixed cyst (both cystic and solid components), then further workup to exclude an underlying neoplasm is necessary.

Occasionally, pheochromocytomas present as cystic-mass lesions. For this reason, the distinction between a pure cyst and a complex, or mixed, cyst is important. Further, FNAB to establish the diagnosis of metastatic disease to the adrenal gland should be considered only when the finding of metastases would alter patient management. Otherwise, the risk of a complication (e.g., pneumothorax, hemorrhage) is unwarranted.

In most cases in which an adrenalectomy is considered, it is necessary to exclude abnormal, but asymptomatic, adrenal function in patients who have an incidentally found adrenal mass. Measurements of free cortisol, 17-hydroxycorticosteroids, 17-ketosteroids, epinephrine, norepinephrine, metanephrine, normetanephrine, and VMA assess adrenocortical and adrenomedullary function. In the normokalemic, normotensive patient, it is unlikely that the adrenal mass is an aldosteronoma causing primary aldosteronism. Therefore, measurements of aldosterone and plasma renin activity are not indicated. An overnight dexamethasone suppression study, with 1 mg dexamethasone given orally at 11:00 pm and plasma cortisol measured at 8:00 am the next morning, will determine whether there is evidence of autonomous (nonsup-pressible) adrenal cortical function. If the 8:00 am plasma cortisol level is less than 5 mg/dL, then the patient does not have nonsuppressible or autonomous adrenal cortical function.

Finally, when it is available, the use of ^{131}I-6b-iodomethyl-norcholesterol (^{59}NP) adrenal scintigraphy is useful in the evaluation of incidentally discovered adrenal masses larger than 2 cm. The imaging pattern on the ^{59}NP scan can direct the management of the adrenal mass by establishing whether the adrenal mass shows increased radiotracer uptake (concordant pattern); decreased, distorted, or absent radiotracer uptake (discordant pattern); or normal, bilateral, symmetric radiotracer uptake despite the presence of a unilateral adrenal mass (nonlateralizing pattern). A concordant pattern implies normal adrenocortical function and a benign etiology. It is usually caused by an adrenocortical adenoma or nodular hyperplasia. A discordant pattern implies a destructive or space-occupying lesion and is usually caused by primary or metastatic carcinoma. A nonlateralizing pattern is consistent with a pseudotumor or small cortical adenoma (< 2 cm).

Treatment

If there is no evidence of excess adrenocortical or medullary function, loss of diurnal rhythm, a suspicious pattern on adrenal scintigraphy, or malignancy on abdominal CT scan, and the adrenal mass is smaller than 3 cm, then the patient can be followed with repeated abdominal CT scans over a 12- to 18-month period. If there is no evidence of enlargement of the adrenal mass during that time, it is reasonable to follow the patient thereafter and to monitor for any changes. If the adrenal mass is larger than 4 cm or has any positive findings, then the patient should undergo unilateral adrenalectomy of the ipsilateral adrenal with perioperative steroid coverage. Lesions that are 3 cm or larger but less than 4 cm are managed on an individual basis depending on the overall assessment of the patient at the time. Careful follow-up is appropriate in any patient with an incidentally discovered adrenal mass who does not undergo adrenalectomy to establish the diagnosis.

Patients who are incidentally found to have an adrenal mass associated with any evidence of adrenocortical or adrenomedullary excess or autonomous function should undergo adrenalectomy regardless of the size of the lesion and the lack or extent of symptoms.

Adrenalectomy is performed with either an open or a laparoscopic technique and either an anterior (transabdominal) or a posterior approach. The surgical technique and approach used depend on the presumed etiology of the mass and the experience of the surgeon.

Treatment Complications

The morbidity and complications associated with adrenalectomy are typically a consequence of the underlying adrenal pathology. For example, among patients who are undergoing adrenalectomy for

Cushing's syndrome, the increased susceptibility to infection, deep venous thrombosis, poor wound healing, and mild glucose intolerance are primarily consequences of hypercortisolism.

Intraoperative complications include hypertension and hemorrhage secondary to inadvertent injury to the adrenal vein, especially during right adrenalectomy. Hemorrhage can be avoided by using meticulous surgical technique. The surgeon should secure control of the venous drainage of the adrenal gland and divide the adrenal vein before manipulating any tumors. The risk of significant changes in blood pressure during adrenalectomy for pheochromocytoma is minimized with adequate preoperative preparation that includes volume replacement and adrenergic blockade. Intraoperative hypertension, usually associated with manipulation of the pheochromocytoma, is managed with nitroprusside.

Perhaps the most important postoperative complication of adrenalectomy is the onset of occult **adrenal insufficiency** or Addisonian crisis as a result of inadequate glucocorticoid (cortisol) replacement. Patients who undergo unilateral adrenalectomy for an adrenal cause of Cushing's syndrome are treated with hydrocortisone perioperatively because the contralateral adrenal gland is assumed to be suppressed until proven otherwise. Patients who undergo bilateral adrenalectomy for Cushing's disease (adrenal hyperplasia) or bilateral pheochromocytomas require lifelong glucocorticoid replacement. Patients who undergo unilateral adrenalectomy for primary aldosteronism, pheochromocytoma, or a nonfunctional adrenal tumor (e.g., adrenal cyst, myelolipoma) do not need cortisol replacement.

Another important cause of adrenal insufficiency is long-term corticosteroid therapy and the ACTH and adrenal suppression that are a result of such treatment for longer than a week. These patients cannot respond normally to the stress of surgery by increasing their secretion of cortisol and become relatively adrenal insufficient in the perioperative period unless adequate replacement is given.

Postural hypotension or dizziness, nausea, vomiting, abdominal pain, weakness, fatigability, hyperkalemia, and hyponatremia are common symptoms and signs of adrenal insufficiency. The patient may not have all of these findings, but the presence of any one of them in a patient in the correct clinical setting raises the index of suspicion. When adrenal insufficiency is suspected in an unstable patient, it is appropriate to draw blood to measure cortisol and then immediately to give the patient parenteral steroids (100–200 mg hydrocortisone IV). Treating a patient with a dose of hydrocortisone that is not needed has no significant consequence; however, missing the diagnosis of adrenal insufficiency could lead to death.

After the surgical resection of any adrenal gland, it is the responsibility of the managing physician to document the presence of an intact or recovered hypothalamic-pituitary-adrenal (HPA) axis before weaning postoperative cortisol replacement. The standard method is to establish that the patient has adequate adrenal reserve

(i.e., demonstrate the ability of the remaining adrenal gland to respond appropriately to ACTH). This can be done with an ACTH stimulation test, which involves administering 250 mg synthetic ACTH by IV bolus or IM injection after a baseline plasma cortisol level is drawn. Plasma cortisol is then measured at 30 and 60 minutes. The test is performed before 9:00 am, and there are no known contraindications. If the baseline cortisol level is 20 mg/dL or greater and increases more than 7 mg/dL, then the HPA axis is normal. If the cortisol level is less than 20 mg/dL and increases less than 7 mg/dL, then the HPA axis is abnormal. Until the HPA axis is normal, the patient needs maintenance hydrocortisone.

Multiple Endocrine Neoplasia Syndromes

These familial endocrine tumor syndromes are inherited as autosomal dominant conditions. They are divided into three types: **MEN-1, MEN-2A, and MEN-2B.** Familial medullary thyroid carcinoma (FMTC) is also inherited as an autosomal dominant condition, but it is associated only with **medullary thyroid carcinoma** and no other endocrine abnormalities.

Multiple Endocrine Neoplasia Type 1

MEN-1 is an inherited endocrine disorder that includes hyperplasia of the parathyroid glands and various tumors, including pancreatic islet cell tumors, anterior pituitary tumors, and occasionally carcinoid tumors and lipomas (Table 20-5). It is an autosomal dominant disorder with variable penetrance (i.e., 50% of the offspring will have the disease, but each one may not express all of the components).

Genetic Defect

The causative gene in MEN-1 has been mapped to the long arm of chromosome 11. Genetic linkage studies are used to determine whether an individual from an affected kindred carries the disease gene. The exact gene defect was recently identified and is called **menin;** however, its function is unknown.

Screening of family members for the presence of disease should begin during the second or third decade. Individuals are questioned and examined for kidney stones, lipomas, hypercortisolism, hypoglycemia, peptic ulcer disease, headaches, acromegaly, and visual field defects. Blood levels of calcium, glucose, prolactin, gastrin, and pancreatic polypeptide are measured.

Parathyroid Hyperplasia

Primary hyperparathyroidism is the most common endocrine disorder in MEN-1.

Table 20-5. Multiple Endocrine Neoplasia Type I: Genetic Characterization and Gland Involvement

Mode of Inheritance	Chromosome	Gene	Glands and Sites Involved [3]	Type of Disease
Autosomal dominant	11	Menin	Papathyroid	Hyperplasia
			Pancreas	Islet cell tumors
			Pituitary	Adenoma
			Thyroid	Adenoma
			Adrenal	Adenoma or carcinoma
			Enterochromaffin system	Carcinoid tumor
			Soft tissue	Lipoma

[3]Not all individuals have all manifestations of the syndrome.

Clinical Presentation and Evaluation

The manifestations are similar to those seen in non–MEN-1 patients with primary hyperparathyroidism. They include asymptomatic hypercalcemia, weakness, fatigue, kidney stones, and bone pain. The prevalence of primary hyperparathyroidism in MEN-1 increases with age and is nearly 100% after 50 years of age. The age of onset is 25 years, which is younger than that in sporadic primary hyperparathyroidism. Primary hyperparathyroidism is diagnosed by measurement of elevated serum levels of total calcium, ionized calcium, and parathyroid hormone. The intact parathyroid hormone assay seldom gives false-positive results and is very specific for primary hyperparathyroidism. These patients always have parathyroid hyperplasia.

Treatment

The operation of choice is either 3½-gland parathyroidectomy or 4-gland parathyroidectomy with forearm transplant. The cervical thymus is also removed because supernumerary glands can occur and are usually within the thymus.

Tumors

Pancreatic Islet Cell Tumors

Patients with MEN-1 also may have pancreatic or duodenal neuroendocrine tumors (islet cell tumors). These tumors may be malignant, and there is a direct correlation between tumor size and the chance of metastases.

Clinical Presentation and Evaluation

Pancreatic islet cell tumors may be nonfunctional or may produce excessive hormones that cause a characteristic clinical syndrome. The most common hormone-secreting pancreatic or duodenal neuroendocrine tumor in MEN-1 is gastrinoma (Zollinger-Ellison syndrome). Moreover, any pancreatic neuroendocrine tumor can occur in patients with MEN-1, including gastrinoma, insulinoma, glucagonoma, vasoactive intestinal peptide tumor (VIPoma), growth hormone–releasing factor tumor, somatostatinoma, pancreatic polypeptide-producing tumor, and foregut or midgut carcinoid tumors.

Symptoms of Zollinger-Ellison syndrome are caused by hypersecretion of gastric acid and include peptic ulcer disease, secretory diarrhea, and esophagitis. The diagnosis is made by detection of abnormally elevated levels of gastric acid output and fasting serum gastrin. For diagnosis, all acid antisecretory medication is discontinued, and the fasting serum level of gastrin and the amount of gastric acid are measured. Fasting serum levels of gastrin greater than 100 pg/mL and basal acid output greater than 15 mEq/hr are diagnostic of Zollinger-Ellison syndrome. A secretin stimulation test may be confirmatory. A positive result is defined as a greater than 200 pg/mL increment in serum gastrin level after secretin.

Patients with insulinoma have neuroglycopenic symptoms during a fast. These symptoms may include personality change, drowsiness, altered mental status, coma, and seizures. Most patients also experience weight gain. Insulinoma is diagnosed by a supervised fast during which levels of glucose, insulin, C-peptide, and proinsulin are measured. Insulinoma is diagnosed if the patient has neuroglycopenic symptoms with serum levels of glucose less than 45 mg/dL and insulin greater than 5 μU/mL. Elevated C-peptide and proinsulin levels are confirmatory and exclude factitious hypoglycemia.

Glucagonoma causes a characteristic red, scaly, pruritic, migratory rash called necrolytic migratory erythema. Patients may also have cachexia, hypoaminoacidemia, anemia, diabetes mellitus, weight loss, and thromboembolic disease. Elevated plasma levels of glucagon (> 500 pg/mL) are diagnostic of glucagonoma. Patients with VIPomas have severe watery diarrhea, dehydration, hypochloremia, achlorhydria, hypercalcemia, and hypokalemia. The diagnosis is dependent on measuring elevated plasma levels of VIP. Nonfunctional islet cell tumors may produce pancreatic polypeptide, which does not cause a clinical syndrome. Serum levels of pancreatic polypeptide are used to screen for the presence of islet cell tumors in MEN-1.

Treatment

After the diagnosis of a clinical syndrome related to an islet cell tumor or an elevated serum level of pancreatic polypeptide, radiologic localization studies are used to image the extent of the islet cell tumor. Radiologic studies include CT scan, endoscopic ultrasound, octreotide scan, angiogram, secretin angiogram, calcium angiogram, and portal venous sampling. Octreotide scans image islet cell tumors based on the density of type 2 somatostatin receptors. Provocative angiograms that use secretin for gastrinoma and calcium for insulinoma can either image the tumor based on a vascular blush during angiography or identify the region of the pancreas that contains the tumor based on the hormone response to the provocative agent. Portal venous sampling measures the concentration of hormone in the portal vein and its tributaries. The concentration of hormone is highest in the vein that drains the tumor. Despite the use of these studies, some patients with biochemical evidence of an islet cell tumor may still have no tumor identified. This situation usually occurs in patients with MEN-1 and Zollinger-Ellison syndrome.

Surgery is indicated to remove potentially malignant islet cell tumors and to provide remission from the hormonal syndrome. Some medications, such as omeprazole for gastric acid hypersecretion in gastrinoma and octreotide (a somatostatin analogue) for the rash in glucagonoma and the diarrhea in VIPoma, may also inhibit hormonal effects. At surgery, these patients commonly have multiple islet cell and duodenal neuroendocrine tumors. Recent studies indicate that the tumors that produce insulin, glucagon, and VIP are more commonly found within the pancreas, whereas the tumors that produce gastrin are usually found within the duodenum. The goal of surgery is to remove these tumors without excessive morbidity and mortality.

Patients with MEN-1 may have concomitant primary hyperparathyroidism and Zollinger-Ellison syndrome. In this setting, studies show that surgery to correct the hyperparathyroidism greatly facilitates the management of Zollinger-Ellison syndrome by reducing serum levels of gastrin, gastric acid secretion, and the amount of medication needed to control gastric acid output. Because of this relation between high levels of calcium and gastrin, experts recommend surgery on the hyperplastic parathyroid glands in these patients before surgery for the gastrinoma.

Pituitary Tumors

Clinical Presentation and Evaluation

The most common pituitary tumor in MEN-1 is prolactinoma, which is associated with galactorrhea and impotence. Elevated serum levels of prolactin are diagnostic and are used as a screening study for pituitary tumors in individuals from kindreds with MEN-1. Pituitary tumors in MEN-1 may also secrete other hormones, including ACTH, growth hormone, and TSH. These tumors are associated with Cushing's disease, acromegaly, and hyperthyroidism, respectively. The biochemical diagnosis of each hormonal syndrome is based on the recognition of the clinical signs and symptoms. MRI or CT scan of the sella and visual field examination are obtained. Bitemporal hemianopsia can occur if very large tumors compress the optic chiasm.

Hypercortisolism in MEN-1 patients may have many etiologies. It can be caused by a pituitary adenoma, an ectopic ACTH-producing carcinoid or islet cell tumor, or an adrenal cortical tumor. Complete evaluation is necessary to determine the precise cause. Studies include a dexamethasone suppression test, petrosal sinus sampling, and imaging studies of the pituitary, adrenals and, if ectopic ACTH is suspected, either CT or MRI scan of the chest and pancreas.

Treatment

Pituitary adenomas that produce prolactin are usually treated with bromocriptine. Pituitary tumors can also be removed surgically. Less commonly, they are treated with irradiation. Patients with hypercortisolism should have the responsible tumor removed surgically.

Less Common Tumors

Less common tumors that appear to be associated with MEN-1 include bronchial or thymic carcinoids, intestinal carcinoids, gastric carcinoids, lipomas, benign adenomas of the thyroid gland, benign adrenocortical adenomas and, rarely, adrenal cortical carcinoma. Carcinoid tumors are malignant and should be removed surgically when identified. Cortical adenomas of the thyroid gland and benign cortical adenomas of the adrenal cortex usually require no treatment unless there is evidence of excessive hormonal function. Lipomas in MEN-1 patients are usually large and are excised when symptomatic.

Multiple Endocrine Neoplasia Type 2A, Type 2B, and Familial Medullary Thyroid Carcinoma

MEN-2A, formerly called Sipple's syndrome, is an autosomal dominant inherited endocrine syndrome that is characterized by MTC, adrenal **pheochromocytoma,** and parathyroid hyperplasia. MEN-2B is an autosomal dominant inherited endocrine syndrome that is characterized by MTC, adrenal pheochromocytoma, and a characteristic phenotype that includes mucosal neuromas, puffy lips, bony abnormalities, marfanoid habitus, intestinal ganglioneuromas, and corneal nerve hypertrophy. The parathyroid disease that is characteristic of MEN-2A is not associated with MEN-2B. FMTC is characterized by an autosomal dominant inheritance of MTC without any other endocrine abnormalities (Table 20-6).

Genetic Defect in MEN-2

The gene for MEN-2A has been localized to the pericentromeric region of chromosome 10. The responsible gene is a transmembrane protein kinase receptor called **RET.** RET is an oncogene in that mutations enhance cellular growth. The exact mechanism by which RET enhances cellular growth is unknown.

Table 20-6. MEN-2A, MEN-2B, and FMTC: Genetic Abnormalities and Associated Diseases

Endocrine Syndrome	Chromosome	Gene	Direct Detection Test Available	Clinical Expression	Percentage Who Have Trait
MEN-2A	10	RET	Yes	MTC	100
				Pheochromocytoma	60
				Parathyroid hyperplasia	40
MEN-2B	10	RET	Yes	MTC	100
				Phenotype	100
				Pheochromocytoma	70
FMTC	10	RET	Yes	MTC	100

MEN, multiple endocrine neoplasia.
RET, a transmembrane protein kinase receptor.
MTC, medullary thyroid carcinoma.
FMTC, familial medullary thyroid carcinoma.

Recent studies detected missense mutations in RET in all patients with MEN-2A, MEN-2B, and FMTC. MEN-2A and FMTC mutations were identified within the extracellular portion of the molecule, whereas MEN-2B mutations were identified within the intracellular domain. Different mutations of the same gene are responsible for different, but similar, clinical syndromes (see Table 20-6).

Medullary Thyroid Carcinoma

MTC occurs in the parafollicular calcitonin-producing C-cells of the thyroid.

Clinical Presentation and Evaluation

Patients with MTC have abnormal plasma levels of calcitonin, both at baseline and after provocative testing with such agents as calcium, pentagastrin, or both. Screening for FMTC is performed by measuring plasma levels of calcitonin after the administration of provocative agents. In patients with MEN-2A, MTC generally appears between the ages of 5 and 25 years, before pheochromocytoma or primary hyperparathyroidism develops.

Recently, detection of RET mutations in the peripheral white blood cells of patients from kindreds with MEN-2A was used as a screening procedure to diagnose an affected individual. Because MTC develops in 100% of individuals with MEN-2A (see Table 20-6), total thyroidectomy is performed when RET mutations are detected (Figure 20-12). Before thyroid surgery, it is necessary to exclude pheochromocytoma by measuring 24-hour urine levels of VMA, metanephrines, and total catecholamines. When total thyroidectomy was performed on these patients based on genetic testing, either premalignant C-cell hyperplasia or in situ MTC was identified in each patient. This is the first instance in which a genetic test was used to diagnose a treatable cancer.

Individuals with MEN-2B have a characteristic phenotype marked by prognathism, puffy lips, poor dentition, mucosal neuromas, corneal nerve hypertrophy,

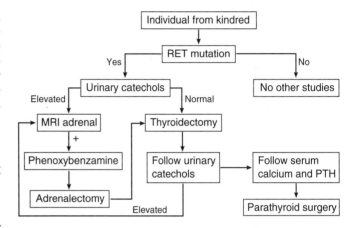

Figure 20-12 Flow diagram for multiple endocrine neoplasia type 2A. *MRI* = magnetic resonance imaging; *PTH* = parathyroid hormone.

and multiple bony abnormalities. MEN-2B is ascertained by the observation of corneal nerve hypertrophy on slit-lamp examination.

Treatment and Prognosis

Total thyroidectomy is indicated for patients with MEN-2A, MEN-2B, and FMTC because each type involves both lobes of the gland. Because patients with MEN-2B usually have locally advanced MTC at presentation, they are seldom cured by thyroidectomy and usually die of disease. Individuals with FMTC have the best prognosis. In these patients, the MTC occurs at an older age and they seldom die. Thus, in the three different familial settings, although the same oncogene is affected, the virulence of the MTC is different. The most virulent form is MEN-2B, the intermediate form is MEN-2A, and the least virulent is FMTC.

Pheochromocytoma in MEN-2A and MEN-2B

Individuals with either MEN-2A or MEN-2B may have bilateral benign intraadrenal pheochromocytomas.

Clinical Presentation and Evaluation

The diagnosis of pheochromocytoma is made by detection of elevated 24-hour urinary levels of VMA, metanephrines, or total catecholamines. Measurement of urinary metanephrines is the single best diagnostic study. Imaging studies can identify which adrenal gland is involved with tumor. CT, MRI, and metaiodobenzylguanidine (MIBG) scans each have utility. MRI scans have some specificity for pheochromocytoma based on signal characteristics of certain sequences. Both MRI and CT scans can image pheochromocytomas as small as 1 cm.

Treatment

Although adrenalectomy is considered the treatment of choice for pheochromocytoma in patients with MEN-2, there is controversy as to its extent. Some recommend bilateral adrenalectomy for all individuals with biochemical evidence of pheochromocytoma because studies show that 70% of cases are bilateral and sudden death can be caused by an unexpected pheochromocytoma. Others remove only the adrenal gland in which a tumor is identified. If unilateral adrenalectomy is performed, careful follow-up is warranted because in some patients, another pheochromocytoma will develop in the contralateral adrenal gland. Because these tumors are relatively small (< 3 cm) and are not malignant in this setting, recent studies show that laparoscopic adrenalectomy is the method of choice to remove them. Resection is performed after the patient is prepared preoperatively with alpha-adrenergic blocking drugs (e.g., phenoxybenzamine).

Parathyroid Disease in MEN-2A

Patients with MEN-2A may also have symptomatic primary hyperparathyroidism. This condition is always caused by multiple gland disease (parathyroid hyperplasia). The diagnosis is ascertained by measurement of elevated serum levels of calcium and parathyroid hormone. The proper surgical treatment is either 3½-gland parathyroidectomy or 4-gland parathyroidectomy with transplant.

Gastrointestinal Manifestations

Some individuals with MEN-2A may also have Hirschsprung's disease. Recent evidence suggests that Hirschsprung's disease is also associated with RET mutations. Individuals with MEN-2B commonly have severe constipation, and they may have megacolon and diverticular disease at a young age. These patients have abnormal gut motility secondary to intestinal ganglioneuromatosis. Constipation should be treated as symptoms arise. As the MTC becomes metastatic, patients with MEN-2B may have severe secretory diarrhea as a result of the secretion of a wide variety of peptide hormones that cause diarrhea. Octreotide is useful in inhibiting the diarrhea secondary to excessive hormone secretion.

Multiple-Choice Questions

Thyroid Gland

1. Which one of the following hormones is associated with medullary carcinoma of the thyroid?
   A. Thyroxine
   B. Thyroid-stimulating hormone (TSH)
   C. Calcitonin
   D. Thyrotropin-releasing hormone (TRH)
   E. Glucagon

2. What is the preferred treatment of medullary carcinoma of the left lobe of the thyroid gland without obvious lymph node or distant metastases?
   A. Left thyroid lobectomy and isthmectomy
   B. Total bilateral thyroidectomy
   C. Left thyroid lobectomy and subtotal right thyroid lobectomy
   D. Total thyroidectomy and central neck dissection
   E. Left thyroid lobectomy and postoperative treatment with L-thyroxine sodium (Synthroid)

3. A firm, solitary, "cold" nodule in the lateral aspect of the left lobe of the thyroid in a 20-year-old woman is best treated by:
   A. Irradiation (radioactive iodine)
   B. Thyroid suppression with thyroxine
   C. Incisional biopsy and enucleation if benign
   D. Total thyroidectomy
   E. Left thyroid lobectomy

4. What is the best initial therapeutic approach in a 60-year-old woman with previously untreated thyroid cancer, skull metastasis, and cervical lymph adenopathy?
   A. Total thyroidectomy and removal of involved lymph nodes
   B. Systemic chemotherapy
   C. ^{131}I radiation therapy
   D. External beam megavoltage radiation therapy to the skull and neck
   E. Suppressive thyroid hormone therapy

5. Graves' disease in a 50-year-old woman is usually treated by:
   A. Radioactive iodine
   B. Early operation
   C. Propranolol
   D. Antithyroid medication, then operation if not effective
   E. Thyroxine suppression

6. Carcinoma of the thyroid in children is most often associated with:
   A. Irradiation
   B. High autoimmune antibody titer in the mother during pregnancy
   C. Viral infection
   D. Iodine-deficient diet
   E. Alteration in serum gamma globulins

7. The most common complication after thyroidectomy is:
   A. Transient hypoparathyroidism
   B. Permanent hypoparathyroidism
   C. Pneumothorax
   D. Paralysis of the laryngeal nerve
   E. Hemorrhage

8. The most common complication after radioactive iodine therapy for hyperthyroidism is:
   A. Tetany
   B. Myxedema
   C. Agranulocytosis
   D. Secondary carcinoma
   E. Riedel's struma

9. All of the following suggest that a thyroid nodule could be malignant EXCEPT:
   A. The nodule scans "hot"
   B. The patient is a child
   C. The patient has a history of x-ray treatment to the head and neck
   D. There is only a single lesion by scan
   E. It is a "cold" nodule of recent onset in a male patient

10. A solitary nodule of the thyroid:
    A. Usually produces pain
    B. Is usually cystic
    C. May be treated with radioactive iodine
    D. Is usually functional on radioactive iodine scan
    E. Requires excision if it is persistent

11. Which patient has the highest possibility of thyroid cancer?
    A. A woman with a single "cold" thyroid nodule
    B. A man with a single "cold" thyroid nodule
    C. A woman with a single "hot" thyroid nodule
    D. A man with diffuse nontoxic goiter
    E. A man with diffuse toxic goiter

12. The inferior thyroid artery commonly comes directly from the:
    A. Thyrocervical trunk
    B. Subclavian artery
    C. Vertebral artery
    D. Common carotid artery
    E. Internal carotid artery

13. In Graves' disease:
    A. Pretibial myxedema is rare
    B. The female:male ratio is 8:1
    C. The initial therapy is total thyroidectomy
    D. The serum level of thyroid-stimulating hormone is very high
    E. The most common cause is struma ovarii

14. Which type of thyroid carcinoma can be specifically diagnosed on the basis of a serum assay?
    A. Follicular carcinoma
    B. Papillary carcinoma

C. Mixed follicular and papillary carcinoma
D. Undifferentiated carcinoma
E. Medullary carcinoma

15. The superior thyroid artery directly originates from the:
    A. Common carotid artery
    B. External carotid artery
    C. Internal carotid artery
    D. Thyrocervical trunk
    E. Subclavian artery

16. The most common malignancy of the thyroid in young (< 40 years of age) patients is:
    A. Follicular carcinoma
    B. Papillary carcinoma
    C. Anaplastic or undifferentiated carcinoma
    D. Medullary carcinoma
    E. C-cell APUDoma

17. What is the most appropriate initial management for a 23-year-old woman with a recent-onset 2-cm thyroid nodule that yields typical follicular cells on fine-needle aspiration?
    A. Observation alone
    B. Radioactive iodine ablation
    C. Thyroid hormone administration to suppress thyroid-stimulating hormone
    D. Thyroid lobectomy
    E. Total thyroidectomy

Parathyroid Glands

18. The most common cause of hypercalcemia is:
    A. Milk-alkali syndrome
    B. Malignancy
    C. Hyperparathyroidism
    D. Prolonged bed rest
    E. Vitamin D intoxication

19. Hypercalcemia as a result of increased gastrointestinal absorption of calcium is associated with:
    A. Pheochromocytoma
    B. Adrenal insufficiency
    C. Vitamin D intoxication
    D. Prolonged bed rest
    E. Metastatic breast cancer

20. Elevated parathyroid hormone levels are seen in all of the following EXCEPT:
    A. Idiopathic hypercalciuria
    B. Tertiary hyperparathyroidism
    C. Furosemide (Lasix) diuresis
    D. Primary hyperparathyroidism
    E. Breast cancer

21. Patients with secondary hyperparathyroidism usually have:
    A. Low serum calcium levels
    B. High serum calcium levels
    C. Low serum phosphate levels

D. Normal serum phosphate levels

E. High 1,25-dihydroxyvitamin D levels

22. Match the following phrase with the best single response. Ectopic calcifications of the arterial tree often occur with:
    A. Primary hyperparathyroidism
    B. Secondary hyperparathyroidism
    C. Both
    D. Neither

23. Match the following phrase with the best single response. Urinary levels of calcium and phosphate are high:
    A. Primary hyperparathyroidism
    B. Secondary hyperparathyroidism
    C. Both
    D. Neither

24. Primary hyperparathyroidism:
    A. Is usually associated with an adenoma
    B. Has elevated serum calcium and phosphate
    C. Is often caused by chronic renal disease
    D. Has low parathormone levels because they are suppressed by elevated calcium levels
    E. Has low calcium levels and high parathormone levels

25. What is the most consistent laboratory finding and best screening test in the diagnostic evaluation of primary hyperparathyroidism?
    A. Low serum phosphorus
    B. Hypercalciuria
    C. Hypocalciuria
    D. Persistent hypercalcemia
    E. High urinary phosphate

26. What is the least likely diagnosis in a patient who has hypercalcemia?
    A. Metastatic cancer
    B. Sarcoidosis
    C. Pancreatitis
    D. Hyperparathyroidism
    E. Vitamin D intoxication

27. Match the following phrase with the best single response. Significant skeletal disease is common in:
    A. Primary hyperparathyroidism
    B. Secondary hyperparathyroidism
    C. Both
    D. Neither

28. Match the following phrase with the best single response. Elevated serum parathormone levels occur in:
    A. Primary hyperparathyroidism
    B. Secondary hyperparathyroidism
    C. Both
    D. Neither

29. Match the following phrase with the best single response. Elevated serum calcium levels occur in:
    A. Primary hyperparathyroidism
    B. Secondary hyperparathyroidism
    C. Both
    D. Neither

Adrenal Glands

30. All of the following features are seen in primary aldosteronism EXCEPT:
    A. Hypertension
    B. Metabolic alkalosis
    C. Hypokalemia
    D. Muscle weakness
    E. Somatic abnormalities

31. The sodium loading test confirms the diagnosis of primary aldosteronism if:
    A. Plasma renin activity and serum aldosterone levels are both elevated after days of loading
    B. Plasma renin levels are reduced and serum aldosterone levels remain elevated
    C. Urinary sodium is decreased from the baseline level
    D. Serum sodium is decreased significantly
    E. Metabolic acidosis worsens dramatically

32. In addition to hypokalemia, the following is noted in primary aldosteronism:
    A. Acidosis
    B. Hyponatremia
    C. Tetany
    D. Edema
    E. Normal or low urine aldosterone

33. Spironolactone (a competitive antagonist of aldosterone) should not be used for:
    A. Confirmation of the diagnosis of primary aldosteronism
    B. Preoperative correction of metabolic and electrolyte abnormalities
    C. Treatment of idiopathic hyperaldosteronism
    D. Treatment of secondary hyperaldosteronism associated with refractory ascites
    E. Definitive treatment of primary aldosteronism

34. The most valuable test to localize an adrenal tumor is:
    A. Computed tomography scan of the abdomen
    B. Selective arteriography
    C. Selective phlebography
    D. Selective adrenal venous sampling
    E. Iodocholesterol scan of the adrenals

35. The treatment of choice in primary "hyperaldosteronism" is:
    A. Surgical excision of the diseased gland
    B. Spironolactone, high potassium intake, and a low-sodium diet
    C. Subtotal adrenalectomy

D. Embolization of the adrenal artery and vein during arteriography and phlebography

E. Antihypertensives with potassium supplements

36. Pheochromocytoma:
    A. Always originates in the adrenal medulla
    B. May originate in the adrenal cortex and extra-adrenal paraganglionic system
    C. Is malignant in most cases
    D. Is often associated with facial pallor, tremor, weight gain, and hypoglycemia
    E. May occur in adults or children

37. Pheochromocytomas are:
    A. Part of the watery diarrhea, hypokalemia, and achlorhydria (WDHA) syndrome
    B. Frequently bilateral (> 30% of the time)
    C. Frequently multiple (> 20% of the time)
    D. Frequently extraabdominal (> 20% of the time)
    E. Occasionally found incidentally

38. Hypertension associated with a pheochromocytoma can be:
    A. Paroxysmal
    B. Characterized by extreme fluctuations superimposed on constant elevation
    C. Associated with severe headache, tachycardia, and pallor
    D. Associated with severe headache, bradycardia, and vomiting
    E. All of the above

39. Paroxysmal attacks of hypertension in pheochromocytoma may be precipitated by all the following EXCEPT:
    A. Exertion or trauma
    B. Drugs or alcohol
    C. Urination
    D. Smoking
    E. Phenoxybenzamine

40. Palpitations, neurofibromatosis, port wine spots, telangiectasis, and excessive sweating are seen in patients with:
    A. Pheochromocytoma
    B. Cushing's disease
    C. Adrenogenital syndrome
    D. Hyperaldosteronism
    E. Graves' disease

41. The diagnosis of pheochromocytoma requires:
    A. Measurement of vanillylmandelic acid (VMA) in the blood
    B. Measurement of catecholamines and their metabolic products in the urine
    C. Demonstration of high norepinephrine levels in the adrenal vein
    D. Blockage with α- and β-blockers
    E. Demonstration of paroxysmal hypertension by provocative tests

42. Cushing's syndrome is least likely to be associated with:
    A. Exogenous prednisone intake in patients with liver disease
    B. Pituitary or extrapituitary tumors
    C. Adrenal carcinoma
    D. Exogenous cortisol administration
    E. Ovulatory menstrual cycles

43. Clinical features of Cushing's syndrome include all of the following EXCEPT:
    A. Weakness
    B. Psychological changes
    C. Truncal obesity
    D. Sexual dysfunction
    E. Osteitis deformans

44. Cushing's syndrome includes all of the following features EXCEPT:
    A. Hypertension
    B. Easy bruisability
    C. Hirsutism
    D. "Buffalo hump"
    E. Ganglioneuromatosis

45. In Cushing's syndrome secondary to adrenal hyperplasia, the source of excess cortisol secretion and the zone of hyperplastic cells is most likely the:
    A. Zona fasciculata
    B. Zona glomerulosa
    C. Zona reticularis
    D. Zona medullaris
    E. Zona pigmentosa

46. The most common cause of Cushing's syndrome is:
    A. Carcinoma of the adrenal cortex
    B. Ectopic adrenocorticotropic hormone (ACTH) secretion
    C. Adenoma of the adrenal cortex
    D. Adrenal medullary hyperplasia
    E. Basophilic tumor of the anterior pituitary

47. The preoperative evaluation of a patient with a suspected pheochromocytoma should include:
    A. Computed tomography (CT) scan of the abdomen
    B. Pituitary tomogram
    C. Urinary 5-hydroxyindoleacetic acid (5-HIAA) assay
    D. Hollander test
    E. Liver scan to identify hepatic metastases

48. All of the following are pertinent in the evaluation of an incidentally discovered adrenal mass EXCEPT:
    A. Serum prolactin level
    B. Careful history and physical examination
    C. Computed tomography (CT) scan of the abdomen
    D. A history of lung carcinoma
    E. Adrenal scintigraphy (^{59}NP scan)

49. All of the following are true of adrenal cortical carcinoma EXCEPT:
    A. Cushing's syndrome is the most common presentation of a functional adrenal cortical carcinoma
    B. They have a predilection for extension into the adrenal vein
    C. They are easily distinguished from pheochromocytomas on magnetic resonance imaging (MRI)
    D. Women with virilizing tumors have hirsutism, temporal balding, increased muscle mass, and amenorrhea
    E. Patients have a median survival of less than 9 months

Multiple Endocrine Neoplasia Syndromes

50. In the surgical treatment of patients with multiple endocrine neoplasia syndrome type 2A (MEN-2A), which tumor should be removed first?
    A. Neuroma
    B. Pheochromocytoma
    C. Medullary carcinoma
    D. Pituitary tumor
    E. Parathyroid adenoma

51. What is the recommended treatment for the parathyroid glands in patients with multiple endocrine neoplasia syndrome type 2B (MEN-2B)?
    A. Removal of 3½ glands
    B. Removal of the parathyroid adenoma
    C. No surgery
    D. Subtotal parathyroidectomy
    E. Removal of only the affected glands

52. Gastrinoma is most commonly associated with which familial endocrine syndrome?
    A. Multiple endocrine neoplasia syndrome type 2A (MEN-2A)
    B. MEN-2B
    C. MEN-1
    D. Familial medullary thyroid carcinoma (FMTC)
    E. von Hippel-Lindau (VHL) syndrome

53. Pheochromocytoma is part of which familial endocrine syndrome?
    A. Multiple endocrine neoplasia syndrome type 2A (MEN-2A)
    B. MEN-1
    C. Familial medullary thyroid carcinoma (FMTC)
    D. Primary hyperparathyroidism
    E. Toxic megacolon

54. Which syndrome is associated with pituitary adenoma?
    A. Multiple endocrine neoplasia syndrome type 2A (MEN-2A)
    B. MEN-2B
    C. Familial medullary thyroid carcinoma (FMTC)

    D. MEN-1
    E. MEN-3

55. Parathyroid gland hyperplasia is associated with all of the following EXCEPT:
    A. Multiple endocrine neoplasia syndrome type 2A (MEN-2A)
    B. MEN-2B
    C. MEN-1
    D. Elevated calcium
    E. Elevated parathyroid hormone

56. Medullary carcinoma of the thyroid is part of all of the following syndromes EXCEPT:
    A. Multiple endocrine neoplasia syndrome type 2A (MEN-2A)
    B. MEN-2B
    C. Familial medullary thyroid carcinoma (FMTC)
    D. von Hippel-Lindau (VHL) syndrome
    E. Sipple's syndrome

57. A RET gene mutation is responsible for the pathologic syndrome associated with all of the following multiple endocrine neoplasia (MEN) syndromes EXCEPT:
    A. MEN-2A
    B. Familial medullary thyroid carcinoma (FMTC)
    C. MEN-2B
    D. MEN-1
    E. Sipple's syndrome

58. In patients with multiple endocrine neoplasia syndrome type 1 (MEN-1) who have primary hyperparathyroidism and Zollinger-Ellison syndrome, which operation should be done first?
    A. Excision of the islet cell tumor
    B. Total parathyroidectomy and forearm transplant
    C. Total gastrectomy
    D. Resection of the pituitary adenoma
    E. Laparotomy

59. Patients with multiple endocrine neoplasia syndrome type 1 (MEN-1) have a greater propensity to each of the following tumors except:
    A. Parathyroid hyperplasia
    B. Pancreatic islet cell tumors
    C. Bronchial or thymic carcinoid tumors
    D. Pheochromocytoma
    E. Lipomas

60. A potentially malignant tumor in a patient with multiple endocrine neoplasia syndrome type 1 (MEN-1) is:
    A. Islet cell tumor
    B. Parathyroid cancer
    C. Pituitary adenoma
    D. Medullary thyroid cancer
    E. Pheochromocytoma

Oral Examination Study Questions Thyroid

CASE 1

A 24-year-old woman has an asymptomatic 3-cm neck mass that she noticed 1 week ago. She is otherwise well.

OBJECTIVE 1

The student describes the initial evaluation of this patient.

A. A family history and a history of radiation exposure are obtained; both are negative.

B. On physical examination, the patient has a 3-cm thyroid nodule. The TSH level is normal.

The student requests an FNA of the thyroid mass.

OBJECTIVE 2

The student lists the different types of thyroid carcinoma and discusses the appropriate therapeutic strategies.

A. Well-differentiated: papillary, follicular

B. Medullary

C. Anaplastic

The FNA is consistent with papillary carcinoma.

OBJECTIVE 3

The student selects an appropriate operation.

A. Total thyroidectomy

B. Total thyroidectomy with central lymph node dissection

C. Thyroidectomy to relieve airway compromise, followed by radiation and chemotherapy

OBJECTIVE 4

The student discusses the follow-up strategies and long-term treatment of the patient.

A. Perform a physical examination and order a radionuclide scan and a thyroglobulin test.

B. Order a calcitonin test.

C. Patients rarely survive long term.

Minimum Level of Achievement for Passing

The student obtains a diagnosis of papillary carcinoma. The student knows the treatment for papillary carcinoma, including follow-up strategies and prognostic variables.

Honors Level of Achievement

The student knows that follicular carcinoma is more aggressive than papillary carcinoma, that there is discussion about the extent of surgical resection for well-differentiated carcinomas, and that small lesions (< 1.0 cm) may be treated with lobectomy. The student knows that Hürthle cell carcinoma is a variant of follicular carcinoma. For follow-up, the student knows that the scan should be performed with ^{131}I rather than ^{99m}Tc and that it should be performed after hormone replacement is discontinued. The student also knows that multicentricity and lymph node metastases are common. The student is familiar with MEN-2 syndrome and can enumerate the components of MEN-1 and MEN-2. The student describes the role of calcitonin in calcium homeostasis. The student also knows that the cell of origin is believed to be the follicular cell, which is almost totally dedifferentiated.

Parathyroid Glands

CASE 1

You are asked to see a 66-year-old woman because her serum calcium was elevated on a routine admission sequential multiplier analyzer (SMA)-12 examination.

OBJECTIVE 1

The student elicits the following important information.

A. The patient had two previous attacks of renal colic, 5 and 8 years previously. She has polyuria, nocturia, and polydipsia.

B. The patient has easy fatigability.

C. The patient had no recent weight loss.

D. Physical examination shows a blood pressure of 180/96 mm Hg and a pulse rate of 84 beats/min, with no other positive physical findings.

OBJECTIVE 2

The student cites a differential diagnosis of hypercalcemia in a 66-year-old white woman.

A. Primary hyperparathyroidism
   1. Parathyroid adenoma
   2. Parathyroid hyperplasia
   3. Parathyroid cancer

B. Malignancy, including the following:
   1. Cancer of the breast
   2. Hematologic malignancy
   3. Multiple myeloma

C. Milk-alkali syndrome, granulomatous disease, thiazide therapy

OBJECTIVE 3

The student lists appropriate x-rays and laboratory studies that are pertinent to the differential diagnosis.

A. Repeat calcium, phosphorus, magnesium, alkaline phosphatase, parathyroid hormone, urine calcium, serum chloride, uric acid levels, and protein electrophoresis.

B. X-rays of the hands, skull, and clavicles; and of the kidney, ureter, and bladder

ADDITIONAL QUESTIONS

1. Elevated parathyroid hormone and calcium levels establish primary hyperparathyroidism as the diagnosis. Does the extent of elevation distinguish adenoma from hyperplasia? (No.)

2. At surgery, a single enlarged red-brown gland is identified. On frozen section, it appears abnormal. Biopsy is performed on two other glands that are believed to be normal on frozen section. A fourth gland is not found. What is the diagnosis? (Adenoma.)

Minimum Level of Achievement for Passing

The student includes the diagnosis of primary hyperparathyroidism and describes adenoma and hyperplasia of the parathyroids as potential causes.

Honors Level of Achievement

The student establishes a treatment plan for parathyroid adenoma and parathyroid hyperplasia. The student also answers one or more of the additional questions.

Adrenal Glands

CASE 1

A 42-year-old man has uncontrolled hypertension of 6 months' duration. He is taking quadruple-drug antihypertensives, and his blood pressure remains at 180/100 mm Hg consistently.

OBJECTIVE 1

The student obtains a pertinent history.

A. The patient has no history of smoking, myocardial infarction, stroke, claudication, diabetes, or other manifestations of atherosclerotic disease.

B. There is no history of frequent sore throats, nephritis, or thyroid disorder.

C. The patient has no symptoms of edema, weight gain, Raynaud's syndrome, or fever.

D. The patient has symptoms of nervousness, flushing, and palpitations.

E. The only medication that the patient is taking is antihypertensives.

F. There is no family history of significant hypertension or thyroid disease.

OBJECTIVE 2

The student performs a pertinent physical examination and forms a differential diagnosis.

A. The pulse is regular at 100 beats/min, blood pressure is 175/100 mm Hg, and temperature is 37.5°C.

B. Examination of the head, eyes, ears, nose, and throat shows no abnormalities. The neck shows no mass or bruit. The chest is clear. The heart has prominent point of maximal impulse (PMI), with a systolic ejection murmur. The abdomen shows no mass or bruit. The results of the peripheral examination are normal. The central nervous system shows deep tendon reflexes and is otherwise normal.

C. Causes of hypertension
   1. Essential hypertension is possible.
   2. Renovascular hypertension must be excluded with measurement of plasma renins, duplex scanning, or arteriogram.
   3. Hyperthyroidism is not likely, but must be ruled out.
   4. Cushing's syndrome is not usually seen with uncontrolled hypertension, but should be considered and ruled out.
   5. Hyperaldosteronism is unlikely with this level of hypertension and normal serum K^+.
   6. Coarctation of the aorta is ruled out by pulses and arteriogram.
   7. Unilateral renal parenchymal disease is ruled out by intravenous pyelogram, CT scan, and IV contrast, or by renal scanning.
   8. Pheochromocytoma is a possibility.

OBJECTIVE 3

The student obtains a pertinent laboratory examination.

A. Complete blood count, electrolytes, blood urea nitrogen, creatinine, calcium, and phosphorus are normal. The glucose level is 240 mg/dL.

B. Results of thyroid function tests are normal.

C. Results of intravenous pyelogram are normal.

D. Peripheral renin activity is normal.

E. Results of 24-hour urine test for catecholamines and VMA show elevated urinary epinephrine, norepinephrine, metanephrine, normetanephrine, and VMA.

F. Chest x-ray and electrocardiogram are normal.

G. CT scan of the chest and abdomen shows a 3-cm mass overlying the aorta, just above the bifurcation.

H. Vena caval catheterization is not necessary, but shows increased norepinephrine above the mass.

I. Duplex scan shows no renal artery stenosis.

OBJECTIVE 4

The student makes the diagnosis of an extraadrenal pheochromocytoma (paraganglionoma of the organ of Zuckerkandl) and plans surgical removal. The student orders the following:

A. Preoperative volume expansion

B. Preoperative alpha-adrenergic blockade (phenoxybenzamine 1–20 mg, 2 to 4 times daily for 7 to 10 days)

C. Propranolol for arrhythmias preoperatively

D. Nitroprusside for the management of intraoperative hypertension with manipulation of the tumor

Minimum Level of Achievement for Passing

The student knows most of the causes of hypertension, including the surgically correctable causes. The student also makes the diagnosis of pheochromocytoma by ruling out the other causes, obtaining a 12- or 24-hour urinary test, or measuring serum metanephrines (if available). The student knows that surgery is the treatment of choice and that preoperative preparation is essential.

Honors Level of Achievement

The student considers the additional diagnosis of MEN-2 (parathyroid adenoma, medullary carcinoma of the thyroid, and bilateral pheochromocytoma or medullary hyperplasia). The student knows which antihypertensives might interfere with 24-hour catecholamine tests (clonidine and Aldomet elevate urinary catecholamines) and should know that alpha (and possibly beta) blockade is necessary before surgery. The student also explains the increased glucose level (catecholamine effect).

Multiple Endocrine Neoplasia Syndromes

CASE 1

A 65-year-old man with a history of peptic ulcer disease with intractable pain and diarrhea of 3 years' duration comes to the office. Please complete the history, physical examination workup, and management.

OBJECTIVE 1

In addition to obtaining the usual ulcer history, the student investigates the possibility of MEN-1 and obtains a positive history of some of the following.

A. The patient has a family history of peptic ulcer disease, diarrhea, renal lithiasis, and pituitary tumors.

B. The patient has a history of renal lithiasis, visual problems, loss of weight, and bone pains.

OBJECTIVE 2

The student suspects MEN-1, including parathyroid hyperplasia, a non-β-cell pancreatic adenoma, or a pituitary adenoma.

OBJECTIVE 3

The student obtains a laboratory workup, including the following.

A. Ca^{2+}, P, alkaline phosphatase, prolactin level, and fasting blood sugar

B. Upper endoscopy, basal acid output, or acidic pH of the gastric contents

C. Serum gastrin levels

D. Serum insulin levels

E. Sella turcica MRI

F. Parathyroid hormone levels

G. CT scan of the pancreas

H. Octreoscan

OBJECTIVE 4

The student initiates medical treatment for Zollinger-Ellison syndrome: omeprazole 20 mg orally twice a day.

OBJECTIVE 5

The student discusses the recommended treatment for the following:

A. Parathyroid hyperplasia

B. Pituitary tumor

C. Insulinoma

D. Zollinger-Ellison syndrome

Minimum Level of Achievement for Passing

The student realizes that MEN-1 is associated with peptic ulcer disease and includes hyperplasia of the parathyroids, adenoma of the pancreas, and adenoma of the pituitary.

Honors Level of Achievement

The student knows the diagnostic workup and treatment of parathyroid hyperplasia, parathyroid adenoma, insulinoma, and Zollinger-Ellison syndrome.

CASE 2

A 28-year-old man is referred for evaluation of a 2-cm nodule in the left upper lobe of the thyroid gland, which is nonfunctioning by scan. Serum T_3 and T_4 levels are normal. The history is remarkable only for hypertension, which is poorly controlled.

OBJECTIVE 1

The student elicits the following important points in the history.

A. The patient has a history of palpitations and diaphoretic episodes.

B. The family history shows that 10 years previously, the patient's father died unexpectedly while undergoing an operative procedure on his thyroid gland.

OBJECTIVE 2

With the historical points obtained earlier, the student pursues the diagnostic workup for MEN-2 syndrome. Steps include:

A. Obtaining a serum calcitonin level

B. Evaluating the patient for pheochromocytoma, including urine metanephrines, normetaephrines, catecholamines, serum epinephrine (and norepinephrine, if desired), and most likely a CT scan of the abdomen to attempt to determine location

C. Evaluating parathyroid gland function, including serum calcium, phosphate, possibly a chloride:phosphate ratio, and serum parathormone levels

D. Measurement of the RET gene mutation in white blood cells

OBJECTIVE 3

After the student establishes the diagnosis of medullary carcinoma of the thyroid gland and pheochromocytoma with the information obtained earlier (assume normal parathyroid function), the student should plan the following therapeutic maneuvers:

A. The initial operative procedure in MEN-2 syndrome is bilateral adrenalectomy with careful exploration of the entire intraabdominal cavity. This exploration should be preceded by preparation of the patient with alpha-adrenergic blocking and possibly beta-adrenergic blocking agents.

B. Subsequent treatment of medullary carcinoma includes total thyroidectomy with formal radical neck dissection if there is involvement of the cervical lymph nodes.

C. Postoperative follow-up includes periodic determinations of serum thyrocalcitonin levels as well as screening of the patient's family for other members who may have occult MEN-2 syndrome.

Minimum Level of Achievement for Passing

The student obtains a diagnosis of medullary thyroid carcinoma and pheochromocytoma and makes the association with MEN-2 syndrome. The student also knows the treatment for medullary carcinoma of the thyroid and pheochromocytoma.

Honors Level of Achievement

The honors student differentiates between MEN-2A and MEN-2B. The student also knows that MEN-2B syndrome is characterized by a marfanoid body habitus, mucosal ganglioneuromas, and an absence of parathyroid gland involvement. The student points out that a medullary carcinoma seen with MEN-2B syndrome appears at an early age and is a particularly aggressive tumor. The student is also familiar with RET.

SUGGESTED READINGS

Thyroid Gland

Hyperthyroidism

Orgiazzi J, Mornex R. Hyperthyroidism. In: Greer MA, ed. *Comprehensive Endocrinology: The Thyroid Gland.* New York: Raven Press, 1990.

Soh Y, Duh Q-Y. Diagnosis and management of hot nodules (Plummer's disease). *Probl Gen Surg* 1997;14:165.

Winsa B, Rastad J, Larrson E, et al. Total thyroidectomy in therapy-resistant Graves' disease. *Surgery* 1994;116:1068.

Thyroid Carcinoma

DeGroot LJ, Kaplan EL, Strauss FH, Shukla MS. Does the method of management of papillary thyroid carcinoma make a difference in outcome? *World J Surg* 1994;18:123.

Gagel RF, Goepfert H, Callender DL. Changing concepts in the pathogenesis and management of thyroid carcinoma. Ca Cancer J Clin 1996:46:261.

Mazzaferri EL, Sissy MJ. Long-term impact of initial surgical and medical therapy on papillary and follicular cancer. *Am J Med* 1994;97:418.

Schlumberger MJ. Papillary and follicular thyroid carcinoma. *N Engl J Med* 1998;338;297.

Schneider AB, Shore-Freedman E, Weinstein RA. Radiation-induced thyroid and other head and neck tumors: occurrence of multiple tumors and analysis of risk factors. *J Clin Endocrinol Metab* 1986;63:107.

Thyroid Nodule

Rojeski MT, Gharib H. Nodular thyroid disease: evaluation and management. *N Engl J Med* 1985;313:428.

Studer H, Gerber H. Non-toxic goiter. In: Greer MA, ed. *The Thyroid Gland.* New York: Raven Press, 1990.

Wool MS. Evaluation of thyroid nodules. In: Cady B, Rossi RL, eds. *Surgery of the Thyroid and Parathyroid Glands,* 3rd ed. Philadelphia, Pa: WB Saunders, 1991.

Parathyroid Glands

Bilezikian JP. Management of acute hypercalcemia. *N Engl J Med* 1992;326(18):1196-1203.

Lafferty FW. Differential diagnosis of hypercalcemia. *J Bone Miner Res* 1991;6 Suppl 2:S51–59.

Ljunghall S, Hellman P, Rastad J, Akerstrom G. Primary hyperparathyroidism: epidemiology, diagnosis and clinical picture. *World J Surg* 1991;15(6):681–687.

Mallette LE. Regulation of blood calcium in humans. *Endocrinol Metab Clin North Am* 1989;18(3):601–610.

Strewler GJ. Indications for surgery in patients with minimally symptomatic primary hyperparathyroidism. *Surg Clin North Am* 1995;75(3):439–447.

Adrenal Glands

Findling JW, Doppman JL. Biochemical and radiologic diagnosis of Cushing's syndrome. *Endocrinol Metab Clin North Am* 1994;23:511–537.

Halpin VJ, Norton JA. Adrenal insufficiency. In: Wilmore DW, et al., eds. ACS Care of the Surgical Patient. *Sci Am* 1997.

Scott HW. Surgery of the adrenal glands. Philadelphia, Pa: JB Lippincott, 1990.

Multiple Endocrine Neoplasia Syndromes

Norton JA. Neuroendocrine tumors of the pancreas and duodenum. *Curr Probl Surg* 1994:77–164.

Veldhuis JD, Norton JA, Wells SA Jr, et al. Therapeutic controversy: surgical versus medical management of multiple endocrine neoplasia (MEN) type I. *J Clin Endocrinol Metab* 1997;82:357–364.

21

Spleen

James C. Hebert, M.D.
Kennith H. Sartorelli, M.D.

OBJECTIVES

1. Discuss the anatomy and functions of the spleen.
2. Discuss the workup and management of a patient with splenic injury.
3. Discuss the role of splenectomy in hematologic abnormalities.
4. Distinguish between splenomegaly and hypersplenism, and discuss their causes.
5. Discuss the consequences of splenectomy and the potential methods to reduce the associated risks.

To many of the ancients, the spleen was an enigma. At one time, functions such as laughter and swiftness were attributed to the spleen. We now realize that the spleen, the largest mass of lymphoid tissue in the body, plays a key role in maintaining the integrity of an individual's immune and hematologic status.

Anatomy

The spleen develops from the dorsal mesogastrium and is present by the sixth week of gestation. The spleen resides in the left upper quadrant of the abdomen, which is bounded by the diaphragm superiorly and the lower thoracic cage anterolaterally. The spleen is intimately associated with the pancreas, stomach, left kidney, colon, and diaphragm by a series of suspensory ligaments (Figure 21-1). The ligaments of the spleen are also derived from the dorsal mesogastrium. The splenorenal, gastrosplenic, splenocolic, and splenophrenic ligaments provide direct fixation of the spleen to the left upper quadrant. The short gastric vessels run through the gastrosplenic ligament. The splenic vessels and the tail of the pancreas traverse the splenorenal ligament. Laxity of the splenic ligaments may cause excessive mobility of the spleen, allowing it access to the lower quadrants of the abdomen (wandering spleen). This condition is treated with splenopexy to the left upper abdomen. The spleen is encased in a capsule that

becomes thin and fibrotic by adulthood. Traction on the spleen or its supporting ligaments by blunt or operative trauma may cause bleeding from capsular avulsion. A normal spleen weighs between 75 and 150 g and is the size of the patient's fist.

The spleen is an extremely vascular organ that receives approximately 5% of the cardiac output. The organ has a dual arterial blood supply. The splenic artery provides the primary inflow, with additional contributions from the short gastric arteries (Figure 21-2). The splenic artery is a branch of the celiac artery and courses along the superior border of the pancreas, dividing into two or more branches before ultimately entering the spleen at its hilum. There are usually four to six short gastric arteries derived from the left gastroepiploic artery. Vexing bleeding from the short gastric vessels can be encountered during splenectomy or operations on the stomach (e.g., fundoplication).

Venous drainage of the spleen occurs through the splenic and short gastric veins. The course of the splenic vein parallels that of the splenic artery. The splenic vein joins the superior mesenteric vein to form the portal vein.

A variety of developmental disorders affect the spleen. The most common developmental anomaly is the presence of **accessory spleens** in addition to a normal spleen. Accessory spleens are found in 10% to 30% of the population and are believed to result from failure of separate splenic masses in the dorsal mesogastrium to fuse. These splenic buds are then carried to various locations by the migration of the splenic ligaments. The most common sites for accessory spleens, in order of decreasing frequency, are the splenic hilum, splenocolic ligament, gastrocolic ligament, splenorenal ligament, and omentum (Figure 21-3). Failure to recognize accessory spleens may lead to relapse of various hematologic disorders after splenectomy.

Polysplenia is the presence of multiple small spleens, with no normal spleen. Polysplenia is associated with multiple anomalies, including severe cardiac defects, situs inversus, and biliary atresia. Absence of the spleen (asplenia), a lethal condition, is also associated with severe cardiac anomalies and situs inversus. Splenogonadal fusion is a rare disorder of development, in which splenic tissue is found in the scrotum, often attached to the testicle.

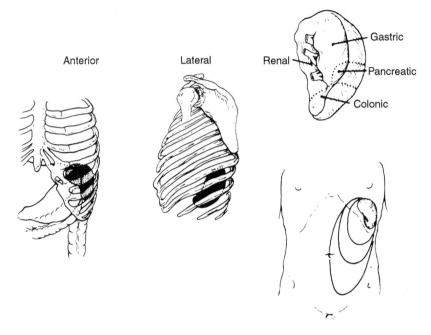

Figure 21-1 Normal external relations of the spleen.

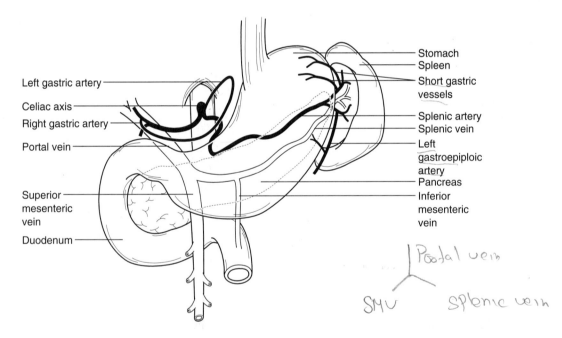

Figure 21-2 Blood supply to the spleen.

Physiology

The spleen has several distinct functions, including hematopoiesis, blood filtering, and immune modulation. The function of the spleen is intimately related to its microstructure. Central to its microstructure is its microcirculation (Figure 21-4). A trabecular meshwork of fibrous tissue joins the fibroelastic capsule to the hilum of the spleen and surrounds the entering blood vessels. Blood enters the splenic parenchyma through central arteries that branch off the trabecular arteries. These central arteries course through the **white pulp**, where they are surrounded by periarterial lymphatic sheaths that consist primarily of T-lymphocytes and macrophages that can process soluble antigens. Some blood flows into the surrounding lymphatic follicles, where B-lymphocytes can proliferate in germinal centers. Mature antibody-producing cells (plasma cells) are found here. Blood that leaves the white pulp flows into a marginal zone, where it is directed either back to the white pulp or through terminal arterioles into the **splenic cords of Billroth** in the **red pulp** (open circulation). In the reticular network of the cords, which have no endothelial cells, blood percolates slowly and comes into contact with numerous macrophages before they enter the endothelial-lined sinuses. The red pulp is the site of removal of antibody-sensitized cells and particulate material. In some pathologic conditions, blood is shunted from the marginal zone directly into the sinuses (closed circulation), bypassing much of the critical filtering function.

The spleen is a site of fetal extramedullary hematopoiesis, but this activity usually ceases by birth in normal humans.

In its capacity as a blood filter, the spleen culls abnormal and aged erythrocytes, granulocytes, and platelets from the nearly 350 L/day of blood that passes through it. As red blood cells near the end of their lives, they lose membrane integrity as a result of declining adenosine triphosphate levels. As a result, they are marked for destruction. Abnormal and senescent red blood cells cannot deform appropriately to enter the splenic sinuses through the fenestrations in the endothelium. Therefore, they are removed in the red pulp. In addition, as red blood cells deform to enter the splenic sinuses as they leave the red pulp, cellular inclusions are pinched off from the cells. This "pitting" function removes nuclear remnants, such as **Howell-Jolly bodies,** from red blood cells. It also removes other red blood cell inclusions, such as **Heinz bodies** (denatured hemoglobin) and **Pappenheimer bodies** (iron inclusions).

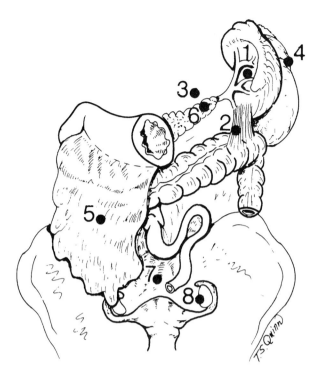

Figure 21-3 Normal internal relations of the spleen (stomach removed) and location of accessory spleens. **1,** Splenic hilum. **2,** Splenocolic ligament. **3,** Gastrocolic ligament. **4,** Splenorenal ligament. **5,** Greater omentum. **6,** Tail of the pancreas. **7,** Mesentery. **8,** Gonadal.

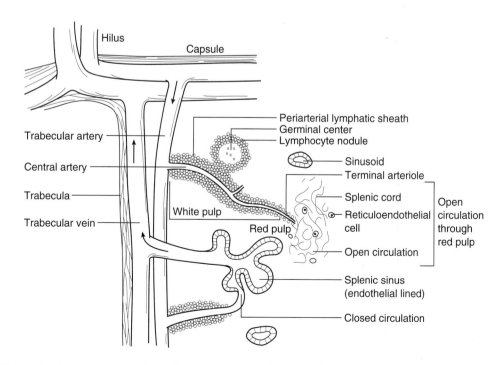

Figure 21-4 Microanatomy of the spleen, with its functional components, showing both open and closed circulations.

The role of the spleen in the sequestration and destruction of granulocytes and platelets under normal circumstances is not well understood. Normally, one-third of the body's platelets are stored in the spleen. Abnormal splenic processing of platelets occurs in several disease processes and causes marked thrombocytopenia. Splenectomy is usually followed by thrombocytosis.

The spleen plays an important role in the immune system and is part of the reticuloendothelial system. It also provides both nonspecific and specific immune responses. A nonspecific response has two arms: (1) clearance of opsonized particles and bacteria by fixed splenic macrophages, and (2) opsonin production. **Opsonins** that are produced by the spleen include properdin, tuftsin, and fibronectin. Properdin activates the alternative pathway of the complement system. Tuftsin facilitates macrophage phagocytosis. The specific immune response of the spleen includes antigen processing and antibody production by splenic lymphocytes that are present in the white pulp. The spleen is the body's largest producer of immunoglobulin M (IgM), and splenectomy causes a marked decrease in IgM and opsonin production. Because of its mass and its position in the circulation, the spleen probably plays a major role in modulating the systemic cytokine response to infection. However, little is understood about this role.

Pathophysiology

General Diagnostic Considerations

Physical Examination

A normal spleen is difficult to palpate because of its size and position. The long axis of the spleen is located behind and parallel to the tenth rib in the midaxillary line. A normal adult spleen is approximately 12 cm long and 7 cm wide. Splenic palpation and percussion are used to determine the size of the spleen. The edge of an enlarged spleen may be palpated at the costal margin and may extend into the left iliac fossa. Rarely, it crosses the midline into the right iliac fossa (see Figure 21-1). An enlarged spleen usually is not tender. Therefore, discomfort on palpation alerts the clinician to the possibility of an infective process, splenic infarction, or splenic trauma. Palpation of the spleen is accomplished either bimanually (Figure 21-5) or with Middleton's method (Figure 21-6). Table 21-1 shows the pathologic conditions that are associated with the need for splenectomy. Percussion of the spleen causes an area of splenic dullness in the left upper quadrant. Feces in the colon or fluid in the stomach may falsely suggest splenomegaly.

Radiographic Imaging

A variety of radiographic techniques are available to aid in the diagnosis and treatment of disorders of the spleen.

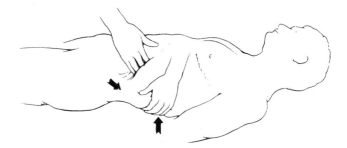

Figure 21-5 Bimanual palpation of the spleen.

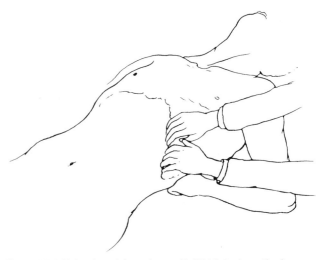

Figure 21-6 Palpation of the spleen with Middleton's method.

Plain Abdominal Roentgenogram

Abdominal x-rays may yield information that suggests splenomegaly as a result of displacement of the colon or stomach, an elevated left diaphragm, or a large splenic shadow (Figure 21-7). Left-sided rib fractures may suggest splenic trauma.

Ultrasound

Ultrasound is a useful tool to evaluate splenomegaly and to show splenic cysts or abscesses (Figure 21-8). Abdominal ultrasound is rapidly gaining acceptance as a means to evaluate patients with traumatic injury for the presence of hemoperitoneum and liver and spleen injuries as well as a means to follow healing splenic injuries. Gas within the intestinal tract may interfere with visualization of the spleen and other structures.

Computed tomography

Computed tomography (CT) scan is the most useful imaging technique to determine splenic size and detect injury (Figure 21-9). CT scans also provide useful information about other potential disease processes or injuries in adjacent organs. Splenic cysts and abscesses are clearly shown by CT scans, and percutaneous drainage can be performed under CT guidance. CT

Table 21-1. Indications for Splenectomy

Splenic rupture (repair of the spleen is preferred in certain patients)
    Trauma
    Spontaneous
    Iatrogenic injury
Hematologic disorders
    Hematolytic anemias
      Hereditary spherocytosis
      Hereditary elliptocytosis
      Thalassemia minor and major (rare)
      Autoimmune hemolytic anemia not responsive to steroid therapy
      Thrombocytopenia
      Idiopathic thrombocytopenic purpura
      Immunologic thrombocytopenia associated with chronic
        lymphocytic leukemia or systemic lupus erythemastosus
      Thrombotic thrombocytopenic purpura
Hypersplenism associated with other diseases
    Inflammation
    Infiltrative diseases
    Congestion
Leukemia and lymphoma
Other diseases
    Splenic abscess (often associated with drug abuse or AIDS)
    Primary and metastatic tumors
    Splenic cysts
    Splenic artery aneurysm

AIDS, Acquired immune deficiency syndrome.

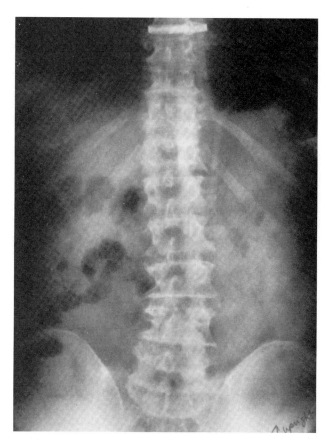

Figure 21-7 Plain film of the abdomen showing an enlarged spleen (radiopaque shadow in the left upper quadrant).

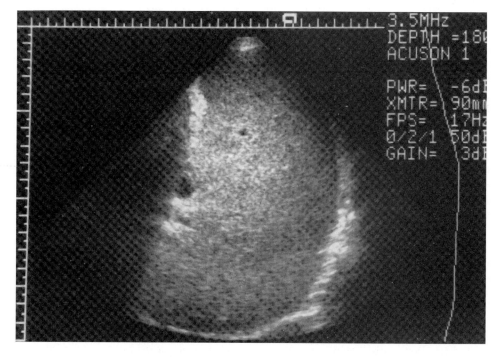

Figure 21-8 Ultrasound of the left upper quadrant showing an enlarged spleen. In this case, splenomegaly is secondary to myelofibrosis.

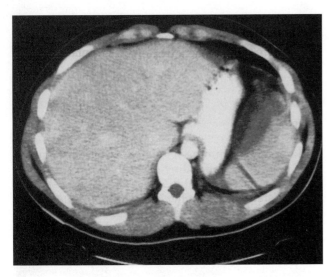

Figure 21-9 Computed tomography scan of the abdomen showing a subcapsular hematoma of the spleen.

Table 21-2. Grades of Splenic Injury

Grade	Description
I	Hematoma: Subcapsular <10% surface area Laceration: <1 cm deep
II	Hematoma: Subcapsular 10%–50% surface area Parenchymal <5 cm diameter
	Laceration: 1–3 cm deep, not involving trabecular vessels
III	Hematoma: Subcapsular > 50 % surface area Parenchymal > 5 cm diameter Any expanding or ruptured
	Laceration: > 3 cm deep or involving trabecular vessels
IV	Laceration: Segmental vessels involved with devascularization <50%
V	Completely shattered spleen or hilar vascular injury with devascularization

scans are useful to follow splenic injuries and to obtain information about the patency of splenic vessels.

Radionuclide scans

Colloid suspensions of technetium are taken up by the reticuloendothelial system and give information about splenic size and function. Radionuclide scans are useful to look for missed accessory spleens after unsuccessful splenectomy to control hematologic disorders.

Angiography

Angiography is useful in showing splenic vein thrombosis and aids in planning portal venous decompressive procedures. Angiography is also helpful in showing splenic tumors. Splenic artery embolization may be a useful adjunct to control bleeding before laparoscopic splenectomy. Partial splenic embolization is used to control hypersplenism in children with portal hypertension and to control bleeding in splenic injuries.

Surgical Disorders of the Spleen

The spleen is subject to a variety of disorders that may require surgical intervention (see Table 21-1). Trauma is the most common reason for splenectomy. Alternatives to splenectomy (e.g., partial splenectomy, embolization, image-guided percutaneous drainage procedures) are often used successfully.

Splenic Trauma

The spleen is the most commonly injured organ after blunt abdominal trauma and the second most commonly injured organ after penetrating abdominal trauma. Traditionally, injuries to the spleen were treated with prompt splenectomy. The recognition of the entity of **overwhelming postsplenectomy infection,** coupled with a better understanding of the immunologic function of the spleen, led to attempts at splenic preservation when feasible.

Clinical Presentation and Evaluation

Three general mechanisms of splenic injury occur: penetrating, blunt compressive, and blunt deceleration. The extent of penetrating injuries depends on the device used to create the injury (firearm vs knife). Penetrating trauma, particularly with firearms, often involves the splenic vasculature as well as adjacent organs. Because of the fixation of the spleen afforded by the splenic ligaments, the spleen is prone to blunt compressive injuries as well as capsular avulsion from rapid decelerations. In adults, the ribs may provide some protection to the spleen. However, rib fractures are present in 20% of spleen injuries, and the rib fragments may contribute to the spleen injury. The compliant thoracic cage of children provides little protection to the spleen from blunt forces. A scale of severity for splenic injuries was devised by the American Association for the Surgery of Trauma (Table 21-2). All patients should be resuscitated according to the guidelines of the Advanced Trauma Life Support Course of the American College of Surgeons.

In evaluating patients for splenic injury, the physician should look for signs and symptoms of local peritoneal irritation and acute hemorrhage. Signs of peritoneal irritation include left upper quadrant tenderness to palpation, pain at the top of the left shoulder **(Kehr's sign),** and percussion dullness of the left flank **(Ballance's sign).** When evaluating patients with penetrating trauma, it must be remembered that the diaphragm and underlying spleen may ascend as high as the fourth intercostal space during inspiration. Any penetrating injury from the level of the nipples down may traverse the peritoneal cavity, and patients with signs of intraperitoneal hemorrhage should undergo prompt celiotomy.

The evaluation of patients with blunt abdominal trauma is complicated by the high incidence of concomitant neurologic and orthopedic injuries. Isolated splenic injury occurs in only 30% of patients. Hemodynamically unstable patients who have signs of blunt abdominal trauma require prompt celiotomy. Stable patients who have signs of abdominal injury and those whose neurologic status is impaired require evaluation with CT scan, ultrasound, or diagnostic peritoneal lavage. If splenic injury is present, several treatment options exist.

Treatment

Splenectomy is performed if the spleen is extensively injured (grade V) or if the patient is profoundly unstable. In stable patients, attempts at splenic preservation with splenorrhaphy or nonoperative management are undertaken.

Splenorrhaphy is operative repair of the spleen. If at least 50% of the splenic volume is preserved, the immune function of the spleen should remain intact. Techniques of splenorrhaphy include debridement of devitalized tissue followed by compression with microcrystalline collagen, pledgeted suture repair, and the creation of polyglycolic acid mesh slings to provide hemostatic compression. Splenorrhaphy is abandoned if the patient has persistent hypotension or extensive additional intraabdominal injuries.

Splenic autotransplantation by placing splenic fragments in the omentum or peritoneal cavity should be avoided. This procedure does not preserve splenic function and may lead to a high risk of bowel obstruction, requiring further surgery associated with troublesome bloody adhesions.

Nonoperative management of splenic injuries is the treatment of choice in hemodynamically stable children. It is also gaining acceptance in adults. For nonoperative therapy to be successful, the patient must be hemodynamically stable, with an isolated splenic injury, usually grades I through III by CT scan. Protocols must be followed. Treatment is undertaken in a very controlled environment by a surgical team experienced in the management of splenic trauma. Protocols vary from institution to institution. Usually, the patient is given bed rest initially in an intensive care unit, and serial physical examinations are performed and hematocrits checked. If the patient shows any signs of shock or has evidence of continued bleeding, then celiotomy is undertaken. Patients who remain hemodynamically stable are followed closely, usually for approximately 1 week in the hospital and then for 6 to 12 weeks of restricted activity. CT or ultrasound is usually obtained to check for splenic healing before the patient is allowed to return to full activity. Nonoperative therapy is successful in more than 85% of children and 70% of adults. Concerns about nonoperative therapy include delayed splenic rupture, risk of transfusions, and missed associated injuries. Although these concerns are real, they are not borne out by experience.

Disorders of Splenic Function

Disorders of the spleen are classified as either functional or anatomic. Functional disorders are considered in terms of too little function (**hyposplenism and asple-**

nia) or excess function (**hypersplenism**). Congenital asplenia or hyposplenism is extremely rare. Splenectomy is the most common reason for the asplenic state, although other conditions (e.g., sickle cell anemia) may lead to a functional asplenic state. The size of the spleen is not related to its hematologic function. Splenomegaly (anatomic enlargement of the spleen) is caused by a variety of conditions (Table 21-3) and should not be confused with hypersplenism (excess function of the spleen). Hypersplenism is characterized by **cytopenia** (anemia, leukopenia, and thrombocytopenia, alone or in combination) and normal or hyperplastic cellular precursors in the bone marrow. Cytopenia results from increased sequestration of the cells in the spleen, increased destruction of cells by the spleen, or production of antibody in the spleen, leading to increased sequestration and destruction of cells. Hyposplenism also occurs with normal or enlarged spleens (multiple myeloma, sickle cell anemia).

There are three hematologic disorders of splenic function for which splenectomy may be helpful: **hemolytic anemia, immune thrombocytopenic purpura** (ITP), and cytopenia associated with splenomegaly from other diseases (secondary hypersplenism).

Hemolytic Anemia

Splenectomy may aid in the management of hereditary hemolytic anemias and some cases of acquired immune hemolytic anemias. Hereditary hemolytic anemias are classified into three broad areas: membrane structural abnormalities, metabolic abnormalities, and **hemoglobinopathies** (Table 21-4).

Hereditary spherocytosis, an autosomal dominant trait, is characterized by abnormally shaped, rigid red cells as a result of a deficiency in spectrin, a membrane component that is essential for deformability. These

Table 21-3. Classification of Splenomegaly (Based on Degree of Enlargement)

Light	Moderate	Great
Chronic passive congestion	Rickets	Chronic myelocytic leukemia
Acute malaria	Hepatitis	Myelofibrosis
Typhoid fever	Hepatic cirrhosis	Gaucher's disease
Subacute bacterial endocarditis	Lymphoma (leukemia)	Neimann-Pick disease
Acute and subacute infection	Infectious mononucleosis	Thalassemia major
Systemic lupus erythematosus	Pernicious anemia	Chronic malaria
Thalassemia minor	Abscesses, infarcts	Leishmaniasis
	Amyloidosis	Splenic vein thrombosis
		Leukemic reticuloendotheliosis (hairy-cell leukemia)

Table 21-4. Hereditary Hemolytic Anemias

Type	Inheritance	Defect	Usefulness of Splenectomy
Abnormal membrane structure			
Spherocytosis	Autosomal dominant	Deficiency in spectrin (membrane component essential for deformability) Rigid erythrocytes cannot pass through splenic vasculature and are sequestered, leading to progressive splenomegaly	Usually
Elliptocytosis	Autosomal dominant	Decreased levels of spectrin; relatively mild in most cases	Rarely
Pyropoikilocytosis	Autosomal recessive	Rare variant of spherocytosis	Usually
Xerocytosis		Water loss leading to increased concentration of hemoglobin	Rarely
Hydrocytosis		Abnormality in erythrocyte Na$^+$/K$^+$ transport	Often
Metabolic abnormalities			
Pyruvate kinase deficiency	Autosomal recessive	Decreased ATP generation leads to membrane destruction	Rarely
Glucose-6-phosphate dehydrogenase deficiency	Sex-linked recessive	Pentose phosphate shunt is blocked and membrane is injured by oxidation injury from certain drugs (e.g., sulfamethoxazole, ASA, phenacetin, nitrofurantoin)	Never
Hemoglobinopathies			
Sickle cell	Autosomal dominant (homozygous more severe)	Valine substitute for glutamic acid at position 6 of β-chain of HbA; rigid, sickle-shaped cells at low O$_2$	Rarely
Thalassemias	Many varieties	Deficits in the synthesis of one or more subunits of Hb	Rarely

ATP, adenosine triphosphate. ASA, Hb

rigid erythrocytes cannot pass into the splenic sinuses and become sequestered in the red pulp. Splenectomy is usually indicated because it allows red cells to survive and hematocrit to reach near-normal values postoperatively. An intraoperative search for an accessory spleen is also performed. The severity of the disease is related to the amount of spectrin produced, and the disease runs in families. Occasionally, the disease is so severe that young children require splenectomy. Splenectomy is deferred if possible, however, until the patient is at least 5 years old because the risk of overwhelming postsplenectomy sepsis is much higher in young children.

Other types of membrane structural abnormalities are less common, but may require splenectomy. A cholecystectomy is performed at the time of splenectomy for hemolytic anemia because pigment gallstones are quite common.

Hemolytic anemias caused by metabolic abnormalities [e.g., pyruvate kinase deficiency, glucose-6-phosphate dehydrogenase (G6PD) deficiency] are not responsive to splenectomy. In G6PD deficiency, the erythrocyte membrane is injured by certain oxidizing drugs, which should be discontinued.

Hemoglobinopathies, which are abnormalities in hemoglobin structure, can lead to red cell deformity and subsequent hemolytic anemia. **Sickle cell disease** is an autosomal dominant disease. The homozygous state is more severe than the heterozygous state. In sickle hemoglobin, valine is substituted for glutamic acid at position six of the beta chain of hemoglobin A. This sub-stitution causes a conformational change in structure that leads to the formation of a rigid sickle-shaped red cell at low oxygen saturations. In addition to hemolytic anemia, sickle cells cause an increase in blood viscosity that leads to stasis and subsequent thrombocytosis. Ischemia occurs as a result and leads to fibrosis in a variety of organs. Most patients with homozygous sickle cell anemia are functionally asplenic because of repeated splenic infarcts and fibrosis. Occasionally, splenectomy is useful in the treatment of patients with splenomegaly in hemolytic crisis. This treatment is usually useful early in the disease.

Thalassemias are characterized by deficits in the synthesis of one or more subunits of hemoglobin. There are many varied types. In thalassemia major (homozygous β-thalassemia), splenectomy is beneficial in reducing the requirements for transfusion, the physical discomfort from massive splenomegaly, and the potential for rupture. In thalassemia minor (heterozygous β-thalassemia), splenectomy can decrease the need for transfusion and the problems associated with iron overload. In general, patients who have thalassemia and undergo splenectomy are at the highest risk for overwhelming postsplenectomy infection. For this reason, alternatives to total splenectomy (e.g., splenic embolization, partial splenectomy) are successful in these patients.

Acquired autoimmune hemolytic anemias are caused by exposure to chemicals, drugs, infectious agents, inflammatory processes, or malignancies. In many cases, a cause is not readily identified. Red blood cells from patients with autoimmune hemolytic anemias are coated with immunoglobulin, complement, or both, which results in a positive direct Coombs' test. Coombs'-negative hemolytic anemia is usually secondary to drugs, toxins, or infectious agents, and is best treated by removing the responsible agent. Patients with Coombs'-positive hemolytic anemia should receive corticosteroid therapy and treatment for any underlying disorders. Splenectomy is indicated when steroids are ineffective, when high doses are required, and when toxic side effects develop during steroid treatment. Splenic sequestration studies and red cell survival may help to select patients who will respond to splenectomy. Further, anemias associated with warm reactive antibodies (usually IgG) do not include complement activation. They are associated with splenic sequestration and usually respond to splenectomy. Hemolytic anemias associated with cold reactive antibodies (usually IgM) are characterized by complement binding and agglutination. Hemolysis occurs in peripheral locations in response to cool environmental temperatures. Splenectomy is usually not helpful in these cases.

Thrombocytopenia

Thrombocytopenia has a variety of causes (Table 21-5). Splenectomy is appropriate only in idiopathic, immune-mediated thrombocytopenias (those in which a cause cannot be found). These platelet disorders are usually characterized by the coexistence of a low platelet count, a normal or increased number of megakaryocytes in the bone marrow, and the absence of other hematologic disorders or splenomegaly. The medication history is important, particularly the history of drugs that interfere with platelet function (e.g., aspirin) or other therapeutic agents that are known to cause thrombocytopenia.

Patients with thrombocytopenia often have multiple petechiae (pinpoint lesions that result from breakage of small capillaries or increased permeability of the arterioles, capillaries, or venules). Petechiae occur in areas of the body that encounter pressure and are characteristic of thrombocytopenia. Purpura causes a confluence of petechiae. Ecchymoses are extensive purpuric lesions that indicate that blood has spread along fascial planes. Ecchymoses are more suggestive of a coagulation disorder than of thrombocytopenia.

If the platelet count is low and coagulation disorders were ruled out by appropriate laboratory tests, then all medications should be discontinued. Antiplatelet antibodies should be measured because they are elevated in 85% of patients with immune cytopenic purpura. The bone marrow is evaluated to determine the number of megakaryocytes. In disorders of platelet destruction (e.g., ITP), the bone marrow shows either normal or increased numbers of megakaryocytes.

Immune Thrombocytopenic Purpura. Acute ITP usually occurs after an acute viral infection. It has an excellent prognosis in children younger than 16 years of age.

Table 21-5. Classification of Thrombocytopenia

Decreased production
  Hypoproliferation (toxic agents, sepsis, radiation, myelofibrosis, tumor involvement of marrow)
  Ineffective platelet production (megaloblastic anemia, Guglielmo's syndrome)
Splenic sequestration (congestive splenomegaly, myeloid metaplasia, lymphoma, Gaucher's disease)
Dilutional loss (after massive transfusion)
Abnormal destruction
  Consumption (disseminated intravascular coagulation)
  Immune mechanisms
    Splenectomy sometimes indicated (idiopathic thrombocytopenic purpura, chronic lymphocytic leukemia, systemic lupus erythematosus)
    Splenectomy not indicated (drug-induced thrombocytopenia, neonatal thrombocytopenia, post-transfusion purpura)

Approximately 80% of these patients have a complete, permanent, spontaneous recovery without therapy. Chronic ITP is primarily a disease of young adults. It affects women more often than men. Patients are best treated initially with a course of corticosteroid therapy. If patients do not respond with an elevated platelet count, splenectomy is performed. In patients who respond to steroid therapy, splenectomy is recommended if thrombocytopenia occurs after steroids are tapered. Patients who initially respond to steroid therapy fare better after splenectomy than those who do not respond to steroids. Patients who have any sign of intracranial bleeding during steroid therapy require emergency splenectomy. Of patients who undergo splenectomy, 75% to 85% respond permanently and require no further therapy. If platelet counts are less than 20,000, platelets should be available for transfusion. Transfusion of platelets is performed after the spleen is removed because transfused platelets are rapidly destroyed in the spleen. For patients who do not respond or who relapse after splenectomy and who do not improve with corticosteroids, treatment with vincristine and γ-globulin shows some success.

Thrombotic Thrombocytopenic Purpura. Thrombotic thrombocytopenic purpura is a disease of the arteries or capillaries. It is characterized by thrombotic episodes and low platelet counts. The constellation of clinical features in virtually all cases consists of fever, purpura, hemolytic anemia, neurologic manifestations, and signs of renal disease. Plasma pheresis, a therapy aimed at removing plasma-derived factors that cause platelet aggregation, is usually successful, either alone or in combination with antiplatelet therapy, whole-blood exchange transfusions, and steroids. Splenectomy is arguably indicated if these measures fail.

Human Immunodeficiency Virus–Associated Thrombocytopenia. Infection with the human immunodeficiency virus (HIV) may lead to HIV-associated thrombocytopenia. HIV-positive patients and those with acquired immune deficiency syndrome (AIDS) and symptomatic HIV-associated thrombocytopenia that is resistant to medical therapy appear to benefit from splenectomy. Sustained resolution of thrombocytopenia is seen in 60% to 80% of these patients. Splenectomy is performed without an undue increase in morbidity and mortality rates. Splenectomy does not appear to accelerate the conversion rate to AIDS in HIV-positive patients.

Hypersplenism Associated with Other Diseases

A number of clinical syndromes are characterized by destruction of various formed elements of the blood. The cardinal features include splenomegaly; some reduction in the number of circulating blood cells affecting granulocytes, erythrocytes, or platelets in any combination; a compensatory proliferative response in the bone marrow; and the potential for correction of these hematologic abnormalities by splenectomy. Both infiltrative and congestive forms of splenomegaly are associated with hypersplenism (Table 21-6). In patients with splenomegaly, sequestration of both red cells and platelets occurs. Red cell transit time through the spleen increases proportionately with splenomegaly. Platelet survival is not usually affected; however, platelet sequestration by the enlarged spleen is increased. For this reason, thrombocytopenia is usually apparent before anemia in patients with hypersplenism associated with splenomegaly.

Hypersplenism is suggested by splenomegaly. Peripheral blood smears may show pancytopenia, isolated thrombocytopenia, anemia, or leukopenia. Most cases of hypersplenism, however, show pancytopenia. The bone marrow is usually hyperplastic. In myelofibrosis, a bone marrow examination shows increased deposition of collagen. The diagnostic approach is dictated by the accompanying features (e.g., hematologic findings, lymphadenopathy, portal hypertension, liver dysfunction, systemic infection). For a variety of reasons, splenectomy is indicated for patients with splenomegaly and hypersplenism. Splenectomy is indicated for hypersplenism if the platelet count is less than 50,000, with evidence of bleeding; if the neutrophil count is less than 2000, with or without frequent intercurrent infections; or if the patient has anemia requiring blood transfusion. In myelofibrosis with myeloid metaplasia as well as other cases of extramedullary hematopoiesis, splenectomy is indicated only when the clinical evidence suggests that the compensatory hematopoietic function of the enlarged spleen is outweighed by accelerated sequestration and destruction of red cells.

In most cases of secondary hypersplenism, splenectomy does not completely alleviate the cytopenia. Postoperatively, however, a dramatic increase in the number of platelets may occur and may be associated with thrombosis and thromboembolism, particularly in myelofibrosis. Close postoperative monitoring of platelets is essential.

Congestive Splenomegaly. Hypersplenism associated with **congestive splenomegaly** as a result of liver failure and the vascular consequences of portal hypertension requires treatment of the hypertension rather than splenectomy. Splenectomy is contraindicated as a primary treatment in this setting because it eliminates the possibility of performing a selective splenorenal shunt procedure, which is a more appropriate treatment for portal hypertension. In this setting, splenectomy may also lead to portal vein thrombosis and complicate potential liver transplantation.

Infiltrative Splenomegaly. In benign cases of **infiltrative splenomegaly** (e.g., Gaucher's disease, an autosomal recessive disorder that causes abnormal accumulation of glucocerebrosides in the reticuloendothelial cells), partial splenectomy and splenic embolization are used instead of splenectomy to treat hypersplenism and abdominal discomfort caused by massive splenomegaly.

Felty's Syndrome. Some patients with rheumatoid arthritis have leg ulcers or other chronic infections, with associated splenomegaly and neutropenia. In these patients, circulating antibodies against neutrophils are found. Splenectomy is controversial because the response is unpredictable. Splenectomy is usually performed for **Felty's syndrome** when severe recurrent infections or intractable leg ulcers occur.

Hematologic Malignancies

Splenectomy is not indicated for acute leukemia. For patients with chronic leukemia, splenectomy is indicated for some cases of hypersplenism and for symptoms associated with massive splenomegaly.

Leukemic reticuloendotheliosis (hairy cell leukemia) is an indolent, progressive form of chronic leukemia. Ongoing hepatomegaly and splenomegaly occur as the disease progresses and the leukemic cells infiltrate the spleen and liver. In the recent past, splenectomy was believed to be an important therapeutic intervention early in the treatment of hairy cell leukemia. Recently, α-interferon and 21-deoxycoformycin were introduced as first-line treatments. Splenectomy is now reserved

---

Table 21-6. Diseases Associated with Hypersplenism

Infiltrative disease of the spleen
 Benign conditions (Gaucher's disease, Niemann-Pick disease, amyloidosis, extramedullary hematopoiesis)
 Neoplastic conditions (leukemias, lymphoma, Hodgkin's disease, primary tumors, metastatic tumors, myeloid metaplasia)
Congestive disease of the spleen
 Portal hypertension
 Splenic vein thrombosis
Miscellaneous diseases
 Felty's syndrome (rheumatoid arthritis, splenomegaly, neutropenia)
 Sarcoidosis
 Porphyria erythropoietica

primarily for palliating cytopenias and symptoms of splenomegaly.

Staging laparotomy is occasionally performed for **Hodgkin's disease** to match the treatment with the extent of disease. Disease that is isolated above the diaphragm and causes no symptoms is sometimes treated with radiation alone. All other stages require systemic chemotherapy. Table 21-7 shows the staging classification for Hodgkin's disease. Patients with Hodgkin's disease who have no systemic symptoms and are classified as preoperative stage I, II, or III are candidates for staging laparotomy. The purpose of staging laparotomy is to determine the extent of disease in the abdomen. Careful systemic examination is required and follows sequential steps, including biopsy of both lobes of the liver, splenectomy, and sampling of nodes from each node-bearing area (hepatoduodenal, celiac, mesenteric, periaortic, iliac). Biopsy is performed on any suspicious nodes that are found on preoperative CT scan and lymphangiogram. Intraoperative plain films that show radiopaque contrast material remaining in the periaortic and iliac lymph nodes after lymphangiogram and intraoperative ultrasonography may be useful in identifying appropriate lymph nodes for biopsy. Often, a bone marrow biopsy specimen is taken from one of the iliac crests. With recent improvements in imaging technologies and changes to more systemic forms of therapy rather than primary radiation therapy for Hodgkin's disease, fewer staging laparotomies are being performed.

Staging laparotomy is rarely performed for patients with non-Hodgkin's lymphoma because the disease does not spread in the orderly progression of Hodgkin's disease. It may be indicated in patients with recurrent disease, relapse after initial remission, massive splenic enlargement that causes local pressure on the abdominal viscera, or symptomatic hypersplenism.

Further Technical Considerations for Splenic Surgery

Splenectomy may be accomplished by traditional open means or by minimally invasive techniques. Open splenectomy is performed with either a midline incision or a left subcostal incision (Kehr's incision). The keys to safe splenectomy are mobilization of the spleen and control of the splenic vasculature. Complete mobilization of the spleen is mandatory for partial splenectomy and to evaluate and repair splenic injuries. It is important not to take the short gastric vessels too close to the stomach to avoid injury of the gastric wall. Care is also taken to avoid injuring the tail of the pancreas at the splenic hilum. Splenectomy for hematologic disease is not complete until a thorough search for accessory spleens is made. Drains are not routinely left after splenectomy.

Increasingly, laparoscopic splenectomy is performed successfully for splenectomy necessitated by ITP, hereditary spherocytosis, and HIV-related thrombocytopenia. The principles for laparoscopic splenectomy are the same as those for open splenectomy. However, it is necessary to morselize the spleen in special bags that are removed through the small incisions. Occasionally, surgeons make a larger lower abdominal incision to remove very large spleens in fragments.

Consequences and Complications of Splenectomy

Hematologic Changes

In a normal patient, after the spleen is removed, the white blood cell count increases by an average of 50% over baseline. In some cases, the number of neutrophils increases to 15,000 to 20,000 mm^3 in the initial postoperative period. The white blood cell count usually returns to normal within 5 to 7 days. Elevation beyond this period suggests infection.

The peripheral smear of a patient who underwent splenectomy routinely shows Howell-Jolly bodies, Pappenheimer bodies, and pitted red cells on phase microscopy. Some red blood cells may show abnormal morphology. The absence of these findings after splenectomy for hematologic disease suggests that an accessory spleen was missed. A radionuclide spleen scan may be useful for identifying retained splenic elements.

The platelet count increases by 30% between 2 and 10 days after splenectomy and usually returns to normal within 2 weeks. **Thrombocytosis** (platelet count > 400,000/mm^3) occurs in as many as 50% of patients. Theoretically, this increase predisposes the patient to thrombotic complications (e.g., pulmonary embolism). However, little evidence supports a correlation between absolute platelet count and thrombosis. Most thromboses and pulmonary emboli occur in patients who have myeloproliferative disorders. Postoperative therapy with platelet inhibitors (e.g., aspirin, dipyridamole) is justified in patients who have myeloproliferative disease and platelet counts greater than 400,000/mm^3 and in all other patients after splenectomy if the platelet count is greater than 750,000/mm^3. Treatment continues until the platelet count returns to normal. Anticoagulation with heparin or warfarin therapy is not beneficial and should be avoided.

Immune Consequences

The risk of postsplenectomy sepsis varies with the age of the patient and the reason for splenectomy. In

Table 21-7. Staging of Hodgkin's Disease

Stage	Description
I	Limited to one lymph node region
II	Two or more regions on the same side of the diaphragm
III	Disease on both sides of the diaphragm limited to lymph nodes, spleen, and Waldeyer's ring
IV	Disease involving bone, bone marrow, lung, liver, gastrointestinal tract, or any organ other than the lymph nodes, spleen, or Waldeyer's ring

otherwise normal children, the potential risk is approximately 2% to 4%. In adults, it is approximately 1% to 2%. Patients who undergo splenectomy for hematologic disorders are at the highest risk. The overall incidence of postsplenectomy sepsis is 40 times that of the general population, and these patients are at risk for fatal sepsis at any time after splenectomy.

Overwhelming infections are usually caused by encapsulated organisms. *Streptococcus pneumoniae* (pneumococcus) is the most common agent (75%), followed in decreasing frequency by *Haemophilus influenzae, Neisseria meningitidis,* beta-hemolytic streptococcus, *Staphylococcus aureus, Escherichia coli,* and *Pseudomonas.* Viral infections, most commonly herpes zoster, may be severe in splenectomized patients. Some parasitic infections (babesiosis, malaria) also overwhelm the splenectomized host.

Overwhelming infections with encapsulated bacteria (e.g., pneumococcus) are insidious in onset, often mimicking a cold or flu. Within a few hours, patients may become septic, and death may ensue rapidly (24–48 hours) despite vigorous antibiotic therapy. Adrenal infarction causing adrenal insufficiency is often associated with these infections (Waterhouse-Friderichsen's syndrome).

Polyvalent pneumococcal polysaccharide vaccines are given after total splenectomy or conservative splenic operation for trauma. Patients with splenic trauma who are managed nonoperatively are also vaccinated. Neither the surgeon nor the patient should consider this vaccine full protection against overwhelming postsplenectomy sepsis. Both clinical and experimental evidence suggests that splenectomized patients may not respond well to pneumococcal polysaccharide antigens. Children who are younger than 2 years of age also do not become effectively immunized. In addition, pneumococcal types that are not contained in the vaccine (or other bacteria) may cause overwhelming sepsis. Patients who undergo elective splenectomy should be immunized well in advance of surgery. The exact timing for immunization is unknown, but longer than 1 week before surgery is probably sufficient. After splenectomy, it is wise to wait until the patient is nutritionally intact and recovers from other injuries before administering the vaccination. Vaccinations against *H. influenzae* type B and *N. meningitidis* are available and should be considered for asplenic patients.

Long-term antibiotic prophylaxis with oral penicillin is a reasonable approach in immunologically compromised patients (e.g., renal transplant recipients), those receiving chemotherapy, and children younger than 6 years of age who undergo splenectomy. This approach does not provide definite prophylaxis for a number of reasons, including lack of compliance, inconvenience, and bacterial resistance.

People who undergo splenectomy should carry identification that explains their medical condition. They should also be instructed to contact their physician at the first sign of any minor infection (e.g., cold, sore throat). Antibiotics should be prescribed and the patient followed closely.

Anatomic Complications After Splenectomy

Morbidity and mortality rates after splenectomy are relatively low. Older patients and those with severe underlying conditions have the highest morbidity and mortality rates.

Atelectasis is the most common problem after splenectomy. It is usually caused by reduced respiratory excursion secondary to high abdominal incisions and irritation of the diaphragm. Atelectasis usually resolves within 2 to 3 days if it is properly treated. Improperly treated, atelectasis can progress to pneumonia. Pleural effusions may be associated with atelectasis, but are more often associated with a subphrenic abscess. Subphrenic fluid may collect in the space left by the spleen. This situation occurs secondary to bleeding, inflammation, or leak of pancreatic fluid as a result of injury to the tail of the pancreas. Abscesses are more likely to occur if the gastrointestinal tract is opened. The placement of prophylactic drains increases the risk of subphrenic abscess. These drains are rarely used unless a pancreatic injury is identified. Subphrenic abscesses are usually apparent within 5 to 10 days after surgery. Signs include fever, pain, pleural effusion, prolonged atelectasis, pneumonia, and prolonged leukocytosis. Ultrasonography and CT scanning are useful for identifying abscesses. Once identified, they are promptly drained, either percutaneously with image guidance or operatively.

Injury to the pancreas occurs in 1% to 3% of patients who undergo splenectomy. It may be clinically unrecognized and cause mild hyperamylasemia or may cause clinical pancreatitis, pancreatic fistula, or pancreatic pseudocysts. Serum amylase or lipase determination on the second to fourth day after surgery may help to identify the pancreatic injury. Symptoms and signs (nausea and vomiting, abdominal distension, abdominal pain and pulmonary complications, such as those seen with a subphrenic abscess) usually develop within 4 to 5 days after splenectomy.

Likewise, injury to the stomach may occur while the short gastric vessels are being divided. This injury may lead to the development of a subphrenic abscess or gastrocutaneous fistula. Some surgeons advocate nasogastric decompression for 2 to 3 days after splenectomy to avoid gastric distension and prevent complications. Care is taken to reinforce the gastric wall, where the short gastric vessels have been clipped or ligated in close proximity to the gastric wall, to prevent problems.

Bleeding at splenectomy usually occurs when it is performed for massive splenomegaly (because of the friability of dilated veins).

Persistent hemorrhage after splenectomy occurs in less than 1% of cases. It usually occurs in patients who undergo splenectomy for thrombocytopenia, especially those in whom the platelet count does not respond to splenectomy. Reoperation to gain hemostasis is considered if bleeding continues after coagulation abnormalities are corrected or if hemodynamic instability occurs.

Multiple-Choice Questions

1. A 28-year-old man comes to the emergency department with fever and weakness. He started to have cold symptoms the day before. His medical history is significant for a splenectomy after a motor vehicle accident 13 years ago. His temperature is 40° C, blood pressure is 80/60 mm Hg, and pulse is 140/min. Physical examination is otherwise unremarkable. The most likely diagnosis is:
   A. Acute dehydration
   B. Overwhelming pneumococcal sepsis
   C. Thyroid storm
   D. Hypothalamic stroke
   E. Viral myocarditis

2. A 23-year-old woman comes to her physician with easy bruising. She had a splenectomy for immune thrombocytopenic purpura 12 months ago. Her platelet count 3 weeks after splenectomy was 175,000/mm^3. Her platelet count today is 40,000/mm^3. A peripheral smear shows normal red cell morphology, with no red cell inclusions. The next best step is:
   A. Platelet pheresis
   B. Bone marrow aspiration for analysis
   C. Radionuclide spleen scan
   D. Corticosteroid therapy
   E. Platelet transfusion

3. A 21-year-old woman is scheduled for splenectomy to treat immune thrombocytopenic purpura. The best time to administer a polyvalent pneumococcal vaccine is:
   A. 2 weeks before splenectomy
   B. 1 day before splenectomy
   C. Immediately after splenectomy
   D. At the time of discharge from the hospital
   E. At the first postoperative clinic visit

4. An 11-year-old boy is involved in a motor vehicle accident in which he was restrained with a lap belt. In the emergency room, his blood pressure is 90/60 mm Hg, pulse is 80/min, and respirations are 14/min. He has mild left upper quadrant tenderness. Computed tomography scan shows a small hematoma in the superior pole of the spleen. No other injuries are identified. The most appropriate next step is to:
   A. Admit the patient for observation
   B. Perform exploratory celiotomy and splenic repair
   C. Perform arteriography and splenic artery embolization
   D. Perform exploratory celiotomy and splenectomy
   E. Discharge the patient and repeat the computed tomography scan in 1 week

5. A 19-year-old woman was involved in a motor vehicle accident 1 hour ago. In the emergency department, blood pressure initially was 90/60 mm Hg, with a pulse of 120/min. After administration of 2 L Ringer's lactate solution, blood pressure is 120/70 mm Hg and pulse is 90/min. The patient remains stable, with a urine output of 40 mL/min. She is alert and oriented. She has abdominal pain. There is tenderness in the left upper abdomen. Chest x-ray and cervical spine films are normal. The next best test is:
   A. Arteriography
   B. Computed tomography scan of the abdomen
   C. Radionuclide liver–spleen scan
   D. Plain films of the abdomen
   E. Intravenous pyelogram

6. A 32-year-old woman with known glucose-6-phosphate dehydrogenase deficiency has fatigue and weakness. She recently treated herself with sulfamethoxazole for a urinary tract infection. Hematocrit is 20%. The most likely mechanism for her hemolysis is:
   A. Sensitization of red blood cells by membrane-bound antibody
   B. Fixation of complement
   C. Intracellular production of hydrogen peroxide
   D. Decreased capacity to generate adenosine triphosphate
   E. Conformational changes in hemoglobin

7. A 24-year-old man was involved in a motor vehicle accident 1 hour ago. Computed tomography scan of his abdomen performed 15 minutes ago shows a severely shattered spleen, with deep lacerations involving the hilum. A large volume of blood is seen in the peritoneal cavity. Blood pressure on admission to the emergency department was 100/70 mm Hg, with a pulse of 110/min. He received 2 L Ringer's lactate solution. Blood pressure is now 90/50 mm Hg, with a pulse of 130/min. In addition to blood transfusion, the most appropriate management is:
   A. Continued close observation in the emergency department
   B. Admission to the intensive care unit
   C. Immediate celiotomy
   D. Arteriography and attempted embolization
   E. Dopamine infusion at 10 μg/kg/min

8. A 23-year-old woman underwent splenectomy for immune thrombocytopenic purpura 4 months ago. She is asymptomatic. The platelet count is 180,000/mm^3. A peripheral smear shows abnormal morphology of some red blood cells as well as the presence of Howell-Jolly bodies. The next most appropriate step is to:
   A. Initiate corticosteroid therapy
   B. Perform a bone marrow aspirate
   C. Perform a radionuclide scan of the spleen
   D. Initiate daily aspirin therapy
   E. Reassure the patient that all is as expected

9. A 25-year-old patient underwent emergency splenectomy for a shattered spleen after a motor vehicle

accident. He is at risk for all of the following complications of splenectomy EXCEPT:

A. Pancreatic fistula
B. Overwhelming pneumococcal sepsis
C. Thrombocytopenia
D. Pleural effusion
E. Subphrenic abscess

10. A 23-year-old woman has severe immune thrombocytopenic purpura. Despite corticosteroid therapy, her platelet count did not rise above 20,000/mm³. She is currently in the operating room undergoing splenectomy. When the abdomen is opened, marked oozing from the skin incision is seen. The most appropriate management is to:

A. Administer fresh frozen plasma
B. Administer vincristine
C. Perform platelet transfusion before splenic artery ligation and splenectomy
D. Proceed with splenectomy
E. Administer γ-globulin

11. A 24-year-old man with known human immunodeficiency virus infection has purpura and thrombocytopenia. After 6 weeks of therapy with corticosteroids, his platelet count is 25,000/mm³ and he continues to have purpura. The most appropriate next step is:

A. Measure the CD4:CD8 ratio
B. Perform splenectomy
C. Perform platelet transfusion
D. Initiate γ-globulin therapy
E. Perform plasma pheresis

12. A 6-year-old boy has purpura after an acute viral illness. His platelet count is 40,000/mm³. Bone marrow aspiration shows a slight increase in the number of megakaryocytes. Except for purpura on his arms and legs and a number of petechiae, physical examination is normal. The most appropriate management is:

A. Platelet transfusion
B. Vincristine therapy
C. Splenectomy
D. Close observation
E. High-dose corticosteroid therapy

13. A 60-year-old man is diagnosed as having immune thrombocytopenic purpura. His bone marrow shows mild megakaryocytosis. No other underlying problems are identified. He takes no medications. Despite high-dose prednisone therapy (80 mg/day) for 8 weeks, his platelet count remains at 20,000/mm³. After splenectomy, his platelet count is unchanged. A peripheral smear shows evidence of Howell-Jolly bodies. The most appropriate next step is to:

A. Reinstitute steroids at higher doses
B. Reexplore the abdomen to look for further splenic tissue
C. Perform platelet transfusion until the platelet count is greater than 50,000/mm³

D. Initiate α-interferon therapy
E. Initiate vincristine therapy

14. A 26-year-old woman has fatigue and weakness. Hematocrit is 20%. She is completing another 2-week course of sulfamethoxazole for a recurrent urinary tract infection. She has no other significant medical history and takes no other medications. A direct Coombs' test is positive. In addition to discontinuing the sulfamethoxazole, the next step in management is:

A. Therapy with corticosteroids
B. Immediate splenectomy
C. Observation
D. Plasma pheresis
E. γ-Globulin therapy

15. A 40-year-old man has thalassemia major (homozygous β-thalassemia). He has massive splenomegaly and abdominal pain and has required transfusions increasingly over the last year. In addition to decreasing transfusion requirements, splenectomy may benefit this patient by:

A. Decreasing the likelihood of overwhelming infection
B. Decreasing the risk of potential rupture
C. Preventing bleeding complications from severe thrombocytosis
D. Decreasing steroid requirements
E. Preventing structural abnormalities of red blood cells

16. A 24-year-old man undergoes splenectomy for a grade V splenic injury that he sustained when he fell while skiing. His platelet count is 450,000/mm³ 2 weeks after splenectomy. The most appropriate next step is:

A. Bone marrow aspiration
B. Aspirin therapy
C. Warfarin therapy
D. Vena cava filter
E. Reassurance

17. A 60-year-old man with myeloid metaplasia underwent splenectomy for massive splenomegaly associated with abdominal pain and progressive hypersplenism. Two weeks postoperatively, his platelet count is 1,200,000/mm³. The next step is:

A. Reassurance
B. Aspirin therapy
C. Intravenous heparin
D. Coumadin
E. Vena cava filter

18. A 22-year-old woman undergoes splenectomy for immune thrombocytopenic purpura through a left subcostal incision. The nest day, her temperature is 38.5° C, blood pressure is 120/80 mm Hg, pulse is 100/min, and respiratory rate is 18/min. Auscultation of the chest shows decreased breath sounds at the left

base, with bronchial sounds. The most likely diagnosis is:
A. Atelectasis
B. Subphrenic abscess
C. Pancreatic injury
D. Stomach injury
E. Colon injury

19. A 22-year-old woman has chronic immune thrombocytopenic purpura. Both antiplatelet antibodies and complement are found on the surface of her platelets. Bone marrow aspirate shows increased megakaryocytes. Her spleen is normal in size. Her platelet count increased from 30,000/mm³ to 120,000/mm³ while she was taking corticosteroids. Which of the following factors will best predict that splenectomy will be successful in treating her immune thrombocytopenic purpura?
A. Increased megakaryocytes
B. Absence of splenomegaly
C. Rise in platelet count with corticosteroid therapy
D. Presence of antiplatelet antibodies
E. Presence of complement on platelet surfaces

20. For which of the following patients with Hodgkin's lymphoma is staging laparotomy most useful?
A. Patients with inguinal nodes and no systemic symptoms
B. Patients with cervical, mediastinal, and inguinal nodes and night sweats
C. Patients with mediastinal nodes and night sweats
D. Patients with mediastinal nodes, positive bone marrow aspirate, and no systemic symptoms
E. Patients with cervical and mediastinal nodes and no systemic symptoms

Oral Examination Study Questions

CASE 1

You are a general surgeon in a community hospital. You are called to the emergency department to evaluate an acutely injured 26-year-old man. He was driving when his car was struck on the driver's door by another car that did not stop at a traffic light. The paramedics report that the patient had left lower chest pain at the scene. The initial vital signs were: blood pressure 115/85 mm Hg, pulse 98/min, and respiratory rate 18/min. On arrival in the emergency department, the patient appears mildly distressed. The nurse reports that his palpable systolic blood pressure is 120 mm Hg, pulse is 102/min, respiratory rate is 16/min, and oral temperature is 37.2° C.

OBJECTIVE 1

A. The student asks the paramedics about vehicular damage (left door caved in, window broken); the status of the other driver (moderate facial lacerations; transported by ambulance to another hospital); and whether the patient was wearing a restraining device (three-point lap–shoulder belt).

B. The student asks the patient about his symptoms in a systematic fashion.
1. Head (no loss of consciousness, no recent alcohol or drug ingestion)
2. Neck (no pain)
3. Chest (left lower posterior chest pain accentuated by deep breath, no other difficulty in breathing)
4. Abdomen (mild nausea, no pain)
5. Extremities (no complaints)
6. Medical history (no previous medical problems, no current medications)

OBJECTIVE 2

The student conducts a system-oriented physical examination. The positive findings are:

A. Chest: abrasion over the left lower posterior chest wall, with marked tenderness in the posterior segments of the ninth and tenth ribs

B. Abdomen: slightly decreased bowel sounds and mild deep left upper quadrant tenderness, with pain referred to the left shoulder

OBJECTIVE 3

The student formulates a differential diagnosis that includes the following:

A. Fractured left lower posterior ribs

B. Left hemopneumothorax

C. Ruptured spleen

D. Renal contusion

Pertinent laboratory tests

A. Chest x-ray shows nondisplaced fractures of the posterior ninth and tenth ribs, with no left hemopneumothorax.

B. Hematocrit is 36%, with white blood cell count of 11,000/mm³.

C. Urinalysis shows no red blood cells.

OBJECTIVE 4

The student suspects ruptured spleen. A nasogastric tube is inserted to decompress the stomach, and at least two large-bore (14-gauge) peripheral intravenous lines are established in case the patient has sudden increased bleeding. The diagnosis is confirmed with peritoneal lavage if the vital signs are labile or with computed tomography of the abdomen if the vital signs are stable. 99mTc sulfur colloid scan does not detect associated intraabdominal injury.

The nurse reports that the patient's systolic blood pressure has dropped abruptly to 90 mm Hg and his pulse has risen to 110/min. The student increases the rate of fluid administration with a colloid solution, orders type and crossmatch of blood, and transfers the patient to the operating room for emergent laparotomy without further diagnostic tests.

OBJECTIVE 5

At midline laparotomy, 1500 mL blood is found in the peritoneal cavity. A thorough abdominal examination confirms that the spleen is the only injured organ, and the patient is now stable hemodynamically. The student mentions that splenorrhaphy is an option in addition to removal of the spleen. The spleen, however, has an extensive central parenchymal fracture that extends into the hilum, precluding safe repair. Splenectomy is performed without incident.

OBJECTIVE 6

The student discusses overwhelming postsplenectomy infection and indicates that the incidence in adults is relatively low (1%–2%). The student reviews the rationale for polyvalent pneumococcal vaccine and the need to give the vaccine in the postoperative period, when nutrition is adequate. Additionally, the student outlines the instructions to the patient regarding early signs of overwhelming postsplenectomy infection and the need to seek medical attention immediately.

Minimum Level of Achievement for Passing

A. The student recognizes the possibility of splenic injury.

B. The student formulates a complete differential diagnosis and orders appropriate laboratory tests.

C. The student knows that surgery is the appropriate treatment.

D. The student requests postoperative treatment with polyvalent pneumococcal vaccine.

Honors Level of Achievement

The honors student categorizes the types of splenic injury and discusses the appropriate treatment for hemodynamically stable patients and those who have continued bleeding or shock.

In addition, the patient discusses the complications of splenectomy.

A. Sepsis

B. Thrombocytosis, thrombosis, and pulmonary embolism

C. Hemorrhage

D. Abscess

E. Injury to the stomach and pancreas

CASE 2

You are a general surgeon in a community hospital. You are asked to evaluate a 66-year-old woman in the emergency department because of ecchymoses involving her lower extremities and forearms. Her medical history is significant for chronic lymphocytic leukemia, diagnosed 5 years earlier, for which she received no specific treatment. The patient is in no acute distress, and the nurse records a blood pressure of 120/80 mm Hg, heart rate of 76/min, and respiratory rate of 15/min. Her temperature is 37.2° C.

OBJECTIVE 1

A. The student asks for more information about the chronic lymphocytic leukemia.
   1. It was discovered on a routine blood test 7 years earlier.
   2. She is followed by a hematologist whom she sees every 6 months, although she missed her last appointment.
   3. She has no other significant medical history and takes no medications.

B. The student pursues the relevant history, which suggests underlying coagulopathy.
   1. The patient says that she bruises easily. She enjoys working in her garden, but finds that minimal trauma causes her arms to bruise.
   2. The bruising has occurred for only the last few months. She does not remember any other bleeding problem.

C. The student pursues the relevant history suggesting any problems with anemia or repeated infections.
   1. The patient says that she gets short of breath quickly during routine daily activities.
   2. The patient recalls having her share of colds, but nothing more than that.

D. The student examines the patient completely.
   1. She has a number of large ecchymoses on her forearms and shins.
   2. She has a large palpable spleen in the upper left quadrant. The inferior tip is at the level of the umbilicus. It is mildly tender.
   3. There are no obvious petechiae. Stool is Hematest negative.

OBJECTIVE 2

A. The student pursues laboratory confirmation of underlying pancytopenia and coagulopathy.
   1. Hematocrit is 32%, and indices are normal.
   2. The white blood cell count is 33,000/mm^3. The differential is 5% neutrophils, 93% lymphocytes, and 2% monocytes.
   3. The platelet count is 56,000/mm^3.
   4. Prothrombin time and partial thromboplastin time are normal.

B. The student concludes that the patient has splenomegaly from chronic lymphocytic leukemia, with corresponding hypersplenism. The patient has no indication for splenectomy at this point.

C. The student refers the patient to her hematologist for further evaluation and monitoring.

OBJECTIVE 3

Fifteen months later, the patient is referred to you by her hematologist. She is having abdominal pain, early satiety, and worsening thrombocytopenia as well as anemia requiring transfusion of both platelets and packed red blood cells at increasingly shorter intervals, despite treatment with prednisone (60 mg/day) and other chemotherapeutic agents. Except for this change, her health has remained the same.

A. The student performs another physical examination. It shows friability of the gums, multiple ecchymoses of the extremities, and a few petechiae over the chest wall. The spleen is palpable below the umbilicus.

B. The student obtains another complete blood count. Hematocrit is 21%; white blood cell count is 35,000, with 4% neutrophils; and platelet count is 24,000/mm³. Results of other clotting studies are normal.

C. The student recommends transfusion of blood and platelets followed by splenectomy.

OBJECTIVE 4

The patient undergoes splenectomy. She has a large spleen that weighs 2100 g. The surgery is difficult, with considerable blood loss. The patient requires transfusion of four units of packed red blood cells intraoperatively. By day 5, she is still in some distress. Blood pressure is 110/60 mm Hg, heart rate is 100/min, respiratory rate is 18/min, and temperature is 38.6° C. Breath sounds are diminished on the left, and no bowel sounds are audible. A nasogastric tube drains a moderate amount of bilious fluid.

A. The student suggests that the patient is experiencing complications from the splenectomy. The student performs further evaluation, including another complete blood count. Hematocrit is 33%; white blood cell count is 33,000/mm³, with 8% neutrophils; and platelet count is 75,000/mm³. Serum lipase is measured (6000 units), and a chest x-ray is taken and shows left lobar collapse, with an effusion.

B. The student follows up with a computed tomography scan. The student suspects subphrenic abscess and injury to the tail of the pancreas, with a pancreatic leak that should be treated by computed tomography–guided (if possible) or operative drainage.

Minimum Level of Achievement for Passing

A. The student recognizes a hematologic disorder and hypersplenism associated with chronic lymphocytic leukemia.

B. The student knows that a large spleen is not an indication for surgery, but recognizes that hypersplenism that causes severe pancytopenia and complications is an indication for splenectomy.

C. The student recognizes that subphrenic abscess is a potential complication of splenectomy, particularly a difficult splenectomy, and must be drained.

Honors Level of Achievement

A. The student knows that other indications for splenectomy include hematologic causes, such as

hemolytic anemia (spherocytosis, elliptocytosis, thalassemia, autoimmune hemolytic anemia), thrombocytopenia (immune thrombocytopenic purpura, thrombotic thrombocytopenic purpura), and hypersplenism.

B. The student knows that splenectomy associated with portal hypertension may be dangerous, even in the face of pancytopenia, and that correcting the portal hypertension is more appropriate than splenectomy.

CASE 3

You are a general surgeon in a community hospital. You are asked to evaluate a 23-year-old woman in the emergency room because of a large ecchymosis of the left flank. The patient slipped on snow this morning and struck the left side of her back on a railing, but did not fall to the ground. She had minimal discomfort and worked throughout the day without difficulty. While showering this evening, however, she noticed a large bruise on her side, where she struck the railing. The patient is in no distress, and the nurse records a blood pressure of 115/75 mm Hg, heart rate of 70/min, respiratory rate of 12/min, and oral temperature of 37.4° C.

OBJECTIVE 1

A. The student asks the patient about her symptoms. The patient denies chest pain, shortness of breath, abdominal pain, nausea, and hematuria. The student pursues a relevant history suggesting underlying coagulopathy. The patient recalls that her gums bled while she brushed her teeth several months ago. She also believes that her last menstrual period was heavier than usual. She denies hematemesis, hematochezia, hematuria, epistaxis, and other trauma-related contusions, and has no family history of bleeding disorders.

B. The student examines the patient thoroughly. A 15 cm ecchymosis on the left flank is the only positive finding. The spleen is not enlarged, and stool is Hematest negative. There are no petechiae.

OBJECTIVE 2

A. The student pursues laboratory confirmation of underlying, but not yet complicated, coagulopathy.
1. Hematocrit is 40%.
2. Findings of urinalysis are normal.
3. Prothrombin time is 11.5 seconds (normal).
4. Partial thromboplastin time is 30.1 seconds (normal).
5. Thrombin time 12.0 seconds (normal).
6. Peripheral smear shows a few large platelets (estimated 58,000/mm³).

B. The student concludes that the patient has pathologic thrombocytopenia and asks further relevant questions. The patient denies drug ingestion, current medication, or recent systemic infection.

C. The student calls a hematologist and refers the patient for office evaluation. The hematologist sends a report on the patient's bone marrow. Findings include "abundant megakaryocytes, many young; erythroid and myeloid precursors are normal." Finally, the patient has elevated antiplatelet antibodies. The student concludes that the patient has idiopathic thrombocytopenic purpura.

OBJECTIVE 3

During follow-up 3 months later, the patient reports increasing bleeding after brushing her teeth.

A. The student refers the patient to the hematologist for immediate evaluation. The hematologist calls the student, reporting a platelet count of 23,000/mm^3, and asks for advice.

B. The student confirms that the patient is not having life-threatening bleeding complications and recommends corticosteroids. The hematologist initiates prednisone at 60 mg/day and sends a copy of office records that indicate a platelet count of 125,000/mm^3 at 3 weeks.

C. The student recommends tapering the corticosteroids when the platelet count normalizes.

OBJECTIVE 4

Four months later, the student is called to the emergency room because the patient has arrived with a syncopal episode and massive vaginal bleeding. The patient is in mild distress. Blood pressure is 95/64 mm Hg, heart rate is 110/min, respiratory rate is 18/min, and oral temperature is 37.2° C.

A. The student initiates standard resuscitation for hemorrhagic shock (two large-bore peripheral intravenous lines, crystalloid infusion, blood type and crossmatch). Hematocrit is 26%, and platelet count is 21,000/mm^3. Despite resuscitative measures, including blood transfusion, the patient continues to have life-threatening vaginal bleeding.

B. The student administers six units of platelets and 100 mg methylprednisolone and performs emergency splenectomy. The patient recovers uneventfully and is given polyvalent pneumococcal vaccine.

OBJECTIVE 5

Six months postsplenectomy, the patient returns to the student with recurrent gum bleeding. Her hemat-

ocrit is 40%, with platelets at 28,000/mm^3. The student evaluates the patient for missed accessory spleen (peripheral smear for target cells, Howell-Jolly bodies, and ^{99m} Tc sulfur colloid scan).

Minimum Level of Achievement for Passing

A. The student recognizes first a hematologic disorder and then immune thrombocytopenic purpura.

B. The student knows that immune thrombocytopenic purpura is chronic and is initially treated with steroids (if it is not associated with life-threatening bleeding). If the patient responds to steroids, but therapy subsequently fails, splenectomy is indicated. Between 75% and 80% of patients who undergo splenectomy are permanently cured.

Honors Level of Achievement

A. The student knows that other indications for splenectomy include hemolytic anemia (spherocytosis, elliptocytosis, thalassemia, autoimmune hemolytic anemia), thrombocytopenia (immunologic changes associated with chronic lymphocytic leukemia), thrombotic thrombocytopenic purpura, and hypersplenism.

B. The student also suspects accessory spleen (see Objective 5) and knows how to diagnose it.

SUGGESTED READINGS

Aksnes J, Abdelnoor M, Mathisen O. Risk factors associated with mortality and morbidity after elective splenectomy. *Eur J Surg* 1995;161:253–258.

Alonso M, Gossot D, Bourstyn E, et al. Splenectomy in human immunodeficiency virus-related thrombocytopenia. *Br J Surg* 1993;80:330–333.

Bond SJ, Eichelberger MR, Gotschall CS, et al. Nonoperative management of blunt hepatic and splenic injury in children. *Ann Surg* 1996;223:286–286.

Bowdler AJ, ed. *The Spleen: Structure, Function and Clinical Significance.* New York, NY: Von Nordstrand Reinhold, 1990.

Cogbill TH, Moore EE, Jurkovich GF, et al. Nonoperative management of blunt splenic trauma: a multicenter experience. *J Trauma* 1989;29(10):1312–1315.

Coon WW. Splenectomy for idiopathic thrombocytopenic purpura. *Surg Gynecol Obstet* 1987;164:225.

Coon WW. Splenectomy in the treatment of hemolytic anemia. *Arch Surg* 1985;120:625–628.

Flowers JL, Lefor AT, Steers, L, et al. Laparoscopic splenectomy in patients with hematological diseases. *Ann Surg* 1996;224:19–28.

Van Wyck DB. Overwhelming postsplenectomy infection (OPSI): the clinical syndrome. *Lymphology* 1983;16:107–114.

22 Diseases of the Vascular System

James F. McKinsey, M.D.
Alan Graham, M.D.
Bruce L. Gewertz, M.D.

OBJECTIVES

Arterial Disease: Atherosclerosis, Aneurysms, Peripheral Arterial Occlusive Disease, and Cerebrovascular Insufficiency

1. Describe five risk factors for the development of atherosclerosis.
2. List three specific sites that have a predilection for atherosclerotic plaque, and explain why this predilection exists.
3. List at least two clinical sequelae of atherosclerosis and three ways to retard the atherosclerotic process.
4. List the common sites and relative incidence of arterial aneurysms.
5. List the symptoms, signs, differential diagnosis, and diagnostic and management plans for a patient with a rupturing abdominal aortic aneurysm.
6. Discuss the indications, contraindications, and risk factors for surgery in patients with chronic abdominal aneurysms.
7. Define and discuss the prevention of the common complications of aneurysm surgery.
8. Compare the presentation, complications (i.e., frequency of dissection, rupture, thrombosis, and embolization), and treatment of thoracic, abdominal, femoral, and popliteal aneurysms.
9. Describe the pathophysiology of intermittent claudication, and differentiate this symptom from leg pain from other causes.
10. Describe the diagnostic approach and medical management of arterial occlusive disease. Discuss the roles of common noninvasive procedures.
11. List the criteria to help differentiate among venous, arterial, diabetic, and infectious leg ulcers.
12. Describe the operative treatment options available for chronic occlusive disease of the distal aorta and iliac arteries, superficial femoral and popliteal arteries, and tibial and peroneal arteries.
13. List four indications for amputation, and discuss the clinical and laboratory methods used to select the amputation site.
14. Describe the clinical manifestations, diagnostic workup, and surgical indications for chronic renal artery occlusion.
15. Describe the natural history and causes of acute arterial occlusion, and differentiate between embolic and thrombotic occlusion.
16. List six signs and symptoms of acute arterial occlusion, and outline its management (e.g., indications for medical vs surgical treatment).
17. Define and differentiate among the following:
    A. Amaurosis fugax
    B. Transient ischemic attacks
    C. Reversible ischemic neurologic defect
    D. Cerebrovascular accident (stroke)
18. Outline the diagnostic methods and the medical and surgical management of a patient with symptomatic carotid artery disease.
19. List the differential diagnoses and outline a management and treatment plan for patients with transient ischemic attacks.
20. Differentiate between hemispheric and vertebrobasilar symptoms.

Venous Disease: Deep Vein Thrombosis and Pulmonary Embolus

1. Identify the usual initial anatomic location of deep vein thrombosis, and discuss the clinical factors that lead to an increased incidence of this problem.
2. Identify the invasive and noninvasive testing procedures used to diagnose venous valvular incompetence and deep vein thrombosis.
3. Outline the differential diagnosis of acute edema associated with leg pain.
4. Describe five modalities to prevent the development of venous thrombosis in surgical patients.

5. Describe the methods used to administer anti-coagulant and thrombolytic agents. Discuss how the adequacy of therapy is evaluated, and describe the contraindications to therapy.
6. Describe the clinical syndrome of pulmonary embolus, and identify the order of priorities in diagnosing and caring for an acutely ill patient with life-threatening pulmonary embolus.
7. List the indications for surgical intervention in venous thrombosis and pulmonary embolus.
8. Outline the diagnostic, operative, and nonoperative management of venous ulcers and varicose veins.

Vasospastic Disorders, Vascular Trauma, and Lymphatic Disorders

1. List five underlying diseases or disorders associated with vasospastic changes in the extremities, and discuss their diagnosis and treatment.
2. Describe the anatomic mechanisms that cause thoracic outlet compression syndrome, and discuss the appropriate diagnostic studies and surgical treatment.
3. List the indications for arteriography in a patient with a possible arterial injury to the extremities.
4. In a patient with recent trauma, outline the physical findings, diagnostic plan, and treatment for suspected arterial injury.
5. Define lymphedema praecox, lymphedema tarda, primary lymphedema, and secondary lymphedema.
6. Explain the pathophysiology of lymphedema, and discuss its treatment.

Diagnostic Radiology in Vascular Disorders

1. Describe the indications and risks for arteriogram and venogram.
2. Define and discuss transluminal angioplasty, and cite the indications for this procedure.
3. Discuss the method, use, and reliability of perfusion and ventilation scans.

Arterial Disease

Anatomy

The three layers of the arterial wall are the intima, media, and adventitia (Figure 22-1). The internal elastic lamina separates the intima from the media, and the external elastic lamina separates the media from the adventitia. The endothelium, which is derived from hemangioblasts, lines the inner aspect of the intima and has a collective mass that is greater than that of the liver. The endothelial layer was previously believed to be an inert interface between blood and the arterial wall, but it is now known that the endothelial cells are highly active metabolically. The endothelium functions as an antithrombotic surface that expresses protein C and protein S and aids in the regulation of vascular tone by both vasodilation and vasoconstriction. The myogenic tone of the blood vessels is further modified by the production of endothelium-derived relaxing factor and prostacyclins, which contribute to arterial vasodilation. Conversely, platelet-derived growth factor and angiotensin II trigger arterial vasoconstriction.

The media is the middle, and thickest, layer of the arterial wall. It is composed chiefly of smooth muscle cells, along with a connective tissue matrix that includes elastin, collagen, and proteoglycans. The strength of the media is derived from collagen. Its elasticity is provided by elastin. The smooth muscle cells and surrounding matrix are organized into discrete circular bundles, or lamellae. Larger vessels, which have more than 28 lamellar units, have vasovasorum that penetrate the adventitia to perfuse the media. Arteries that have fewer than 28 lamellar units are oxygenated directly from the blood within the vessel. The adventitia is the outermost layer. It extends beyond the external elastic lamina and is composed of loose connective tissue, fibroblasts, capillaries, and neural fibers. The adventitia provides little strength to the artery, but may be important in containing hemorrhage after trauma or aneurysmal rupture.

Atherosclerosis

The most common cause of arterial stenosis and occlusion is **atherosclerosis,** a degenerative disease that is characterized by endothelial cell dysfunction, inflammatory cell adhesion and infiltration, and the accumulation of cellular and matrix elements, leading to the formation of fibrocellular plaques. In the end stages of the disease, advanced plaques impede blood flow and lead to the well-known ischemic syndromes of angina pectoris, **claudication,** and renovascular hypertension. More sudden events (e.g., myocardial infarction, stroke, atheroembolism) may be caused by disturbances within plaques, including rupture of the fibrous cap into the lumen, hemorrhage in the substance of the plaque, and **embolism.**

Risk factors for the development of atherosclerosis include cigarette smoking, hypertension, abnormalities in cholesterol metabolism (elevated levels of low-density lipoprotein and depressed levels of high-density lipoprotein), diabetes mellitus, obesity, coagulation disorders, and regions of turbulence within the arterial circulation. The first signs of atherosclerosis may appear as early as childhood or adolescence. They are manifested by lipid- and macrophage-laden fatty streaks that form on the endothelial surface. These lesions progress to fibrous plaques that are usually located at areas of flow disturbance. Fibrous plaques

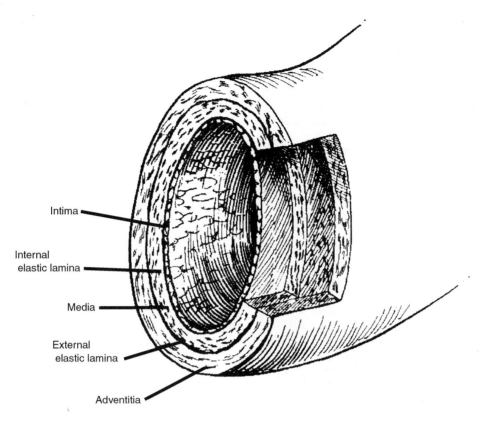

Figure 22-1 Layers of the arterial wall.

generally consist of lipid-laden macrophages encapsulated by collagen and elastin. As the fibrous plaque matures, regions within the plaque become necrotic and eventually rupture, leading to plaque ulceration. Within these complex plaques, regions of microcalcification develop that can progress to significant calcium deposits. Although atherosclerosis is usually considered a systemic disease, plaques tend to localize in specific regions. The most common sites of atherosclerotic plaques are within the coronary arteries, the carotid bifurcation, the proximal iliac arteries, and the arteries of the legs. Regions of arterial bifurcation are most predisposed to the development of atherosclerotic plaques because of turbulence at the flow divider that results in regions of low shear stress and flow stagnation (Figure 22-2). This stasis allows greater contact time between the atherogenic factors in the blood (e.g., lipids) and the vessel wall. It appears that smoking is a greater risk factor for peripheral atherosclerosis (incidence nine times that of the normal population) than for coronary atherosclerosis (incidence four times that of the normal population).

The common sequelae of atherosclerosis are: (1) myocardial infarction or angina pectoris as a result of coronary atherosclerosis; (2) transient ischemic attack (TIA) or stroke as a result of carotid bifurcation atherosclerosis; and (3) lower extremity ischemia that causes difficulty in walking, **rest pain,** or gangrene. Less common clinical presentations are renal hypoperfusion and small bowel ischemia. The symptoms of arterial stenosis are caused by either gradual progressive occlusion

from an enlarging plaque that limits distal perfusion or a sudden **thrombosis** of the artery at a region of stenosis. Sudden arterial occlusion does not allow for the development of collateral arterial channels, but gradual stenosis of the artery allows for the development of arterial collaterals to maintain distal perfusion. The result is either sudden ischemia or more gradual-onset chronic ischemia. Plaque ulcerations often become a nidus for thrombus formation or platelet deposition. Distal embolization of this material may produce an acute occlusive event and sudden onset of symptoms.

Atherosclerosis is a progressive event. The best way to retard its progression is to modify the atherosclerotic risk factors (discussed earlier). Cessation of cigarette smoking, control of hypertension, and diet modification may have the greatest effect on reducing atherosclerotic risk. Exercise has a protective effect by increasing the level of high-density lipoproteins, which enhance the transport and metabolism of other lipids.

Aneurysms

Anatomy and Epidemiology

An **aneurysm** is a focal dilation of an artery to more than 1.5 its normal diameter. Aneurysms may be either true aneurysms, which are generally associated with atherosclerosis and include all three layers of the arterial wall, or false aneurysms (pseudoaneurysms), which occur secondary to trauma or infection and are covered by only a thickened fibrous capsule. Aneurysms are also

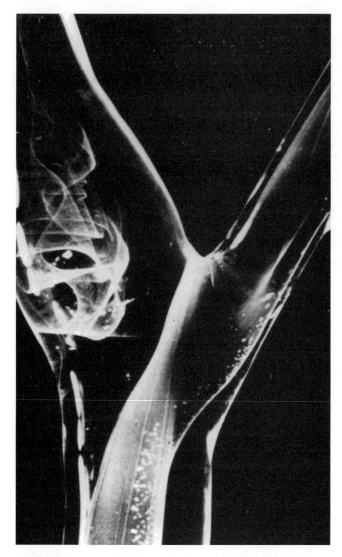

Figure 22-2 Glass model of the carotid bifurcation. Hydrogen gas bubbles show the streamlining of flow fields at the carotid flow divider and the complex counterrotating helical pattern at the arterial wall opposite the flow divider. (Reprinted with permission from Zarins CK, Glagov S. Arterial wall pathology in atherosclerosis. In Rutherford RB, ed. *Vascular Surgery*, 4th ed. Vol. 1. Philadelphia, Pa: WB Saunders, 1996:214.)

classified by their shape. A fusiform aneurysm is diffusely dilated and irregular, whereas a saccular aneurysm is an eccentric outpouching of an otherwise normal-appearing artery (Figure 22-3).

Aneurysms may occur in any location within the arterial tree, but are most common in the infrarenal aorta, iliac arteries, and popliteal arteries (Table 22-1). It is estimated that 2% to 3% of men older than 70 years of age have an aortic aneurysm, but patients with high-risk factors may have an incidence of up to 10%. Aneurysmal formation is a systemic and familial disease. A patient with one popliteal aneurysm has a 60% chance of having an aneurysm in the contralateral popliteal artery and a 50% chance of harboring an abdominal aortic aneurysm (AAA). Approximately 20%

of patients with AAAs have a first-degree relative with the same disease.

Pathophysiology

Approximately 90% of all aneurysms are associated with atherosclerosis. Atherosclerosis probably impairs the diffusion of nutrients and allows for metalloproteinase-mediated arterial wall degeneration, although the exact mechanisms are unknown. Less common causes of aneurysm formation include connective tissue disease (Marfan's syndrome, Ehlers-Danlos syndrome), infection (mycotic aneurysm), medial degeneration, disruption of anastomotic connections (anastomotic pseudoaneurysm), and trauma (traumatic pseudoaneurysm) [Table 22-2].

The most serious complication of aneurysms is their propensity for enlargement and rupture. The growth rate of aneurysms is unpredictable. Although most AAAs enlarge at an average rate of approximately 0.3 cm/year, the range of expansion rates is wide; some aneurysms double in size over a few months. The size of an aneurysm is critically important because the risk of rupture is diameter-dependent. According to a modification of the law of Laplace, the larger and thinner an aneurysm grows, the higher its tangential wall stress (*J*):

$$J = \frac{P \times r}{t}$$

where *P* = intraluminal pressure, *r* = aneurysm radius, and *t* = wall thickness.

Clinical Presentation and Evaluation

Aneurysms are usually discovered as asymptomatic masses on routine physical examination or during radiologic tests for other conditions. Approximately 20% of aneurysms cause symptoms, including localized pain or tenderness, thrombosis or distal embolization that causes peripheral ischemia, and rupture (Figure 22-4). The clinical presentation reflects the location of the aneurysm. Abdominal and thoracoabdominal aortic aneurysms tend to be discovered during routine examination or, if ruptured, as a clinical catastrophe that causes acute back pain, hypotension, and hemodynamic collapse. Popliteal and femoral aneurysms rarely rupture, but a laminated thrombus often develops and can dislodge, embolize to the arteries of the calf and foot, and cause acute arterial ischemia. Carotid artery aneurysms may cause either asymptomatic pulsatile neck masses or cerebrovascular ischemia, including **TIAs** or stroke.

The diagnosis of aortic and peripheral artery aneurysms is often made by a careful physical examination. If an aneurysm is suspected, the patient undergoes confirmatory radiologic evaluations. The best screening tool for aortic and peripheral aneurysms is ultrasonography. A well-performed ultrasound assesses the size and general location of the aneurysm with more than 95% accuracy. If the diagnosis of AAA is established, the patient undergoes either computed tomography (CT) scanning or

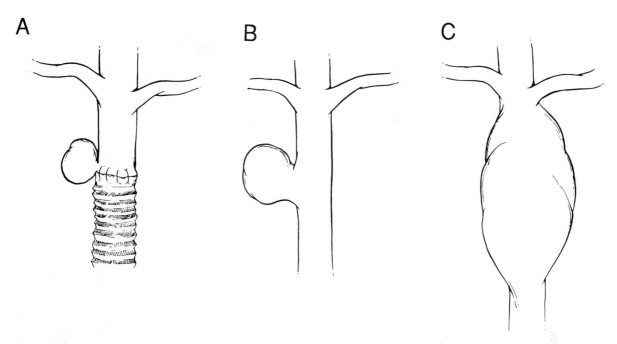

Figure 22-3 Classification of aneurysms. **A,** Pseudoaneurysm. **B,** Saccular atherosclerotic aneurysm. **C,** Fusiform atherosclerotic aneurysm.

Table 22-1. Localization and Incidence of Abdominal Aneurysms

Location of Aneurysm	Incidence
Abdominal aortic artery	1.5%–3.0%
Common iliac artery	20%–40% present with AAA
	0.03% isolated, without AAA
Splenic artery	0.8%
	60% of all splanchnic artery aneurysms
Renal artery	0.1%
Hepatic artery	0.1%
Superior mesenteric artery	0.07%
Celiac axis	0.05%

AAA, abdominal aortic artery.

Table 22-2. Etiology of Aneurysmal Disease

Congenital
  Idiopathic
  Tuberous sclerosis
  Turner's syndrome
  Poststenotic dilation
Inherited abnormalities of connective tissue
  Marfan's syndrome
  Ehlers-Danlos syndrome
  Cystic medial necrosis
Dissection
Infections
  Mycotic
  Posttraumatic
  Infection of existing aneurysm
Inflammatory
Aneurysms associated with pregnancy
  Splenic artery
  Mesenteric vessels
  Renal artery
Aneurysms associated with arteritis
  Takayasu's disease
  Giant cell arteritis
  Polyarteritis nodosa
  Systemic lupus erythematosus
Pseudoaneurysm
Nonspecific aortic aneurysms: "atherosclerotic"

magnetic resonance imaging (MRI) to evaluate the full extent of the aneurysm and better assess the need for intervention. In the past, most AAAs were further evaluated with invasive contrast angiography. Because of improvements in the performance and interpretation of CT scans, however, many patients proceed to operation without angiography if they are relatively free of atherosclerotic arterial occlusive disease. Routine angiography is still advised for peripheral artery aneurysms to plan the arterial reconstruction.

Treatment

The natural history of AAAs is to enlarge and rupture. Patients with AAAs have a greatly decreased life expectancy compared with age-matched controls. Aneurysm rupture is expected to cause as many as 60% of deaths. As stated earlier, the risk of rupture is directly related to the diameter of the aneurysm. Most clinical studies show that a 4-cm AAA has an annual risk of rupture of less than 5% (5-year risk of rupture is 25%), but the annual rate increases to 15% when the AAA reaches 6 cm (Figure 22-5). Because the current surgical mortality rate

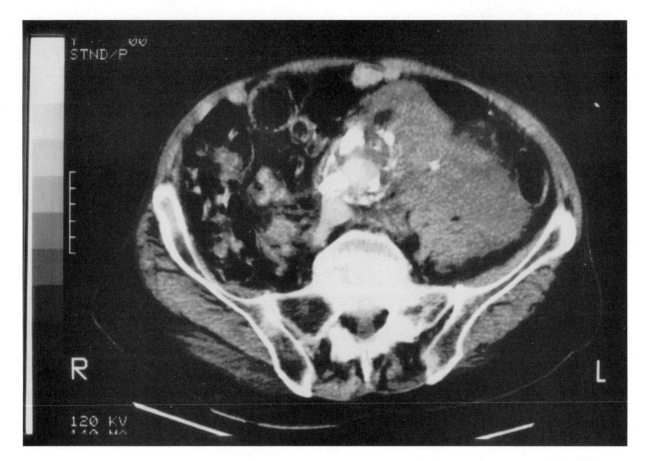

Figure 22-4 Computed tomography scan of a calcific abdominal aortic aneurysm with a contained rupture into the left retroperitoneum.

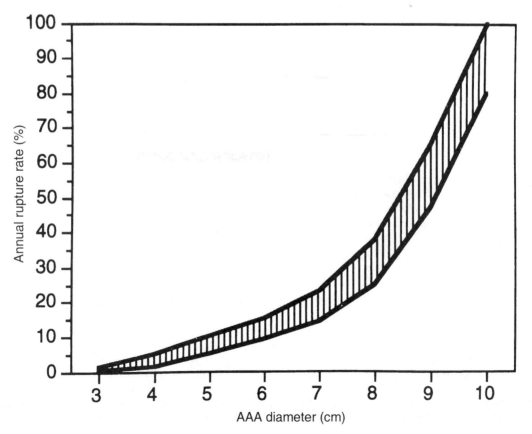

Figure 22-5 The annual risk of aneurysm rupture according to size. (Reprinted with permission from Sampson LN, Cronenwett JL. Abdominal aortic aneurysm. *Probl Gen Surg* 1995;2:385–417.)

for elective repair of AAAs is 2% to 4%, it is reasonable to offer good-risk patients repair for most aneurysms that are larger than 5 cm in diameter. Patients with serious risk factors (e.g., coronary artery disease, renal insufficiency, pulmonary disease) are managed more conservatively. Nonetheless, most clinicians believe that repair should be undertaken whenever the anticipated risk of rupture exceeds the risk of surgery.

The elective surgical treatment of AAAs is usually accomplished with an abdominal incision. The normal proximal aorta and distal arteries are dissected and isolated. After heparinization, the aorta is clamped and the aneurysm incised. A prosthetic graft is sewn in place and covered with the residual aneurysm sac (Figure 22-6). Aneurysms that involve the iliac arteries or the more proximal portions of the abdominal or thoracic aorta are technically more challenging, but good results were obtained in modern series.

The evolution of sophisticated catheter techniques and devices led to the development of the endovascular graft as an alternative to traditional operative AAA repair. The procedure involves placing a combination of stents and grafts through the femoral or iliac arteries. Deployment into the proximal infrarenal aorta and bifurcation allows exclusion of the aneurysm sac. Although experience is limited, endovascular grafts were successfully placed in more than 200 patients and may become the standard therapy for a subset of aneurysms with favorable anatomic conditions.

Patients who have rupture of an aneurysm associated with severe acute back pain and hypotension have a dismal prognosis unless they are immediately treated. These patients must be taken to the operating room for repair. They should be carefully resuscitated with fluid and blood products while being prepared for operation. Even in the best of hands, the success rate

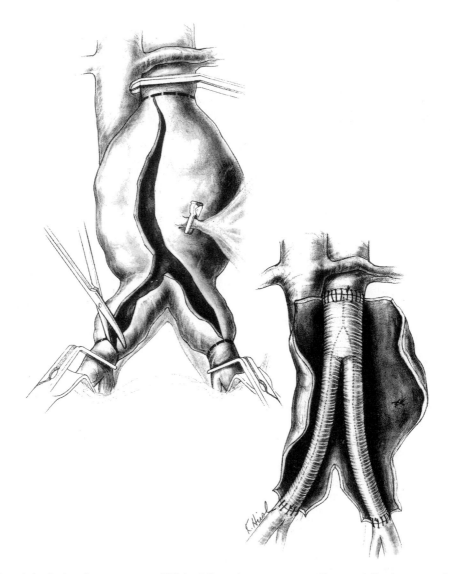

Figure 22-6 Repair of an abdominal aortic aneurysm and bilateral iliac artery aneurysms with an aortoiliac bypass graft. (Reprinted with permission from Zarins CK, Gewertz BL. Aneurysms. In: *Atlas of Vascular Surgery.* New York, NY: Churchill Livingstone, 1989:51.)

for operations for AAA rupture is less than 50%, and many survivors have major complications, including renal dysfunction, myocardial infarction, extremity amputation, and cerebrovascular accident.

Popliteal aneurysms are generally repaired if they exceed 2 cm in diameter or if there is evidence of thrombus formation or distal embolization. As stated earlier, preoperative angiography is essential for planning the reconstruction and, occasionally, for delivering thrombolytic (clot busting) therapy to recanalize thrombosed distal vessels. In contrast to AAA repair, in which the aneurysm is opened directly, popliteal aneurysm repair is generally accomplished with bypass surgery. An important component of the procedure is ligation of the proximal or distal popliteal artery to prevent embolization downstream. The preferred conduit is saphenous vein graft because of its superior patency record for below-the-knee revascularization.

Complications

Immediate complications after elective repair of aortic aneurysms include myocardial infarction (3%–16%), renal failure (3%–12%), colonic ischemia (2%), distal emboli, and hemorrhage. Long-term complications include aortic graft infection, graft thrombosis, and **pseudoaneurysm** formation. Aortic graft infection can occur 5 to 7 years later as a pseudoaneurysm because of the breakdown of the graft-to-artery anastomosis. Gradual disruption of the proximal or distal anastomotic suture lines, unassociated with infection, may cause anastomotic pseudoaneurysms to form. They are usually amenable to repair with interpositional grafting.

After aortic repair, colonic ischemia can result from the disruption of pelvic arterial collateral flow, ligation of the inferior mesenteric artery, or perioperative hypotension. The patient with postoperative colonic ischemia can have colonic emptying, guaiac-positive diarrhea, or abdominal pain. Patients who have diarrhea immediately postoperatively, with or without blood, should undergo sigmoidoscopy to further evaluate the viability of the sigmoid colon and rectum. If the colon is frankly infarcted, then the affected colonic portion is resected and a colostomy performed. However, if the colon appears dusky, but without frank necrosis, then the patient is treated with blood pressure support, broad-spectrum antibiotics, and frequent repeat sigmoidoscopy to follow the ischemic repair.

Graft infection, with or without a fistula between the aorta and duodenum (**aortoenteric fistula**), is a devastating long-term complication with a mortality rate that exceeds 50%. It should be suspected in any patient with an indwelling aortic graft who has sepsis, abdominal pain, or gastrointestinal bleeding. The diagnosis is often difficult to establish, but may be confirmed with a combination of CT scanning, blood cultures, endoscopy, and surgical exploration. Some patients are managed with antibiotics and in situ graft replacement, but most undergo graft excision with concomitant duodenal repair and extraanatomic bypass to restore extremity perfusion.

Popliteal artery aneurysms classically cause either distal emboli or thrombosis. Distal emboli may cause "blue toe syndrome," in which a mural thrombus embolizes to the digital vessels of the foot, resulting in localized thrombosis and gangrene. Thrombosis of the popliteal artery aneurysm itself has a grim prognosis and a 50% amputation rate. The morbidity rate is so high because the popliteal artery aneurysm generally thromboses only after it has showered multiple emboli to the lower extremity, thrombosing the outflow vessels. This finding prompted an interest in the use of preoperative thrombolytic therapy to lyse the obstructed outflow vessels and facilitate arterial reconstruction.

Aortic Dissection

Aortic dissection results from a tear in the intima, with extension of a pulsatile blood column traveling through the media distally throughout the thoracic and abdominal aorta. These lesions classically begin in the thoracic aorta, but can extend into the abdominal aorta and compromise the arterial blood supply to the mesenteric circulation, renal circulation, spinal cord, or distal extremities. Complications from an ascending aortic dissection are related to either retrograde or antegrade propagation of the dissection. With retrograde dissection toward the aortic valve, the origins of the coronary arteries can be obstructed, resulting in acute myocardial ischemia. The dissection can also extend into the aortic valve leaflets and result in acute aortic valve insufficiency. The most devastating complication is proximal extension of the dissection into the aortic root and free rupture into the pericardial sac, which results in cardiac tamponade. Dissection can also extend into the brachiocephalic vessels and cause stroke. The diagnosis of an aortic dissection is confirmed by transesophageal echocardiography, CT scan, or angiography. Acute management of aortic dissection is directed at lowering the blood pressure and heart rate to decrease the stress on the arterial wall. Acute surgical intervention is reserved for dissections that involve the ascending aorta or those that begin in the descending thoracic aorta and occlude the mesenteric, renal, or iliac vessels and result in sudden ischemia. Enlargement of a chronic dissection with aneurysm formation is the main indication for elective repair.

Peripheral Arterial Occlusive Disease

Occlusion or stenosis of the arteries of the lower extremities is usually called peripheral vascular disease (PVD). Common sites that are predisposed to the development of atherosclerotic plaques include the iliac, superficial femoral, and tibial arteries. Specific symptoms are dictated by the number and severity of occlusions, the degree of collateralization, and the patient's tolerance for limitation in walking distance. Stenosis or occlusion of the aorta and iliac arteries (aortoiliac occlusive disease) is more common in adults between 40 and 60 years of age. The predilection to aortoiliac disease is increased by a family history of arterial occlusive disease, cigarette smoking, and hyperlipidemia. Disease confined below the inguinal ligament is known as femoropopliteal occlusive disease. The most common pattern of occlusion is disease of the distal superficial femoral artery within the adductor (Hunter's) canal. Femoropopliteal occlusive disease is often asymptomatic without extensive exercise as a result of collateralization from the profunda femoris artery. Involvement of the arteries below the popliteal trifurcation is called tibial occlusive disease or simply distal disease. Tibial occlusive disease is common in patients with diabetes, end-stage renal failure, and advanced age.

Physiology

Large atherosclerotic plaques occlude the arterial lumen, impede blood flow, and diminish blood pressure distal to the stenosis. The loss of pressure (for steady flow of a Newtonian liquid) is described by Poiseuille's law:

$$\Delta P = \frac{8Q\,L\,\eta}{\pi\,r^4}$$

where ΔP = change in pressure, Q = volume of blood flow, L = arterial length, η = density, and r = arterial radius. As noted, the loss in pressure is directly proportional to the volume of blood flow and the arterial length, but inversely proportional to the fourth power of the radius. A decrease in radius has the most profound effect on ΔP. In general, ΔP is small until the reduction in diameter is approximately 50% (75% reduction in cross-sectional area), when it increases exponentially with greater narrowing.

The enlargement of an atherosclerotic plaque is the leading cause of peripheral vascular arterial occlusive disease. Previous studies showed that the vessel initially adapts to the atherosclerotic plaque and enlarges its overall diameter. Once maximal enlargement is attained, this compensation is exhausted, and the luminal area is progressively decreased by the atherosclerotic process (Figure 22-7). Other potential causes of arterial occlusive disease are Buerger's disease (thromboarteritis obliterans) and cystic adventitial disease. Although it is much less common, extraluminal compression of the arterial system can occur as a result of compression of the artery by aberrant muscular bands (e.g., popliteal artery entrapment syndrome).

Clinical Presentation

Ischemia of the lower extremity can cause intermittent claudication, rest pain, skin ulceration, and gangrene. The degree of ischemia determines the type or extent of presentation. Claudication, from the Latin *claudatio* (to limp), is characterized by reproducible pain in a major muscle group that is precipitated by exercise and relieved by rest. The joints and foot are generally spared. Although these patients maintain adequate arterial perfusion at rest, arterial occlusions prevent the augmentation of blood flow that is necessary to meet the metabolic demands of active muscles during exercise. The result is conversion to anaerobic metabolism and local metabolic acidosis. The muscle groups that are affected by claudication are always distal to the level of arterial obstruction. Hence, aortoiliac occlusion classically causes Leriche syndrome, which is defined by impotence, absence of femoral pulses, lower extremity claudication, and muscle wasting of the buttocks. Occlusion of the superficial femoral artery causes calf claudication.

The natural history of untreated claudication is generally benign. In the prominent Framingham study, the risk of major amputation was only 5% for gangrene within 5 years if claudications were treated conservatively. With cessation of cigarette smoking and an organized exercise program, as many as 50% of patients with claudication improve and their symptoms completely resolve. The most common cause of death in patients with claudication is a cardiac or cerebral event.

Rest pain indicates more advanced peripheral ischemia, just as rest angina is a more advanced form of exertional angina. Most commonly, patients have pain in the toes and metatarsal heads while lying down at night. Temporary relief is achieved by dangling the legs over the side of the bed or standing and walking around the room. By making the feet more dependent, gravitational hydrostatic pressure increases venous pressure, slows capillary flow, and temporarily enhances oxygen delivery. Rest pain is caused by nerve ischemia because these tissues are most sensitive to hypoxia. Nocturnal cramps in the calf muscle, unassociated with impairment of blood flow, can usually be distinguished from true rest pain by the location of the pain (calf vs distal foot) and the absence of advanced ischemic changes in the skin.

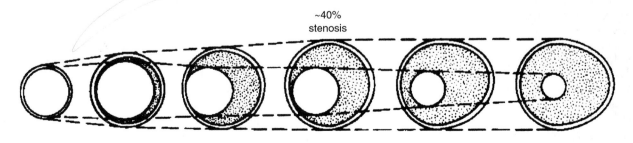

~40% stenosis

Figure 22-7 Proposed arterial adaptation to enlarging atherosclerotic plaques. Initially, the artery enlarges to maintain the luminal diameter despite the enlarging plaque. After the plaques create a stenosis of more than 40%, the artery can no longer adapt, and a luminal stenosis develops. (Reprinted with permission from Glagov S, Weisenberg E, Zarins CK, et al. Compensatory enlargement of human atherosclerotic coronary arteries. *N Engl J Med* 1987;316:1371.)

Ulceration of the skin of the toes, heel, or dorsum of the foot can occur as a result of arterial insufficiency. Even minor trauma (e.g., friction from an ill-fitting shoe), incorrect nail care, or a small break in the skin can lead to chronic, progressive ulceration as a result of insufficient arterial perfusion to allow for healing. Ulcerations usually cause pain, except in patients with diabetes, who often have associated peripheral neuropathy. Ischemic ulcers may have a punched-out appearance and a pale or necrotic base.

By comparison, venous ulcerations usually occur at the level of the medial or lateral malleolus. They are usually associated with venous pooling and red blood cell extravasation that leads to an orange–brown skin discoloration secondary to hemosiderin deposition. The ulcers are located at the level of the medial and lateral malleoli because of the presence of perforating veins that connect the superficial and deep venous systems at the level of the ankle. Venous ulcerations may have a granulating base and are usually associated with significant edema. Treatment of venous stasis ulcerations is generally conservative (discussed later).

Diabetic ulcerations are painless and are located on the plantar or lateral aspect of the foot. They are a direct result of the neuropathy of diabetes. Because of the injury to the autonomic motor and sensory nerves, the skin becomes dry and the foot can become deformed (Charcot's foot). The changes associated with diabetes are worsened by the arterial occlusive process that usually accompanies diabetes.

The outlook for patients with rest pain is far worse than that for patients with claudication. Persistent nocturnal pain and disruption of sleep cycles can lead to irritability and chronic fatigue. In addition, if untreated, nearly 50% of patients with rest pain need amputation for intractable pain or gangrene within a short period.

Dry and wet gangrene are differentiated clinically. Dry gangrene is mummification of the digits of the foot without associated purulent drainage or cellulitis. Wet gangrene is an ongoing infection. The severely ischemic foot is an excellent nidus for the colonization and growth of bacteria and is generally malodorous, with copious purulent drainage. The outlook is ominous, with potential sepsis and immediate limb loss.

Physical Examination

Routine evaluation of patients with PVD includes a thorough physical examination and noninvasive vascular testing. A search for cervical **bruits,** precordial murmurs, and pulsatile masses or bruits in the abdomen is mandatory. Examination of the lower extremity includes inspection, palpation, and auscultation. Inspection of the legs and feet in a patient with PVD may show loss of hair on the distal aspect of the leg, muscle atrophy, color changes in the leg, and ulcers or gangrene. Patients with severe PVD often have Buerger's sign (dependent rubor). With dependency of the foot, pooling of oxygenated blood in the maximally dilated arteriolar bed distal to an arterial occlusion causes the foot to appear ruborous (red). When the extremity is elevated, hydrostatic pressure decreases, allowing drainage of pooled blood, and the foot becomes white (pallor). Palpation should include investigation of the presence and character of the arterial pulsations at the groin (femoral artery), at the popliteal fossa (popliteal artery), at the dorsum of the foot (dorsalis pedis artery), and posterior to the medial malleolus (posterior tibial artery).

Patients who do not have palpable pulses in any of these positions are examined with continuous-wave Doppler ultrasound. The Doppler probe emits 2- to 10-MHz ultrasonic waves that are reflected by flowing red blood cells and detected by a receiving crystal. The frequency shift between the transmitting and the receiving crystals is proportional to the velocity of the moving particles and provides a qualitative assessment of the degree of stenosis. Normally, a triphasic waveform is seen, representing the forward flow of systole, reversal of the arterial velocity waveform against the relatively high-resistance vascular bed, and resumption of forward flow during diastole. If proximal stenosis is present, the pulse volume from cardiac contraction loses kinetic energy crossing the area of stenosis and does not have enough energy to recoil against the vascular outflow bed. As a result, the Doppler signal becomes biphasic. With further progression of proximal arterial stenosis, the waveform becomes more blunt and widened, and it eventually becomes monophasic (Figure 22-8).

In addition to this qualitative assessment of disease, the systolic pressure within the arteries of the foot can be determined. A blood pressure cuff is inflated on the calf and then slowly deflated while the Doppler signal is monitored. The pressure at which a signal reappears is the systolic pressure within the artery. The pressure is normalized for all patients by dividing the ankle pressure by the systolic blood pressure in the arm and calculating the **ankle–brachial index** (ABI). In general, an ABI less than 0.8 is consistent with claudication, whereas an ABI less than 0.4 is usually associated with rest pain or tissue loss.

Advances in ultrasound technology have led to better anatomic correlation with arterial duplex scanning. Duplex scanners provide visualization of blood flow within the artery in two dimensions and calculate the velocity of flowing blood. In regions of significant stenosis, high-velocity jets are seen as blood travels through the narrow lumen.

Patients with severe lifestyle-limiting claudication, rest pain, or gangrene should undergo diagnostic arteriography. Arteriography is performed with a percutaneous femoral artery puncture, advancement of a wire and catheter into the abdominal aorta, and injection of radiopaque contrast agent for visualization of the distal arterial tree. Complications of these tests, including idiosyncratic dye reactions, contrast agent nephropathy, and puncture site hemorrhage, are infrequent, but mandate careful patient selection.

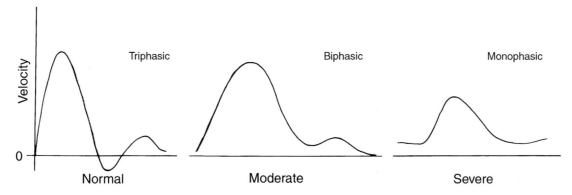

Figure 22-8 A Doppler ultrasound instrument provides an analog display of blood flow velocity (waveform). With progressive occlusion, the waveform changes from triphasic to biphasic to monophasic.

Differential Diagnosis

Intermittent claudication can be differentiated from musculoskeletal or neurogenic pain by a careful history, physical examination, and noninvasive vascular evaluation. Neurogenic lower extremity pain is usually not located in major muscle groups and is not precipitated by exercise. Straight raised leg lifts and findings of sensory examinations may be abnormal. Musculoskeletal pain is often present at rest. Pain secondary to spinal stenosis is relieved by bending forward while walking. It often radiates down the limb and is not relieved immediately (< 5 minutes) by resting.

Treatment
Medical

As many as 50% of patients with intermittent claudication obtain significant relief with cessation of smoking and a regimented exercise program. Treatment with pentoxifylline (Trental) is of uncertain benefit, although a small percentage of patients respond favorably. Some patients with painless ischemic ulcers respond to careful local therapy if they are followed closely for progression or the development of gangrene.

Many discrete areas of arterial lesions, especially in the iliac arteries, are amenable to percutaneous transluminal **angioplasty** (PTA) [Figure 22-9*A* and *B*]. PTA is performed at the time of diagnostic arteriography and involves advancement of an intraarterial balloon-tipped catheter across the stenotic lesion. Inflation of the balloon disrupts the plaque and stretches the arterial wall, resulting in luminal enlargement. The development of endovascular stents allowed stenoses to be dilated and held open within the arterial wall. The results of PTA strongly depend on the location of the lesion, its length, the degree of arterial occlusion, the amount of calcification within the plaque, and the tortuosity of the vessel. In the iliac region, more than 90% of short stenotic lesions can be successfully dilated, and the 2-year patency rate is 70%. Angioplasty of the superficial femoral arteries is less durable. The initial success rate of 75% decreases to approximately 50% at 2 years,

depending on patient selection. Angioplasty of the infrapopliteal and tibial vessels is reserved for patients who are poor surgical risks because only 40% to 50% remain patent after 1 year.

Surgical or chemical lumbar sympathectomy is rarely effective in patients with diabetes or those with profound ulcerations and gangrene. Improvement is reported in patients with rest pain alone.

Surgical
Endarterectomy. Endarterectomy (excision of the diseased arterial wall, including the endothelium, the occluding plaque, and a portion of the media) is the standard operative treatment for carotid bifurcation atherosclerosis. Endarterectomy has more limited usefulness in the treatment of lower extremity occlusive diseases because lower extremity atherosclerotic disease is often extensive, with no discrete starting or ending points. Few patients with aortoiliac disease are candidates for aortoiliac endarterectomy, but many surgeons use local endarterectomy of the common femoral artery and profunda femoral arteries to improve outflow for an aortofemoral bypass graft.

Bypass Procedures. Bypass procedures are the principal operative treatment for PVD. Aortoiliac occlusive disease is usually treated with aortobifemoral bypass. With a combination of midline abdominal and groin incisions, a prosthetic graft is sutured to the infrarenal aorta and tunneled through the retroperitoneum to both femoral arteries (Figure 22-10). In cases of concomitant superficial artery occlusion, the profunda femoral artery is the primary outflow bed. Aortofemoral bypass grafting is a durable procedure with a 5-year patency rate of greater than 90%. Aortofemoral bypass graft limb occlusion is usually caused by the progression of distal outflow disease, which limits blood flow through the graft, causing stasis and thrombosis.

If the patient is a prohibitive surgical risk for an intraabdominal procedure or has had multiple intraabdominal procedures or infections (hostile abdomen),

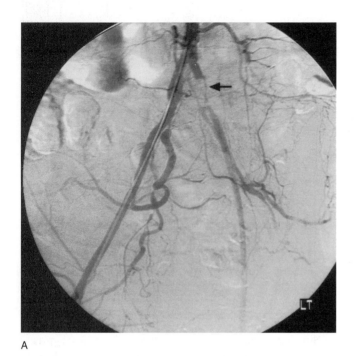

A

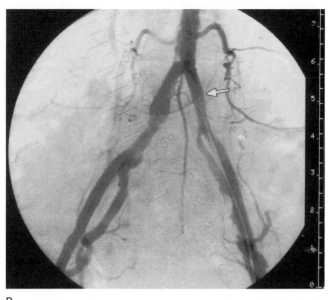

B

Figure 22-9 A, Angiogram showing a short segment occlusion of the proximal left common iliac artery *(solid arrow).* **B,** Successful percutaneous balloon angioplasty of the iliac lesion *(open arrow).*

extraanatomic bypasses are considered. Extraanatomic bypasses include axillary artery–femoral artery bypass grafts and femoral artery–femoral artery bypass grafts tunneled in the subcutaneous tissue. In critically ill patients, this procedure is performed with local anesthesia and intravenous sedation. The patency rates for extraanatomic bypasses are lower than those for aortofemoral bypass grafts, especially in the presence of superficial femoral artery occlusion. Occlusions can also occur secondary to the longer length of the bypass graft. Graft compression or kinking also may occur within the subcutaneous tunnels.

In patients with rest pain and occluded superficial femoral arteries with proximal profunda femoral artery stenoses, opening the stenoses (profundaplasty) can assist by increasing perfusion through the collaterals. However, if the ischemia has progressed to tissue loss or gangrene, it is unlikely that the profundaplasty can adequately increase arterial inflow into the leg to heal the ulcerative lesions. In this case, arterial bypass is performed.

Patients who have femoropopliteal occlusive disease are best treated with bypass of the occluded segment. Preoperative diagnostic arteriography is used to assure that the patient has adequate arterial inflow into the femoral arteries as well as to identify the distal target vessel, usually the popliteal or tibial artery. Bypass to the popliteal artery above the knee is performed with either the patient's own veins (autologous vein) or polytetrafluoroethylene with equivalent initial results. In contrast, prosthetic bypasses to arteries below the knee function poorly. These distal bypass procedures are best accomplished with autologous vein (Table 22-3). Saphe-

nous vein bypass grafts can be reversed so that the venous valves are in the same direction as arterial flow. The disadvantages of this orientation are the complete removal of the vein from its nutrient bed as well as a potential size mismatch between the proximal aspect of the saphenous vein and the small distal artery. Alternatively, in situ bypasses can be performed in which the saphenous vein is left in its normal anatomic position and the vein valves are disrupted with a valvulotome. This approach allows a better size match between the artery and the vein. In addition, the vasovasorum of the vein is undisturbed. Disadvantages of in situ bypass include endothelial injury during passage of the valvulotome and the possibility of missing a valve cusp (retained valve).

Postoperative duplex graft surveillance of saphenous vein bypass grafts is effective in identifying regions of anastomotic and graft stenosis that, if uncorrected, could lead to graft failure. The combination of duplex graft surveillance and surgical reintervention with repair of stenotic lesions, which occurs in 20% of grafts, results in higher long-term patency of the saphenous vein bypass graft. The primary assisted patency rates of these vein grafts approach 90%. In contrast, if a stenosis of a saphenous vein graft is allowed to progress to occlusion and then is revised, the patency rate at 2 years is only 30%.

Immediate complications of arterial bypass graft procedures are often caused by technical problems (e.g., postoperative bleeding from the anastomotic site, graft thrombosis, hematoma in the region of the incision, lymphatic leakage that results in a lymphocele). Because many patients with peripheral vascular occlusive

Table 22-3. Outcomes of Infrainguinal Arterial Bypasses

Graft Type	2-yr Patency (%) Primary/Secondary	4-yr Patency (%) Primary/Secondary
Above-knee femoropopliteal, PTFE	75	60
Above-knee femoropopliteal, vein	80	70
Below-knee femoropopliteal, PTFE	60	40
Below-knee femoropopliteal, vein	75–80 / 90	70–75 / 80
Femoral-tibial bypass, PTFE	30	20
Femoral-tibial bypass, vein	70–75 / 80–90	60–70 / 75–80

PTFE, polytetra fluroethylene.

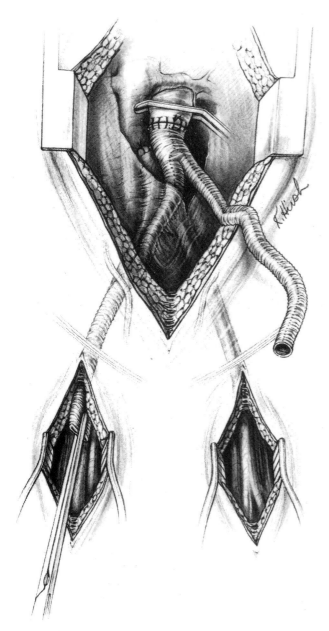

Figure 22-10 Aortobifemoral bypass graft showing the creation of the retroperitoneal tunnels to the groins. (Reprinted with permission from Zarins CK, Gewertz BL. Aneurysms. In: *Atlas of Vascular Surgery.* New York, NY: Churchill Livingstone, 1989:125.)

circumstance, the arterial anastomosis is weakened, and massive bleeding can occur into the bowel.

Amputation. Amputation may be the only option in patients with severe rest pain or gangrene who are not candidates for surgical revascularization or who do not have a suitable target vessel for a distal bypass. Partial foot amputation, with removal of areas of gangrene, may be required to augment a successful distal bypass. Other indications for amputation include trauma, with severe nerve and vascular injury, and neoplasm. An amputation is virtually never performed for venous disease without coexisting arterial insufficiency. In general, the more distal the amputation, the better the rehabilitation potential.

These distal amputations include toe, transmetatarsal, and Syme's (ankle) amputations. If arterial inflow is inadequate and an arterial bypass cannot be performed, then a below-the-knee or above-the-knee amputation may be required.

It is important to choose the appropriate site for amputation to assure adequate wound healing. If there is an occluded and unreconstructable superficial femoral artery and if there are no distal vessels below the knee, a below-the-knee amputation is often the lowest level that will heal. If the perfusion pressure is greater than 50 mm Hg at the popliteal artery and the ABI is greater than 0.6, then healing is expected in more than 70% of cases. It is important to attempt to preserve the knee joint because significantly more energy is required to ambulate with an above-the-knee prosthesis.

Above-the-knee amputation is required when profound ischemia and gangrene extend almost to the knee. At this higher amputation level, healing is likely, even in advanced cases. Above-the-knee amputation is

disease have concomitant coronary artery disease, renal insufficiency, or pulmonary obstructive disease, postoperative complications are always a concern.

A long-term problem associated with arterial bypass graft procedures is progressive arterial occlusive disease of the outflow vessels that results in graft thrombosis, graft infection, and pseudoaneurysm formation. Aortoduodenal fistula is one of the most devastating complications of aortofemoral bypass grafting. If it is not properly covered, the aortic graft anastomosis can erode into the third portion of the duodenum and contaminate the aortic graft with duodenal contents. In this also indicated in patients who are bedridden or at high risk because of other medical conditions.

Chronic Intestinal Ischemia

Pathophysiology

The visceral arterial supply includes the celiac axis, superior mesenteric artery, and inferior mesenteric artery. If one of the major visceral vessels becomes stenotic or occluded, the gastroduodenal artery and marginal artery can supply significant collateral flow (Figure 22-11). After there is significant occlusion of two of the three major arterial pathways to the visceral organs, patients often have visceral ischemic symptoms.

Clinical Presentation

The clinical manifestations of chronically decreased blood supply to the intestine (chronic intestinal ischemia) include postprandial abdominal pain and weight loss. Postprandial pain usually occurs 1 to 2 hours after meals and ranges from a persistent epigastric ache to severe, disabling, cramping pain. Other symptoms include early satiety and abdominal bloating. Many patients have a fear of food because of postprandial pain and limit their oral intake. This factor accounts for the significant weight loss seen in many patients. The typical age at presentation is older than 45 years. Associated comorbid atherosclerotic symptoms are often present (e.g., coronary artery disease, claudication, cerebrovascular accident). The malnutrition associated with chronic visceral ischemia suggests a differential diagnosis that includes disseminated carcinomatosis and primary visceral malignancies.

Diagnosis

Many patients see a surgeon only after an extensive gastrointestinal workup. The diagnosis is based on an accurate history and physical examination as well as

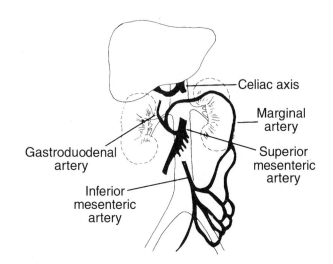

Figure 22-11 The intestinal circulation is characterized by three main vessels: the celiac axis, superior mesenteric artery, and inferior mesenteric artery. Collaterals connect these vessels so that chronic occlusion of one vessel is well compensated.

mesenteric angiography and noninvasive duplex ultrasound studies of the visceral vessels. The noninvasive duplex scan assesses the flow within the visceral vessels as well as the presence of a proximal arterial stenosis. The limitation of the duplex scan is its inability to evaluate the visceral vessels if a significant amount of bowel gas is present. To confirm the diagnosis, arteriograms should show hemodynamically significant lesions of at least two of the three major visceral vessels and evidence of collateral flow circumventing the stenotic mesenteric vessel. Evaluation of the proximal superior mesenteric artery and celiac axis is made by a lateral arteriogram because of the anterior positioning of the origin of these blood vessels off the aorta.

Treatment

Mesenteric revascularization should be considered in patients who have a history that is consistent with mesenteric ischemia as well as angiographic evidence of significant arterial occlusive disease of the visceral vessels. In these cases, mesenteric revascularization usually provides symptomatic improvement and prevents catastrophic mesenteric infarction.

Surgical revascularization options include endarterectomy of the proximal visceral vessels or bypass with vein or synthetic bypass conduits. Most patients have symptomatic improvement with revascularization of a single mesenteric vessel. However, many experienced surgeons routinely revascularize at least two of the visceral vessels to maximize the durability of the repair. Proximal mesenteric artery balloon angioplasty is being evaluated, but is more difficult than iliac artery angioplasty because of the acute angle of the origin of the visceral vessel.

Renal Artery Stenosis

Renal artery stenosis is the most common cause of surgically correctable hypertension. Stenoses can result from atherosclerosis, fibromuscular dysplasia, or posttraumatic subintimal dissections. Although renovascular hypertension accounts for approximately 5% of the total incidence of hypertension, this mechanism is responsible for a disproportionate fraction of hypertension in children and young adults and for new-onset hypertension in the elderly. Renal vascular hypertension is often refractory to medical management, and patients usually require multiple antihypertensive medications to partially control their hypertension. Other causes of surgically correctable hypertension include pheochromocytoma, aldosterone-secreting tumors, and descending thoracic aortic coarctation.

Anatomy

Atherosclerotic renal artery lesions usually occur in the proximal to middle portion of the renal artery and often represent an extension of an aortic plaque into the renal artery ostium. In contrast, fibromuscular dysplasia most commonly involves the middle to distal portion of the renal artery, with sparing of the proximal aspect of the renal artery (Figure 22-12). **Fibromuscular**

dysplasia is a hyperplastic, fibrosing process of the intima, media, or adventitia. It is three times more common in women than in men, and it usually occurs in the second to fourth decade. Bilateral involvement is seen in as many as 50% of cases.

Pathophysiology

Critical stenosis of the renal artery causes decreased blood pressure and flow to the kidney as well as decreased glomerular filtration. This change stimulates the renal juxtaglomerular apparatus to produce renin, which catalyzes the conversion of angiotensinogen to angiotensin I. Angiotensin-converting enzyme then converts angiotensin I to angiotensin II, a potent vasoconstrictor. Angiotensin II also stimulates the production of aldosterone, causing sodium retention and increased plasma volume. This combination of vasoconstriction and sodium retention causes a profound hypertensive state.

Physical Examination

Most untreated patients have profound diastolic hypertension exceeding 120 mm Hg. An epigastric or flank bruit may be noted on auscultation of the abdomen and suggests turbulent flow within the renal artery.

Diagnosis

Renal scan, renal function studies, and intravenous urography are used as screening studies to separate patients with renal vascular hypertension from the general hypertensive population. The high incidence of false-negative results limits reliance on these studies.

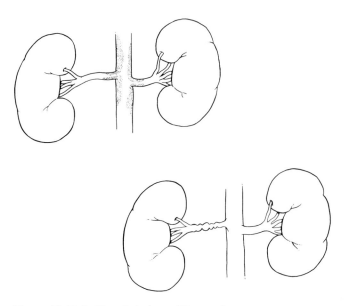

Figure 22-12 A, Stenotic lesions of the renal artery cause hypoperfusion of the kidney and activation of the renin-angiotensin system. As a result, significant hypertension occurs. Atherosclerotic lesions usually involve the origin to the middle portion of the renal artery. **B,** Fibromuscular hyperplasia involves the middle to the distal portion of the renal artery.

Urograms may contribute to the diagnosis of renal ischemia by showing: (1) a decrease in renal size secondary to hypoperfusion; (2) ureteral notching as a result of compression by collateral blood vessels; and (3) a delayed nephrogram with hyperconcentration of contrast. More important, urography may exclude other primary renal parenchymal pathology.

A functional test for renal vascular hypertension is the captopril challenge test. Captopril, an angiotensin II–converting enzyme inhibitor, prevents the conversion of angiotensin I to angiotensin II. Because of the blockage of synthesis of angiotensin II, more renin is produced and plasma renin levels are elevated after captopril administration. A positive captopril test also leads to a decrease in the glomerular filtration rate because of the blockage of the effect of angiotensin II on the efferent arteriole of the renal glomeruli. There was early enthusiasm for renal vein renin samplings as an accurate diagnostic test for renal vascular hypertension. Unfortunately, in patients with bilateral renal artery stenosis, the ratio may be 1, with both renal arteries producing higher levels of renin.

Renal duplex ultrasonography can assess the flow velocity profile in both renal arteries as well as the juxtarenal aorta. A significant difference in renal artery velocities (renal artery:aorta ratio > 3.5:1) suggests the presence of a hemodynamically significant renal artery stenosis. The duplex scan can also determine the renal parenchymal size to determine whether one of the kidneys is atrophying as a result of ischemia. The sensitivity and specificity of renal artery duplex ultrasonography for detecting significant renal artery stenosis are greater than 90%.

The definitive diagnosis of renal artery stenosis is confirmed by angiography. Renal arteriogram not only detects renal artery stenoses but also assists in determining kidney size by evaluating the postinjection nephrogram.

Treatment

Antihypertensive medications are usually ineffective in controlling renovascular hypertension. In particular, angiotensin II–converting enzyme inhibitors are avoided in cases of bilateral renal artery stenosis because these drugs decrease the glomerular filtration rate and may cause renal failure.

In patients with severe hypertension and hemodynamically significant renal artery stenosis, some form of renal revascularization should be considered. Fibromuscular dysplasia responds exceptionally well to percutaneous transluminal balloon angioplasty in all agegroups. Current experience with fibromuscular disease in pediatric patients and young adults suggests that more than 95% of patients are cured or significantly improve with renal artery angioplasty. Atherosclerotic lesions of the proximal renal artery are less responsive to angioplasty because the renal artery plaque is usually an extension of an aortic plaque. These lesions are more likely to return to their original degree of stenosis. Preliminary findings suggest that the use of a metallic stent after angioplasty provides better results in these cases.

Surgical treatment for renal vascular hypertension is performed in patients who have recurrent stenosis after angioplasty. It is also performed when lesions are not correctable with angioplasty. Surgical interventions include endarterectomy of the atherosclerotic lesions and bypass to the renal artery from the aorta, the hepatic arteries, or the splenic arteries.

Acute Arterial Occlusion

Clinical Presentation

Acute occlusion of an extremity or visceral vessel can cause limb, intestinal, or life-threatening ischemia. Etiologies of acute arterial occlusion include in situ thrombosis of preexisting atherosclerotic occlusive disease, arterial emboli, vascular trauma (either penetrating or blunt), and thrombosis of a preexisting arterial aneurysm. Patients with preexisting arterial occlusive disease may have a history of claudication or intestinal angina before arterial thrombosis occurs and acute symptoms of ischemia develop. These patients may already have a moderate collateral bed and therefore may have less acute symptoms. In contrast, patients with arterial emboli, vascular trauma, or thrombosis of a preexisting aneurysm are asymptomatic before new arterial occlusion occurs and may have more profound ischemic symptoms.

The great majority (80%) of arterial emboli originate in the left side of the heart. Thrombi form in the left atrium in cases of atrial fibrillation and at akinetic or hypokinetic regions of previous myocardial infarction. These thrombi can dislodge and embolize to the peripheral circulation. Nonthrombotic emboli can also occur from atherosclerotic lesions of the aorta and aortic valve. Mural thrombi within thoracic, abdominal aortic, and popliteal aneurysms can also cause distal embolization.

The most common site of embolic occlusion is the femoral artery. Other common sites are the axillary, popliteal, and iliac arteries; the aortic bifurcation; and the mesenteric vessels.

The classic presentation of limb-threatening acute arterial occlusion includes the "six Ps": pallor, pain, paresthesia, paralysis, pulselessness, and poikilothermia (change in temperature). These changes are limited to the area distal to the region of acute arterial occlusion. For example, with femoral artery occlusion, the ischemic changes (one or more of the six Ps) occur in the distal thigh, calf, or foot.

Acute mesenteric ischemia results from arterial occlusion (embolus or thrombosis), mesenteric venous occlusion, or nonocclusive mesenteric ischemia (especially vasospasm). Embolization to the superior mesenteric artery accounts for approximately 50% of all cases of acute mesenteric ischemia; 25% of cases occur secondary to thrombosis of a preexisting atherosclerotic lesion. Most superior mesenteric artery emboli lodge just distal to the origin of the middle colic artery, approximately 3 to 10 cm from the origin of the superior

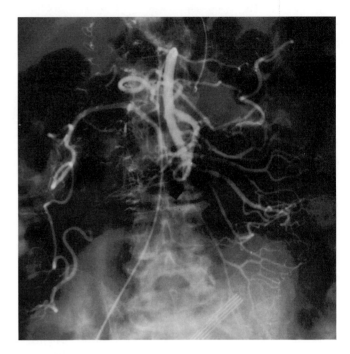

Figure 22-13 Acute embolus of the proximal superior mesenteric artery *(solid arrow).*

mesenteric artery (Figure 22-13). Nonocclusive mesenteric ischemia accounts for an additional 25% of cases of acute mesenteric ischemia. The etiology of nonocclusive mesenteric ischemia is multifactorial, but usually involves moderate to severe mesenteric atherosclerotic lesions in association with a low cardiac output state or the administration of vasoconstricting medications or digitalis.

Treatment

Patients with acute arterial occlusion require rapid evaluation and diagnosis to prevent limb-, bowel-, or life-threatening ischemia. Anticoagulation with intravenous heparin is administered to prevent further propagation of the thrombus. Contraindications to anticoagulation include a history of gastrointestinal bleeding, a new neurologic deficit, head injury, ongoing sites of active bleeding, and antibodies to heparin. Aggressive fluid resuscitation and correction of ongoing systemic acidosis should be performed. Patients who are in critical condition may require inotropic support. Dextran and mannitol offer advantages as part of the treatment of acute arterial occlusion. Dextran enhances the electronegativity of the red blood cells and the vessel wall and leads to a decrease in the propagation of thrombus. Dextran and mannitol function as an oncotic load to draw free water back into the bloodstream and hemodilute the blood. Surgical interventions should not be significantly delayed to allow for correction of the acidosis because the ongoing ischemia is the primary contribution to the acid–base disturbance.

In cases of limb-threatening ischemia, immediate surgical thrombectomy or embolectomy is performed.

Preoperative arteriogram may be of benefit in patients who have a history of arterial occlusive disease. In patients with sudden acute ischemia, arteriograms should be avoided and immediate surgical revascularization performed, based on physical examination and the level at which the pulse is absent.

The surgical approach is directed toward rapidly reperfusing the threatened extremity or organ. This reperfusion can be accomplished by embolectomy, endarterectomy, or surgical bypass. The results of revascularization are variable and depend on the extent of the occlusive disease and the duration of ischemia. In embolic occlusion, embolectomy is performed through peripheral vessels with specialized balloon-tipped catheters. Careful, complete thrombectomy is performed both proximally and distally. Distal thrombectomy is essential because nearly one-third of patients with arterial occlusions have additional thrombus past the point of occlusion. Pathologic evaluation should be performed of all emboli, especially in the absence of atrial fibrillation, to assure that the embolus is not of tumor origin. If the embolus is of thrombotic origin, its shape may give a good indication of its origin.

After extremity or organ revascularization, the reperfused organ is examined to determine the extent of tissue damage and the potential for edema. If there was lengthy lower extremity ischemia (> 4 hours), fasciotomy is often required to decompress the muscular compartments and prevent compression of the arteries, nerves, and veins (i.e., compartment syndrome). Unfortunately, the mortality rate from acute arterial occlusion is relatively high. This high rate is related to the advanced age of the patient population as well as to comorbid factors (e.g., myocardial disease). In the case of embolic arterial occlusion, postoperative anticoagulation should be considered because as many as one-third of patients have recurrent embolus or thrombosis without anticoagulation within 30 days.

In patients who have acute arterial ischemia without signs of profound ischemia to either the limb or the intestine, thrombolytic therapy can be considered. The goal of thrombolysis is to reperfuse the limb gradually, causing fewer systemic effects and a lower probability of compartment syndrome than a surgical approach. This approach requires arterial cannulation of the area proximal to the area of occlusion and administration of a thrombolytic agent (urokinase, streptokinase, or tissue plasminogen activator). However, if there are signs of critical ischemia, thrombolytic therapy is aborted and surgical revascularization is performed emergently.

Cerebrovascular Insufficiency

Cerebrovascular insufficiency can result from arterial occlusive, ulcerative, or aneurysmal disease of the carotid or vertebral arteries. The most devastating complication of cerebral vascular insufficiency is stroke. Stroke is the third leading cause of death in North America. Each year, more than 500,000 new strokes and 200,000 stroke-related deaths occur. The medical cost of managing patients after stroke is estimated at $15 to 20 billion per year.

Strokes are caused by infarction or hemorrhage within the cerebral hemispheres. Approximately 75% of cerebral infarctions are caused by embolism from atherosclerotic plaques in the carotid arteries of the neck. Although medical management, including antihypertensive, hypocholesterolemic, and antiplatelet agents, may help to prevent carotid atheroembolism, the most effective strategy is removal of the plaque through carotid endarterectomy (CEA).

Anatomy

Blood reaches the brain through the paired carotid and vertebral arteries. The right and left carotid arteries originate from the innominate artery and the aortic arch, respectively. The vertebral arteries arise from the proximal portions of the subclavian arteries. The common carotid arteries in the midneck bifurcate into the external carotid arteries (which supply the muscles of the face) and the internal carotid arteries. The internal carotid arteries have no branches in the neck, but they enter the petrous portion of the skull and give rise to the ophthalmic artery of the retina and the anterior and middle cerebral arteries that serve the cerebral cortex. The paired vertebral arteries form a single blood vessel within the brain stem (basilar artery) and then give rise to the posterior cerebral arteries and the arteries of the cerebellum. The arteries of the anterior and posterior circulation are part of a rich collateral network of vessels (circle of Willis) that is composed of the P1 segments of the posterior cerebral arteries, the posterior communicating arteries, the A1 segments of the anterior cerebral arteries, and the anterior communicating artery. Theoretically, an intact circle of Willis allows cerebral perfusion to be maintained in the face of occlusion or stenosis of one or more of the main branches. Unfortunately, this collateral network is complete in less than 25% of people.

Physiology

Approximately 15% of the cardiac output is directed to maintain cerebral perfusion. The resting total cerebral blood flow is 50 to 60 mL/min/100 g brain matter, with as much as 100 mL/min/100 g directed to the more cellular gray matter and 20 mL/min/100 g to the less cellular white matter. Cerebral ischemia can result once the total perfusion is less than 18 mL/min/100 g brain matter. Cerebral infarction can occur after the cerebral perfusion decreases to less than 8 mL/min/100 g.

A number of mechanisms maintain cerebral blood flow in the face of systemic hypotension or fixed lesions in the named arteries. Baroreceptors located at the carotid sinus sample and regulate blood pressure and heart rate. Further, cerebral vessels dilate in response to decreased perfusion pressure (autoregulation). This change is probably mediated by local receptors in the vascular smooth muscle and by autoregulatory autocoids (e.g., nitric oxide).

Pathophysiology

Although cerebral ischemia occasionally results from decreased blood flow, atheroembolism is by far the most common cause of cerebral infarction. Cerebral embolism may originate from any source between the left atrium and cerebral arteries, including the atrial appendage, left ventricle, aortic valve, aortic arch, carotid bifurcation, and carotid siphon. The most common source is an atherosclerotic lesion at the carotid bifurcation. Experimental models show that the carotid bifurcation contains areas of low and oscillatory shear stress. This finding may account for the transfer of circulating cellular elements to predisposed segments of the arterial wall and the development of occlusive plaques. Like any lesion in the body, most plaques are eventually covered with a fibrous cap, or scar, and separated from the circulation. Occasionally, however, the fibrous cap is disrupted, allowing embolism of exposed plaque elements or laminated thrombus. Less common causes of carotid arterial occlusive disease include fibromuscular dysplasia, Takayasu arteritis, arterial dissection, and trauma.

Hypoperfusion can cause neurologic deficits in the watershed areas between the perfused territories of the main cerebral arteries, where collateral flow is marginal. Sudden thrombosis of the carotid artery can cause massive cerebral infarction or may be asymptomatic if there is adequate collateral circulation from the contralateral carotid artery and the basilar artery (silent occlusion).

Clinical Presentation and Evaluation

Symptoms of cerebral vascular insufficiency are classified according to the location of the deficit, its duration, and the presence of cerebral infarction. These symptoms can be either transient or permanent. **Amaurosis fugax** (fleeting blindness) is a transient monocular blindness that is caused by emboli to the ipsilateral ophthalmic artery. Classically, amaurosis fugax is described as a curtain of blindness being pulled down from superior to inferior and involving the eye ipsilateral to the carotid lesion. TIAs are short-lived, often repetitive changes in mentation, vision, or sensorimotor function that are completely reversed within 24 hours. Most TIAs last seconds to minutes before they resolve completely. Because TIAs often involve the middle cerebral artery distribution, patients often have contralateral arm, leg, and facial weakness. Symptoms consistent with TIA that last longer than 24 hours, but less than 72 hours, are called **reversible ischemic neurologic deficits.** A stroke-in-evolution is a rapid progressive worsening of a neurologic deficit. A cerebral infarction, or **cerebrovascular accident,** is a permanent neurologic deficit, or stroke. Cerebral CT scan or MRI of a patient who had a stroke shows a region of nonviable cerebral tissue. Atherosclerotic carotid artery disease is not the only etiology of these clinical presentations. TIAs are also caused by migraines, seizure disorders, brain tumors, intracranial aneurysms, and arteriovenous malformations.

The severity of the neurologic deficit is determined by the volume and location of the ischemic area of the brain. The most commonly involved area is the perfused territory of the middle cerebral artery (parietal lobe), which is the main outflow vessel of the carotid artery. Hypoperfusion of the middle cerebral artery causes contralateral hemiparesis or hemiplegia and, occasionally, paralysis of the contralateral lower part of the face (central seventh nerve paralysis). Difficulty with speech (aphasia) is noted if the dominant hemisphere is involved. The left hemisphere is dominant in nearly all right-handed people and most left-handed people.

Patients with ischemia of the brain tissue that is supplied by the anterior cerebral artery have contralateral monoplegia that is usually more severe in the lower extremity. Posterior cerebral artery ischemia may result from carotid artery occlusive disease, but is also related to obstruction of both vertebral arteries or the basilar artery. Dizziness or syncope may be accompanied by visual field defects, palsy of the ipsilateral third cranial nerve, and contralateral sensory losses.

Diagnosis of Cerebrovascular Disease

As with most syndromes of vascular insufficiency, the diagnosis is usually suggested by the history alone. A carefully elicited history may also localize the neuroanatomic deficit and the offending arterial lesion. Physical examination should include a thorough neurologic examination as well as a search for evidence of arterial occlusive disease in other vascular beds. The classic finding in a patient with carotid stenosis is a cervical bruit (high-frequency systolic murmur) heard during auscultation with a stethoscope placed at the angle of the jaw. Unfortunately, there is little correlation between the degree of stenosis and the pitch, duration, or intensity of the bruit. A minimal stenosis can produce a loud bruit, but a near-total occlusion may not produce a bruit at all. A bruit can also be produced from other cervical blood vessels or transmitted from the aortic valve. Because of the close proximity of the carotid artery to the ear, some patients actually note a buzzing or heartbeat in their ear referred from the carotid stenosis. During ophthalmologic examination, small, yellow refractile particles (Hollenhorst plaques) are seen at the branch point of the retinal vessels. These plaques are cholesterol emboli from a carotid artery, aortic arch, or aortic valve plaque.

Noninvasive tests can characterize the extent of carotid artery stenosis without the use of arteriography. Candidates for noninvasive testing include patients with cerebrovascular symptoms, those with cervical bruit and, in some cases, those who are undergoing major vascular procedures (e.g., coronary artery bypass grafting). Noninvasive, yet direct, evaluation of the extracranial and carotid arterial vessels is obtained with Doppler ultrasound. The nature of the plaque (soft, calcific, or ulcerated) and its precise location (common vs external vs internal carotid artery) can be determined with both carotid arterial systems. The accuracy of imaging is enhanced by combining B-mode ultrasound with Doppler-derived assessments of blood flow velocity (duplex scan). A limitation of duplex scanning is the inability to assess the intracranial circulation and the origins of the common carotid arteries from the aortic arch. Occasionally, visualization of the bifurcation is impaired by calcification of the vessels.

The definitive study of the extracranial carotid arterial system is arteriography. Arterial injections offer the clearest definition of carotid plaques and potential ulcerations (Figure 22-14). Arteriography is indicated in patients who have a potential aortic arch or intracranial lesion, those with uncertain symptoms, and those in whom the carotid stenosis cannot be clearly visualized on duplex ultrasonography. Complications are rare, but can be devastating. They include cerebrovascular accident (approximately 0.5% of cases).

Recent improvements in cerebral MRI and magnetic resonance angiography (MRA) led to increased application in patients with carotid occlusive disease. MRI is useful for evaluation of the brain for infarction, tumor, arteriovenous malformation, and hemorrhage. MRA provides detailed visualization of the carotid arterial system without requiring arterial puncture and injection (Figure 22-15).

Treatment

Medical therapy for cerebrovascular disease is directed at the control of risk factors (e.g., hypertension, hyperlipoproteinemia) and anticoagulation or administration of antiplatelet drugs (e.g., aspirin, dipyridamole, ticlopidine). Anticoagulation and antiplatelet therapy are most commonly used in patients with ulcerative nonstenotic lesions or severe intracranial disease because surgical therapy would not change the natural history of the disease process. A recent prospective randomized study [North American Symptomatic Carotid Endarterectomy Trial (NASCET)] evaluated the treatment of patients with 50% to 70% and more than 70% internal carotid artery stenosis and cerebrovascular symptoms in the distribution of the affected carotid artery. After 2 years of follow-up, researchers found that in symptomatic patients who had more than 70% ipsilateral stenosis and were managed with antiplatelet therapy alone, the risk of cerebrovascular accident or death was approximately 26% compared with 9% in patients who were treated with CEA. The risk in patients with 50% to 69% stenosis was also reduced with CEA. More recently, asymptomatic patients with documented 60% or greater carotid stenosis were studied [Asymptomatic Carotid Atherosclerosis Study (ACAS)]. The risk of stroke in the medically managed group was calculated at 11% in 5 years. CEA reduced the risk to 5%. These findings firmly established the role of CEA in the prevention of stroke in patients with significant carotid stenosis.

In experienced hands, the morbidity and mortality rates for CEA are less than 2%. Recurrent lesions may occur in as many as 10% of endarterectomized arteries, so long-term follow-up with serial ultrasonogra-

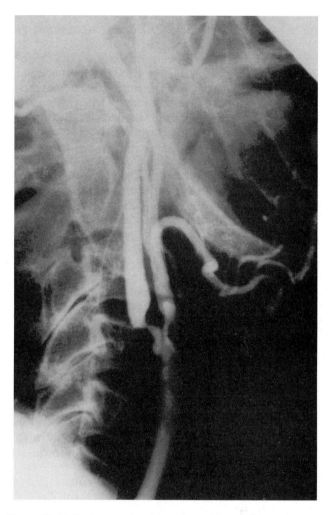

Figure 22-14 Angiogram of an internal carotid stenosis showing an ulcerative and stenotic atherosclerotic lesion at the carotid bifurcation in a patient who has transient ischémic attacks.

phy is advised. Restenosis within 2 years usually represents intimal hyperplasia, whereas recurrence in the long term is usually a manifestation of recurrent atherosclerosis.

Carotid angioplasty with placement of a metallic stent is being investigated in the treatment of cerebrovascular disease. This procedure allows percutaneous treatment of carotid stenosis without the risk of surgical intervention. The incidence of distal embolization (stroke) and recurrent stenosis is higher than with CEA, but the procedure is less invasive. The results of long-term follow-up and the incidence of restenosis are not yet available.

Vertebral Basilar Disease

The classic syndrome of vertebral basilar insufficiency (subclavian steal syndrome) is associated with subclavian or innominate artery occlusive disease. Symptoms occur when an occlusive lesion that is located proximal to the origin of the vertebral vessel decreases perfusion pressure in the subclavian artery.

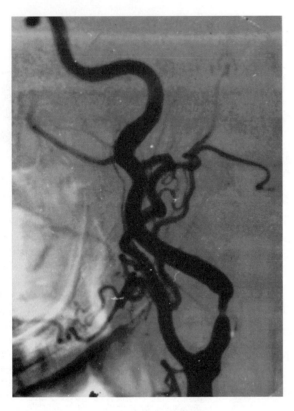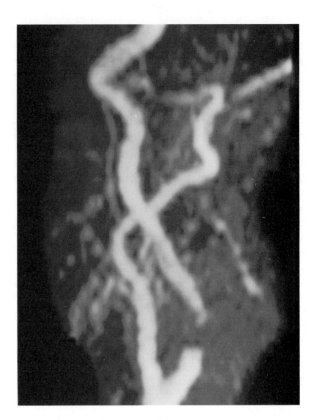

Figure 22-15 A, A conventional cerebral angiogram. **B,** A magnetic resonance angiogram in the same patient.

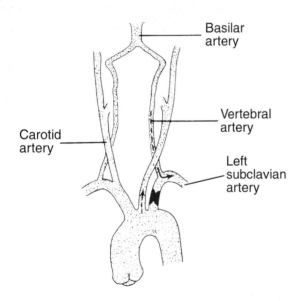

Figure 22-16 Subclavian steal syndrome. Proximal occlusion of the left subclavian artery causes retrograde flow of blood through the left vertebral artery, "stealing" blood from the basilar circulation and causing transient dizziness and syncope with arm exercise.

The vertebral artery then functions as a collateral pathway to the arm circulation. During arm exercise, vascular resistance in the arm decreases, and flow is reversed in the vertebral artery. As a result, basilar arterial blood flow and perfusion pressure are decreased (Figure 22-16). Symptoms of posterior cerebral and cerebellar ischemia are common and include light-headedness, syncope, and nausea correlated with arm exercise. Supraclavicular bruits are often detected, and blood pressure in the ipsilateral brachial artery is usually reduced by at least 40 mm Hg. Because of the increased length of the left subclavian artery relative to the right, there is a three to four times increased incidence of left subclavian stenosis and subclavian steal syndrome.

In patients with associated carotid artery disease, CEA alone may relieve the symptoms of vertebral basilar insufficiency by increasing collateral flow to the posterior cerebral artery and cerebellum. However, in most symptomatic patients with subclavian steal syndrome, the most commonly performed procedures are carotid–subclavian bypass and reimplantation of the subclavian artery into the proximal common carotid artery. These procedures restore normal blood flow to the subclavian artery and allow antegrade perfusion of the vertebral artery.

Venous Disease

The recognition and treatment of venous disease were documented as early as 1500 BC. The treatment of varicose veins was described in 400 AD as: cut the skin, expose the varix, insert a probe under it, pull out the varix, and cut. Interestingly, there has been little change in the method of treatment since that time.

Anatomy

The venous system is divided into peripheral and central systems. The central venous system includes the inferior and superior vena cava, iliac veins, and subclavian veins. The peripheral venous system includes the upper and lower extremity venous systems as well as the venous drainage of the head and neck region. The extremity veins are further classified as either superficial or deep. The superficial system of the lower extremity is composed of the greater and lesser saphenous veins and their tributaries. The deep venous system is composed of the large veins that travel with the major named arteries of the extremity. The common femoral, superficial femoral, and profunda femoral veins parallel the arteries of the same names. The anterior tibial, posterior tibial, and peroneal veins are almost always paired. The calf actually has six primary deep veins in contrast to three primary arteries. Unidirectional flow back to the heart is maintained by a series of bicuspid vein valves. These vein valves prevent reflux of blood back toward the lower extremity during standing. The superficial and deep venous systems communicate through perforating veins that direct blood from the superficial system to the deep system. Incompetency of the valves and perforating veins as a result of scarring or distension allows retrograde flow from the deep system into the superficial system and can cause varicosities and venous ulcerations.

Physiology

The muscular compartments of the calf are critically important in the venous circulation. Muscular contraction increases pressure within the compartments, thereby forcing blood back to the heart. Unlike the deep veins, the superficial veins are not surrounded by muscular compartments and therefore are not emptied by muscular contraction. Thrombosis of a superficial vein causes swelling, erythema, and tenderness along its course. Patients who have superficial thromboses are managed with nonsteroidal anti-inflammatory agents and warm compresses. They do not require bed rest. The pathophysiology of venous disease is generally caused by obstruction of the venous system, venous valvular insufficiency, or elements of both.

Deep Vein Thrombosis

Approximately 500,000 patients per year have deep vein thrombosis. If pulmonary thromboembolism occurs, in-hospital fatality rates exceed 10%. In 1856, Virchow identified a triad of risk factors for deep vein thrombosis. It included stasis, venous endothelial injury, and hypercoagulable states. Other risk factors include pregnancy, the use of oral contraceptives, a history of deep vein thrombosis, surgical procedures, sepsis, and obesity. Bony and soft tissue trauma to the legs is a common cause of endothelial injury. Stasis and venous distension may also injure the venous endothelium.

Clinical Presentation

As many as 50% of episodes of hospital-acquired deep vein thrombosis are asymptomatic. The remaining patients have local pain secondary to inflammation and edema. Deep vein thrombosis of the left iliac venous system is four times more common than that of the right iliac venous system because of the potential for compression of the left iliac vein by the aortic bifurcation. Unfortunately, in a small percentage of patients, the first symptom of deep vein thrombosis is pulmonary embolism.

Diagnosis

Physical examination of a patient with a lower extremity deep vein thrombosis may show unilateral extremity swelling or pain. Calf pain precipitated by dorsal flexion of the foot (Homan's sign) is present in fewer than 50% of cases. Because the accuracy of diagnosis based on clinical and physical examination alone is only 50%, more objective diagnostic studies are needed to confirm the presence of deep vein thrombosis before treatment. In addition to deep vein thrombosis, the differential diagnosis of acute edema and leg pain includes congestive heart failure, trauma, ruptured plantaris tendon, acute or chronic arterial insufficiency, infection, lymphangitis, lumbosacral strain, sciatica, muscle hematoma, and renal failure.

Noninvasive diagnostic studies increase the accuracy of diagnosis to 95%. A Doppler ultrasound probe can document the loss of the normal augmentation of venous flow with distal compression and the variation of venous flow with respiration. Normally, lower extremity venous flow decreases with inspiration as a result of increased intraabdominal pressure. Although indirect tests, including impedance plethysmography and ^{125}I-labeled fibrinogen scanning, have a role in the detection of deep vein thrombosis, the most common noninvasive test is duplex ultrasonography. Its accuracy is greater than 95% because it can characterize venous blood flow and visualize the venous thrombus. The accuracy of duplex scanning is decreased in the tibial veins because of the occasional difficulty encountered when visualizing these small veins within the muscular compartments. In unusual cases, CT scans of the abdomen and pelvis, with intravenous contrast material, may aid in the diagnosis of pelvic and vena caval thrombosis. If the results of noninvasive diagnostic tests are not definitive, venography is performed.

Treatment

The goals of treatment include decreasing the risk of pulmonary embolus and preventing further propagation of the venous thrombus. Primary therapy includes anticoagulation with intravenous heparin and elevation of the extremity. Anticoagulation is maintained with continuous infusion of heparin and monitoring of the partial thromboplastin time to twice the normal level. After the patient is adequately anticoagulated with heparin, long-term anticoagulation is begun with sodium warfarin (Coumadin). Coumadin therapy is monitored to maintain a therapeutic prothrombin time. Sodium warfarin inhibits the vitamin K–dependent factors for both the procoagulant factors (II, VII, IX, X) and the anticoagulant factors (protein C and protein S). Because the half-lives of protein C and protein S are less than those of the procoagulant factors, for a short time after the initiation of Coumadin therapy, the patient may become hypercoagulable. Coumadin skin necrosis is a catastrophic complication of this rare hypercoagulable state. It can cause significant loss of skin, especially skin overlying poorly vascularized regions (i.e., adipose tissue). For this reason, heparin anticoagulation is maintained during the beginning of Coumadin therapy. Contraindications to anticoagulation therapy include bleeding diathesis, gastrointestinal ulceration, recent stroke, cerebral arteriovenous malformations, recent surgery, hematologic disorders (e.g., hemophilia), and bone marrow suppression as a result of chemotherapy.

Anticoagulation therapy prevents further propagation of the thrombus, but does not actually dissolve or lyse the existing thrombus. Fibrinolysis occurs gradually, through the endogenous plasminogen system, or may be stimulated by the administration of exogenous streptokinase or urokinase. Definite indications for thrombolytic therapy include subclavian vein thrombosis, acute renal vein thrombosis, and acute superior vena cava occlusion by the thrombus. Its application is also being investigated for routine use in lower extremity deep vein thrombosis. It is uncertain whether venous valvular function can be preserved despite successful thrombolytic therapy. Initial reports show no difference in the incidence of **postthrombotic syndrome** with thrombolytic therapy compared with anticoagulation alone.

Surgical thrombectomy is usually reserved for cases of limb-threatening ischemia. Even in complete iliofemoral thrombosis with massive edema (phlegmasia cerulea dolens or phlegmasia alba dolens), venous thrombectomy has limited usefulness because more than 50% of thromboses recur.

Prophylaxis for Deep Vein Thrombosis

Deep vein thrombosis with a potential for pulmonary embolus is a significant risk for patients undergoing major surgery. Preoperative prophylaxis has the greatest potential for prevention. Prophylactic measures include mechanical therapy (intermittent segmental compression device, early ambulation, and passive range of motion) and pharmacologic therapy (subcutaneous heparin, dextran, aspirin, or Coumadin).

Pulmonary Embolism

Pulmonary embolism results from the migration of venous clots to the pulmonary arteries. Clots may originate in any peripheral vein, especially the iliac, femoral, and large pelvic veins.

Clinical Presentation

Patients with pulmonary embolism may have no specific clinical findings or may have massive cardiovascular collapse. The classic clinical presentation (Table 22-4) includes pleuritic chest pain, dyspnea, tachypnea, tachycardia, cough, and hemoptysis. Right-sided heart strain is seen on electrocardiogram. Patients with hypercoagulable conditions are predisposed to deep vein thrombosis and pulmonary embolism.

Diagnosis

Chest x-ray is rarely diagnostic for pulmonary embolus. A pleural effusion is present in as many as one-third of patients with pulmonary embolus. The classic wedge-shaped region of atelectasis from a pulmonary embolus (Westermark sign) is rarely noted. Chest x-ray is most useful for ruling out other potential pulmonary pathology. The definitive diagnosis of pulmonary embolism is made by ventilation–perfusion lung scan or pulmonary angiogram. A wedge-shaped or lobar defect seen on perfusion scan without a ventilation deficit indicates a high probability of pulmonary embolism. Pulmonary angiogram has a specificity and a sensitivity of greater than 98%, but it is an invasive procedure.

Treatment

The primary therapy for pulmonary embolism is anticoagulation in an attempt to prevent further pulmonary emboli. If the patient is hemodynamically unstable, inotropic support may be required. If the patient remains stable, but is compromised as a result of the pulmonary embolus, thrombolytic therapy is considered. There is no direct correlation among clot size, cardiopulmonary dynamics, and other risk factors and survival in patients with acute embolism. Multiple small emboli cause cardiovascular collapse as often as massive emboli.

Percutaneous pulmonary embolectomy suction devices aid in the removal of large clots from the pulmonary artery. If the patient becomes profoundly hypotensive and hypoxic despite intubation and vasopressor support, pulmonary artery embolectomy (Trendelenburg operation) may be considered. Unfortunately, direct surgical removal of the embolus is associated with a mortality rate of more than 80%. If a patient with lower extremity or pelvic venous thrombus has a contraindication to anticoagulation or has a pulmonary embolism while anticoagulated (failure of anticoagulation), a mechanical filter device can be placed in the inferior vena cava. This device traps emboli before they reach the pulmonary artery.

Table 22-4. Clinical Presentations of Pulmonary Embolus

Pleuritic chest pain (70%)
Dyspnea and tachypnea (80%)
Tachycardia (45%)
Hemoptysis (25%–30%)
Associated findings
Cough and rales
Right heart failure

Chronic Venous Insufficiency

Chronic venous insufficiency is a direct result of local venous hypertension. Causes of venous hypertension include venous valvular incompetence, venous obstruction as a result of intrinsic or extrinsic compression, muscular calf pump failure, and reflux from perforating veins.

Clinical Presentation

The clinical manifestations of chronic venous insufficiency are chronically swollen legs, hyperpigmentation, and venous stasis ulcerations.

Diagnosis

Physical examination shows an orange–brown skin discoloration at the level of the ankle as a result of hemosiderin deposition, lower extremity edema, venous varicosities, or ulcerations. Venous stasis ulcerations usually occur at the medial and lateral malleoli of the ankle. These chronic changes in the lower extremity as a result of venous hypertension are postthrombotic, but may also be caused by congenital primary deep valvular incompetence.

Noninvasive vascular laboratory evaluation includes venous duplex ultrasonography, which allows visualization of venous flow as well as reflux through incompetent venous valves. Likewise, a duplex scan can directly visualize a deep vein chronic occlusion or note the inability of the vein to be compressed secondary to the mass of the venous thrombus. If the noninvasive duplex scan is not diagnostic, venography may be necessary.

Treatment

The initial management of lower extremity edema and potential ulceration of chronic venous insufficiency is elevation of the lower extremity and the use of gradient compression stockings. In patients with venous ulceration, meticulous wound care is required to prevent infection during healing. In the patient who is noncompliant with leg elevation and local wound care, a medicated tightly applied dressing (Unna's boot) may be required. If the wound does not heal, but the edema is controlled, split-thickness skin grafting may accomplish wound healing. Occasionally, surgical interruption of perforating veins is necessary to heal venous ulcers.

The preferred initial treatment of varicose veins is compression stocking therapy to alleviate the venous hypertension. If further therapy is required for small varicosities, sclerotherapy can be used. Sclerotherapy entails the injection of an irritating solution into the varicose vein to promote an inflammatory response, scarring, and obliteration of the lumen. For larger varicosities, the superficial venous system is surgically removed (stripped) and the associated varicosities excised. This procedure is performed only after confirmation that the deep venous system is patent and has no evidence of deep vein thrombosis.

Arteriovenous Malformations

Arteriovenous malformations result from abnormal embryologic development of the maturing vascular spaces, producing pathologic arteriovenous connections that involve small and medium-sized vessels. There is an equal male:female ratio, and the lower extremities are involved two to three times as often as the upper extremities. Although lesions are present at birth, most are identified only in the second and third decade as they gradually enlarge. On palpation, a vibration, or **thrill,** is often noted over the level of the fistula. In larger arteriovenous malformations, skin ulceration and bleeding are troublesome complications. Rarely, congenital arteriovenous fistulae produce cardiac enlargement and heart failure as a result of increased blood flow to the right side of the heart.

The management of symptomatic, localized congenital arteriovenous malformations is surgical excision. However, the treatment of large or diffuse lesions can be extremely difficult and is associated with a high recurrence rate. An alternative is percutaneous intraarterial sclerosis of the main feeding artery to decrease the amount of blood that is shunted from the arterioles to the venules.

Acquired arteriovenous fistulae are also abnormal communications between the arteries and veins, but they usually result from iatrogenic injuries (arterial catheterizations) or penetrating trauma (gunshot or knife wounds). These fistulae are often associated with a false aneurysm and involve large vessels (common femoral artery–common femoral vein fistula). A palpable thrill or bruit may be present. Venous hypertension and venous stasis changes occur with long-standing arteriovenous fistulae.

All acquired traumatic arteriovenous fistulae should be repaired to prevent the development of complications (e.g., cardiac failure, local pain, aneurysmal formation, limb length discrepancy in children, chronic venous hypertension). Direct compression of post-catheterization arteriovenous fistulae is often effective, especially if anticoagulants are not used. Operative intervention requires complete dissection and separation of the involved vessels and appropriate vascular repair. To exclude some arteriovenous communications nonoperatively, coated metallic stents are also used.

Vasospastic Disorders, Vascular Trauma, and Lymphatic Disorders Syndrome

Episodic digital vasospasm involving the hands and feet was first described by Maurice Raynaud in 1862. Raynaud's syndrome is cold- or emotion-induced episodic digital ischemia. As many as 90% of patients are female, and 50% have an associated autoimmune disease (e.g., scleroderma, lupus erythematosus, rheumatoid arthritis, Sjögren's syndrome). Some appear to have a work-related syndrome caused by the use of vibratory machinery. Unilateral Raynaud's syndrome is more common in men and is often associated with proximal arterial disease of the large vessels (e.g., subclavian stenosis, occlusion).

The clinical aspects may vary, but the classic Raynaud's attack has three distinct phenomena (white, blue, red syndrome). Exposure to cold initially causes profound vasospasm and blanching of the digits (white). After 15 minutes, cyanosis is evident, presumably from venous filling with delayed venous emptying (blue). Later, the digits and hands become hyperemic as vasospasm lessens and flow to the digits is restored (red).

The diagnosis of Raynaud's syndrome is made from the history and physical examination. Coexistent symptoms of connective tissue disorders are often elicited. Laboratory tests (e.g., sedimentation rate, complement assay, antinuclear antibody assay) often confirm the immunologic disorders associated with the syndrome.

Treatment consists of discontinuing any medications that cause reduced cardiac output or vasospasm and that are associated with Raynaud's syndrome (e.g., ergotamines, oral contraceptives, beta-blockers). Other pharmacologic agents, especially calcium channel–blocking agents, are used to decrease the tendency toward vasospasm. Surgical sympathectomy is not an effective treatment. Revascularization of an ischemic extremity may markedly improve the symptoms in patients with arterial occlusive disease.

Thoracic Outlet Syndrome

Symptoms that mimic a vasospastic disorder may occur in thoracic outlet syndrome. This syndrome is also seen in young and middle-aged women. Symptoms are caused by compression or irritation of the brachial plexus and, to a much lesser extent, the subclavian artery as they pass through the thoracic outlet and the costoclavicular space.

Anatomic causes of the syndrome include: an elongated transverse process of the seventh cervical vertebra; a fully developed cervical rib; congenital bands in the outlet related to the cervical rib, middle scalene muscle, or anterior scalene muscle; and a narrowed costoclavicular space, often because of a previously fractured rib or clavicle, with callus formation.

Paresthesias of the arm and hand reflect neurologic compression and are much more common than arterial symptoms. When arterial symptoms occur, they include coldness of the hand and arm, pallor, and muscle fatigue. In rare cases, stenosis of the subclavian artery causes emboli to the hand.

Evaluation of these patients involves a detailed history and a thorough physical examination to document localized scalene muscle tenderness and radicular phenomena. Adson's test (disappearance of the radial pulse on abduction and external rotation of the shoulder), said to be indicative of thoracic outlet syndrome in the early literature, is now considered relatively nonspecific. Cervical spine x-rays are obtained to identify cervical ribs or bands. Nerve conduction velocity across the outlet has little value. Angiography is recommended only if a bruit is present or embolization is suspected.

After the diagnosis is confirmed, nonsurgical treatments, including postural training, are attempted. If symptoms persist, surgical decompression of the outlet may be warranted. The most commonly used procedure is resection of the first thoracic rib, removal of any cervical ribs, and division of the anterior scalene muscle.

Vascular Trauma

Blood vessels are injured directly by penetrating trauma (e.g., stab wounds, gunshot wounds) and blunt trauma, especially fractures of the long bones. In high-speed collisions involving motor vehicles or aircraft, vessels may be partially or totally disrupted by the shearing stress of sudden acceleration and deceleration. Patients with arterial injuries may have obvious signs (e.g., external hemorrhage, absence of distal pulses), but the signs of vascular injury are often subtle. Hemorrhage may be occult and confined to soft tissue or body cavities. Other findings that indicate vascular injury include acute arteriovenous fistulae (associated with to-and-fro murmurs or palpable thrills), neurologic deficits and paresthesias (as a result of nerve compression by adjacent hematomas), or organ-specific deficits that reflect obstruction of the main arterial supply (e.g., cerebral infarction with carotid artery injuries). Injury to the endothelial surface (intimal flaps) may not cause thrombosis for hours or days and therefore cannot be diagnosed by physical examination until the complication occurs. A common misconception is that a patient who has an arterial injury must have a reduced or absent distal pulse. This problem occurs only if the injury is hemodynamically significant.

Immediate diagnosis and treatment of arterial injuries is indicated to avoid excessive blood loss and to restore extremity or organ blood flow. If the diagnosis is missed on initial evaluation, late complications may be much more difficult to treat. These late complications include pseudoaneurysms, gradual enlargement of small lacerations in vessels, high-volume arteriovenous fistulae with venous insufficiency and high-output cardiac failure, and delayed thrombosis from untreated intimal flaps or dissections.

The poor reliability of physical diagnosis in accurately assessing the location and extent of vascular injury mandates investigation when penetrating trauma occurs near blood vessels, even if no overt signs of injury are present. If the patient has a viable extremity with an ABI of approximately 1.0, then the vessels that are near the region of trauma can be further evaluated by noninvasive duplex studies. If the extremity is ischemic, then angiography is indicated. Because of the tremendous concussive energy of high-velocity missiles, extensive damage can result, even from near-misses. Specific types of blunt trauma (especially dislocation of the knees and elbows) are so often associated with arterial contusions and intimal disruption that arteriography is prudent, even if no symptoms are present.

Although the consequences of venous injury are not as severe as those of arterial trauma, venous laceration must be considered in any patient who has evidence of excessive blood loss and no arterial lesion on angiography. Venography can usually confirm and localize the injury. Venous injury also predisposes the patient to the development of deep venous thrombosis.

Immediate vascular repair may be as simple as ligation or lateral suture. In some cases, bypass grafts are needed to resect the vessel completely. In these cases, it is preferable to use an autologous vein from an uninjured extremity because this conduit has a high patency rate and a low infection rate, even in the face of contamination. Repair of a concomitant major venous injury in an extremity results in a higher patency rate for the arterial repair.

Lymphatic Disorders

The lymphatic system serves a number of functions, including drainage of proteins and extracellular fluid that are lost from the capillary circulation and removal of bacteria and foreign materials. Lymphedema occurs when lymph transport and transcapillary fluid exchange are impaired. In these situations, the production of lymph continues at a constant rate, but drainage is inadequate, and protein-rich fluid accumulates. The high osmolality of the lymphatic fluid attracts even greater amounts of extracellular fluid.

Primary lymphedema is classified as congenital lymphedema (present at birth), lymphedema praecox (starting early in life, usually at 10–15 years of age), and lymphedema tarda (starting after 35 years of age). The lymphangiographic appearance further divides primary lymphedema into hyperplasia (numerous large, dilated lymphatic vessels are present; usually associated with lymphedema tarda) and hypoplasia (lymphatics are few in number and small in caliber; usually associated with lymphedema praecox). Acquired lymphedema occurs after recurrent infection, radiation, surgical excision, or neoplastic invasion of regional lymph nodes.

Patients with lymphedema usually have diffuse painless enlargement of the extremities. With time, the soft "pitting" edema becomes "woody" as progressive fibrosis of the connective tissue occurs.

Treatment includes both medical and surgical management, neither of which can cure the process. The use of proper support hosiery, avoidance of prolonged standing, elevation of the bed at night, administration of diuretics, and meticulous foot care to minimize lymphangitis are the primary medical therapies. Lymphangitis is treated aggressively with antibiotics, elevation, and bed rest. Patients with recurrent inflammation should be considered candidates for continuing antibiotic therapy. Patients with long-standing acquired lymphedema are at a small increased risk of lymphosarcoma and should be examined frequently.

Surgical intervention is considered only if medical management fails. Surgical approaches fall into two categories: reconstruction of the lymphatic drainage (lymphangioplasty) and excision of varying amounts of subcutaneous tissue and skin. Unfortunately, the results of surgery are disappointing.

Diagnostic Radiology in Vascular Disorders

Arteriograms (angiograms) and venograms (phlebograms) are invasive procedures and should be used cautiously. Specific indications for each procedure were discussed previously. These studies are generally performed to localize disease, not to diagnose it. The history, physical examination, and noninvasive laboratory studies are adequate for medical management in most situations. Contrast studies are the "road map" for the surgeon after vascularization is elected. The most commonly used technique for arteriography involves puncture of a peripheral artery, with passage of an intravascular catheter for selective injection of arteries (Seldinger technique). The femoral artery is often used; axillary and brachial arteries are also used. Lower extremity venograms are performed by cannulating a foot vein and then injecting contrast material.

The principal complications of arteriography include bleeding around the puncture site, thrombosis at the puncture site from an intimal flap caused by passage of the catheter, formation of a pseudoaneurysm, hypersensitivity reaction to the iodinated dye, and contrast-related renal toxicity, especially in diabetic patients. Bleeding may be immediate or delayed and may cause a pseudoaneurysm later. The initial presentation of local bleeding includes paresthesias in the involved limb because of compression of adjacent nerves. Thrombosis usually occurs within 6 hours of arterial puncture, but may occur days later. Pseudoaneurysms secondary to catheter trauma may be thrombosed by duplex-directed compression, especially in patients who are not undergoing anticoagulation therapy. If compression therapy is not successful, then surgical exposure, with closure of the puncture site and repair of the injured intima, is appropriate.

In patients with known hypersensitivity to iodinated contrast material, steroids and antihistamines can be administered before the procedure to decrease the incidence and severity of reactions. All patients should be questioned carefully about previous allergic reactions before arteriogram or venogram is performed. Hydration before and after arteriography is important in all patients, particularly those with renal insufficiency. Judicious use of diuretics also decreases nephrotoxicity.

Venograms are less risky procedures. A low incidence of phlebitis (< 3%) is expected if the injected contrast material is dilute and is flushed from the veins with heparinized saline after the study is completed. Newer nonionic contrast agents are associated with a decreased incidence of postvenography thrombophlebitis.

Multiple-Choice Questions

1. A middle-aged woman comes to your office with an ulcerated area that has surrounding induration and inflammation in the area of the medial malleolus. She has superficial varicosities in the greater saphenous distribution. Your diagnosis is:
   A. Diabetes mellitus
   B. Venous stasis ulcer
   C. Spider bite
   D. Scleroderma
   E. Deep venous thrombosis

2. Pulmonary embolism is least commonly seen with:
   A. Pregnancy
   B. Pancreatic cancer
   C. Pelvic trauma
   D. Antithrombin III deficiency
   E. Factor XI deficiency

3. The most efficient method to prevent pulmonary embolism is:
   A. Low–molecular-weight heparin
   B. Aspirin
   C. Dipyridamole (Persantine)
   D. Subcutaneous heparin
   E. Early ambulation

4. Pulmonary emboli arise most commonly from the:
   A. Deep femoral veins
   B. Tibial veins
   C. Popliteal veins
   D. Axillary veins
   E. Iliac veins

5. The most common symptom of pulmonary embolus is:
   A. Leg pain
   B. Dyspnea
   C. Hemoptysis
   D. Retraction of one side of the chest
   E. Cardiac murmur

6. A 30-year-old woman had recent onset of diastolic hypertension and a normal intravenous urography with a creatinine of 1.2 mg/dl. The most likely diagnosis is:
   A. Atherosclerotic renovascular disease
   B. Medial cystic necrosis
   C. Fibromuscular dysplasia
   D. Aldosterone-secreting tumors
   E. Pheochromocytoma

7. The best treatment for a 45-year-old male smoker with a two-block intermittent claudication is:
   A. Femoral popliteal bypass
   B. Aortofemoral bypass
   C. Medical therapy
   D. Transluminal angioplasty
   E. Femoral endarterectomy

8. The best initial treatment for a 23-year-old woman with a swollen, red, tender, painful saphenous vein is:
   A. Heat, analgesics, and continued ambulation
   B. Elevation, elastic stockings, and bed rest
   C. Heparin, bed rest, and subsequent Coumadin administration
   D. Streptokinase
   E. Venous division and stripping

9. A 60-year-old man with a history of hypertension has an 8-cm pulsatile abdominal mass and back pain. Blood pressure is 100/70 mm Hg, pulse is 120/min, and respiration rate is 20/min. The best course is to:
   A. Take the patient to the operating room
   B. Order an angiogram immediately
   C. Order a computed tomography scan immediately
   D. Order an ultrasound immediately
   E. Admit and observe the patient

10. Three days after emergency aneurysm resection, the patient has several episodes of guaiac-positive diarrhea. The next step in the management of this patient is to:
    A. Discontinue the antibiotics
    B. Administer diphenoxylate (Lomotil)
    C. Add gentamicin
    D. Perform sigmoidoscopy
    E. Perform further exploratory surgery

11. Risk factors for atherosclerosis include all of the following EXCEPT:
    A. Smoking
    B. Diabetes mellitus
    C. Hypertension
    D. Poor nutrition
    E. Hereditary factors

12. Leriche syndrome is associated with all of the following EXCEPT:
    A. Buttocks atrophy
    B. Impotence
    C. Aortoiliac occlusive disease
    D. Embolization to the toes
    E. Claudication

13. Signs and symptoms of chronic intestinal ischemia include all of the following EXCEPT:
    A. Postprandial pain
    B. Weight loss
    C. Diarrhea
    D. Food fear
    E. Abdominal bruit

14. Transient ischemic attacks as a result of carotid atherosclerosis usually involve the perfusion territory of the:
    A. Middle cerebral artery
    B. Anterior cerebral artery
    C. Posterior cerebral artery
    D. Vertebral artery
    E. Lateral cerebral artery

15. Subclavian steal is usually associated with occlusion of:
    A. The left carotid artery
    B. The right carotid artery
    C. Both vertebral arteries
    D. The subclavian artery
    E. The posterior communicating artery

16. The main advantage of below-the-knee amputation versus above-the-knee amputation is:
    A. Below-the-knee amputation is more likely to heal primarily
    B. After below-the-knee amputation, less effort is required to walk with a prosthesis
    C. Below-the-knee amputations cause less distortion of the patient's body image
    D. Below-the-knee amputations are technically easier
    E. Below-the-knee amputation requires less operative time

17. A surgically correctable cause of hypertension is:
    A. Abdominal aortic aneurysm
    B. Pheochromocytoma
    C. Zollinger-Ellison syndrome
    D. Hypernephroma
    E. Acute tubular necrosis of the kidney

18. The most probable diagnosis in a 72-year-old man with severe abdominal postprandial pain, weight loss of 40 lb in 3 months, an abdominal bruit, and guaiac-positive stool is:
    A. Occult carcinoma of the colon
    B. Abdominal angina (mesenteric ischemia)
    C. Gastrointestinal arteriovenous malformation
    D. Malabsorption syndrome
    E. Peptic ulcer disease

19. The "six Ps" of acute arterial insufficiency include:
    A. Palpitations
    B. Paroxysmal nocturnal dyspnea
    C. Pancytopenia
    D. Paresthesia
    E. Paramusia

20. Cell survival in compartment syndrome is determined by:
    A. Compartment pressure alone
    B. Duration of preexisting hypoxia
    C. Patient age
    D. Duration of increased pressure
    E. Both time and pressure

Oral Examination Study Questions

CASE 1

A 49-year-old man has acute onset of pain in the right leg. His symptoms began 4 hours ago and include pain, pallor, paresthesias, absent pulses in the right foot, and coolness of the leg. He has decreased ability to move his foot. He has no history of claudication, vascular disease, or cardiac disease. He does not smoke and does not have diabetes.

On physical examination, the patient has a prominent left popliteal pulse and a prominent midepigastric abdominal pulse. All of his other pulses are normal, except the ones in the right popliteal, dorsalis pedis, and posterior tibial arteries. These are absent. There are no stigmata of chronic peripheral vascular disease. He has no evidence of cardiac arrhythmia.

OBJECTIVE 1

The student lists a differential diagnosis that includes the following:
    A. Popliteal aneurysm
    B. Thrombosis of superficial femoral or popliteal artery
    C. Occlusive disease
    D. Embolism from the heart or aorta

The student discusses the difference between popliteal occlusion thrombosis and embolism. The student also describes the bilateral nature of popliteal aneurysms and their association with other aneurysms. The student explains that popliteal aneurysms embolize or thrombose and are often diagnosed by ultrasound in addition to physical examination.

OBJECTIVE 2

The student outlines the therapy for both diagnoses.
    A. Immediate anticoagulation with heparin is initiated.
    B. The patient undergoes emergency bypass surgery. If the diagnosis of popliteal aneurysm is not made, the student may entertain the possibility of thrombectomy or lytic therapy.
    C. A postoperative search is made for other aneurysms.

Minimum Level of Achievement for Passing

The student makes the diagnosis of acute occlusion of the popliteal artery and entertains the possibility of thrombosis or embolism. The student recognizes the urgent nature of the process, with possible limb loss if no action is taken to relieve the obstruction within 8 hours after occurrence.

Honors Level of Achievement

The student recognizes that the patient has a popliteal aneurysm and proceeds with surgical bypass. In addition, the student looks for other aneurysms in the postoperative period and plans prophylactic repair.

CASE 2

A 45-year-old accountant comes to your clinic with left leg pain of 2 months' duration.

OBJECTIVE 1

The student asks questions to characterize the complaint.

A. The onset was gradual, with decreasing ambulatory distance over the last 2 months.

B. The pain is located in the left calf.

C. The patient has pain when he walks 2 blocks. The pain goes away when he stops walking.

D. The patient denies rest pain, ulcer, trauma, injury, edema, diabetes, myocardial infarction, stroke, and family history of vascular or cardiac disease.

The patient is an accountant and has not pushed himself to exercise. He smokes 2 packs a day and is not very active, although he hunts. However, the pain bothers him so much that he cannot hunt. He is overweight and has no other illnesses.

On physical examination, the only pertinent findings are:

A. Loss of hair on both feet

B. Pulses

	C	R	F	P	PT	DP
Left	2	2	2	0	0	0
Right	2	2	2	2	2	2

C. Bilateral iliac artery bruits, but no superficial femoral bruits

OBJECTIVE 2

The student makes the diagnosis of left iliac artery stenosis and left superficial femoral artery occlusion with probable right iliac artery stenosis.

OBJECTIVE 3

The student describes the noninvasive documentation of arterial occlusive disease and orders a Doppler examination. This test corroborates the diagnosis with mildly decreased thigh pressures bilaterally and decreased above-the-knee and below-the-knee pressures on the left.

OBJECTIVE 4

The student outlines a medical treatment plan, including an exercise plan for 2 to 3 months, that includes:

A. Walking to the pain threshold daily, resting, and repeating four to five times a session

B. Losing weight

C. Stopping smoking

D. Pentoxifylline

OBJECTIVE 5

The patient's condition does not improve after 2 to 3 months of compliant medical therapy. The student describes the indications for surgical therapy.

A. Pain that significantly interferes with lifestyle

B. Pain that interferes with occupation

C. Impending or actual tissue loss

D. Rest pain

The student describes the available surgical procedures. They include angioplasty and vascular surgery.

The student outlines the risks of surgery, including myocardial infarction, cerebrovascular accident, infection, occlusion of the graft, and hemorrhage.

Minimum Level of Achievement for Passing

The student obtains a good history and performs a physical examination. The student makes the anatomic diagnosis, which is corroborated by segmental Doppler pressures. Arteriography is not indicated. The student outlines the proper medical therapy and the indications for surgical intervention.

Honors Level of Achievement

The student discusses the possible invasive interventions for therapy and their attendant risks and complications.

CASE 3

You are an emergency room physician. A 70-year-old man with a history of mild hypertension and a myocardial infarction 18 years ago is brought by ambulance to the emergency department of your medical center. He had an episode of acute epigastric pain and fainting while dining with his family at a local restaurant.

OBJECTIVE 1

The student performs a rapid first assessment, obtaining the following history and physical examination findings.

A. The patient is alert, diaphoretic, and somewhat obese. He has severe epigastric pain radiating to the left groin and back. He has never had this type of pain before. He is taking clonidine for high blood pressure.

B. The initial vital signs are: respirations 22/min, blood pressure 110/80 mm Hg, pulse 120/min, and temperature 37.5 °C.

C. Other physical findings include a rigid upper abdomen and tenderness in the midepigastrium. No organomegaly or masses are felt because of rigidity. The abdomen is rounded, but no fluid is present. Bowel sounds and femoral pulses are present, the chest is clear, and there is no cardiac murmur.

OBJECTIVE 2

The student recognizes that diaphoresis, tachycardia, and relative hypotension constitute an acute surgical emergency. The student initiates appropriate treatment.

A. Place two large-bore intravenous lines, and hang Ringer's lactate solution wide open.

B. Send blood for a complete blood count, sequential multiple analyzer (SMA)-18, and amylase. Perform type and crossmatch for six units of blood. Order urinalysis.

C. Order an electrocardiogram, a chest x-ray, and a flat plate of the abdomen.

D. Place a Foley catheter (30 mL urine found).

E. Formulate a differential diagnosis that includes the following:
   1. Myocardial infarction
   2. Pancreatitis
   3. Leaking aneurysm
   4. Perforated ulcer
   5. Renal stone
   6. Appendicitis

F. Call the surgeons.

OBJECTIVE 3

The student institutes treatment. The nurse reports that the patient's blood pressure initially responded to the fluid push. However, while the chest x-ray and flat plate were being performed, the blood pressure fell to 90 mm Hg systolic. The student calls the surgeons immediately and notifies the anesthetists and the operating room that there is a patient with abdominal catastrophe.

OBJECTIVE 4

The patient is emergently brought to the operating room, where a ruptured abdominal aortic aneurysm (AAA) is found and repaired with a tube graft. The student knows the possible postoperative complications of AAA repair.

A. Perioperative renal failure

B. Colonic ischemia

C. Myocardial infarction

D. Embolism and possible limb loss

E. Mortality rate of at least 25% in an emergency situation

F. Paraplegia

Minimum Level of Achievement for Passing

The student recognizes that this patient has a possible abdominal catastrophe and requires rapid workup. The student formulates a quick differential diagnosis. When the patient's condition deteriorates, the student sends the patient to the operating room. The student lists the postoperative complications.

Honors Level of Achievement

The student also knows the mechanisms behind the complications associated with AAA repair and how to avoid them.

SUGGESTED READINGS

Atherosclerosis

Zarins CK. Hemodynamics factors in atherosclerosis. In: Moore W, ed. *Vascular Surgery: A Comprehensive Review.* Philadelphia, Pa: WB Saunders, 1991:86–96.
Zierler RE, Strauduers DE. Haemodynamics for the vascular surgeon. In: Moore W, ed. *Vascular Surgery: A Comprehensive Review.* Philadelphia, Pa: WB Saunders, 1991:141–168.

Aneurysm

Brewster DC. Clinical and anatomical considerations for surgery in aortoiliac disease and results of surgical treatment. *Circulation* 1991;82(2):142–152.
Brewster DC, Franklin DP, Cambria RP, et al. Intestinal ischemia complicating abdominal aortic surgery. *Surgery* 1991;109(4):447–454.
Clark ET, Gewertz BL, Bassiouny HS, Zarins CK. Current results of elective aortic reconstruction for aneurysmal and occlusive disease. *J Cardiovasc Surg* 1990;31:438–441.
Estes JE Jr. Abdominal aortic aneurysm: a study of one hundred and two cases. *Circulation* 1950;2:258–264.
Halloran BG, Baxter BT. Pathogenesis of aneurysms. *Semin Vasc Surg* 1995;8(2):85–92.
Hollier LH, Taylor LM, Ochsner J. Recommended indications for operative treatment of abdominal aortic aneurysms: report of a sub-committee of the Joint Council of the Society for Vascular Surgery and the North American Chapter of the International Society for Cardiovascular Surgery. *J Vasc Surg* 1992;15:1046–1056.

Arterial Occlusive Disease

Blair JM, et al. Percutaneous transluminal angioplasty versus surgery for limb-threatening ischemia. *J Vasc Surg* 1989; 9:698–703.
Fillinger MF, Cronenwett JL. Anatomic distribution and natural history of aorto-iliac and infrainguinal atherosclerosis. In: Ernst CB, Stanley JC, eds. *Current Therapy in Vascular Surgery.* St. Louis, Mo: Mosby 1995:328–332.
Moore WM Jr, Hollier L. Mesenteric artery occlusive disease. *Card Clin* 1991;9(3):535–541.
Stanley JC. Abdominal visceral aneurysms. In: Haimovici H, ed. *Vascular Emergencies.* New York, NY: Appleton-Century-Crofts, 1981:387–397.
Taylor LM, et al. Natural history and non-operative treatment of chronic lower extremity ischaemia. In: Rutherford RB, ed. *Vascular Surgery,* 4th ed. Philadelphia, Pa: WB Saunders, 1996:751–765.
Taylor LM, et al. Present status of reversed vein bypass grafting: five-year results of a modern series. *J Vasc Surg* 1990;11:193–206.

Cerebrovascular Insufficiency

Executive Committee for the Asymptomatic Carotid Atherosclerosis Study. Endarterectomy for asymptomatic carotid artery stenosis. *JAMA* 1995;273:1421–1461.
Gewertz BL, McCaffrey MT. Intraoperative monitoring during carotid endarterectomy. *Curr Probl Surg* 1987;24:481–532.
Hobson RW II, Weiss DG, Fields WS, et al. Efficacy of carotid endarterectomy for asymptomatic carotid stenosis. *N Engl J Med* 1993;328:221–227.
McKinsey JF, Desai TR, Bassiouny HS, et al. Mechanisms of neurologic deficits and mortality with carotid endarterectomy. *Arch Surg* 1996;131(5):526–531.
North American Symptomatic Carotid Endarterectomy Trial Collaborators. Beneficial effect of carotid endarterectomy in symptomatic patients with high-grade carotid stenosis. *N Engl J Med* 1991;325: 445–453.
Riles TS, Imparato AM, Jacobowitz GR, et al. The cause of perioperative stroke after carotid endarterectomy. *J Vasc Surg* 1994;19:206–216.

Venous Disease

Collins R, Scrimgeour A, Yusuf S, Phil D, Peto R. Reduction in fatal pulmonary embolism and venous thrombosis by perioperative administration of subcutaneous heparin. *N Engl J Med* 1988;May: 1162–1173.
Greenfield LJ, Peyton R, Crute S, Barnes R. Greenfield vena cava filter experience: late results in 156 patients. *Arch Surg* 1981;116:1451.
Lensing Anthonie WA, Prandoni P, Brandjes P, et al. Detection of deep vein thrombosis by real-time B-mode ultrasonography. *N Engl J Med* 1989;February:342–345.
Raju S, Fredericks R. Valve reconstruction procedures for nonobstructive venous insufficiency: rationale, techniques, and results in 107 procedures with 2–8 year follow-up. *J Vasc Surg* 1988; February:301–310.

23

Transplantation

Mitchell H. Goldman, M.D.
Stephen B. Leapman, M.D.

The concept of tissue replacement, or transplantation, is based on the idea that patients who have end-stage disease of critical organs can be kept alive beyond the useful life of these organs and tissues. Until the middle of the 20th century, the failure of any organ that is essential to life was uniformly fatal. However, technologies to sustain life despite transient organ failure were slowly developed. Two examples are early dialysis for acute renal failure and the refinement of respirators for respiratory insufficiency. The experimental techniques of organ and tissue transfer were attempted in humans, mostly in the form of kidney transplantation and skin grafting. Early attempts at kidney transplantation failed because the understanding of immunology did not evolve as rapidly as did the idea of organ replacement.

Now, because of improved understanding of immunology and of organ and tissue preservation, end-stage failure of several organs essential to life no longer dooms the patient. In addition, tissues that are not vital to life (e.g., cornea, bone, skin, dura) can be transplanted, improving the quality of many lives.

Organ and Tissue Donation

Organs and tissues for transplantation come from either cadaver donors or living donors (usually relatives of the transplant recipient). Even though grafts from living related donors have the advantages of increased graft survival, ready availability, and immediate graft function, cadaver donors are the major source of graft tissues. Kidney, segmental pancreas, segmental liver, lung, small bowel, and bone marrow grafts can be taken from living donors. All other organs and tissues are procured from cadavers.

The recognition of a potential cadaver donor is the initial step in organ donation. Solid organs can be transplanted if they remain perfused in situ until the time of retrieval. Therefore, any patient who has normal cardiac function and has been pronounced "brain dead" is a potential donor. To increase the supply of noncardiac organs, the use of donors whose hearts are no longer beating has gained increased attention, especially when the donor organ can be rapidly cooled in situ after cardiac function ceases.

The diagnosis of **brain death** must be made before organ harvest is performed. This diagnosis is usually made by the primary care physician or a neurologist. Donors are previously healthy people who have irreversible central nervous system injury as a result of trauma, cerebrovascular accident, central nervous system tumors, or cerebral anoxia. Contraindications to donation include most chronic medical problems, pre-existing hypertensive cardiovascular disease, malignancy other than primary brain tumors, cardiac arrest that causes prolonged warm ischemia of organs, and uncontrolled infection. Additionally, human immunodeficiency virus or hepatitis C or B usually precludes donation. The federal Centers for Disease Control also advise against using individuals as donors whose history or behavior makes them high risk for having transmissible disease. The President's Commission for the

Table 23-1. Criteria to Determine Cessation of Brain Function

Clinical Signs	Confirmatory Tests
Absence of spontaneous respirations	Sustained apnea when disconnecting respirator
Absence of pupillary light reflex	
Absence of corneal reflex	Electroencephalogram
Absence of oculocephalic or oculovestibular reflex	Radionuclide brain scan
	Cerebral angiography
Unresponsiveness to stimuli	
Known cause for condition	
Duration of condition over time	
Known irreversibility	

Table 23-2. Laboratory Studies Used to Determine Acceptability of Organs for Transplantation

Laboratory Study	Evaluated Organ
Cardiac catheterization, echocardiogram	Heart, heart–lung
Electrocardiogram	Heart, heart–lung
Chest x-ray	Heart, lung, heart–lung
Creatinine phosphokinase with MB bands	Heart, heart–lung
Bronchoscopy	Lung
BUN, creatinine	Kidney
Glucose	Pancreas
Liver function tests	Liver
Blood, urine, sputum culture	All
Hepatitis screen	All
Serologic test for syphilis	All
Human immunodeficiency virus	All

BUN, blood urea nitrogen.

Study of Ethical Problems in Medicine and Biochemical and Behavioral Research defined brain death and endorsed criteria that are used as guidelines. These guidelines are separated into clinical criteria and confirmatory objective studies. Clinical criteria indicate that the individual is totally unresponsive to stimuli (Table 23-1). Clinical situations that mimic complete unresponsiveness (e.g., barbiturate or opiate overdose, profound hypothermia) must be excluded. Patients who are being considered as donors should be as close to normothermia as possible. Confirmatory studies support the diagnosis of brain death, but this diagnosis may be made by clinical criteria only. Evaluation of the potential donor requires serial observations over a period of 6 to 24 hours. During this time, referral by the primary hospital staff to the organ procurement organization is initiated.

For specific organs and tissues, age is a relative contraindication to donation. Acute or chronic diseases that affect certain organs may exclude them from consideration. A history of hepatic disease excludes liver donation, and a history of hepatitis B excludes most organ and tissue donation. Preexisting renal disease excludes kidney donation, and diabetes mellitus precludes pancreatic donation. Cardiac trauma, coronary artery disease, pneumonia, and advanced age exclude cardiac and heart–lung donation. Donors who are older than 35 to 40 years of age may require coronary catheterization to rule out significant cardiac disease. Pulmonary trauma, pneumonia, and respiratory compromise preclude lung donation. Bronchoscopy may be required to rule out infection. Minimal hypertension may not be a contraindication to kidney donation, although severe hypertension is an absolute contraindication to cardiac or renal donation. Laboratory studies are useful to determine the acceptability of donor organs (Table 23-2).

Consent for organ or tissue donation is obtained through a signed donor card, the appropriate driver's license designation (usually a consent sticker), a consent statement, or a will, or by permission of the next of kin or suitable legal guardian. If a medical examiner is involved, permission may also be required from both the medical examiner and the legal guardian. The opti-

mal situation for organ donation occurs when the family has previously discussed and agreed on organ donation.

After the donor is declared brain dead, treatment is directed toward optimizing organ function. Ventilation is maintained with a mechanical respirator, and arterial blood gases are monitored. Because many patients who have closed head injuries are purposely dehydrated to decrease cerebral edema, vigorous rehydration may be necessary. If vigorous hydration with crystalloid or colloid is inadequate to maintain perfusion, a vasopressor (dopamine or dobutamine) is used. Vasoconstrictors are avoided because of their vasospastic effect on the renal and splanchnic beds. Donors who have massive diuresis because of diabetes insipidus may require vasopressin. Although oliguria is often corrected with hydration, diuretics (e.g., furosemide, mannitol) may help to initiate and maintain urinary output. Monitoring of cardiac and pulmonary function is imperative when a heart, heart–lung, or lung donation is considered. Bone, skin, dura, fascia, and eye donors do not need a functioning cardiovascular system, and the corresponding tissue can be procured as many as 12 to 24 hours after the cessation of cardiac and respiratory function.

Organ Preservation

Effective preservation of whole organs after harvest enhances the success of cadaveric transplantation by providing time for distant transplant centers to retrieve the needed organs, perform precise tissue typing and crossmatching between donor and recipient, prepare the recipient, and work with national and international organ-sharing programs. The most critical steps in the preservation of solid organs are rapid organ cooling and sterile storage in a cold environment (Table 23-3).

The kidney, heart, lung, liver, and pancreas are routinely flushed in situ with a cold solution to stop metabolism rapidly. Usually, hyperosmotic (325–420 mOsm/L) or

Table 23-3. Preservation Methods and Useful Durations

Organ	Preservation Method	Typical Solution	Useful Duration
Kidney	Ice slush	Hyperosmotic Hyperkalemic	24–96 hr
	Hypothermic pulsatile perfusion	Colloid solution	96 hr
Heart	Ice slush	Crystalloid with cardioplegia	6 hr
Liver	Ice slush	Hyperosmotic Hyperkalemic	12–24 hr
Pancreas	Ice slush	Hyperosmotic Hyperkalemic	24 hr 24 hr
Heart–lung	Ice slush	Crystalloid with/without cardioplegia	3–6 hr
Lung	Ice slush	Pulmonoplegia	6–10 hr
Small bowel	Ice slush	Hyperosmotic	Hours
Eyes			
Scleral grafts	Freezing	With/without glycerin	Several months
Cornea	Refrigeration Cryopreservation	Storage media	3–14 days Several months
Skin	Cryopreservation Lyophilization	Glycerin, DMSO	Indefinitely
Skeletal tissue	Cryopreservation Lyophilization	Glycerin, DMSO	Indefinitely

DMSO, dimethyl sulfoxide.

hyperkalemic solutions are used. In some situations, a colloid is added. The organs are subsequently removed, individually packaged in sterile containers, and placed in ice. Hypothermic (7°–10° C) continuous pulsatile perfusion with a colloid solution is used to extend renal preservation time. Pulsatile perfusion is administered with an apparatus that includes a pulsatile pump, a membrane oxygenator, and tubing connected to the renal artery. The colloid solution is continuously recirculated. Cryopreservation with cryoprotectants (e.g., glycerin, dimethyl sulfoxide) and **lyophilization** are useful in preserving skin, skeletal, and scleral tissues. Nutrient media and normothermic or hypothermic preservation are used with cornea, skin, cartilage, and bone.

Organ and Tissue Allocation

After organs and tissues are recovered from the cadaver donor, a national allocation system is used to distribute these lifesaving and health-restoring resources appropriately. Tissues and cornea are distributed through appropriate local and national banking systems. Organ allocation is regulated through a contract from the federal government by the **United Network for Organ Sharing (UNOS)** in Richmond, Virginia. UNOS is the national headquarters for the listing of patients who need an organ for transplantation (Table 23-4). All organs that are recovered from donors are registered with UNOS, and the patients who need organs are matched by the computer listing process. All organs are usually matched according to ABO compatibility. In addition, kidneys and kidney–pancreas combinations are distributed according to human leukocyte

antigen (HLA) match and waiting time. Hearts, livers, and lungs are primarily shared on the basis of ABO match. However, the seriousness of the recipient's condition, distance from the donor center, size match, and waiting time are used to determine which ABO-matched recipient has priority. The national program allows sharing of these scarce resources equitably while balancing medical and ethical issues. The numerous committees of UNOS, which represent all aspects of organ donation, procurement, and transplantation, oversee this process. UNOS attempts to increase donation and to ensure that organs are distributed fairly, with the best possible results.

The allocation of musculoskeletal tissue is different because several tissues can be banked for long periods. Therefore, tissue allocation is managed through well-organized tissue banks that have a variety of tissues "on the shelf." Centers that perform tissue transplantation can obtain the necessary tissues as specific needs arise. There is no national computer system similar to UNOS for tissue allocation. For bone marrow, a national computer network of living donors is being developed to allow volunteers to donate perfectly matched bone marrow to those in need. Distribution of corneal grafts is based on local waiting lists.

Immunology

Transplantation involves a surgical procedure that transfers tissue from one site to another in the same individual or between different individuals. An **autograft** is tissue that is transplanted from one site of the

Table 23-4. Number of Patients on UNOS Waiting Lists by Organ Needed and ABO Blood Group, August 1996

Organ	O	A	B	AB	Total
Kidney	17,295	9456	5865	783	33,399
Cornea	—	—	—	—	4098[a]
Heart	1929	1268	405	91	3693
Heart–lung	115	84	20	8	227
Liver	3634	2364	721	207	6926
Lung	1019	825	240	73	2157
Pancreas	135	117	44	11	307
Total	24,127	14,114	7295	1173	50,807

[a]Number of patients on the waiting list at the end of 1995.
UNOS, United Network of Organ Sharing.

body to another in the same individual (e.g., skin graft removed from the leg and placed on a wound elsewhere). An **isograft** is tissue that is transferred between genetically identical individuals (e.g., renal transplant between monozygotic twins). An **allograft** is tissue that is transplanted between genetically dissimilar individuals of the same species (e.g., cadaver donor renal transplant). A **xenograft** is tissue that is transferred between individuals of different species (e.g., porcine skin grafted onto a human burn victim). An **orthotopic graft** (orthograft) involves placement of an organ in the normal anatomic position. An orthotopic graft usually necessitates removal of the native organ (e.g., cardiac transplantation). A **heterotopic graft** involves placement of an organ at a site different from the normal anatomic position (e.g., renal transplantation).

The success of a graft depends on the degree of genetic similarity between the organ and the host and on the effectiveness of the immunosuppressive means used to alter host response. In vitro testing can identify favorable donor–recipient genetic combinations. In addition, the discovery of new immunosuppressive agents led to better graft survival, fewer and less severe episodes of rejection, and less risk of infection. The result is an improved outlook for patients who require transplantation.

Immune competence in humans is based primarily on preformed humoral antibody responses. Antibodies may be present at birth (e.g., ABO blood group antibodies), or they may be acquired. Successful transplantation requires ABO blood group compatibility for organs that express ABO antigens (e.g., kidney, heart). If ABO blood group–directed antibodies are present in the blood that is perfusing an organ that contains one or more of these antigens, antibody-mediated killing of the endothelium occurs. The result is thrombosis and organ necrosis, as seen in **hyperacute rejection.** Acquired antibodies directed against **human leukocyte antigens** (HLA system) may form in response to blood transfusions, pregnancy, or previously transplanted organs. These antibodies are complement-dependent and are cytotoxic to tissue that has similar surface antigens. Recipient serum must be tested for the presence of these antibodies with a microcytotoxicity test that uses donor lymphocytes as

target antigens. If recipient antibodies are present, lymphocyte killing takes place, with a resultant positive **crossmatch.** If certain organs are transplanted in the presence of a positive crossmatch, circulating antibodies attach to the endothelium of the donor organ. If complement is present, these antibodies destroy the organ. The presence of an incompatible ABO blood group or a preformed complement-dependent antibody directed toward the donor tissue is usually a contraindication to transplantation.

The genetic loci for both humoral and cellular immune responses are located on the short arm of the sixth chromosome. These loci are responsible for two classes of histocompatibility molecules. Class I antigens are single-chain glycoproteins and are cataloged as HLA, B, or C. These antigens are present on all nucleated cells and are inherited in an autosomal codominant fashion. The subloci are genetically transferred as haplotypes on a single segment of chromosome. Thus, a recipient shares one of two haplotypes with each parent. According to Mendelian genetics, a recipient has a 25% chance of sharing two haplotypes, a 50% chance of sharing one haplotype, and a 25% chance of not sharing a haplotype with a sibling. Unrelated individuals randomly share similar antigens. Class I antigens play an important role in the antigen-recognition phase of cellular immunity. They are detected by a serologic evaluation that uses lymphocytes and a known panel of antisera in a complement-dependent microcytotoxicity test. In living related donor kidney transplants, these antigens have a very strong correlation with graft success.

Class II antigens are glycoproteins that have two polymeric chains, each with a common subunit. These antigens are present on B-lymphocytes, dendritic cells, activated **T-cells,** endothelial cells, and monocytes. Several series are found within this HLA locus, including the HLA-D locus and the HLA-Dr, Dq, and Dp loci. The antigens form the cellular arm of the immune response and are defined by the mixed lymphocyte culture test (MLC). The MLC is a strong predictor of success in living related renal transplants. Because this test takes 5 to 7 days to perform, it is not useful in cadaver transplants, especially cardiac, liver, and pancreatic transplants. The HLA-Dr locus correlates with the D locus and can be evaluated serologically. In renal transplants, the graft success rate is approximately 20% higher with Dr-matched cadaver donors compared with Dr-unmatched donors. Heart, liver, and lung transplants require cadaver donors, and preservation time is significantly shorter than in renal transplantation. For these reasons, ABO matching and crossmatching are the most common tests performed before transplantation. In some cases, even crossmatching is disregarded when an emergency transplant is performed. Bone, skin, dura, and other cryopreserved or lyophilized tissues usually do not require typing and crossmatching before transplantation because their immunogenic activity is very weak after preservation. Better results are reported with corneal transplants after HLA matching.

Immunologic Events After Transplantation

Rejection is an immunologic attempt to destroy foreign tissue after transplantation. It is a complex and incompletely understood event. Four types of clinically identified rejection occur. They are classified according to the time of occurrence and the immune mechanism involved.

Hyperacute Rejection

Hyperacute rejection occurs soon (minutes to several hours) after graft implantation. The organ becomes flaccid, cyanotic, and, in the case of the kidney, anuric. Histologically, polymorphonuclear leukocytes are packed in the pericapillary area, and endothelial necrosis with vascular thrombosis occurs. Hyperacute rejection is associated with preformed antibodies directed toward either ABO blood group or HLA antigens. It rarely occurs today because of the practice of crossmatching and blood group matching (Table 23-5).

Accelerated Acute Rejection

Accelerated acute rejection occurs during the first several days after transplantation. In the kidney, it is characterized by oliguria and may be accompanied by disseminated intravascular coagulation, thrombocytopenia, and hemolysis. The organ becomes swollen, tender, and congested. Histologically, extensive arteriolar necrosis and perivasculitis are present. Immunologically, this type of rejection is believed to represent a second set of anamnestic responses that are mediated by both antibodies and lymphocytes. Usually, the antibody crossmatch is negative, but may become positive after rejection occurs. A preformed antibody may be present at a low or undetectable level that produces a negative pretransplant crossmatch. This type of rejection is rare, and there is no effective treatment.

Acute Rejection

Acute rejection occurs in as many as 90% of cadaver donor transplants. It may even occur in well-matched living related donor transplants. This type of rejection causes organ failure. Microscopically, T-lymphocyte infiltration occurs into vascular and interstitial spaces. Organs that have severe acute rejection show evidence of endotheliitis. In the kidney, glomeruli are often spared relative to other regions. In the heart, the infiltrate is usually pericapillary and is associated with interstitial edema and myonecrosis. In the liver, the infiltrate is often seen in the area of the vascular triad. In the lung, bronchiolitis occurs. Acute rejection is treated with increased doses of immunosuppression. If it is reversed, the patient has an excellent chance of retaining the graft. Repeated acute rejection may ultimately damage the organ.

Table 23-5. Rejection: General Pathology

Rejection Type	Time	Pathology	Treatment	Prognosis
Hyperacute	Immediately to hours after transplant	Swollen, edematous organ Antibody-mediated vascular thrombosis and necrosis Polymorphonuclear infiltrates	Usually prevented by crossmatching and blood group matching	Poor
Accelerlated	2–5 days	Swollen, edematous organ Arterial necrosis Vasculitis Lymphocyte infiltration	No effective treatment	Poor
Acute	7–10 days; may recur during subsequent years	Mononuclear cell infiltration into vascular and interstitial spaces Endotheliitis, bronchiolar inflammation (lung) Myocyte injury (heart) Bile duct injury (liver)	Increased immunosuppression or change to different regimen	80%–90% reversal
Chronic	Years	Obliterative vasculopathy Myocardial fibrosis and coronary obliteration (heart) Progressive bile duct loss (liver) Bronchiectasis, pleural thickening (lung)	No effective treatment At best, prevention of acute deterioration	Relentless deterioration

Chronic Rejection

Chronic rejection is a slow, progressive immunologic process that occurs over a period of months to years. It is characterized by vascular intimal hyperplasia, lymphocytic infiltration, and atrophy and fibrosis of renal, cardiac, or hepatic tissue. Immunologically, **chronic rejection** is mediated by both humoral and cellular elements through poorly understood mechanisms. It is unaltered by increased immunosuppression.

Immunosuppressive Drug Therapy

All recipients of allografts require immunosuppressive therapy. The sole exception is a patient who receives a transplanted organ from an identical twin (isograft). The role of immunosuppression is twofold: (1) to provide maintenance suppression of the immune system to prevent rejection and (2) to treat episodes of rejection if the recipient "breaks through" the maintenance program. Immunosuppressive agents are classified as biologic or pharmacologic. They are the main components of immunosuppressive programs. Immunosuppressive modalities (e.g., radiation therapy, plasmapheresis, thoracic duct drainage) are of historic interest only in solid-organ transplantation. Complications include gastrointestinal intolerance and neutropenia. Because the eyes are an immune-privileged site, matching and systemic immunosuppression are rarely required for corneal transplants. However, when rejection occurs, topical steroids are used.

Immunosuppressive agents are always used in combination (Table 23-6) because no single agent or technique provides adequate therapy. For this reason, agents are often chosen to attack the immune system at various times after transplantation and to complement each other by suppressing the immune system at different levels or by different mechanisms. Some agents prevent the recognition of antigens. Others depress cellular clonal expansion. Some agents affect cellular cytotoxicity during an episode of rejection, and others prevent the formation or release of cytokine. All agents reduce the recipient's resistance to infection and increase the recipient's susceptibility to both routine and opportunistic organisms (e.g., fungi, viruses, parasites, protozoa). These agents also reduce the recipient's ability to provide immunosurveillance against tumors. As a result, transplant recipients have a tenfold to hundredfold increase in the incidence of tumors, especially lymphomas and skin cancers (Table 23-7).

Table 23-6. Clinically Available Immunosuppressive Agents and Techniques in Organ Transplantation

Pharmacologic	Biologic
Azathioprine	Polyclonal sera
Cyclosphosphamide	Monoclonal sera
Cyclosporine	Blood transfusions
FK-506	
Rapamycin	
Steroids	
Mycophenolate mofetil	

Table 23-7. Drugs Used for Immunosuppression

Name	Use	Mechanism of Action	Side Effects
Corticosteroids (prednisone, Medrol)	Maintenance, rejection therapy	Lympholysis, inhibition of IL-1 release	Cushing's syndrome, dyspepsia, osteonecrosis, cancer
Azathioprine (Imuran)	Maintenance	Inhibition of nucleic acid synthesis	Bone marrow depression, veno-occlusive hepatic disease, arthralgia, pancreatitis, red cell aplasia, cancer
Cyclosporine (Sandimmune, Neoral)	Maintenance	Inhibition of secretion and formation of IL-2 (by inhibiting calcineurin)	Nephrotoxicity, hypertension, hyperkalemia, hepatotoxicity, hirsutism, gingival hyperplasia, tremors, breat fibroadenomas, cancer
FK-506 [tacrolimus (Prograf)]	Maintenance, treatment of refractory rejection	Inhibition of production of IL-2	Nephrotoxicity, glucose intolerance, neurotoxicity, cancer
Mycophenolate mofetil (CellCept)	Maintenance	Inhibition of inosine monophosphate dehydrogenase	Gastrointestinal intolerance, neutropenia
OKT3 (monoclonal antibody)	Treatment of rejection	Depletion of T-cells, modulation of CDS receptor from surface of T-cells	Fever, chills, pulmonary edema, cerebritis, lymphoproliferative disorders
Polyclonal antilymphocyte preparations	Treatment of rejection	Depletion of lymphocytes	Anaphylaxis, fever, leukopenia, thrombocytopenia, lymphoproliferative disorders

IL, interleukin.

Pharmacologic Agents

The most commonly used immunosuppressive agents are corticosteroids (prednisone, methylprednisolone). These compounds are used to provide maintenance immunosuppression and, in higher doses, to treat rejection. Their mechanism of action is poorly understood, but steroids are lympholytic and inhibit the release of interleukin-1 from macrophages. Prednisone is the most common steroid preparation used in transplantation. Initial doses start at 1 to 2 mg/kg, tapering to 0.1 to 0.25 mg/kg 1 year after transplant. The complications of steroid use are protean and include dyspepsia, cataracts, osteonecrosis, Cushing's syndrome, acne, capillary fragility, and glucose intolerance.

Azathioprine (Imuran) is an antimetabolite. It is metabolized to its active form, 6-mercaptopurine, by the liver. It acts principally to inhibit the synthesis of nucleic acid. Therefore, it is a relatively nonspecific agent, and it affects all replicating cells of the body. Its major side effect is bone marrow depression manifested by leukopenia and thrombocytopenia. These effects are dose-dependent. Other side effects include veno-occlusive hepatic disease, arthralgias, pancreatitis, and red cell aplasia. It is used for baseline immunosuppression, but never to treat rejection directly. It is always used with other immunosuppressants.

Cyclosporine (Sandimmune, Neoral) is an undecapeptide that blocks the secretion of interleukin-2, a T-cell growth factor. It prevents the proliferation and maturation of cytotoxic T-cells that cause graft rejection. This drug is a potent immunosuppressant and is used for maintenance therapy in combination with other agents. It is not effective in the treatment of rejection. Complications include dose-dependent nephrotoxicity, hepatotoxicity, hyperkalemia, hypertension, gingival hyperplasia, tremors, and breast fibroadenomas. Whole blood levels of cyclosporine are routinely monitored to assure maximal therapeutic benefit and minimize complications.

Tacrolimus (FK-506, Prograf) is a macrolide antibiotic. Its mechanism of action is similar to that of cyclosporine (inhibiting the production of interleukin-2 and other cytokines). It is more potent than cyclosporine, and it suppresses both B- and T-cell activity. It is used for maintenance immunosuppression in combination with steroids and azathioprine (or mycophenolate mofetil). Tacrolimus is effective in the treatment of refractory rejection. Its side effects include dose-dependent nephrotoxicity, glucose intolerance, infections, and a higher incidence of lymphoproliferative disorders. As with cyclosporine, drug monitoring is essential.

Mycophenolate mofetil (CellCept) was approved for clinical transplantation in 1995. Its mechanism of action differs from that of the other compounds; it is a noncompetitive, reversible inhibitor of inosine monophosphate dehydrogenase (the enzyme necessary to convert inosine monophosphate to guanosine monophosphate). Because only lymphocytes require the de novo synthesis of guanosine monophosphate, mycophenolate mofetil profoundly inhibits T- and **B-cell** function. This drug is used in combination with steroids and cyclosporine or tacrolimus for maintenance therapy. Its use for chronic rejection is under review. The compound is particularly effective in transplant populations that are at high risk for rejection (e.g., African-Americans, children, previously transplanted patients).

Biologic Agents

Biologic agents are either polyclonal or monoclonal sera that are prepared by immunizing an animal (e.g., horse, rabbit, mouse, rat) with human lymphocytes. The polyclonal sera antithymocyte globulin and antilymphocyte globulin are beneficial when used as induction therapy for solid-organ transplant recipients or to treat acute cellular rejection. These preparations are usually given intravenously and are never used for maintenance therapy. Monoclonal antibodies have been prepared against various cell-surface receptors on the T-cell. Therefore, the compounds are directed against specific T-cell subsets, and not against the entire T- or B-cell population. One of these antibodies, OKT3, is directed against the CD3 receptor on the T-cell and is used for prophylactic induction therapy as well as for treatment of acute cellular rejection.

Blood transfusions, either donor-specific or random, are still believed to provide protection against rejection. Donor blood transfusion is carried out in living donor transplantation. The mechanism is still poorly understood, but may be related to the formation of blocking antibodies. These antibodies cover up recognition antigens on the donor cells and prevent them from being recognized as nonself. Infusion of donor marrow into the recipient of a solid organ is a similar manipulation of the immune system that may encourage specific immunosuppression and prevent rejection.

End-Stage Renal Disease and Kidney Transplantation

Dialysis

Treatment of end-stage renal failure often involves long-term hemodialysis or peritoneal dialysis to maintain life. Because of the availability of maintenance dialysis, kidney transplantation is usually a nonemergency procedure that allows tissue typing and matching, long-term survival without transplant, and survival after transplant rejection. The principle of dialysis is simple: on one side of the semipermeable membrane is the extracellular fluid of the patient; on the other side of the membrane is the material that is to be discarded. Products of normal metabolism that are not excreted by the failed kidney accumulate in the extracellular fluid, pass through the semipermeable membrane to the dialysate solution, and are discarded. Hemodialysis requires connection of the patient's vascular space to a dialysis machine. In acute situations, large cannulae are inserted into the venous circulation through the femoral, jugular, or subclavian veins. For long-term hemodialysis, permanent access to the circulation is achieved by connecting an artery to a vein in an easily accessible and reusable area (e.g., radial artery and cephalic vein just above the anteromedial elbow joint). A vascular bridging conduit of polytetrafluoroethylene graft may be placed in a subcutaneous tunnel, with one end sewn to an artery and the other to a vein to provide a large-caliber fistula for hemodialysis. In peritoneal dialysis, access to the peritoneal membrane requires a transabdominal indwelling catheter that is used for infusion and drainage of dialysate fluid. Most procedures to place hemodialysis and peritoneal catheters are performed under local anesthesia.

Postoperative complications involve infection of synthetic or foreign material, clotting or aneurysm of the vascular conduit, dysfunction of the peritoneal dialysis catheter, and peritonitis. Infectious complications are treated with appropriate antibiotics or removal of the graft or catheter. The large numbers of patients who receive long-term dialysis (> 100,000 in the United States) attest to the efficacy of the surgical procedures that permit this therapy.

Indications for Transplant

A patient who has end-stage renal failure from any cause may be a candidate for transplant, regardless of the type or duration of dialysis support required. The acceptable age range for kidney recipients is 1 to 70 years, although infants and patients who are older than 70 years of age can be successfully transplanted. The patient should be currently free of infections and free of cancer for at least 5 years. Patients with localized cancers (e.g., skin cancer) may undergo retransplantation after successful excision of the lesion. Other chronic disease processes should be minor, self-limited, or under control (e.g., a patient with known coronary artery disease should be optimally treated and show cardiovascular stability before undergoing renal transplantation).

Transplant Procedure

Kidney transplantation is nearly always a heterotopic allograft, placed in the extraperitoneal iliac fossa (Figure 23-1). The renal artery and vein are sewn to a corresponding iliac vessel, and the ureter is implanted in the urinary bladder. Technical variations are common and include intraabdominal graft placement in infants and small children as well as donor-to-recipient ureter-to-ureter anastomosis instead of donor ureter-to-recipient bladder ureteroneocystostomy.

Treatment of the renal transplant recipient involves methods used for any operative procedure as well as those specific to the patient. Ambulation, diet, and medication orders are much the same as for patients who undergo operations such as herniorrhaphy or appendectomy. Early postgraft care involves hourly monitoring of vital signs and urine output. Immunosuppression for renal transplantation varies from center to center.

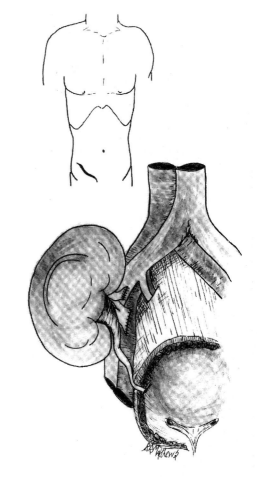

Figure 23-1 A heterotopic human renal allograft in the right extraperitoneal iliac fossa. The renal artery and vein anastomoses are end to side, respectively, to the external iliac artery and vein. A tunneled ureteroneocystostomy allows normal micturition.

Signs and symptoms of acute rejection include increasing serum creatinine, proteinuria, hypertension, fever, decreasing urine output and, occasionally, low-grade abdominal pain. Acute rejection is treated by modulation of the immune response to prevent graft loss while allowing for suitable host defense mechanisms to allay severe, acute infection. Usually, intravenous methylprednisolone, OKT3, or antithymocyte globulin therapy is given for several days. Acute rejection is usually reversible.

Complications

Two types of complications occur: transplant and nonrenal (Table 23-8). Both types of complications have early and late components. Early complications of kidney transplantation include excessive diuresis, urinary leak or fistula, hemorrhage, vascular anastomotic leak or thrombosis, formation of perigraft lymphocele, graft rupture, and severe rejection. Late graft complications include stenosis of the ureter or renal artery and recurrent disease in the transplanted kidney. Fortunately, the latter problem, which is most common with focal glomerular sclerosis and systemic disease (e.g., diabetes) is uncommon (< 5%). Perigraft infection occurs both early and late. Nonrenal early complications include infections and cardiovascular events (e.g., postoperative myocardial infarction, cerebrovascular accident, deep vein thrombophlebitis). Late problems unrelated to the kidney include infection, peptic ulcer disease, aseptic joint necrosis, cataracts, diabetes mellitus, hypertension, liver disease, and the risk of neoplasia that accompanies immunosuppression. Kidney transplant recipients are usually treated prophylactically for ulcer disease with an H_2 receptor blocker. Infections are the most common complications. They may be common (e.g., pneumococcal pneumonia) or unusual

(e.g., necrotizing fasciitis from a rare fungus). Organisms that cause clinical infection in the immunosuppressed host include cytomegalovirus, common bacteria, fungi, and protozoa such as *Pneumocystis carinii*.

Prognosis

The results of kidney transplantation have improved since 1975. Functional graft survival rates of 75% to 85% for cadaveric kidneys and 95% for living related donor organs at 1 year are now common (Table 23-9). In addition, patient survival now exceeds 95% at 1 year. Rates of infection-related deaths have fallen drastically. These improvements are the result of better preparation of patients with end-stage renal failure and recognition of the limits of antirejection therapy. Overuse of immunosuppressive therapy does not result in better graft survival and is detrimental to patient survival. The loss of a renal allograft requires a return to dialysis, but second and subsequent renal allografts are often performed successfully.

Although complications occur, kidney transplantation is the model of solid-organ replacement therapy. In the United States, more than 8000 patients undergo this procedure annually.

Liver Transplantation

Indications

The patient who is considered a candidate for liver transplant has a life expectancy of 1 year or less and is free of malignancy and infection. Transplantation is best carried out before the onset of terminal events associated with end-stage liver failure. Table 23-10 shows

Table 23-8. Complications of Renal Transplantation

Type	Early	Late
Renal	Massive diuresis	Ureteric stenosis
	Ureter anastomotic leak	Vascular anastomotic
	Hemorrhage	stenosis (aneurysm)
	Lymphocele	Recurrent primary renal
	Rejection	disease
	Rupture	Neoplasia
	Thrombosis	
Nonrenal	Infection	Infection
	Myocradial infarction	Progressive
	Peptic ulcer disease	atherosclerotic vascular
	Thromboembolic disorders	disorders, hypertension
	Steroid-induced acne	Diabetes mellitus
		Aseptic joint necrosis
		Cataract
		Cushing's syndrome
		Hepatic disease

Table 23-9. UNOS Data of Graft and Patient Survival Rates at 1, 2, 3, and 5 years, October 1987 Through December 1994 (US Transplants, All Orgrans)

Organ	Survival Type	N	Length of Survival			
			1 yr (%)	2 yr (%)	3 yr (%)	5 yr (%)
Cadaveric donor kidney	Graft	55,312	81.1	75.4	69.8	59.2
	Patient	55,330	93.4	90.5	87.5	80.6
Living donor kidney	Graft	16,851	91.5	88.0	84.1	75.6
	Patient	16,855	97.3	95.9	94.2	90.3
Liver	Graft	19,964	70.2	65.6	62.4	57.0
	Patient	19,964	80.0	76.3	73.6	68.8
Pancreas	Graft	3922	73.8	68.6	63.7	56.0
	Patient	3922	90.5	87.2	84.1	79.2
Heart	Graft	14,665	81.8	77.4	73.4	65.7
	Patient	14,665	82.8	78.6	75.0	67.8
Lung	Graft	2616	71.1	61.6	53.9	39.6
	Patient	2616	72.7	64.3	57.1	42.6
Heart–lung	Graft	424	62.5	53.6	50.0	39.8
	Patient	424	62.7	54.6	50.9	41.4

diseases that are treated by liver transplantation. Table 23-11 shows the indications to proceed with the procedure. The decision to proceed can be based on subtle findings and usually requires the judgment of an experienced clinician. Waiting times before transplantation may be 1 year or longer, depending on the availability of organs and the condition of the recipient. Patients whose condition is urgent (e.g., those with fulminant liver failure) receive priority. Those whose condition is less urgent receive priority based on waiting time.

Procedure

Liver transplantation uses the whole liver from a cadaver donor. An orthotopic graft is nearly always used. Removal of the recipient native liver begins while the donor liver is being removed. After native hepatectomy is completed, the new liver is implanted by sewing the suprahepatic vena cava to the cuff of the remaining suprahepatic vena cava and performing an infrahepatic vena caval anastomosis (Figure 23-2). The donor hepatic artery is sewn to the recipient artery, and the donor portal vein is sewn to the recipient portal vein. Biliary drainage is commonly achieved by duct-to-duct anastomosis in the adult and by Roux-en-Y choledochojejunostomy in the child. One requirement for hepatic transplantation is size match between the donor and recipient livers. This match is particularly difficult to obtain in a timely manner in small children. This problem led to the use of **reduced-size livers** (larger livers that are surgically resected during preservation after removal). The resulting segment of liver, its blood supply, and the bile duct are reimplanted into the recipient. The success rate with this procedure is equivalent to that of whole-liver grafts, and it is even used for adult recipients. In fact, split livers are used to provide transplants to two recipients. Additionally, liver segments can be resected from living related donors (parents) and successfully reimplanted into small children.

Complications

Complications of liver transplantation include perioperative hemorrhage, bleeding disorders, vascular thrombosis, and leaks or strictures of the biliary tract. After transplantation, perihepatic infection and transient respiratory, renal, or cardiac failure often occur. Acute rejection may also occur, but it is usually less

Table 23-10. Diseases Treated with Liver Transplantation

Benefit	Diseases

Proven	End-stage liver failure from:
	  Cirrhosis: postnecrotic resulting from hepatitis C, autoimmune hepatitis, cryptogenic cirrhosis, alcoholic cirrhosis
	  Primary biliary cirrhosis
	  Primary sclerosing choloangitis
	  Metabolic disease with and without cirrhosis: Wilson's disease, α-1-antitrypsin disease, primary hemochromatosis, and others
	  Congenital biliary atresia (children)
	  Congenital hepatic fibrosis

Possible	Acute liver failure, resulting from fulminant or acute toxic liver damage Budd-Chiari syndrome Cirrhosis, resulting from hepatitis B virus Certain rare primary hepatic tumors: fibrolamellar hepatocellular carcinoma, epithelioid hemangioendothelioma, endrocrine tumors
Questionable	Primary hepatic tumor confined to liver: hepatocellular carcinoma Mestastic carcinoma Alcoholic hepatitis

Table 23-11. Indications for Liver Transplantation

Progressive end-stage liver failure secondary to chronic disease
  Gastrointestinal hemorrhage associated with coagulopathy and esophageal varices
  Progressive encephalopathy
  Progress malnutrition and muscle wasting
  Symptomatic progression of liver deterioration (e.g., pruritis, bony fractures, malaise)
  Recurrent infections, especially spontaneous bacterial peritonitis, pneumonia, septicemia, or intrahepatic abscess seen with progressive biliary strictures
Acute liver failure
  Encephalopathy progressing to stage III or IV coma (semicomatose or comatose, requiring mechanical ventilation)
  Progressive coagulopathy with gastrointestinal bleeding

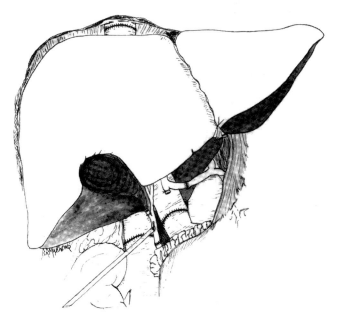

Figure 23-2 An orthotopic human hepatic allograft. End-to-end vascular anastomoses connect the donor and recipient hepatic artery, portal vein, and vena cava both suprahepatically and infrahepatically. The most commonly used common bile duct-to-duct anastomosis is shown.

common and milder than that seen in kidney transplantation. Cyclosporine is more successful in preventing liver rejection than it is for other organs. Late complications of liver transplantation include stenosis of the biliary tree, recurrent hepatitis, ongoing chronic rejection, and toxicity from cyclosporine or other immunosuppressive drug therapy. Chronic rejection is often managed by retransplantation, with excellent results.

Prognosis

Patient and graft survival rates in liver transplantation approach 85% at 1 year for patients who are operated on before the terminal phase of their disease. In patients who are in hepatic coma, survival statistics for both the operation and the postoperative period are poor. Approximately one-half of these patients live 1 year beyond the time of transplant because of complications associated with major surgery in the face of acutely life-threatening hepatic failure.

Heart, Heart–Lung, and Lung Transplantation

Heart Transplantation

Indications

The indication for heart transplantation is end-stage cardiac failure in a patient who is expected to die of cardiac disease within 6 months. Age is not a contraindication. The patient must be free of infection and neoplasm and have full potential for rehabilitation. Specific indications for heart transplantation include idiopathic cardiomyopathy, viral cardiomyopathy, ischemic cardiac disease, postpartum cardiomyopathy, terminal cardiac valvular disease, and hypertensive cardiomyopathy. Cardiac transplantation is most often performed in adults because many congenital cardiac defects can be corrected surgically. However, neonatal and pediatric cardiac transplantation is also performed successfully.

Procedure

The usual cardiac transplant is a size-matched orthotopic allograft. The recipient heart is removed, and the donor heart is sewn into place by attaching the left and right atria of the donor heart to the left and right atria of the recipient. The pulmonary artery and aortic anastomoses are completed (Figure 23-3). The heart is resuscitated and allowed to take over support of the recipient.

Some centers use heterotopic grafts. These grafts allow the recipient's heart to remain as a safety net if the donor heart is rejected. In heterotopic grafts, the donor heart is placed alongside the recipient heart, and the donor and recipient atria and aorta are anastomosed. A graft is used to connect the donor pulmonary artery to the recipient pulmonary artery.

Complications

The complications of cardiac transplantation are largely infection and rejection, with ensuing progressive

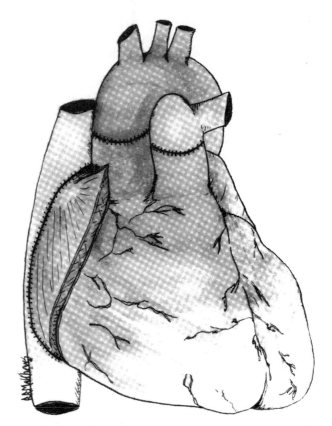

Figure 23-3 An orthotopic human cardiac allograft. The left and right atria of the graft are sutured to the posteriormost atrial walls, which remain intact in the recipient. End-to-end anastomoses of the pulmonary artery and aorta are completed before the transplanted heart is resuscitated and cardiopulmonary bypass support is terminated.

cardiac failure. In heart–lung transplants, restrictive fibrosis of the lung is also described. Early postoperative problems, in addition to infection, include respiratory, renal, and cerebrovascular complications. Late problems are limited to chronic allograft rejection and the long-term effects of immunosuppressive therapy. Accelerated coronary artery disease occurs in some patients and may be related to chronic rejection. Retransplantation and percutaneous transluminal angioplasty are performed for this problem.

Prognosis

Newer immunosuppressive agents (e.g., cyclosporine) and the safe use of endomyocardial biopsy to diagnose rejection have improved the outcome of cardiac transplantation. The current 1-year graft and patient survival rate is 80% or higher, and the 5-year rate is 60% to 70%.

Heart–Lung Transplantation

Heart–lung transplantation is performed when severe pulmonary hypertension accompanies cardiac disease. It is also performed for congenital heart disease. In addition to the complications of cardiac transplantation, complications of heart–lung transplantation include restrictive fibrosis of the lung. Acute and chronic rejection of the lung may be manifested by bronchiolitis. The 1-year survival rate for heart–lung transplant recipients is 63%.

Lung Transplantation

Indications

Single- and double-lung transplantations are performed for patients with α_1-antitrypsin deficiency, interstitial pulmonary fibrosis, primary pulmonary hypertension, and cystic fibrosis and emphysema. Single- or double-lung transplantation can provide total pulmonary function to patients with end-stage pulmonary disease without suppuration and concomitant cardiac failure. Lung cancer is a contraindication to lung transplantation. Recipients must be free of infection and are usually younger than 65 years of age. The donor and the recipient must be of equivalent height and weight.

Complications

Rejection is the most common complication. It is diagnosed by the appearance of infiltrates on chest x-ray and is confirmed with transbronchial or transthoracic needle biopsy. Breakdown of the bronchial anastomosis is a dreaded complication that occurs in 5% of transplants. For this reason, the dose of steroids is kept as low as possible to enhance healing. In lung transplantation, acute and chronic rejection of the lung may be manifested by bronchiolitis.

Procedure

The surgery is performed through a posterolateral thoracotomy for single-lung transplants and through a transverse thoracotomy for double-lung transplants. The donor pulmonary veins are sewn to a left atrial recipient cuff after the sleeve bronchial anastomosis is performed. Finally, the pulmonary arteries are anastomosed.

Prognosis

Patient survival rates for lung transplantation are 73% at 1 year and 57% at 3 years.

Pancreas and Islet Transplantation

Indications

Pancreatic transplantation is the only form of treatment of type I diabetes mellitus that establishes a long-term insulin-dependent, normoglycemic state. To achieve this end, either whole-organ, segmental, or islet cell transplantation is offered to patients who have this disease. According to the International Pancreatic Transplant Registry, more than 4000 patients have undergone transplantation with whole-organ or segmental pancreatic grafts. Through December 1994, nearly 150 patients with type I diabetes received adult islet allografts. Although successful whole-organ or islet-only transplantation affords the patient normo-

glycemia, the effect of pancreatic transplantation on the chronic complications of diabetes mellitus is less clear. However, peripheral neuropathy may improve, and diabetic retinopathy may stabilize. In patients who undergo simultaneous renal transplants, the kidney may be protected because glomerular and mesangial changes (signs of early diabetic damage) are absent from the kidney after simultaneous kidney–pancreas transplantation. Unfortunately, the effects of pancreatic transplantation on the main causes of morbidity and mortality in diabetic patients (e.g., vascular disease, infection) are missing. The last two decades of work in this field showed that patients who have diabetes and functioning pancreatic grafts can enjoy perfect metabolic control and the freedom from dietary restrictions.

Whole-Organ Pancreas Transplantation

In the past, a variety of techniques were used for this operation. Today, the procedure is mostly standardized.

Procedure

The donor pancreas and duodenal C-sweep are transplanted together in the false pelvis of the recipient. The operation is performed intraperitoneally. The arterial supply of the pancreas, including the splenic and superior mesenteric arteries, is anastomosed to the recipient iliac artery. The pancreatic venous drainage (donor portal vein) is attached to the recipient iliac vein. The donor duodenal C-sweep is attached to the dome of the recipient bladder to provide an outlet for the exocrine secretions of the pancreas. Pancreatic function is monitored as urinary amylase concentrations in the postoperative period. Alternatively, the pancreas is anastomosed to the small bowel to provide exocrine drainage into the bowel.

Complications

The postoperative course of combined whole-organ pancreatic–kidney transplantation is more complicated than that of kidney transplantation alone. More episodes of rejection occur, and they require more immunosuppression. Subsequently, these patients have more infectious complications and longer hospital stays. The frequency of vascular complications is similar to that of renal transplant patients, but urinary complications (e.g., infection, leakage, minor bleeding) are greater in pancreas transplant patients. Pancreas-alone transplants have similar complications, including anastomotic leak, vascular thrombosis, and urinary complications when the pancreas is attached to the bladder.

Prognosis

The success rates for whole-organ pancreas transplantation approach those for other solid-organ transplantations. Some series report patient survival rates of 95% and graft survival rates of more than 80%. These rates are comparable to those for renal transplantation. Patients who undergo successful pancreatic transplants report an increased sense of well-being and better overall rehabilitation.

Islet Cell Transplantation

Islet cell transplantation offers the potential for long-lasting strict glucose control. This technique, although perfected in murine systems, has not found its way into practical clinical use. Recent strides were made by increasing the number of viable islets from donor pancreata with the use of new, gentler digesting agents. Techniques to culture or freeze the islets may eventually provide an islet banking system for elective transplantation. The proper delivery system for islets is still debatable. Current options include injection into the portal vein, placement under the renal capsule, and encapsulation into immunoisolated chambers. The success rate for achieving insulin independence approaches 20% at 1 year. The increased rejection rate, the need for large numbers of islets, and the small number of donors relative to the large potential recipient pool have held back the widespread implementation of islet cell transplantation.

Intestinal Transplantation

Indications

Short-gut syndrome, the prime indication for small intestinal transplantation, has an incidence of 2 to 3 per million population. The syndrome is the result of many intestinal disorders, including intestinal strangulation or infarction from midgut volvulus, obstruction, or internal hernias; trauma; and vascular accidents of the mesenteric vessels. Other associated diseases include Crohn's disease, low-grade tumors, and necrotizing enterocolitis. Candidates for transplantation must depend on parenteral nutrition. Some transplant centers perform cluster-graft transplantation, including liver, pancreas, and small bowel, after upper abdominal exenteration to treat otherwise unresectable tumors.

Procedure

The donor bowel may come from a living relative or from a cadaver. A segment of small bowel at least 100 to 150 cm long is necessary to provide an adequate absorptive surface. The allograft may be heterotopic or orthotopic. It is preferable to provide for venous drainage into the recipient's portal system. The ends of the bowel may be anastomosed to the recipient's remaining bowel or brought up to the abdominal wall as an ostomy. The latter approach allows easy observation and biopsy to monitor rejection or ischemia.

Complications

Complications include rejection, graft-versus-host disease, and sepsis from the translocation of bacteria through the bowel mucosal barriers.

Prognosis

The results of small-bowel transplantation are tenuous. The procedure is considered experimental and should be performed at centers that have specific protocols. Graft survival is typically less than 3 years, and in many cases, less than 1 year.

Transplantation of Other Organs and Tissues

Occasionally, allografts of parathyroid tissue, bone, and skin are successful. The use of cyclosporine and matching for bone marrow transplantation added to the success of these procedures. Allografts of skin, bone, fascia, dura, endocrine organs, eyes, and blood vessels are used clinically in a variety of situations or are being studied in several centers. Most of the musculoskeletal tissues that are used for transplantation are either lyophilized, fresh frozen, or fresh grafts. Lyophilized bone is used to replace deficits that are created surgically, to fill spaces, and to aid in posttraumatic reconstruction. Lyophilization significantly reduces the immunogenicity of the tissue while leaving a matrix for bony regrowth (osteotransduction) or promoting new bone growth (osteoinduction). Either particles or larger pieces of bone are used. Allograft fascia and whole joints are also used in reconstructive orthopedic surgery. When available, cryopreserved human allograft valves are used for aortic valve replacement. These valves do not require postoperative anticoagulation. Allograft veins are used in peripheral vascular surgery when no autogenous veins are available for limb salvage. The results are significantly poorer than with autogenous material.

Multiple-Choice Questions

1. Which of the following organs cannot be obtained from a living relative?
   A. Pancreas
   B. Kidney
   C. Liver
   D. Lung
   E. Heart

2. Clinical criteria that are used to determine the cessation of brain function for organ donation include:
   A. Absence of deep tendon reflexes
   B. Absence of spontaneous respirations
   C. Decerebrate response
   D. Decorticate response
   E. Severe head injury

3. What drug is most useful in maintaining blood pressure in an organ donor?
   A. Norepinephrine
   B. Aramine
   C. Epinephrine
   D. Dopamine
   E. Pitocin

4. The 1-year graft survival rate for cardiac transplantation is:
   A. 10%
   B. 25%
   C. 50%
   D. 75% to 85%
   E. 98%

5. A tissue that is transplanted between genetically dissimilar individuals of the same species is:
   A. An autograft
   B. An allograft
   C. An isograft
   D. A xenograft
   E. An orthotopic graft

6. Immunologic testing for a match in cadaver kidney transplantation includes all of the following EXCEPT:
   A. ABO blood group match
   B. Human leukocyte antigen (HLA)-B
   C. Mixed lymphocyte culture
   D. Crossmatch
   E. HLA-Dr

7. Hyperacute rejection:
   A. Occurs 10 to 14 days after transplantation
   B. Is often the result of preformed antimonocyte antibodies
   C. Is treated with high doses of cyclosporine
   D. Can be prevented by pretreatment with steroids
   E. Is associated pathologically with endothelial necrosis and vascular thrombosis

8. In a perfectly matched living related renal transplant between an 18-year-old and his 8-year-old brother:
   A. Cyclophosphamide is the immunosuppressive drug of choice
   B. No immunosuppression is needed
   C. Antilymphocyte globulin is the primary form of immunosuppression
   D. Immunosuppression is used to prevent rejection
   E. Cyclosporine is used in high doses to prevent rejection

9. When used for immunosuppression, cyclosporine:
   A. Induces the generation of an anti–T-cell antibody
   B. Has a high incidence of ocular cataracts
   C. Simplifies the diagnosis of rejection because a biopsy specimen shows classic cellular infiltrates
   D. Permits the concurrent use of a lower dose of steroids
   E. Induces the production of interleukin-1

10. A heart transplant is usually:
    A. A heterotopic allograft
    B. An isotopic autograft
    C. An orthotopic allograft
    D. An orthotopic isograft
    E. A heterotopic xenograft

11. The best candidates for liver transplantation are patients who have all of the following EXCEPT:
    A. Postnecrotic cirrhosis from hepatitis C
    B. Primary biliary cirrhosis
    C. α_1-Antitrypsin disease
    D. Hepatocellular carcinoma
    E. Congenital biliary atresia

12. Cardiac transplantation is LEAST likely to be indicated for:
    A. Hypertensive cardiomyopathy in a 40-year-old man
    B. Idiopathic cardiomyopathy discovered 6 months after a full-term normal pregnancy in a 26-year-old woman
    C. Coronary artery disease with a history of multiple myocardial infarcts in a 48-year-old man
    D. Idiopathic cardiomyopathy in an otherwise healthy 38-year-old man
    E. Transposition of the great vessels in an otherwise healthy 9-month-old infant

13. Pancreas transplantation:
    A. Is the treatment of choice for type II diabetes mellitus
    B. Causes rejection less often than transplantation of most other organs
    C. Has increased perioperative complications
    D. Has a 1-year graft survival rate of more than 90%
    E. Produces the best results when islets are used alone

14. Immunosuppressive drug therapy causes an increased incidence of all of the following EXCEPT:
    A. Lymphoma
    B. Cytomegalovirus infection
    C. Atherosclerosis
    D. Herpes infection
    E. Carcinoma

15. Which of the following is a contraindication to liver donation?
    A. Diabetes mellitus
    B. Hypertension
    C. Treated pneumococcal meningitis
    D. Prolonged warm ischemia
    E. Coronary artery disease

16. Systemic immunosuppression is not usually necessary in:
    A. Corneal transplant
    B. Islet transplant
    C. Cardiac transplant
    D. Lung transplant
    E. Liver transplant

17. What is the longest safe preservation time for liver transplantation?
    A. 4 hours
    B. 18 hours
    C. 36 hours
    D. 72 hours
    E. Indefinitely

18. Indications for lung transplantation include all of the following EXCEPT:
    A. Interstitial pulmonary fibrosis
    B. α_1-Antitrypsin deficiency
    C. Cystic fibrosis
    D. Squamous cell carcinoma
    E. Pulmonary hypertension

19. Leukopenia is associated with:
    A. Azathioprine
    B. Prednisone
    C. Cyclosporine
    D. FK-506
    E. OKT3

20. Hypertension, tremors, and elevated liver function test results are associated with:
    A. Azathioprine
    B. Prednisone
    C. Cyclosporine
    D. Antilymphocyte globulin
    E. OKT3

Oral Examination Study Questions

CASE 1

You are a general surgery intern. A 30-year-old man comes to the emergency room with a 45-caliber gunshot wound to the head. He is in shock and in a coma. The neurosurgeon determines that the amount of brain damage makes this situation nonoperative. The outlook is dismal. An endotracheal tube is placed. The neurosurgeon asks you whether this patient is a potential organ donor.

OBJECTIVE 1

The student knows the criteria for brain death, including clinical criteria and confirmatory tests.
   A. Clinical criteria
      1. No spontaneous respiration
      2. No pupillary light reflex
      3. No corneal reflex
      4. No oculocephalic or oculovestibular reflex
      5. No response to stimuli
   B. Confirmatory tests
      1. Discontinuation of respirator support with normal PCO_2 and PO_2
      2. Electroencephalogram
      3. Radionuclide brain perfusion scan
      4. Cerebroangiography
   C. Consent from the medical examiner and the family if a donor card is not signed
   D. Evaluation of the patient for 6 to 24 hours
   E. Exclusion of confounding factors (e.g., hypothermia, drug overdose)

OBJECTIVE 2

The student knows the criteria for the donation of specific organs and tissues.
   A. For whole-organ donation, maintenance of adequate donor perfusion and ventilation is of paramount importance. Prolonged absence of perfusion is a contraindication to whole-organ donation, but may not be a contraindication to tissue donation (e.g., cornea, bone, skin).

   B. Donors must have no evidence of acute infection or malignancy other than primary central nervous system tumors. A positive hepatitis B test is a contraindication, as is a positive human immunodeficiency virus antibody test.

   C. Preexisting renal disease, diabetes mellitus, and severe hypertension are contraindications to renal donation. Oliguria and elevated blood urea nitrogen and creatinine values secondary to appropriate treatment of the neurosurgical injury are not usually contraindications.

   D. Cardiac trauma, coronary artery disease, pneumonia, severe hypertension, and age older than 40 years usually precludes heart or heart–lung donation. Donors may require cardiac catheterization to rule out coronary artery disease and bronchoscopy to rule out pulmonary disease. Diabetes mellitus excludes pancreatic donation.

   E. Routine tests performed on a potential multiple-organ donor include electrocardiogram, chest x-ray, hepatitis screen, blood urea nitrogen, creatinine, creatine phosphokinase with MB bands, blood glucose, liver function tests, Venereal Disease Research Laboratories tests, human immunodeficiency virus antibody, blood and urine cultures, and arterial blood gases. Tissues such as eye, bone, dura, fascia, and skin may be obtained up to 12 hours after cardiorespiratory function ceases.

OBJECTIVE 3

The student discusses the methods used to obtain consent for donation, including who may give consent.
   A. A signed donor card or indication of organ donation consent on a driver's license is a legal document and may be considered consent for donation.

   B. The spouse is the next person who may give consent.

   C. Parents or guardians are next.

   D. Siblings follow.

   E. Consent from the medical examiner often must be obtained.

OBJECTIVE 4

The student describes the maintenance of a donor until organ donation is performed.

A. Maintenance of donor perfusion and ventilation with a mechanical respirator is of paramount importance. Arterial blood gases are monitored.

B. Rehydration is usually necessary to improve perfusion. Crystalloid (half- or quarter-normal saline) and Ringer's lactate may be used. Occasionally colloid or blood is necessary.

C. A vasopressor (e.g., dopamine, dobutamine) may be used. Vasoconstrictive agents are avoided.

D. Massive urinary volumes from diabetes insipidus may occur, and vasopressin may be necessary.

OBJECTIVE 5

The student knows the limits of organ preservation.

A. Kidney: 24 to 96 hours

B. Heart: 4 to 6 hours

C. Heart and lung: 4 to 6 hours

D. Lung: 6 to 12 hours

E. Liver: 12 to 24 hours

F. Pancreas: 12 to 24 hours

G. Cornea: 3 to 14 days

H. Skin, bone, fascia, and dura: indefinitely

Minimum Level of Achievement for Passing

The student knows most of the criteria for brain death and the usefulness of confirmatory tests. In addition, the student knows the criteria and exclusionary criteria for heart, liver, and kidney donation. The student knows that an organ donation card or indication of consent on a license is a legal document and that the spouse is the initial person required to give consent. Finally, the student describes the basic management of an organ donor.

Honors Level of Achievement

The student knows the criteria for all organs. The student also knows how to treat the complications that occur during basic management (e.g., diabetes insipidus).

CASE 2

A 25-year-old woman who has diabetes has a creatinine clearance of 6 mL/min. Her nephrologist asks you to evaluate her to identify possible methods to treat end-stage renal disease.

OBJECTIVE 1

The student identifies the methods used to treat end-stage renal disease and discusses the advantages and disadvantages of each, including possible complications.

A. Diet and fluid management are the initial steps in therapy.

B. In-center hemodialysis is the most common mode of therapy for end-stage renal disease. Access to the circulation is obtained either through an atriovenous fistula that involves a cephalic vein and a radial artery or through placement of a graft in the forearm with synthetic material, the brachial or radial artery, and an upper vein.

C. Home hemodialysis is less expensive than in-center hemodialysis, but it requires a sophisticated family environment.

D. Acute peritoneal dialysis is provided by the placement of an acute peritoneal catheter. Chronic ambulatory peritoneal dialysis may also be used. Access to the peritoneal lining is obtained through a catheter placed in a subcutaneous tunnel in the abdominal wall, into the peritoneal cavity.

E. Cadaver transplantation is an option, as is renal transplantation from a living related donor. A living related transplant from a full-matched sibling is preferable. In patients with diabetes, this option is considered before dialysis is initiated. The complications of hemodialysis include anemia; secondary hyperparathyroidism; accelerated vascular disease; a sense of ill-being; dietary, travel, weight, and fluid restrictions; and infection of the access site. The atherosclerotic complications are accelerated in patients who have diabetes. Transplantation offers some respite from these complications and seems to curtail the progress of diabetic neuropathy and eye problems.

F. Combined pancreas–kidney transplantation may offer attenuation of neuropathic and ophthalmologic complications, in addition to freedom from insulin.

OBJECTIVE 2

The patient decides to undergo a renal transplant. She has three brothers and a sister. There is no family history of diabetes. The student discusses the criteria for living related organ donation. They are:

A. ABO typing compatibility

B. Human leukocyte antigen (HLA) compatibility. A simple Mendelian autosomal heredity is associated with the HLA system: 25% of siblings are full, or two-haplotype, matches; 50% are single-haplotype matches; and 25% are no match.

C. The donor has no history of malignancy or infections.

D. The donor is willing to donate.

The patient has a brother who is a two-haplotype match and is mixed lymphocyte culture unreactive. Renal transplantation is performed. What immunosuppressive regimens are available, and which should be tried?

Minimum Level of Achievement for Passing

A. The student knows that good renal function (indicated by normal creatinine clearance) and normal renal anatomy in the donor are necessary for donation.

B. The student knows that cyclosporine, steroids, and azathioprine are one mode of therapy. The student describes the potential complications of this therapy.

C. The student describes the complications associated with cyclosporine (i.e., hypertension, infection, nephrotoxicity, hepatotoxicity, hirsutism, lymphoma); azathioprine (i.e., bone marrow suppression); and steroids (i.e., dyspepsia, cataracts, osteonecrosis, Cushing's syndrome, acne, capillary fragility, glucose intolerance). The student also knows the availability of tacrolimus, mycophenolate mofetil, and biologic agents (antithymocyte globulin, antilymphocyte globulin, OKT3).

D. The student knows the immediate complications of transplantation (e.g., urinary fistula, graft thrombosis, hemorrhage, perigraft infection). The student also describes some of the late complications of transplantation.

E. The student describes the events associated with hyperacute, accelerated, acute, and chronic rejection and the treatment of each. Hyperacute rejection is antibody-mediated rejection that occurs within hours after transplant. It is associated with intravascular thrombosis and is usually untreatable. Accelerated rejection is both antibody-mediated and cellularly mediated and is associated with previous sensitization to antigen and the development of antibodies against the kidney. It is associated with endothelial injury and perivascular infiltrates and is usually untreatable. Acute rejection is the most common type. It occurs in as many as 90% of cadaveric transplant recipients. It is both humorally and cellularly mediated, is associated with perivascular infiltrates of round cells, and is treated with high-dose steroids, antilymphocyte globulin, or anti–T-cell antibodies. This treatment has a success rate of 70% to 80%. Chronic rejection is antibody-mediated and occurs over a long period. It is usually untreatable and is associated with interstitial fibrosis, perivascular fibrosis, and endothelial thickening.

F. The student states the 1-year graft survival rates for cadaveric (70%–80%), one-haplotype (90%), and two-haplotype living related renal transplants (95%).

Honors Level of Achievement

A. The student describes the different HLA loci and their apparent effect on graft survival.

B. The student knows that cyclosporine acts on T-cells. It inhibits the production of interleukin-2 receptors and the generation of cytotoxic T-lymphocytes. The student accurately describes the pathologic events associated with rejection. The student knows the graft survival rates for hepatic, pancreatic, cardiac, lung, and bowel transplantation.

CASE 3

A 40-year-old man had four previous myocardial infarctions. He was admitted three times in the last 6 months for congestive heart failure and is now receiving maximum medical therapy. His current ejection fraction is 10%.

OBJECTIVE 1

The student gives the indicators for cardiac transplantation:

A. Age (not a contraindication)

B. Expectation of imminent death from cardiac disease

C. Cardiomyopathy, end-stage ischemic disease, or valvular cardiac disease

D. Absence of pulmonary vascular disease manifested by high pulmonary vascular resistance (indication for heart–lung or lung transplantation); absence of infection, pulmonary infarction, and malignancy

E. Potential for rehabilitation

OBJECTIVE 2

A. State the 1-year survival rate for cardiac transplantation (80%).

B. Describe the method used to diagnose rejection in cardiac transplants (endomyocardial biopsy).

C. Describe the complications of cardiac transplantation.
   1. Rejection
   2. Infection
   3. Renal failure
   4. Cerebrovascular accident
   5. Effects of immunosuppression, including cyclosporine toxicity and steroid toxicity
   6. Accelerated atherosclerosis, which may be related to chronic rejection

Minimum Level of Achievement for Passing

The student recognizes that the patient is a candidate for cardiac transplantation and lists the criteria for transplant candidates. The student knows the results of cardiac transplantation.

Honors Level of Achievement

The student knows the complications of cardiac transplantation and knows how to diagnose and treat rejection.

SUGGESTED READINGS

Bonnefoy-Berard N, Revillard J-P. Mechanisms of immunosuppression induced by antithymocyte globulins and OKT3. *J Heart Lung Transplant* 1996;15:435–442.

Gordon RD, Todo S, Tzakis AG, et al. Liver transplantation under cyclosporine: a decade of experience. *Transplant Proc* 1995; 23:1393–1396.

Halloran PF. Aspects of allograft rejection: Part IV. Evaluation of new pharmacologic agents for prevention of allograft rejection. *Transplant Rev* 1995;9:138–146.

Henry ML, Ferguson RM, eds. Vascular access for hemodialysis: Part IV. Chicago, IL: WL Gore & Associates and Precept Press, 1995.

Hosenpud JD, Novick RJ, Breen TJ, Keck B, Daily P. The registry of the international society for heart and lung transplantation: Twelfth official report. 1995. *J Heart Lung Transplant* 1995;14:805–815.

Mihalov ML, Gattuso P, Abraham K, Holmes EW, Reddy V. Incidence of post-transplant malignancy among 674 solid-organ-transplant recipients at a single center. *Clin Transplant* 1996;10:248–255.

Smith CM, Ellison MD, Daily OP, White R, eds. 1995 Annual Report of the U.S. Scientific Registry of Transplant Recipients and the Organ Procurement and Transplantation Network. Rockville, Md: Health Resources and Services Administration, 1995.

Sutherland DER, Gruessner RWG, Gores PF. Pancreas and islet transplantation: an update. *Transplant Rev* 1994;8:185–206.

Williams KA, Coster DJ. Clinical and experimental aspects of corneal transplantation. *Transplant Rev* 1993;7:44–64.

Wood RFM, Pockley AG. Small bowel transplantation. *Transplant Rev* 1994;8:64–72.

24 Surgical Oncology

Malignant Diseases of the Skin

Nicholas P. Lang, M.D.
Pablo R. Duran, M.D.

Malignant Diseases of the Lymphatics and Soft Tissue

Kirby I. Bland, M.D.
Stephen M. Gemmett, M.D.

OBJECTIVES

Malignant Diseases of the Skin

1. Describe the etiology and incidence of basal and squamous cell carcinomas.
2. Discuss the clinical characteristics, treatment methods, and prognosis for basal and squamous cell carcinomas.
3. List the predisposing factors for and the four categories of melanoma.
4. List four signs and symptoms of a malignant nevus.
5. Outline the steps to confirm a diagnosis and determine the extent of malignant melanoma.
6. On the basis of the extent of a malignant nevus, describe the malignant potential and prognosis.
7. Outline the local, regional, and systemic therapies for malignant melanoma.

Malignant Diseases of the Lymphatics and Soft Tissue

1. List the signs and symptoms of Hodgkin's disease and non-Hodgkin's lymphoma.
2. Describe the workup for a patient with biopsy-proven lymphoma.
3. Describe the role of the surgeon in the staging of Hodgkin's disease and non-Hodgkin's lymphoma.
4. List the clinical features of a sarcoma in the trunk or abdomen and in the extremity.

5. Describe the considerations in the evaluation of sarcoma, including the techniques, biopsy, and studies to localize and adequately stage the disease.
6. Discuss the treatment of sarcomas, including surgery, radiation therapy, and chemotherapy.

Malignant Diseases of the Skin

Nearly every individual has 9 to 15 freckles, moles, or other aberrations of the skin. Although the most common malignant tumor in the United States is skin cancer, it is impractical to remove every lesion from every individual. Fortunately, the vast majority of lesions are benign, and many lesions are of only cosmetic importance. Many patients, however, raise questions about the malignant potential of skin lesions and whether removal is necessary. For this reason, every physician should be aware of the characteristics of malignant skin lesions so that appropriate therapy can be instituted in a timely fashion. Table 24-1 lists the general characteristics of malignant lesions. They should be committed to memory.

Basal Cell and Squamous Cell Carcinoma

Incidence and Etiology

In the United States, the increase in the number of participants in outdoor fitness activities and the preoccupation with maintaining an attractive appearance with a suntan are accompanied by a rise in the number of cases of skin cancer. Unfortunately, just as the link between cigarette smoking and carcinoma of the lung is firmly established, there is clear evidence that one etiology of skin cancer is chronic exposure to sunlight.

Approximately one-third of all new cancers in humans are skin cancers. The vast majority of these are either **squamous cell carcinoma** (SCC) or **basal cell carcinoma** (BCC). Approximately 800,000 new cases of nonmelanoma skin cancers are diagnosed annually,

Table 24-1. Characteristics of Malignant Skin Lesions

Change in pigmentation (darker or lighter)

Rapid growth

Bleeding

Crusting

Serous exudate

Loss of skin appendages, hair follicles, etc.

Satellite nodules

Regional lymphadenopathy

Raised borders

Central ulceration

Pain, itching, or other discomfort

Inflammatory areolae

Rubbery texture

compared with 38,300 cases of **melanoma.** These figures show an increase of 15% to 20% over the incidence reported only a decade earlier by the National Cancer Institute. Of the two most common lesions, BCC occurs in 80% of cases and SCC in 20%. Fortunately, the cure rate for the these nonmelanoma neoplasms is as high as 97% with current therapeutic modalities. However, approximately 2130 people die annually from nonmelanoma skin cancers. The skin is the most easily accessible portion of the body for diagnostic observation, and early diagnosis of skin malignancies facilitates treatment and cure. For these reasons, the physician must recognize these tumors and their potentially premalignant precursors early and institute prompt therapy. Although skin cancers may remain curable as they increase in size, the cosmetic and functional deformity that results from the excision of a large tumor makes reconstruction of the defect a formidable challenge (Figures 24-1 to 24-5). Further, although BCCs rarely metastasize, large SCCs clearly have metastatic potential.

Tumor incidence increases with age. Most patients are older than 65 years of age at the time of diagnosis. There is a 3:1 predominance of these tumors in men, possibly because of employment patterns that require greater sun exposure.

A variety of etiologic factors are implicated in the development of BCC and SCC. The most common factor is solar radiation, especially ultraviolet B light in the spectrum of 290 to 320 nm. For this reason, physicians who practice in sunny climates tend to see more patients with BCC and SCC. The cumulative effect of solar radiation causes irreversible epidermal damage. These tumors are often seen in association with other skin changes caused by solar radiation, including wrinkling, telangiectasis (dilated blood vessels), actinic keratosis (erythematous, gritty-surfaced lesions), and solar elastosis (yellow papules). Given this relation to sun exposure, it is not surprising that approximately 80% to 90% of tumors are found in the head and neck area and on the back of the hands.

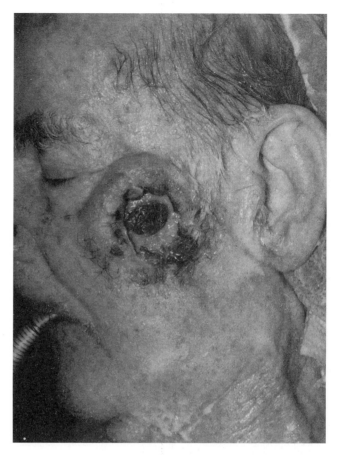

Figure 24-1 Large, neglected squamous cell carcinoma of the left cheek of a man who is approximately 79 years old. The tumor extends nearly to the periosteum of the zygomatic bone.

Chemical carcinogens are also implicated in the development of skin cancer. Examples include arsenic, paraffin oil, creosote, pitch, fuel oil, coal, and psoralens, plus ultraviolet A photochemotherapy. Cigarette smoking is also associated with SCC of the lip, mouth, and nonmucosal skin. Human papilloma virus is strongly associated with SCC. Human papilloma virus is seen in both SCC of the genital area and **Bowen's disease.**

Genetic and ethnic factors, as reflected in skin complexion, play an important predisposing role in the development of SCC and BCC. Fair-skinned Caucasians with light hair and eye color are at greater risk than those with darker pigmentation. Because these tumors are unusual in black patients, melanin may afford protection against the damage caused by solar radiation. Another example of genetic influence is **xeroderma pigmentosum,** which is a rare, genetically transmitted disease that is characterized by faulty DNA repair of ultraviolet damage. Patients who have this abnormality eventually have numerous cutaneous neoplasms (Figure 24-6). Albinism, epidermodysplasia verruciformis, and basal cell nevus syndrome are other genetically determined skin diseases that are associated directly with an increased risk of cutaneous SCC.

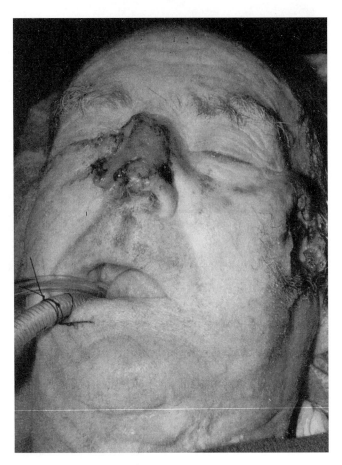

Figure 24-2 Synchronous squamous cell carcinoma of the nose in the patient shown in Figure 24-1. The tumor is eroding through the entire nasal skin and portions of the cartilage.

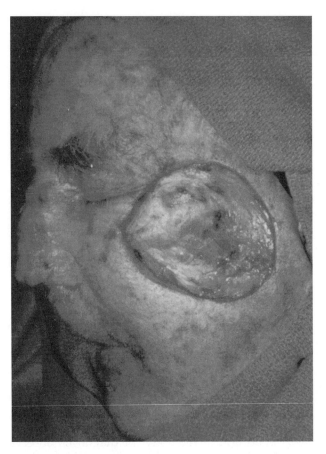

Figure 24-3 After the tumor is excised, portions of the zygoma are seen near the lateral aspect of the eye.

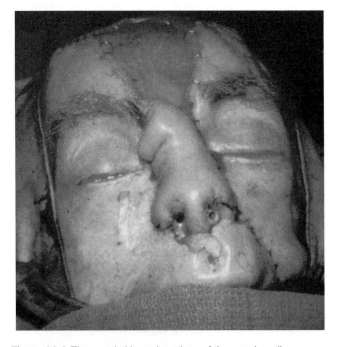

Figure 24-4 The nasal skin and portions of the nasal cartilage were removed. The nose was reconstructed with a forehead flap and a left nasolabial flap. The resulting forehead defect was covered with a split-thickness skin graft. The cheek defect was also repaired with a skin graft.

Certain chemicals (e.g., arsenicals) are associated with skin cancers. The first finding of a specific cause for cancer is credited to Pott in 1775. Pott showed the relation between soot and carcinoma of the scrotum in chimney sweeps. SCC, or epidermoid carcinoma, also arises in chronic burn scars. Marjolin (1828) described the process of malignant ulceration in burn scars **(Marjolin's ulcers).** Carcinomas that develop in burn scars are aggressive and can be rapidly lethal. Epidermoid carcinoma also develops within chronically draining skin sinuses and fistulae (e.g., at the site of a chronic osteomyelitis infection). These tumors also tend to be highly malignant.

The frequency of skin cancer is increased in patients who are immunosuppressed for organ transplantation. Because the kidney is the most commonly transplanted organ, kidney transplant patients make up the majority of the at-risk group. However, patients who undergo heart transplantation have a higher incidence of premalignant and malignant nonmelanoma skin cancers. In general, patients who undergo heart transplantation are older, receive more immunosuppressive treatment, and have the shortest interval from transplantation to the development of the first lesion. Skin cancers in trans-

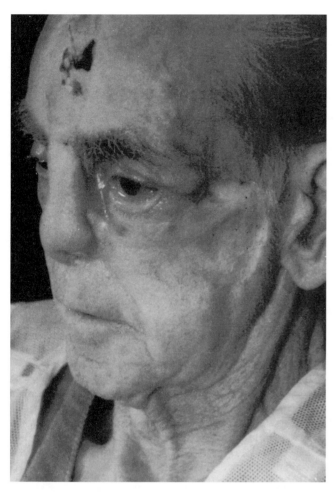

Figure 24-5 The patient's appearance approximately 1 month after completion of the reconstruction.

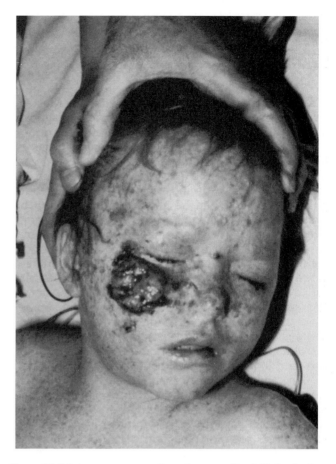

Figure 24-6 Large squamous cell carcinoma on the right cheek of a 4-year-old child with xeroderma pigmentosum.

plant patients are more virulent. The local growth rate and the metastatic rate are both increased.

Although less common today, radiation is another physical agent that is responsible for the development of malignant skin tumors, usually SCC. This phenomenon is particularly true for dentists and physicians who use x-ray equipment without appropriate protection and in patients who received radiation treatment for benign skin conditions (e.g., acne).

Basal Cell Carcinoma

Clinical and Histopathologic Characteristics

BCC arises from the basal layer of germinating cells of the skin epithelium or from epithelial appendages (e.g., hair follicles, sebaceous glands). Usually, these lesions grow slowly and are nonaggressive. However, if the tumor is left untreated, it destroys normal tissue, including cartilage, in its growth path. These tumors also spread microscopically a significant distance beyond the visible lesion. Although a number of descriptive forms were proposed based on appearance, only three major varieties are discussed here.

Nodular BCC typically begins as a smooth, dome-shaped, round, waxy, or pearly papule (Figure 24-7). The lesion may take as long as 1 year to double in size. It may have telangiectases on the surface that bleed readily when traumatized. As the tumor enlarges, the center tends to undergo necrosis, forming a central ulcer with invasion into deep structures (rodent ulcer) [Figure 24-8]. The rodent ulcer is more difficult to eradicate, and if it is not adequately treated, it may erode into the deep structures, including the skull, orbit, or brain.

Pigmented BCC is similar to the nodular form, except that it contains melanocytes that impart a dark brown or blue-black color. Understandably, it may be confused with melanoma.

Morphea-like or **fibrosing BCC** is an indurated, yellow plaque with ill-defined borders. The overlying skin remains intact for a long time. The skin looks shiny and taut because the tumor causes an intense fibroblastic response that gives it a scar-like appearance (Figure 24-9). This variety is less common than the nodular form and is more often initially overlooked. The margins of this form of BCC are very difficult to identify because the tumor cells invade normal tissue well beyond the visible margins.

Histologically, BCC consists of masses of darkly stained cells that extend downward from the basal layer

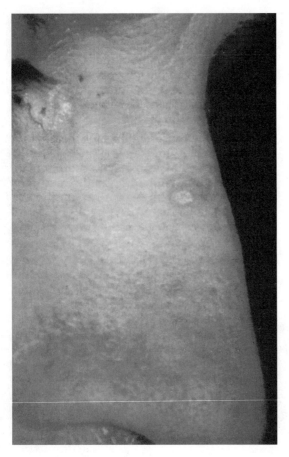

Figure 24-7 Small, early basal cell carcinoma on the lateral bridge of the nose of a woman who is approximately 50 years old. The lesion was elliptically excised, with clear margins.

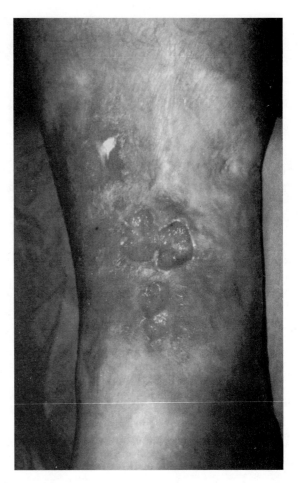

Figure 24-8 Recurrent basal cell carcinoma on the leg of a 63-year-old man. These ulcers form as the lesion penetrates more deeply, outstrips its blood supply, and undergoes central necrosis.

of epithelium and into the dermis and subcutaneous tissue. The peripheral nuclei have a palisading configuration. The tumor rarely shows rapid early growth. It causes no pain or discomfort, and the patient may defer seeking medical attention until the lesion is well advanced. Alternatively, the patient may first seek care because of troublesome bleeding from the tumor when it is traumatized (e.g., shaving).

Treatment

Effective therapy for both BCC and SCC centers on two major principles: histologic confirmation of the diagnosis and complete removal or destruction of the tumor. For small lesions (≤ 0.5 cm), after histologic confirmation is obtained by needle biopsy, many dermatologists recommend cryotherapy (freezing the tumor) or electrodesiccation and curettage (using a sharp spoon-like instrument with electrocautery to remove the bulk of the tumor). Both of these treatments take several weeks to heal. Radiation therapy and radium implants are no longer used. The disadvantage of the current treatment modalities is that complete tumor excision is not guaranteed because tissue surrounding the tumor is destroyed and is not examined microscopically for tumor cells. Most surgeons recommend excision for the management of BCC. To ensure complete tumor

removal, a 1-cm margin of normal tissue is included in the resected specimen. A minimum margin of 0.5 cm is included for a lesion that is located near a critical anatomic feature (e.g., eyelid). With a morphea-like, or fibrosing, tumor, a 1.5-cm margin is preferable. At the time of removal, the specimen is carefully labeled to show its orientation (e.g., superior margin, anterior). A diagram of the position of the specimen in relation to the surrounding structures is also useful. Frozen sections are carefully examined. If the margins are clear of tumor, the surgical wound is closed primarily, skin is grafted, or a flap is turned to provide coverage. If there is uncertainty about the margin of the specimen, additional tissue is sent for frozen-section examination. If the wound is large, it is covered with a sterile dressing until the results are obtained, at which point a graft or flap is applied. Closure is postponed to prevent the harvest of an insufficient graft or flap if additional resection is necessary.

Patients with many small BCCs are treated with topical therapy (e.g., 5-fluorouracil).

Prognosis

With adequate surgical excision, approximately 95% of patients are cured. Recurrence at the site of tumor

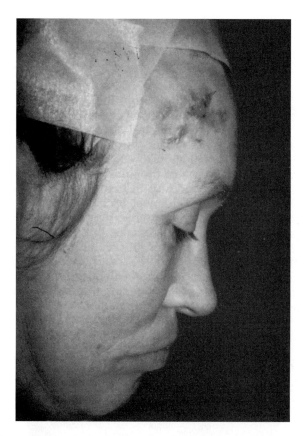

Figure 24-9 Large morphea-type basal cell carcinoma of the forehead. The fibrous tissue reaction causes a scar-like appearance.

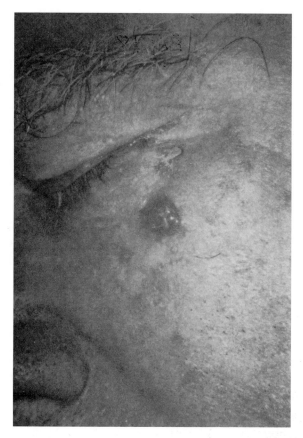

Figure 24-10 Ulcer-like appearance of a small squamous cell carcinoma of the cheek of a 56-year-old man.

removal is usually caused by tumor cells left at the margins. However, 20% of patients who have a single BCC have a second lesion within 1 year. Of patients who have multiple tumors, 40% have an additional BCC within 1 year. Some patients experience a field change within the skin that increases their susceptibility to the further development of BCC tumors. Therefore, long-term skin surveillance at 6-month to 1-year intervals is imperative after tumor resection in all patients with BCC.

Squamous Cell Carcinoma

Clinical and Histopathologic Characteristics

SCC differs from BCC in a number of ways, the most important of which is the potential of SCC for metastatic spread. Usually, the lesions reach considerable size before metastases occur, but this potential emphasizes the need for careful examination of the lymphatic drainage of the area at the time of initial physical examination. Approximately 75% of SCC tumors occur in the head and neck. The lower lip is the most common site. The tumor may arise de novo or from an area with pre-existing skin damage, burn scars, chronic ulcers, osteomyelitic sinuses, or chronic granulomas. SCC is also seen in scars from chronic discoid lupus erythematosus. For any chronic nonhealing ulcer of the leg that is increasing in size and is not responding as expected to appropriate therapy, biopsy should be per-

formed in four quadrants to rule out SCC. Bowen's disease, a skin condition that is characterized by chronic scaling and occasionally by a crusted, purple, or erythematous raised lesion, is considered carcinoma in situ that has not yet broken through the epidermal–dermal junction. Over time, this lesion may become frankly invasive SCC.

It is not clear how often metastatic spread occurs from SCC, although, considering all SCC tumors, the rate of metastasis is probably low (approximately 1%–2%). However, tumors that arise as a result of thermal injury, draining osteomyelitic sinuses, chronic ulcers, and Bowen's disease tend to metastasize more often than tumors that arise in sun-damaged skin. Tumors that arise either de novo or in sun-damaged skin and penetrate 8 mm or more from the surface are more likely to metastasize.

Clinically, the tumor arises as an erythematous firm papule on normal or sun-damaged skin. It grows relatively slowly and is, at first, difficult to distinguish from a hyperkeratotic lesion. As the tumor enlarges, it forms a nodule, with central ulceration surrounded by firm induration. Beneath the area of ulceration is a white or yellow necrotic base. When this base is removed, a crater-like defect remains (Figure 24-10). It does not have the pearly, raised margins of BCC tumors (see Figure 24-7). SCC tumors often have crusts or scabs as a result of repetitive trauma, bleeding, or leakage of the serous exudate (Figure 24-11). As with BCC lesions, SCC lesions may enlarge and erode through adjacent tissue, causing considerable destruction (Figure 24-12).

Microscopically, the tumors are irregular nests of epidermal cells that infiltrate the dermis to varying depths and show varying degrees of differentiation. The more differentiated the tumor, the greater the number of epithelial pearls (keratinous material) seen in the depths of the tumor.

Treatment

The considerations for the treatment of SCC lesions are essentially the same as those for BCC lesions. The standard margin of resection is 1 cm, and the same criteria apply for skin grafting and flap coverage. A major difference is the occasional need for lymph node dissection, with excision of the primary lesion.

Prognosis

As with BCC, the prognosis for small lesions is excellent, with a cure rate of 95%. In larger lesions that penetrate the subcutaneous tissue, the risk of nodal metastasis increases substantially. After lymph node involvement occurs, the prognosis is poor. Two-thirds of patients with SCC may die after the disease penetrates into subcutaneous tissues. Nearly all patients with lymph node involvement eventually die of their disease. Follow-up in patients with excised SCC lesions should be as rigorous as in patients with BCC. The patient is examined every 6 months for local recurrence, evidence of regional nodal metastasis, or new lesions.

Melanoma

Incidence and Etiology

In 1995, melanoma accounted for approximately 3% of cases of cancer in the United States (approximately 34,000 cases) and approximately the same proportion of cancer deaths. It represents only 5% of cutaneous neoplastic growth, but its malignant potential is more aptly represented by the fact that melanoma causes 74% of deaths from skin cancer. The incidence among blacks is 0.8 per 100,000 population. Among whites, the incidence is 4.5 per 100,000 population. The age-adjusted incidence is 4.2 per 100,000 population. The age varia-

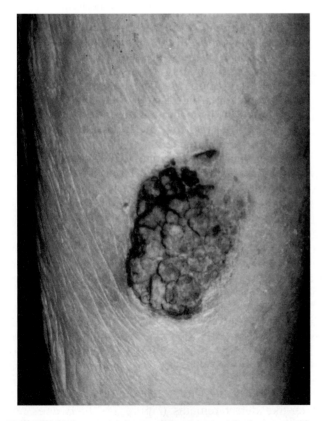

Figure 24-11 Large squamous cell carcinoma of the leg covered by a crust of congealed serous fluid and blood. When the crust is removed, the underlying lesion bleeds considerably.

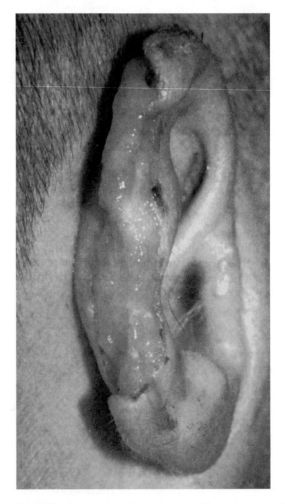

Figure 24-12 Posterior aspect of an ear eroded by squamous cell carcinoma that extends into the ear cartilage. This patient came to the emergency room after his ear was bitten by a dog. Careful examination of the lesion raised the index of suspicion for a skin malignancy. A frozen-section biopsy confirmed the lesion as squamous cell carcinoma.

tion progresses from 0.4 cases per 100,000 people who are 10 to 19 years old to 16 cases per 100,000 people who are older than 80 years old. In addition, statistics collected on the incidence of this disease show an apparent doubling of occurrence approximately every 15 years. This increase does not appear to be the result of more complete reporting or an alteration in the pathologic criteria for diagnostic inclusion because the increase in incidence is accompanied by a parallel rise in mortality rates.

Several studies in Australia, New Zealand, and the United States show an increased incidence of melanoma near the equator. Melanomas occur with increased incidence on the lower legs in women and on the trunk in men. These data suggest that exposure to sunlight has a role in the etiology of melanoma, but they do not explain the occurrence of melanoma in areas of the body that have minimal exposure to sunlight.

The incidence of melanoma is higher in people with a light complexion and blue eyes. In Australia and New Zealand, the incidence of melanoma in the Celtic population is the highest in the world (14 per 100,000 in men; 17 per 100,000 in women). In the United States, the incidence is 4 to 5 per 100,000.

Approximately one-fourth of cutaneous melanomas occur in the head and neck area. Of these, 88% occur outside the protected area (hair-bearing scalp). This area is one-half covered with hair and constitutes only 9% of the total body surface area. Even so, this anatomic site has the highest incidence of melanoma. This situation suggests, but does not prove, a solar etiology for melanoma in this area. The site distribution of malignant melanoma in blacks is strikingly different from that in whites. In Uganda, approximately 70% of melanomas are found on the plantar surface compared with 6% in whites. Likewise, 8% of melanomas in Uganda occur in the nasopharynx, an extremely rare site in the white population. All of these factors seem to influence the development of melanoma, but no single explanation is satisfactory for all locations and frequencies of melanoma.

The etiology of melanoma is not known. However, 50% to 60% of melanomas arise from or near benign nevi. The triggering event for malignant transformation is not known. Benign nevi are extremely common, and very few become malignant. The one exception is **congenital giant hairy nevus** (bathing trunk nevus), which undergoes malignant transformation to melanoma in 10% to 30% of untreated lesions.

Familial malignant melanomas account for 8% to 12% of all melanomas. As many as 44% of patients who have multiple primary melanomas have a family history of this tumor. Familial melanomas tend to occur at a younger age than sporadic tumors. Of patients who have a melanoma, 3% to 5% have a second primary melanoma. In these patients, the risk is calculated at 900 times that of the population at large.

A third recognized risk factor for hereditary melanoma is **familial atypical mole and melanoma syndrome (FAM-M),** previously called dysplastic nevus syndrome. Hereditary melanoma and FAM-M represent an autosomal dominant gene with high penetrance. These lesions are associated with genetic alterations in chromosomes 1p, 6q, 7, and 9 and are implicated in the pathogenesis of familial melanoma. A tumor suppresser gene in chromosome 9p21 is probably involved in familial melanoma as well as sporadic melanoma. Several kindreds with familial melanoma have large premalignant nevi, predominantly in the horse-collar distribution over the upper trunk. Genetic predisposition to malignant melanoma is also associated with the hereditary syndrome xeroderma pigmentosum.

Embryology of Melanocytes

Melanocytes are derived from neural crest tissue. During early gestation, the cells migrate to the skin, uveal tract, meninges, and ectodermal mucosa. Melanocytes reside in the skin (in the basement layer of the epidermis) and elaborate melanin pigment under a variety of stimuli.

The number of melanocytes per unit area of skin surface does not correlate with the propensity for melanoma to develop. The density of melanocytes in Caucasians and African-Americans is approximately the same for any skin site. Differences in skin pigmentation are determined by the melanosome–pigment package that is passed out of the melanocyte, by way of its dendritic processes, and phagocytized by surrounding keratinocytes. These cells then migrate up to the epidermis, where they cause the phenotypic patterns and degrees of skin coloration observed in people.

Clinical and Histopathologic Characteristics

As many as 11 types of melanoma are described, excluding ocular lesions. For this discussion, melanoma is classified as **lentigo maligna melanoma, superficial spreading melanoma, nodular melanoma,** and **acral lentiginous melanoma.** Melanoma has two distinct growth patterns. The horizontal, or lateral, growth phase indicates increasing lesion size, but little risk of distant spread. The deep, or vertical, growth phase is much more dangerous because it indicates invasion and potential metastatic spread.

Lentigo maligna melanoma occurs in a Hutchinson's freckle. This type of melanoma is characterized by a long period of development and by its tendency to occur on the face, head, and neck of older people. The median age at diagnosis is approximately 70 years. This type of melanoma constitutes 10% to 15% of cutaneous melanomas and is the most benign cutaneous melanoma (Figures 24-13 and 24-14). It commonly occurs in areas that are heavily exposed to the sun. Women are affected more often than men. The lesions are large, flat, and tan or brown. As the vertical growth phase begins to develop, the lesions become focally elevated. The basic tan-brown pattern of the radial growth phase persists during this period. The elevation is either lighter or darker than the surrounding radial growth phase. The rarity of rose and pink colors in the radial growth phase distinguishes lentigo maligna melanoma from superficial spreading melanoma.

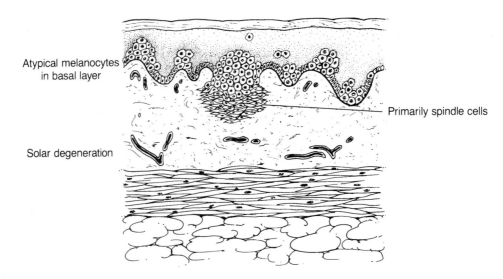

Atypical melanocytes
in basal layer

Primarily spindle cells

Solar degeneration

Figure 24-13 Lentigo maligna melanoma develops when invasion occurs in a lentigo maligna.

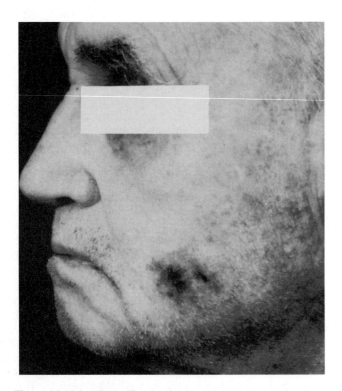

Figure 24-14 Lentigo maligna melanoma.

Superficial spreading melanoma accounts for approximately 70% of all cutaneous melanomas. It is intermediate in malignancy and affects the sexes equally. The legs are most commonly affected in women, and the back is most commonly affected in men. The peak incidence of superficial spreading melanoma occurs in the fifth decade (Figures 24-15 and 24-16). This tumor has both radial and vertical growth phases. The radial growth phase is characterized by melanoma cells within the epidermis and papillary dermis and by a host response of inflammatory cells,

fibroblasts, and the formation of new blood vessels. The radial growth phase of superficial spreading melanoma is more obviously elevated than the radial growth phase of lentigo maligna melanoma. The vertical growth phase of superficial spreading melanoma seems to develop more rapidly than that in lentigo maligna melanoma and is heralded by the appearance of a palpable nodule. The vertical growth phase seems to be the source of metastatic disease and, depending on the depth of invasion, produces metastases in as many as 85% of cases. Early superficial spreading melanoma lesions are a haphazard combination of colors (usually tan, brown, blue, and black). Most lesions also have areas of rose and pink. The common characteristics of variation in color, marginal notching, and loss of skin creases distinguish this lesion from the more common intradermal junctional nevus. More advanced lesions have palpable nodularity, which indicates the development of a vertical growth phase. They also may be surrounded by satellite nodules. Many of these tumors have white sections that represent areas of spontaneous regression.

Nodular melanoma is the most malignant type, involving almost exclusively a vertical growth phase. It accounts for approximately 12% of all cutaneous melanomas. Nodular melanoma occurs twice as often in men as in women (Figures 24-17 and 24-18). The host cellular response is usually less than that seen with other types of melanoma. Clinically, these lesions develop quickly and have a palpable nodular component in their earliest stages. Nodular melanoma is blue-black. The variability in coloration and margins that is seen with superficial spreading melanoma is rare in the nodular type.

Acral lentiginous melanoma occurs on the palms and soles and in subungual sites. This melanoma has some of the growth characteristics of both superficial spreading and nodular melanoma. The exact prognostic significance of these different characteristics has not been

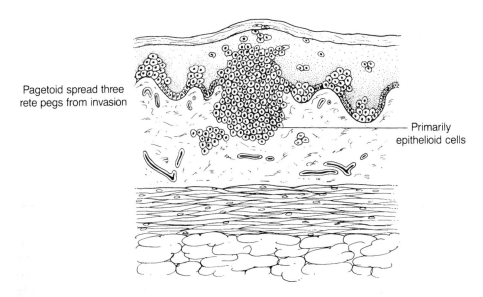

Pagetoid spread three rete pegs from invasion

Primarily epithelioid cells

Figure 24-15 Superficial spreading melanoma is characterized by radial growth (pagetoid spread) and vertical growth (invasion).

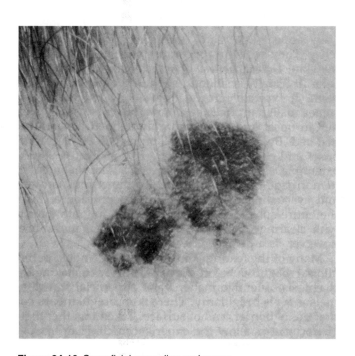

Figure 24-16 Superficial spreading melanoma.

determined in a large series. Acral lentiginous melanoma (Figure 24-19), however, seems to have a worse prognosis than superficial spreading melanoma, but it is not as severe as nodular melanoma. This melanoma has both a radial and a vertical growth phase. In the subungual location, the radial growth phase may simply be a streak in the nail associated with irregular tan-brown staining of the nail bed.

In addition to the types listed earlier, melanoma may arise in a giant hairy nevus; in the oral, vaginal, and anal mucous membranes; in a blue nevus; or in a visceral organ. Melanoma occasionally occurs as a metastatic lesion without a demonstrable primary site.

Diagnosis

Lesions that are occasionally confused with cutaneous melanoma are **junctional nevi, compound nevi, intradermal nevi, blue nevi,** BCCs, **seborrheic keratoses, dermatofibromas,** and subungual hemorrhage. These types can often be differentiated clinically by an expert. However, if there is any question about the type, histologic examination provides the necessary confirmatory evidence. Junctional nevi usually appear during the early years of life and are particularly apparent during adolescence. They vary in size from a few millimeters to several centimeters. They are light to dark brown, with a flat, smooth surface and irregular edges. Compound nevi are usually brown or black, with a raised nodular surface that often contains hair. They are usually smaller than 1 cm and occur in all age-groups. Intradermal nevi can be very large, although they are usually less than 1 cm in diameter. Their color varies from light to dark brown, and they may have a raised warty or smooth surface. The presence of coarse hairs distinguishes them from other nevi. Blue nevi are smooth blue-black lesions that are smaller than 1 cm, with well-defined, regular margins. They usually occur on the face, the dorsum of the feet and hands, and the buttocks. They are rarely associated with malignant melanoma. BCCs are most common in middle-aged people. A pigmented BCC tumor is usually blue-black, with raised edges and capillary neovascularity. Initially, the lesion is smooth, but it can become ulcerated. Seborrheic keratoses are occasionally black. They are usually 1 cm or larger and typically appear as raised and warty, with a greasy consistency. They appear to be stuck onto the skin. Dermatofibromas are occasionally dark brown. They are usually smooth, slightly raised, and without hairs. They typically grow very slowly and never become malignant. Subungual hemorrhage is usually sudden in onset and is sharply defined beneath the nail bed. By comparison, melanoma has a gradual

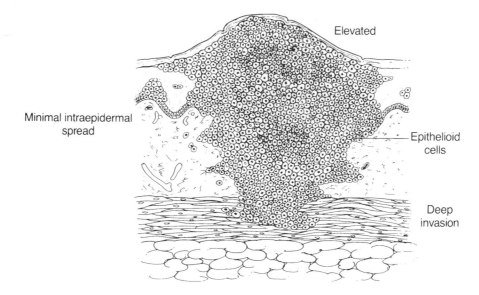

Figure 24-17 Nodular melanoma usually appears as uniform malignant cells with deep invasion and little intraepithelial growth.

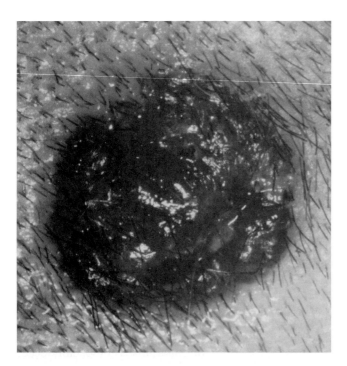

Figure 24-18 Nodular melanoma.

onset and has poorly demarcated streaks that extend along the axis of the nail. The diagnosis of hemorrhage is confirmed by puncturing the nail and evacuating the blood. In time, the entire subungual hemorrhage migrates distally, and the nail bed clears. Subungual melanoma, however, is a persistent lesion.

Many of the features of cutaneous melanoma permit clinical diagnosis before biopsy. The key to making the diagnoses of lentigo maligna and superficial spreading melanoma is irregularity (e.g., coloration, border, and surface). Taken together, these characteristics allow the experienced clinician to diagnose most melanomas.

Patients, however, have many other types of pigmented lesions that require diagnosis. Although it is possible to be quite certain about some pigmented lesions, many others require biopsy for histologic examination before therapy can be planned. Nodular melanoma does not have the border variability seen in lentigo maligna and superficial spreading melanoma. However, it does have the variability of color and does cause a raised nodule. Its coloration, thickness, and rapid growth permit easy clinical diagnosis.

Accurate microstaging is very important in the management of melanoma. The person who performs the biopsy must provide the pathologist with adequate and satisfactory material. The pathologist cannot be expected to reconstruct the lesion from multiple fragments of tissue with no information regarding orientation. The physician who performs the biopsy must maximize its value by direct communication with the pathologist and by properly planning the biopsy. If possible, a biopsy includes complete excision of the lesion, with a small margin of normal tissue, so that the pathologist can accurately stage the lesion. If this procedure is not feasible, the second choice is to perform an incisional biopsy. To help the pathologist stage the lesion correctly, the specimen must include the thickest portion of the lesion.

Staging

In the last 15 years, a better understanding of the growth and development of primary melanoma lesions has allowed surgeons to design treatment tailored to the characteristics of the primary lesion and to predict outcome on the basis of these characteristics. The two features of the tumor that seem most important in determining prognosis are the radial and vertical growth phases. Three of the four common varieties of melanoma (lentigo maligna, superficial spreading, and acral lentiginous melanoma) have an indolent radial growth phase that may last for several years. The radial

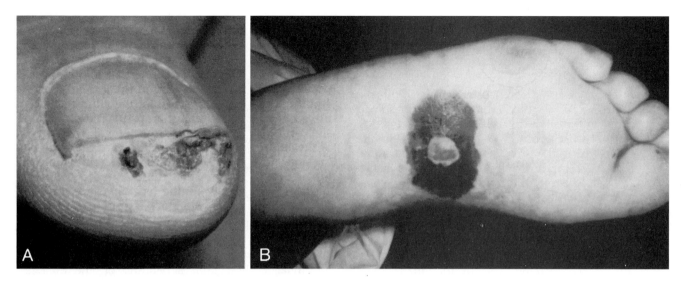

Figure 25-19 A and **B,** Acral lentiginous melanoma.

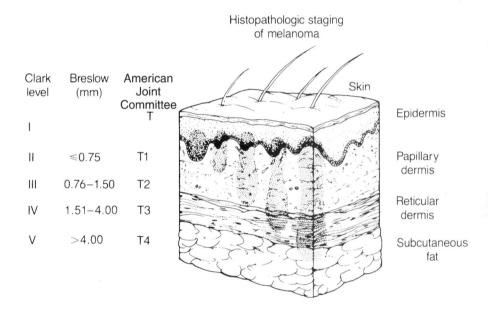

Figure 24-20 The American Joint Committee staging system uses both the Clark and the Breslow classifications.

growth phase is characterized by abnormal melanocytes that extend centrifugally in the epidermis, with minimal invasion of the papillary dermis. In superficial spreading melanoma, these large epithelioid cells occur in nests and as an intradermal component at least three rete pegs away from the area of invasion. These cells have relatively uniform nuclei, with an abundance of dusky cytoplasm. The vertical growth phase consists of malignant cells that invade the dermis for variable distances. Cells may vary in appearance from one cluster to another. Lymphocyte infiltration is fairly common around these invading cells.

Two systems are used for microstaging malignant melanomas. The **Clark system** for primary melanoma is based on the level of invasion of the tumor. Level I lesions are confined to the epidermis, level II lesions

invade the papillary layer of the dermis, level III lesions reach the junction of the papillary and reticular layers, level IV lesions invade the reticular dermis, and level V lesions invade the subcutaneous fat. Survival is related to the depth of invasion; it is best for level I lesions and worst for level V lesions. A disadvantage of this system is that different pathologists may interpret the levels of invasion variably (Figure 24-20).

The disadvantage of the Clark microstaging system is addressed by the **Breslow system,** which uses an ocular micrometer to measure the thickness of the tumor in millimeters at the deepest point of its vertical growth. The thicker the tumor, the worse the prognosis (see Figure 24-20). The Breslow system allows more objective evaluation and easier comparison among pathologists.

The TNM (tumor, node, metastasis) system combines information from the Clark and Breslow systems as well as information about the status of lymph nodes and distant metastases to provide a comprehensive staging (Table 24-2).

Malignant melanoma can spread through both the lymphatic route and the blood route. Lymphatic spread can occur as in-transit metastases or as enlarged nodes. In-transit metastases occur when melanoma cells are trapped between the primary tumor and regional lymph nodes and produce a region of cutaneous metastases more than 3 cm from the primary site. Mechanical blockage of afferent lymph drainage by either metastatic disease or lymph node dissection is believed to be the cause of these in-transit metastases. Regional lymph nodes may filter metastatic melanoma cells, but they do not stop all metastatic cells. After melanoma becomes metastatic, it has striking tropism for small bowel mucosa and distant cutaneous sites. The most common cause of gastrointestinal bleeding in a patient with melanoma is small bowel metastases. These metastases can also cause obstruction and intussusception. The lung, liver, and brain are other common metastatic sites.

Treatment

The two questions about local therapy concern the proper width of excision and the proper depth of excision. Current recommendations are 1-cm margins of resection for melanomas less than 1 mm thick and 2-cm radial margins of excision for intermediate-thickness melanomas (1–4 mm). The previous recommendation for 4-cm lateral margins in every direction is difficult to achieve in certain locations. Also, when compared with 2-cm margins in randomized prospective studies, 4-cm margins provide no statistical difference in the recurrence rate or 5-year survival rate. The need for skin graft for closure is also significantly reduced (46% with 4-cm lateral margins vs 11% with 2-cm lateral margins). In most cases, the excision extends through the subcutaneous tissue to the level of the underlying fascia. Excision of the fascia with the lesion does little to prevent the spread of melanoma.

There is general agreement that if regional lymph nodes are abnormal on physical examination (clinical stage III), regional node dissection is performed. There is also agreement that if these nodes are not palpable and the primary lesion is less than 0.76 mm thick (clinical stage I), regional node dissection is not indicated because the incidence of metastatic disease from these lesions is extremely low. The management of regional lymph nodes in other cases of stage I and II melanoma is controversial, however. Some authorities recommend elective lymph node dissection (ELND) only if regional nodes are palpable on follow-up. Others recommend prophylactic dissection, depending on the thickness and other characteristics of the primary lesion. A prospective multi-institutional randomized surgical trial was performed by the Intergroup Melanoma Surgical Program. In this study, ELND provided significant improvement in the 5-year survival rate for patients whose tumor was 1 to 2 mm thick, patients without tumor ulceration, and patients 60 years of age or younger who had melanomas that were 1 to 2 mm thick or who did not have ulceration. This finding is supported by the evidence of a 20% incidence in microscopic involvement of regional lymph nodes in patients with intermediate-thickness melanoma and a 30% improvement in the survival rate in patients who underwent ELND of microscopically involved nodes versus those who underwent therapeutic lymph node dissection for palpable nodes.

A recent development in intraoperative lymphatic mapping and sentinel node biopsy for early-stage melanoma was pioneered by Dr. Don Morton. It uses selective-technique visible blue dye (blue-V) or

Table 24-2. TNM Classification: AJCC-UICC Melanoma Staging System

Stage	Criteria		5-yr Survival
I	pT1	Primary melanoma < 0.75 mm thick and/or Clark's level II (N0, M0)	98%–100%
	pT2	Primary melanoma 0.76–1.50 mm thick and/or Clark's level III	90%–92%
II	pT3	Primary melanoma 1.51–4.00 mm thick and/or Clark's level IV	66%
III	pT4	Primary melanoma > 4 mm thick and/or Clark's level V and/or satellites within 2 cm of the primary tumor	41%
		pT4a—Tumor > 4 mm thick and/or invading the subcutaneous tissue	
		pT4b—Satellite(s) within 2 cm of the primary tumor	
		Regional lymph node and/or in-transit metastases; any pT, N1 (regional nodes < 3 cm), or N2 (tergional nodes > 3 cm) an/or in-transit metastasis	
		N2a—Metastasis > 3 cm in greatest dimension in any regional lymph node(s)	
		N2b—In-transit metastasis	
		N2c—Both N2a and N2b	
IV		Systemic metastases; any pT, any N, M1 (distant metastases)	32%
		M1a—Metastasis in skin or subcutaneous tissue or lymph node(s) beyond the regional lymph nodes	
		M1b—Visceral metastasis	

isosulfan blue dye injected intradermally at the site of the melanoma on either side of the biopsy scar. An incision is made over the regional lymph basin. The blue-stained sentinel node is identified and submitted for frozen-section examination and immunohistochemical studies. If the sentinel node is negative, there is a 99% chance that the remaining lymph nodes are not involved with metastatic melanoma, as shown by long-term follow-up. If the sentinel node is positive, then a complete node dissection is required because the probability of finding other positive lymph nodes is 37%.

Sentinel node biopsy can also be performed based on lymphoscintigraphy with intradermal injections of radiolabeled material (often ^{99m}Tc sulfur colloid). After injection, dynamic imaging (10 sec/frame), static imaging (> 30 minutes), and late imaging (1–2 hours) are used to identify the location of draining nodes. This technique is used to check the lymphatic bed intraoperatively with a handheld gamma counter probe. The best results occur when the vital blue dye and lymphoscintigraphy methods are combined.

The management of distant disease is determined primarily by its location and symptoms. Metastatic disease to the brain is usually treated with either radiation therapy alone or with a combination of surgical removal and whole-brain radiation. Pulmonary nodules, if few in number, may be resected, but this practice is not generally followed. These patients usually undergo chemotherapy. Distant spread to an extremity that involves in-transit metastases is managed by regional limb perfusion with a chemotherapeutic agent (e.g., L-phenylalanine mustard) and hyperthermia. This treatment is beneficial only if the disease is confined to that extremity. It often provides a satisfactory result (salvaging the extremity and prolonging the patient's life). Dacarbazine is the most active single agent for the treatment of metastatic melanoma. It is also used in combination with other agents. Regardless of the protocol, the response rate is low (20%), even when partial and complete responses are combined. No effective chemotherapy is available for either primary or metastatic melanoma. Most patients who have recurrent metastatic melanoma are treated according to a protocol so that data collection can continue and treatment be improved.

Radiation is rarely used as the single treatment for melanoma. However, it is used to treat metastatic disease (e.g., whole-brain radiation after brain metastasis). New fractionation methods, with higher single doses given less often, increased the response rate from 35% to 75%. This improvement made radiation therapy useful in the management of patients with metastatic disease.

Prognosis

In stages I and II (disease limited to the primary site), both the Clark and Breslow systems of microstaging allow patients to be subdivided into different risk categories for recurrent disease and eventual death (see Table 24-2). In general, the risk of recurrence after excision of a primary melanoma is extremely low if the

melanoma is less than 0.76 mm thick. On the other hand, if the melanoma is 4 mm or thicker, the probability of both recurrence and death is extremely high. Overall, the 5-year survival rate for patients with stage I disease is 75%. For patients with stage II disease, it is 66%.

In stage III (disease spread to the draining lymph nodes), the presence of metastatic disease in the regional lymph nodes is an ominous prognostic sign. The clear finding that melanoma has spread beyond the primary site decreases the 5-year disease-free survival rate to between 20% and 40%. This prognosis is even worse as the number of involved lymph nodes increases.

In stage IV (disease spread to distant sites), patients survive an average of 6 months. Patients who have only skin and lymph node metastases fare better (median survival of 14 months) than those with visceral metastases (median survival of 4 months). A review by Balch et al. showed five factors that seem to affect the prognosis in melanoma: pathologic stage, ulceration, surgical treatment, thickness, and location of the primary site (upper extremities vs other sites). Although these data were developed from a retrospective analysis of a large group of patients, most clinicians agree that these factors are important in predicting outcome in patients with melanoma.

Excisional Biopsy

A biopsy is considered whenever a patient has a lesion with the following symptoms: color change, size change, itching, bleeding, or oozing. A biopsy is also done if a patient has a lesion with the following signs: irregular color, nodularity, scab formation, ulceration, or irregular notched margins. Excisional biopsy is preferred when possible because the entire lesion is available for step-section histopathologic analysis to determine the depth of penetration. This information is critical for further management. Before local anesthesia is initiated, the physician outlines an ellipse around the lesion with 2- to 4-mm margins. The long axis of the ellipse is placed to permit easy therapeutic reexcision of the site. In general, the long axis of the ellipse is directed toward the node-bearing area. In addition, the physician confirms that the planned defect can be closed easily without undue tension. After the ellipse is outlined, field block local anesthesia is administered with a single injection at either end of the ellipse, infiltrating into normal tissue rather than into the tumor. Full-thickness skin and subcutaneous tissue are excised as part of the biopsy. After the bleeding points are controlled, the skin is reapproximated with alternating simple and vertical mattress stitches to give a smooth, straight closure (Figure 24-21). If the size or location of the primary site prevents excisional biopsy, then an incisional biopsy is performed.

Incisional Biopsy

The prognosis is not compromised by the use of incisional biopsy as long as definitive therapy is initiated

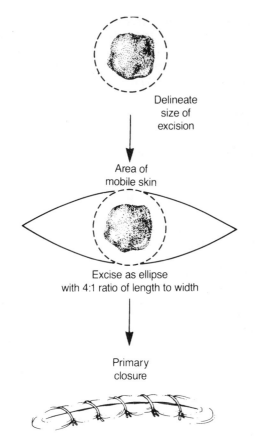

Delineate
size of
excision

Area of
mobile skin

Excise as ellipse
with 4:1 ratio of length to width

Primary
closure

Figure 24-21 Scalpel excision with primary closure is used for smaller lesions.

promptly. Selection of the biopsy site is critical because of the effect of tumor thickness on prognosis. An incisional biopsy must include some of the thickest part of the pigmented lesion to allow correct microstaging. The placement of the incisional biopsy should not compromise definitive surgical therapy. Field block anesthesia is used, with a single puncture near the site of the planned biopsy in normal skin so that the infiltration is in normal skin and underneath, rather than into, the melanoma. The normal skin involved in the biopsy site is reapproximated. Some authors recommend leaving the biopsy defect in the pigmented lesion open to avoid introducing melanoma cells into the subcutaneous tissue by passage of a needle.

The frequency of melanoma is increasing. Although it is much less common than BCC or SCC, it is the cause of 74% of deaths from skin cancer. The risk factors for melanoma are easily identified, even by the layperson. Consequently, early detection is a reasonable goal that should result in improved cure rates. Randomized prospective trials are underway to address questions about the treatment of certain groups of patients with stage I and II melanoma. To ensure maximum benefit to the patient, the physician should assist the patient with early diagnosis, correct staging, and treatment.

Malignant Diseases of the Lymphatics and Soft Tissue

Hodgkin's Lymphoma and Non-Hodgkin's Lymphoma

Lymphomas are malignancies that arise in the lymphoid tissues of the body. Collections of lymphoid cells occur in the lymph nodes, the white pulp of the spleen, Waldeyer's ring, the thymus gland, and lymphoid aggregates in the submucosa of the respiratory and gastrointestinal tracts **(Peyer's patches)**. The two major subgroups of malignant lymphoma are **Hodgkin's lymphoma** (20%) and **non-Hodgkin's lymphoma** (80%). Lymphomas are classified based on immunohistopathologic standards (Table 24–3). Lymphomas originate from **B-cells, T-cells,** histiocytes, or other lymphoid cells.

Hodgkin's Lymphoma
Incidence and Etiology

The incidence of Hodgkin's lymphoma follows a bimodal curve, with peaks in young adulthood (late 20s) and in older adults (mid-70s). The average age of a patient with Hodgkin's lymphoma is 32 years. The incidence in the United States was relatively stable over the last few decades, with approximately 4 cases per 100,000 as of the mid-1980s.

The etiology of Hodgkin's lymphoma is unknown. Various theories are postulated, including infectious causes (e.g., Epstein-Barr virus). The cellular origin of Hodgkin's lymphoma is also uncertain, although it may involve the monocyte-macrophage cell line.

Clinical Presentation and Evaluation

Hodgkin's lymphoma usually causes asymptomatic cervical lymphadenopathy (60%–80%). Supradiaphragmatic disease occurs initially in 90% of young adults who have Hodgkin's lymphoma. In older adults, however, the likelihood of subdiaphragmatic disease is 25%. Systemic (B) symptoms include fever, night sweats, malaise, and loss of more than 10% of body weight. Hodgkin's lymphoma may be localized or disseminated. Patients also may have signs and symptoms because of the mass effect of mediastinal or retroperitoneal disease.

All patients must undergo a thorough evaluation, including a complete physical examination. Particular attention is paid to the peripheral lymph node regions. A chest x-ray is also needed. The next step is excisional biopsy of an enlarged, abnormal lymph node. Biopsy is performed on cervical rather than axillary or inguinal nodes, which are more likely to show reactive changes and therefore be nondiagnostic. After the histologic diagnosis is made, a bone marrow biopsy is obtained. Finally, the liver, spleen, and retroperitoneal nodes are evaluated with computed tomography (CT) scan.

Staging laparotomy plays a critical role in the evaluation of most patients with limited (minimal) stage

Table 24-3. Lymphoid Neoplasms Recognized by the International Lymphoma Study Group

B-cell neoplasms

I. Precursor B-cell neoplasm: precursor B-lymphoblastic leukemia/lymphoma
II. Peripheral B-cell neoplasms
   1. B-cell chronic lymphocytic leukemia, prolymphocytic leukemia or small lymphocytic lymphoma
   2. Lymphoplansmacytoid lymphoma or immunocytoma
   3. Mantle cell lymphoma
   4. Follicle center lymphoma, follicular
      Provisional cytologic grades: I (small cell), II (mixed small and large cell), III (large cell)
      Provisional subtype: diffuse, predominantly small cell type
   5. Marginal zone B-cell lymphoma
      Extranodal (MALT-type with or without monocytoid B cells)
      Provisional subtype: nodal (with or without monocytoid B cells)
   6. Provisional entity: splenic marginal zone lymphoma (with or without villous lymphocytes)
   7. Hairy cell leukemia
   8. Plasmacytoma or plasma cell myeloma
   9. Diffuse large B-cell lymphoma[a]
      Subtype: primary mediastinal (thymic) B-cell lymphoma
  10. Burkitt's lymphoma
  11. Provisional entity: high-grade B-cell lymphoma, Burkitt-like[a]

T-cell and putative NK-cell neoplasms

I. Precursor T-cell neoplasm: precursor T-lymphoblastic lymphoma or leukemia
II. Peripheral T-cell and NK-cell neoplasms
   1. T-cell chronic lymphocytic leukemia or prolymphocytic leukemia
   2. Large granular lymphocyte leukemia
      T-cell type
      NK-cell type
   3. Mycosis fungoides or Sezary syndrome
   4. Peripheral T-cell lymphomas, unspecified[a]
      Provisional cytologic categories: medium cell, mixed medium and large cell, large cell, or lymphoepithelioid cell
      Provisional subtype: hepatosplenic γδ T-cell lymphoma
      Provisional subtype: subcutaneous panniculitic T-cell lymphoma
   5. Angioimmunoblastic T-cell lymphoma
   6. Angiocentric lymphoma
   7. Intestinal T-cell lymphoma (with or without associated enteropathy)
   8. Adult T-cell lymphoma or leukemia
   9. Anaplastic large cell lymphoma, CD30+, T- and null-cell types
  10. Provisional entity: anaplastic large-cell lymphoma, Hodgkin's-like

Hodgkin's lymphoma

I. Lymphocyte predominance
II. Nodular sclerosis
III. Mixed cellularity
IV. Lymphocyte depletion
V. Provisional entity: lymphocyte-rich classical Hodgkin's lymphoma

[a] These categories probably include more than one disease entity.
Adapted with permission from Harris NL, Jaffe ES, Stein H, et al. A revised European-American classification of lymphoid neoplasms: a proposal from the International Lymphoma Study Group. *Blood* 1994; 84(5): 1361–1392.
MALT, mucosa-associated lymphoid tissue; NK, natural killer.

Table 24-4. Histopathologic Types of Hodgkin's Disease

Classification (Rye)	Relative Frequency (%)
Nodular sclerosis	50
Mixed cellularity	37
Lymphocyte predominance	5
Lymphocyte depletion	8

Hodgkin's disease. Staging laparotomy includes splenectomy and biopsy of the splenic hilar, celiac, porta hepatis, mesenteric, paraaortic, and iliac nodes. Bilateral wedge and needle biopsies of the liver are also performed. To attempt to maintain fertility after radiation treatment in premenopausal women, the ovaries are positioned in a retrouterine site and sutured to presacral fascia (oophoropexy). Staging laparotomy may not be necessary in patients who have a large mediastinal mass and older patients who have mixed or lymphocyte-depleted histology. These patients require systemic therapy, and laparotomy does not alter the course of treatment.

Staging

The Rye classification system groups Hodgkin's lymphoma histologically into four categories: lymphocyte predominant, nodular sclerosis, mixed cellularity, and lymphocyte depleted (Table 24-4). Nodular sclerosis is the most common histologic type (relative frequency of 50%). Histologically, Hodgkin's lymphoma appears as a tumor with a large reactive background of lymphocytes, eosinophils, and plasma cells, with a few malignant mononuclear cells and multinuclear giant cells (Reed-Sternberg cells). The Reed-Sternberg cell has a classic "owl eye" appearance (Figure 24-22). This cell must be present for the diagnosis of Hodgkin's lymphoma to be made. Reed-Sternberg cells are also present in other disorders, including mononucleosis and other inflammatory conditions, and with phenytoin (Dilantin) therapy.

The Ann Arbor classification is used to stage Hodgkin's lymphoma (Table 24-5). This classification identifies patients as stage A (asymptomatic) or stage B (fevers, night sweats, and weight loss). Stage classification is based on the involvement of single, multiple, or disseminated sites of one or more extralymphatic organs.

Treatment

The treatment of Hodgkin's lymphoma is determined by staging. Radiation therapy plays a major role in the treatment of limited-stage disease (stages I and II). Chemotherapy, with or without radiation therapy, is recommended for advanced disease. Radiation is administered in doses of 3000 to 4000 rad to areas of known involvement and to neighboring nodal basins that are likely to represent the next area of spread.

Chemotherapy significantly alters the prognosis of patients with Hodgkin's lymphoma, with cure achieved in 80% of cases. The most common regimen is nitrogen

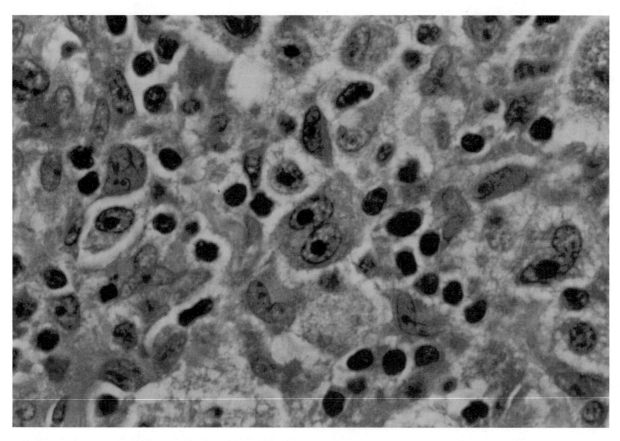

Figure 24-22 Hodgkin's lymphoma, mixed cellularity subtype. A classic, diagnostic bilobulated Reed-Sternberg cell is surrounded by a variety of cell types, including malignant Hodgkin's cells and benign small lymphocytes and histiocytes (hematoxylin and eosin × 1000). Courtesy of Dr. Rogers Griffith, Department of Pathology, Rhode Island Hospital, Providence, Rhode Island.

Table 24-5. Ann Arbor Staging Classification for Hodgkin's Lymphoma

Stage	Findings
I	Involvement of a single lymph node region (I) or a single extralymphatic organ or site (I^E)
II	Involvement of two or more lymph node regions on the same side of the diaphragm (II) or localized involvement of an extralymphatic organ or site (IIE)
III	Involvement of lymph node regions on both sides of the diaphragm (III) or localized involvement of an extralymphatic organ or site (IIIE), spleen (III^S), or both (III^{SE})
IV	Diffuse or disseminated involvement of one or more extralymphatic organs with or without associated lymph node involvement (involved organs should be identified by a symbol)
A	Asymptomatic
B	Fever, sweats, weight loss > 10% of body weight

mustard, vincristine, procarbazine, and prednisone (MOPP). Another common regimen is doxorubicin (Adriamycin), bleomycin, vinblastine, and dacarbazine (ABVD).

Prognosis

The prognosis for patients with Hodgkin's lymphoma is excellent. Risk factors include the stage of disease at the time of treatment and the histology. The lymphocyte-predominant group appears to have the best prognosis, followed by the nodular-sclerosis group. With adequate staging and therapy, 80% of patients are cured. The risk of a second tumor after treatment continues to increase with time. The risk of leukemia reaches a plateau of approximately 3% at 10 years.

Non-Hodgkin's Lymphoma

Non-Hodgkin's lymphomas are a diverse group that represent a large spectrum of malignancies. Their histology, immunology, and clinical characteristics are heterogeneous.

Incidence and Etiology

Since 1970, the incidence of non-Hodgkin's lymphoma has increased dramatically by 65%. In 1996, approximately 52,000 new cases were expected to be diagnosed. Non-Hodgkin's lymphoma appears to be associated with human immunodeficiency virus, although the increased incidence is not entirely explained by the rise in the number of cases of acquired immune deficiency syndrome (AIDS).

As with Hodgkin's lymphoma, the etiology of most types of non-Hodgkin's lymphoma is unclear. The incidence appears to increase in association with immunosuppression. Both patients with AIDS and those who undergo renal transplantation are at increased risk for this disorder. Viruses can cause specific lymphomas. Burkitt's lymphoma is associated with Epstein-Barr virus infection, and human T-cell lymphoma virus-1 is associated with a T-cell lymphoma that is found in the Caribbean Islands.

Clinical Presentation and Evaluation

Most patients with non-Hodgkin's lymphoma are asymptomatic at presentation, although 20% have B symptoms. Patients may have enlarged lymph nodes, with gastrointestinal symptoms that include nausea, vomiting, and bleeding. Unlike Hodgkin's lymphoma, non-Hodgkin's lymphoma tends to spread in a disseminated fashion. Patients may have symptoms secondary to the extent of spread. Some dramatic presentations include superior vena cava syndrome, acute spinal cord compression, and meningeal involvement.

The evaluation of patients with non-Hodgkin's lymphoma begins with a complete history and physical examination. Next, diagnostic studies are performed, including complete blood count, liver function tests, chest x-ray, and CT scan of the chest, abdomen, and pelvis. Bone marrow biopsy is then performed. Patients with intermediate-grade non-Hodgkin's lymphoma with bone marrow involvement and those with high-grade non-Hodgkin's lymphoma may require lumbar puncture because central nervous system involvement is increased in these groups. Staging laparotomy is usually not indicated because these patients tend to have disseminated disease.

Staging

Many histologic classification systems are used for non-Hodgkin's lymphoma. The most widely used are the Rappaport and the Working Formulation systems (Table 24-6). The Rappaport system groups tumors by architecture (diffuse vs nodular) and cell type. In the Working Formulation system, the terms follicular and large cell replace the terms nodular and histiocytic in the Rappaport system. The grade is classified as high, intermediate, or low based on histology. The stage is determined with the Ann Arbor system, although this system is somewhat limited because non-Hodgkin's lymphoma tends to occur in disseminated form. In 1993, the International Non-Hodgkin's Lymphoma Prognostic Factors Project devised a new classification system (Table 24-7) that groups patients based on risk of relapse. This system aids in determining which patients will benefit from more aggressive treatment.

Table 24-6. Histologic Groups in Non-Hodgkin's Lymphoma

Working Formulation Grade	Rappaport Classification
Low	
Small lymphocytic	Well-differentiated lymphocytic lymphoma
Follicular small cleaved lymphocytic	Nodular, poorly differentiated lymphocytic lymphoma
Mixed follicular small cleaved cell and large cell	Nodular, mixed lymphoma
Intermediate	
Follicular, predominantly large cell	Nodular, histiocytic lymphoma
Diffuse small cleaved cell	Diffuse, poorly differentiated lymphocytic lymphoma
Diffuse large cell (cleaved or uncleaved)	Diffuse histiocytic lymphoma
High	
Diffuse large cell immunoblast B-cell T-cell Polymorphic Epithelial cell component	Diffuse histiocytic lymphoma
Lymphoblastic Convoluted Nonconvoluted	Lymphoblastic lymphoma
Small noncleaved Burkitt's Non-Burkitt's	Diffuse undifferentiated lymphoma

Adapted with permission from Rosenthal D, Eyre H. Hodgkin's disease and non-Hodgkin's lymphomas. In:*Textbook of Clinical Oncology,* 2nd ed. Atlanta, Ga: American Cancer Society, 1995:451–469.

Treatment

The treatment of non-Hodgkin's lymphoma is variable, depending on the histologic subtype and the stage. Surgery, radiation therapy, and chemotherapy are the treatment options. The primary role of surgery is for diagnosis, although it is sometimes an important aspect of treatment. Localized gastric and small-bowel non-Hodgkin's lymphoma may be effectively treated with resection. Radiation therapy is useful in localized non-Hodgkin's lymphoma, although this presentation is unusual. Radiation therapy is also used for complications related to mass effect (e.g., superior vena cava obstruction, spinal cord compression).

Non-Hodgkin's lymphoma tumors are primarily treated with chemotherapy. A variety of agents and treatment protocols are used. The response to chemotherapy and the duration of remission are related to tumor grade and stage.

Prognosis

To determine the prognosis, tumor grade and stage are considered. Low-grade tumors tend to follow an indolent course, and if left untreated, patients often survive 5 years or longer. On the other hand, high-grade tumors may progress rapidly if they are not treated, and may result in death. These tumors respond well to chemotherapy. Factors that affect responsiveness in

Table 24-7. International Non-Hodgkin's Lymphoma Prognostic Factors Project

Category	Risk Factors[a] (n)	Complete Response Rate (%)	2-yr Survival (%)	5-yr Survival (%)
Low risk	≤1	87	84	73
Low–intermediate risk	2	67	66	50
High–intermediate risk	3	55	54	43
High risk	4 or 5	44	34	26

[a]Risk factors include age (≥ 60 yr), Stage (I/II versus III/IV), extranodal sites (≤ I or > I), performance status (Eastern Cooperative Oncology Group ≤ I vs 2), and lactic dehydrogenase level (normal vs abnormal).
Adapted with permission from The International Non-Hodgkin's Lymphoma Prognostic Factors Project. A predictive model for aggressive non-Hodgkin's lymphoma. *N Engl J Med* 1993;329:987–994. Copyright 1993 Massachusetts Medical Society. All rights reserved.

patients with high- and intermediate-grade tumors have been defined. The prognosis is poor in patients who are older than 50 years of age and have B symptoms and bulky disease and those who have extranodal disease and bone marrow or gastrointestinal involvement.

Sarcoma

Soft Tissue Sarcomas

Soft tissue sarcomas are malignant tumors that are derived from mesenchymal tissue. Although they are distributed throughout the body, they predominate in connective and supportive tissues within the abdomen and extremities. These tumors are relatively uncommon, accounting for 1% of all malignant tumors in adults.

Soft tissue sarcomas are further classified according to their histopathologic tissue of origin (Table 24-8). The most common site is the extremity (52%), with 37% found in the lower extremity and 15% in the upper extremity. Intraabdominal and retroperitoneal tumors occur in 14% of cases (Figure 24-23). The rest are located within the viscera (13%), trunk (9%), thoracic region (5%), head and neck (5%), and genitourinary tract (2%).

Incidence and Etiology

Soft tissue sarcoma in adults is relatively uncommon. However, in children younger than 15 years of age, the incidence is approximately 6%. In this age-group, soft tissue sarcoma ranks fifth as a cause of death. In adults, the incidence of soft tissue sarcoma is approximately 2 cases per 100,000. In the United States, 5000 to 6000 cases of soft tissue sarcoma are diagnosed each year. Approximately half of these patients die of their disease. Death results from uncontrollable local recurrence invading adjacent tissue, from metastasis to the lung from extremity or torso lesions (Figure 24-24), or from metastasis to the liver from intraabdominal lesions.

The etiology of soft tissue sarcoma is unclear. Many factors are implicated, including genetic defects, radiation, chemical exposure, and trauma. Li-Fraumeni syndrome is a group of tumors that includes breast cancer and soft tissue sarcoma. Within this group, there is an

Table 24-8. Soft Tissue Tumors and Their Tissue of Origin

Tissue	Benign	Malignant
Fibrous tissue	Fibroma	Fibrosarcoma
Adipose tissue	Lipoma	Liposarcoma
Striated muscle	Rhabdomyoma	Rhabdomyosarcoma
Smooth muscle	Leiomyoma	Leiomyosarcoma
Synovial mesothelium	Mesothelioma	Synovial sarcoma
Blood vessels	Angioma	Angiosarcoma[a]
Lymph vessels	Lymphangioma	Lymphangiosarcoma
Peripheral nerve	Neuroma	Malignant neurolemmoma, schwannoma
Myofibroblast		Malignant fibrous histiocytoma

[a]See text for discussion of Kaposi's sarcoma.

increased incidence of mutation of the p53 tumor suppressor gene. Patients with familial syndromes [e.g., Gardner's syndrome, von Recklinghausen's disease (neurofibromatosis)] are also at increased risk for sarcoma. Gardner's syndrome increases the risk of desmoid tumors, and von Recklinghausen's disease increases the risk of malignant peripheral nerve sheath tumors. The incidence of lymphangiosarcoma increases after surgery and radiation therapy for breast cancer (Stewart-Treves syndrome). Lymphangiosarcoma also occurs in extremities with a history of chronic edema of congenital or traumatic origin or with a history of filariasis.

Clinical Presentation and Evaluation

Most malignant soft tissue tumors are relatively slow-growing and do not cause symptoms until they become large (Figures 24-25 to 24-27). Tumors within the extremity are detected early, but tumors within the retroperitoneum can attain considerable size before they are detected (see Figure 24-23). Approximately 75% of patients with extremity sarcoma have a painless mass, and pain is the initial symptom in 25%. Patients who have a retroperitoneal tumor often have vague pain. Paresthesias, weight loss, and nausea or vomiting

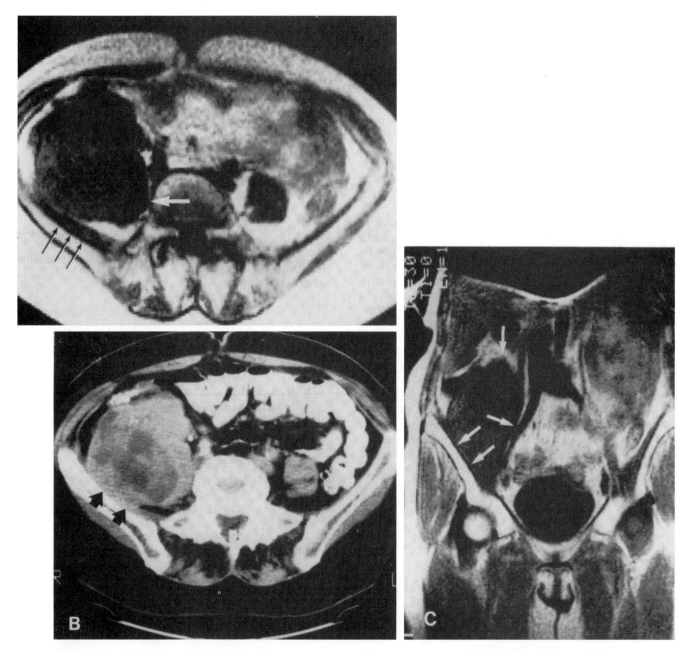

Figure 24-23 Large mesenchymoma of the retroperitoneum and iliac fossa with intraabdominal extension. **A,** Axial magnetic resonance imaging scan showing noninvolved cortical bone *(arrow)* and a patent right iliac venous system. **B,** Transaxial computed tomography scan with intravenous contrast showing a necrotic tumor of the right iliac fossa. The mass appears to invade the iliac bone *(arrows)*. Involvement of the iliac vein cannot be determined. **C,** Coronal magnetic resonance imaging scan of the mesenchymoma showing uninvolved cortical bone *(arrows)* and complete visualization of the right iliac vein without contrast. The lesion was resected en bloc.

also occur. Pain, intestinal obstruction, and chronic blood loss are also associated with intestinal sarcoma.

Staging

The most commonly used staging system for soft tissue sarcoma is that of the American Joint Committee on Cancer (Table 24-9). This system uses tumor grade, tumor size, and the presence of nodal or distant metastasis for staging.

Tumor grade is the most important prognostic indicator. Factors such as cellularity, the number of mitotic fig-

ures, vascularity, pleomorphism, anaplasia, the presence of tumor necrosis, and invasive characteristics determine tumor grade (Table 24-10). According to this system, there are four grades of sarcoma. Most well-differentiated tumors are considered low grade, and the other three grades are considered high. This distinction is important in determining the likelihood of metastasis, which can affect the decision regarding adjuvant therapy.

A tumor larger than 5 cm increases the likelihood of metastasis and mortality. Nodal spread and distant metastases increase the stage and worsen the prognosis.

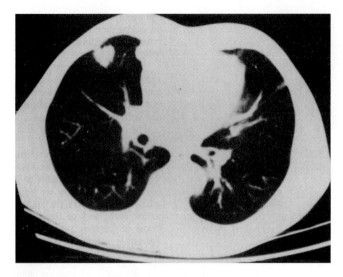

Figure 24-24 Computed tomography scan of a patient with lung metastasis as a result of extremity sarcoma.

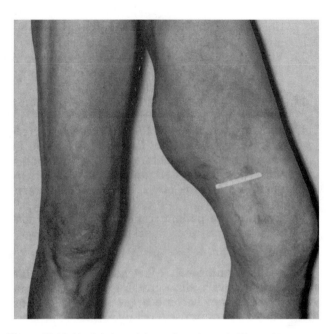

Figure 24-26 Medial view of the patient shown in Figure 24-25.

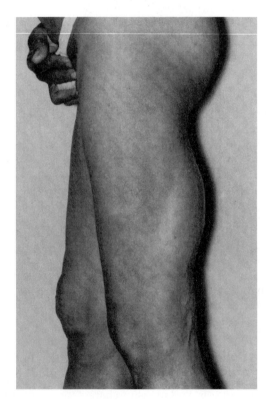

Figure 24-25 A 56-year-old patient with a large, painless thigh mass *(lateral view)*. The final diagnosis was liposarcoma.

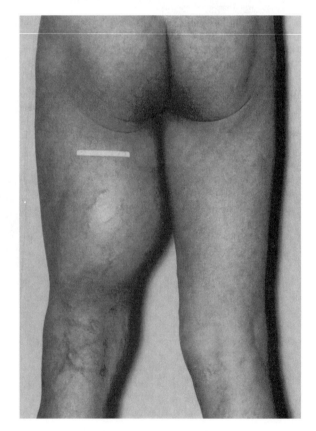

Figure 24-27 Posterior view of the patient shown in Figure 24-25.

Table 24-9. TNM Staging for Soft Tissue Sarcomas

Primary tumor (T)
TX   Primary tumor cannot be assessed
T0   No evidence of primary tumor
T1   Tumor ≤ 5 cm in greatest dimension
T2   Tumor > 5 cm in greatest dimension

Regional lymph nodes (N)
NX   Regional lymph nodes cannot be assessed
N0   No regional lymph node metastasis
N1   Regional lymph node metastasis

Distant metastasis (M)
MX   Presence of distant metastasis cannot be assessed
M0   No distant metastasis
M1   Distant metastasis

Histopathologic grade (G)
GX   Grade cannot be assessed
G1   Well differentiated
G2   Moderately differentiated
G3   Poorly differentiated
G4   Undifferentiated

Stage grouping

Stage grouping				
Stage IA	G1	T1	N0	M0
Stage IB	G1	T2	N0	M0
Stage IIA	G2	T1	N0	M0
Stage IIB	G2	T2	N0	M0
Stage IIIA	G3, 4	T1	N0	M0
Stage IIIB	G3, 4	T2	N0	M0
Stage IVA	Any G	Any T	N1	M0
Stage IVB	Any G	Any T	Any N	M1

Adapted with permission from Beahrs OH, Henson DE, Hutter RVP, Kennedy BJ, eds. *American Joint Committee on Cancer Manual for Staging of Cancer*, 4th ed. Philadelphia, Pa: JB Lippincott, 1992: 131–133.

Table 24-10. Guidelines to Histologic Grading of Sarcomas

Low Grade	High Grade
Good differentiation	Poor differentiation
Hypocellular	Hypercellular
Increased stroma	Minimal stroma
Hypovascular	Hypervascular
Minimal necrosis	Much necrosis
<5 mitoses/10 high-power fields	>5 mitoses /10 high-power fields

Adapted with permission from Hadju SI, Shiu MH, Brennan MF. The role of the pathologist in the management of soft tissue sarcomas. *World J Surg* 1988; 12: 326–331.

An alternative staging system was devised by Memorial Sloan-Kettering Cancer Center. This system considers size, depth, and grade, and identifies them as favorable or unfavorable. The sum of favorable and unfavorable characteristics determines the stage (Table 24-11).

Table 24-11. Memorial Sloan-Kettering Clinical Staging System for Sarcomas

Factors	Favorable	Unfavorable	Stage Grouping	
Size	<5 cm	≥ 5 cm	0	3 favorable signs
Depth	Superficial	Deep	I	2 favorable signs; 1 unfavorable sign
Grade	Low	High	II	1 favorable sign; 2 unfavorable signs
			III	3 unfavorable signs
			IV	Evidence of metastasis

Arca MJ, Sondak VK, Chang AE. Diagnostic procedures and pretreatment evaluation of soft tissue sarcomas. *Semin Surg Oncol* 1994; 10(5): 323–331. Copyright 1994 John Wiley & Sons, Inc. Reprinted by permission of Wiley-Liss, Inc, a subsidiary of John Wiley & Sons, Inc.

Clinical evaluation begins with the history. If the patient has a lump or mass, a careful and complete history is taken. Attention is paid to factors such as previous trauma, infection, and growth characteristics. The physical examination includes an accurate, detailed assessment of the mass, including size, position, consistency, depth with respect to skin, and mobility. Although sarcomas rarely metastasize to regional lymph nodes, fewer than 5% disseminate in this manner, so regional nodes must be inspected for evidence of disease.

After a complete physical examination, biopsy of a large mass is deferred until diagnostic imaging is performed. Biopsy techniques vary worldwide among clinics and according to the experience of the clinician. Fine-needle aspiration often provides inadequate tissue for histopathologic typing and determination of grade. Tru-cut biopsy (a technique that uses a large-diameter needle that allows sampling of a core of tissue), however, is an excellent technique for diagnosis. Open biopsy is the benchmark diagnostic approach. Excisional biopsy is indicated for lesions smaller than 3 cm and involves removal of the entire mass. Incisional biopsy is the procedure of choice for lesions larger than 3 to 5 cm, and involves removal of a portion of the mass. The incision is carefully placed at the apex of the mass, where the tumor is believed to be closest to the skin, avoiding extensive dissection of normal tissue planes. The incision is oriented to facilitate subsequent wide excision. In the extremity, the incision is made along the long axis. On the trunk, the incision follows Langer's lines. Fresh tissue is sent to the pathology laboratory for immunohistochemistry, cytogenetic studies, and electron microscopic examination.

After the diagnosis and tumor grade are determined, the tumor size, depth, and relation to major neurovascular and skeletal elements are assessed. CT scan and magnetic resonance imaging studies (Figure 24-28) are used to evaluate the characteristics of the sarcoma as well as the presence of metastatic disease. The workup also includes a chest x-ray to rule out metastatic spread to the lungs.

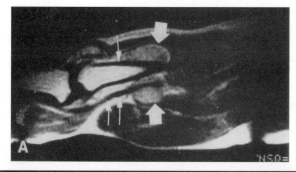

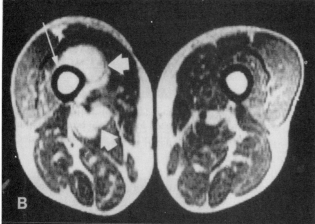

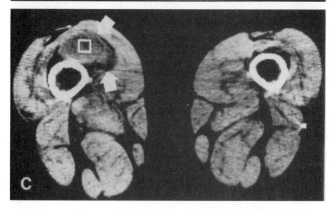

Figure 24-28 High-grade liposarcoma of the distal thigh. **A,** Coronal magnetic resonance imaging scan in a mixed T1- and T2-weighted image confirms the margin of the femur, neurovascular bundle *(double arrows)*, and two separate loci of liposarcoma. **B,** Transaxial magnetic resonance imaging scan of the thigh differentiates noncontiguous liposarcoma adherent to, but not invading, the cortical bone *(small arrow)* of the femur or the neurovascular bundle. **C,** Axial computed tomography scan of the distal thigh shows the nondistinct relation of the liposarcoma to the femur and the neurovascular bundle. A single anterior tumor mass is seen *(arrows)*.

Sarcomas grow in a three-dimensional manner, taking the path of least resistance and compressing the surrounding tissue. This compression gives the appearance of encapsulation. However, the surrounding tissue has formed a pseudocapsule, and microscopic extensions of malignant tissue project beyond it. Because of the presence of this pseudocapsule, marginal resection or enucleation of the tumor results in local recurrence rates of

65% to 90%. Wide excision of these tumors, including 2- to 3-cm of normal tissue, improves local control, with recurrence rates of 30%.

Treatment

The management of these malignancies has evolved considerably. Surgery is the mainstay of treatment, and increasing numbers of patients are treated with adjuvant radiation and chemotherapy. In the past, recurrence rates after amputation were improved over those with local resection, although deformity and significant loss of function occurred. More recently, limb-sparing procedures that combine wide excision (Figures 24-29 and 24-30) and adjuvant radiation therapy produced excellent results. Approximately 90% of patients with extremity sarcoma can now be treated with limb-sparing techniques.

Surgical resection is the procedure of choice for intraabdominal sarcomas. Involvement of adjacent structures is common, and wide en bloc resection is necessary. Lymphadenectomy is not required because the likelihood of lymphatic spread is low. The role of palliative surgery for patients with unresectable tumors is controversial. This surgery is usually reserved for tumors that are believed to be symptomatic as a result of intestinal or urinary tract obstruction. Routine adjuvant radiation therapy does not appear to be indicated. The benefit of this therapy is not clear, and there is a clear risk of radiation enteritis. Studies are underway to evaluate the role of chemotherapy.

Prognosis

The 5-year actuarial survival rate for patients with extremity sarcoma is 60%. Superficial lesions smaller than 3 cm have an excellent prognosis (5-year patient survival rate of 90%). Patients with larger high-grade tumors have a 5-year survival rate of only 30%. These tumors usually metastasize to the lung, usually within 2 years of initial diagnosis.

For patients who have intraabdominal tumors and undergo complete resection, the 5-year survival rate is 75%. Patients who undergo partial resection have a far worse prognosis (5-year survival rate of 30%). These tumors recur locally, with extensive intraabdominal spread, and usually metastasize to the liver.

Kaposi's Sarcoma

In the past, Kaposi's sarcoma was largely limited to elderly Jewish men of Mediterranean descent and to people from sub-Saharan Africa. With the AIDS epidemic, the incidence of Kaposi's sarcoma has increased. Kaposi's sarcoma is the most common neoplastic complication of AIDS. Homosexual and bisexual men are much more likely to have Kaposi's sarcoma than others with AIDS. This finding suggests a sexually transmitted etiology in this patient population.

Kaposi's sarcoma lesions initially appear as flat, blue patches that resemble a hematoma. Later, they become raised, rubbery nodules. Non-AIDS Kaposi's sarcoma is typically found on the lower extremities. AIDS-related

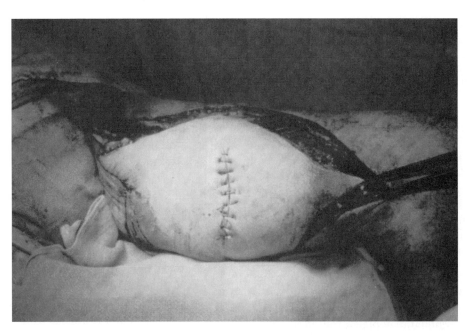

Figure 24-29 High-grade malignant fibrous histiocytoma of the medial thigh. The elliptical incision for a limb-sparing resection includes the previous biopsy site. A limited longitudinal biopsy incision is preferred over the incorrectly positioned transverse incision that is shown. These transversely placed scars necessitate a wider ellipse of skin excision, which technically limits conservative approaches for resection.

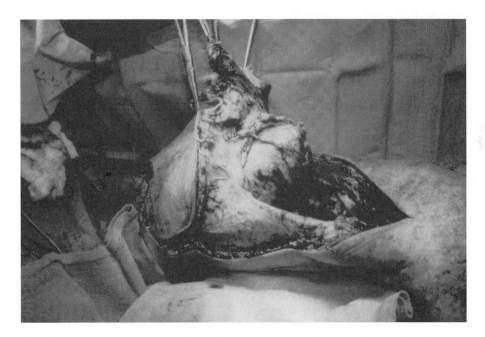

Figure 24-30 Wide excision of the sarcoma from the medial thigh. The specimen includes the malignant fibrous histiocytoma and the adductor magnus muscle group. The semitendinosus and semimembranosus muscles were approximated to the rectus femoris muscle to provide tissue coverage of the femoral vessels. The defect is covered by a skin graft. The patient had an uneventful postoperative course, with no neuromuscular disability.

Kaposi's sarcoma often begins in the perioral mucosa. The palate is the most common site. AIDS-related Kaposi's sarcoma is often multifocal, with rapid spread to the lymph nodes. It often involves the gastrointestinal tract. Biopsy shows endothelial cells, with fibroblasts, spindle cells, and increased capillary growth. These malignancies are considered angiosarcomas.

Surgical excision or local radiation is effective for small, localized lesions. Agents such as vinblastine, bleomycin, and doxorubicin produce responses in more advanced cases. Patients with AIDS-related Kaposi's sarcoma have a far worse prognosis because of immunodeficiency, the presence of opportunistic infection, and the inability to use conventional multidrug regimens. Local radiation shrinks these lesions and provides palliation. Treatment includes single-drug regimens with vinblastine or VP-16. There is also interest in the use of α-interferon.

Multiple-Choice Questions

Malignant Diseases of the Skin

1. Differences in skin color are determined by the:
   A. Concentration of melanocytes
   B. Thickness of the skin
   C. Melanosome content of the keratinocytes
   D. Concentration of amelanotic melanocytes
   E. Concentration of melanin pigment in the melanocytes

2. Which statement about melanoma is correct?
   A. Its causes are known and well understood.
   B. Exposure to sunlight may play a role in its development.
   C. Between 10% and 20% of patients who have melanoma will have a secondary primary melanoma.
   D. Basal cell nevus syndrome is unrelated to heredity.
   E. Xeroderma pigmentosum is unrelated to the development of malignant melanoma.

3. What is the most common type of malignant melanoma?
   A. Lentigo maligna
   B. Nodular
   C. Acral lentiginous
   D. Superficial spreading
   E. Ocular

4. Subungual melanoma:
   A. Has a worse prognosis than superficial spreading melanoma
   B. Is not a type of acral lentiginous melanoma
   C. Is treated by local excision rather than finger amputation
   D. Rarely metastasizes to the lungs
   E. Is usually diagnosed early

5. Clark's staging system for primary malignant melanoma is based on the:
   A. Surface area of the tumor
   B. Thickness of the lesion
   C. Depth of invasion of the skin and subcutaneous tissue
   D. Presence of nodal metastases
   E. Absence of distant metastases

6. Clark's level II melanoma:
   A. Is confined to the epidermis
   B. Invades the papillary layer of the dermis
   C. Reaches the subcutaneous tissues
   D. Invades the reticular layer of the dermis
   E. Has a comparatively poor prognosis

7. Breslow's classification of primary malignant melanoma is based on the:
   A. Level of invasion by the tumor
   B. Total volume of the tumor
   C. Thickness of the lesion
   D. Presence of distant metastases
   E. Absence of nodal involvement

8. Which anatomic site has the highest incidence of malignant melanoma?
   A. Extremities
   B. Torso
   C. Fingernail beds
   D. Head and neck
   E. Vagina

9. A melanoma that is 0.00 to 0.75 mm thick:
   A. Has an excellent prognosis
   B. Will never metastasize
   C. Must be treated with prophylactic node dissection
   D. Should not be treated with wide local excision
   E. Is treated with a course of postoperative radiation therapy

10. Which lesions are most likely to be confused with malignant melanoma?
    A. Acrochordon, sebaceous cyst, and basal cell carcinoma
    B. Seborrheic keratosis, rodent ulcer, and xanthelasma
    C. Benign nevus, basal cell carcinoma, seborrheic keratosis, and subungual hematoma
    D. Benign nevus, seborrheic keratosis, and intradermal inclusion cyst
    E. Seborrheic keratosis, tinea capitis, and subungual hematoma

11. Biopsy of a lesion that is suspected of being a malignant melanoma should:
    A. Be incisional
    B. Be performed under general anesthesia
    C. Include the thinnest portion of the lesion
    D. Involve a wide excision
    E. Be excisional whenever possible

12. Local excision of a cutaneous melanoma includes:
    A. A 2-cm skin margin and underlying subcutaneous fat
    B. A 5-cm skin margin and underlying subcutaneous fat
    C. A 2-cm skin margin, subcutaneous tissue, and underlying fascia
    D. A 4-cm skin margin and subcutaneous tissue down to the fascia
    E. A 3-cm skin margin, subcutaneous tissue, and underlying fascia

13. A patient who has a primary cutaneous melanoma and a palpable regional lymph node should undergo:
    A. Wide excision of the primary site
    B. Wide excision of the primary site and regional lymph node dissection if the regional lymph node enlarges during a period of observation
    C. Wide excision of the primary site and regional lymph node dissection
    D. Wide excision of the primary site and radiation therapy to the regional lymph nodes
    E. Wide excision of the primary site and biopsy of the regional nodes

14. A patient who has a malignant melanoma that is less than 0.75 mm thick and no palpable regional nodes should undergo:
    A. Wide excision of the primary site only
    B. Wide excision of the primary site and prophylactic regional lymph node dissection
    C. Excisional biopsy of the primary site followed by radiation therapy
    D. Wide local excision and eventual regional lymph node biopsy
    E. Wide local excision and radiation therapy to the primary lesion site

15. Which statement about the use of chemotherapy to treat recurrent or disseminated malignant melanoma is correct?
    A. Several chemotherapeutic agents are effective against this tumor.
    B. Dacarbazine may be effective in 20% of the patients treated.
    C. Chemotherapy is used in conjunction with surgical treatment of stage I tumor.
    D. Complications caused by chemotherapy are unusual.
    E. Chemotherapy usually controls this tumor.

16. What is the most common cancer in humans?
    A. Melanoma
    B. Basal cell carcinoma
    C. Squamous cell carcinoma
    D. Adenocarcinoma
    E. Sarcoma

17. What is the most important risk factor for skin cancer?
    A. Chemical (arsenic) exposure
    B. Sun exposure
    C. Burn scar tissue
    D. X-ray exposure
    E. Skin thickness

18. Treatment of basal cell carcinoma includes all of the following EXCEPT:
    A. Surgical excision
    B. Electrodesiccation and curettage
    C. Radium implants
    D. Cryotherapy
    E. Topical chemotherapy

19. What is the most common site of squamous cell carcinoma?
    A. Arms
    B. Legs
    C. Trunk
    D. Head and neck
    E. Perineum

20. Squamous cell carcinoma may have all of the following features EXCEPT:
    A. Pearly, raised margins
    B. Central ulceration
    C. Firm induration
    D. Crust
    E. Irregular borders

Malignant Diseases of the Lymphatics and Soft Tissue

21. Which histologic subtype of Hodgkin's lymphoma has the best prognosis?
    A. Lymphocyte predominant
    B. Nodular sclerosis
    C. Mixed cellularity
    D. Lymphocyte depleted
    E. Prognosis is not related to histologic subtype

22. According to the Ann Arbor staging classification, what is the correct stage for a patient who has Hodgkin's lymphoma involving only the cervical and mediastinal lymph nodes?
    A. Stage I
    B. Stage II
    C. Stage III
    D. Stage IV
    E. Stage IVB

23. According to the Ann Arbor staging classification, what is the correct stage for a patient who has involvement of the cervical lymph nodes, mediastinal lymph nodes, and spleen?
    A. Stage I
    B. Stage II
    C. Stage III
    D. Stage IV
    E. Stage IVB

24. Staging laparotomy for a patient with Hodgkin's lymphoma includes all of the following EXCEPT:
    A. Splenectomy
    B. Biopsy of the splenic hilar lymph nodes
    C. Biopsy of the paraaortic lymph nodes
    D. Biopsy of the omental lymph nodes
    E. Biopsy of the liver

25. The preferred method for biopsy of a lymph node in a patient who is suspected of having lymphoma is:
    A. Fine-needle aspiration cytology
    B. Core-needle biopsy
    C. Incisional biopsy
    D. Excisional biopsy
    E. Radical lymphadenectomy

26. What is the primary method of therapy for limited-stage Hodgkin's lymphoma (stages I and II)?
    A. Radiation therapy
    B. Chemotherapy
    C. Chemotherapy and radiation therapy
    D. Observation
    E. Immunotherapy

27. The incidence curve for Hodgkin's lymphoma shows that the incidence of the disease is:
    A. Maximal in young patients and decreasing with age
    B. Maximal in elderly patients
    C. Bimodal
    D. Unrelated to age
    E. Determined only by heredity

28. What is the most common site of lymphadenopathy in a patient who has Hodgkin's lymphoma?
    A. Cervical
    B. Axillary
    C. Mediastinal
    D. Inguinal
    E. Retroperitoneal

29. According to the Ann Arbor classification, a patient who has cervical and mediastinal lymph node involvement, fever, and night sweats is classified as:
    A. Stage IA
    B. Stage IB
    C. Stage IIA
    D. Stage IIB
    E. Stage IIIB

30. Which histologic subtype of Hodgkin's lymphoma is the most common?
    A. Lymphocyte predominant
    B. Nodular sclerosis
    C. Mixed cellularity
    D. Lymphocyte depleted

31. Most sarcomas have a common embryologic origin in the primitive:
    A. Endoderm
    B. Ectoderm
    C. Mesoderm
    D. Endoderm and ectoderm
    E. Ectoderm and mesoderm

32. In the adult population in the United States, soft tissue sarcomas account for what percentage of all cancers?
    A. 0.01%
    B. 1%
    C. 6%
    D. 10%
    E. 25%

33. Soft tissue sarcomas:
    A. Have no proven genetic predisposition
    B. Usually cause a painful mass
    C. Are more common in children
    D. Never metastasize

34. What is the most common site of soft tissue sarcoma?
    A. Head and neck
    B. Chest
    C. Trunk
    D. Upper extremity
    E. Lower extremity

35. According to the Memorial Sloan-Kettering clinical staging system for sarcoma, which factor is NOT favorable?
    A. Size less than 5 cm
    B. Low grade
    C. Superficial depth
    D. High grade
    E. Absence of metastases

Questions 36–40

Match the following diseases with their associated malignancy.
    A. Li-Fraumeni syndrome
    B. Gardner's syndrome
    C. Von Recklinghausen's disease
    D. Stewart-Treves syndrome
    E. Kaposi's sarcoma

36. Peripheral nerve sheath tumors

37. Lymphangiosarcoma after mastectomy and radiation

38. Palate tumors

39. Breast cancer and soft tissue sarcoma

40. Desmoid tumors

Oral Examination Study Questions

CASE 1
A 65-year-old man has an ulcer on his lower lip that will not heal.

OBJECTIVE 1
The student formulates a differential diagnosis.
A. Herpetic ulcer

B. Injury

C. Skin cancer (typical presentation for squamous cell carcinoma of the lip)

OBJECTIVE 2
The student establishes a diagnosis.
A. Punch biopsy

B. Incisional biopsy

OBJECTIVE 3

The student initiates appropriate therapy.
A. Radiation therapy
B. Surgery: v-lip excision

OBJECTIVE 4

The student provides appropriate follow-up.
A. The patient should avoid sun exposure.
B. The patient should use sunscreen.

Minimum Level of Achievement for Passing

The student includes skin cancer in the differential diagnosis and recommends a biopsy to establish diagnosis. The student also knows that sun exposure is an important etiology of skin cancer.

Honors Level of Achievement

The student lists punch biopsy as an option. In addition, the student mentions that nodal spread is possible for larger lesions.

CASE 2

An 80-year-old woman has a 2-cm fungating mass on the back of the hand. The lesion is freely movable. Results of axillary examination are normal.

OBJECTIVE 1

The student formulates a differential diagnosis.
A. Injury
B. Keratoacanthoma
C. Skin cancer

OBJECTIVE 2

The student establishes a diagnosis.
A. Punch biopsy
B. Incisional biopsy (edge of the lesion)

OBJECTIVE 3

The student initiates appropriate therapy.
A. Radiation therapy is not usually used.
B. Surgery includes excision and split-thickness skin graft.

OBJECTIVE 4

The student provides appropriate follow-up.
A. The patient should avoid sun exposure (probably not critical in an 80-year-old patient).
B. The patient should return for follow-up at 3-month intervals to check for new primary skin cancers as well as nodal spread to the axilla.

Minimum Level of Achievement for Passing

The student establishes a tissue diagnosis of squamous cell carcinoma and recommends surgery or radiation therapy.

Honors Level of Achievement

The student lists the problems associated with radiation therapy (e.g., reduced joint range of motion) and recognizes that a skin graft is required to close the defect. The student also recognizes the need for follow-up to check for nodal spread or new skin cancers.

CASE 3

A 50-year-old forest ranger has a 6-mm nodule on the right cheek. Physical examination shows a freely movable, raised lesion with pearly borders.

OBJECTIVE 1

The student formulates a differential diagnosis.
A. Sebaceous cyst
B. Squamous cell carcinoma
C. Basal cell carcinoma

OBJECTIVE 2

The student establishes a diagnosis.
A. Punch biopsy
B. Excisional biopsy
C. Incisional biopsy

OBJECTIVE 3

The student initiates appropriate therapy.
A. Surgery
B. Radiation therapy
C. Cryosurgery

OBJECTIVE 4

The student provides appropriate follow-up.
A. The patient should use sunscreen.
B. The patient should avoid sun exposure.
C. The patient should return for periodic follow-up to check for new skin cancer.

Minimum Level of Achievement for Passing

The student establishes a diagnosis of basal cell carcinoma and recommends treatment with surgery or cryosurgery.

Honors Level of Achievement

The student compares cryosurgery with surgical excision. Points to consider include the freezing time for cryotherapy versus the need for an incision. Cryotherapy is fast, whereas surgery takes longer. In addition, the healing time differs (3–4 weeks for cryosurgery vs 1 week for surgery). The student recommends follow-up because of the risk of new skin cancers.

CASE 4

A 40-year-old woman was born in Australia, immigrated to the United States 10 years ago, and has worked on a farm in New Mexico for the last 10 years.

She has had a mole in the middle of her upper back for many years and believes that it has increased in size during the last few months.

Physical examination shows a 2-cm lesion that is flat, has irregular borders, and exhibits a variety of colors (white, blue, purple, and black).

OBJECTIVE 1

The student suspects that the patient has a malignant melanoma.

A. Identify the lesion as likely superficial spreading melanoma.

B. Identify other varieties of melanoma (nodular, lentigo maligna, and acral lentiginous).

C. Describe the characteristics of each variety.

OBJECTIVE 2

A. Identify the predisposing factors in the patient's history, including exposure to sunlight and a likely Celtic origin.

B. Identify additional predisposing factors, including heredity and a history of malignant melanoma.

OBJECTIVE 3

The student identifies the signs and symptoms of melanoma.

A. Identify the signs and symptoms of melanoma, including increase in size, irregular border, and variegated color.

B. List additional symptoms and signs, including pruritus, color change, scab formation, ulceration, "weeping," hemorrhage, nodularity, and satellitosis.

OBJECTIVE 4

The student describes how an excisional biopsy is performed.

A. Explain why an excisional biopsy is preferable, and identify when it is necessary.

B. Describe an elliptical incision that has 2- to 3-mm skin margins and a long axis toward the regional lymph nodes, if possible.

C. Describe field block anesthesia.

D. Verify that the biopsy specimen includes a full thickness of the skin and some subcutaneous tissue.

E. Describe acceptable closure of the defect.

Minimum Level of Achievement for Passing

The student accurately diagnoses the patient's melanoma, describes the predisposing factors, describes the signs and symptoms of melanoma, recognizes the need for excisional biopsy, and describes the procedure for excisional biopsy.

Honors Level of Achievement

The student discusses the diagnosis and treatment of melanoma. The student also provides additional information (e.g., discusses the evidence for and against the proposition that ultraviolet light is of etiologic significance).

CASE 5

A patient has a lesion on the anterior aspect of the right thigh. There are no palpable inguinal nodes. You suspect a melanoma and perform an excisional biopsy. The findings confirm your suspicion. No distant metastases are found. The pathology report is consistent with a superficial spreading melanoma that invades the reticular dermis and is 2.5 mm thick.

OBJECTIVE 1

The student is familiar with the classification and microstaging of melanomas.

A. Identify this tumor as clinical stage I.

B. Define clinical stages II (palpable regional nodes) and III (distant metastases).

C. Identify this lesion as Clark's level IV.

D. Discuss the definition of Clark's levels of tumor invasion:
1. Level I: Confined to the epidermis
2. Level II: Invading the papillary dermis
3. Level III: Invading the junction of the papillary and reticular dermis
4. Level IV: Invading the reticular dermis
5. Level V: Invading the subcutaneous fat

E. Discuss Breslow's method to determine tumor thickness (use of an ocular micrometer), and explain why this method is superior to Clark's approach (difficulties involved in identifying the junction of the papillary and reticular dermis and defining invasion of the reticular dermis).

OBJECTIVE 2

The student describes relations among clinical stages, Clark's levels of invasion, Breslow's classification of tumor thickness, and survival.

A. State that survival decreases with higher clinical stages, deeper levels of invasion, and greater tumor thickness.

B. Identify the approximate 5-year survival rate for each stage:
1. Stage I: 75%
2. Stage II: 66%
3. Stage III: 41%

Minimum Level of Achievement for Passing

The student describes the staging methods and explains the relation between clinical stage and survival.

Honors Levels of Achievement

The student also knows the 5-year survival rate for each stage.

CASE 6

A 35-year-old homosexual man has an 8-month history of multiple blue-red, 0.3- to 1.0-cm nodules on the skin of the left lower extremity. These lesions are more distal initially and progress superiorly.

OBJECTIVE 1

The student establishes a diagnosis of Kaposi's sarcoma. Excisional biopsy of a lesion shows undifferentiated mesenchymal cells.

OBJECTIVE 2

The student recognizes the following predisposing factors:

A. Immunosuppression. The student suspects that this patient has acquired immune deficiency syndrome. This condition also occurs in patients who undergo transplantation.

B. Ethnic background, including Jewish, Italian, and African

OBJECTIVE 3

The student institutes appropriate treatment.

A. Radiation (primary type of treatment)

B. Chemotherapy (sometimes helpful)

C. Surgery (sometimes helpful)

OBJECTIVE 4

The student recognizes the natural history of the disease.

A. Risk of other neoplasms, especially lymphoreticular neoplasm

B. Multifocal, rather than metastasizing, nature

Minimum Level of Achievement for Passing

The student establishes a diagnosis by biopsy.

Honors Level of Achievement

The student suggests the diagnosis of Kaposi's sarcoma. The student knows the relation of this disease to immunosuppression and ethnic background.

CASE 7

A 50-year-old man has a 6-cm mass in the right anterior thigh. The mass has been present for approximately 2 weeks. He struck his right thigh on a table edge approximately 6 weeks before he came to the clinic. The mass appears very firm, is fixed to the muscle fascia, and is nontender. Femoral and inguinal lymph nodes are 0.5 to 1.0 cm bilaterally.

OBJECTIVE 1

The student formulates a differential diagnosis.

A. Organizing hematoma

B. Sarcoma

C. Soft tissue neoplasm (typical age and location)

OBJECTIVE 2

The student establishes a diagnosis.

A. Ultrasound, computed tomography scan, and soft tissue x-rays

B. Incisional biopsy, which shows a high-grade malignant fibrous histiocytoma

OBJECTIVE 3

The student initiates appropriate therapy.

A. Wide local excision, including adjacent normal tissue

B. Role of a pseudocapsule as a misleading factor in the extent of excision; extension of tumor beyond the pseudocapsule

OBJECTIVE 4

The student provides appropriate follow-up. The student knows:

A. The risk of local recurrence (33%)

B. The likelihood of pulmonary metastasis through hematogenous spread (50%)

C. The low frequency of regional nodal metastasis (< 5%)

D. The single most important prognostic factor (histologic grade of the sarcoma)

Minimum Level of Achievement for Passing

The student establishes a histologic diagnosis. The student knows that metastasis occurs primarily through the bloodstream.

Honors Level of Achievement

The student recognizes the likelihood of sarcoma and suggests open biopsy followed by wide local excision. The student suggests local recurrence and pulmonary metastases as areas for particular vigilance. The student knows that the overall 5-year survival rate in this patient is approximately 30%.

CASE 8

A 23-year-old man who was previously in good health has Hodgkin's lymphoma. At diagnosis, the patient had no fever, night sweats, or weight loss. Biopsy of an anterior cervical lymph node showed nodular sclerosing Hodgkin's lymphoma.

OBJECTIVE 1

The student evaluates the patient.

A. The student discusses the initial evaluation, including chest x-ray, liver function tests, and abdominal studies, including computed tomography scan.

B. The student discusses the clinical stage of this patient, assuming that the results of these studies are normal (stage IA).

OBJECTIVE 2

The student initiates appropriate therapy.

A. Discuss the management options, including staging laparotomy. If the results are negative, the patient is treated with radiation. The 5-year survival rate is 90% to 95%.

B. Discuss the stage after a staging laparotomy shows involvement of the spleen and two celiac nodes (stage III^s).

C. Discuss the treatment of this patient, including the options of radiation therapy and chemotherapy. Radiation therapy and chemotherapy offer a 5-year survival rate of 60% to 70%.

D. Discuss the prognosis for this patient and the complications of therapy, including second malignancies and recurrence. The risk of secondary malignancy is increased when radiation and chemotherapy are combined.

Minimum Level of Achievement for Passing

The student performs a thorough initial evaluation and staging laparotomy. The student stages the tumor in all cases.

Honors Level of Achievement

The student has a thorough knowledge of clinical staging, appropriate therapy for the stage, and prognosis.

SUGGESTED READINGS

Malignant Diseases of the Skin

Balch CM, Houghton AN, Milton GW, et al. *Cutaneous Melanoma.* Philadelphia, Pa: JB Lippincott, 1992.

Balch CM, Houghton AN, Peters L. Cutaneous melanoma. In: DeVita VT, Hellman S, Rosenberg SA, eds. *Cancer: Principles and Practice of Oncology,* 4th ed. Philadelphia, Pa: JB Lippincott, 1993:1499–1542.

Fleming ID, Cooper JS, Henson DE, et al. *American Joint Committee on Cancer Staging Manual,* 5th ed. Philadelphia, Pa: Lippincott-Raven, 1997.

Patterson JAK, Geronemus RG. Cancers of the skin. In: DeVita VT, Hellman S, Rosenberg SA, eds. *Cancer: Principles and Practice of Oncology,* 4th ed. Philadelphia: JB Lippincott, 1993:1612–1650.

Sober AJ. Diagnosis and management of skin cancer. *Cancer* 1983;51:2448–2452.

Malignant Diseases of the Lymphatics and Soft Tissue

Brennan MF, Casper ES, Harrison LB, Shiu MH, Gaynor J, Hajdu SI. The role of multimodality therapy in soft tissue sarcoma. *Ann Surg* 1991;214(3):328–338.

Conlon B. Soft tissue sarcomas. In: Murphy GP, Lawrence W Jr, Lenhard RE, eds. *Textbook of Clinical Oncology,* 2nd ed. Atlanta, Ga: American Cancer Society, 1995:435–450.

Hartge P, Devesa S, Fraumeni J Jr. Hodgkin's and non-Hodgkin's lymphomas. Cancer Surveys 19/20. Trends in Cancer Incidence and Mortality, 1994.

Lawrence W Jr. Operative management of soft tissue sarcomas: impact of anatomic site. *Semin Surg Oncol* 1994;10:340–346.

Mazanet R, Antman KH. Adjuvant therapy for sarcomas. *Semin Oncol* 1991;18(6):603–612.

Rosenthal D, Eyre H. Hodgkin's disease and non-Hodgkin's lymphomas. In: Murphy GP, Lawrence W Jr, Lenhard RE, eds. *Textbook of Clinical Oncology,* 2nd ed. Atlanta, Ga: American Cancer Society, 1995:451–469.

25

Ethical Issues in Surgical Practice

Peter Angelos, M.D., Ph.D.

OBJECTIVES

1. Describe the components of informed consent, and explain how it is obtained from surgical patients.
2. Discuss the underlying principles of successful physician–patient communication.
3. List the types of advance directives used. Describe how physicians respond to advance directives and "do-not-resuscitate" orders.
4. Discuss the central goals of end-of-life care.

Ethical issues have become increasingly important in medicine and surgery over the last 35 years. During this period, both the expectations of patients and the behaviors of physicians have changed. The belief that physicians can best make decisions for patients (paternalistic approach), which was accepted for hundreds of years, became suspect. For many reasons, the authority of physicians was challenged and the need to respect patient autonomy became increasingly important. For example, at one time, physicians often did not tell patients that they had cancer. Now, physicians not only discuss diagnoses with their patients, but they also engage them in detailed discussions about options and alternatives for treatment.

This change in medical care is evident in all fields of medicine, but is most profound in surgery. The need to obtain **informed consent** for procedures has greatly influenced the daily activities of every surgeon. In addition, the growth of new fields of surgery has created new ethical challenges. For example, the development of transplant surgery has raised questions about brain death as well as how to equitably distribute the scarce number of organs available. A student on a surgical service must strive to understand the most important ethical issues that affect surgical patients. This chapter explores four issues that are central to the care of surgical patients: (1) informed consent, (2) physician–patient communication, (3) **advance directives** and do-not-resuscitate (DNR) orders, and (4) end-of-life care.

Although these issues are not unique to surgical patients, they are often emphasized because of the nature of surgery and the needs of surgical patients. In this chapter, the examples primarily concern patients with surgical problems, but the issues extend to all areas of medical care.

Informed Consent

For surgeons, obtaining informed consent is a central part of patient care. No operation or invasive test can be undertaken without the patient's informed consent. To obtain informed consent, two issues must be addressed. First, the patient must have the mental capacity **(competency)** to allow him or her to decide whether to participate in a procedure. The criteria for competency are difficult to define. However, a person is usually considered competent when he or she understands his or her condition and the consequences of the choices and the person's reasons for making the choices make sense to the medical and surgical staff. Second, the patient must be given sufficient information to make an informed decision. In most cases, a patient must be told the indications, risks, benefits, and alternatives before being asked to consent to a procedure. Although the requirements for informed consent seem straightforward, numerous questions can arise during the process.

Questionable Competency

In many cases, the competency of surgical patients to make informed choices is questioned. For example, a patient who recently used drugs or alcohol may not be able to make informed choices. If a patient needs surgery, but is intoxicated when he or she is brought to the emergency room, the procedure is delayed if possible until the patient can give consent. In an emergency, a **surrogate** gives consent for the patient. In most cases, the surrogate decision-maker is the next of kin. However, if no such person is available and the procedure is required to save the patient's life, the surgeon must record these facts and obtain consent in another fashion because of medical necessity. If adequate time is available, consent is usually obtained from a legally designated surrogate. However, this approach requires time and the involvement of legal counsel to obtain a judicial order naming a guardian to give consent for the patient. In most cases, there is not adequate time to proceed down this legal path. These situations are addressed in the next section. When a patient shows evidence of drug use, a physician need not try to obtain informed consent because the patient, who is not in control of all of his or her faculties, cannot make a choice. Just as a patient cannot be asked to give consent to an elective surgical procedure after being given narcotics for pain, an intoxicated patient cannot refuse consent for an urgent, potentially lifesaving procedure.

Emergency Situations

In a traumatically injured patient who needs emergency care, the stress and shock of the injury may be sufficient to prevent the patient from having the capacity to make decisions. As a general rule, when traumatically injured patients require urgent treatment for potentially life-threatening injuries, physicians can do whatever is urgently required to save the patient's life, even when informed consent is not obtained. This exception to the requirement for informed consent does not apply when there is no urgent need for intervention. In other words, in an emergency situation, after appropriate documentation is obtained, the surgeon may perform potentially lifesaving treatment without informed consent. The ethical basis for proceeding with surgery in these situations is presumed consent. The assumption that underlies this exception is that if the urgent intervention is undertaken and the patient survives, at a later time, when the patient has full decision-making capacity, the patient can decline medical care.

Hospitals have their own specific policies for the documentation that is necessary to operate on patients emergently without consent. In some institutions, if a patient cannot give consent, no family members can be reached, and the procedure is urgently required, documentation of these facts by the surgeon is adequate. In other hospitals, a hospital administrator must be notified and must give the consent that is documented in the chart. Regardless of the policy, the underlying principle is the same: in emergency situations, the physician should proceed without consent if necessary to attempt to save the patient's life.

Patients Who Refuse to Hear the Risks of a Procedure

Some patients who need surgical intervention do not want to be informed of the risks and possible complications. These patients often believe that if the procedure is recommended by the surgeon, following that advice is the best course. They would rather not worry about potential complications. Students and surgical residents sometimes believe that they must discuss these issues with a patient to obtain informed consent. In fact, patients need only to have the opportunity to be informed about a procedure. A patient who chooses to make a decision without this information should not be forced to hear the information. In this situation, the medical student or physician should record in the chart that the patient was offered information about the risks and complications, but declined to hear them. The ethical requirement to obtain informed consent should never be used as an excuse to give a patient potentially upsetting information if the patient declines this information.

Patients Who Request a Procedure That Is Not Indicated

Occasionally, a patient is convinced that a surgical procedure is required when there is no medical reason to perform it. In this case, the surgeon has no ethical or legal imperative to provide it. For example, a 50-year-old woman undergoes routine colonoscopy and removal of three benign adenomatous polyps, each smaller than 1.0 cm. The patient has no significantly increased risk of colon cancer. However, she goes to a surgeon and requests a total colectomy. In this situation, the surgeon need not respond to the patient's wishes because a colectomy is not indicated. In other words, patients should be given a choice of appropriate surgical options, but not a choice of inappropriate options.

Patients Who Refuse Life-Sustaining Treatment

Situations in which patients refuse life-sustaining treatments are especially difficult. The basic premise of informed consent is that patients are not operated on or treated against their will. However, as noted in the discussion on competency, sometimes patients are not competent to make decisions about their care. Often more difficult for surgeons are situations in which a patient seems competent, but refuses a procedure that is necessary to save his or her life. In this situation, another physician (preferably a psychiatrist) should determine whether the patient's reasoning capacity is adequate to refuse the life-sustaining procedure. As difficult as it is for a surgeon to see a patient die as a result of a reversible process because surgery was refused, it is important to remember that rational people can make irrational choices. A patient who makes a "bad" choice is not necessarily incompetent to make decisions. If a patient is clearly competent, but refuses a life-sustaining procedure, the medical record should reflect the fact that the patient was told of the risks of not having the surgery (including death), yet refused the procedure.

Conclusions

Informed consent for surgery is a process that extends beyond simply obtaining a patient's signature on a form. This process requires time for the patient to be educated about the procedure and to ask questions. The procedure must be explained in language that is understandable to the patient. The patient must be told specifically why the surgery is needed as well as the potential risks and benefits. Whenever possible in elective situations, it is helpful to have a family member or close friend present with the patient during this discussion because patients may have difficulty processing all of the information. The consent process should be undertaken no more than a few weeks before surgery. This process should be undertaken by someone who is well versed in the procedure and who understands and can clearly explain the risks and potential complications to the patient. The ideal person is the attending surgeon. In some cases, a senior surgical resident may have ade-

Table 25-1. Need for Written Informed Consent for Procedures

Procedure	Written Consent
Any operating room procedure	Required
Placement of chest tubes	Likely required
Placement of Swan-Ganz catheter	Likely required
Paracentesis	Likely required
Placement of arterial catheter	Possibly required
Placement of peripheral intravenous line	Unlikely required
Drawing blood	Not required

Table 25-2. Key Points in Giving Bad News

1. Select appropriate setting (e.g., quiet, private, no interruptions).
2. Assess patient's baseline knowledge.
3. Determine level of information patient is seeking.
4. Present information in clear, lay language, repeating key points and allowing time for questions.
5. Allow patient to respond, and acknowledge patient's response.
6. Summarize discussions, and make plans for further discussion.

Adapted with permission from Buckman R., How to break bad news: a guide for health care professionals.
Baltimore, Md: Johns Hopkins University Press, 1992.

quate knowledge and experience to undertake this discussion.

Hospitals often place great emphasis on the informed consent form. In many cases, little attention is given to the process as long as the patient signs the appropriate generic surgical consent form. Students and house staff should remember that the consent form is a hospital policy that is meant to ensure that the patient has completed the consent process. Often the consent process occurs in the surgeon's office several weeks before the surgery. Most hospital regulations require that the informed consent form be signed within 30 days of the procedure. Many hospitals require that the signing of the consent form be witnessed by someone other than the physician. This witness may be a nurse, resident, medical student, or family member. Who actually obtains the patient's signature on the form is of little importance as long as the informed consent process is undertaken before the patient signs the form.

Individual hospitals vary with respect to which procedures require written informed consent. Operating room procedures uniformly require written consent. Other invasive procedures usually need written consent as well. For example, a written consent form is usually required before placement of a chest tube. Written consent is less likely to be needed for less invasive procedures (Table 25-1).

The issues of informed consent are essential for medical students on surgery clerkships to understand. Nowhere beside surgery is the importance of informed consent as great. Although other physicians must obtain informed consent for certain tests and interventions, surgeons must clearly understand the requirements of informed consent when treating any patient who needs an operation. Every patient who is competent to make decisions about his or her own care must have the opportunity to make an informed choice. To be informed, a patient must have the opportunity to be told the indications, risks, benefits, and alternatives to the proposed procedure.

Physician–Patient Communication

Communication with patients is a challenging area for both medical students and young physicians. As with many other interactions, more experience leads to greater comfort. Although there is no substitute for experience, a few principles of effective communication are useful. First, communication requires that both parties participate and respond to each other. This principle is easy to forget because the physician must often provide a great deal of information that may be difficult for the patient to understand. Consider the case of a woman who recently underwent a breast biopsy. The physician reviewed the pathology report and now must discuss the diagnosis of breast cancer with the patient. When giving bad news, the physician must remember that communication involves being sensitive to the patient's needs and preferences as well as providing the patient with accurate information.

Delivering bad news is both an educational process and a receptive, responsive process. The appropriate setting is critical. Ideally, this conversation should occur in person, in a quiet setting that offers privacy. The physician must allow adequate time for an unhurried discussion. If possible, the conversation should be held in the presence of a family member or close friend with whom the patient will be discussing the news. The physician should assess the patient's underlying knowledge and the level of detail that the patient wishes to discuss. The information should be presented in clear, nonmedical terms, and the patient should be allowed to respond and ask questions. Repetition of key points is helpful. When a patient asks a question that cannot be answered, the physician should acknowledge that there is not yet an answer. When a patient asks a question about which there is tremendous uncertainty, the physician should acknowledge the uncertainty and avoid making unfounded predictions. At the end of the discussion, the physician should summarize the important points and plan for future discussions to address additional questions and concerns. This final step is critical because many patients are shocked by bad news and do not think of questions until later. Table 25-2 outlines this approach. Although the table suggests a sequence of steps, these steps are closely intertwined and may not proceed in a temporal fashion.

Communication between patients and other members of the health care team can be just as important as physician–patient communication. Students sometimes feel left out of discussions about patient communication; however, students often have more opportunity than other members of the team to develop a personal relationship with a patient. Medical students on surgical rotations must clearly understand the significance of their communication with patients to provide the most effective medical care and to be the most helpful to patients.

Patient Confusion about the Role of the Medical Student

Given the large numbers of health care providers with whom hospitalized patients come into contact, it is not surprising that patients often mistake medical students for residents or attending physicians. The only real ethical issue in this case is whether the medical student is clearly introduced as a medical student. Any other euphemism (e.g., student doctor, colleague of the attending physician) may be misleading. Medical students have the responsibility not to misrepresent their role. However, a student need not feel an ethical obligation to continuously correct a patient who refers to the student as "Doc." A patient may use the term loosely or as a sign of respect. Patients need not be faulted for this behavior; however, care must be taken to ensure that patients are not misled into believing that a medical student is a physician.

Families Who Request That the Patient Not Be Told of the Diagnosis

The relationship between a patient and members of the health care team can be stressed by any situation that deliberately impedes communication. One stressful situation occurs whenever family members request that a patient not be told of a diagnosis. For example, during exploratory laparotomy for a bowel resection, multiple liver metastases are unexpectedly found in a 42-year-old man. After the procedure, the surgeon discusses the findings with the family. The family requests that the patient not be told of the metastatic disease so that the patient "does not lose hope." If the attending surgeon honors this request, all communication between the patient and members of the health care team is compromised. Consider the medical student who is assigned to this patient. If the medical student is bound by a decision not to be truthful with the patient, little meaningful communication can occur. This situation is particularly onerous for a student or resident because patients often ask questions of these "junior" members of the team that they would not ask of an attending surgeon.

The impediments to communication among family members in this situation are illustrated by Tolstoy's story, *The Death of Ivan Ilych:*

> What tormented Ivan Ilych most was the deception, the lie, which for some reason, they all accepted, that he was not dying but was simply ill, and that he only need keep quiet and undergo a treatment and then something very good would result . . . this deception tortured him—their not wishing to admit what they all knew and what he knew, but wanting to lie to him concerning

his terrible condition and wishing and forcing him to participate in that lie.

It is the responsibility of the attending surgeon to avoid a situation in which information is withheld from a patient. The attending surgeon must explain the unfortunate consequences of withholding information from patients. These consequences should also be explained to the patient's family. Ultimately, the surgeon's primary responsibility is to the patient, and all information must be shared with the patient. Likewise, other members of the health care team should discourage family from avoiding a discussion of a patient's impending death.

Patients Who Refuse to Hear Negative Information

Students and physicians are sometimes frustrated by patients who seem to be oblivious to a poor prognosis and actively refuse to discuss a poor prognosis. This situation may be difficult for the health care team because it seems to run counter to the ideal of truthful communication with patients. However, as in the case of a patient who refuses to hear the risks of an operation, there is no absolute requirement that a patient be given information if the patient declines to listen. Members of the health care team should not purposefully withhold information, but once it is offered, if the patient declines to hear it, the patient's wishes should be honored.

Patients Who Request That the Family Not Be Told

The situation in which a patient requests that medical information not be shared with family members is both similar to and different from the situation in which the family requests that information be withheld from the patient. If a patient requests that family members not be told of his or her impending death, the impediments to communication within the family are similar to those described earlier. However, the physician's primary responsibility is to the patient. Unless there is a significant risk to others, the physician is not required to communicate information about the patient that the patient wants kept private.

Advance Directives and Do-Not-Resuscitate Orders

One of the greatest changes in patient care over the last 20 years is the increasingly common use of advance directives and DNR orders. Advance directives are instructions given by patients, before they become ill or incapacitated, that describe the care they wish to receive should they become unable to express their wishes. Informal advance directives are verbal expressions of these wishes. Formal advance directives are documents that provide evidence of the patient's wishes. Formal advance directives (referred to here simply as advance directives) usually take the form of a **living will** or a

durable power of attorney for health care. These documents extend patients' control over their decision making into the period after they are no longer competent. A living will describes a patient's preferences for treatment decisions if specific conditions are met. A durable power of attorney for health care names a specific person as the proxy decision-maker if the patient is not competent to make decisions.

A DNR order allows a patient (or surrogate) to choose not to undergo cardiopulmonary resuscitation (CPR) in the event of cardiac arrest. DNR orders are grounded in the respect for patient autonomy because they give patients (or surrogates) the chance to refuse consent for CPR.

Although advance directives and DNR orders are usually considered advances in an ethical approach to patient care, they can create dilemmas for the medical student or resident on a surgical service. Because many critically ill patients and many patients with known malignancies are treated on surgical services, the issues of advance directives and DNR orders are increasingly addressed by surgeons.

Conflicts Between the Wishes of Surrogate and Patient

If a patient has a durable power of attorney for health care and refuses treatment, but the named surrogate wants the patient to have the treatment, the conflict between the patient's wishes and the surrogate's wishes may appear to be difficult to resolve. However, a durable power of attorney for health care does not take effect until the patient is incompetent to make decisions. If the patient is fully able to make decisions, the wishes of the surrogate have no bearing. The surrogate assumes decision-making responsibility only if the patient is unable to make decisions.

A conflict may arise between the patient's wishes and the surrogate's decisions when the patient is incompetent to make decisions, but is conscious and able to express wishes. When a student or physician sees the expressed wishes of a patient overridden by a surrogate, the discomfort may be great. However, it is important not to give too much weight to the wishes of a patient who is not competent. When a surrogate makes decisions that are in direct conflict with the patient's stated wishes, all members of the health care team must strongly consider how much moral weight to grant to the patient's apparent wishes. Only if the physician is clearly acting in the patient's best interests can an argument be made to overrule the surrogate's decisions. Judicial intervention is required to overrule a surrogate in this situation, and it may be difficult to obtain.

Surrogates Who Refuse a Life-Sustaining Procedure for a Potentially Reversible Condition

The conflicts between beneficence and respect for patient autonomy are most apparent when an appropriate surrogate for an incompetent patient refuses to consent to treatment for a life-threatening, but potentially reversible condition. Beneficence is the principle of wanting to do good for (benefit) patients. Respect for patient autonomy (including the autonomy of surrogates) may contradict beneficence when the patient or surrogate defines the benefit for the patient differently than the health care provider. Although it may be difficult for the health care team to see a patient die of a potentially reversible condition, the patient or surrogate may define benefit in broader terms than strictly medical benefit. Although a student or resident may find this situation challenging, the decisions of patients or their surrogates must be respected.

Surgery Consultations for a Patient with a DNR Order

DNR orders are a recent phenomenon. Before the widespread use of CPR, DNR orders were not a concern. Now, as the ability to treat cardiac or pulmonary arrest has increased, more and more patients choose not to have CPR. A major problem with DNR orders in hospitals, however, is that they can mean different things to different people. One patient may have long-standing objections to CPR and therefore requests a DNR order every time she is admitted to the hospital. Another patient may have spent months in an intensive care unit and now has multiple-system organ failure. In this patient, the DNR order may be part of a broad withdrawal of supportive care.

The possibility that a DNR order may have multiple meanings is critical for the student or resident on a surgical service to realize. Often a request for a surgical consultation on a patient with a DNR order is met with the superficial response that a patient who has a DNR order certainly will not want surgery. Because DNR orders can be interpreted so differently by both patients and physicians, every patient who has a DNR order must be approached as an individual. In other words, knowing that a patient has a DNR order is not enough information to permit any conclusions to be drawn about what the patient might want if surgery were needed. The historical fact that a DNR order is in the chart should prompt additional questions about what the DNR order means to the patient and to the primary physician. Only by probing these issues further is it possible to determine whether having an operation, if needed, is congruent with the DNR order.

DNR Orders in the Perioperative Period

When a patient who has a DNR order requires an operation and consents to one, additional issues must be addressed. Foremost among these issues is how to treat the DNR order during the perioperative period. The difficulty in maintaining a DNR order in the operating room and the perioperative period is that the distinction between resuscitation and a general anesthetic cannot be clearly drawn. A general anesthetic often involves intubation, mechanical ventilation, fluids or pressors, and even cardiac drugs. Outside the operating room, any of these interventions would meet the definition of resuscitation, but under a general anesthetic, these interventions are part of routine care. Largely because of the difficulty in defining resuscitation in the operating room, many hospitals have policies that routinely cancel all DNR orders in patients who go to the operating room. This type of blanket policy inappropriately limits patients' opportunities to make choices about their care.

Because of the problems associated with DNR orders in surgical patients, both the American College of Surgeons and the American Society of Anesthesiologists endorse an approach called required reconsideration. This approach sets a definition of resuscitation individually for each patient who receives a general anesthetic. The surgeon or anesthesiologist negotiates the goals of the procedure and the patient's wishes relative to an agreed-on definition of resuscitation.

End-of-Life Care

In recent years, patients and physicians have paid increasing attention to end-of-life care. The growth of the hospice movement and the field of palliative medicine are evidence of the need to continue this focus on how to care for patients when a cure is no longer possible. Although medical students spend large amounts of time in hospitals that emphasize highly technical curative medicine, a consideration of issues at the end of life is necessary.

Discussing Death with a Dying Patient

Discussing impending death with a patient and family is a difficult, but important task of the surgeon. Medical students on surgical services should attempt to observe these discussions whenever possible because there is no easy way to learn how to have such a discussion. As the locus of medical care moves out of the hospital and into the outpatient setting, medical students have less opportunity to witness these critical interactions. The goal in any discussion of impending death is to provide accurate information while sustaining the ongoing relationship with the patient and family. Although there is no right way to have such a conversation, a rule of thumb is to offer information and be prepared to provide more detail if the patient requests it. It is best to avoid predicting how long a patient is likely to survive unless the uncertainty of these predictions is emphasized. Predicting how long a patient has to live often establishes an adversarial relationship with the patient or family (who may want to prove the doctor wrong). The goal for students is to observe as many such interactions as possible so that the student can consider alternative approaches to the discussion, depending on the patient's wishes.

Surrogates Who Request a "Futile" Procedure

Futility is a concept that is often raised in end-of-life care. Occasionally, a patient is believed to have so many medical problems that continued treatment is an exercise in futility. In this case, physicians may want to limit interventions because they are believed to be futile. According to this line of argument, physicians have no obligation to provide futile treatment. The problem is that futility often cannot be objectively determined.

Whenever futility is raised as the basis for opposing treatment, it is important to ask, "Futile in relation to what?" In other words, futility is based on an assumption about a person's values. To say that a treatment is futile is really to say that its burdens significantly outweigh its benefits. However, health care providers may be poorly positioned to decide what will benefit a patient because benefit applies to more than the patient's medical state.

Some authors define futility in strictly numeric terms. Schneiderman and colleagues suggest that when a treatment is not effective in 100 consecutive cases, it is considered futile. In other words, if the chances of success of a medical intervention are sufficiently remote, the intervention is considered futile. The problem with this approach is that deciding which cases are sufficiently similar to meet this criterion is difficult. Further, a physician's willingness to recommend a medical intervention that has little chance of success seems dependent on how much pain, suffering, time, expense, and effort are involved. Therefore, futility implies more than just the unlikelihood of success. It also implies that even the remote potential benefits are outweighed by the burdens to the patient.

Rather than relying on futility to provide a medical reason why certain treatments should not be undertaken, health care givers should discuss with the patient the benefits and burdens of the proposed treatment. In this way, the complexity of the decision is acknowledged and discussed. Avoiding the use of the concept of futility helps to combat the misconception by both patients and physicians that futility can be defined by physicians, independent of the patient's values.

Patients or Surrogates Who Request Discontinuation of Mechanical Ventilation

The request to withdraw mechanical ventilation by a critically ill patient or appropriate surrogate can be unsettling, especially when there is reason to believe that the patient's medical condition is reversible. Despite the psychological difficulty caused by this situation, however, it is analogous to that described in the section on informed consent. Competent patients or their surrogates can refuse consent for any intervention, including mechanical ventilation.

Further, there is no moral difference between discontinuing mechanical ventilation and refusing to initiate it. In other words, the outdated view that once started, certain medical interventions (e.g., mechanical ventilation) cannot be stopped, is patently false from both legal and moral standpoints.

Treatment of Patients After Life Support Is Withdrawn

Physicians are trained primarily in the curative model of medical care: the goal of medicine is to conquer disease and cure patients. Given this model, whenever the goal of medical care moves away from cure, physicians and medical students may feel uncomfortable with continued interaction with the patient and family. The recent emphasis on palliative care is an attempt to shift the focus of medicine away from the predominant cure model. Nevertheless, extra efforts are often necessary to maintain a relationship with a patient when cure is no longer considered an option.

When life-sustaining treatment is withdrawn, the goal of medical intervention shifts to caring for the patient in a broader sense. Attempts are made to meet the physical, psychological, and social needs of the patient and family. The best way to meet these needs is often to continue to maintain a relationship with the patient and family. Only by continuing to engage the patient and family, even during the dying process, can the health care team effectively provide care after life support is withdrawn.

Conclusion

This chapter examined important ethical issues in the care of surgical patients. The topics chosen are not exhaustive of the field of medical ethics, nor are they unique to surgical patients. However, they are areas of particular importance to the care of surgical patients, and they provide opportunities for the medical student to observe important interactions. Although many other ethical issues arise in relation to rare conditions and experimental procedures, the issues presented in this chapter are commonly encountered by surgeons in clinical practice. Students who pay close attention to these issues will have greater confidence when addressing them as a resident and an attending physician.

Multiple-Choice Questions

1. Informed consent is not required of patients who are undergoing surgery when:
   A. The patient is intoxicated, and no family members are available to provide consent for elective surgery
   B. The patient is intoxicated, and no family members are available to provide consent for emergency surgery
   C. The patient is intoxicated, and family members are present at the time of elective surgery
   D. The patient is intoxicated, and family members are present at the time of emergency surgery
   E. The patient is not intoxicated, but is refusing a lifesaving operation

2. A living will:
   A. Cannot be rescinded by the patient once it is drawn up
   B. Takes effect whenever the patient is admitted to the hospital, regardless of whether the patient is competent
   C. Takes effect when the patient is no longer competent to make decisions
   D. Increases the influence of paternalism over patient choices
   E. Can be used to justify overriding a competent patient's wishes

3. Durable power of attorney for health care documents:
   A. Name surrogate decision-makers for patients who are not competent to make decisions
   B. Cannot be used to provide consent for surgery
   C. Cannot be used to justify a do-not-resuscitate (DNR) order in a comatose patient
   D. Take effect only in patients who have terminal conditions
   E. May cause problems when a competent patient disagrees with the wishes of the named surrogate

4. Which of the following statements is true of do-not-resuscitate (DNR) orders?
   A. They may be written only for patients with terminal conditions.
   B. They may be written only for patients who have acquired immune deficiency syndrome or cancer.
   C. They may be written only for competent patients.
   D. They may be written for competent patients or incompetent patients who have a surrogate.
   E. They may be written against the wishes of competent patients.

5. A do-not-resuscitate (DNR) order in a patient's chart means:
   A. The patient is not a surgical candidate
   B. The patient should not have expensive diagnostic tests
   C. The patient wishes to die
   D. All of the above
   E. None of the above

6. Which statement is true of do-not-resuscitate (DNR) orders in the operating room?
   A. Patients with DNR orders should never have surgery.
   B. Limits to intraoperative care by surgeons and anesthesiologists should be reviewed with the patient preoperatively.
   C. Resuscitation is easily distinguished from routine intraoperative care.
   D. Patients with DNR orders should never have general anesthesia.
   E. DNR orders in the operating room are relevant only to surgeons and are of no concern to anesthesiologists.

7. Which description of informed consent is true?
   A. The patient must be told all major risks of any procedure, even if he or she prefers not to hear them.
   B. Patients are not told of risks of procedures that will likely cause them major concern.
   C. Patients are given the opportunity to hear the indications, risks, and benefits of a surgical procedure.
   D. The standards for informed consent do not apply when a patient is incompetent, even if a surrogate is available.
   E. Informed consent is not required if the patient needs the operation to survive.

8. If a patient appears to be competent, but refuses a life-sustaining treatment, what step is taken next?
   A. Intravenous sedation is given and emergency surgery is performed so that informed consent is not required.
   B. No further steps are needed because any patient may refuse any procedure.
   C. Psychiatric consultation is provided to determine the patient's ability to competently refuse surgery.
   D. The chairman is called and asked to override the patient's refusal of surgery.
   E. The hospital attorney is asked to obtain a court order for surgery.

9. When used as an argument against further treatment, which statement about the concept of futility is true?
   A. Futility is a precise medical term that is well defined and accepted by most physicians.
   B. Futility clearly defines the limits of what physicians must provide.
   C. Futility is determined by physicians on an individual basis by carefully reviewing the patient's chart and determining the overall prognosis.
   D. Futility is a complex concept that is related to the benefits and burdens of the intervention under discussion and that requires exploration of the patient's values.
   E. None of the above

10. Which of the following statements about communication with patients and family members is true?
    A. Family members are encouraged to openly discuss even a poor prognosis with the patient.
    B. Patients are encouraged not to discuss a poor prognosis with their families to avoid upsetting them.
    C. Physicians carefully avoid mentioning a poor prognosis to avoid diminishing all hope.
    D. Patients and families are given as little information as possible so that they need not feel burdened by a bad prognosis.
    E. Physicians should share a poor prognosis only with family members and keep this information from patients.

Oral Examination Study Questions

CASE 1

A 30-year-old woman comes to the emergency room with signs and symptoms that suggest acute appendicitis. The patient is hesitant to have the operation and declines to give consent. Discuss the ramifications of this decision with the patient.

OBJECTIVE 1

The student conducts a standard informed consent discussion. The student describes the indications, risks, and benefits of appendectomy in the face of presumed acute appendicitis.

OBJECTIVE 2

The student describes situations in which a patient can refuse a potentially lifesaving procedure. The patient's competency is addressed by assessing the patient's ability to reason and to understand the potential consequences of refusing treatment.

OBJECTIVE 3

The student describes the elements that must be included in the patient's chart to document the discussion. A psychiatry consultation should be considered.

Minimum Level of Achievement for Passing

The student describes the specific issues that must be covered when obtaining informed consent (indications, risks, and benefits). The student describes situations in which a patient can refuse lifesaving procedures.

Honors Level of Achievement

The student describes the steps that are necessary to allow a patient to refuse life-sustaining treatment. These steps include a formal assessment of the patient's competency to make decisions about health care and complete documentation of the discussion in the chart.

CASE 2

A 78-year-old man was diagnosed 3 months ago with metastatic adrenocortical carcinoma. He has been in a coma for the last 2 weeks, with an overall worsening condition. He is now intubated and ventilated. The family wants to withdraw support.

Review the important issues relevant to this decision. Provide a cogent ethical argument for discontinuing ventilator support.

OBJECTIVE 1

The student reviews with the family the patient's formal or informal advance directives. The student explains the difference between a living will and a durable power of attorney for health care. An advance directive should be used correctly to make treatment decisions.

OBJECTIVE 2

The student describes acceptable ethical arguments for withdrawing treatment, regardless of whether the patient has a formal advance directive.

Minimum Level of Achievement for Passing

The student describes the different types of advance directives and explains how each is applied in this case.

Honors Level of Achievement

The student provides thoughtful arguments for withdrawing treatment, regardless of whether the patient has an advance directive.

CASE 3

A 60-year-old woman was recently diagnosed with colon cancer. She has multiple metastases in the liver and lungs. She has considered her poor long-term prognosis and wants to discuss having a do-not-resuscitate (DNR) order formalized in case she is admitted to the hospital. She requests an explanation of a DNR order and its implications for her future medical care.

OBJECTIVE 1

The student explains the difference between a DNR order and an advance directive. The student explains cardiopulmonary resuscitation (CPR) in lay terms and describes the concept of presumed consent as the basis for providing CPR.

OBJECTIVE 2

The student explains the limitations of a DNR order in directing medical care. The student also compares the implications of a DNR order with those of a durable power of attorney for health care.

Minimum Level of Achievement for Passing

The student understands and explains the difference between an advance directive and a DNR order.

Honors Level of Achievement

The student explains the limitations of a DNR order or a living will compared with a durable power of attorney for health care.

SUGGESTED READINGS

Buckman R. *How to Break Bad News: A Guide for Health Care Professionals.* Baltimore, Md: Johns Hopkins University Press 1992.

Cohen CB, Cohen PJ. Do-not-resuscitate orders in the operating room. *N Engl J Med* 1991;325:1782–1797.

Edwards WS, Yahne C. Surgical informed consent: what it is and is not. *Am J Surg* 1987;154:574–578.

Haeckler C, Moseley R, Vawter D, eds. *Advance Directives in Medicine: Legal, Ethical, and Medical Considerations.* New York, NY: Praeger Press, 1989.

Schneiderman LJ, et al. Medical futility: its meaning and ethical implications. *Ann Intern Med* 1990;112:949–954.

Truog RD, Brett AS, Frader J. The problem with futility. *N Engl J Med* 1992;326:1560–1564.

Weir RF, Gostin L. Decisions to abate life-sustaining treatment for nonautonomous patients. *JAMA* 1990;264:1846–1853.

26 Surgical Procedures, Techniques, and Skills

Richard M. Bell, M.D.

The Operating Room

The surgical theater can be an uncomfortable place for the novice. The intensity of the environment and the regulations that govern the maintenance of sterile technique add to the awkwardness and anxiety. Fortunately, the code of conduct is straightforward and easily learned. The operating room is the arena where the student physician can actually see and touch the pathology. Surgeons use this opportunity to demonstrate how surgical therapy affects the disease process, to demonstrate living human anatomy, and to discuss normal and pathologic physiology.

Attire

Knowledge of the surgical environment and the meticulous practice of **asepsis** and **sterile technique** are required. Infectious complications increase hospital stay, patient discomfort, costs, and the risk of death and disfigurement. For the student, participation in the care of the surgical patient and admission to the surgical suite are privileges.

Proper design of facilities and regulations for attire and conduct in the surgical suite are important factors in preventing the transportation of microorganisms into the operating room. To minimize the transportation of virulent hospital pathogens directly into the surgical arena, street clothes are never worn within restricted areas of the surgical suite and operating room attire is not worn outside of the operating area. All persons who enter restricted areas are required to wear clean surgical apparel, including hats, scrub clothes, shoe covers, and face masks. Each item of surgical garb is designed to protect the patient from contamination from hair, fomites (objects, such as clothing, that might harbor a disease agent), and microorganisms in the air.

The hat, or hood, covers and contains all hair. It fits snugly, and the edges are secured by elastic or drawstrings. Personnel with long hair can wear hoods that tie under the chin.

Scrub clothes are made of a closely woven fabric that is flame resistant, lint-free, cool, and comfortable. A large variety of scrub suits are available. They should fit closely, and shirts and drawstrings should be tucked into the pants.

All persons who enter the restricted areas of the surgical suite wear shoe covers. They are changed between operative procedures and are never worn outside the operating area.

High–filtration-efficiency disposable masks are worn at all times in the operating room. These masks are tied securely to cover the mouth and nose entirely. To prevent cross-infection, masks are handled only by the strings. They are never lowered to hang loosely around the neck. Masks are changed frequently and promptly discarded after use.

Protective glasses or face shields are worn to prevent inoculation of the eyes with body fluids or irritant solutions.

Scrubbed team members also wear sterile gowns and gloves. Most institutions use water-repellent disposable gowns. Although the entire gown is sterilized, neither the back nor any area below the waist or above the chest is considered sterile after the gown is donned. The cuffs are made of stockinette to fit the wrist tightly. Sterile gloves cover the wrists.

Scrubbing

Sterilization of the skin is not possible. However, every effort is made to reduce the bacterial count and minimize the possibility of microbial contamination. The surgical scrub is a process of mechanical scrubbing with a chemical antiseptic solution. General preparations for the surgical scrub include ensuring that the fingernails are short and unpolished, removing all hand jewelry, cleaning under each fingernail, and performing a short prescrub of the hands and arms.

The following anatomic pattern of scrubbing is suggested: the fingernails, the four surfaces of each finger, the dorsal surface of the hand, the palmar surface of the hand, and the area over the wrists and up the arm, ending 2 inches above the elbow (Figure 26-1). Because the hands are in most direct contact with the **sterile field,** all steps of the scrub procedure begin with the hands and end at the elbows. After the scrub, the hands and forearms are held higher than the elbows. In this way, contaminated water can roll off at the elbow and not run down the arms to contaminate the hands (Figure 26-2). The hands and arms are also held away from the body.

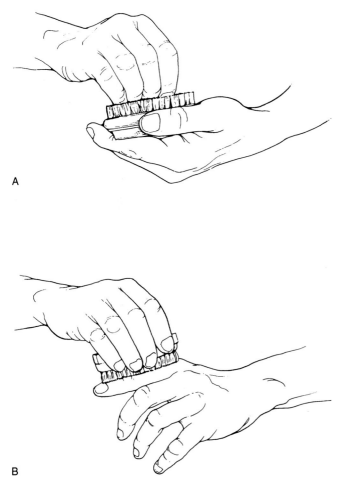

A

B

Figure 26-1 A, Use of a bristle brush to scrub the fingernails. **B,** The anatomic pattern of scrubbing. Four surfaces of each finger are scrubbed.

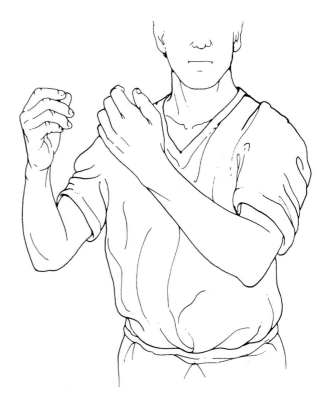

Figure 26-2 The arms and forearms are held away from the body and higher than the elbows.

To dry the hands, a folded sterile towel is grasped with one hand. The towel is allowed to unfold without touching any sterile object. One arm is dried by holding the towel in the opposite hand. Drying is begun at the fingers and hand. The arm is then rotated, and the towel is drawn up to the elbow. The used portion is never brought back into the dry area. The towel is then reversed, and the opposite hand and arm are dried with the unused part of the towel. The towel is discarded in the appropriate container.

Gowning and Gloving

A person who is gowning unassisted picks up the gown, taking care to touch only the inner surface. The gown is held by the inside and allowed to unfold, with the inside of the gown toward the body. With the hands at shoulder level, the arms are inserted into the sleeves. The arms remain extended, and the **circulating nurse** assists by pulling the gown over the shoulders and tying it in the back.

If a **closed-gloving technique** is used (gowning and gloving without assistance), the hands are advanced to the edge of the cuff, but not through it (Figure 26-3A).

With this method, the gloves are handled through the fabric of the gown sleeves. The hands are pushed through the cuff openings as the gloves are pulled on. With this technique, the glove is placed palm down onto the pronated forearm of the matching hand, with the fingers of the glove pointing toward the elbow and the glove cuff on the gown wristlet (Figure 26-3B). The glove is held securely by the hand on which it is placed. The other hand is used to stretch the cuff over the sleeve opening to cover the gown wristlet (Figure 26-3C). The cuff is drawn back onto the wrist, and the fingers are adjusted (Figure 26-3D). The gloved hand is used to position the other glove on the opposite sleeve in the same fashion (Figure 26-3E).

If an **open-gloving technique** is used, the hands are advanced completely through the cuffs of the gown (Figure 26-4). The left glove is removed from the package by placing the fingers of the right hand on the folded-back cuff, touching only the inner surface of the glove. The left hand is inserted into the glove, but the cuff is not turned up. The right glove is taken from the package by slipping the gloved left fingers under the inverted cuff and pulling the glove into the right hand. The cuffs are pulled over the gown wristlet by rotating the arm slightly.

If the **scrub nurse** assists with gowning and gloving, the nurse holds the gown open with the inner side toward the person who is gowning. The arms are inserted into the gown. The circulating nurse reaches inside the gown, grasps the sleeve seam, pulls the gown

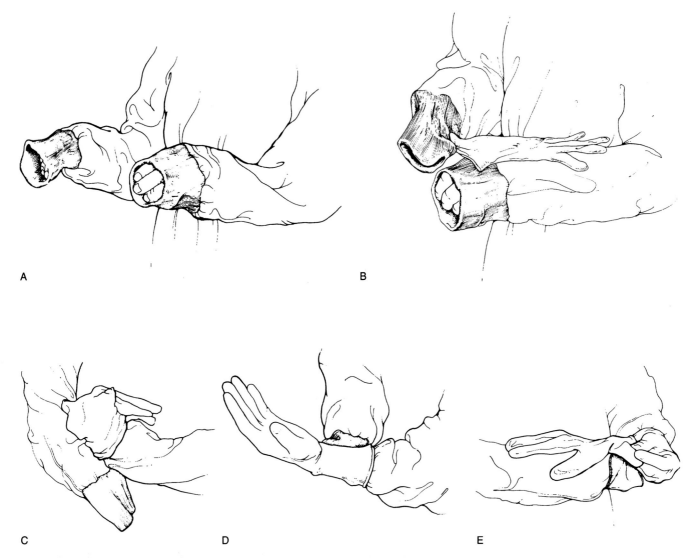

A

B

C

D

E

Figure 26-3 The closed-gloving technique. **A,** The hands are advanced to the edge of the cuff, but not through the cuff. **B,** The glove is placed down on the forearm, with the fingers pointed toward the elbow. **C,** The other hand stretches the glove over the gown wristlet (through the gown fabric). **D,** The cuff is drawn back onto the wrist. **E,** The gloved hand is used to pull on the remaining glove in the same way.

on, and ties the back closure. After the gown is on, the scrub nurse holds the gloves open, and the hands are slipped into them.

After gloving, the exterior ties in the front of the gown are untied. The tie that is attached to the back of the gown is handed to another person who is gowned and gloved. The other tie is held securely, and the person turns in the opposite direction to close the back panel of the gown. The tie is retrieved and tied securely at the side.

A glove that becomes contaminated is changed immediately. If a question about contamination arises, it is best to change gloves or both gown and gloves. The hand with the contaminated glove is extended to the circulating nurse, who grasps the outside of the glove cuff and pulls it off inside out. Surgical personnel should not attempt to remove a glove unassisted because the other hand may become contaminated. The sleeve wristlet is pulled down over the hand when the

glove is removed because the new glove could be contaminated by the gown sleeve. If possible, another sterile team member assists with the regloving. If this assistance is not possible, the person steps aside and applies the new glove with the open-gloving technique.

To remove the gown and gloves properly, the gown is removed first by pulling it down from the shoulders and turning the sleeves inside out while the arms are pulled from the sleeves. The gloves are removed by turning them inside out and protecting the hands by not touching the outer, soiled surface (Figure 26-5). As a matter of courtesy and to contain contaminants, the gown and gloves are discarded in the receptacles provided.

Some procedures that are associated with large concentrations of bacteria pose additional risk of infection. These procedures are known as dirty, contaminated, or septic. Special practices may be necessary to confine potentially infectious material (e.g., intraabdominal

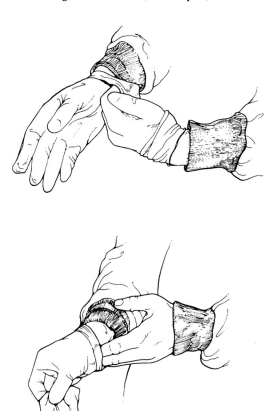

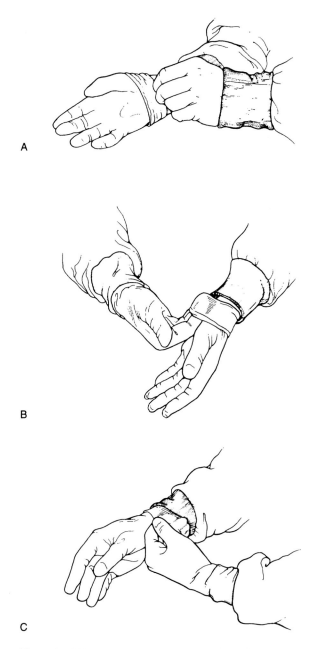

Figure 26-5 Gloves are removed by turning them inside out without touching the soiled part with the hands.

Figure 26-4 The open-gloving technique. **A,** The left ungloved hand pulls on the right glove, touching only the inner surface. **B,** The gloved fingers of the right hand are inserted under the cuff, and the glove is pulled onto the left hand. **C,** The glove cuffs are pulled over the gown wristlets.

sepsis, empyema, gross fecal contamination, perirectal abscesses). Personnel should remove the gown, gloves, shoe covers, hat, and mask before leaving the operating room.

Principles of Asepsis and Sterile Technique

A simple definition of asepsis is the absence of any infectious agents. However, the term is also used broadly to describe a wide variety of procedures that reduce the incidence of infection in patients and hospital personnel. These practices include sterilization of goods and supplies, disinfection of the hospital environment, **antisepsis** of animate objects, and environmental control of the operating room.

Sterilization is the process that kills all forms of living matter, including bacteria, viruses, yeast, and mold. Special equipment for this process uses **moist heat, dry heat,** or **ethylene oxide gas.**

Moist heat destroys all forms of microbial life, including spores, through denaturation and coagulation of intracellular protein. The essential factors are temperature, time, and pressure. A temperature of 250°F, a time exposure of 15 to 30 minutes, and a pressure of 15 to 17 pounds per square inch are required to kill all microorganisms. Other variables are the size, contents, and packaging methods of the materials to be sterilized.

A high-speed instrument sterilizer, the autoclave (flash sterilizer), is used for moist-heat sterilization in the operating room. The autoclave functions rapidly at a high temperature and increased pressure. To sterilize unwrapped instruments, the requirements are 270°F, 27 pounds of pressure, and minimum exposure time of 3 minutes.

Dry-heat sterilization is used only for articles that cannot tolerate the corrosive action of steam or for products that cannot be penetrated by steam or gas (e.g., petroleum products, powders, glassware, delicate instruments). In the absence of moisture, higher temperature and longer exposure times are required: 340°F for 1 hour, 280°F for 3 hours, and 250°F for 6 hours.

Sterilization with ethylene oxide gas kills bacteria by reacting with the chemical components of the cell protein. This type of sterilization is particularly useful for items that cannot withstand moisture or high heat (e.g., lensed instruments, air-powered instruments, glassware, paper or rubber products). This type of sterilization depends on gas concentration, temperature, humidity, and exposure time.

A biologic control test provides assurance of sterilization. Process monitors (e.g., heat-sensitive tape) indicate exposure to sterilization conditions, but do not assure sterility. Packaged items are marked with a sterilization date. The time that a sterile package may be kept in storage without compromising its sterility is its shelf life. Shelf life depends on the conditions of storage, the packaging materials, the seal of the package, and the integrity of the package. Any package that is outdated, exposed to moisture, dropped on the floor, or punctured is considered contaminated.

The hospital environment is disinfected with chemical agents that destroy pathogenic bacteria on inanimate surfaces. The operating room and all furniture (e.g., operating table, instrument tables, lights) are cleaned with chemical disinfectants after each operation.

Antisepsis is the use of chemical agents to destroy bacteria on animate surfaces. Before an operative procedure is begun, personnel perform the surgical scrub on the hands and arms with antiseptic soaps. The patient's skin is also carefully prepared to create an area with reduced levels of bacteria.

Environmental control of the surgical suite is essential to minimize contamination and provide maximum protection for the patient. These factors include maintaining greater air pressure in the room than in the hallway so that air is forced out of the surgical area. Additional measures include restricting traffic, controlling the room temperature (68–72°F), controlling the humidity (50%), and maintaining an air change rate of 18 to 25 times per hour.

A variety of measures and controls are used to maintain an environment that is as sterile and free of bacteria as possible. The integrity of this environment depends on strict adherence by all personnel to sterile technique. To minimize the risk of infection, attention to the following principles of sterile technique is essential.

1. Only sterile items are used within a sterile field. The sterility of these items is provided by proper packaging, sterilization, and handling.

2. Parts of a gown that are considered sterile are the sleeves and the front from the waist to the shoulder level.
3. Tables are sterile only at table level (top). The edges and sides below table level are not sterile.
4. The edges of anything that encloses sterile contents (e.g., packaging) are not sterile.
5. Persons who are sterile touch only items that are sterile. Persons who are not sterile touch only items that are not sterile.
6. Sterile persons stay within the sterile area. Persons who are not sterile avoid entering the sterile area.
7. Sterile persons avoid leaning over an area that is not sterile. Persons who are not sterile avoid reaching over a sterile area.
8. Sterile persons minimize contact with an area that is not sterile.
9. A sterile field is created immediately before use.
10. Sterile areas are continuously kept in view.
11. If the integrity of the microbial barriers is destroyed, contamination occurs.
12. Microorganisms are kept to a minimum.

A sterile field is created by the placement of sterile sheets and towels in a specific position to maintain the sterility of the operative surfaces. The patient and the operating table are covered with drapes so that the site of incision is exposed, yet isolated (Figure 26-6). Objects that are draped include instrument tables, basins, the Mayo stand, and trays. Sterile team members function within this limited area and handle only sterile items. All members of the operating team constantly safeguard the sterility of the operative field.

Surgical Preparation

A wide area of skin around the operative incision is meticulously prepared by shaving and scrubbing. Shaving is performed just before the procedure and ideally outside the operative theater. Skin preparation cleanses the operative site of transient and resident microorganisms, dirt, and skin oil.

Skin preparation is usually carried out from a separate table (prep table). After the patient is positioned on the operating table, one member of the surgical team prepares the patient's skin with antiseptic solution. Sterile gloves are worn. The incision line is scrubbed first, and the team member works outward, toward the periphery of the field (Figure 26-7). Theoretically, the incision line is the cleanest area. The number of organisms increases with increasing distance from the incision site. After the lateral limits of the operative field are reached, the sponge is discarded. The process is repeated with a new sponge. The sponge is never brought from the outside of the field to repeat the scrub of the central incision area. Areas that are likely to contain large numbers of bacteria (e.g., perineum, groin, axilla) are washed last. Cleansing is done vigorously, with particular attention given to difficult areas (e.g., umbilicus). Cotton-tipped applicators may be used in the umbilical area. Towels are used to absorb excess

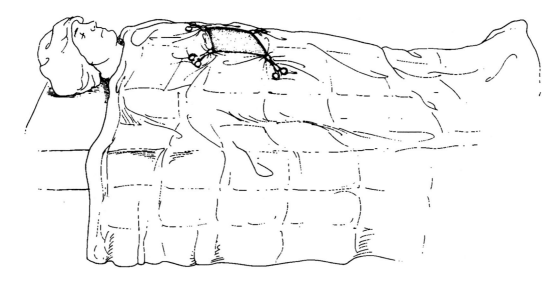

Figure 26-6 The incision site is exposed, yet isolated.

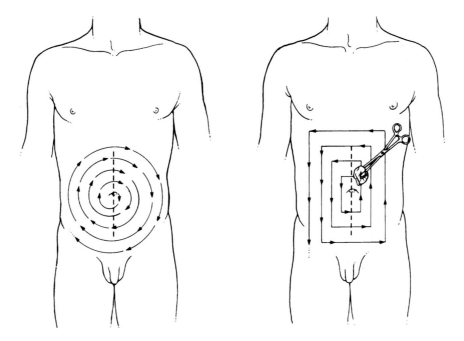

Figure 26-7 Preparation of the operative site. Movement is from the center toward the periphery.

solution and prevent the solution from pooling under the patient.

The procedure for applying antiseptic solution to various parts of the body may vary, depending on the site and the surgeon's preference. Painting of the operative area with antiseptic solution follows the same principles as the scrub (i.e., from the center toward the periphery). After the skin is prepared, the patient is ready for draping.

Draping involves covering the patient and the surrounding areas with a sterile barrier to create a sterile area. Drapes are fluid resistant, antistatic, abrasive-free,

lint-free, and flexible enough to fit contours. The following standard principles for draping are followed:

1. Place drapes on a dry area.
2. Handle the drapes as little as possible. Avoid shaking them because air currents carry contaminants.
3. Make a cuff over the gloved hand to protect the hand from contacting an area that is not sterile.
4. Never reach across the table to drape the opposite side; instead, go around the table.
5. Hold the drape high enough to avoid touching areas that are not sterile.

6. After a drape is placed, do not adjust it. If a drape is placed incorrectly, discard it.
7. Unfold the drape toward the feet first.
8. Place the folded edge toward the incision to provide a smooth outline of the field. Prevent instruments or sponges from falling between the layers.
9. Any part of the drape below waist level or table level is considered contaminated and should not be handled.
10. Towel clips that are fastened through the drapes have contaminated points. Remove them only if necessary, and discard them.
11. If a hole is found after a drape is placed, cover that area with another barrier.

Draping procedures may vary from one hospital to another; however, standardized methods of application are followed.

Assisting in the Operating Room

A student is often asked to assist during an operative procedure. Assisting can produce a spectrum of emotional responses that varies from elation to fear and trepidation. Usually, undergraduates are asked to hold retractors or provide other measures to gain exposure for the operating surgeon. The assistant is often excluded from the field of view and asked to maintain an uncomfortable position while pulling on a retractor with strength that has long been spent. In addition, the assistant may feel ill, exhausted, or worried, and may anticipate a barrage of questions about regional anatomy, physiology, or surgical technique. Most surgeons respond positively to students who show an interest and some evidence of independent study about the patient or the operation. Because most surgical procedures are elective, students usually have time to become familiar with the basic operative steps.

The following checklist may help the student prepare for the role of assistant or observer in the operating room. A well-prepared student is more likely to have a positive experience and to make a contribution to the team's effort.

- What procedure is planned?
- What is the regional anatomy?
- What are the normal physiology and the pathophysiology of the organ?
- What are the surgical and nonsurgical treatment options?
- What is the effect of the procedure on the pathophysiology?
- What are the potential complications?

In most cases, the operative plan is clear (e.g., cholecystectomy for cholelithiasis). A review of the regional anatomy is always beneficial. The blood supply to the organs involved, the lymphatic drainage, and the proximity to other vital structures (e.g., relation of the common bile duct to the portal vein or hepatic artery) are important. A surgical atlas may be the best reference for anatomic detail because this type of text approaches the subject from a surgeon's perspective.

Most surgeons assume that students can describe the normal physiology of the organ or organ systems involved. An understanding of the abnormal, or pathophysiologic, process is the goal of most undergraduate clerkships.

Most problems have more than one surgical approach in addition to nonsurgical approaches (e.g., treatment for breast cancer, approach to the solitary thyroid nodule). Knowledge of how the surgical procedure reverses or changes the pathophysiologic process enhances the student's understanding of the operating room experience.

Every surgical procedure carries a risk of complication. Some complications are related to the technical aspects of the procedure (e.g., anastomotic leak or stenosis, pseudoaneurysm, common duct injury during laparoscopic cholecystectomy). Others involve physiologic or anatomic alterations caused by surgery (e.g., marginal ulcers at the site of gastrojejunostomy, dumping syndrome, afferent loop syndrome). Many surgical atlases list the common complications of each procedure. The risks of anesthesia, pulmonary compromise, atelectasis, thrombophlebitis, and wound infection are complications of many procedures.

Functioning as a good assistant can be as demanding as serving as the primary surgeon. Assisting effectively is learned behavior that requires experience and knowledge of the procedure. A good assistant anticipates the steps in the procedure and helps, rather than competes with, the operating surgeon. Keeping the field dry, anticipating the cutting of sutures, and providing adequate exposure are within the capabilities of even the novice in the operating room. Most surgeons recognize that the undergraduate student is in unfamiliar territory, and senior members of the team usually provide instruction on how to help. The assistant pays attention to the procedure and avoids distractions. For example, conversation should be limited to the case. Care is taken not to lean on the patient inadvertently while standing at the operative table because nerve damage or interference with ventilation could occur.

The surgical technician passes the requested instruments. A student who attempts to retrieve or replace instruments on the Mayo stand may disrupt the organization and flow of the operation. Many surgical technicians consider the Mayo stand hallowed ground, and trespassers are often chastised. The ability to provide the requested instruments, ties, or suture material quickly is hampered by extra hands or disorganized instruments.

The operative field is kept as tidy as possible. To contain contamination, simplify the accounting of sponges, and provide a rough estimate of blood loss, sponges that are used during the procedure are dropped into the container that is provided. Searching for a misplaced sponge tries everyone's patience.

The members of the surgical team remain in the room until the patient leaves or the surgeon grants permission to leave. The student should remain available to assist with application of the dressing, transfer of the patient to the stretcher, or other tasks.

Proper positioning of the patient for the operation is determined by the surgeon. The following principles are considered.

- Proper maintenance of respiration
- Unimpaired circulation
- Protection of muscles and nerves from pressure
- Accessibility and exposure of the operative field
- Uninterrupted administration of anesthetic agents
- Accessibility for administration of intravenous fluids
- Comfort and safety of the patient

The following important safety measures are observed when a patient is transferred or positioned.

- The table is securely locked in position.
- The patient's head is protected from movement by the anesthesiologist.
- Uninterrupted flow of intravenous fluids is maintained.
- Care is taken not to hyperextend the arms.
- Slow, gentle movement is used to avoid circulatory or respiratory compromise.
- The placement of pressure on nerves is avoided. Steps include ensuring that the legs are not crossed while the patient is in the supine position and placing pillows or rolls under the chest if the patient is prone.
- Nothing is allowed to obstruct tubing.

Operating tables are divided into three or more hinged sections that are flexed or extended to obtain the desired position. This procedure is often called "breaking" the table. The joints of the table are called "breaks." The operative table can be placed in a number of positions, including **Trendelenburg** (head down) and reverse Trendelenburg (head up). The table can also be rotated laterally, fixed, raised, or lowered. Special equipment and table attachments (e.g., safety belts, arm straps, arm boards, braces, supports, stirrups, bandage rolls) are used to stabilize the patient on the table. Although the circulating nurse assumes the major responsibility for positioning the patient, the safety of the patient during the operative procedure is a responsibility that is shared by every member of the surgical team.

Classification of Operative Wounds

Operative wounds are classified, according to the risk of contamination or infection, as **clean, clean-contaminated, contaminated,** or **dirty.** This classification allows prediction of the risk of subsequent wound infection and allows comparison of the techniques of different surgical teams.

In clean wounds, the gastrointestinal, respiratory, or urinary tract is not entered. In addition, inflammation is not present, and no break in technique occurs. The risk of infection is negligible.

In clean-contaminated wounds, the gastrointestinal, respiratory, or urinary tract is entered without significant spillage or break in operative technique. The risk of infection is minimal.

Contaminated wounds involve gross spillage of the contents of the gastrointestinal or urinary tract or a major break in operative technique. This category includes fresh traumatic wounds because of the potential for contamination. The risk of infection approaches 5%.

A wound is considered dirty if pus or a perforated viscus is encountered. Old traumatic wounds with necrotic tissue, wounds that require the excision of a foreign body, or wounds that have gross fecal contamination are also considered dirty. Because the infection rate is high if these wounds are closed primarily, they are often left open.

The prevention of wound infection in the surgical patient requires the following steps:

- Control of endogenous infection
- Strict adherence to sterile technique
- Careful operative technique and wound closure
- Reduction of exogenous or environmental sources of contamination
- Thorough, prompt cleansing and debridement of traumatic wounds
- Prevention of intraoperative wound contamination
- Use of prophylactic antibiotics in selected patients
- Adherence to sterile technique for dressing changes
- Documentation of wound infection statistics

Wound infections lead to prolonged hospitalization, significant patient discomfort, incisional hernias, and unsightly scars. Adherence to the principles described in this chapter minimizes the morbidity associated with wound infection.

A Short Atlas of Common Surgical Procedures

This section describes some common surgical procedures. See a complete surgical atlas for more details.

Appendectomy
Indications

Right lower quadrant pain
Peritoneal signs on physical examination
Fever (usually low grade)
Anorexia
Occasional nausea or vomiting
Right lower quadrant pain on rectal or vaginal examination
Occasional palpable mass

Leukocytosis
Incidental finding (usually performed after another planned procedure)

Differential Diagnosis

Gastroenteritis
Mesenteric adenitis
Pelvic inflammatory disease
Ovarian accident
   Ruptured cyst
   Torsion
   Mittelschmerz
Ectopic pregnancy
Meckel's diverticulum
Inflammatory bowel disease

Complications

Wound infection
Pelvic abscess
Enterocutaneous fistula
Pylephlebitis
Appendiceal perforation

Procedure

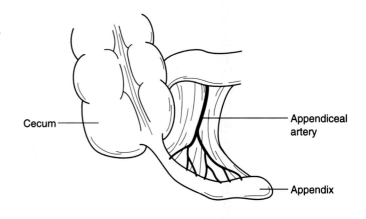

2. The cecum is mobilized into the surgical incision.

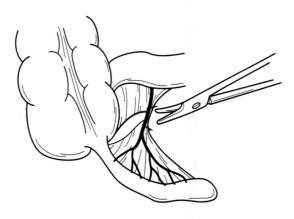

3. The mesoappendix, which contains the appendiceal artery, is divided, and the vessels are ligated.

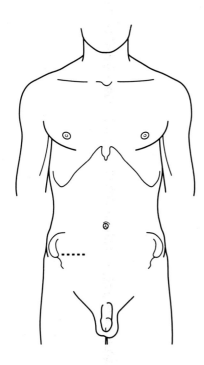

1. A transverse or oblique incision is made, usually over McBurney's point.

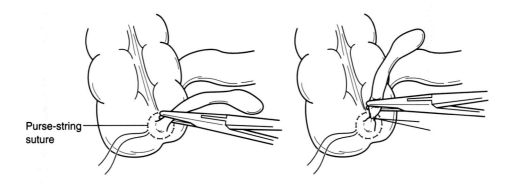

Purse-string
suture

4. A purse-string suture is placed in the cecum near the base of the appendix. The base of the appendix is crushed and tied.

Laparoscopic Appendectomy
Procedure

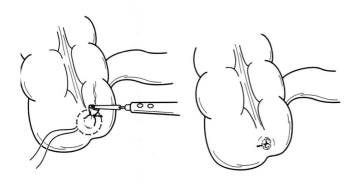

5. The mucosa of the appendiceal stump is cauterized to prevent bacterial spillage and mucocele formation. The stump is inverted, and the purse-string suture is tied securely.

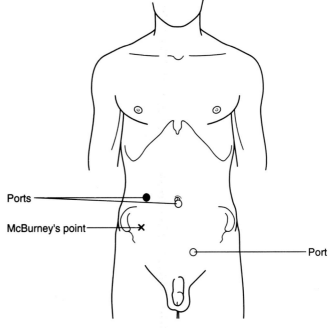

Ports

McBurney's point

Port

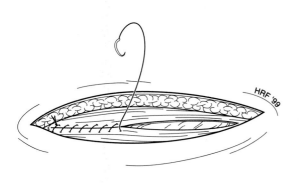

HRF '99

1. Ports are placed for the camera and operative tools.

6. The cecum is returned to its normal position in the celomic cavity, and the wound is irrigated and closed in layers. The skin may be left open if the appendix is perforated.

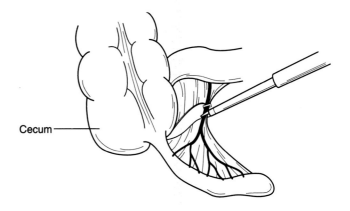

Cecum

2. The cecum is mobilized, and the appendiceal vessels are clipped and divided.

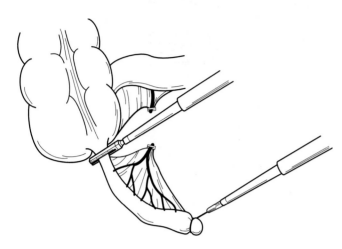

3. A stapling device is used to transect the appendix. The appendiceal stump is cauterized.

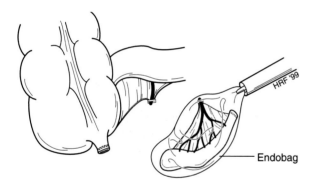

Endobag

4. The appendix is placed in a plastic bag and removed. The ports are withdrawn.

Cholecystectomy

Indications

Acute or chronic cholecystitis
Cholelithiasis
Choledocholithiasis

Differential Diagnosis

Peptic ulcer disease
Pancreatitis
Gastroenteritis
Acute appendicitis
Right lower lobe pneumonia

Complications

Wound infection
Subhepatic or subphrenic abscess
Bile peritonitis
Common bile duct injury
Hollow viscus injury
Postoperative hemorrhage
Retained common duct stone
Pancreatitis (postoperative)

Procedure

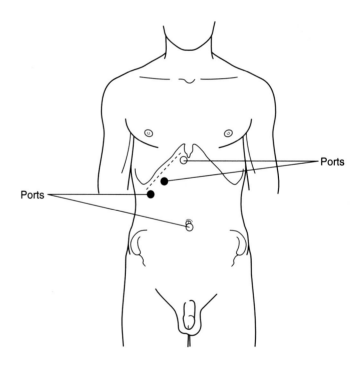

Ports

Ports

1. The gallbladder is approached through a right subcostal incision. Whether the procedure is performed open or laparoscopically, the approach to removing the gallbladder is the same. Operative and camera ports are placed.

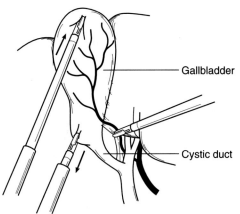 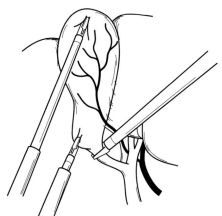

2. Dissection is performed to isolate the cystic duct and artery. The cystic duct is clipped or tied proximally to prevent the migration of stones into the common duct.

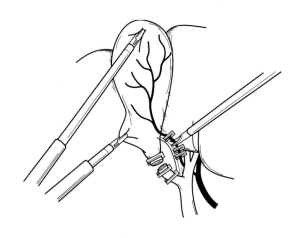

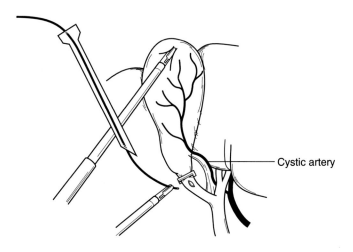

3. A cholangiogram is performed.

4. The cystic artery and cystic duct are tied or clipped and divided.

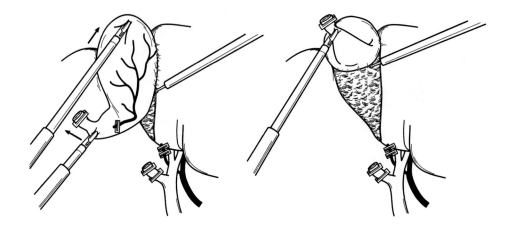

5. The gallbladder is removed from the liver bed with blunt, sharp, or electrocautery dissection.

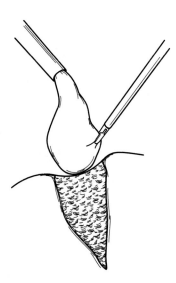

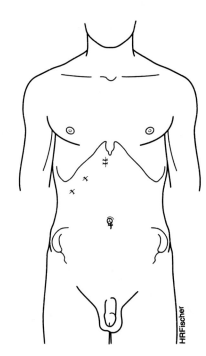

6. The gallbladder is removed through a large port.

7. The wounds are closed.

Open Cholecystectomy

Procedure

1. Open cholecystectomy is performed in essentially the same fashion. The major difference is that different instruments are used.
2. The incision is larger and requires closure in layers.

Colectomy/Small Bowel Resection

Indications

Malignancy
Diverticular disease
   Hemorrhage
   Perforation
   Stricture
   Obstruction
Malignancy
Inflammatory bowel disease
Trauma
Volvulus

Complications

Wound infection
Pelvic abscess
Anastomotic leak
Enterocutaneous fistula
Anastomotic stricture
Recurrent disease

Procedure

1. The colon/small bowel is approached through a midline incision or laparoscopically through the ports indicated.
2. The segment of the colon/small bowel to be resected is mobilized. Additional mobilization may be required to perform an anastomosis without tension. The blood supply to the resected segment is isolated and divided.
3. The mesentery is divided sharply or with electrocautery.

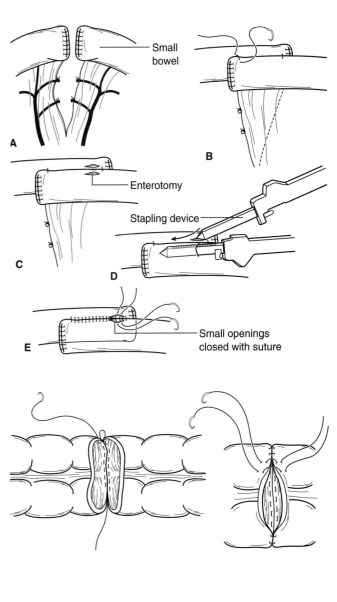

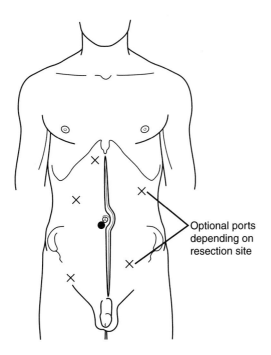

4. Reapproximation is performed by sewing or with a stapling device.

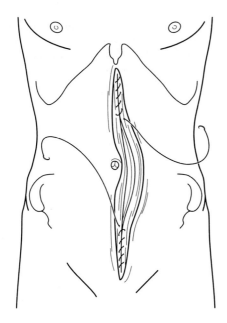 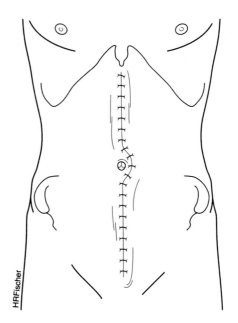

5. The incision is closed according to the surgeon's preference.

Splenectomy

Indications

Trauma or hemoperitoneum
Hemolytic anemia
Thrombocytopenia
Hypersplenism
Leukemia or lymphoma
Splenic abscess
Splenic cyst
Splenic aneurysm
Metastatic disease

Complications

Subphrenic abscess
Postoperative hemorrhage
Gastric wall necrosis
Thrombocytosis
Overwhelming postsplenectomy sepsis syndrome

Procedure

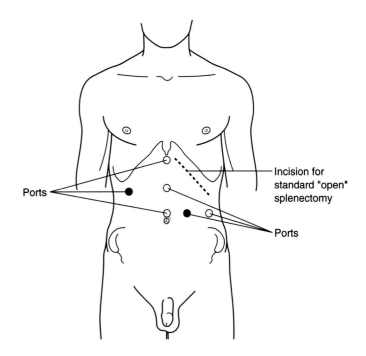

1. The celomic cavity is entered through a left sub-costal incision, or ports are placed for a laparoscopic approach.
2. The lesser sac is entered by dividing the short gastric vessels between clips or ties and the lienogastric ligament.

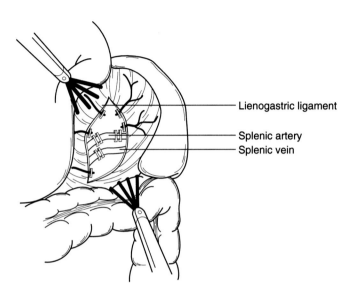

- Lienogastric ligament
- Splenic artery
- Splenic vein

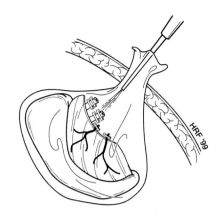

4. If the procedure is done laparoscopically, it may be necessary to puree the spleen in a bag to facilitate removal.
5. The abdomen is closed in layers according to the surgeon's preference.

Surgical Procedures on the Breast

Biopsy

Indications

Breast mass
Mammographic abnormality

Complications

Wound infection
Breast hematoma

Procedure

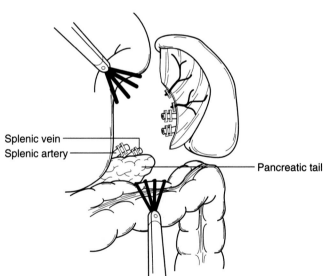

Splenic vein
Splenic artery

Pancreatic tail

3. The splenic artery and vein may be ligated near the superior border of the pancreatic tail.

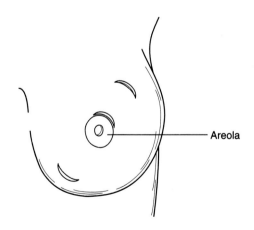

- Areola

1. Biopsy is performed under general or local anesthesia. A circumareolar or skin-line incision is made.

Procedure

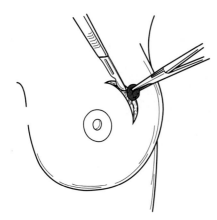

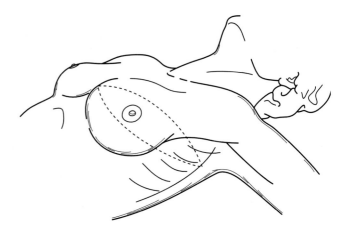

1. A transverse incision is usually used.

2. The mass may be grasped with a clamp and excised sharply with gentle traction.

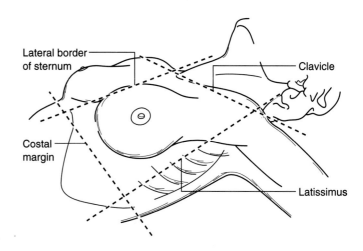

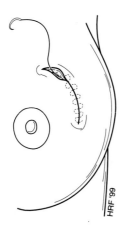

3. After hemostasis is achieved, the incision is closed with a subcuticular stitch.

Mastectomy

Indications
Malignant disease
High-risk histopathology

Complications
Hematoma or seroma
Flap necrosis
Axillary vein injury
Long thoracic nerve injury
Thoracodorsal nerve injury
Lymphedema or lymphadenitis
Recurrent disease

2. The limits of the dissection include the clavicle superiorly, the latissimus dorsi posteriorly, the sternum medially, and the sixth rib inferiorly.

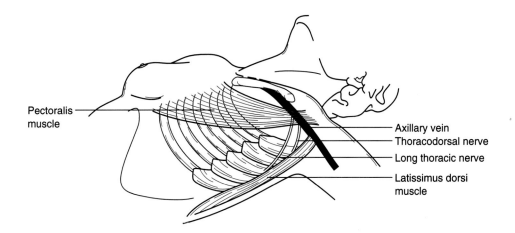

Pectoralis muscle

Axillary vein
Thoracodorsal nerve
Long thoracic nerve
Latissimus dorsi muscle

3. Axillary dissection preserves the long thoracic and thoracodorsal nerves. The axillary vein is cleaned of node-bearing from its inferior surface.

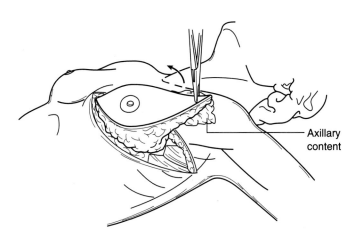

Axillary content

4. The breast is removed from the chest wall, from the axillae medially. The pectoralis fascia is taken, but the pectoralis muscle is left.

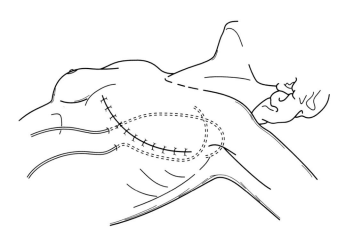

5. Drains are placed beneath the skin flaps. The subcutaneous tissue and skin are closed directly over the chest wall.

Partial Mastectomy (Breast Preservation)
Procedure

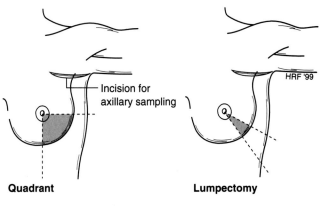

Incision for axillary sampling

HRF '99

Quadrant

Lumpectomy

1. Breast conservation preserves the breast mound.
2. A sampling of axillary lymph nodes is usually performed with these procedures.

Vascular Procedures
Abdominal Aortic Aneurysm
Indications
Aneurysm larger than 5 cm
Rupture or leak
  Back pain
  Syncope
  Shock

Complications

Death
Renal failure
Ischemic colitis
Graft infection
Graft thrombosis
Distal embolization of atherosclerotic debris
Myocardial infarction
Aortoduodenal fistula
Pseudoaneurysm

Procedure

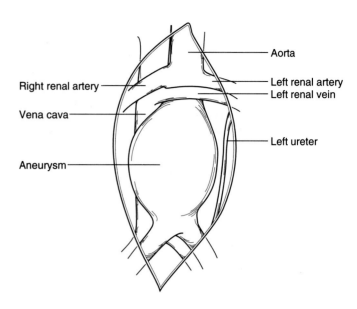

2. The small bowel is mobilized to the right side to expose the aorta. If rupture occurs, the aorta may be approached directly through the mesentery of the bowel.

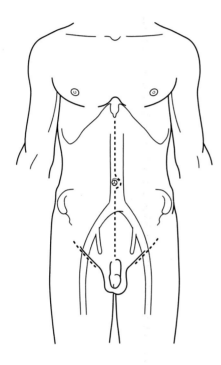

1. The aorta is approached through a generous midline incision. Both groins are prepared to allow access to the femoral vessels.

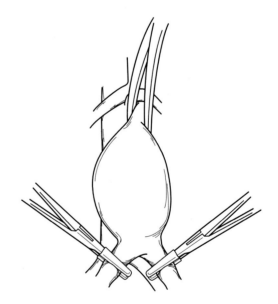

3. Proximal control of the aorta is gained either above or below the renal arteries, depending on the clinical situation. Distal control is gained below the aneurysm.

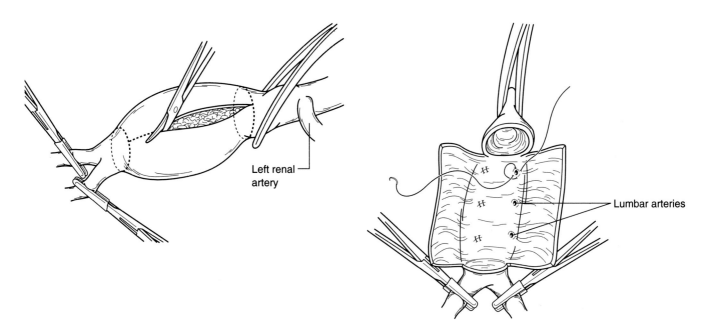

Left renal artery

Lumbar arteries

4. The aneurysm is opened after the aorta is cross-clamped, preferably below the renal arteries.

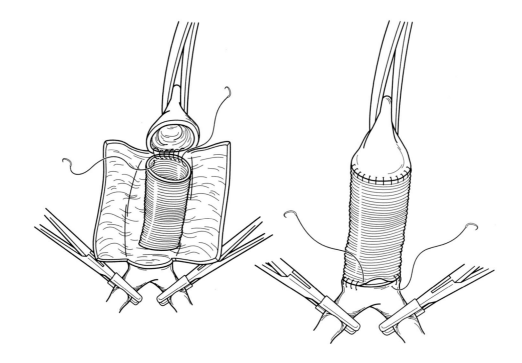

5. A prosthetic graft is sewn into place. The graft may be either tubular or bifurcated. The inferior mesenteric artery may be reimplanted into the graft.

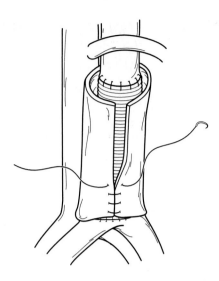

Aortobifemoral Graft

Indications

    Aortoiliac occlusive disease
    Incapacitating claudication
    Ischemic rest pain
    Impending tissue loss

Complications

    Death
    Renal failure
    Ischemic colitis
    Graft infection
    Graft thrombosis
    Distal embolization of atherosclerotic debris
    Myocardial infarction
    Aortoduodenal fistula
    Pseudoaneurysm

Procedure

6. A cuff of the wall of the aneurysm is sewn over the graft.

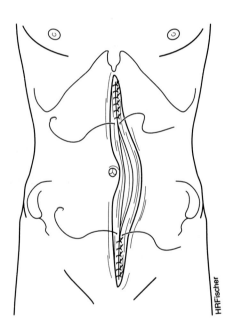

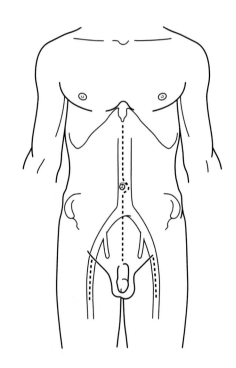

7. The abdominal cavity is irrigated and closed in a standard fashion.

1. The aorta is approached in a similar fashion to the aneurysm repair. Both groins must be surgically prepared.

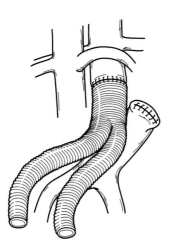

2. The proximal anastomosis is completed.

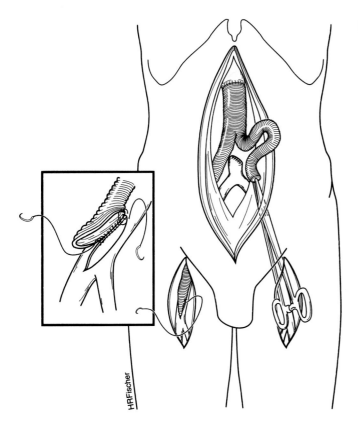

3. The femoral arteries are exposed through groin incisions. The limbs of the graft are tunneled through the retroperitoneum to lie on top of the femoral arteries.
4. Distal anastomoses are performed.

5. Abdominal closure is performed in a standard fashion. Groin wounds are closed in layers.

Femoropopliteal Bypass with Saphenous Vein

Indications
Symptomatic femoral occlusive disease
Adequate inflow
No profundus stenosis at the origin

Complications
Death
Renal failure
Ischemic colitis
Graft infection
Graft thrombosis
Distal embolization of atherosclerotic debris
Myocardial infarction
Aortoduodenal fistula
Pseudoaneurysm

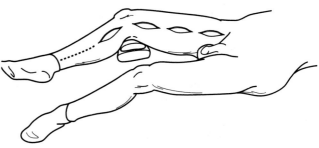

1. Both lower extremities are prepared for surgery.

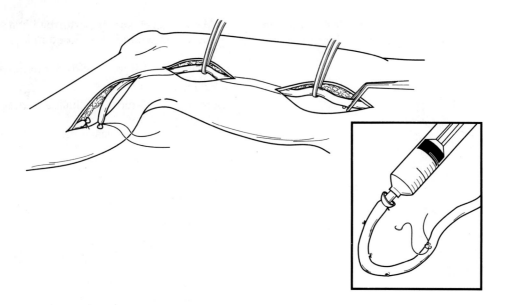

2. Saphenous vein is harvested from the ipsilateral leg. The branches are tied, and the vein is carefully dilated hydrostatically.

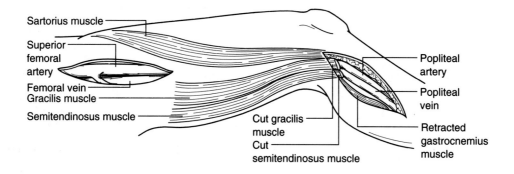

Sartorius muscle

Superior femoral artery

Femoral vein

Gracilis muscle

Semitendinosus muscle

Cut gracilis muscle

Cut semitendinosus muscle

Popliteal artery

Popliteal vein

Retracted gastrocnemius muscle

3. The femoral artery is exposed in the groin. The popliteal artery is exposed below the site of occlusion as determined by preoperative angiography.

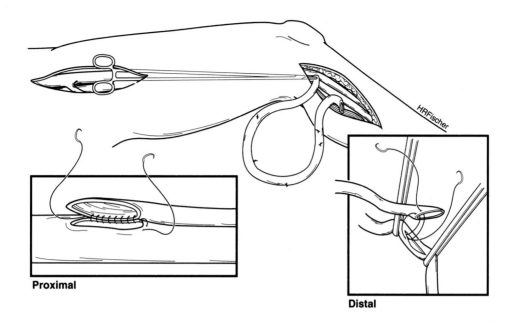

Proximal

Distal

4. The vein is usually reversed, but it may be left in situ or not reversed. The valves are cut. The distal anastomosis is performed first, then the proximal anastomosis. Anastomoses are performed with fine monofilament permanent suture.

5. The leg incisions are closed.

Carotid Endarterectomy

Indications

Transient ischemic attacks
Critical carotid stenosis

Complications

Bleeding or hematoma
Stroke
Embolic event
Thrombosis
Nerve injury
  Hypoglossal
  Vagus
  Marginal mandibular
  Superior laryngeal

Procedure

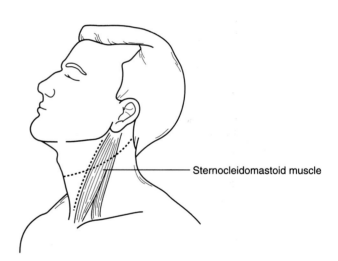

Sternocleidomastoid muscle

1. An incision is made over the anterior border of the sternocleidomastoid muscle. Some surgeons use a more transverse incision.

2. The carotid artery is exposed by retraction of the sternocleidomastoid muscle laterally.

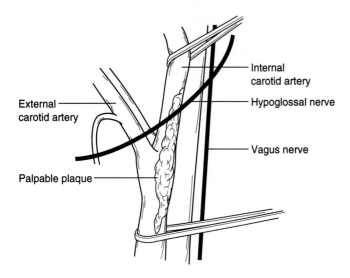

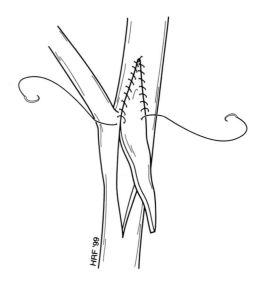

4. A vein patch is used to close the arteriotomy, or the vessel wall is reapproximated primarily. The incision is closed in layers.

Vascular Access for Dialysis

Indications

Long-term hemodialysis

Complications

Graft thrombosis
Graft infection
Erosion of graft through the skin
Pseudoaneurysm
Congestive heart failure

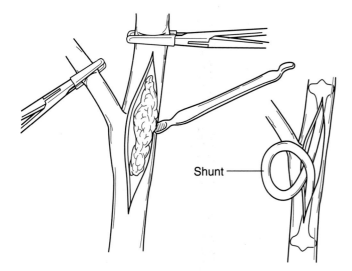

3. An arteriotomy is performed, and the plaque is exposed. It is dissected from the vessel lumen with a small periosteal elevator, and removed. Some surgeons place a shunt to maintain blood flow.

Procedure

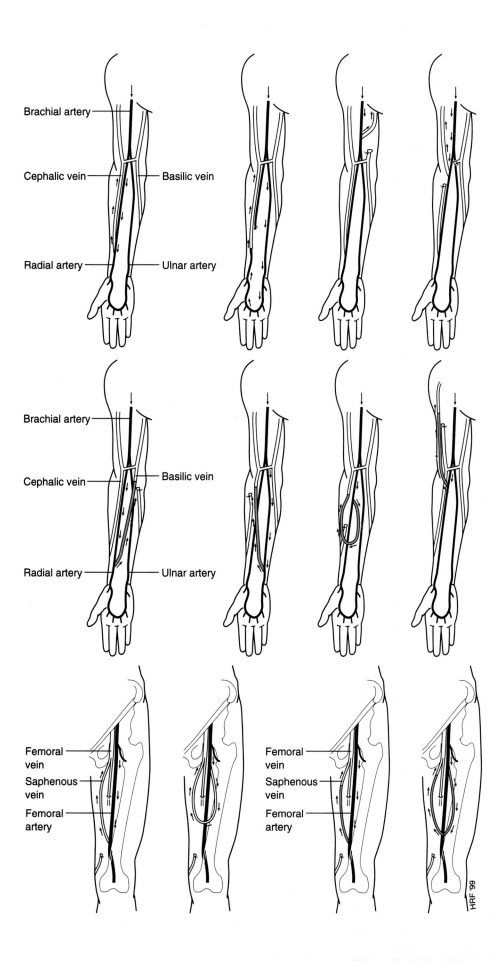

1. General, regional, or local anesthesia is used. After the arm is prepared, an incision is made over the artery and vein.
2. Usually, an end (of vein)-to-side (of artery) anastomosis is performed. Alternatively, a prosthetic graft is sewn between the artery and vein. These grafts are usually "looped" in the forearm.
3. If inadequate vascular structures are present in the upper extremities (usually inadequate veins), the proximal thigh vessels can be used.

Central Venous Access

Indications

Acute venous access
Resuscitation from shock or placement of pulmonary artery catheter
Long-term venous access
   Chemotherapy
   Nutritional support
   Phlebotomy
Dialysis

Complications

Hemothorax or pneumothorax
Subclavian or carotid artery injury
Arrhythmia
Mediastinal hemorrhage
Venous thrombosis
Catheter malposition or malfunction
Sepsis
Skin erosion

Procedure

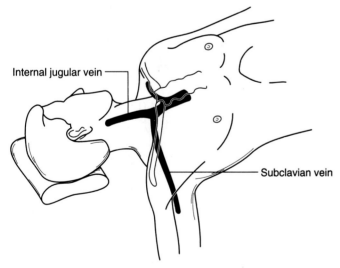

1. The subclavian or internal jugular vein is selected. The patient is placed in the Trendelenburg position, with the head turned to the opposite side.

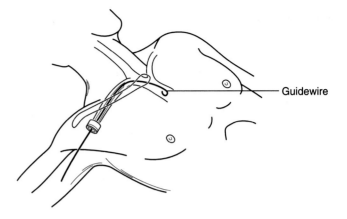

2. The vein is punctured and the guidewire inserted. The electrocardiogram monitor is observed for signs of cardiac dysrhythmia.

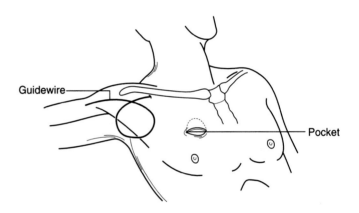

3. If a chronic port is to be inserted, local anesthesia is infiltrated along the path for the catheter tunnel. A pocket for the reservoir is made.

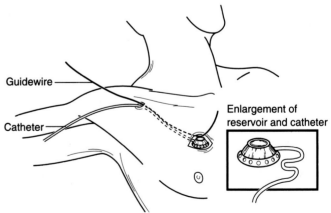

4. The device is assembled, flushed with heparinized saline, and positioned in the reservoir pocket. The catheter is brought out of the skin at the site of the guidewire.

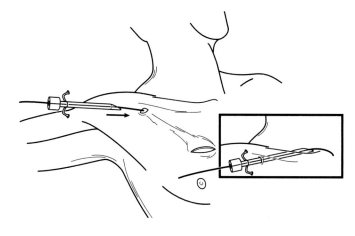

Gastrostomy

Conventional Gastrostomy

Indications

Chronic gastric decompression
Gavage
Comfort

Complications

Intraperitoneal leak
Wound infection
Tube malposition
Clogging
Inadvertent tube removal

Procedure

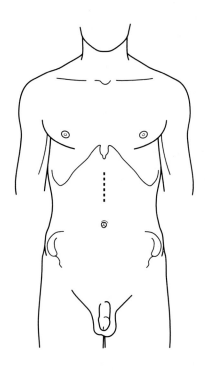

5. The final length of the catheter is measured, and the tear-away sheath over the vein dilator is inserted. The dilator and guidewire are removed.

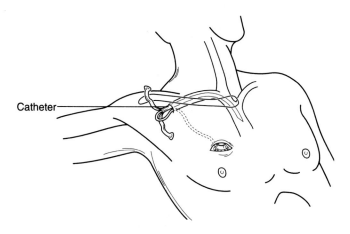

Catheter

6. The catheter is inserted into the sheath, which is removed by tearing.

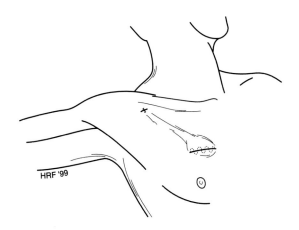

HRF '99

7. Wounds are closed. A chest x-ray is obtained to exclude pneumothorax and confirm proper positioning. This procedure may be performed with portable fluoroscopy.

1. The abdominal cavity is entered through a small upper midline incision.

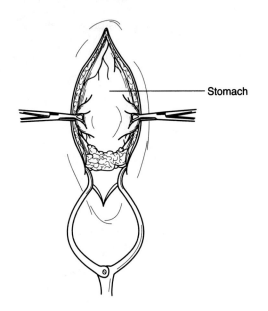

Stomach

2. The stomach is mobilized into the operative wound.

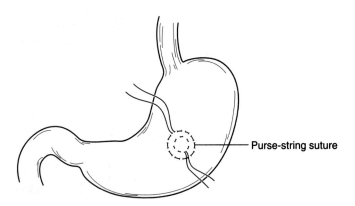

Purse-string suture

3. Two purse-string sutures are placed in the anterior wall of the stomach.

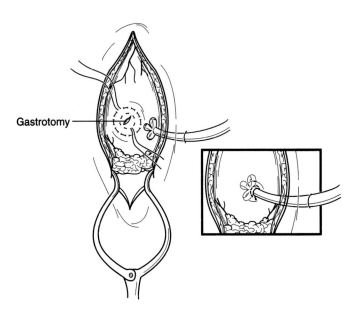

Gastrotomy

4. The gastric tube is brought through a separate incision in the abdominal wall. It is placed in the stomach through a small gastrotomy in the center of the sutures. The sutures are tied securely.

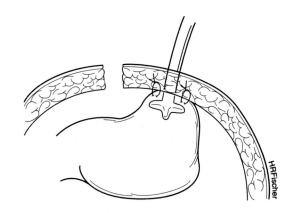

5. The stomach is tacked to the anterior abdominal wall.
6. The wound is closed.

Percutaneous Endoscopically Guided Gastrostomy
Procedure

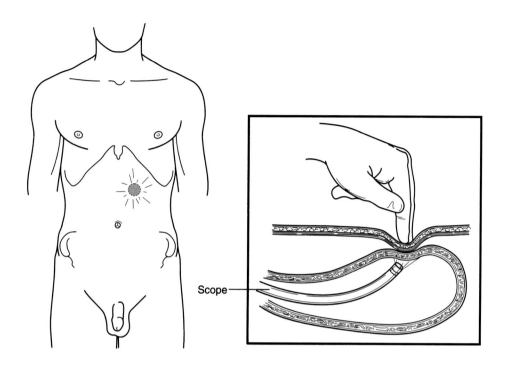

1. The endoscope is passed into the stomach. Palpation over the transilluminated spot on the abdominal wall indicates the site of percutaneous gastric puncture.

2. The stomach is punctured with a needle. A guidewire is passed into the stomach and snared while the wire is visualized through the scope.

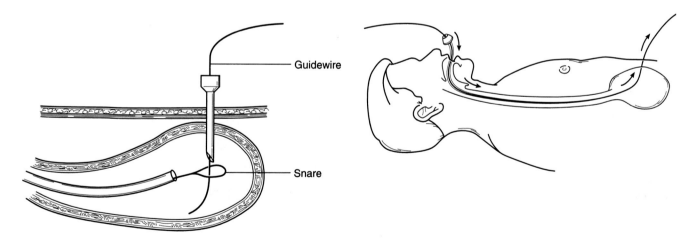

3. The scope and guidewire are removed. The gastrostomy tube is threaded over the guidewire. The tube is long and tapered, and it acts as a dilator as it passes through the anterior abdominal wall.

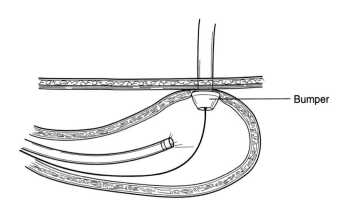

Bumper

4. The gastrostomy tube is drawn retrograde (i.e., from mouth to stomach). The bumper is positioned after the endoscope is reintroduced into the stomach.

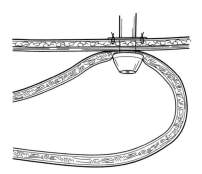

5. The guidewire is removed. The tube is fixed to the abdominal wall with a suture or with bumpers that are contained in the kit.

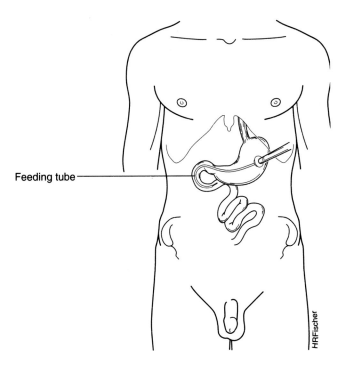

Feeding tube

HRFischer

6. An enteral feeding port may be placed through the gastrostomy tube, with endoscopy assistance if necessary.

Inguinal Herniorrhaphy
Conventional Herniorrhaphy
Indications
Inguinal hernia

Complications
Wound infection
Recurrence
Spermatic duct injury
Ilioinguinal nerve entrapment
Testicular swelling
Femoral vein injury

Procedure

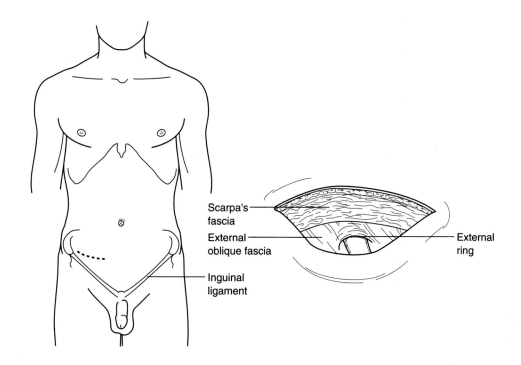

Scarpa's fascia
External oblique fascia
Inguinal ligament
External ring

1. A transverse inguinal skinfold incision is made and carried through Scarpa's fascia to the fascia of the external oblique muscle.

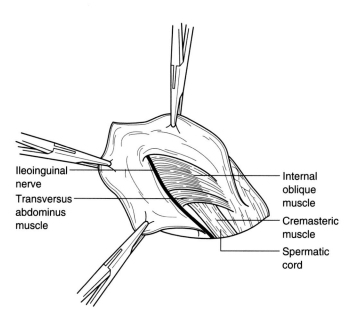

Ileoinguinal nerve
Transversus abdominus muscle
Internal oblique muscle
Cremasteric muscle
Spermatic cord

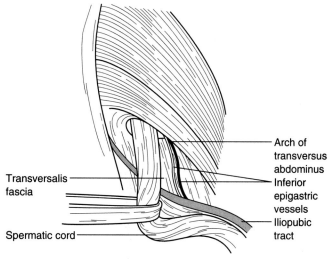

Transversalis fascia
Spermatic cord
Arch of transversus abdominus
Inferior epigastric vessels
Iliopubic tract

3. The spermatic cord is mobilized, and a sling is passed around the cord for traction. In women, the round ligament may be divided between ties.

2. The external oblique fascia is opened in the direction of the fibers through the external ring, avoiding the nerves.

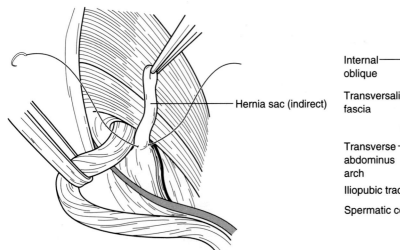

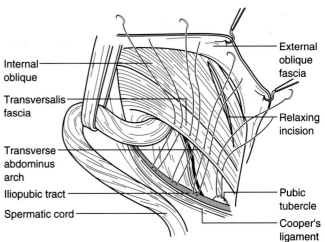

4. An indirect hernia sac is located adjacent to the cord, anteriomedially, originating lateral to the inferior epigastric vessels. Direct hernias are located medially to these vessels, through a defect in the transversalis fascia. It is dissected from the cord structures and ligated at its base. It is not necessary to dissect the direct hernia sac.

5. An anatomic repair is performed to reinforce the inguinal floor and internal ring. A relaxing incision may be required to perform the repair without tension.

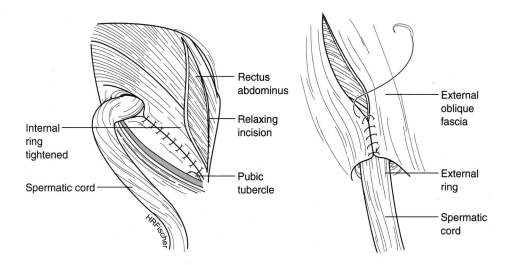

6. Closure is performed in layers.

Laparoscopic Herniorrhaphy
Procedure

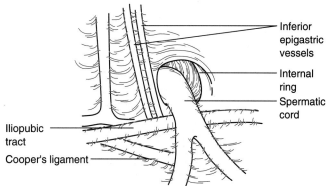

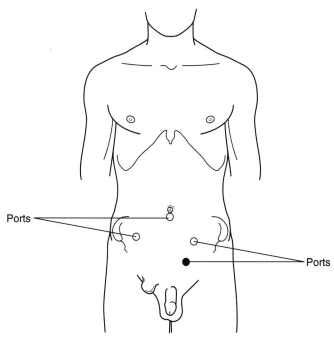

1. Operative and camera ports are placed.

2. The anatomy of the inguinal floor is identified, and the peritoneum is opened.

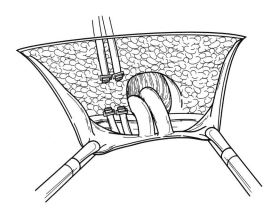

3. The indirect inguinal hernia sac is removed from the defect.

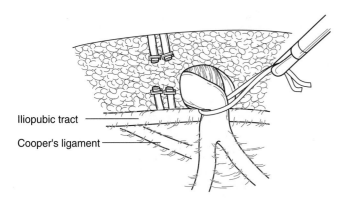

4. The inferior epigastric artery and vein may be divided. The spermatic cord is encircled with a sling.

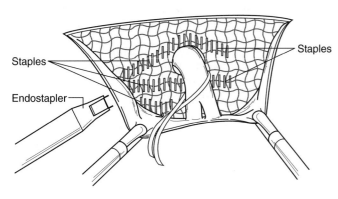

5. Polypropylene mesh is fashioned to fit around the spermatic cord and form a new inguinal floor.

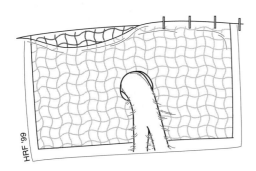

6. The peritoneum is repositioned over the mesh.
7. Ports larger than 5 mm are closed.

Anal Procedures

Indications

Infectious anal process refractory to medical management
Bleeding
Abscess
Prolapse

Complications

Stenosis
Incontinence
Recurrence

Procedures

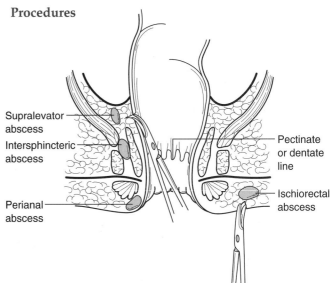

1. Incision or drainage of perirectal abscess

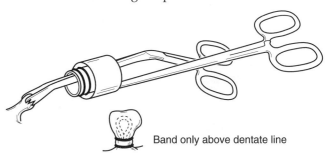

Band only above dentate line

2. Rubber band ligation of hemorrhoid

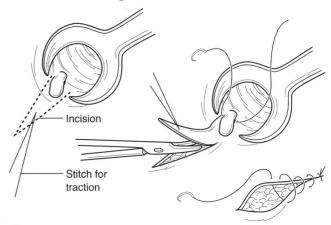

3. Hemorrhoidectomy

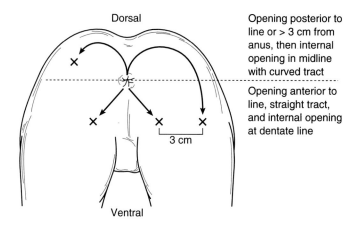

Opening posterior to line or > 3 cm from anus, then internal opening in midline with curved tract

Opening anterior to line, straight tract, and internal opening at dentate line

4. Goodsall's rule of anal fistulae

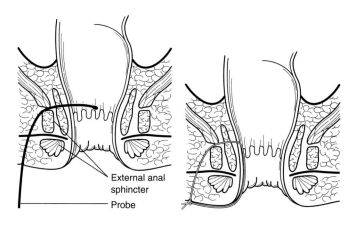

External anal sphincter

Probe

5. Placement of seton

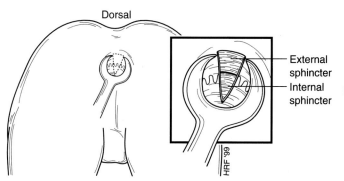

Dorsal

External sphincter

Internal sphincter

HRF '99

6. Internal sphincterotomy

Thyroid and Parathyroid Procedures

Indications

Thyroid nodule
Graves' disease (hyperparathyroidism)
Metastatic disease
Hyperparathyroidism
    Adenoma
    Second or third degree

Complications

Skin flap necrosis
Cellulitis
Recurrent laryngeal nerve injury
    Unilateral: hoarseness
    Bilateral: inspiratory stridor (may require trache-
    ostomy)
Hematoma
Hypocalcemia

Procedure

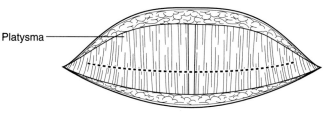

1. A transverse neck incision is made for procedures on both the thyroid and the parathyroids.

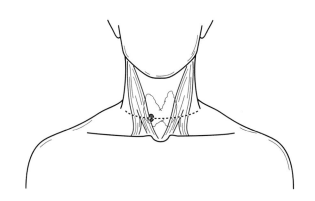

Platysma

2. The platysma is transected.

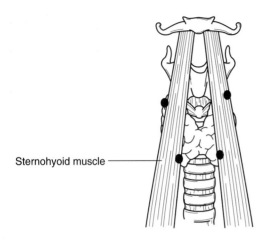

Sternohyoid muscle

3. Strap muscles are divided in the midline.
4. The thyroid is mobilized to expose the blood supply.
5. The recurrent laryngeal nerve is identified and preserved. The position of the parathyroid glands is variable.

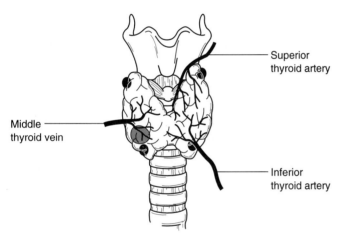

Middle thyroid vein

Superior thyroid artery

Inferior thyroid artery

6. The inferior parathyroids (IIIs) are identified in proximity to the inferior thyroidal vessels. Nearly 60% of the time, they are located behind the lower third of the gland or within 1 cm of the lower pole.

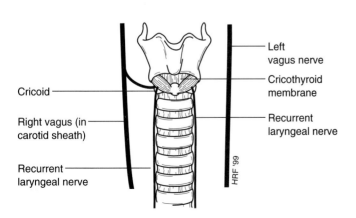

Cricoid

Right vagus (in carotid sheath)

Recurrent laryngeal nerve

Left vagus nerve

Cricothyroid membrane

Recurrent laryngeal nerve

HRF '99

7. The superior parathyroids (IVs) are found behind the middle portion of the gland (near the area where the recurrent laryngeal nerve enters the larynx) in three-fourths of cases.
8. Operations on the thyroid preserve the parathyroids with their native blood supply. If a parathyroid is devascularized, it may be minced and reimplanted in a neck muscle.
9. During operations for hyperparathyroidism, all four parathyroid glands must be identified.

Thyroidectomy
Indications
Solid thyroid nodule
Goiter
Hyperthyroidism
Graves' disease
Thyroid malignancy

Complications
Hypothyroidism
Persistent hyperthyroidism
Hypocalcemia
Recurrent laryngeal nerve injury
Superior laryngeal nerve injury
Hemorrhage or airway compromise

Procedure

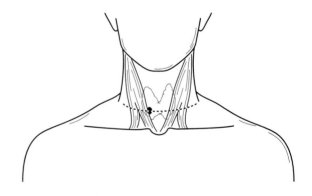

1. The neck is slightly hyperextended. An incision is made approximately two finger-breadths above the sternal notch, usually in a natural skin crease.

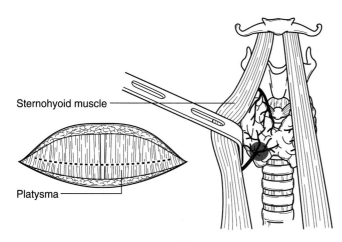

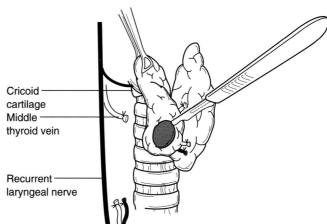

2. The platysma muscle is divided, and the strap muscles are separated in the midline. Adequate exposure is usually achieved, but the strap muscles can be divided if necessary.

4. The middle thyroid vein is ligated and divided. The recurrent laryngeal nerve is found in the tracheoesophageal groove and must be preserved. The superior parathyroids may be located near the middle thyroidal vein or in the area where the recurrent laryngeal nerve enters the larynx.

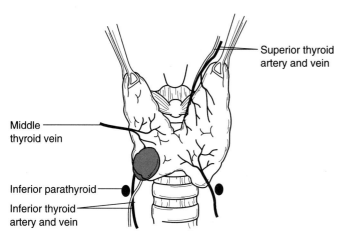

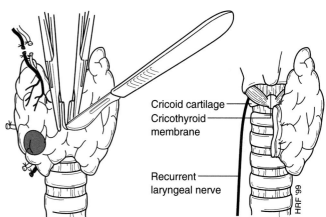

3. The thyroid gland is exposed. Dissection is usually begun inferiorly, and the inferior thyroidal artery and vein are ligated and divided. The inferior parathyroid glands are identified and preserved with their blood supply. The position of the parathyroids is variable, but 60% of the time, the inferior parathyroid glands are located behind the lower one-third of the gland or within 1 cm of the lower pole.

5. The superior thyroidal artery and vein are ligated. The isthmus is divided between clamps, and the remaining thyroid tissue is ligated with suture to ensure hemostasis. The lobe of the thyroid gland is bluntly dissected from the trachea. If a total thyroidectomy is planned, the procedure is completed on the opposite lobe.

Tracheostomy

Indications

Chronic airway access
  Mechanical ventilation
  Tracheal suctioning
Proximal obstruction or stenosis
  Laryngeal carcinoma
  Bilateral vocal cord paralysis
  Acute epiglottitis (children)

Complications

Laryngeal or tracheal fracture
Esophageal injury
Bleeding pneumothorax
Tracheoesophageal fistula
Tracheoinominate artery fistula
Tracheal stenosis
Tracheomalacia
Subcutaneous emphysema
Pneumomediastinum
Recurrent laryngeal nerve injury
Tube displacement
Tracheitis

Procedure

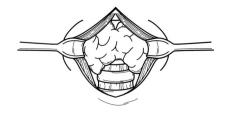

1. A transverse or vertical incision is used.

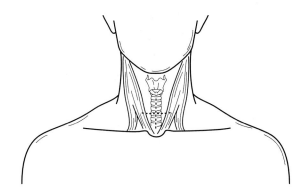

2. Strap muscles are separated in the midline.

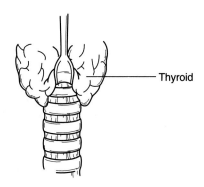

3. The thyroid isthmus is retracted or divided.

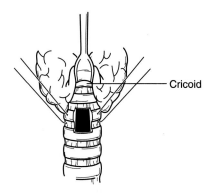

4. Traction sutures are placed laterally. A window is cut in the anterior surface of the trachea, approximately at the level of the second or third tracheal ring. Some surgeons prefer a simple vertical incision.

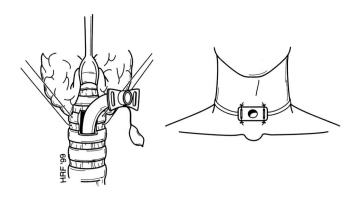

5. The tracheostomy appliance is inserted into the tracheotomy site without excessive force. It is fixed firmly to the neck to prevent dislodgement.

Common Ward Procedures

Nasogastric Intubation

Indications

Gastric decompression
Gavage (feeding)
Lavage (irrigation or dilution of the gastric contents)
Sampling of the gastric contents for analysis

Contraindications

Basilar skull fracture
Facial fractures
Obstructed nasal passage (if needed, orogastric intu-
bation is considered)

Procedure

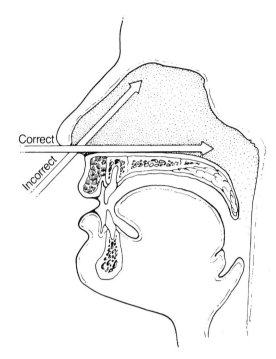

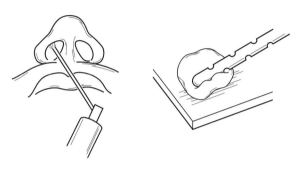

1. The nasal passage is anesthetized with a topical
   anesthetic. The nasogastric tube is lubricated with
   jelly.

3. The tip of the tube is directed toward the hypopharynx, not toward the base of the skull. The patient is
   asked to swallow. Small sips of water through a
   straw may be helpful.
4. The tube is advanced as the patient swallows until
   the estimated length of tubing is inserted.

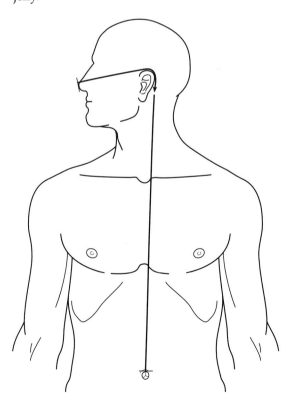

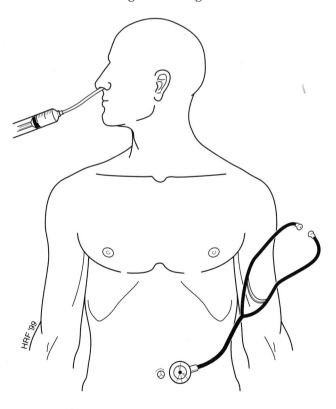

2. The length of tubing necessary to reach the stomach
   is estimated.

5. Auscultation over the stomach as air is injected
   through the tube confirms proper tube placement.
   The return of gastric contents or bile also confirms
   proper placement.

Bladder Catheterization

Indications
Bladder decompression
Measurement of urine output
Relief of obstruction
Diagnosis
Lavage

Contraindications
Suspected urethral injury
Stricture (more experience necessary)

Complications
False passage
Hemorrhage
Urethral disruption
Bladder spasm
Bladder contamination

Procedure
1. The meatus is cleaned with antiseptic solution.

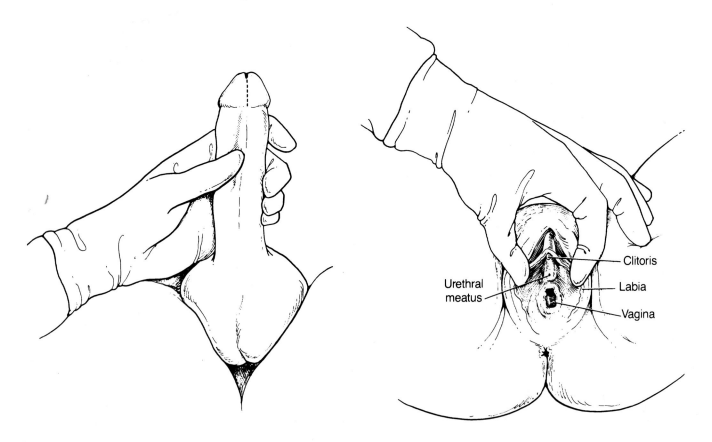

2. The penis is held upright, and the lubricated catheter is inserted into the urethra. Urine must be identified in the collection system before the balloon is inflated. In women, the labia are not allowed to reapproximate until the catheter is positioned in the bladder and the balloon is inflated.

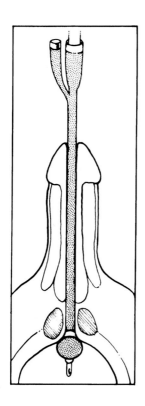

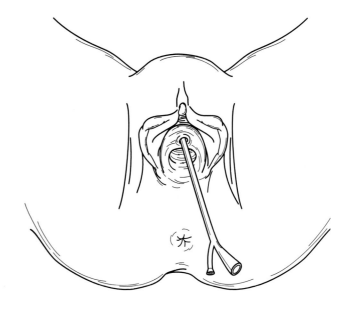

3. The catheter is taped to the lower abdomen in men and to the medial thigh in women.

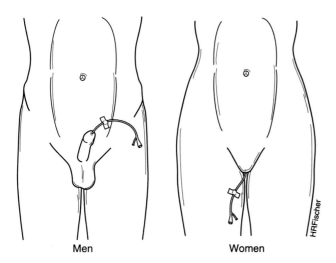

Men   Women

Answers to Multiple-Choice Questions

Note: The parenthetical reference following each explanation indicates the section or subsection of the chapter in which the answer is found.

Chapter 3

1. Correct: E. In a young man, total body water is approximately 60% of body weight. In a young woman or an elderly man, the total body water would be less, approximately 50% to 55% of total body weight. (Normal Physiology)

2. Correct: B. Aldosterone release is triggered by a decrease in renal perfusion, which is seen in extracellular depletion. Antidiuretic hormone (ADH) secretion is dependent on plasma osmolarity, but also on volume receptor activity in the right and left atria. Decreased volume leads to ADH release. Renin release is part of the aldosterone release mechanism in that when the juxtaglomerular apparatus senses a decrease in renal perfusion, it is stimulated to secrete renin. This renin promotes the secretion of angiotensin I and its subsequent conversion to angiotensin II, which stimulates the release of aldosterone. Although controversial, adrenocorticotropic hormone (ACTH) is not thought to be a potent stimulator of aldosterone. (Normal Physiology)

3. Correct: C. Plasma osmolality can be estimated by the following formula:

   Osmolarity = 2 × serum sodium + [glucose mg/dL ÷ 18] + [BUN ÷ 2.8].

   Plugging the values given into the question gives an estimate of serum osmolality in this patient of approximately 323 mOsm. (Normal Physiology)

4. Correct: D. When hyperosmolar fluid is infused, the body equalizes the osmolarity across the cellular membranes. This process causes water to leave the cells and interstitial space and enter the intravascular space. There is an increase in both intracellular and extracellular fluid osmolarity because of the infusion of the hypertonic solution. In addition, extracellular fluid volume increases because water moves out of the cells and into the extracellular fluid. Serum sodium concentration decreases because more water is located in the intravascular space. Intracellular fluid volume decreases because the water moves out of the cells. (Normal Physiology)

5. Correct: E. Magnesium deficiency is often seen with hypokalemia, and when hypokalemia appears to be refractory to treatment, the magnesium level should be measured and corrected if necessary. Insulin drives potassium into the cells and therefore can produce a state of hypokalemia. Aldosterone causes sodium resorption in exchange for potassium and hydrogen ion in the distal tubules and therefore can be associated with hypokalemia. Metabolic alkalosis is often associated with hypokalemia, whereas metabolic acidosis is associated with movement of potassium from the intracellular to the extracellular compartment, thereby causing hyperkalemia. (Potassium)

6. Correct: D. Hypokalemia is often associated with paralytic ileus and muscular weakness. On the other hand, hyponatremia has more neurologic consequences. The signs and symptoms of hypernatremia include those of dehydration as well as those of neuromuscular and neurologic disorders, ranging from twitching and restlessness to delirium and coma. Hypocalcemia initially causes perioral numbness and tingling, along with hyperactive deep-tendon reflexes. If it is severe, it can lead to seizures. Hyperchloremia has no specific symptoms, but there are usually signs and symptoms of accompanying disorders. (Hypokalemia)

7. Correct: B. Patients with gastric outlet obstruction and persistent vomiting most likely have hypochloremic hypokalemic metabolic alkalosis. An attempt should be made to replace what they have lost. The most important ion to replace in these patients is chloride. Also, because of the hypokalemia, these patients need potassium replacement. (Normal Physiology)

8. Correct: B. Using the two rules in the text, arterial pH and Paco$_2$ can be used to determine whether the patient has compensated or uncompensated alkalosis or acidosis. (Normal Physiology)

9. Correct: E. Hypochloremia impairs renal bicarbonate excretion. If serum bicarbonate remains high, the metabolic alkalosis persists until the chloride deficit is repleted. Although replacement of the potassium deficit is important, the metabolic alkalosis may persist until the chloride deficit is repleted. (Hypochloremia)

10. Correct: A. The fluid that is lost through the gut is usually isotonic. Therefore, the volume deficit is also isotonic. Metabolic acidosis occurs because of a loss of bicarbonate in the diarrhea. Metabolic alkalosis with

isotonic volume contraction is more common in gastric outlet obstruction. Hypertonic extracellular volume contraction requires a loss of hypotonic fluid (e.g., sweat). Hypotonic extracellular volume contraction requires a loss of hypertonic or isotonic fluid, with replacement of isotonic or hypotonic fluid. (Metabolic Acidosis)

11. Correct: D. Hypomagnesemia is often caused by dietary deficiency as a result of chronic alcoholism or gastrointestinal losses (e.g., diarrhea). Improperly constituted hyperalimentation or prolonged intravenous therapy without adequate oral intake can also cause hypomagnesemia. It can also be caused by the administration of some diuretics. It is not caused by hyperparathyroidism. Hypomagnesemia can produce severe hypocalcemia because of its effect on parathyroid hormone (PTH). (Hypomagnesemia)

12. Correct: D. Patients with severe hypercalcemia can be treated with oral or intravenous phosphate supplements. However, when given intravenously, phosphates may cause precipitous declines in serum calcium. Therefore, phosphate supplements should not be used in this patient. Her hypercalcemia is life-threatening because it is causing somnolence. Intravenous saline is the initial therapeutic measure, followed by diuretics once urine output is established and then by mithramycin or corticosteroids, which take 24 to 48 hours to act. Insulin and glucose infusions are appropriate in severe hyperkalemia. (Hypercalcemia)

13. Correct: E. Hypophosphatemia is common in surgical patients. These patients may also have losses of potassium and magnesium. These losses often result from inadequate uptake because of inadequate intake or losses from the gastrointestinal tract. Hypophosphatemia can cause respiratory failure. (Hypophosphatemia)

14. Correct: B. One of the first signs of acute renal failure is the inability of the kidney to conserve sodium. Therefore, a urine sodium concentration of 70 mEq/L without the administration of diuretics indicates acute renal failure rather than extracellular volume depletion, which would cause near-total conservation of sodium by the kidney. The other answers are all consistent with extracellular fluid depletion, although decreased urine output is common in both disorders. (Volume Depletion)

15. Correct: B. Chloride is the most common anion in the interstitial fluid. Sodium and potassium are cations. Bicarbonate and phosphate come in second and third in concentration in the interstitium. (Normal Physiology)

16. Correct: C. Sodium concentration of lactated Ringer's solution is 130 mEq/L. Normal saline is 154/mEq/L, half-normal saline is 77 mEq/L, and quarter-normal saline is 34 mEq/L. (Normal Physiology)

17. Correct: A. Secretion of both antidiuretic hormone (ADH) and aldosterone is increased in the first 24 hours postoperatively. These increased levels cause a direct increase in sodium reabsorption in the kidney. Potassium excretion is increased, and urine sodium levels are decreased because of the increased hormonal levels. (Normal Physiology)

18. Correct: D. The most reliable indicator of the level of resuscitation in any patient is the hourly urinary output. This value is best measured with an indwelling catheter. Although pulmonary capillary wedge pressure and central venous pressure are helpful in this area, they can be misleading in certain instances (e.g., heart failure). Heart rate and blood pressure often do not change with small changes in volume status. (Normal Physiology)

19. Correct: E. The first step is to note which values are abnormal. This patient's P_{O_2} is low, but probably not low enough to cause him to pass out. The pH is low and P_{CO_2} is high, implying a respiratory cause. If the cause of his acidosis were metabolic, a lower HCO_3 would be expected. The next step is to determine whether any compensation has occurred. Using rule 1 from advanced cardiac life support (ACLS), with an increase in P_{CO_2} from 40 to 70 mm Hg (30 mm Hg), a decrease in pH of $0.08 \times 3 = 0.24$ is expected. This patient's pH is 7.16, a decrease of 0.24 from 7.4, so he has uncompensated respiratory alkalosis, as might be expected from too much narcotic. (Respiratory Acidosis)

20. Correct: B. This patient has partially compensated metabolic acidosis, probably from lactic acidosis as a result of hypovolemia. His decreased P_{CO_2} shows that he is attempting to compensate for the acidosis. Using advanced cardiac life support (ACLS) rule 2, a decrease of 0.15 in pH is expected for each 10 mEq/L decrease in HCO_3. This patient has a decrease in HCO_3 of 15 mEq/L (25 – 10), which should translate into a pH of $7.4 - (0.15 \times 1.5) = 7.18$. His pH is 7.2, which shows that he has compensated partially. To determine his bicarbonate deficit, use the equation:

$$mEq\ HCO_3\ needed = mEq/L\ [HCO_3]\ deficit \times (kg\ wt \times 0.25)$$
$$(25 - 10) \times (60 \times 0.25)$$
$$15 \times 15 = mEq$$

(Metabolic Acidosis)

Chapter 4

1. Correct: D. None of the liver function enzyme concentrations (e.g., alkaline phosphatase) correlate with nutritional status. Anthropometric, immunologic (e.g., delayed hypersensitivity skin tests, absolute lymphocyte count), and biochemical (e.g., serum transferrin or prealbumin, nitrogen balance, urine urea nitrogen excretion) tests relate to nutritional status. (Assessment of Nutritional Status/Anthropometric

Measurements, Biochemical Measurements, and Immunologic Measurements)

2. Correct: B. Injured, inflamed, or infected tissues release mediators that promote a catabolic response. This response is marked by increased levels of catecholamines, protein breakdown rates, lipolysis, and excretion of urea. Glutamine and alanine are released in the periphery (from skeletal muscle) for increased hepatic gluconeogenesis and oxidation by the intestinal mucosa and kidneys. (Metabolic Patterns That Affect Nutrition/Catabolic)

3. Correct: C. Patients who cannot eat because of coma, critical illness, or multiple injuries require nutritional support to maintain weight and body composition. Those with significant weight loss by history or increased protein losses by disease (high-output fistula) need nutritional support to replace and correct losses. Gangrenous appendicitis is a brief, acute illness. A short fast associated with appendectomy does not require support. (Assessment of Nutritional Status/History; Table 4–4; Table 4–9; Nutritional Support in Selected Surgical Situations/Inflammatory Bowel Disorders)

4. Correct: A. Hypokalemic, hypochloremic metabolic alkalosis is caused by uncompensated external loss of chloride and proton-containing fluids. Electrolyte and glucose abnormalities are caused by variances in supply, changes in the effectiveness of monitoring, and endocrine changes in different disease states. (Complications of Parenteral Nutrition; Table 4–8)

5. Correct: A. Proximal bowel fistulas may heal with bowel rest (provided by parenteral nutritional support). Diabetes mellitus requires close monitoring of blood sugar, regardless of the route of nutritional support. Although a major burn of the anterior torso may preclude subclavian vein access, the internal jugular vein can be used. Malignancy is not a contraindication to support. A jejunal feeding tube placed after operative drainage of a pancreatic abscess allows nutritional support at least as safely as total parenteral nutrition (TPN). (Techniques of Nutritional Support; Table 4–4; Table 4–5; Table 4–9)

6. Correct: A. Prophylactic antibiotics have no role in reducing catheter sepsis rates. Heparin-bonding, antibiotic-bonding, and antiseptic-bonding catheters generally reduce catheter sepsis, as does the use of a single-lumen catheter that is devoted to delivering total parenteral nutrition (TPN) in comparison with multiple-lumen catheters. However, aseptic technique at the time of catheter insertion and during site care is the most important method to reduce catheter-related sepsis. (Table 4–11; Complications of Parenteral Nutrition)

7. Correct: B. Zinc is an essential trace element, but it is not involved in high-energy bond formation, insulin activity, or red blood cell production. (Basic Nutritional Needs/Micronutrients: Trace Elements; Table 4–2)

8. Correct: D. The short half-life of prealbumin allows its weekly measurement to reflect acute changes in nutritional status. Albumin is affected by too many nonnutritional variables, and the creatinine-height index is too slow-changing. Nitrogen balance reflects the effectiveness of replacement of nitrogen losses. (Assessment of Nutritional Status; Table 4–1)

9. Correct: C. To increase the estimate of resting energy expenditure in a nonstressed person to the level associated with the hypercatabolic levels associated with the septic state, the best factor is 1.75. The other choices are wrong (0.9), sufficient for a nonstressed or mildly stressed person (1.24), or too great, which may lead to overfeeding. (Basic Nutritional Needs/Energy Needs)

10. Correct: D. Only linoleic acid is an essential fatty acid, and it must be supplied exogenously to persons who are receiving long-term total parenteral nutrition (TPN). (Techniques of Nutritional Support)

11. Correct: A. Alanine is released from skeletal muscle for transport to the liver, and it enters the gluconeogenic pathways. The branched-chain amino acids isoleucine and valine are oxidized in muscle itself. Arginine has immune-enhancing properties, and tyrosine is a substrate for (among other things) thyroxine. (Metabolic Patterns That Affect Nutrition/Catabolic; Basic Nutritional Needs/Protein and Amino Acid Needs)

12. Correct: E. Lipid emulsions contain linoleic acid and are relatively calorie-dense; therefore, they are useful in clinical situations that require volume restriction, and they do not produce CO_2. Hyperchloremic metabolic acidosis is caused by an excess of chloride ions (as a result of protein hydrolysis) in amino acid solutions. (Techniques of Nutritional Support/Parenteral Nutrition with Lipid Emulsion; Table 4–10)

13. Correct: D. Hypophosphatemia is associated with impaired myocardial contractility, decreased seizure threshold, paresthesias, weakness, and death. Reduced adenosine triphosphate content impairs red blood cell formation and decreases leukocyte chemotaxis, phagocytosis, and bactericidal functions. It does not cause bone pain. (Techniques of Nutritional Support/Complications of Parenteral Nutrition; Table 4–11)

14. Correct: C. The production of five or more loose, watery stools per day may be caused by contaminated tube feedings, excessive osmolar loads as a result of hypertonicity of the solution, or excessively rapid administration. Persons who have lactase deficiency cannot digest lactose from milk-based formu-

las. Concurrent broad-spectrum antibiotic treatment can also induce infectious diarrhea caused by *Clostridium difficile*. Fat content in commercial formulations does not cause diarrhea. (Enteral Nutritional Support/Implementation and Administration of an Enteral Feeding Program; Table 4–6)

15. Correct: A. Body fat is the greatest storehouse of energy in the body; carbohydrate is stored as glycogen, and is sufficient for only 24 to 48 hours. No proteins serve as storage forms of oxidative (energy) substrate. Bioimpedance assessment or triceps skinfold thickness measurements gauge body fat stores. Arm-muscle circumference and nitrogen balance deal with lean body mass and protein status. Liver biopsy is not an appropriate means of assessing body composition or energy stores. (Assessment of Nutritional Status; Basic Nutritional Needs)

16. Correct: B. Investigators report that levels of protein intake for nitrogen balance in normal, active persons vary from 1.0 to 1.5 g amino acids/kg/day. The additional stresses of operation, injury, burns, or infection increase these requirements to 2.5 g/kg/day. (Basic Nutritional Needs/Protein and Amino Acid Needs)

17. Correct: E. Glucose-dependent tissues include brain, bone marrow, red blood cells, peripheral nerves, and renal medullary cells. Intestinal epithelium uses glutamine as substrate. (Metabolic Patterns That Affect Nutrition)

18. Correct: B. Adaptation to prolonged fasting (starvation-adapted state) maximally reduces total body protein breakdown and nitrogen excretion to as little as 2 to 3 g/day. The other patterns are associated with accelerated protein breakdown rates. (Metabolic Patterns That Affect Nutrition)

19. Correct: D. In a sense, chemically defined diets are "predigested" to the elemental components of whole foods, minimizing the need for digestion. Lactose is not used, and fat content is usually low. (Techniques of Nutritional Support/Enteral Nutritional Support)

20. Correct: B. Nasogastric tubes may cause discomfort, even to the point of self-discontinuance of the tube, and they are associated with the rare complication of tracheoesophageal fistula. However, any type of formula can be given, and diarrhea is related more to the choice of formula, rate, and osmolarity than to the type of tube used. Aspiration pneumonitis is the most serious and unpredictable complication of prepyloric feeding. (Enteral Nutritional Support; Table 4–5; Table 4–6)

21. Correct: B. Copper deficiency impairs iron uptake in hemoglobin synthesis and is also associated with leukopenia. Zinc deficiency is associated with failure to heal wounds, cerebellar dysfunction, alopecia, and facial dermatitis. Chromium is necessary as an insulin cofactor, selenium deficiency causes cardiomyopathy and myositis, and magnesium deficiency causes weakness, neuromuscular hyperexcitability, and anorexia. (Basic Nutritional Needs/Micronutrients: Trace Elements; Table 4–2)

22. Correct: A. Only in adynamic ileus is the gastrointestinal tract unavailable to receive and absorb nutrients. Spontaneous oral intake is not possible in coma and is hazardous in severe dysphagia. Patients with exacerbations of Crohn's disease may benefit therapeutically from enteral nutrition. Enteral feeding is not excluded by pancreaticocutaneous fistulas, especially if access is through the jejunum. (Techniques of Nutritional Support; Table 4–4; Table 4–5)

23. Correct: E. Both equations require knowledge of the patient's age, sex, height, and weight to calculate the resting energy expenditure. This number is multiplied by a factor to account for activity. Body habitus does not play an independent role. (Basic Nutritional Needs/Energy Needs; Table 4–1)

24. Correct: B. When long-term infusion of highly concentrated glucose solutions is suddenly discontinued, the increased endogenous insulin levels precipitate hypoglycemia. A blood transfusion more likely elevates than depresses serum potassium. Transfusion reactions cause fever, back pain, hemolysis, and hypotension, but not coma. Bacteremia induces a febrile response. Air embolus may cause both shock and unconsciousness, but is not usually associated with blood transfusion. (Techniques of Nutritional Support; Table 4–11)

25. Correct: C. Recovery from major injury and burns is enhanced by enteral nutritional support compared with fasting and parenteral nutrition. Early use (after hemodynamic stabilization) increases its benefits. Because of increased proteolysis, more protein than usual is needed, and an enhanced supply of arginine may have particular benefit as a positive immunomodulator. No more than 40% of nonprotein calories should be supplied by fats. (Techniques of Nutritional Support)

26. Correct: C. Of all injuries and illnesses, thermal injuries cause the greatest increase in energy requirements in proportion to the depth and extent of the burn. The maximum estimated amount of calories is 200% of the resting energy expenditure calculated by the Harris-Benedict or World Health Organization equations. Underfeeding depletes the body's energy stores (fat) and lean body mass (proteins), whereas excessive calorie feeding increases the burden of removing oxidative byproducts, particularly carbon dioxide. (Basic Nutritional Needs)

Chapter 5

1. Correct: A. Factor XII influences the partial thromboplastin time. The activation of factor XIII is involved in the stabilization of fibrin much later in the coagulation process. The prothrombin time (PT) measures the rate of conversion of fibrinogen to fibrin. Dysfibrinogenemia does not influence the activation of the extrinsic pathway. (The Hemostatic Process)

2. Correct: C. The clotting factors of the intrinsic and extrinsic pathways and plasminogen deficiencies do not have a direct influence on the bleeding time, nor do increases in any of the clotting factors. (Evaluation of the Patient/Tests for Evaluation of Hemostasis)

3. Correct: D. The prothrombin time (PT) assay measures the adequacy of clotting factors in the extrinsic and common pathways. Factors of the intrinsic pathway (factors VIII, IX, XI, XII, and von Willebrand) do not influence PT. Platelet function also does not influence PT because a platelet substitute is added in the test tube. Protein C levels do not have any effect on PT because protein C is not a part of the extrinsic or common pathway. (Evaluation of the Patient/Tests for Evaluation of Hemostasis)

4. Correct: A. The activated partial thromboplastin time (APTT) measures the integrity of the clotting factors in the intrinsic and common pathways. Tissue thromboplastin and factors V, VII, and X and are measured by the prothrombin time (PT). Platelet function is excluded as a part of this test by adding platelet substitutes in the test tube. Protein S has no direct effect on the intrinsic and common pathways. (Evaluation of the Patient/Tests for Evaluation of Hemostasis)

5. Correct: B. Warfarin (Coumadin) depresses the functional adequacy of factors II, VII, IX, and X, and this depression causes prolongation of both the prothrombin time (PT) and the activated partial thromboplastin time (APTT). It does not alter the thrombin time, and it has no influence on factors V and VIII. The pharmacologic effect of Coumadin is independent of calcium, and it is not influenced by antithrombin III levels. (Causes of Excessive Surgical Bleeding/Preexisting Hemostatic Defects/Acquired Bleeding Disorders)

6. Correct: A. The most likely diagnosis is hemolytic transfusion reaction leading to disseminated intravascular coagulation. Thrombotic thrombocytopenic purpura generally has a somewhat slower onset and is associated with thrombocytopenia, fever, transient neurologic changes, and other organ dysfunction. A two-unit blood transfusion is not enough to dilute clotting factors. Von Willebrand's disease would have caused bleeding from the initiation of surgery. Fibrinolysis secondary to malignancy is unusual in carcinoma of the colon. It is more common in carcinoma

of the genitourinary tract. (Causes of Excessive Surgical Bleeding/Intraoperative Complications)

7. Correct: E. Shock, extensive trauma, sepsis, and acute hemolytic transfusion reactions are all associated with disseminated intravascular coagulation (DIC). Immunosuppression does not lead to DIC, although if patients become septic in association with immunosuppression, DIC can occur. (Common Bleeding Disorders in the Surgical Patient/Disseminated Intravascular Coagulation)

8. Correct: D. Although disseminated intravascular coagulation (DIC), von Willebrand's disease, and vitamin K deficiency can be associated with postoperative bleeding, the most common cause of postoperative bleeding is bleeding from an unligated vessel. Antithrombin III deficiency is associated with a hypercoagulable state. (Causes of Excessive Surgical Bleeding/Postoperative Bleeding)

9. Correct: B. Treatment of the precipitating cause is the best approach to disseminated intravascular coagulation (DIC). When the cause cannot be treated and chronic DIC persists, warfarin (Coumadin) may slow the process, but will not completely eradicate it. Cryoprecipitate is used to support patients with severe fibrinogenemia as a result of DIC, but this therapy is supportive and does not directly correct or eliminate the DIC. Factor VIII and red cell transfusions may also be given as supportive therapy, but they should be viewed as support only and not as corrective treatment. (Common Bleeding Disorders in the Surgical Patient/Disseminated Intravascular Coagulation)

10. Correct: E. All of the other materials (platelet concentrates, factor IX concentrates, cryoprecipitative plasma, and whole blood) may be used in selected cases to provide patient support if bleeding occurs, but ε-amino caproic acid blocks the fibrinolytic process and provides further fibrinolysis. (Common Bleeding Disorders in the Surgical Patient/Bleeding Disorders Caused by Increased Fibrinolysis)

11. Correct: B. Platelet concentrates may be stored for 3 to 5 days at room temperature. The number of platelets per bag depends on the platelet count of the donor. Platelets have a shortened survival time when they are refrigerated. To date, cryopreservation, glycerinization, and dimethyl sulfoxide preservation of platelets have not been successful. (Blood Replacement Therapy/Collection and Storage of Blood and Blood Products)

12. Correct: E. Cryoprecipitate is a rich source of fibrinogen and thus is used to treat hypofibrinogenemia. It can be used as part of the treatment for disseminated intravascular coagulation (DIC), for selected cases of von Willebrand's disease, and for occasional cases of hemophilia A. It is not used as volume support

because it is a very small volume blood product and is available in limited supply. There are safer and much more readily available blood products for volume support. (Blood Replacement Therapy/Plasma Component Therapy)

13. Correct: C. Because one administered unit of packed red cells raises the hematocrit by approximately 4%, the patient will need 6.25 units of packed red cells to raise the hematocrit from 15% to 40% (i.e., by 25%); 7 full units should be administered. (Blood Replacement Therapy/Blood Component Therapy/Estimating Red Blood Cell Transfusion Needs)

14. Correct: A. The bleeding time measures the number and function of platelets. Answers B, C, and D all measure coagulation factor levels, and fibrin split products measure the activity of the fibrinolytic pathway. (Evaluation of the Patient/Tests to Evaluate Hemostasis)

15. Correct: C. The activated partial thromboplastin time (APTT) measures these coagulation factors. The bleeding time measures platelet number and function. The prothrombin time (PT) measures the extrinsic and common pathways. Thrombin time measures the conversion of fibrinogen to fibrin. Fibrin split products indicate fibrinolytic pathway activity. (Evaluation of the Patient/Tests to Evaluate Hemostasis)

16. Correct: D. Fibrinogen-to-fibrin conversion is measured by the thrombin time. The bleeding time measures platelet number and function. The prothrombin time (PT) measures the extrinsic and common pathways. The activated partial thromboplastin time (APTT) measures factor V, VIII, IX, X, XI, and XII levels. Fibrin split products indicate fibrinolytic pathway activity. (Evaluation of the Patient/Tests to Evaluate Hemostasis)

17. Correct: B. Factors V, VII, and X are best measured by the prothrombin time (PT), which measures the extrinsic and common pathways. The bleeding time measures platelet number and function. The activated partial thromboplastin time (APTT) measures factor V, VIII, IX, X, XI, and XII levels. Fibrinogen-to-fibrin conversion is measured by the thrombin time. Fibrin split products indicate fibrinolytic pathway activity. (Evaluation of the Patient/Tests to Evaluate Hemostasis)

18. Correct: A. The bleeding time can be influenced by vessel wall integrity. This problem is most commonly seen in patients with fragile skin syndrome (e.g., the elderly) and in patients who receive long-term corticosteroid therapy. The prothrombin time (PT), activated partial thromboplastin time (APTT), and thrombin time measure various clotting factor levels, and fibrin split products measure fibrinolytic activity. (Evaluation of the Patient/Tests to Evaluate Hemostasis)

19. Correct: A. Banked blood has a progressive loss of red cell viability depending on the duration of storage before transfusion. Platelet function is decreased; in fact, platelets become relatively dysfunctional quickly in banked blood because it is refrigerated. As the red cells die off in the banked blood, potassium levels increase. There is also increased hydrogen ion concentration as blood is stored, and the coagulation factors decay relatively rapidly with blood storage, although today, because most blood is stored as packed red blood cells, there are almost no coagulation factors in the packed red blood cells that are transfused to patients. (Blood Replacement Therapy/Collection and Storage of Blood and Blood Products)

20. Correct: E. Factor VIII is made and stored principally in the vascular endothelium. In patients with liver failure, factor VIII levels are normal. (Causes of Excessive Surgical Bleeding/Preexisting Hemostatic Defects/Acquired Bleeding Disorders)

Chapter 6

1. Correct: C. All of the other answers can result in hypovolemia, but it is usually not as severe as that seen after hemorrhage. (Etiologies, Diagnosis, and Management of Hypoperfusion States; Table 6–8)

2. Correct: B. Increased systemic and pulmonary arterial resistance reduces ventricular function directly, as does myocardial ischemia, independent of intravascular volume. A low hemoglobin value does not usually impair cardiac function. (Etiologies, Diagnosis, and Management of Hypoperfusion States; Table 6–8)

3. Correct: C. A 20% intravascular volume loss in a 70-kg man is estimated at 1000 mL. The 3:1 rule for crystalloid resuscitation would result in the administration of 3000 mL. (A Practical Guide to the Patient in Shock/Provide an Excellent Circulation)

4. Correct: B. Agitation is characteristic of hypoperfusion states. The use of sedatives, restraints, and nasal oxygen does not affect the primary etiology of the agitation, and (if sedatives are used) may precipitate more severe hemodynamic embarrassment. (Etiologies, Diagnosis, and Management of Hypoperfusion States/Decreased Venous Return: Hypovolemia/Physical Examination in Hypovolemic Hypoperfusion)

5. Correct: C. Blood pressure alone is an inadequate monitor; a measure of tissue perfusion is more useful. Usually, urinary output greater than 0.5 mL/kg is sufficient information to indicate adequate renal perfusion. However, other clinical data (e.g., mental status, color and temperature of the extremities), although not as easily measured, should not be ignored. (Etiologies,

Diagnosis, and Management of Hypoperfusion States/Endpoints for Resuscitation of the Circulation)

6. Correct: D. Cardiogenic hypoperfusion secondary to severe inflammation causes decreased cardiac output and increased atrial pressures, lactate levels, and respiratory rate. (Severe Inflammatory States/Effects of Severe Inflammation on the Circulation)

7. Correct: E. The primary treatment of hypoperfusion secondary to severe inflammation is improvement of venous return, not the use of inotropes, vasodilators, or steroids. (Diagnosis and Management of Severe Inflammation/Treatment/Supporting Organ Function: Cardiovascular and Pulmonary)

8. Correct: B. (Table 6–1)

9. Correct: E. Hypovolemic hypoperfusion is indistinguishable from cardiogenic shock by all of the parameters listed, except that ventricular filling pressures are high in cardiogenic shock and low in severe hypovolemic hypoperfusion. (Etiologies, Diagnosis, and Management of Hypoperfusion States/Cardiogenic Hypoperfusion and Cardiogenic Shock)

10. Correct: C. (Hypoperfusion States/The Neurohumoral Response to Hypoperfusion)

11. Correct: B. (Hypoperfusion States/The Neurohumoral Response to Hypoperfusion)

12. Correct: D. Both severe hypovolemic hypoperfusion and severe inflammation may increase arterial lactate and blood glucose levels. (Severe Inflammatory States/Effects of Severe Inflammation on Cellular Function)

13. Correct: D. Oxygen consumption and intrapulmonary shunt increase, and peripheral resistance decreases. Vasoactive drugs are used only in select cases. (Diagnosis and Management of Severe Inflammation/Treatment/Supporting Organ Function: Cardiovascular and Pulmonary)

14. Correct: A. Only epinephrine and norepinephrine have major acute circulatory effects. (Hypoperfusion States/The Neurohumoral Response to Hypoperfusion)

15. Correct: E. Elevated blood glucose is secondary to increased gluconeogenesis associated with increased glucocorticoid release, increased epinephrine levels, and decreased glycogen stores. (Hypoperfusion States/The Neurohumoral Response to Hypoperfusion)

16. Correct: A. Normal oxygen consumption is approximately 250 mL/min, with a range of 130 to 160 mL/min/m^2 when adjusted for body surface area.

The other values are much too low or too high. (Table 6–1)

17. Correct: D. The calculation of oxygen consumption is based on the difference in oxygen content between arterial and mixed venous blood. (Table 6–1)

18. Correct: B. Although attention to the circulation is important during severe inflammation, the primary principle is to locate and treat the underlying inflammatory disease. Steroid administration does not usually treat the underlying disease process. (Diagnosis and Management of Severe Inflammation/Treatment)

19. Correct: D. Inflammation can cause all of the effects listed, except increasing intrathoracic pressure. (Severe Inflammatory States/Effects of Severe Inflammation on the Circulation)

20. Correct: A. Although it is possible to translocate and activate the coagulation cascade during severe hypovolemic hypoperfusion, ischemia and reperfusion is the primary mechanism for hypoperfusion-induced inflammation. Lactic acid increases as a consequence of anaerobic metabolism or stimulation of inflammatory cells, and does not stimulate inflammation directly. Macrophages are activated primarily by inflammatory stimuli, not by ischemia. (Hypoperfusion States/The Effects of Hypoperfusion on Inflammation)

Chapter 7

1. Correct: B. Any disruption of the normal tissue anatomy can be classified as a wound. A wound may close spontaneously without suturing, and if it has fewer than 10^5 bacteria, it is usually considered a noninfected wound. (Introduction)

2. Correct: B. Granulation tissue has four important components: fibroblasts, capillaries, bacteria, and inflammatory cells. Bacteria are also contained in granulation tissue. Mature collagen fibers are present in the remodeling phase of wound healing after the wound is closed. Epithelial cells and skin appendages are present only in healed wounds. (Classification of Healing Wounds/Secondary Healing)

3. Correct: B. During the maturation phase of wound healing, no net collagen production occurs because collagen synthesis is equal to collagen destruction. (Phases of Wound Healing/Maturation Phase)

4. Correct: A. A clean wound is a wound that has fewer than 10^5 organisms/g tissue; it will often take a skin graft. Granulation tissue contains bacteria and may have greater than 10^5 bacteria/g; it usually will not take a skin graft. (Factors That Affect Wound Healing)

5. Correct: A. During the inflammatory phase of wound healing, there is an influx of inflammatory cells into

the wound. However, during this phase, there is no significant amount of collagen production. (Phases of Wound Healing/Substrate Phase)

6. Correct: C. An infected granulating wound has greater than 10^5 bacteria/g. Because of the high bacteria count, a skin graft usually would not take over an infected granulating wound. Multiple organisms can be cultured from an infected granulated wound. (Factors That Affect Wound Healing)

7. Correct: D. A dressing serves all of these functions, except decrease bacteria growth. In certain occlusive dressings, fluid collection underneath the dressing may promote increased growth of bacteria. (Technique of Wound Debridement and Closure/Dressings)

8. Correct: A. The proliferative phase is the second phase of wound healing. During this phase, there is an abundance of collagen synthesis in the wound, and the wound is erythematous and raised. (Phases of Wound Healing/Proliferative Phase)

9. Correct: C. The layers that have the greatest strength in wound closure are the dermis and fascia. Therefore, stitches can be removed at any time if appropriate dermal sutures were placed. (Wound Debridement and Closure)

10. Correct: C. For maximum wound strength, the dermal and the fascia layers must be approximated separately because they are the strength layers. (Technique of Wound Debridement and Closure/Suture Removal)

11. Correct: D. To decrease bacteria load in the wound, the dead space is eliminated and the debris removed. Topical antibiotics decrease bacteria load in a contaminated wound in preparation for coverage with well-vascularized tissue. (Technique of Wound Debridement and Closure/Wound Debridement and Closure)

12. Correct: E. Catgut sutures derived from sheep intestines are biologic sutures that last 7 to 10 days. (Technique of Wound Debridement and Closure/Suture Material)

13. Correct: C. Silk sutures are not commonly used today. Silk sutures are polyfilament nonabsorbable sutures. (Technique of Wound Debridement and Closure/Suture Material)

14. Correct: D. Nylon suture is a monofilament nonabsorbable suture, and it is commonly used for skin closure because it induces low inflammatory response. (Suture Material)

15. Correct: A. Polyglycolic suture is commonly used to approximate the dermal layer. It is a polyfilament absorbable suture. (Technique of Wound Debridement and Closure/Suture Material)

16. Correct: C. The maturation phase is the third phase of wound healing, and is characterized by cross-linking of collagen. There is no net increase in collagen production. Once the wound has matured, the scar appears flat and soft. (Phases of Wound Healing/Maturation Phase)

17. Correct: E. In a contaminated wound, monofilament sutures are better than polyfilament sutures because they cause less inflammatory reaction and a decrease in bacteria trapping. (Technique of Wound Debridement and Closure/Suture Material)

18. Correct: C. Wounds are allowed to heal by secondary intention because the increased bacteria count in certain wounds may lead to wound infection if they are closed primarily. (Classification of Healing Wounds/Secondary Healing)

19. Correct: C. During the proliferative phase of wound healing, there is net increase in collagen production because collagen synthesis is greater than collagen destruction. (Phases of Wound Healing/Proliferative Phase)

20. Correct: C. In an infected wound from a perforated appendix, primary closure inevitably leads to infection. Therefore, the wound may be packed with gauze, and on the fifth postoperative day, it is closed with sterile strips. (Management of the Contaminated and Infected Wound/The Infected Wound)

Chapter 8

1. Correct: A. Prophylactic antibiotics are routinely used in clean procedures in which a foreign body is implanted, in clean-contaminated cases, and in contaminated cases. Drainage or age is not a criterion for the selection of antibiotic prophylaxis. Antibiotics are indicated for drainage of a pelvic abscess. (Prevention of Surgical Infection/Perioperative Antibiotics)

2. Correct: D. When an infection follows a clean procedure, a break in "technique" is usually the identified problem. A short operative time is of primary importance in this process. Prophylactic antibiotics and air laminar flow are seldom used for routine clean surgical procedures. (Prevention of Surgical Infection/Surgical Asepsis)

3. Correct: C. All of the listed nosocomial infections are seen after surgical procedures; however, because of the frequent and almost ubiquitous use of mechanical urinary drainage in patients who are undergoing major surgical procedures, the urinary tract is the most common site of infection. Removal of the

catheter and induced diuresis are usually the only steps that are needed to effect cleansing of the bladder. (Management of Established Infection/Hospital-Acquired Infections/Urinary Tract Infection)

4. Correct: E. The area as described is consistent with a furuncle. Incision and drainage are the essential management techniques for all localized infections in which pus is present. (Table 8–4)

5. Correct: B. A paronychia is an infection at the margin of the nail that may extend beneath the nail. A felon is an infection of the soft tissue pulp space of the digit. Both require incision and drainage of the localized infection. A felon rarely extends to the synovial spaces. (Management of Established Infection/Community-Acquired Infections/Hand Infections)

6. Correct: A. Necrotizing fasciitis is an infection of mixed aerobic and anaerobic organisms that have a synergistic relation. This relation provides an invasive character to the process. Death is the outcome if adequate debridement of the necrotic and infected tissue is not performed. This process is seen after trauma of any sort. Hyperbaric oxygen is of no benefit in the absence of adequate debridement. (Management of Established Infection/Community-Acquired Infections/Skin and Soft Tissue Infections)

7. Correct: A. The most common cause of early postoperative fever is infection of the pulmonary tract. Atelectasis is seen most often. Because of the proximity of the left hemidiaphragm to the spleen, some degree of left lower lobe infiltrate is a distinct possibility in this patient. Computed tomography (CT) scan, intravenous pyelogram, and venogram are not indicated at this point because the complications that they would potentially identify usually develop later in the course. (Management of Established Infection/Hospital-Acquired Infections/Pulmonary Infection)

8. Correct: D. All of the tests or examinations listed, except the upper gastrointestinal series, are used to evaluate postoperative patients for intraabdominal sepsis. Because of intestinal ileus and the potential for anastomotic leak, an upper gastrointestinal series is rarely effective in this setting and is potentially dangerous if barium should leak into the peritoneal cavity. (Management of Established Infection/Hospital-Acquired Infections/Intraabdominal Infection)

9. Correct: C. Clearly, the most useful test to localize an intraabdominal infection is the computed tomography (CT) scan. This technique is therapeutic in selected patients when the area identified is amenable to percutaneous aspiration and drainage. The other diagnostic techniques are indirect methods for localization. Sonography has limited applicability in the postoperative patient because of bowel ileus

and distension. (Management of Established Infection/Hospital-Acquired Infections/Intraabdominal Infection)

10. Correct: D. The clinical scenario described is typical for patients with perforated colonic diverticulitis with established peritonitis, which is a surgical emergency. In this case, antibiotics are therapeutic, not prophylactic, and should be directed toward the mixed and anaerobic bacterial population found in the colon. Oral antibiotics are only effective when combined with a mechanical bowel preparation in the elective setting. (Management of Established Infection/Hospital-Acquired Infections/Intraabdominal Infection)

11. Correct: E. Prophylactic antibiotics are used in selected clean, clean-contaminated, and contaminated elective cases. The antibiotics should have an extended half-life, be relatively free of toxic effects, and be effective against the pathogens that are most likely to be encountered. The antibiotics should be administered immediately before the procedure so that tissue levels are present at the time of the incision. They are only continued for several doses postoperatively. (Prevention of Surgical Infection/Perioperative Antibiotics)

12. Correct: B. Young age is not a factor in the development of an infection after surgery. All of the other listed variables alter the local or systemic host environment in favor of the pathogen. (Pathogenesis of Infection; Table 8–1)

13. Correct: C. Adequate debridement and cleansing is the foundation for managing traumatic soft tissue wounds. Depending on the extent of injury and the degree of contamination, antibiotics are used, either systemically or, more effectively, topically. Unless complete debridement is accomplished, primary closure of the wound is also performed. (Prevention of Surgical Infection)

14. Correct: B. *Streptococcus* species is a frequent pathogen that is responsible for early cellulitis after a laceration. *Staphylococcus* causes local inflammation and pus formation. The other three species are rarely isolated after a laceration, but are encountered after intraabdominal procedures, especially if the colon is involved. (Table 8–4)

15. Correct: D. Synergistic gangrene is an infection that involves both aerobic and anaerobic pathogens. The cornerstone of treatment involves a change in the local microenvironment where these organisms are present. This goal is easily accomplished with debridement. Other treatment modalities are helpful only after the local environment is excised. (Table 8–7)

16. Correct: A. Suppurative thrombophlebitis usually develops in a vein that is used for intravenous cannulation. The process of pus formation is occult at times. For this reason, a close physical examination of all intravenous sites is necessary when fever, leukocytosis, and bacteremia occur. Impetigo is a skin infection that rarely causes bacteremia. Atelectasis causes fever, but seldom results in prolonged leukocytosis or bacteremia. Systemic signs of infection seldom accompany a local furuncle. Hashimoto's thyroiditis is an autoimmune disease. (Management of Established Infection/Hospital-Acquired Infections/Foreign Body–Associated Infection)

17. Correct: D. Both suppurative thrombophlebitis and associated bacteremia in the intravascular cannulae are the result of an infective focus in proximity to the percutaneous site of device entry. To effectively treat the source, the foreign body is removed and the area debrided. Antibiotics are rarely needed if the local site of infection is adequately cleaned. (Management of Established Infection/Hospital-Acquired Infections/ Foreign Body–Associated Infection)

18. Correct: B. Clearly, the hallmark of treatment for intraabdominal abscess in drainage. When abscess occurs secondary to continued intestinal soilage, repair or exteriorization of the bowel segment is indicated. Systemic antibiotics are adjuncts to surgical intervention, but are not effective as a sole form of therapy. Hot soaks, elevation, and immobilization are of little benefit for intraabdominal infections. (Management of Established Infection/Hospital-Acquired Infections/Intraabdominal Infection)

19. Correct: A. Hidradenitis is an infection of the sweat glands in the axilla or groin regions. Wide debridement is the most effective form of therapy to prevent frequent recurrence. A sebaceous cyst may become secondarily infected. This infection occurs anywhere as an isolated subcutaneous mass. A furuncle or a felon is a subcutaneous abscess that is located primarily on the trunk. A pilonidal cyst is the result of a sinus between the buttocks that becomes secondarily infected. (Table 8–7)

20. Correct: C. Human immunodeficiency virus (HIV), hepatitis B, hepatitis C, and cytomegalovirus are transmitted by blood and body fluids. Therefore, they pose an occupational risk to the surgeon. There is a highly effective vaccine for hepatitis B that affords immunity to the host. No such vaccine is currently available for the other virus particles. Hepatitis A is transmitted by the fecal–oral route and does not usually present a threat to the health care provider unless he or she regularly dines at the friendly corner pub. (Management of Established Infection/Community-Acquired Infections/Viral Infections)

Chapter 9

1. Correct: B. The first priority in treating the trauma patient is to perform the primary survey, which is defined as the diagnosis and treatment of all immediately life-threatening injuries. A, C, D, and E are all performed in the secondary survey. (Algorithm)

2. Correct: D. The first step in the primary survey is D. A is performed in the secondary survey. B, C, and E occur later in the primary survey. Remember the "ABCDEs" of trauma management. (Algorithm; Airway Obstruction)

3. Correct: E. In the sleeping, lethargic, or unconscious patient, the jaw muscles are relaxed. As a result, the jaws fall posteriorly, and in the supine patient, the tongue can prolapse into the hypopharynx and obstruct the airway. Signs of supraglottic airway obstruction are stridor, snoring, and gurgling. The oropharyngeal and nasopharyngeal airways are designed to prevent the tongue from obstructing the airway. The oropharyngeal airway can cause gagging or vomiting in a patient who has an intact gag reflex. The nasopharyngeal airway is a soft, flexible tube with a trumpet-like flange on the external end. It is well tolerated in the patient who has an intact gag reflex. B, the chin-lift, is functionally the same maneuver as the jaw-thrust. A and C refer to intubating the trachea, which is not at risk of being compromised in this patient. (Airway Obstruction; Figure 9–10)

4. Correct: B. This patient's airway is at risk of compromise. The trachea can be deviated, compressed, and occluded by the rapidly expanding pulsatile hematoma. Therefore, this patient needs tracheal intubation. The patient is breathing, which makes her a candidate for nasotracheal intubation. In this procedure, an endotracheal tube is passed blindly through one of the nostrils into the trachea. Orotracheal intubation is an option, but would likely require the patient to be sedated or paralyzed because a laryngoscope would have to be placed behind the tongue or epiglottis to visualize the vocal cords. In an awake patient, this procedure can stimulate gagging, coughing, and vomiting. C and E do not prevent airway compromise. A cricothyroidotomy is indicated only if orotracheal intubation fails. (Tracheal Intubation: The Definitive Airway; Figure 9–10)

5. Correct: C. A trauma patient who is hypotensive and tachycardic has usually lost at least 30% of the blood volume. This patient fits the criteria for class III hemorrhage. Acutely, hematocrit is not a reliable indicator of the volume of hemorrhage because not enough time has passed to permit equilibration with the extravascular space. (Hemorrhagic Shock; Table 9–1)

6. Correct: D. A general rule of thumb is that 3 mL crystalloid fluid is needed to replace 1 mL blood. This

3:1 ratio allows for the redistribution of crystalloid into the interstitial and intracellular spaces. (Hemorrhagic Shock/Treatment of Hemorrhagic Shock)

7. Correct: E. Hypovolemia and the adrenergic response to hemorrhage appear to empty the venous capacitance vessels in the early stages of shock. Therefore, inflation of the pneumatic antishock garment (PASG) displaces little additional blood. Compression of the arterioles in the lower extremities increases systemic vascular resistance. Inflation of the abdominal compartment of the garment compresses the inferior vena cava and thereby impedes venous return to the heart. Elevation of the diaphragm also occurs with inflation of the abdominal compartment. This elevation may interfere with ventilation. The PASG stabilizes fractures by acting as a splint to prevent movement of fractured bones. (Treatment of Hemorrhagic Shock)

8. Correct: A. Hypotension, distended neck veins, tracheal deviation to the right, and a hyperresonant left chest are signs of a left tension pneumothorax. This immediately life-threatening thoracic injury must be treated without delay. A left needle thoracostomy is a temporizing maneuver that allows time to insert a chest tube, which is the definitive treatment of tension pneumothorax. Waiting for chest x-ray confirmation could lead to the patient's death. Pericardiocentesis is not indicated because the patient does not have cardiac tamponade. Cardiac tamponade does not cause tracheal deviation or a hyperresonant chest. (Immediately Lethal Thoracic; Table 9–3)

9. Correct: D. This patient is at risk for traumatic aortic rupture and great vessel injury. Often, there are no specific symptoms or signs. A high index of suspicion in patients with deceleration injuries may be the only indication for further evaluation. Arteriography is the diagnostic procedure of choice. Computed tomography (CT) is not an optimal study to diagnose this condition. Other useful diagnostic studies include transesophageal echocardiography and spiral CT arteriography. Fractures of the scapula and ribs 1 and 2 require significant forces. As a result, they are associated with major injuries to the head, neck, cervical spine, lung, and aorta and its major branches. To look for a delayed pneumothorax, a repeat chest x-ray is obtained within 6 hours. Nothing suggests that A and B are indicated in this patient. (Potentially Lethal Thoracic Injuries; Nonlethal Thoracic Injuries)

10. Correct: A. This patient has a pelvic fracture with an associated urethral injury. Before a Foley catheter is inserted, the perineum and rectum must be examined. The presence of blood at the urethral meatus, a perineal hematoma, or an abnormal prostate examination requires that a retrograde urethrogram be performed to assure continuity of the urethra. A suprapubic bladder catheter is normally required if the urethra is injured. Urethral injuries are commonly associated with pelvic fractures in men. (Abdominal Trauma/Gastric and Bladder Catheters)

11. Correct: B. In trauma patients, unrecognized intraabdominal hemorrhage is one of the leading causes of preventable deaths. Patients with significant abdominal trauma often have no significant physical findings to indicate intraabdominal injury. The classic signs of abdominal pain, tenderness, and rebound are often camouflaged by other extraabdominal injuries or masked by an altered level of consciousness as a result of head trauma, drugs, or alcohol. In hypotensive trauma patients with normal breath sounds and no external signs of blood loss, the abdomen is a likely source of occult hemorrhage. Diagnostic peritoneal lavage is an excellent way to evaluate a patient for intraabdominal bleeding. In view of the normal chest x-ray, a spiral computed tomography (CT) scan is not indicated. This patient is not fully resuscitated, and decreasing the intravenous rate would only make the situation worse. D and E are not indicated. (Abdominal Trauma/Diagnostic Evaluation; Figure 9–14)

12. Correct: E. Gunshot wounds to the abdomen have a high incidence of significant intraabdominal injury. Therefore, prompt laparotomy is required. A, B, and D are not indicated. An intravenous pyelogram is not indicated because this patient's urine is pale yellow and negative for blood. (Abdominal Trauma/Diagnostic Evaluation; Figure 9–14)

13. Correct: B. This patient has an acute epidural hematoma, which usually results from a tear in the middle meningeal artery. Classic signs are loss of consciousness (concussion), followed by a lucid interval, and then depressed consciousness and contralateral hemiparesis. The prognosis is usually excellent because the underlying brain injury is minimal. The lucid interval seen in this patient is not seen in patients with the diagnoses in A, C, D, and E. (Head Injury; Table 9–8)

14. Correct: D. This patient is hypotensive and tachycardic. In the trauma patient, these findings indicate blood loss until proven otherwise. Hypotension in a patient with a head injury should prompt a search for hemorrhage. Isolated closed head or brain injuries do not cause hypotension. The physiologic response to increased intracranial pressure (e.g., intracranial hemorrhage, cerebral edema) is systemic hypertension. This process is known as the Cushing reflex. Septic shock rarely occurs immediately after acute injury. Spinal cord injury patients have bradycardia associated with hypotension. Patients with cardiac injury usually have distended neck veins. (Head Injury)

15. Correct: A. This patient has a basal skull fracture and increased intracranial pressure (ICP). Normal ICP is less than 10 mm Hg. When ICP increases, the body attempts to maintain cerebral perfusion pressure by increasing the systemic blood pressure. This early response to increased ICP is the Cushing reflex. In addition to hypertension, this reflex is associated with bradycardia and decreased respiratory rate. Patients with the diagnoses in B, C, and E have hypotension. (Head Injury/Cerebral Anatomy and Physiology)

16. Correct: B. This patient has a zone II injury. Zone I is the base of the neck and extends from the sternal notch to the top of the clavicles or cricoid cartilage. Injuries in this zone carry a high mortality rate because they involve major vascular and tracheal damage. Zone II is the central portion of the neck and extends from the top of zone I to the angle of the mandible. Injuries in zone II carry a lesser mortality rate because they are obvious and operative exposure is not difficult. Zone III is the distal portion of the neck and extends from the angle of the mandible to the base of the skull. Zone II injuries can be explored without further evaluation. Injuries in zones I and III usually require further evaluation. D is incorrect because if these endoscopic procedures were normal, the patient would still require arteriography. E is incorrect because the esophagus, trachea, and carotids could also be injured. (Penetrating Neck Injuries)

17. Correct: C. This patient has a spinal cord injury. Hypotension associated with bradycardia is suggestive of neurogenic shock. This situation is seen in high thoracic and cervical cord injuries (usually above the level of T-5). Other findings that suggest cervical spine injury include flaccid areflexia; diaphragmatic breathing; the ability to flex, but not extend the elbow (injury involving the C-7 nerve root, which supplies the triceps); grimaces to pain above, but not below the clavicles; and priapism. Sepsis, hemorrhage, and cardiac injury cause hypotension with tachycardia. Cardiac injury causes pump failure and distension of the neck veins. Brain injury associated with increased intracranial pressure causes hypertension. (Spine and Spinal Cord Injury)

18. Correct: E. Airway management in the child differs from that in the adult. The child's larynx is more cranial and anterior, and the trachea is shorter. Orotracheal intubation is the preferred route. A, B, C, and D can all be used in children. Nasotracheal intubation is contraindicated in children because of the anatomic factors that increase the risk of injury to the nasopharynx or the risk of penetration of the calvarium. (Pediatric Trauma)

19. Correct: C. Ultrasound is an excellent choice because, in addition to providing information about the presence of intraperitoneal blood, it can provide information about the fetus, placenta, and uterus. Diagnostic peritoneal lavage is invasive. The indications are the same as in the nonpregnant patient. However, the incision is properly made above the apex of the uterine fundus. Abdominal x-rays and arteriography expose the fetus to radiation. Unlike abdominal ultrasound, serial physical examinations do not provide information about the presence of intraperitoneal blood. (Trauma in Women)

20. Correct: B. This patient has a compartment syndrome. This condition results from an increase in the fascial compartmental pressure. This increase causes interstitial tissue pressure to become higher than capillary perfusion pressure. The result is ischemia to the muscles and nerves within the fascial compartment. The syndrome usually takes hours to develop, but it may develop rapidly, as when there is an arterial bleed into the compartment. It typically occurs in the calf and forearm, but can also occur in the thigh, arm, foot, and hand. Muscular swelling and compartmental bleeding are the usual etiologic factors. Initiating events include arterial injuries, crush injuries, fractures, prolonged compression, and restoration of blood flow to a previously ischemic extremity. An early sign is decreased sensation, caused by neural ischemia, in the distribution of the compartmental nerves. Other signs and symptoms include pain, especially pain exacerbated by passive stretch of the involved muscles; a tense, swollen compartment; and weakness of the involved muscle. Decreased pulses and capillary filling are not reliable findings because they usually do not occur until late in the evolution of this condition. The diagnosis is usually made clinically. Treatment is surgical fasciotomy. A, D, and E will do nothing to treat the syndrome. Amputation is not indicated. (Extremity Trauma)

Chapter 10

1. Correct: B. This patient illustrates the danger that health care workers face when dealing with hazardous material spills. Unwary physicians and nurses who attempt to help this man could suffer serious burns from the acid on his clothing, which is continuing to burn the patient as well. This chemical must be neutralized before a primary survey can be conducted safely. (Initial Care of the Patient With Burns/Stop the Burning Process)

2. Correct: A. This patient's history and physical findings suggest significant inhalation injury. Carbon monoxide poisoning, hypoxia, and impending airway obstruction may all be present. In any trauma patient, a compromised airway requires treatment before the rest of the primary survey can be undertaken. Chest x-ray may be normal despite significant injury. His coma is almost certainly caused by hypoxia. (Initial Care of the Patient With Burns/Primary Survey)

3. Correct: C. This woman demonstrates the "five Ps" of ischemic compression: pain, pallor, pulselessness, paralysis, and poikilothermia (coolness). She is at risk for irreversible necrosis of her forearm if the compression is not relieved quickly. Her history is inconsistent with inhalation injury. Fracture is unlikely. Skin grafting is not a priority at this point, and enteral nutrition is probably not needed for such a small wound. (Definitive Care of Burn Patients/Resuscitation Period)

4. Correct: E. Burns can heal only if some epidermis remains alive. When burns are very deep, even the deepest epidermal appendages are destroyed. Deep injuries are usually relatively pain-free because many of the pain sensors are also destroyed. Dermis that is destroyed by burning never regenerates. Deep burns can form scar tissue, but this outcome may not be desirable. Skin grafting is almost always performed after resuscitation is completed. (Pathophysiology of Burn Injury/Full-Thickness Burns)

5. Correct: D. Fluid losses, which complicate burn wounds, occur at the expense of intravascular volume, a phenomenon known as burn shock. Swelling is progressive over the first 24 hours after injury, and can cause cardiovascular collapse. Appropriate fluid resuscitation, according to the Parkland formula and other regimens, does not prevent swelling, but maintains blood volume at an acceptable level. These formulas are helpful in predicting fluid requirements, but must be adjusted according to continued reevaluation of the patient. (Definitive Care of Burn Patients/Resuscitation Period)

6. Correct: B. Inhalation injury produces chemical damage to the airways that may cause no symptoms for hours or days after exposure. Normal oxygenation and chest x-ray do not exclude this type of injury. Facial burns, singed nasal hair, carbonaceous sputum, and other physical findings can suggest the diagnosis, but are not always present. Even if the diagnosis is made, endotracheal intubation is performed only if it is clinically indicated. (Initial Care of the Patient With Burns/Primary Survey)

7. Correct: C. Bacteria readily colonize avascular burn eschar, but do not necessarily invade the viable tissue below. When they do, bacteremia and systemic sepsis result. The use of topical and systemic antibiotics, including silver sulfadiazine, and early burn wound excision have helped to reduce the incidence of burn wound sepsis. However, increasingly virulent microbial strains continue to emerge, making this complication a continued threat to burn patients. (Wound Coverage Period/Infection Control)

8. Correct: E. The combination of early excision and skin grafting has gained widespread popularity as a way of reducing the risks of burn wound infection, as well as the pain, metabolic stress, and length of hospitalization for patients with major injuries. Although blood loss and pain can be problems, even very large procedures can be performed safely by experienced teams. In most burn centers, excision and skin grafting are performed only after successful resuscitation is completed. Tangential, or "layered," excision is now the most widely performed procedure. (Wound Coverage Period/Excision and Skin Grafting)

9. Correct: D. This patient was injured in a manner that frequently produces multiple trauma. His primary survey is essentially completed, and resuscitation is underway. He is very likely to have other injuries, which can prove life-threatening long before the burn injury becomes a problem. All other aspects of burn treatment should wait until after a thorough trauma evaluation is performed. (Initial Care of the Patient With Burns/Secondary Survey)

10. Correct: B. Patients with large injuries must be given aggressive nutritional support before weight loss and inanition occur. Total parenteral nutrition is difficult to manage in patients with large burns, and is associated with many more complications than enteral feeding. Prophylactic antibiotics are not helpful in preventing burn-associated infections, and systemic corticosteroids are probably deleterious to patients. (Wound Coverage Period/Nutritional Support)

11. Correct: E. This patient fits many criteria for referral to a specialized burn care facility. She has a high anticipated likelihood of mortality and will require costly specialized care. (Table 10–2)

12. Correct: A. Burn wounds begin to contract soon after injury. In addition, the pain and swelling that accompany an acute burn interfere with circulation and healing. The functional result obtained from such a small, but serious injury will probably depend more on physical therapy than on surgical care. Waiting longer than a day or two to begin therapy gives contracture time to start, and makes eventual recovery more difficult. Remember: rehabilitation begins at the time of injury. (Definitive Care of Burn Injuries/Rehabilitation Period)

13. Correct: E. In recent years, the use of broad-spectrum antibiotics has favored the emergence of multiply resistant strains of many organisms. The use of topical as well as systemic agents has not solved the problem of burn wound infection, but has selected the most troublesome organisms as causative agents. (Wound Coverage Period/Infection Control)

14. Correct: B. Although inhalation injury can cause immediate death from carbon monoxide poisoning and hypoxia, patients who survive the initial event should survive this problem. Similarly, airway obstruction is usually a treatable problem with a

limited time course. Pneumonia is the most worrisome complication of smoke inhalation because it is often persistent, recurrent, and difficult to treat. Persistent infection, including pneumonia, often leads to the development of the multiple organ failure syndrome, which is usually fatal. (Initial Care of the Patient With Burns/Primary Survey; Table 10–1)

15. Correct: C. This patient illustrates the importance of the secondary survey in victims of burn injury. This man's burns are too limited in extent to cause severe shock, especially so soon after injury. Smoke inhalation is doubtful, especially with good blood gas values. There is no evidence of ethanol intoxication or closed head injury. Unless a second injury (i.e., abdominal trauma) is considered, it cannot be diagnosed. (Initial Care of the Patient With Burns/Secondary Survey)

Chapter 11

1. Correct: E. The hallmark of an indirect hernia is protrusion of the abdominal contents through the internal (deep) ring and into a peritoneal sac, which is the persistent processus vaginalis on the anterior medial aspect of the spermatic cord. The internal ring is superior to the inguinal ligament; the mass is not caudal to it, nor is it protruding through an epigastric (upper abdominal) defect. An indirect hernia may be hard to reduce, but this difficulty is not a feature of a "simple" one. (Indirect Inguinal Hernia/Anatomy and Pathophysiology)

2. Correct: D. A direct hernia protrudes through the floor of the inguinal canal. The defect is large and is unlikely to incarcerate. The other choices are small hernia defects, which are surrounded with fascia or muscle that constricts the opening and tends to incarcerate the contents of the hernia sac. (Direct Inguinal Hernia/Treatment)

3. Correct: C. Umbilical hernias are dangerous because they can incarcerate or strangulate abdominal tissues. Because most umbilical hernias in infants close spontaneously, they are not repaired until the child is 4 or 5 years of age. Putting cotton or a coin in a defect does not help and may delay its spontaneous closure. The adult with hepatomegaly and ascites has increased abdominal pressure; an umbilical hernia in this patient should not be closed because it may not heal and has a high recurrence rate. (Umbilical Hernias/Treatment)

4. Correct: D. Wound infection separates the edges of the wound, interferes with wound healing, and produces an incisional hernia. Although poor surgical technique can cause a hernia, it is uncommon because of the carefulness of the surgeon. Obesity does not increase the risk of incisional hernia, but may make it harder for the surgeon to close the wound. Transverse incisions result in fewer hernias than vertical incisions. Early ambulation speeds patient recovery, but does not increase the number of hernias. (Other Hernias/Incisional Hernia)

5. Correct: B. A sliding hernia is one in which the hernia sac itself is formed by one of the intraabdominal structures. The bowel, omentum, or bladder slides into the internal ring and forms part of the peritoneal sac. A Richter's hernia is one that incarcerates or strangulates a portion of the intestinal wall. A Littre's hernia is an inguinal hernia that contains a Meckel's diverticulum. A spigelian hernia occurs at the junction of the semilunar line of the lateral border of the rectus muscle and the posterior rectus sheath at the posterior semicircular line of Douglas. A pantaloon hernia is an indirect inguinal hernia that occurs with a direct inguinal hernia, which results in an indirect and a direct hernia with the inferior epigastric vessels in between. (Other Hernias/Sliding Hernia)

6. Correct: E. The external oblique aponeurosis is the most superficial aponeurosis of the abdominal wall. It forms the external ring that allows the spermatic cord to pass from the inguinal canal, anterior to the pubic tubercle, into the scrotum. The conjoined tendon is the combination of the transversus muscle, aponeurosis, and internal oblique muscle on the medial side of Hesselbach's triangle. The inguinal ligament is the reflection of the external oblique aponeurosis. (Layers of the Abdominal Wall/External Oblique Muscle)

7. Correct: B. The processus vaginalis is the peritoneum that advances into the scrotum and becomes the tunica vaginalis of the testicle. None of the other structures listed has any peritoneum on its surface. The vas deferens extends from the testicle to the urethra within the spermatic cord without any peritoneum. (Layers of the Abdominal Wall/Peritoneum)

8. Correct: A. No posterior rectus fascia is found below the line of Douglas. Only transversalis fascia and peritoneum are found between the rectus muscle and the abdominal cavity. The other four answers are muscles and fascia of the abdomen that could be the source of the posterior rectus sheath, but not below this line. (Anatomy of the Abdominal Wall/Midline Structures)

9. Correct: C. Indirect inguinal hernia is the most common hernia and the most likely to incarcerate. Femoral hernia is uncommon, but is likely to incarcerate. Although the other types listed can incarcerate, they most often have a wide opening that decreases the risk of incarceration. (Indirect Inguinal Hernia/Clinical Presentation)

10. Correct: C. Because the midline aponeurosis has few large blood vessels or other structures, making and closing a vertical midline incision is much faster than making and closing a transverse incision. The other

answers are all advantages of making a transverse incision. (Abdominal Incisions)

11. Correct: D. The adult umbilical scar is subject to stretching and defects that enlarge and produce a hernia. These hernias do not close spontaneously. They occur in all races and are covered only by skin and scar. When the cord infection in infancy heals, any resulting hernia usually closes. (Umbilical Hernias/Anatomy and Pathophysiology)

12. Correct: D. Because a persistent processus vaginalis is the cause of all indirect inguinal hernias, the etiology is congenital, regardless of whether the patient is a child or an adult. The other answers do not cause this hernia. The peritoneal sac is present at birth. (Indirect Inguinal Hernia/Anatomy and Pathophysiology)

13. Correct: A. Gastroschisis is a failure of the abdominal wall and umbilicus to close. The defect is lateral to the umbilicus and has no covering. The intestines usually protrude through the defect, not the stomach. The intraabdominal organs are usually normally developed. (Umbilical Hernias/Anatomy and Pathophysiology)

14. Correct: D. An omphalocele is a herniation of abdominal contents through the middle of the umbilicus. The abdominal contents are covered by a thin membrane of peritoneum and the amnion (no skin covering). An omphalocele is much more complicated than an umbilical hernia because of the threat of infection and the protrusion of abdominal contents. (Umbilical Hernias/Anatomy and Pathophysiology)

15. Correct: E. Hesselbach's triangle is the posterior inguinal wall through which a direct hernia protrudes. The sides of the triangle are formed by the rectus sheath. The superior portion is the conjoined tendon (internal oblique and transverse abdominal muscles), and the inferior portion is the inguinal ligament. The external oblique is not a part of this triangle. (Other Hernias/Hesselbach's Hernia)

16. Correct: B. The contents of the abdomen protrude through the muscle or through a fascial defect in the abdominal wall. Distension, a mass, or a sac in the abdomen or in the skin and subcutaneous tissue does not constitute a hernia. (Hernias)

17. Correct: C. Because a direct inguinal hernia is acquired from pressure and tension on muscle and fascia, it occurs in older men. A femoral hernia is also caused by injury to these tissues, but it occurs infrequently. Indirect hernias are congenital and occur at a younger age. Incarceration and strangulation are infrequent complications of hernias.
(Inguinal Hernias/Direct Inguinal Hernia)

18. Correct: D. If a hernia becomes incarcerated, the abdominal contents become trapped in the sac and cannot be reduced into the abdomen. The other answers are types of hernias that may be incarcerated. (Indirect Inguinal Hernia/Clinical Presentation)

19. Correct: A. Because an indirect hernia occurs through a small abdominal defect, the contents of the sac are much more likely to become incarcerated than the direct hernia, which has no sac. (Indirect Inguinal Hernia/Clinical Presentation)

20. Correct: D. A bulge indicates that the abdominal contents are protruding through an abdominal wall defect. A bulge is a common finding in both types of hernia. (Direct Inguinal Hernia/Clinical Presentation)

21. Correct: A. Only an indirect hernia has a true sac, which is the remnant of the processus vaginalis. This true hernia sac is excised as part of the repair. The direct hernia has a layer of peritoneum as part of the bulging defect, but it is not a true hernial sac and seldom needs to be opened or excised. (Direct Inguinal Hernia/Anatomy and Pathophysiology)

22. Correct: A. Because an indirect hernia is congenital, it is the type that occurs in infants. A direct hernia is acquired and occurs in older persons. (Indirect Inguinal Hernia/Anatomy and Pathophysiology)

23. Correct: B. An umbilical hernia often closes spontaneously up to the age of 5 years. An indirect hernia sac is composed of peritoneum and seldom closes spontaneously. (Umbilical Hernias/Clinical Presentation)

24. Correct: B. A femoral hernia bulges through the floor of the inguinal canal, into the femoral ring, and projects below the inguinal ligament into the femoral canal of the upper thigh. An inguinal hernia occurs above the inguinal ligament. A spigelian hernia occurs at the lateral border of the rectus sheath, 4 to 6 cm superior to the groin. A Richter's hernia is a portion of the bowel wall incarcerated in a hernia rather than a hernia at a specific location. For this reason, a femoral hernia with this type of incarceration could also be a Richter's hernia. (Femoral Hernia/Clinical Presentation)

25. Correct: C. The transversalis fascia is an envelope outside the peritoneum. The external oblique and transversus muscles are part of the abdominal wall, but are not a preperitoneal envelope. Scarpa's fascia is the deep layer of subcutaneous fascia that lies between the skin and the anterior abdominal fascia and muscles. The fascia of the rectus muscle and the linea alba are strong structures of the anterior abdominal wall. (Layers of the Abdominal Wall/Transversalis Fascia)

26. Correct: D. A truss is a leather, plastic, or metal rounded plate that is strapped across the hernia bulge. Although a truss may reduce the hernia bulge, it does not produce closure of a hernia defect. Instead, it often encourages an increase in its size. (Indirect Inguinal Hernia/Treatment)

27. Correct: E. Hesselbach's triangle defines the floor of the inguinal canal, which is medial to the inferior epigastric vessels and the site of the bulging direct hernia. Choice A refers to an incisional hernia located in a scar from a previous abdominal incision. Choice B describes Petit's hernia through the inferior lumbar triangle above the iliac crest. Choice C refers to the sac through the internal ring, which causes an indirect hernia. Choice D describes the location of the spigelian hernia.

28. Correct: A. A strangulated hernia is an incarcerated hernia that causes compromise of venous drainage and arterial blood flow. It produces gangrene and perforation of the bowel wall. The remaining answers are all types of hernias, but none of these types results in perforation of the bowel, unless it becomes a strangulated hernia. (Indirect Inguinal Hernia/Clinical Presentation)

Chapter 12

1. Correct: A. Hiatal hernias of the paraesophageal type should be surgically repaired when found because they are prone to incarceration or strangulation. Otherwise, the mere presence of a hiatal hernia does not require operative intervention. (Hiatal Hernia and Gastroesophageal Reflux Disease)

2. Correct: A. Zenker's diverticula are closely related to dysfunction of the cricopharyngeal muscle. They are pulsion diverticula that occur over years. Symptoms include regurgitation, aspiration, or dysphagia. Symptomatic diverticula require operative correction. (Esophageal Motility Disorders/Esophageal Diverticula/Pathophysiology)

3. Correct: D. Spontaneous esophageal perforation occurs in the distal third of the esophagus secondary to a sudden increase in intraesophageal pressure. The resulting pain from mediastinitis closely mimics the pain of myocardial infarction. Through-and-through perforation of the esophagus is best managed operatively, whereas the mucosal tear of Mallory-Weiss syndrome is managed expectantly. (Traumatic Esophageal Disorders)

4. Correct: C. Manometric studies allow for the assessment of the motility of the esophagus, which can be abnormal in achalasia, and the function of the lower esophageal sphincter, which is abnormal in both achalasia and reflux esophagitis. (Examination of the Esophagus)

5. Correct: E. A history of emesis followed by chest pain and subcutaneous emphysema points to little less than esophageal perforation. In acute myocardial infarction and ruptured aortic aneurysm, the pain generally comes first, followed by emesis. Subcutaneous emphysema is seen in patients with spontaneous pneumothorax, but rarely with emesis. (Traumatic Esophageal Disorders/Esophageal Perforation)

6. Correct: C. Vomiting should not be induced after alkaline ingestion, nor should neutralization be attempted. These maneuvers may make the injury worse. Early endoscopy is needed to assess the degree of injury, rule out perforation, and help plan future therapy. Steroids and antibiotics may or may not be helpful in grade II and III injuries. (Traumatic Esophageal Disorders/Caustic Ingestion/Evaluation; Treatment)

7. Correct: B. A high-pressure zone is seen manometrically at the level of the diaphragm; however, no distinct muscle fibers with specialized sphincter function can be identified. The lower esophageal sphincter functions best when it is in its normal subdiaphragmatic position and when it is hormonally responsive. (The Esophagus/Anatomy; Pathophysiology)

8. Correct: A. Operative myotomy with fundoplication relieves the symptoms of achalasia in 95% of affected individuals. Dilation carries a 60% to 80% success rate, with a high rate of recurrence. Diverticula can occur secondary to the disturbance in motility. Vomiting is clearly positional, and calcium channel blockers can provide temporary relief of symptoms. (Esophageal Motility Disorders/Achalasia/Treatment)

9. Correct: B. A left hydropneumothorax is seen in Boerhaave's syndrome because the esophagus tends to rupture at the most unprotected site, just above the diaphragm on the left side. The syndrome is a through-and-through perforation of the esophagus that is often successfully treated by primary repair and drainage without resection. The diagnosis is made most successfully with barium swallow. (Traumatic Esophageal Disorders/Esophageal Perforation)

10. Correct: C. Operative intervention is indicated when stenosis is present or when esophagitis does not respond to medical therapy. Celestin tubes provide palliation for carcinoma of the esophagus and have no place in the treatment of gastroesophageal reflux disease. Lye ingestion, Schatzki ring, and peptic ulcer disease are unrelated disease processes. (Hiatal Hernia and Gastroesophageal Reflux Disease)

11. Correct: A. Barrett's esophagus is associated with a 10% incidence of adenocarcinoma of the esophagus. Squamous carcinoma of the esophagus accounts for approximately 85% of the primary cancers of the

esophagus. It is not associated with Barrett's esophagus. (Malignant Tumors/Epidemiology)

12. Correct: E. The other choices are all associated with an increased incidence of carcinoma of the esophagus. Low levels of folate are associated with anemia and spinal cord defects, but not with esophageal cancer. (Malignant Tumors/Epidemiology)

13. Correct: E. Computed tomography scan of the chest, magnetic resonance imaging scan of the chest, and transesophageal ultrasound can be used to help stage esophageal cancer, but will not confirm the diagnosis. Esophagram or an upper gastrointestinal series may lead to a high index of suspicion. Esophagoscopy with biopsy and bronchoscopy will confirm the diagnosis and indicate whether the trachea or bronchus has been invaded. (Malignant Tumors/Clinical Presentation and Evaluation)

14. Correct: D. Patients who present late have a 75% or greater chance of widespread metastatic disease. (Malignant Tumors)

15. Correct: A. Lugol's solution reacts with the high glycogen content of the normal esophagus and changes to a black or green color. Early neoplasms lack this high concentration of glycogen and remain unstained. (Malignant Tumors)

16. Correct: C. Multiple biopsies of the lesion or brush cytology of the unstained area yields a diagnosis in nearly 100% of cases. The patient may be advised to stop the consumption of alcohol and tobacco, but this step will not confirm the diagnosis. Barium swallow and esophagram ultrasound will not confirm the histopathology. An acid perfusion test (Bernstein) is helpful for evaluating reflux esophagitis, but not neoplasms of the esophagus. (Malignant Tumors/Clinical Presentation and Evaluation)

17. Correct: A. Expansive endoesophageal tubes are associated with lower rates of morbidity and mortality than the more rigid endoesophageal tubes. (Malignant Tumors/Prognosis)

18. Correct: B. Computed tomography scan of the chest and abdomen confirms mediastinal and abdominal nodes and liver metastasis, and it is less expensive than magnetic resonance imaging. Magnetic resonance imaging confirms the extent of disease, but is more costly. Esophageal ultrasound may confirm local invasion of the tumor, but not distant metastasis. Laparoscopy confirms abdominal spread, but not spread within the chest. Sputum cytology is helpful in identifying carcinoma of the lung. (Malignant Tumors/Clinical Presentation and Evaluation)

19. Correct: C. Consumption of fat is not related to an increase in esophageal cancer. Heavy alcohol intake, low levels of vitamin A, and severe reflux esophagitis with Barrett's esophagus are all associated with an increased incidence of esophageal cancer. (Malignant Tumors/Epidemiology)

20. Correct: A. Complications from this procedure can be severe, and the procedure is difficult to learn. Consequently, it is not widely practiced. Surgical treatment is the most reliable approach, with more than 95% of patients having complete relief of symptoms. (Esophageal Motility Disorders/Achalasia/Treatment)

Chapter 13

1. Correct: D. The right and left gastroepiploic arteries are derived from the gastroduodenal and splenic arteries, respectively, and supply blood to the greater curvature of the stomach. The common hepatic artery supplies the lesser curvature through the right gastric artery. The superior mesenteric artery makes no contribution to gastric circulation. (Anatomy/Stomach)

2. Correct: D. The vagus nerves enter the abdomen through the esophageal hiatus and give off gastric branches that originate at the lesser curvature of the stomach. Vagal stimulation is partially responsible for parietal cell secretion of hydrochloric acid. In addition, branches of the right vagus innervate the pancreas, small bowel, and proximal colon. Left vagal branches innervate the liver and biliary system. Sympathetic innervation is composed of preganglionic fibers, mainly in the thoracic splanchnic nerves, and postganglionic fibers that arise in the celiac plexus. (Anatomy/Stomach)

3. Correct: C. Gastric chief cells secrete pepsinogen, G-cells produce the hormone gastrin, delta cells produce somatostatin, and goblet cells secrete mucus. Parietal cells secrete hydrochloric acid as well as intrinsic factor. (Anatomy/Stomach)

4. Correct: D. G-cells are found in the duodenum and the proximal small intestine, but the vast majority are confined to the gastric antrum. Parietal cells and chief cells are found mainly in the fundus of the stomach. Mucus-secreting cells are located throughout the gastric mucosa. (Anatomy/Stomach)

5. Correct: C. The release of secretin is initiated when acid in the duodenum causes the intraluminal pH to fall below 4.5. Although the products of fat digestion also stimulate secretin release, this release occurs only at high luminal fat concentrations. Gastric distension causes antral release of gastrin, as does the presence of polypeptides and amino acids in the stomach. Secretin is not released in response to the products of carbohydrate digestion. (Physiology/Physiology of Hydrochloric Acid Secretion)

6. Correct: E. Most duodenal ulcers occur within 5 cm of the pylorus. They occur more frequently on the

anterior wall. Because no viscera or other structures are located adjacent to the anterior surface of the duodenum at this point, ulcer erosion through the wall allows fluid and air to escape through a free perforation. Ulcer erosion through the posterior duodenal wall can involve the gastroduodenal artery and result in massive hemorrhage, or the ulcer can erode into the head of the pancreas and produce pancreatitis. Recurrent ulceration, with subsequent healing and scar formation, can lead to obstruction of the duodenal lumen, but the incidence is lower than that of perforation. Duodenal ulcers that form as the result of acid hypersecretion do not undergo malignant degeneration, although the rare carcinoma of the duodenum can occur as an ulcerating lesion. (Duodenal Ulcer Disease/Clinical Presentation and Evaluation)

7. Correct: A. Chronic duodenal ulcer disease with cicatrix formation leads to gastric outlet obstruction, with subsequent postprandial vomiting and gastric dilation as the stomach attempts to propel ingested food past the point of obstruction. The inability to maintain adequate caloric intake leads to progressive weight loss and malnutrition. Sudden, severe abdominal pain, accompanied by signs of peritoneal irritation, is characteristic of a perforated ulcer. Constant, dull epigastric pain, accompanied by weight loss and a palpable abdominal mass, suggests malignancy. Massive hemorrhage from a posterior penetrating ulcer causes hematemesis, melena, and hypotension as the patient loses intravascular volume. The persistence of symptoms despite appropriate medical management is known as intractability, and it suggests the diagnosis of Zollinger-Ellison syndrome. (Duodenal Ulcer Disease/Acute Ulcer Disease/Clinical Presentation and Evaluation)

8. Correct: C. Air that escapes through a duodenal perforation floats to the top of the abdominal cavity and becomes trapped under the diaphragm. This occurrence is best demonstrated by a chest x-ray taken with the patient standing. Front and upright abdominal x-rays are unreliable because a film taken with the patient supine usually does not detect air that rises to the anterior abdominal wall, and the upright abdominal film inadequately shows the patient's diaphragm. An upper gastrointestinal series with water-soluble contrast agent (e.g., Gastrografin) shows extravasation of contents through a duodenal perforation. This test is more time-consuming, requires fluoroscopy or multiple images, and is more cumbersome for a patient who is already under great stress as the result of an intraabdominal catastrophe. Abdominal ultrasound is nonspecific in detecting free air or fluid early after perforation occurs. Although abdominal computed tomography detects free intraperitoneal air, it is inefficient in terms of both time and cost. (Duodenal Ulcer Disease/Acute Ulcer Disease/Clinical Presentation and Evaluation)

9. Correct: E. Fiberoptic endoscopy allows visualization of the esophageal, gastric, and duodenal mucosa, along with any underlying pathology. In addition, endoscopy can be used as a therapeutic modality, allowing injection of bleeding vessels in an ulcer base with vasoconstricting agents, thermal coagulation of similar vessels, or biopsy of a slowly bleeding gastric tumor. The dual role of endoscopy in both diagnosis and treatment makes it a valuable tool in the management of upper gastrointestinal hemorrhage. A barium contrast study can delineate normal anatomy and show intraluminal masses, mucosal abnormalities, or points of obstruction. Sites of hemorrhage, however, generally go undetected. For this reason, this test is ineffective in the setting of acute hemorrhage. Selective angiography and bleeding scans with radioactively tagged red blood cells rely on active hemorrhage, with visualization of intravenous contrast material or a radioactive red blood cell mass as it leaves the circulation and pools at the site of hemorrhage. Because bleeding can be intermittent, these tests have a significant false-negative rate and are not a substitute for endoscopy. Angiography plays a role in the patient with a documented bleeding ulcer who poses an unacceptable surgical risk. The site of hemorrhage can be localized with selective angiography and the responsible vessel embolized with small foam pads or coils to achieve hemostasis. Computed tomography scan with intravenous contrast does not identify the site of hemorrhage and is inappropriate in the management of these patients. (Chronic Ulcer Disease/Clinical Presentation and Evaluation/Endoscopy)

10. Correct: B. Modification of diet plays a minor role in the nonsurgical management of peptic ulcer disease, with the exception of limiting the intake of caffeine, alcohol, and chocolate. These substances, known as secretagogues, stimulate the release of hydrochloric acid. Antacids, histamine antagonists, and proton pump inhibitors are the mainstay of medical therapy. Anticholinergics can inhibit vagal stimulation of parietal cells, but may cause unpleasant side effects. (Chronic Ulcer Disease/Medical Treatment)

11. Correct: C. Although the prevalence of *H. pylori* infection in the general population is greater than 50% by 60 years of age, peptic ulcers develop in only a small percentage of patients who harbor the organism. The diagnosis is established by any one of several quick, inexpensive tests. The most common is endoscopic biopsy of the gastric mucosa, which on examination appears chronically inflamed. Multiple-treatment regimens exist, and most require a 2-week course of therapy. After ulcers are adequately treated, recurrence rates are significantly reduced.

(Chronic Ulcer Disease/Medical Treatment/*H. pylori* Eradication)

12. Correct: D. Truncal vagotomy involves division of the vagus nerves at the esophageal hiatus. As a result, the cephalic phase of gastric acid production is eliminated. Basal acid output is markedly diminished, and the negative feedback mechanism for gastrin release, caused by low gastric pH, is abolished. Truncal vagotomy denervates the entire stomach, including the parietal cell mass, the antrum and pylorus, and most of the abdominal viscera. This procedure also affects the motility of the stomach and can lead to gastric atony, necessitating a concomitant gastric emptying procedure. (Chronic Ulcer Disease/Surgical Treatment/Truncal Vagotomy)

13. Correct: D. Of the listed procedures, truncal vagotomy and antrectomy has the lowest incidence of recurrent ulcer formation. See the text for comparison of recurrence and complication rates. (Table 13–1)

14. Correct: C. Zollinger-Ellison syndrome is suspected in patients who have refractory or extensive peptic ulceration that is unresponsive to conventional treatment. The syndrome results from the independent production of gastrin by a tumor that is most commonly found in the pancreas or duodenum. Administration of intravenous secretin causes an unexplained paradoxical rise in serum gastrin concentration in patients with gastrinomas. This rise is diagnostic. Of gastrinomas, 60% to 90% are malignant, with an overall 5-year survival rate of 50%. Medical therapy is directed at treating gastric acid hypersecretion with conventional drugs or suppressing gastrin production with synthetic analogues of somatostatin. The goal of surgery is to resect the tumor, if it is localized, and to address the complications of ulcer disease. Resection of the gastrin-producing G-cell mass in the antrum of the stomach has little effect on the ulcer disease because the gastrinoma independently produces gastrin, which stimulates the production of hydrochloric acid by the parietal cells. (Duodenal Ulcer Disease/Zollinger-Ellison Syndrome/Clinical Presentation and Evaluation)

15. Correct: D. Duodenal ulcers occur in the face of acid hypersecretion, but gastric ulcers are associated with normal or diminished acid output. Most gastric ulcers develop on the lesser curvature of the stomach, at the junction between the body and the antrum of the stomach. Gastric ulcers respond to medical management in approximately 50% of patients. The rest require surgical intervention. (Gastric Ulcer Disease/Medical Treatment)

16. Correct: B. Prepyloric (type III) ulcers and gastric ulcers that occur along with duodenal ulcers (type II) are considered and treated as variants of duodenal ulcer disease. They require an acid-reducing procedure. Total gastrectomy eliminates the source of acid production, but the complication rate is unacceptable. Truncal vagotomy alone is not an option because drainage for the relatively atonic stomach would be necessary. Simple excision of the ulcer does not solve the problem of acid hypersecretion. Distal gastrectomy eliminates the G-cell stimulation of parietal cell activity by gastrin, but does not address the cephalic phase of acid production from uninterrupted vagal tone. Therefore, of the options listed, truncal vagotomy and antrectomy is the best answer. (Gastric Ulcer Disease/Surgical Treatment)

17. Correct: D. The symptoms of early dumping syndrome are alleviated by limiting the osmolar load presented to the small intestine. This goal can be accomplished by minimizing carbohydrate intake, avoiding fluid intake at mealtime, and increasing the number of fat calories in the diet. (Gastric Ulcer Disease/Postgastrectomy Syndromes/Early Dumping Syndrome)

18. Correct: E. Surgical alterations of normal gastric anatomy that allow free reflux of duodenal contents into the stomach (pyloroplasty, gastroduodenostomy, or gastrojejunostomy) predispose to the development of alkaline reflux gastritis. Bile and pancreatic secretions significantly increase intraluminal pH and cause chronic irritation of the gastric mucosa, with associated epigastric pain and nausea. The symptoms are relatively constant compared with those of the other postgastrectomy syndromes listed, which produce episodic and dramatic complications. (Gastric Ulcer Disease/Postgastrectomy Syndromes/Alkaline Reflux Gastritis)

19. Correct: B. The patient is considered to have a gastric malignancy until proven otherwise. Although an ulcer crater is shown radiographically, it cannot be assumed to be benign, and the patient's age and history of weight loss place cancer at the top of the differential diagnosis. Confirmation of the diagnosis is obtained by endoscopy and multiple biopsies of the lesion. A true benign gastric ulcer may be amenable to medical management, with the caveat that repeat endoscopy is mandatory to evaluate ulcer healing or progression. Failure to heal should prompt the clinician to consider neoplasm again as the etiology for the ulcer and to perform repeat biopsies. (Malignant Diseases of the Stomach/Gastric Carcinoma/Clinical Presentation and Evaluation)

20. Correct: C. Determination of the malignant potential of a lesion should not be based on radiographic findings, which are no substitute for endoscopy with direct visualization and tissue biopsy. Benign and malignant gastric ulcerations can appear as mucosal defects that radiate rugal folds. This appearance can be attributed to the changes that accompany a site of chronic inflammation with surrounding scar contracture.

(Malignant Diseases of the Stomach/Gastric Carcinoma/ Clinical Presentation and Evaluation)

Chapter 14

1. Correct: B. Because of the high concentration of lymphoid follicles in the appendix in this age-group, a gastrointestinal virus that causes swelling of the follicles and, hence, obstruction of the appendiceal lumen can lead to appendicitis. (Acute Appendicitis/ Anatomy)

2. Correct: C. Acute appendicitis is caused by obstruction of the appendiceal lumen, most often by swollen lymphoid follicles. (Acute Appendicitis/Pathophysiology)

3. Correct: C. Surgical appendectomy is the most reliable treatment for acute appendicitis, with a morbidity rate of less than 5% and a mortality rate of less than 1%. Complications greatly increase in cases of perforation, with resulting mortality rates of 5% to 10%. However, if localized perforation occurs, treatment with antibiotics and an interval appendectomy 6 weeks later may be considered. (Acute Appendicitis/ Treatment)

4. Correct: B. The most common location of carcinoid tumors is the appendix. These tumors, 50% of which are asymptomatic, are often found at the time of appendectomy for right lower quadrant pain. They can increase in size and cause partial obstruction of the appendiceal lumen. This obstruction leads to acute appendicitis and necessitates removal of the appendix. (Diseases of the Appendix/Tumors of the Appendix)

5. Correct: B. Meckel's diverticulum develops from the vitelline duct, a midgut structure. (Meckel's Diverticulum/Anatomy)

6. Correct: A. Meckel's diverticulum often contains two types of ectopic tissue, gastric and pancreatic. Because these tissues are prone to gastrointestinal bleeding, the most common presenting symptom is gastrointestinal bleeding. (Meckel's Diverticulum/ Clinical Presentation and Evaluation)

7. Correct: D. The mucosa found in Meckel's diverticulum is related to midgut or hindgut mucosa, not foregut mucosa (i.e., esophagus). (Meckel's Diverticulum/Anatomy)

8. Correct: E. Crohn's disease may occur anywhere from the mouth to the anus. It characteristically has "skip lesions," as opposed to the contiguous disease pattern observed in ulcerative colitis. (Crohn's Disease/Pathophysiology)

9. Correct: B. Approximately 50% of patients with Crohn's disease have ileocolic involvement. Approxi-

mately 30% to 40% have small intestinal involvement only. In contrast, only approximately 20% of patients have isolated involvement of the colon. (Crohn's Disease/Clinical Presentation)

10. Correct: E. Crohn's disease cannot be cured by any medical or surgical therapy. For this reason, it is a major therapeutic challenge to the physician. (Crohn's Disease/Significance and Incidence/ Treatment)

11. Correct: D. The goals of therapy are to alleviate the symptoms of Crohn's disease, provide nutritional support, suppress the inflammatory process, and use broad-spectrum antibiotics to treat the septic complications. The efficacy of continued corticosteroids to maintain patients in remission has not been proven. (Crohn's Disease/Treatment/Medical Therapy)

12. Correct: C. Acute terminal ileitis precipitated by *Yersinia* produces an inflammatory response in the terminal ileum in 20% of patients with Crohn's disease. Although this problem resolves spontaneously in 90% of cases, the appendix should be removed if the cecum is normal. This procedure eliminates the possibility of appendicitis in the differential diagnosis in any future attacks of right lower quadrant abdominal pain. (Crohn's Disease/Treatment/Surgical Therapy)

13. Correct: D. Postoperatively, almost 40% of all patients have a recurrence within 5 years. These recurrences are usually found proximal to the anastomosis after resection. For example, in patients with ileitis or ileocolitis, the most common site of recurrent disease is the neoterminal ileum. (Crohn's Disease/Complications)

14. Correct: D. Volvulus and tumor are relatively unusual causes of small bowel obstruction in adults. Gallstone ileus is quite unusual. In industrialized nations, postoperative adhesions are the most common cause of small bowel obstruction, but worldwide, the most common cause is hernia. (Small Bowel Obstruction/ Significance and Incidence)

15. Correct: E; 16. Correct: D. Fluid and electrolyte repair is often the most important aspect of care for patients with small bowel obstruction. The volume of fluid administered must take into account the calculated maintenance rate for the patient. However, the losses sustained before presentation must also be replaced. There is no way to calculate exactly the losses from vomitus and third-space loss (into the lumen and wall of the bowel). These losses must be estimated based on when the symptoms began, the volume and frequency of vomiting, and the estimated level of bowel obstruction. Half of the estimated volume should be administered in the first 8 hours after arrival, and the remainder administered over the next

16 hours. Urine output can be used to evaluate the adequacy of replacement. Finally, ongoing abnormal losses from the nasogastric tube must be replaced on a volume-for-volume basis. (Small Bowel Obstruction/ Treatment)

17. Correct: E. By definition, there must be an abnormal communication between the biliary tree and the gastrointestinal tract in order for a gallstone to cause intestinal obstruction. (Small Bowel Obstruction/ Significance and Incidence)

18. Correct: A. Small bowel malignancies can arise from any layer of the bowel wall. They are much less common than their benign counterparts and, unlike their benign counterparts, they generally become symptomatic. Because of their relatively advanced stage at diagnosis, their prognosis is poorer than that of tumors arising in the colon. When found, they are best treated by wide resection with en bloc resection of the mesentery draining the involved segment. (Small Bowel Tumors/Malignant Tumors/Adenocarcinomas; Carcinoid Tumors)

19. Correct: E. The substances that cause the carcinoid syndrome are largely deactivated by the liver. Thus, the carcinoid syndrome usually occurs only when tumor products enter the systemic circulation directly. Primary carcinoid tumors in the bronchus and low rectum can cause the syndrome. The output from tumors in the midgut are all carried to the liver by the portal vein and deactivated there. Hepatic metastases of carcinoid tumors (regardless of the site of the primary) can cause the syndrome because their products enter the hepatic vein and, thus, the systemic circulation. (Small Bowel Tumors/Malignant Tumors/Carcinoid Tumors)

20. Correct: A. Villous adenoma of the small bowel is malignant in approximately 30% of cases. The other tumors are considered to have essentially no malignant potential. (Small Bowel Tumors/Adenomas)

21. Correct: B. Occult bleeding can be seen with any small bowel tumor. However, with carcinoids, villous adenomas, and Brunner's gland adenomas, it is rare. Adenocarcinomas can ulcerate and bleed, but the tumor that is most commonly associated with bleeding is leiomyosarcoma. Two-thirds of leiomyosarcomas of the small intestine cause bleeding, and that bleeding can be massive. (Small Bowel Tumors/ Leiomyomas)

Chapter 15

1. Correct: D. Colon cancer and familial polyposis syndrome are associated with blood streaking or oozing, but rarely is the bleeding massive. Ulcerative colitis is occasionally associated with brisk bleeding, but this bleeding is rarely high volume. Colonic varices are associated with massive lower gastrointestinal bleeding, but they are much less common than diverticulosis. (Colon and Rectum/Diverticular Disease/ Diverticulosis)

2. Correct: E. Perforation, fistula formation, obstruction, and hemorrhage are all associated with diverticular disease. However, there is no evidence that diverticular disease predisposes to carcinoma of the colon. Although they may coexist, there does not appear to be a causal relation. (Colon and Rectum/Diverticular Disease/Diverticulosis)

3. Correct: B. Gardner's syndrome and familial polyposis syndrome are inherited conditions that are characterized by the formation of hundreds to thousands of polyps. Cancer will develop in virtually 100% of patients with these syndromes if they are not treated. Villous adenomas are malignant in 30% to 35% of cases. Even tubular adenomas may be premalignant. Only the polyps associated with Peutz-Jeghers syndrome carry no risk of malignancy because they are hamartomas. (Colon and Rectum/Polyps and Carcinoma of the Colon and Rectum/Colorectal Polyps)

4. Correct: D. Adhesions of the large intestine rarely cause large bowel obstruction. Similarly, fecal impaction can usually be resolved with enemas and digital disimpaction. Of the remaining three answers, all are associated with large bowel obstruction, but in retrospective studies, carcinoma was the most common cause of large bowel obstruction. (Colon and Rectum/Colonic Obstruction and Volvulus/Obstruction of the Large Intestine)

5. Correct: E. Tumors in the sigmoid region usually cause obstructive symptoms or bleeding. Tumors in the rectum often cause a change in the physical appearance of stools as well as some blood streaking. Malignant tumors of the splenic flexure and transverse colon are also associated with guaiac-positive stools and low-grade obstruction. However, tumors in the cecum characteristically become quite large before they cause symptoms. As a result, patients often lose weight, have anemia, and frequently have a palpable mass in the right lower quadrant. (Colon and Rectum/Polyps and Carcinoma of the Colon and Rectum/Carcinoma of the Colon and Rectum/Clinical Presentation and Evaluation; Table 15–3)

6. Correct: C. The management of a perforated diverticulum with peritoneal soiling almost always involves resection of the perforated area with a diverting colostomy and Hartmann's pouch. Simply creating a loop colostomy does nothing for the abscess and infection that are already present. A sigmoid colon resection with primary anastomosis should not be attempted in this setting because it is doomed to failure in the presence of such contamination and edema. Similarly, merely performing a laparotomy to drain the infection is inadequate treatment because it

does nothing for the perforation itself. Intravenous antibiotics and hydration are clearly inappropriate for a patient with peritonitis and fecal soiling. (Colon and Rectum/Diverticular Disease/Diverticulitis/Treatment)

7. Correct: B. This patient has an obvious perianal abscess. Diverting colostomy is inappropriately aggressive for this straightforward problem. Similarly, hemorrhoidectomy and fissurectomy are the wrong operations for this disease. Although antibiotics and warm soaks provide temporary relief, they never represent definitive treatment of this abscess. Incision and drainage is required to prevent extension and dissection of the abscess. (Anus and Rectum/Perianal Infection/Abscess/Treatment)

8. Correct: B. Hemorrhoids cause some itching and pressure, but bright, aching pain is most commonly associated with anal fissure. Anal fistulae are rarely accompanied by pain. Low rectal cancers may cause pain, but they are less common than anal fissures. Similarly, Crohn's proctitis may be associated with fissures and perirectal abscesses, but it is not as common as anal fissures. (Anus and Rectum/Anal Fissure/Clinical Presentation and Evaluation)

9. Correct: D. This question clearly describes a second-degree internal hemorrhoid. Hemorrhoidectomy is generally reserved for grade IV and advanced grade III hemorrhoids. Incision and drainage is not an appropriate choice unless the hemorrhoids are actually thrombosed. Similarly, aspiration of the hemorrhoid accomplishes little. The correct choice is the use of suppositories and stool softeners to provide symptomatic relief. Most hemorrhoids spontaneously resolve with conservative management. (Anus and Rectum/Hemorrhoids/Treatment)

10. Correct: B. Subtotal colectomy with ileoproctostomy is an inappropriate choice because it involves retaining the rectum with active disease in the mucosa. Complications can occur, and the risk of cancer increases over time. A proctocolectomy with Brooke ileostomy was appropriate treatment in years past, but consigning a young patient to a permanent ileostomy when there are better options available is no longer appropriate. Similarly, abdominoperineal resection is an inappropriate operation because it involves leaving most of the colon, removing the rectum, and giving the patient a permanent colostomy. The Kock pouch was the operation of choice more than 20 years ago, but it fell out of favor when the continent nipple had a high failure rate. The operation of choice today for most patients with ulcerative colitis is colectomy, mucosal proctectomy, and ileoanal pullthrough. (Colon and Rectum/Ulcerative Colitis and Crohn's Disease of the Colon/Treatment)

11. Correct: E. The patient who has volvulus has substantial abdominal distension, obstipation, and x-rays that show massive dilatation of the sigmoid region. Nasogastric suction and intravenous hydration may be used in the initial management of the patient, but they do not represent therapy. Similarly, placement of a Cantor tube and intravenous hydration offer little advantage over simple nasogastric suction. Subtotal colectomy is excessively aggressive management of this problem. Placement of a loop colostomy is inappropriate treatment because it subjects the patient to the risks of laparotomy, but does not take care of the underlying problem. Sigmoidoscopic decompression as initial treatment of volvulus is the correct answer. At some point, operative therapy may be required, either colopexy or resection of the involved area of the sigmoid. (Colon and Rectum/Colonic Obstruction and Volvulus/Volvulus of the Large Intestine/Treatment)

12. Correct: E. An "apple core" lesion caused by adenocarcinoma of the colon is associated with obstruction in a moderate percentage of cases. For this reason, most surgeons believe that, even in the presence of metastatic liver tumors, the primary lesion should be removed to prevent obstruction and emergency surgery in the near future. Closing the abdomen and doing nothing subjects the patient to the risk of laparotomy with none of the advantages. Performing a biopsy on the liver or the primary lesion, again, helps to make a diagnosis, but does not take care of the incipient obstruction. (Colon and Rectum/Carcinoma of the Colon and Rectum/Treatment)

13. Correct: D. Only one of these systems drains into the systemic venous system. The right, middle, superior hemorrhoidal, and left colic systems all drain into the portal vein. Only the inferior hemorrhoidal system drains principally into the caval system. (Anatomy)

14. Correct: B. A Dukes' stage B2 colon cancer is a lesion that has penetrated the full thickness of the colon wall, but is not associated with lymph nodes. Clearly, the survival rate of a patient with a Dukes' stage B2 tumor is superior to that of a patient who has either positive lymph nodes (Dukes' stage C1 or C2) or metastatic disease (Dukes' stage D). On the other hand, patients with tumors that involve just the mucosa or muscularis (Dukes' stage A or B1) have a higher survival rate than those who have tumors with full-thickness involvement. (Table 15-4)

15. Correct: E. The finding of a "bird's beak" on barium enema is associated with volvulus. Carcinoma more commonly causes either an apple core–type lesion or irregularity of the bowel wall. Diverticular disease is associated with multiple small mucosal outpouchings. Crohn's disease is associated with mucosal irregularity and narrowing over a long segment of colon. Chronic ulcerative colitis is associated with a "lead pipe" appearance. (Colon and Rectum/Colonic

Obstruction and Volvulus/Volvulus of the Large Intestine/Clinical Presentation and Evaluation)

16. Correct: B. The finding of a long, narrowed segment of the terminal ileum ("string sign") is associated with Crohn's disease. None of the other lesions are associated with long, narrowed areas in the terminal ileum. Occasionally, diverticular disease is associated with stricture, but it usually involves a short segment of the bowel and is virtually never as long or as narrow as the string sign associated with Crohn's disease. (Table 15–3)

17. Correct: B. A lateral subcutaneous sphincterotomy is the operative procedure of choice for intractable anal fissure. The correct treatment of a fistula-in-ano is fistulotomy with curetting. A perirectal abscess is best treated by incision and drainage, whereas hemorrhoids are treated by hemorrhoidectomy. Anal cancer is usually treated by radiation and chemotherapy; occasionally, it is treated by abdominoperineal resection. (Anus and Rectum/Anal Fissures/Treatment)

18. Correct: C. A digital rectal examination tells little about the diagnosis of colitis because the disease tends to be mucosal and there is usually little palpable. Similarly, a bowel obstruction pattern on an x-ray film is rarely associated with ulcerative colitis. An anorectal abscess is more likely to be associated with Crohn's colitis, and microcytic anemia is too nonspecific to suggest a specific diagnosis. Accordingly, endoscopy is clearly the most accurate and definitive modality in making the diagnosis of ulcerative colitis. (Colon and Rectum/Ulcerative Colitis and Crohn's Disease of the Colon/Clinical Presentation and Evaluation/Treatment)

19. Correct: E. A tumor in the descending colon is most commonly associated with crampy abdominal pain, with a change in bowel habits. Abdominal pain on defecation is more likely associated with an obstructing rectal carcinoma. Most sigmoid and descending colon cancers do not cause a palpable left lower quadrant mass; that is seen more commonly in cecal cancers. Anemia, with bloody, mucus-containing stool is again nonspecific, but is more common in right colon cancers. High-volume, high-frequency diarrhea is nonspecific and does not suggest the diagnosis of any type of colon cancer. (Colon and Rectum/Carcinoma of the Colon and Rectum)

20. Correct: D. The depth of penetration of the primary lesion corresponds with the prognosis better than any of the other descriptors. Although the size of the primary lesion may correlate with the prognosis, it is still of less importance than the depth of penetration. The age of the patient, the amount of hematochezia, and the blood supply of the segment do not correlate well with the prognosis. (Colon and Rectum/Carcinoma of the Colon and Rectum/Prognosis)

Chapter 16

1. Correct: C. The most common gallstones found in western society are of the mixed variety, which contain a high proportion of cholesterol. These stones tend to form in lithogenic bile, which is supersaturated with cholesterol. The relative concentrations of cholesterol, bile salts, and lecithin must be maintained within a fairly limited range to keep the cholesterol soluble in bile. A decrease in the concentration of bile salts favors precipitation of cholesterol. Most mixed stones do not contain enough calcium to render them radiopaque. Increased levels of bilirubin in bile are associated with the formation of pigment stones, but not mixed stones. (Pathogenesis of Gallstones)

2. Correct: B. An increased incidence of gallstones is associated with a number of conditions. In patients with regional enteritis (Crohn's disease) involving the terminal ileum or with resection of the terminal ileum, there is a decrease in the bile acid pool, which increases the likelihood of cholesterol precipitation and gallstone formation. Prolonged total parenteral nutrition favors gallstone formation as a result of hyperconcentration of bile and gallbladder stasis. Patients with sickle cell anemia and other hemolytic disorders tend to form pigment stones. The incidence of gallstones is extremely high among Native Americans; more than 50% of men and 80% of women harbor mixed stones by the age of 60. Although obesity is associated with an increased incidence of gallstones, there is no evidence that essential hypertension increases the risk of gallstone formation. (Epidemiology of Gallstones)

3. Correct: A. Biliary colic results from transient obstruction of the cystic duct by a gallstone. It tends to occur postprandially and may awaken the patient at night. The pain is visceral and thus poorly localized. Inflammation of the gallbladder results in constant pain accompanied by other clinical features of acute cholecystitis. Passage of stones through the ampulla of Vater may cause acute biliary pancreatitis. (Chronic Calculous Cholecystitis)

4. Correct: E. The patient has a clinical picture that suggests acute cholecystitis. In this condition, the abdominal pain is constant, and the examination may show tenderness and guarding in the right upper quadrant, a positive Murphy's sign, and possibly a tender mass in the abdomen. Results of the laboratory findings are also consistent with the diagnosis of acute cholecystitis. Ultrasonography and radionuclide biliary (HIDA) scan are helpful in establishing a definitive diagnosis. Compared with acute cholecystitis, acute hepatitis is generally associated with less pronounced abdominal findings and higher levels of aspartate aminotransferase (AST) and alanine aminotransferase (ALT). Acute pancreatitis is usually accompanied by high levels of serum amylase, although

mild elevation does not rule out the disease. This presentation is not typical for acute duodenal ulcer. (Acute Cholecystitis)

5. Correct: A. The clinical picture is characteristic of biliary colic resulting from chronic calculous cholecystitis. The initial diagnostic study of choice is ultrasonography, which is very sensitive and specific for gallstones. Ultrasonography also provides information about the liver and pancreas. It is noninvasive, quick, relatively inexpensive, and does not entail the use of radiation. Oral cholecystogram is useful as a backup study in situations where gallstones are suspected clinically, but are not visualized on ultrasonography. The radionuclide biliary (HIDA) scan is the optimum test to confirm the diagnosis of acute cholecystitis, but it does not show gallstones. Compared with ultrasonography, a computed tomography (CT) scan is less sensitive for the detection of gallstones. A barium upper gastrointestinal series may be performed to further evaluate a symptomatic patient after biliary pathology is ruled out through the use of appropriate studies. (Chronic Calculous Cholecystitis)

6. Correct: C. The appropriate approach to a patient with asymptomatic gallstones that are found incidentally on a study done for another reason is continued observation. Of individuals with asymptomatic gallstones, approximately 1% to 2% per year have symptoms or complications of the gallstone disease; thus, two-thirds of these people remain free of symptoms or complications after 20 years. Also, the likelihood of complications decreases as the length of time the gallstones remain silent increases. An exception to this conservative approach is made in a patient with a calcified gallbladder ("porcelain" gallbladder) because these patients have a significantly higher risk for carcinoma of the gallbladder. None of the interventional approaches are justified at this time. (Asymptomatic Gallstones)

7. Correct: D. The patient has a history that is consistent with obstructive jaundice, and on examination is found to have a palpable, nontender gallbladder. The clinical picture suggests malignant disease (e.g., carcinoma of the pancreas) as the cause of the obstructive jaundice (Courvoisier's law). The gallbladder is passively distended because of back pressure caused by the distal malignant obstruction. If the obstruction were caused by a stone in the common duct, the chronically diseased gallbladder (the most likely source of the stone) would be thick-walled and thus incapable of distension. Acute hepatitis does not cause obstructive jaundice or a palpable gallbladder. The picture is not compatible with acute cholangitis or acute cholecystitis in view of the lack of signs of acute inflammation. Further, if the gallbladder is palpable in acute cholecystitis, it is tender. (Obstructive Jaundice)

8. Correct: A. Gallstones are present in nearly 80% of patients with gallbladder cancer. The presenting symptoms include vague right upper quadrant pain, weight loss, and malaise. Jaundice is present in approximately 50% of cases. The abdominal examination may show a mass in the right upper quadrant, but it is generally nontender. Appropriate management includes cholecystectomy, wide resection of the gallbladder fossa and liver bed, and regional lymphadenectomy, if technically feasible. The overall 5-year survival rate is generally less than 5%. (Gallbladder Cancer)

9. Correct: E. This patient has the classic Charcot's triad: abdominal pain, jaundice, and fever. Laboratory studies are consistent with the clinical diagnosis of acute cholangitis. The patient needs intravenous fluids, intravenous antibiotics, and nasogastric intubation (for the paralytic ileus). Administration of vitamin K is indicated to correct the coagulopathy that results from malabsorption of vitamin K. Ultrasonography should be performed to support the diagnosis; typically, gallstones with intrahepatic and extrahepatic ductal dilatation are found. Endoscopic retrograde cholangiopancreatography (ERCP) or percutaneous transhepatic cholangiography (PTC) would help to define the site and the cause of the obstruction to the common duct. Approximately 70% of patients with cholangitis respond to the treatment described earlier and may be scheduled for a definitive operation subsequently. If patients do not respond to this therapy, urgent decompression of the ducts with PTC or ERCP can be lifesaving. Emergency celiotomy is not part of the initial management plan. (Acute Cholangitis)

10. Correct: D. Extrahepatic bile duct malignancies occur most commonly in individuals who are 50 to 70 years old, and with equal frequency in both sexes. Two-thirds of bile duct carcinomas are located above the junction of the cystic duct with the common hepatic duct. The tumors are generally slow-growing and locally invasive. They rarely metastasize to distant sites. The 5-year survival rate after resection of lesions in the distal third of the common duct (by a Whipple procedure) is approximately 30%. Although the overall prognosis associated with the proximal lesions is poor, resection offers the best chance of survival. (Extrahepatic Bile Duct Malignancies)

11. Correct: D. Microorganisms commonly associated with acute cholecystitis are *Escherichia coli, Klebsiella pneumoniae, Streptococcus faecalis,* and *Clostridium welchii* or *Clostridium perfringens. Helicobacter pylori* is not associated with acute cholecystitis; however, it is found in patients with duodenal ulcer, gastric ulcer, gastric cancer, and gastritis. (Acute Cholecystitis)

12. Correct: B. Although gallstone ileus accounts for only 1% to 3% of all cases of intestinal obstruction, it is

the cause of nonstrangulated small intestinal obstruction in approximately 25% of patients who are older than 70 years of age. Gallstone ileus results from the erosion of a large stone through the gallbladder directly into the small intestine, through an internal fistula, usually between the gallbladder and the duodenum. The clinical picture and radiologic findings on plain x-rays are consistent with mechanical small bowel obstruction. Plain x-rays may show air in the biliary tree. Jaundice and fever are not typically found in these patients. Appropriate management includes celiotomy and enterolithotomy (extraction of the stone from the small intestine to relieve the obstruction). Cholecystectomy and definitive correction of the internal fistula are often deferred because of the existing comorbid conditions. They are sometimes performed during a second procedure. (Gallstone Ileus)

13. Correct: E. More than 90% of bile duct strictures occur as a result of iatrogenic injury during an operative procedure. Approximately 75% of bile duct injuries occur during simple cholecystectomy. The incidence of injuries associated with laparoscopic cholecystectomy is higher than that associated with open cholecystectomy, but it should decrease with the surgeon's experience. A large number of iatrogenic injuries go unrecognized until they result in complications from delayed stricture formation. These patients typically have obstructive jaundice and recurrent cholangitis. Long-standing strictures may result in biliary cirrhosis and portal hypertension. With the operative repair of strictures, excellent outcomes are achieved in 70% to 90% of patients in the hands of experienced surgeons. (Bile Duct Injury and Stricture)

14. Correct: D. In most elective and many emergency situations, laparoscopic cholecystectomy is the preferred approach for the management of gallstone disease. Advantages of this procedure over open cholecystectomy include minimal postoperative pain, shorter hospitalization and the possibility of ambulatory surgery, minimal wound complications, and more rapid recovery, with earlier return to normal activity. The incidence of bile duct injury is slightly higher with laparoscopic cholecystectomy than with open cholecystectomy, but is directly related to the surgeon's experience with this procedure. (Laparoscopic Cholecystectomy)

15. Correct: E. Initial management of acute cholecystitis includes a regimen of giving the patient nothing by mouth, administering intravenous fluids, and starting intravenous antibiotics. The bacteria commonly associated with acute cholecystitis are *Escherichia coli, Klebsiella pneumoniae, Streptococcus faecalis,* and *Clostridium welchii* or *Clostridium perfringens.* Parenteral analgesic may be administered judiciously, after the diagnosis is confirmed and further plans for

therapy have been made. A nasogastric tube is inserted if the patient has abdominal distension or is vomiting. Early cholecystectomy, within 3 days of the onset of symptoms, is recommended. (Acute Cholecystitis)

16. Correct: C. Acute biliary (gallstone) pancreatitis is usually caused by the passage of small stones and biliary sludge through the ampulla of Vater, rather than by the impaction of a large stone at the ampulla. Patients with acute biliary pancreatitis have the classic clinical picture of pancreatitis. However, serum amylase levels may be higher than in patients with alcoholic pancreatitis. After the initial management, a definitive operation is performed during the same hospitalization (after the patient shows clinical improvement). If this procedure is not done, recurrence of acute pancreatitis occurs in 25% to 60% of patients. If the disease continues to progress despite conservative management, urgent endoscopic retrograde cholangiopancreatography (ERCP) and sphincterotomy may be indicated. However, the latter procedure should not be performed as part of the initial management. (Acute Biliary Pancreatitis)

17. Correct: A. Radionuclide biliary (HIDA) scan includes the intravenous injection of a ^{99m}Tc-labeled derivative of iminodiacetic acid, which is excreted by the liver into the bile in high concentrations. The radionuclide then enters the gallbladder if the cystic duct is patent, and the gallbladder begins to fill within 30 minutes. Visualization of the common bile duct and duodenum, without filling of the gallbladder, after 4 hours indicates cystic duct obstruction and supports the diagnosis of acute cholecystitis. HIDA scan is also of value in identifying a suspected bile leak after surgery. The scan does not show stones in the gallbladder or the common bile duct. (Acute Cholecystitis)

18. Correct: B.

19. Correct: C.

20. Correct: C. Radiologic visualization of the biliary ductal anatomy is often helpful in making the diagnosis and planning therapy for patients with extrahepatic bile duct obstruction. Percutaneous transhepatic cholangiogram (PTC) and endoscopic retrograde cholangiopancreatogram (ERCP) are complementary studies that can provide valuable information. The performance of PTC is facilitated by the presence of dilated bile ducts, yielding a success rate of more than 95%. This study is particularly valuable for visualization of the proximal ductal system. ERCP requires a skilled endoscopist and is particularly useful in patients with bile ducts that are of normal size and in those with suspected ampullary lesions because biopsy of the ampulla can also be obtained. Cytologic specimens may be obtained with either PTC or ERCP. Also, either approach may be used for extraction of biliary calculi. (Obstructive Jaundice)

Chapter 17

1. Correct: A. Because acute pancreatitis is analogous to a retroperitoneal burn injury, maintenance of adequate intravascular volume is the main component of initial treatment. The other therapies may have a role, but are less important than assuring adequate tissue perfusion. (Acute Pancreatitis/Treatment)

2. Correct: D. White blood cell count, glucose, calcium, and aspartate aminotransferase are components of Ranson's criteria. Serum amylase has no prognostic value. (Acute Pancreatitis/Prognosis)

3. Correct: B. Treatment of persistent pain that does not respond to medical therapy is the main indication for operative intervention in chronic pancreatitis. Operation has no effect on the progression of exocrine and endocrine insufficiency. Patients with chronic pancreatitis are not at increased risk for pancreatic carcinoma, although differentiating masses caused by chronic pancreatitis and carcinoma can be difficult. (Chronic Pancreatitis/Treatment)

4. Correct: D. The only risk factors identified for pancreatic carcinoma are increasing age and cigarette smoking. There is a slight male predominance. (Pancreatic Neoplasms/General Considerations)

5. Correct: B. In response to duodenal acidification, secretin stimulates the secretion of bicarbonate-rich pancreatic fluid. The other responses are not caused by secretin. (Physiology/Exocrine)

6. Correct: C. Alcohol and gallstones are the etiologic agents in more than 85% of cases of acute pancreatitis. The other causes are less common, but should be considered after the most common etiologies are ruled out. (Acute Pancreatitis/Etiology)

7. Correct: B. When operation is indicated, drainage of the pseudocyst into the stomach or a loop of jejunum has the best result. Cholecystojejunostomy is used to relieve obstructive jaundice. Sphincteroplasty has no role in the treatment of pseudocyst. External drainage by a sump tube is indicated if the pseudocyst is infected (i.e., pancreatic abscess). Resection is reserved for small distal pancreatic pseudocysts and cystic neoplasms. (Pseudocysts/Treatment/Surgical)

8. Correct: E. Adenocarcinoma of the pancreatic ductal epithelium accounts for 90% of pancreatic neoplasms. (Pancreatic Neoplasms/General Considerations)

9. Correct: B. Unrelenting abdominal pain that radiates to the back is the most characteristic symptom of acute pancreatitis. The other symptoms are associated with complications of acute pancreatitis or with chronic pancreatitis. (Acute Pancreatitis/Clinical Presentation and Evaluation)

10. Correct: A. Painless jaundice in an elderly patient suggests pancreatic cancer. Although pancreatic cancer is often associated with abdominal pain, it is not as acute in onset or as severe as the other etiologies. (Pancreatic Neoplasms/Clinical Presentation and Evaluation)

11. Correct: D. Insulinomas are associated with fasting hypoglycemia. Because the majority are benign, metastases are rare. Gastrinomas cause recurrent ulcers and can be associated with intermittent diarrhea. (Pancreatic Neoplasms/Islet Cell Tumors of the Pancreas)

12. Correct: A. Pancreatic carcinoma occurs in the head of the gland in approximately 70% of cases. Carcinomas of the body and tail are usually unresectable at the time of diagnosis. (Pancreatic Neoplasms/General Considerations)

13. Correct: C. Because of the development of obstructive jaundice, periampullary lesions present earlier than more distal lesions. The median survival of patients with metastatic disease is less than 6 months; attempts at pancreatic resection are contraindicated in these patients. Weight loss is a grave prognostic sign. (Pancreatic Neoplasms/Clinical Presentation and Evaluation)

14. Correct: A. Although more than 27,000 people die as a result of pancreatic carcinoma each year, no reliable screening tests exist. (Pancreatic Neoplasms/General Considerations)

15. Correct: D. A high-quality, contrast-enhanced computed tomography scan of the abdomen is the most accurate test to assess pancreatic masses. Vascular invasion and liver metastases can be detected with this study. Arteriography and endoscopic retrograde cholangiopancreatography are useful adjunctive tests. (Pancreatic Neoplasms/Clinical Presentation and Evaluation)

16. Correct: B. The release of cholecystokinin is stimulated by duodenal free fatty acids, peptides, and amino acids. Protein digestion products in the stomach and gastric distension stimulate gastrin release. Secretin release is stimulated by acid in the duodenum. (Physiology/Exocrine)

17. Correct: E. Although peptic ulcer disease is common, gastrinoma accounts for fewer than 1% of cases of this disease. Patients with recurrent ulcers after definitive therapy, ulcers distal to the duodenal bulb, multiple ulcers, or ulcers and severe secretory diarrhea should be evaluated for gastrinoma. (Pancreatic Neoplasms/Zollinger-Ellison Syndrome)

18. Correct: D. Pancreatic enzyme secretion must decrease to less than 10% before malabsorption,

which manifests as steatorrhea, becomes apparent. (Chronic Pancreatitis)

19. Correct: D. Most acute fluid collections associated with acute pancreatitis resolve. Those that persist for more than 4 to 6 weeks (pseudocysts) require drainage, preferably into adjacent stomach or a loop of small intestine. By definition, a pseudocyst is not lined by epithelial tissue. (Pseudocysts/Treatment/Surgical)

20. Correct: A. The pancreas receives portions of its blood supply from the splenic, gastroduodenal, and superior mesenteric arteries. The anterior pancreaticoduodenal arcade is formed by branches of the superior mesenteric and gastroduodenal arteries. The proper hepatic artery provides no branches to the pancreas. (Anatomy/Arterial Blood Supply)

Chapter 18

1. Correct: D. Most hepatic adenomas occur in women between the ages of 30 and 50 years. Most women with these tumors have a history of taking oral contraceptives. If the patient is fit for operation and the size and location of the adenoma allow safe resection, these tumors are excised because of the risks of rupture, bleeding, and malignant transformation. The central stellate pattern seen radiographically and pathologically in some cases of focal nodular hyperplasia is not present in hepatic adenomas. Hemangiomas are the most common benign tumor of the liver. (Hepatic Tumors, Cysts, and Abscesses/Benign Tumors/Hepatic Adenoma)

2. Correct: A. Hepatocellular carcinoma accounts for more than 90% of all primary liver cancers. It usually occurs in the setting of some form of chronic liver disease, most commonly hepatitis B or C. Because the host liver is usually cirrhotic, resection of even small hepatocellular carcinomas is often precluded by a lack of hepatic reserve. In patients who undergo resection, more than 50% of recurrences are in the liver. (Hepatic Tumors, Cysts, and Abscesses/Malignant Tumors/Hepatocellular Adenoma)

3. Correct: D. The liver is a common site for metastatic deposits from colorectal cancers. Rising levels of carcinoembryonic antigen (CEA) often prompt liver imaging studies that show the metastases. If there is no extrahepatic spread, if margins of at least 1 cm are obtained, and if there is adequate hepatic reserve after resection, removal of the hepatic metastasis is considered. Long-term cure is reported with resection of as many as five metastatic nodules from the liver. Resection can be curative, but chemotherapy is not known to be so. (Hepatic Tumors, Cysts, and Abscesses/Malignant Tumors/Metastatic Tumors)

4. Correct: A. Simple cysts of the liver have thin walls, are not septate, and contain clear, serous fluid. They are commonly diagnosed incidentally by radiographic studies and rarely require excision. Polycystic liver disease is an autosomal dominant disorder that is often associated with polycystic kidney disease. Despite the presence of innumerable cysts, hepatic function is usually well preserved. (Hepatic Tumors, Cysts, and Abscesses/Hepatic Cysts/Simple Cysts and Polycystic Liver Disease)

5. Correct: D. Simple hepatic cysts occur with equal frequency in men and women, but cystic neoplasms are more common in women. Thickened walls, septations, and calcifications should prompt consideration of a neoplastic cyst. Neoplasia is uncommon in polycystic liver disease. Cystadenomas are resected if feasible because of their malignant potential. (Hepatic Tumors, Cysts, and Abscesses/Hepatic Cysts/Cystic Neoplasms)

6. Correct: E. Echinococcal cysts are considered in patients who have lived in endemic areas and have daughter cysts or wall calcifications on imaging studies. When echinococcus is suspected, serologic testing is performed because needle aspiration or surgery may result in spillage of protoscolices, with disastrous results. (Hepatic Tumors, Cysts, and Abscesses/Hepatic Cysts/Hydatid Cysts)

7. Correct: C. Pyogenic abscesses are almost always associated with an identifiable primary source. Common primary sources are the gastrointestinal tract (i.e., diverticulitis, appendicitis), biliary sepsis, and dental or other remote abscesses. Percutaneous drainage, specific antibiotic therapy, and treatment of the primary infection are the mainstays of therapy. (Hepatic Tumors, Cysts, and Abscesses/Hepatic Abscesses/Pyogenic Abscesses)

8. Correct: B. Portal vein occlusion accounts for an estimated 50% of cases of portal hypertension in children. Although this condition is often called a congenital portal vein occlusion, it is probably not really congenital. Most cases are believed to be secondary to omphalitis. One clearly identifiable cause of omphalitis is umbilical vein catheterization in the neonate. The umbilical vein communicates directly with the left portal vein. With portal vein occlusion, there is often a network of portoportal collateral veins. This network gives rise to the term cavernous transformation of the portal vein. (Portal Hypertension)

9. Correct: B. The serum ammonia level is often elevated in patients with hepatic encephalopathy. However, this test is nonspecific and is prone to laboratory error. Certain electroencephalographic and psychomotor findings are consistent with, but not specific for, encephalopathy. An increased ratio of the

aromatic to the branch chain amino acids is one of the postulated causes of encephalopathy. However, few laboratories are equipped to analyze serum amino acid ratios, and these analyses are too expensive and cumbersome for clinical use. The best way to diagnose hepatic encephalopathy is clinical evaluation. (Portal Hypertension/Hepatic Encephalopathy)

10. Correct: E. Transjugular intrahepatic portacaval shunting (TIPS) is technically possible in the vast majority (> 90%) of patients with portal hypertension. Although TIPS is occasionally used for uncontrolled ascites, its value in this setting has not been tested in proper clinical trials. Even if it effectively controls ascites in a given patient, there is a real risk of inducing another complication of portal hypertension, encephalopathy. The incidence of encephalopathy with a patent TIPS is as great as 30%, which is more than double the incidence after splenorenal shunt. For this reason and because the operative risk is relatively low, operative shunts are the treatment of choice to prevent recurrent variceal bleeding in Child's A or B patients in whom endoscopic therapy fails. (Portal Hypertension/Ascites)

11. Correct: E. The distal splenorenal shunt decompresses esophagogastric varices by shunting blood across the short gastrics through the spleen, out the splenic vein, and into the left renal vein. This operation is technically much more demanding than either a standard or a small-bore portacaval shunt. Because it both disrupts the retroperitoneal lymphatic channels and maintains portal hypertension in all but the gastrosplenic compartment, this operation can be ascitogenic. Still, it results in a very low incidence of bleeding from varices and is associated with a statistically significant lower incidence of encephalopathy than a portacaval shunt. (Portal Hypertension/Variceal Bleeding/Surgical Therapy)

12. Correct: C. In any patient with massive upper gastrointestinal bleeding, endoscopy is performed as soon as possible. Only after the source of the bleeding is correctly identified can rational treatment be instituted. Endoscopy can be performed in encephalopathic patients, although consideration may be given to first placing an endotracheal tube to protect the airway. Pharmacologic therapy may be instituted before endoscopy when variceal bleeding is suspected, but endoscopy is performed as quickly as possible thereafter. (Portal Hypertension/Variceal Bleeding/Endoscopic Therapy)

13. Correct: D. A Sengstaken-Blakemore tube stops variceal bleeding in approximately 90% of patients when properly applied. Because it can cause esophageal rupture and a number of other serious complications, its use is generally reserved for patients who have proven variceal bleeding and in whom both pharmacologic and endoscopic therapy have failed. Further, it is used only by experienced personnel in accordance with a strict protocol. The Sengstaken-Blakemore tube neither causes nor worsens hepatic encephalopathy. Although bleeding is effectively controlled by a properly placed Sengstaken-Blakemore tube, it often recurs when tamponade is released. Therefore, a more definitive treatment is often required after the Sengstaken-Blakemore tube is removed. (Portal Hypertension/Variceal Bleeding/Cessation of Acute Bleeding/Luminal Tamponade)

14. Correct: C. The percentage of patients with cirrhosis who have varices is unknown. There is reasonably good evidence, however, that only approximately 30% of patients with varices ever have clinically significant variceal bleeding. The risk of death per admission for variceal bleeding is estimated at 25% to 50%. Lactulose is used to treat hepatic encephalopathy, but has no known effect on the mesenteric vasculature. (Portal Hypertension/Variceal Bleeding/Cessation of Acute Bleeding)

15. Correct: D. More than one-half of all episodes of upper gastrointestinal bleeding in patients with cirrhosis are from sources other than varices. When variceal bleeding is suspected, good intravenous access, with two large-bore lines, is established. Crystalloid solutions can be administered until blood products are available, but blood products should constitute the majority of volume resuscitation. Lactulose helps to correct encephalopathy in two ways. It acts as a cathartic, and it alters the intraluminal pH of the colon so that the bacteria produce less nitrogen. The distal splenorenal shunt is associated with a fairly high operative mortality rate in Child's C patients. Therefore, in that population, transjugular intrahepatic portacaval shunting (TIPS) or an operative portacaval shunt is probably a better treatment. Somatostatin is slightly more effective than vasopressin in stopping variceal hemorrhage. Additionally, because somatostatin is associated with fewer complications, it is the preferred pharmacologic treatment for acute variceal bleeding. (Portal Hypertension/Variceal Bleeding/Cessation of Acute Bleeding/Pharmacologic Therapy)

16. Correct: D. Historically, transplantation for chronic hepatitis B led to early, severe hepatocellular injury, frequently with loss of the graft and death of the patient. New strategies may make transplantation for chronic hepatitis B possible. Reinfection of the graft in patients who undergo transplantation for chronic hepatitis C is almost universal, but these infections are usually indolent and well tolerated, at least in the short term. (Liver Transplantation/Indications for Transplantation/Chronic and Progressive Advanced Liver Disease/Chronic Hepatitis C)

17. Correct: B. Ascites, variceal bleeding, and encephalopathy are all manifestations of advanced liver disease that may be seen in the patient with a failing liver. Children can successfully undergo transplantation if a suitable donor is found. Liver transplantation is technically more difficult in obese patients, but obesity is not a contraindication. Hepatitis B is no longer an absolute contraindication to liver transplantation. In addition to extrahepatic malignancy, human immunodeficiency–positive status, and uncontrolled sepsis, active alcohol or substance abuse and advanced cardiac or pulmonary disease are absolute contraindications to liver transplantation. (Liver Transplantation/Table 18–2)

18. Correct: E. Variceal bleeding, encephalopathy, and ascites are all manifestations, but not causes, of liver failure. Hemochromatosis is not corrected by transplantation. Patients with a history of alcohol or substance abuse who are carefully selected for transplantation have a low rate of recidivism and usually do not cause graft loss by their former habits. Autoimmune hepatitis, Wilson's disease, and alpha$_1$-antitrypsin deficiency are corrected by liver transplantation. (Liver Transplantation/Indications for Transplantation)

19. Correct: D. Acute rejection is seen in 40% to 70% of liver transplants. It usually occurs 5 to 30 days after operation and is first manifested by rising transaminase levels. These patients are successfully treated by bolus corticosteroid therapy. Nonresponders are effectively treated by OKT3. (Liver Transplantation/Complications of Liver Transplantation/Liver Allograft Dysfunction)

20. Correct: E. People are usually excluded from donation if they are hepatitis B–, hepatitis C–, or human immunodeficiency virus– positive. The allowable cold ischemia time for livers is 12 to 18 hours. Liver dysfunction from technical complications usually appears in the first 7 days after transplantation. Hepatorenal syndrome in the recipient is often reversed after transplantation. Immunosuppression of the recipient usually begins before or during the transplant. (Liver Transplantation/Technical Aspects)

Chapter 19

1. Correct: C. The intercostal branchial nerve provides sensation to the upper inner arm. The other three nerves all provide motor innervation. Thrombosis of the axillary vein may result in lymphedema. (Anatomy; Complications of Surgery)

2. Correct: C. Localization of the site of discharge is necessary to proceed with duct excision in the operating room. Ductography does not eliminate the need for surgery or aid the ductal excision if the localization is done on physical examination. Cytology of ductal discharge has no significant clinical benefit.

Breast ultrasound is not useful as a screening test in ductal discharge. Additional mammographic views are unlikely to aid in the diagnosis and do not eliminate the need for surgery. (Physical Examination; Benign Conditions of the Breast/Nipple Discharge)

3. Correct: A. Atypical hyperplasia is a major risk factor and requires yearly screening in a 36-year-old patient who otherwise would be advised to begin annual screening at 40 years of age. None of the other conditions change the usual recommendations appropriate for age. (Clinical Presentation and Evaluation)

4. Correct: C. The wide excision must have clear microscopic margins. The addition of radiation therapy in this setting decreases local recurrence significantly. Modified radical mastectomy is unnecessary, particularly because axillary dissection is not appropriate for localized ductal cancer in situ. There is no proven benefit for radiation treatment as the only therapy or for tamoxifen as adjuvant therapy. (Treatment of Breast Cancer/Surgery)

5. Correct: D. Intraductal papilloma is the most common cause of bloody nipple discharge in this age-group. Breast cancer occurs in 10% to 15% of patients with bloody discharge, and must be excluded. Other common causes include duct ectasia, fibrocystic changes, and breast cysts. (Benign Conditions of the Breast/Nipple Discharge)

6. Correct: D. The presence of an involved supraclavicular node makes the classification stage IV because the disease is considered metastatic. The other descriptions represent lower stages. (Breast Cancer/Clinical Staging)

7. Correct: A. Because cysts do not increase the risk of breast cancer, it is appropriate to treat an asymptomatic patient with observation only. Mammography cannot distinguish between solid and cystic lesions. Symptomatic cysts are best treated with aspiration, but cyst fluid cytology has no significant benefit in management. (Benign Conditions of the Breast/Breast Cyst)

8. Correct: C. Although the physical examination and ultrasound findings are consistent with fibroadenoma, observation is safe only after the diagnosis is confirmed. The least invasive method is fine-needle aspiration cytology. Mammography has little role in the evaluation of patients younger than 30 years of age who have benign findings. (Benign Conditions of the Breast/Fibroadenoma)

9. Correct: B. Lobular cancer in situ increases the relative risk tenfold to twelvefold. All of the other risk factors increase the relative risk onefold to twofold. (Clinical Presentation and Evaluation)

10. Correct: B. Most patients presenting with breast pain rather than seeking treatment for the pain are seeking reassurance that it does not represent cancer. If, after reassurance, the pain remains a significant concern, treatment should begin with the least risky modalities (e.g., elimination of caffeine, vitamin E) and progress to oil of evening primrose capsules, oral contraceptives, and finally danazol, the treatment with the highest incidence of side effects. Mammography and ultrasound are not indicated in the absence of significant physical findings (e.g., breast mass). (Benign Conditions of the Breast/Breast Pain)

11. Correct: A. Prospective randomized trials show no difference in the chance for cure and survival or in recurrence rates between patients undergoing breast conservation and those undergoing mastectomy. Axillary dissection is necessary to provide lymph node information so that the appropriate adjuvant therapy can be chosen. Radiation is necessary, regardless of lymph node status, because it reduces the incidence of local recurrence in the breast. (Treatment of Breast Cancer/Choosing a Surgical Option)

12. Correct: B. Standard treatment for a premenopausal patient with node-positive breast cancer is combination chemotherapy. Usually, radiation of the chest wall and axilla is added to mastectomy only if the patient has T3 tumors or extensive nodal involvement. Hormonal therapy may supplement chemotherapy in the premenopausal patient, but is more commonly used in the postmenopausal group. Bone marrow transplantation is usually reserved for patients with ten or more positive lymph nodes. (Treatment of Breast Cancer/Adjuvant Treatment)

13. Correct: B. Erythema and exfoliation are expected complications in patients undergoing radiation therapy. Radiation pneumonitis is a rare complication of radiation therapy, and lung cancer has not been reported. Lymphoma, anorexia, and hair loss are not seen with radiation therapy. (Treatment of Breast Cancer/Complications of Radiation Therapy)

14. Correct: B. Approximately 60% of patients who take tamoxifen have hot flashes. Although endometrial cancer is reported as a complication of tamoxifen therapy, it is extremely rare. Osteoporosis may be prevented by the peripheral estrogenic effects of tamoxifen. Thrombocytopenia and breast tenderness are not associated with tamoxifen therapy. (Treatment of Breast Cancer/Complications of Treatment with Tamoxifen)

15. Correct: D. In patients with inflammatory breast cancer, the 5-year survival rate is approximately 25%. This rate is even worse than that for patients with node-positive infiltrating ductal or infiltrating lobular cancer. Patients with medullary cancer have a prognosis similar to and perhaps slightly better than that

of those with infiltrating ductal cancer. (Histologic Types of Breast Cancer)

16. Correct: C. Fine-needle aspiration cytology is the least invasive method for diagnosing a palpable breast mass, allowing definitive operative therapy in a single trip to the operating room. Core biopsy is another alternative for office-based biopsy. An attempt is made to make a diagnosis before definitive operative intervention rather than going to the operating room without a diagnosis so that the operative course of action depends on an intraoperative frozen section. (Diagnostic Evaluation/Biopsy Techniques)

17. Correct: B. Current indications for a metastatic survey before the initiation of treatment include symptoms referable to metastasis (e.g., bony pain) and the presence of a T3 tumor (> 5 cm) or inflammatory breast cancer. A metastatic survey is not performed routinely because of the low yield and high cost of the studies. (Diagnostic Evaluation/Studies to Evaluate Metastatic Breast Disease)

18. Correct: B. In pregnancy, estrogen and progesterone levels remain quite high, so there is continued hypertrophy and budding of the ductal system as well as increased acinar development. During each cycle, preovulatory estrogen production stimulates ductal proliferation. The onset of lactation is secondary to the sudden postpartum decrease in hormone levels that is associated with the onset of prolactin secretion. Postmenopausally, the lack of hormonal stimulation results in replacement of breast parenchyma with adipose tissue. (Physiology)

19. Correct: C. The ordering of factors that predict prognosis, from most predictive to least predictive, is as follows: tumor size, lymph node status, estrogen receptor status, and other factors, including ploidy, cathepsin D, her-2-neu oncogene expression, and S-phase. (Breast Cancer/Prognosis)

20. Correct: C. Both mastectomy and radiation therapy provide whole breast treatment. For this reason, radiation therapy is not necessary after mastectomy, except in cases of advanced disease. The local recurrence rate and 5-year survival rate are not statistically significantly different between patients undergoing breast conservation and those undergoing mastectomy. The need for subsequent adjuvant therapy (e.g., chemotherapy, tamoxifen) is unaffected by the choice of surgical therapy. (Treatment of Breast Cancer/Choosing a Surgical Option)

Chapter 20
Thyroid Gland

1. Correct: C. Medullary carcinomas are derived from the C-cell component of the thyroid that secretes calcitonin. Thyroxine, thyroid-stimulating hormone

(TSH), thyrotropin-releasing hormone (TRH), and glucagon levels are normal. (Thyroid Carcinoma/Medullary Carcinoma)

2. Correct: D. Because of the tendency for multicentricity, the aggressive nature of medullary lesions, and the likelihood for nodal metastatic spread, total thyroidectomy with at least central neck lymph node dissection should be performed. Lesser operations result in a lower survival rate and a higher rate of recurrence. (Thyroid Carcinoma/Medullary Carcinoma)

3. Correct: E. A solitary nodule, especially in a male, suggests carcinoma. A benign result on fine-needle aspiration might allow observation with suppression with thyroid hormone. However, with an indeterminate result, a formal biopsy in the form of a thyroid lobectomy should be performed. If the result is positive, completion to a total thyroidectomy is necessary. Radioactive iodine therapy is inappropriate and would be ineffective because the isotope is preferentially taken up by the normal thyroid and not by the lesion. Total thyroidectomy without confirmation of the diagnosis of carcinoma is too radical, and incisional biopsy and enucleation do not allow adequate pathologic evaluation of the relation of the nodule to the rest of the thyroid. (Thyroid Nodule)

4. Correct: A. Thyroid is the only tissue that concentrates iodine. Although thyroid cancers are often thought of as "cold," in most cases, these cells take up iodine, but to a lesser degree than normal thyroid tissue. Therefore, the best treatment for this patient is radioiodine to ablate the metastases. Before ablation can be achieved, however, all thyroid tissue must be excised, including any obviously involved nodes. Otherwise, the radioactive iodine will be taken up by the thyroid and not by the metastases. There is no effective systemic chemotherapy. External beam radiation is less effective than radioactive iodine therapy, but may be used if radioactive iodine therapy is ineffective. Suppression with thyroid hormone is part of the treatment, but is not effective as a primary modality. (Thyroid Carcinoma/Papillary Carcinoma)

5. Correct: A. Radioactive iodine is the treatment that carries the lowest morbidity and mortality for the treatment of Graves' disease. Propranolol and thyroxine suppression have a role in the treatment, but are not definitive. If antithyroid medication is used and is ineffective, radioactive iodine therapy is the next step, not operation. Operative management of Graves' disease is generally reserved for specific indications, such as patients who are pregnant, are noncompliant with antithyroid drugs, are allergic to iodine, or who refuse radioactive iodine therapy after antithyroid drugs fail. (Hyperthyroidism/Graves' Disease/Treatment)

6. Correct: A. There is a clear association between sublethal radiation exposure and the development of thyroid cancer. There is no known association with the other options. (Thyroid Nodule/Clinical Presentation and Evaluation)

7. Correct: A. Because of the close association between the parathyroid and the thyroid, dissection of these glands off the thyroid during thyroidectomy often causes transient hypoparathyroidism. In skilled hands, hemorrhage, pneumothorax, and permanent injury to the parathyroid or the recurrent laryngeal nerves are uncommon (< 1%). (Thyroid Nodule/Treatment)

8. Correct: B. Radioactive iodine therapy is extremely safe and does not result in secondary cancers, agranulocytosis, or injury to the parathyroids. It does, however, cause hypothyroidism in 50% to 70% of patients after 10 years. (Hyperthyroidism/Graves' Disease/Treatment; Table 20–2)

9. Correct: A. A thyroid nodule is more likely to be malignant in a child younger than 7 years of age, a man older than 40 years of age, or a woman older than 50 years of age. Radiation exposure is a recognized risk factor. A solitary lesion suggests malignancy. Multiple "cold" nodules suggest a multinodular goiter. Toxic, or "hot," nodules are rarely malignant. (Thyroid Nodule/Clinical Presentation and Evaluation)

10. Correct: E. Thyroid nodules that do not shrink with adequate thyroid suppression and are not clearly benign should be excised. In general, thyroid nodules are not painful. Toxic nodules and cysts are significantly less common than solid, nontoxic nodules. Because the nodule usually takes up radioiodine to a lesser degree than normal thyroid tissue (i.e., "cold" nodule), treatment with radioactive iodine is inappropriate. (Thyroid Nodule)

11. Correct: B. A solitary "cold" nodule is more likely to be a carcinoma when it occurs in a man. Toxic nodules and diffuse goiters, whether toxic or not, are highly unlikely to be malignant. (Thyroid Nodule/Clinical Presentation and Evaluation)

12. Correct: A. The thyrocervical trunk, a branch of the subclavian artery, gives rise to the inferior thyroid artery. The vertebral, common carotid, and internal carotid arteries have no branches in the neck. (Thyroid Gland/Anatomy)

13. Correct: B. Graves' disease is much more common in women than in men. Pretibial myxedema, although not common, is not rare. The initial therapy is antithyroid drugs, not surgery. The thyroid-stimulating hormone (TSH) level is extremely low, not high. Struma ovarii (thyrotoxicosis arising from thyroid tissue in an

ovarian teratoma) is an extremely rare condition. (Hyperthyroidism)

14. Correct: E. Medullary carcinoma secretes calcitonin, which can be assayed in the serum and is specific to that tumor. Although thyroglobulin may be elevated in other types of thyroid malignancy, this finding is not specific. (Thyroid Carcinoma/Medullary Carcinoma/ Clinical Presentation and Evaluation)

15. Correct: B. The superior thyroid artery is the first branch of the external carotid artery. The thyrocervical trunk, which arises from the subclavian artery, gives rise to the inferior artery. The common and internal carotid arteries have no branches in the neck. (Thyroid Gland/Anatomy)

16. Correct: B. Papillary carcinoma is significantly more common than follicular carcinoma. Anaplastic carcinoma is uncommon, especially in this age range. Medullary carcinoma and lymphoma are uncommon. (Thyroid Carcinoma/Papillary Carcinoma; Table 20–3)

17. Correct: C. The most likely diagnosis in this low-risk patient is follicular adenoma. Therefore, excision by lobectomy or total thyroidectomy is inappropriate. Radioactive iodine therapy would be ineffective because the isotope will go to the normal thyroid, not to the lesion. Observation is an acceptable alternative, but is less appealing than suppression, the opportunity to induce regression, and relief of the patient's symptoms. (Thyroid Nodule/Treatment)

Parathyroid Glands

18. Correct: C. Hypercalcemia is most commonly caused by hyperparathyroidism, less commonly by malignancy, and rarely by the other causes listed. (Parathyroid Glands/Pathophysiology)

19. Correct: C. The metabolites of vitamin D regulate intestinal calcium absorption. (Parathyroid Glands/ Pathophysiology)

20. Correct E. Lytic metastases to bone from breast cancer release calcium. Parathyroid hormone is not involved. (Parathyroid Glands/Pathophysiology)

21. Correct: A. In secondary hyperparathyroidism, the increased production of parathyroid hormone occurs in response to hypocalcemia. (Parathyroid Glands/ Pathophysiology)

22. Correct: B. Extensive soft tissue calcification is a feature of tertiary hyperparathyroidism. (Parathyroid Glands/ Pathophysiology)

23. Correct: A. Although parathyroid hormone stimulates calcium resorption in the distal tubules of the kidney,

it also inhibits renal tubular resorption of phosphate. (Parathyroid Glands/Pathophysiology)

24. Correct: A. Adenoma is the most common cause of hyperparathyroidism. (Parathyroid Glands/Pathophysiology)

25. Correct: D. An elevated serum calcium level (total or ionized) is the simplest, least expensive screening test for hyperparathyroidism. (Parathyroid Glands/Pathophysiology)

26. Correct: C. Acute pancreatitis may cause transient hypocalcemia. The other conditions cause hypercalcemia. (Parathyroid Glands/Pathophysiology)

27. Correct: B. Severe bone disease because of the resorption of calcium is common in both secondary and tertiary hyperparathyroidism. (Parathyroid Glands/ Pathophysiology)

28. Correct: C. Elevated serum parathormone levels occur in all forms of hyperparathyroidism. (Parathyroid Glands/Pathophysiology)

29. Correct: A. Secondary hyperparathyroidism occurs in response to a decreased serum calcium level. (Parathyroid Glands/Pathophysiology)

Adrenal Glands

30. Correct: E. Hypertension, metabolic alkalosis, hypokalemia, and muscle weakness are all clinical features of primary aldosteronism, although they may not all be seen in the same patient at the same time. Somatic abnormalities are not specific features of hyperaldosteronism (primary or secondary). (Adrenal Glands/Primary Aldosteronism)

31. Correct: B. The sodium loading test is designed to show that the elevated serum aldosterone level cannot be suppressed in patients with primary aldosteronism, even by loading the patient with sodium and expanding the circulating plasma volume (normally potent inhibitors of aldosterone secretion). An elevated serum aldosterone level in the presence of elevated plasma renin activity is secondary hyperaldosteronism. A decreased urinary sodium level is not specific for primary aldosteronism. A significant decrease in serum sodium or metabolic acidosis is not seen in primary aldosteronism. (Adrenal Glands/Primary Aldosteronism/Diagnosis)

32. Correct: C. Hypokalemia, hypomagnesemia, and metabolic alkalosis can lead to tetany in patients with primary aldosteronism. Alkalosis causes a decrease in the ionized calcium fraction and shifts the distribution of serum calcium toward the protein-bound fraction. As a result, the patient becomes relatively hypocalcemic. Acidosis, hyponatremia, edema, and normal or low urine aldosterone are not seen in

primary aldosteronism. (Adrenal Glands/Primary Aldosteronism/Clinical Presentation)

33. Correct: E. The definitive treatment of primary aldosteronism is surgical excision of the responsible adrenal tumor. Spironolactone (a competitive antagonist of aldosterone) is used with varying success in the other clinical settings described, and may be the treatment of choice for idiopathic hyperaldosteronism. (Adrenal Glands/Primary Aldosteronism/Treatment)

34. Correct: A. Selective arteriography and phlebography are no longer indicated to evaluate adrenal tumors because of the risks of associated complications (hemorrhage and thrombosis) without the benefit of any increase in sensitivity or specificity over computed axial tomography (CT) and other less invasive modalities. Selective adrenal venous sampling is indicated in only a select group of patients who have either no obvious adrenal tumor or ambiguous adrenal tumors (e.g., bilateral adrenal masses) that have overt clinical findings and diagnostic biochemical evidence of autonomous, excess adrenal function. In this case, it cannot be assumed that either or both adrenal masses are responsible for the patient's clinical syndrome. Iodocholesterol scans are primarily supplementary imaging modalities used to evaluate adrenal tumors. (Adrenal Glands/Cushing's Syndrome [Diagnosis], Primary Aldosteronism [Diagnosis], Pheochromocytoma [Diagnosis], and Incidentally Discovered Adrenal Mass [Diagnosis])

35. Correct: A. The treatment of choice for primary "hyperaldosteronism" is surgical excision of the diseased gland. Spironolactone is indicated for the treatment of idiopathic hyperaldosteronism, and it may be used to preoperatively prepare and facilitate the correction of metabolic abnormalities in primary aldosteronism before adrenalectomy. The other options either are not as correct or are contraindicated. (Adrenal Glands/Primary Aldosteronism/Treatment)

36. Correct: E. Pheochromocytomas may originate from the adrenal medulla or from chromaffin tissue in the peripheral autonomic nervous system, located anywhere from the base of the skull to the pelvis. They never originate from the adrenal cortex. Only 10% of pheochromocytomas are malignant. Weight gain and hypoglycemia are not features of pheochromocytomas, but may be coincidentally present. (Adrenal Glands/Pheochromocytoma)

37. Correct: E. Pheochromocytomas are bilateral in 10% of cases, multiple in 10% of cases, extraadrenal in 10% of cases, and extraabdominal in only 2% of cases. They are occasionally found incidentally, but are never part of the watery diarrhea, hypokalemia, and achlorhydria (WDHA) syndrome. The WDHA (Verner-Morrison) syndrome is caused by a vasoac-

tive intestinal peptide (VIP)-secreting pancreatic neuroendocrine tumor, and although it can be associated with pheochromocytoma (as well as with ganglioneuroma, medullary thyroid carcinoma, neuroblastoma, and carcinoma of the lung), it is not part of the syndrome. (Adrenal Glands/Pheochromocytoma)

38. Correct: E. The hypertension that is associated with pheochromocytoma can be paroxysmal, characterized by extreme fluctuations superimposed on constant elevation, and associated with severe headaches, pallor, tachycardia or bradycardia, nausea, and vomiting. (Adrenal Glands/Pheochromocytoma/Clinical Presentation)

39. Correct: E. Paroxysmal attacks of hypertension in pheochromocytoma may be precipitated by exertion, trauma, certain drugs, alcohol, micturition (urination), smoking, or any change in position. Phenoxybenzamine is the alpha-blocking (antagonistic) agent that is most often used to block the alpha-adrenergic effects of the norepinephrine and epinephrine secreted by the pheochromocytoma. (Adrenal Glands/Pheochromocytoma/Clinical Presentation, Diagnosis)

40. Correct: A. Palpitations, neurofibromatosis, port wine spots, telangiectasis, and excessive sweating may be present in a patient with pheochromocytoma because of associated syndromes. None of the other conditions account for all of the symptoms and findings. (Adrenal Glands/Pheochromocytoma/Clinical Presentation, Diagnosis)

41. Correct: B. The diagnosis of pheochromocytoma requires the measurement of catecholamines and their metabolic products in the urine or blood. Some centers can now measure serum metanephrine. Normetanephrine and metanephrine provide the best specificity and sensitivity. Vanillylmandelic acid (VMA) is excreted in the urine and not in the blood. High levels of norepinephrine in the adrenal vein are seen in a patient under "stress" conditions who is not harboring a pheochromocytoma. Everyone has blockage of alpha- and beta-adrenergic receptors when given the appropriated antagonists. Provocative tests are contraindicated in patients who are suspected of harboring a pheochromocytoma because they may precipitate a catecholamine crisis. Further, false-positive results are associated with the finding of paroxysmal hypertension by a provocative test. (Adrenal Glands/Pheochromocytoma/Diagnosis)

42. Correct: E. Cushing's syndrome is least likely to be associated with ovulatory menstrual cycles. Liver disease compromising hepatic function can interfere with the excretion of exogenous prednisone and result in the accumulation of prednisone and excess steroids, causing Cushing's syndrome. Pituitary tumors are the most common cause of Cushing's syn-

drome. Extrapituitary tumors can cause Cushing's syndrome by secreting adrenocorticotropic hormone (ACTH)-like peptides that stimulate adrenocortical hyperplasia and hyperfunction. Adrenal cortical carcinomas are functional in approximately 50% to 60% of cases, the overwhelming majority of which secrete glucocorticoids that cause Cushing's syndrome. Exogenous cortisol administration can also cause Cushing's syndrome when it is excessive or when the process of steroid elimination is sufficiently impaired (e.g., liver failure) so that the corticosteroid accumulates. However, normal menstrual cycles do not affect cortisol levels or influence adrenocortical function. (Adrenal Glands/Cushing's Syndrome/Clinical Presentation, Diagnosis)

43. Correct: E. Weakness, psychological changes, truncal obesity, and sexual dysfunction are features of Cushing's syndrome, although all of these features may not be present in any one patient. Osteitis deformans is a disease of bone that is marked by repeated episodes of increased bone resorption followed by excessive attempts at repair (e.g., Paget's disease). It is not associated with Cushing's syndrome. (Adrenal Glands/Cushing's Syndrome/Clinical Presentation)

44. Correct: E. Hypertension, easy bruisability, hirsutism (especially in women), and the presence of a "buffalo hump" are all consequences of the excess glucocorticoids found in Cushing's syndrome. Ganglioneuromatosis is seen in multiple endocrine neoplasia (MEN) syndrome type 2B. It is not associated directly with Cushing's syndrome. (Adrenal Glands/Cushing's Syndrome/Clinical Presentation)

45. Correct: A. The zona glomerulosa is responsible for the production of aldosterone. The zona reticularis is responsible for the production of androgens and related precursors. The zona medullaris and zona pigmentosa do not exist in the adrenal cortex. (Adrenal Glands/Physiology)

46. Correct: E. The most common cause of Cushing's syndrome is a basophilic tumor of the anterior pituitary (Cushing's disease). It is seen in 60% of cases. Carcinoma of the adrenal cortex is an infrequent cause of Cushing's syndrome; combined with benign adenoma of the adrenal cortex, it accounts for approximately 15% of cases. Ectopic adrenocorticotropic hormone (ACTH) secretion by a primary malignancy (e.g., oat cell carcinoma of the lung) occurs in 10% to 15% of cases. Adrenal medullary hyperplasia does not cause Cushing's syndrome, but causes hypercatecholaminemia (i.e., pheochromocytoma). (Adrenal Glands/Cushing's Syndrome/Pheochromocytoma/Diagnosis)

47. Correct: A. The preoperative evaluation of a patient with a suspected pheochromocytoma should include a computed tomography (CT) scan of the abdomen.

Tomograms of the pituitary are not used to evaluate patients with suspected pituitary neoplasms and would have nothing to do with a suspected pheochromocytoma. Urinary 5-hydroxyindoleacetic acid (5-HIAA) is used to evaluate patients with suspected carcinoid tumors. The Hollander test is used to measure the completeness of gastric vagal denervation after vagotomy [measure of the extent of increase in hydrogen concentration in gastric juice after the administration of insulin to induce hypoglycemia (a potent gastric acid secretagogue)]. A liver scan is less effective than a CT scan in identifying hepatic metastases from a malignant pheochromocytoma or any other primary malignancy that can metastasize to the liver. (Adrenal Glands/Pheochromocytoma/Diagnosis)

48. Correct: A. Serum prolactin levels are used to consider the presence or absence of a pituitary adenoma (prolactinoma) in the appropriate clinical setting. The remaining choices play a potential role in establishing the likely etiology of an incidental adrenal mass lesion. A careful history and physical examination will alert the physician to the possibility of a hyperfunctioning adrenal mass or to another etiology of adrenal pathology. A computed tomography (CT) scan of the abdomen provides evidence of the benign or malignant nature of the lesion. A history of lung carcinoma raises the possibility that the adrenal lesion represents metastasis. Finally, an NP-59 adrenal scan provides additional information about the nature and function of the respective adrenal mass lesion. (Adrenal Glands/Incidentally Discovered Adrenal Mass/Diagnosis)

49. Correct: C. Adrenal cortical carcinomas and pheochromocytomas both give bright images on magnetic resonance imaging (MRI) scans (i.e., they both have high T2-weighted images compared with the liver on MRI). Therefore, because of the overlap of MRI findings between these two lesions, they are not easily distinguishable on the basis of this imaging modality alone. The rest of the choices are true. (Adrenal Glands/Adrenal Cortical Carcinoma/Diagnosis)

Multiple Endocrine Neoplasia Syndromes

50. Correct: B. Studies show that sudden death can be caused by pheochromocytoma, especially during the induction of anesthesia. Therefore, in any patient with multiple endocrine neoplasia syndrome type 2A (MEN-2A) who is undergoing surgery for another condition, pheochromocytoma should be excluded by obtaining a 24-hour urinalysis for catecholamines. If found, a pheochromocytoma should be removed first. (MEN/MEN-2A, MEN-2B, and Familial MTC/Pheochromocytoma in MEN-2A and MEN-2B)

51. Correct: C. Parathyroid disease is associated with multiple endocrine neoplasia syndrome type 1

(MEN-1) and MEN-2A, but not with MEN-2B. (MEN/MEN-2A, MEN-2B, and Familial MTC)

52. Correct: D. Gastrinoma is found in patients with multiple endocrine neoplasia syndrome type 1 (MEN-1), but not in those with MEN-2, familial medullary thyroid carcinoma (FMTC), or von Hippel-Lindau (VHL) syndrome. (MEN/MEN-1/Tumors in MEN-1/ Pancreatic Islet Cell Tumors)

53. Correct: A. Patients with either multiple endocrine neoplasia syndrome type 2A (MEN-2A) or MEN-2B may have bilateral pheochromocytoma. (MEN/ MEN-2A, MEN-2B, and Familial MTC/Pheochromocytoma in MEN-2A and MEN-2B)

54. Correct: D. Medullary thyroid carcinoma, adrenal pheochromocytoma, and parathyroid hyperplasia are associated with multiple endocrine neoplasia syndrome type 2A (MEN-2A) and 2B. Pituitary adenoma is found in patients with MEN-1. (MEN/MEN-2A, MEN-2B, and Familial MTC; MEN-1)

55. Correct: B. Parathyroid gland hyperplasia is associated with multiple endocrine neoplasia syndrome type 1 (MEN-1) and MEN-2A and is diagnosed by elevated serum levels of calcium and parathyroid hormone. It is not associated with MEN-2B. (MEN/ MEN-2A, MEN-2B, and Familial MTC)

56. Correct: E. Medullary thyroid carcinoma is found in patients with multiple endocrine neoplasia syndrome type 2A (MEN-2A), MEN-2B, and familial medullary thyroid carcinoma (FMTC). Sipple's syndrome is another name for MEN-2A. MTC is not part of von Hippel-Lindau (VHL) syndrome (MEN/MEN-2A, MEN-2B, and Familial MTC)

57. Correct: D. Studies show a mutation in the RET gene in all individuals with multiple endocrine neoplasia syndrome type 2A (MEN-2A), MEN-2B, and familial medullary thyroid carcinoma (FMTC). MEN-1 is caused by a menin gene mutation. (MEN/MEN-2A, MEN-2B, and Familial MTC/Genetic Defect in MEN-2)

58. Correct: B. Studies show that patients who have multiple endocrine neoplasia syndrome type 1 (MEN-1) with Zollinger-Ellison syndrome and primary hyperparathyroidism should undergo surgical therapy (total parathyroidectomy and forearm transplant or 3–1/2–gland parathyroidectomy) for primary hyperparathyroidism first because it lessens the acid secretion, serum gastrin level, and symptoms of Zollinger-Ellison syndrome. (MEN/MEN-1/Parathyroid Hyperplasia)

59. Correct: D. Although patients with multiple endocrine neoplasia syndrome type 1 (MEN-1) have a greater propensity to parathyroid hyperplasia, lipo-

mas, pancreatic islet cell tumors, bronchial or thymic carcinoid tumors, and others, only patients with MEN-2 are at risk for pheochromocytoma. (MEN/ MEN-2A, MEN-2B, and Familial MTC)

60. Correct: A. Patients with multiple endocrine neoplasia syndrome type 1 (MEN-1) often have parathyroid hyperplasia and tumors of the anterior pituitary, but only the pancreatic islet cell tumors are likely to be malignant. (MEN/MEN-1/Tumors in MEN-1/Pancreatic Islet Cell Tumors)

Chapter 21

1. Correct: B. The onset of overwhelming pneumococcal infection in postsplenectomy patients is insidious, with symptoms that resemble those of upper respiratory infection. Rapid progression to overwhelming sepsis is the rule. The mortality rate is 75% despite antibiotic therapy. (Consequences and Complications of Splenectomy/Immune Consequences)

2. Correct: C. A normal peripheral smear that shows no evidence of Howell-Jolly bodies or red cell abnormalities after splenectomy is unusual. Patients who have recurrent symptoms of immune thrombocytopenic purpura after splenectomy, with a normal smear, should have a radionuclide spleen scan to rule out a missed accessory spleen. (General Diagnostic Considerations/Radiographic Imaging; Consequences and Complications of Splenectomy/Hematologic Changes)

3. Correct: A. The spleen is probably necessary for an optimal response to pneumococcal vaccine. Immunization is performed well in advance of elective splenectomy to allow for optimal response. (Consequences and Complications of Splenectomy/Immune Consequences)

4. Correct: A. The blood pressure is normal for an 11-year-old boy. The pulse may be slightly elevated. The child is hemodynamically stable. A protocol for nonoperative management of the splenic injury should be followed. Surgery is not necessary unless there is evidence of hemodynamic deterioration. The patient must be followed according to a strict protocol, and should not be discharged until he shows evidence of no further bleeding from his spleen. (Splenic Trauma/Treatment)

5. Correct: B. The patient is hemodynamically stable, although there is evidence of some early blood loss. Computed tomography scan of the abdomen provides the most useful information for management, including information about the spleen, liver, and kidneys, and potentially other organs, such as the pancreas and bowel. (Splenic Trauma/Treatment)

6. Correct: C. Hemolytic anemia occurs in patients who have glucose-6-phosphate dehydrogenase deficiency when certain drugs (e.g., sulfamethoxazole) cause oxidation injury by intracellular production of hydrogen peroxide. The other mechanisms are not working in this case. (Disorders of Splenic Function/Hemolytic Anemia)

7. Correct: C. The patient shows signs of hemodynamic instability. He has evidence of splenic trauma and needs an immediate operation. (Splenic Trauma/Treatment)

8. Correct: E. This patient had an excellent response to splenectomy. The platelet count is satisfactory. The peripheral smear shows evidence of a complete splenectomy, with no evidence of retained splenic tissue. (Consequences and Complications of Splenectomy/Hematologic Changes)

9. Correct: C. Thrombocytosis usually occurs after splenectomy. The other choices are all recognized complications of splenectomy. (Consequences and Complications of Splenectomy/Hematologic Changes; Immune Consequences; Anatomic Complications After Splenectomy)

10. Correct: D. Platelets that are transfused before splenectomy are rapidly sequestered and destroyed and would not be of value. Likewise, the other therapies are ineffective in this setting. (Thrombocytopenia/Immune Thrombocytopenic Purpura)

11. Correct: B. Sustained resolution of thrombocytopenia occurs in 60% to 80% of patients with medically resistant human immunodeficiency–associated thrombocytopenia. (Thrombocytopenia/HIV-Associated Thrombocytopenia)

12. Correct: D. In children, acute immune thrombocytopenic purpura usually resolves spontaneously without therapy. (Thrombocytopenia/Immune Thrombocytopenic Purpura)

13. Correct: E. Patients who do respond or who have a relapse after splenectomy and do not improve with corticosteroids show some response to therapy with vincristine or gamma globulin. Platelet transfusions are ineffective for long-term maintenance because platelets are rapidly destroyed. (Thrombocytopenia/Immune Thrombocytopenic Purpura)

14. Correct: A. Drug-associated hemolytic anemia is usually Coombs' negative. These patients are treated by discontinuing the offending drug. Coombs'-positive hemolytic anemia, as in this case, is associated with red cells that are coated with immunoglobulin, complement, or both. Corticosteroid therapy should be initiated. Splenectomy is indicated when steroids are ineffective. (Disorders of Splenic Function/Hemolytic Anemia)

15. Correct: B. Patients with thalassemia major have massive splenomegaly and are at risk for rupture secondary to minor trauma. Splenectomy is beneficial in reducing transfusion requirements, physical discomfort from splenomegaly, and the potential for rupture. (Disorders of Splenic Function/Hemolytic Anemia)

16. Correct: E. Thrombocytosis usually occurs after splenectomy. Values are usually within normal limits within a few weeks. Antiplatelet therapy is indicated for otherwise normal patients if the platelet count exceeds 750,000/mm^3. (Consequences and Complications of Splenectomy/Hematologic Changes)

17. Correct: B. Patients who have myeloproliferative disease with platelet counts greater than 400,000/mm^3 are at risk for thrombosis and pulmonary emboli. Platelet inhibitors (e.g., aspirin, dipyridamole) are justified until the platelet count returns to normal. (Consequences and Complications of Splenectomy/Hematologic Changes)

18. Correct: A. The findings of physical examination suggest atelectasis at the left base. Although the other options are associated with atelectasis, it is unusual for it to be clinically apparent so soon after surgery. (Consequences and Complications of Splenectomy/Anatomic Complications After Splenectomy)

19. Correct: C. Patients who have immune thrombocytopenic purpura and an increase in platelet count while receiving steroids have the best chance for long-term response to splenectomy. (Thrombocytopenia/Immune Thrombocytopenic Purpura)

20. Correct: E. Because early stages of Hodgkin's disease involving one or two nodal groups above the diaphragm may be treated with radiation therapy alone, staging laparotomy may be useful to determine the extent of disease in the abdomen. Patients who have disease below the diaphragm or systemic symptoms require systemic chemotherapy. (Hematologic Malignancies)

Chapter 22

1. Correct: B. Venous stasis ulcerations classically occur at the level of the medial and lateral malleoli. The most distal communication between the superficial and deep venous systems (Cockett perforators) occurs in this region. The presence of superficial varicosities further implicates venous valve incompetence and venous hypertension. Diabetic ulcerations usually occur secondary to arterial occlusive disease at the heel or distal foot. Similarly, scleroderma usually involves the distal fingers as well as the toes, but does not usually involve the ankle. Deep vein thrombosis can cause superficial varicosities, but ulcers are

usually secondary to venous hypertension or venous stasis. (Venous Disease/Chronic Venous Insufficiency/Diagnosis)

2. Correct: E. Pulmonary embolism results from the breaking free of a preexisting deep vein thrombus that lodges in a pulmonary arterial branch. Deep vein thrombosis can be precipitated by a hypercoagulable state (e.g., pancreatic cancer), antithrombin III deficiency, or pregnancy. Trauma directly to the vein or prolonged bed rest can precipitate deep vein thrombosis. Because factor XI plays a role in thrombus formation, a deficiency of factor XI would not increase the likelihood of venous thrombosis or pulmonary embolus. (Venous Disease/Pulmonary Embolism/Clinical Presentation)

3. Correct: E. The most effective way to prevent pulmonary embolus is to prevent deep vein thrombosis. Early ambulation has the greatest potential to prevent deep vein thrombosis. If early ambulation is not possible, then the next best prophylactic measures are prophylaxis with subcutaneous heparin twice a day, the use of a segmental compression device, and warfarin. Low–molecular-weight heparin, dextran, aspirin, and dipyridamole (Persantine) have limited ability to prevent deep vein thrombosis. (Venous Disease/Deep Vein Thrombosis/Prophylaxis for Deep Vein Thrombosis)

4. Correct: E. Thrombi within the iliac veins and inferior vena cava are the most common sources for pulmonary embolus. The second most common sources are the common femoral vein and external iliac vein. The more peripheral veins are less likely to cause a significant pulmonary embolus. The thrombus from veins below the level of the popliteal vein are unlikely to cause a pulmonary embolus. (Venous Disease/Pulmonary Embolism)

5. Correct: B. The most common symptom of pulmonary embolus is dyspnea, which is also associated with tachypnea. Leg pain is caused by the inflammatory response and subsequent swelling associated with iliac or femoral deep vein thrombosis. In approximately 25% to 30% of cases, pulmonary embolus may cause hemoptysis. Asymmetric chest wall movement is more consistent with a tension pneumothorax or collapse of one entire lung field. A new cardiac murmur may be related to right-sided heart failure and hemodynamic changes, but is not usually associated with pulmonary embolus. (Venous Disease/Pulmonary Embolism/Clinical Presentation)

6. Correct: C. In patients who have profound diastolic hypertension, normal intravenous urography, and normal to moderately elevated renal function, the differential diagnosis includes renal vascular hypertension. In patients who are older than 50 years of age, the leading cause of renal vascular hypertension is atherosclerosis, but in the younger age group, the leading cause is fibromuscular dysplasia. Medial cystic necrosis can result in the formation of aneurysms, but is unlikely to cause renal artery stenosis. Pheochromocytoma can cause episodic profound systolic and diastolic hypertension. For this reason, it is included in the differential diagnosis of patients with new onset of hypertension. The surgically correctable causes of hypertension include renal vascular hypertension, pheochromocytoma, aldosterone-secreting tumors, and descending thoracic aortic coarctation. (Arterial Disease/ Renal Artery Stenosis)

7. Correct: C. The best treatment for a 45-year-old male smoker with two-block intermittent claudication is cessation of cigarette smoking and initiation of an exercise program of progressive ambulation. With this therapy, 50% of patients can increase their ability to ambulate, and no further intervention is required. If this therapy fails, then further evaluation is indicated. Aortogram with runoff further defines the areas of atherosclerotic occlusive disease. These lesions are treated with either arterial bypass graft or angioplasty. Femoral endarterectomy has little role because of the high recurrence rate for claudication. (Arterial Disease/Peripheral Arterial Occlusive Disease/Clinical Presentation)

8. Correct: A. This patient has the classic signs and symptoms of superficial venous thrombophlebitis, a local inflammation and thrombosis of a superficial vein that is best treated with nonsteroidal anti-inflammatory agents, local warm compresses, and continued ambulation. This condition is not treated in the same way as a deep vein thrombosis, for which therapy includes elevation, anticoagulation, and bed rest. If the thrombosis extends to the level of the saphenous vein, to the femoral vein junction, then saphenous vein ligation is considered to prevent propagation of the thrombus into the deep venous system. (Venous Disease/Physiology)

9. Correct: A. The classic triad for a ruptured abdominal aortic aneurysm includes a pulsatile abdominal aortic mass, back pain, and hypotension. This patient has all three elements of the triad and should be taken emergently to the operating room for surgical exploration and repair. Delay in treatment can lead to further blood loss from the aneurysm. Angiogram has extremely limited usefulness, and evaluation of abdominal aortic aneurysms with angiogram will visualize only the luminal area and not areas occupied by mural thrombus. Computed tomography scan provides the best evaluation of the size and location of the abdominal aortic aneurysm. Unstable patients should not undergo computed tomography scan or angiogram, where access to the patient and treatment is extremely limited. Patients also should not undergo significant fluid resuscitation or administration of blood pressure–elevating agents because of the

potential for increased blood loss from the ruptured abdominal aortic aneurysm. The patient's pressure should be maintained at a level that provides adequate mentation, but the patient should not be overly resuscitated. (Arterial Disease/Aneurysms/Treatment)

10. Correct: D. One of the complications of abdominal aortic aneurysm repair with ligation of the inferior mesenteric artery is left colonic and sigmoid ischemia. In patients who have early return of bowel function, diarrhea, or bloody diarrhea, colonic ischemia is always considered. The best diagnostic tool is sigmoidoscopic visualization of the mucosal surface of the colon. Other causes of diarrhea include potential overgrowth of normal colonic bacteria, which can be related to antibiotic administration. Simply treating the diarrhea with diphenoxylate (Lomotil) is not indicated because it could mask the symptoms of colonic ischemia. Reexploration may be required if peritoneal signs consistent with colonic ischemia or infarction develop. (Arterial Disease/Aneurysms/Complications)

11. Correct: D. There is a strong association between atherosclerosis and smoking, diabetes, and hypertension. These factors may be additive. Patients who have diabetes, who smoke, or who have hypertension are at markedly increased risk for atherosclerosis. Atherosclerosis also has a strong hereditary component. Poor nutrition is not implicated in atherosclerotic disease. (Arterial Disease/Atherosclerosis)

12. Correct: D. Leriche syndrome is associated with aortoiliac arterial occlusion. Its components include muscular atrophy of the buttocks and thigh, impotence, and claudication. It is unlikely to be associated with embolization to the toes. Partially obstructing irregular plaques usually cause toe embolization of atherosclerotic or hematologic material from the ulcer or lesion. Emboli can originate from cardiac mural thrombus or from the mural thrombus of an aneurysm. (Arterial Disease/Peripheral Artery Occlusive Disease/Clinical Presentation)

13. Correct: C. The classic syndrome of chronic mesenteric ischemia includes postprandial pain, weight loss, food fear because of postprandial pain, and an abdominal bruit on physical examination. Diarrhea is associated with colonic ischemia, but is less common in small bowel chronic ischemia. (Arterial Disease/Chronic Intestinal Ischemia/Clinical Presentation)

14. Correct: A. Transient ischemic attacks are usually caused by atherosclerotic or hematologic emboli from a stenotic lesion in the carotid bifurcation or proximal internal carotid artery. The intestinal carotid artery supplies the middle cerebral artery and then the anterior cerebral artery. The posterior cerebral artery is perfused by the basilar and vertebral arteries, which are separate vessels that originate at the aortic arch. (Arterial Disease/Cerebrovascular Insufficiency/Clinical Presentation and Evaluation)

15. Correct: D. Subclavian steal syndrome is associated with occlusion of the subclavian artery proximal to the origin of the vertebral artery. It causes low flow in the distal subclavian artery, with a subsequent low-pressure region. Flow is reversed within the vertebral artery from the basilar artery that goes to the lower-resistance subclavian artery. This reversal essentially steals blood from the posterior circulation to supplement blood flow to the extremity. Occlusion of the carotid or vertebral system does not affect flow in the subclavian artery or the subclavian steal syndrome. (Arterial Disease/Vertebral Basilar Disease)

16. Correct: B. The main advantage of below-the-knee amputation is that significantly less effort is required to walk with a below-the-knee prosthesis than with an above-the-knee prosthesis. Below-the-knee amputation causes more wound complications than above-the-knee amputation because of the potential for atherosclerotic occlusion at the level of the popliteal artery and the potential for more distal ischemia. Below-the-knee amputation is technically more challenging because of previous operative incisions and the need to create a posterior flap to help cover the anteriorly positioned tibia. (Arterial Disease/Peripheral Arterial Occlusive Disease/Treatment/Surgical/Amputation)

17. Correct: B. Surgically correctable causes of hypertension include renal vascular hypertension, descending thoracic aortic coarctation, pheochromocytoma, and aldosterone-secreting tumors. Abdominal aortic aneurysms can occur because of hypertension, but do not precipitate hypertension. Zollinger-Ellison syndrome can cause refractory gastrointestinal ulcerations and bleeding, but does not cause hypertension, hypernephromas, or acute tubular necrosis of the kidney. (Arterial Disease/Renal Artery Stenosis)

18. Correct: B. In patients who have the triad of postprandial pain, weight loss, and abdominal bruit, the most probable diagnosis is chronic mesenteric ischemia. Occult colonic carcinoma cannot be ruled out, however, especially with a history of guaiac-positive stools. Postprandial pain and abdominal bruit are not associated with colon carcinoma, malabsorption syndromes, or peptic ulcer disease. Gastrointestinal arteriovenous fistula can cause abdominal bruit and blood in the stools, but is unlikely to cause weight loss or postprandial pain. (Arterial Disease/Chronic Intestinal Ischemia/Clinical Presentation)

19. Correct: D. The "six Ps" of arterial insufficiency are pulselessness, pain, paresthesia, paralysis, pallor, and poikilothermia (change in temperature). (Arterial

Disease/Acute Arterial Occlusion/Clinical Presentation and Evaluation)

20. Correct: E. The chance of cell survival is a factor of both the pressure and the duration of the elevated compartment pressure. Preexisting hypoxia and chronic ischemia can help to prevent cell death through conversion to a more anaerobic environment. Patient age has little effect on the potential for cell survival in association with compartment syndrome. (Arterial Disease/Acute Arterial Occlusion/Treatment)

Chapter 23

1. Correct: E. All of the organs, except the heart, may be obtained from a living relative. Pancreas and liver are taken as segments. Lung is taken as a lobe. (Organ and Tissue Donation)

2. Correct: B. The absence of spontaneous respiration indicates loss of brain stem function, which is a terminal event. Deep tendon reflexes are spinal reflexes and do not indicate brain injury. Severe head injury may leave a patient without brain function and decerebrate and decorticate responses that indicate persistent brain function. (Organ and Tissue Donation/Table 23–1)

3. Correct: D. A standard dose of dopamine has minimal vasoconstrictive effects and some beneficial effect on renal perfusion. The others have significant vasoconstrictive effects. (Organ and Tissue Donation)

4. Correct: D. The 1-year graft survival rate for cardiac, liver, and cadaver kidney transplants is 75% to 85%. (Heart, Heart–Lung, and Lung Transplantation/Heart Transplantation)

5. Correct: B. An allograft is a graft between genetically dissimilar individuals of the same species. Autografts, isografts, and xenografts are grafts from the self, from genetically identical members of the same species, and from other species, respectively. An orthotopic graft is one that is placed in the normal anatomic position. (Immunology)

6. Correct: C. All of the tests except mixed lymphocyte culture (MLC) can be performed within 4 to 8 hours and affect the final results of the allograft. Because MLC takes 3 to 5 days to perform, it is not useful for cadaver transplants, which must be performed in less than 72 hours. (Immunology)

7. Correct: E. Hyperacute rejection that occurs minutes to hours after transplantation is mediated by anti-ABO or anti–human leukocyte antigen antibodies. It is untreatable with either high doses of cyclosporine or pretreatment with steroids. (Immunology/Immunologic Events After Transplantation)

8. Correct: D. Even with perfectly matched renal transplants between siblings, immunosuppression is used. Cyclophosphamide and antilymphocyte globulin are not the first-line drugs used to prevent rejection. Cyclosporine can be used in normal doses. (Immunology/Immunosuppressive Drug Therapy)

9. Correct: D. Cyclosporine inhibits the production of interleukin-2 in T-lymphocytes. It is not associated with cataracts and does not have a significant effect on cellular infiltrates on biopsy. In combination with other drugs, it allows steroid doses to be lowered without affecting graft survival. (Immunology/Immunosuppressive Drug Therapy/Pharmacologic Agents)

10. Correct: C. Heart transplants are usually orthotopic (normal position) allografts (from a member of the same species). (Heart, Heart–Lung, and Lung Transplantation/Heart Transplantation/Procedure)

11. Correct: D. Long-term results with hepatocellular carcinoma are not as good as those with the other diseases. (Liver Transplantation/Table 23–7)

12. Correct: E. Transposition of the great vessels is a surgically correctable condition. The rest of the conditions, at end stage, are not correctable. (Heart, Heart–Lung, and Lung Transplantation/Heart Transplantation/Indications)

13. Correct: C. Type II diabetes mellitus is treated medically. Whole pancreas transplants are rejected at least as often as other organ transplants. Approximately 75% survive for at least 1 year despite an increased incidence of perioperative complications. With islet transplants, the rate of insulin independence is only 20% at 1 year. (Pancreas/Islet Transplantation/Whole Organ Transplantation/Complications)

14. Correct: C. An increased incidence of viral infection and cancer, including lymphomatoid skin carcinoma, is associated with immunosuppression. Although elevated cholesterol levels are reported with cyclosporine, the incidence of atherosclerosis does not appear to be increased. The atherosclerosis that occurs with cardiac transplants is more likely to be related to rejection than to the immunosuppressive drugs. (Immunology/Immunosuppressive Drug Therapy)

15. Correct: D. Prolonged warm ischemia is likely to result in a nonfunctioning organ. The other conditions would not prevent liver donation. (Organ and Tissue Donation)

16. Correct: A. Because the cornea is a privileged site, no immunosuppression is necessary for corneal transplant. All of the other types of transplant require

lifelong immunosuppression. (Immunology/Immunosuppressive Drug Therapy/Pharmacologic Agents)

17. Correct: B. Livers are usually transplanted within 18 hours after procurement. (Organ and Tissue Donation/Organ Preservation)

18. Correct: D. Lung transplantation is not indicated in patients who have cancer that has a high propensity to recur. The other diseases are indications for pulmonary transplantation. (Heart, Heart–Lung, and Lung Transplantation)

19. Correct: A. Leukopenia is a complication associated with azathioprine, an antimetabolite. Prednisone may cause leukocytosis, and cyclosporine and FK-506 have no effect on white blood cell count. OKT3 may affect lymphocyte count. (Immunology/Immunosuppressive Drug Therapy/Pharmacologic Agents)

20. Correct: C. Cyclosporine is associated with these complications. The rest of the immunosuppressive agents are not. (Immunology/Immunosuppressive Drug Therapy/Pharmacologic Agents)

Chapter 24
Malignant Diseases of the Skin

1. Correct: C. Skin pigmentation is determined by phagocytosis of the melanosome–pigment package by keratinocytes, which then migrate to the epidermis. (Melanoma/Embryology of Melanocytes)

2. Correct: B. The incidence of melanoma is increased in sun-exposed areas, such as the head and neck for men and women and the legs for women. (Melanoma/Incidence and Etiology)

3. Correct: D. Superficial spreading melanoma accounts for 70%, lentigo maligna melanoma for 10% to 15%, nodular melanoma for 12%, and acral lentiginous and ocular melanoma for the remainder. (Melanoma/Clinical and Histopathologic Characteristics)

4. Correct: A. The prognosis for acral lentiginous melanoma is intermediate between superficial spreading melanoma and nodular melanoma. (Melanoma/Clinical and Histopathologic Characteristics)

5. Correct: C. Clark's staging of primary melanoma is based on the layer of the epidermis, dermis, or subcutaneous tissue that is involved with tumor cells. (Melanoma/Staging)

6. Correct: B. Clark divided microstaging into five categories. In level II, melanoma invades the papillary dermis. (Melanoma/Staging)

7. Correct: C. Breslow modified Clark's microstaging system by improving objectivity through the use of an ocular micrometer to determine tumor thickness. (Melanoma/Staging)

8. Correct: D. Sun exposure is associated with an increased incidence of melanoma. The most highly exposed area (and therefore the area with the highest incidence of melanoma) is the head and neck. (Melanoma/Incidence and Etiology)

9. Correct: A. The thinner the primary lesion, the better the prognosis. Metastases are rare, but they can occur, even with thin melanomas. (Melanoma/Prognosis)

10. Correct: C. Only this group contains all lesions that have some likelihood of being pigmented and therefore of being confused with melanomas. (Melanoma/Diagnosis)

11. Correct: E. Incisional biopsy is rarely indicated because most lesions are small enough to be easily excised without compromising treatment. Local anesthesia is standard. The biopsy specimen obtained during the rarely indicated incisional biopsy should include the thickest portion of the lesion because of the effect of thickness on risk. (Melanoma/Diagnosis)

12. Correct: A. Randomized trials are underway to establish wide local excision (local excision with a 2-cm margin) as the standard of care. (Melanoma/Treatment)

13. Correct: C. A patient who has clinical stage III disease (positive regional nodes) should undergo treatment of the primary tumor and regional nodes. The regional lymph nodes should undergo surgical excision, not biopsy. (Melanoma/Treatment)

14. Correct: A. A thin melanoma in a patient with no palpable lymph nodes is treated with local excision of the tumor with a 2-cm margin (wide local excision). (Melanoma/Treatment)

15. Correct: B. Chemotherapy for melanoma is still toxic and has a low yield. With the best regimen (dacarbazine), the response rate is only 20%. (Melanoma/Treatment)

16. Correct: B. One-third of new cancers are skin cancers, and 80% of these are basal cell cancers. Each year, 800,000 new cases of nonmelanoma skin cancer are diagnosed. (Basal Cell and Squamous Cell Carcinoma/Incidence and Etiology)

17. Correct: B. Exposure to sunlight is the most important risk factor for skin cancer. (Basal Cell and Squamous Cell Carcinoma/Incidence and Etiology)

18. Correct: C. Radium implants would result in long-term radiation of the skin and would cause much

damage even as they eradicate the skin cancer. The other four treatments are very successful. (Basal Cell Carcinoma/Treatment)

19. Correct: D. As with melanoma, the area that is most often and most intensely exposed to sunlight has the highest incidence of squamous cell carcinoma. (Squamous Cell Carcinoma/Clinical and Histopathologic Characteristics)

20. Correct: A. Pearly, raised margins are characteristic of basal cell carcinoma. The other choices are typical of squamous cell carcinoma. (Squamous Cell Carcinoma/Clinical and Histopathologic Characteristics)

Malignant Diseases of the Lymphatics and Soft Tissue

21. Correct: A. The lymphocyte-predominant group has the best prognosis, followed by nodular sclerosis. The lymphocyte-depleted group has the worst prognosis. (Hodgkin's Disease/Prognosis)

22. Correct: B. Stage II Hodgkin's disease involves two or more lymph node regions on the same side of the diaphragm or an extralymphatic organ or site. (Table 24–5)

23. Correct: C. Stage III Hodgkin's disease involves lymph node regions on both sides of the diaphragm or an extralymphatic organ or site, the spleen, or both an extralymphatic site and the spleen. (Table 24–5)

24. Correct: D. Staging laparotomy involves splenectomy and biopsy of the splenic hilar, celiac, porta hepatis, mesenteric, paraaortic, and iliac nodes, as well as liver biopsy. The omentum is not included. Staging laparotomy is used for Hodgkin's disease, but not for non-Hodgkin's lymphoma. (Hodgkin's Disease/Clinical Presentation and Evaluation)

25. Correct: D. Diagnosis requires removal of the entire abnormal, enlarged node. Biopsy is performed on cervical nodes rather than inguinal or axillary nodes, which are more likely to show reactive changes. (Hodgkin's Disease/Clinical Presentation and Evaluation)

26. Correct: A. Radiation therapy is used for limited-stage Hodgkin's disease. Chemotherapy, with or without radiation therapy, is recommended for advanced (stages III and IV) disease. (Hodgkin's Disease/Clinical Presentation and Evaluation)

27. Correct: C. The incidence of Hodgkin's disease is bimodal, with peaks in young adulthood and again in the older years (mid-70s). (Hodgkin's Disease/Incidence and Etiology)

28. Correct: A. Cervical adenopathy is the most common sign of this malignancy (60%–80%). (Hodgkin's Disease/Incidence and Etiology)

29. Correct: D. Stage IIB includes involvement of two or more lymph node regions on the same side of the diaphragm, with fever and night sweats. (Table 24–5)

30. Correct: B. Nodular sclerosis occurs in 50% of cases. The next most common type is mixed cellularity (37%). (Table 24–4)

31. Correct: C. Sarcomas are a group of malignant tumors derived from the mesoderm. (Soft Tissue Sarcomas)

32. Correct: B. Sarcomas are relatively uncommon. They account for approximately 1% of all malignant tumors in adults. (Soft Tissue Sarcomas)

33. Correct: C. Sarcomas are more common in children (6%) than in adults (1%). Sarcomas usually cause a painless mass and metastasize to the lung and liver. (Soft Tissue Sarcomas/Incidence and Etiology)

34. Correct: E. The lower extremity is the most common site for sarcomas (37%). (Soft Tissue Sarcomas)

35. Correct: D. This system considers tumor size, depth, and grade. It characterizes high-grade sarcomas as unfavorable because they are likely to metastasize. (Table 24–11)

36. Correct: A. (Soft Tissue Sarcomas/Incidence and Etiology)

37. Correct: B. (Soft Tissue Sarcomas/Incidence and Etiology)

38. Correct: C. (Soft Tissue Sarcomas/Incidence and Etiology)

39. Correct: D. (Soft Tissue Sarcomas/Incidence and Etiology)

40. Correct: E. (Kaposi's Sarcoma)

Chapter 25

1. Correct: B. Informed consent is required from a patient or surrogate (e.g., family member). If a patient is intoxicated and no surrogate is available, the procedure is postponed. Only an emergency procedure can be undertaken without consent in this situation. (Informed Consent/Questionable Competency)

2. Correct: C. Living wills allow patient choice to extend into a time when the patient is incompetent. In this way, paternalism is restricted. A living will takes effect only when a patient is not competent to make decisions. It can be changed or rescinded whenever

a patient wishes. (Advance Directives and Do-Not-Resuscitate Orders)

3. Correct: A. A durable power of attorney for health care document names a surrogate to make decisions if a patient is not competent to do so. The surrogate can then make any choices that the competent patient could have made. A disagreement cannot arise between a competent patient and the surrogate because the durable power of attorney has no effect when the patient is competent. (Advance Directives and Do-Not-Resuscitate Orders/Conflicts Between the Wishes of Surrogate and Patient)

4. Correct: D. Do-not-resuscitate (DNR) orders simply limit cardiopulmonary resuscitation. They are not restricted by the patient's diagnosis or competency (as long as a surrogate is involved if the patient is incompetent). However, a DNR order should not be written against a competent patient's wishes. (Advance Directives and Do-Not-Resuscitate Orders/Surgery Consultations for a Patient with a DNR Order)

5. Correct: E. Because a do-not-resuscitate (DNR) order can apply in many situations, it cannot be assumed to have any meaning beyond refusal of cardiopulmonary resuscitation without a careful assessment of the situation. (Advance Directives and Do-Not-Resuscitate Orders/Surgery Consultations for a Patient with a DNR Order)

6. Correct: B. Do-not-resuscitate (DNR) orders in the operating room and during the perioperative period can pose a problem because of the difficulty involved in distinguishing between resuscitation and standard intraoperative care of patients receiving general anesthetics. An individual approach that includes consultation with the patient (or surrogate), surgeon, and anesthesiologist is necessary to clarify definitions and discuss limitations of treatment before surgery. (Advance Directives and Do-Not-Resuscitate Orders)

7. Correct: C. Informed consent allows patients to participate in their own care by making decisions about their treatment. Patients must have the opportunity to be informed when making these choices, but there is no minimum information that must be provided if the patient prefers not to hear it. (Informed Consent/Patients Who Refuse to Hear the Risks of a Procedure)

8. Correct: C. Competent patients may refuse any procedure, even a life-sustaining one. Before a patient's refusal is accepted, however, confirmation that the patient is competent to make decisions should be sought through a psychiatrist's consultation and evaluation. Neither a surgery department chairman nor a hospital attorney can override a competent patient's choice. (Informed Consent/Patients Who Refuse Life-Sustaining Treatment)

9. Correct: D. Futility is a difficult concept to define because it involves weighing the benefits and burdens of treatment. Therefore, it depends on the patient's values. Physicians should not discuss futility as though it were a clear, precise term. (End-of-Life Care/Surrogated Who Request a "Futile" Procedure)

10. Correct: A. Withholding information about a lethal condition or a poor prognosis should never be encouraged. In facing impending death, patients and family members are best served by open communication that allows full use of support systems and allows appropriate grieving to occur. (Physician–Patient Communication/Families Who Request That the Patient Not Be Told of the Diagnosis)

Glossary

abrasion – wound that has superficial loss of epithelial elements; dermis and deeper structures remain intact.

absorbable sutures – surgical suture material prepared from a substance that is digested by body tissues and therefore is not permanent; available in various diameters and tensile strengths; can be treated to modify its resistance to absorption; can be impregnated with antimicrobial agents.

achalasia – esophageal motility disorder characterized by failure of the circular esophageal muscle in the distal 2 cm of the esophagus to relax.

acidemia – elevation of blood hydrogen ion.

acidosis – primary increase in Pco_2 or primary decrease in HCO_3.

acral lentiginous melanoma – malignant melanoma that occurs in areas with no hair follicles (e.g., palms, nail beds, soles of feet).

activated partial thromboplastin time (APTT) – clotting test used to detect deficiencies in the intrinsic coagulation pathway; a prolonged APTT indicates deficiencies in factor I, II, V, VIII, IX, X, XI, or XII.

adenoma – mucosal tumor of the small and large intestine; tubular, villous, and mixed cell types are seen.

adenoma, hepatic – benign tumor that consists of unencapsulated sheets of hepatocytes without ductular elements; apparently hormonally responsive; risk of spontaneous rupture.

adenoma, parathyroid – benign tumor of a parathyroid gland.

adenoma, toxic – solitary autonomous hyperactive thyroid nodule.

adenoma, villous – polyp characterized by sessile morphology; relatively high incidence of malignant degeneration.

adhesion – fibrous tissue that often occurs after abdominal surgery; can lead to bowel obstruction.

adhesion, platelet – sticking of platelets to surfaces other than another platelet; collagen is the common in vivo surface to which platelets adhere.

adrenal incidentaloma – incidentally discovered adrenal mass that is not associated with any symptoms that overtly suggest adrenal abnormality.

adrenal insufficiency (Addisonian crisis) – result of inadequate circulating glucocorticoids; common signs and symptoms are postural hypotension, dizziness, nausea, vomiting, abdominal pain, weakness, fatigability, hyperkalemia, and hyponatremia; if not treated promptly, causes complete cardiovascular collapse and death.

adrenal scintigraphy – use of a radiolabeled isotope of cholesterol [^{131}I-6b-iodomethyl-norcholesterol (NP-59)] to image the adrenal glands with a method that directly correlates the normal function of the gland with its scanned image; the scanned image is correlated with the anatomic computed tomography image to gain a better understanding of the etiology of the mass.

adrenocorticotropic hormone (ACTH) stimulation test – administration of synthetic ACTH to stimulate the secretion of cortisol and evaluate the adequacy of adrenal reserve and the integrity of the hypothalamic-pituitary-adrenal axis.

advance directive – a mentally capable patient's instructions regarding his or her medical care if he or she becomes incapacitated and unable to make decisions.

afterload – resistance to ventricular ejection; may be increased by obstruction (i.e., aortic stenosis) or vascular constriction (i.e., increased systemic vascular resistance).

aggregation, platelet – platelet-to-platelet sticking; a white clot is formed that is composed almost exclusively of platelets.

airway – in trauma management and basic cardiac life support, the process of maintaining patency of the upper airway, specifically the mouth, oropharynx, larynx, and trachea.

airway compromise – airway obstruction; loss of airway patency from any cause.

airway, nasopharyngeal (nasal) – device, usually made of rubber, designed to prevent the tongue from obstructing the nasopharynx; placed through a nostril into the nasopharynx (see Figure 9-4D); well tolerated in the patient with an intact gag reflex.

airway, oropharyngeal (oral) – device, usually made of plastic, designed to prevent the tongue from obstructing the oropharynx; placed through the mouth and over the tongue (see Figures 9-4E and 9-5); should not be used in a conscious patient with an intact gag reflex because it can cause gagging, vomiting, and aspiration.

aldosterone – hormone produced by the zona glomerulosa in the adrenal gland; secreted as part of the renin–angiotensin system in response to decreased blood flow in the kidneys; causes sodium retention and potassium and hydrogen loss in the distal tubule.

alkalemia – depression of blood hydrogen ion.

alkalosis – primary decrease in Pco_2 or primary increase in HCO_3.

allograft (homograft) – tissue transferred between genetically dissimilar members of the same species (e.g., most human transplants).

alpha$_1$-antitrypsin deficiency – inherited autosomal dominant disorder that causes varying degrees of liver and lung injury over a patient's lifetime; some patients have predominantly pulmonary dysfunction; others have liver disease that leads to cirrhosis and the need for liver transplantation.

amaurosis fugax – transient monocular blindness as a result of emboli to the ipsilateral ophthalmic artery; classically described as a curtain of blindness being pulled down from the superior to the inferior aspect of the affected eye.

AMPLE history – mnemonic for taking a quick history: Allergies, Medications, Past illnesses, Last meal, and the Events surrounding the injury are noted.

anal fissure – painful linear tear in the lining of the anal canal below the dentate line.

aneuploid – having an abnormal number of chromosomes, not an exact multiple of the haploid number, in contrast to having abnormal numbers of complete haploid sets of chromosomes (e.g., diploid, triploid); prognostic factor used to estimate the risk of recurrence of breast cancer; ploidy is measured with flow cytometry, which permits analysis of DNA content per cell and allows determination of ploidy levels within a tumor cell population; diploid indicates a good prognosis; aneuploid indicates a poorer prognosis.

aneurysm – dilation of an artery to greater than 1.5 to 2 times its normal size; may be saccular (sac-like bulging on one side of the artery) or fusiform (elongated, spindle-shaped diffuse dilation of the arterial wall).

angioplasty – reconstruction of a blood vessel, either surgically or by balloon dilation; surgical angioplasty entails reconstruction of the artery, usually with a patch; balloon angioplasty involves percutaneous placement of an intraarterial balloon; the balloon is then inflated, thereby disrupting the arterial plaque as well as a portion of the media and consequently enlarging the artery.

ankle–brachial index – comparison of the systolic blood pressure at the level of the ankle divided by the brachial arterial pressure; this ratio provides an assessment of the degree of lower extremity arterial occlusive disease, with the brachial arterial pressure used as a control.

annular pancreas – ring of pancreas encircling the duodenum; caused by a failure of the embryonic primordia to unite completely; each portion has its own duct.

antibiotic resistance – resistance to a previously effective antibiotic by a microbial pathogen through changes in its DNA structure.

antidiuretic hormone (vasopressin) – hormone produced by the supraoptic and paraventricular nuclei of the hypothalamus; secreted in response to increased osmotic pressure and decreased effective plasma volume; also released in response to stress; regulates water balance by stimulating resorption in the distal renal tubule.

antisepsis – prevention of infection by inhibiting the growth of infectious agents.

antrectomy – distal gastric resection that removes the gastrin-producing cells of the stomach.

aponeurosis – flat tendon; broad, fibrous sheet of tendinous fibers that provides attachment to broad muscles (e.g., oblique muscles of the abdominal wall).

appendicitis – inflammation of the appendix.

asepsis – absence of living pathogenic organisms; state of sterility.

asplenism – complete loss of splenic function.

atherosclerosis – degenerative change of the arterial wall; characterized by endothelial dysfunction, inflammatory cell adhesion, and infiltration and accumulation of cellular and acellular elements within the arterial wall; lipid deposition is associated with fibrosis and calcification and can lead to severe arterial occlusive disease.

autograft – graft (e.g., skin) that consists of the patient's own tissue.

autologous bone marrow transplant – technique that allows harvest of a patient's bone marrow cells before the administration of very high-dose chemotherapy; after chemotherapy, the cells are transplanted back into the patient; currently recommended for patients with 10 positive lymph nodes; used investigationally for patients with metastatic disease; large prospective trials do not substantiate a survival benefit in these two settings.

AVPU – mnemonic for quickly assessing the level of consciousness in a patient with traumatic injury: is the patient Alert, responsive to Vocal stimuli, responsive to Painful stimuli, or Unresponsive?

avulsion – tearing away or forcible separation of tissue; may be partial or total.

B-cells – immunocytes derived from bone marrow stem cells; commonly, B-cells produce circulating antibodies and are responsible for the humoral response to foreign tissues.

bacteremia – presence of viable bacteria in the blood.

Ballance's sign – percussion dullness of the left flank; occurs with a ruptured spleen.

Barrett's esophagus – presence of columnar epithelium in the esophagus; results from a metaplastic change caused by repeated inflammation of normal squamous epithelium; small, but significant tendency toward the development of cancer.

basal cell carcinoma – carcinoma of the skin that arises from the basal cells of the epidermis or hair follicles.

basal cell carcinoma, morphea-like – tumor with an indurated, yellow plaque with ill-defined borders; overlying skin remains intact for a long period; less common than nodular basal cell carcinoma.

basal cell carcinoma, nodular – most common variant of basal cell carcinoma; characterized by a central depression and a rolled border; usually located on the head and neck.

basal cell carcinoma, pigmented – similar to nodular basal cell carcinoma, except that tumors contain melanocytes; may be confused with melanoma.

Beck's triad – three classic clinical signs of cardiac tamponade: (1) muffled (distant) heart sounds, (2) elevated central venous pressure (jugular venous distension), and (3) hypotension.

bezoar – accumulation of a large mass of undigested material in the stomach.

biliary colic – episodic epigastric or right upper quadrant abdominal pain; associated with nausea and vomiting; secondary to transient cystic duct obstruction with a gallstone; tends to occur postprandially; usually lasts 1 to 4 hours.

Billroth I procedure – gastrointestinal reconstruction that creates an anastomosis between the distal end of the stomach and the duodenum (gastroduodenostomy).

Billroth II procedure – gastrointestinal reconstruction that creates an anastomosis between the stomach and a loop of jejunum (gastrojejunostomy).

bleeding disorder, acquired – hemostatic defect caused by a nongenetic factor (e.g., liver disease, anticoagulation therapy); more common than congenital bleeding disorders.

bleeding disorder, congenital – inherited hemostatic defect (e.g., hemophilia, von Willebrand's disease); fairly uncommon.

bleeding history – important part of the presurgical evaluation; a personal or familial bleeding problem is the most important predictive factor of operative and perioperative bleeding complications.

bleeding time test – interval between the appearance of the first drop of blood and the removal of the last drop after incision of the forearm or puncture of the ear lobe or finger; bleeding time is prolonged in cases of thrombocytopenia, diminished prothrombin, abnormal platelet function, phosphorus or chloroform poisoning, and in some liver diseases; it is normal in hemophilia.

blood cell, red (erythrocyte) – cellular portion of the blood that contains hemoglobin; responsible for carrying oxygen to the tissues.

blood cell, white (leukocyte) – cellular portion of the blood that does not contain hemoglobin; classified as granular (i.e., neutrophils, eosinophils, basophils) and nongranular.

Boerhaave's syndrome – full-thickness rupture of the esophagus (in contrast, Mallory-Weiss syndrome is a bleeding mucosal rupture at the same site); associated with loss of gastroesophageal contents (typically into the left side of the chest) and acute sepsis; may cause a syndrome similar to myocardial infarction.

Bowen's disease – skin condition characterized by chronic scaling and occasionally a crusted, purple, or erythematous raised lesion; may become invasive squamous cell carcinoma.

brain death – irreversible cessation of all brain function.

BRCA-1 gene – BRCA-1 and BRCA-2 are the two major genes responsible for the inherited predisposition to breast cancer; BRCA-1 is also related to ovarian cancer; in patients who have mutations in either gene, the risk of breast cancer is approximately 80% by age 70; in contrast, the lifetime risk is approximately 12% in the general population.

Breslow system – system for microstaging malignant melanomas based on the thickness of the tumor in millimeters; survival is related to tumor thickness.

bruit – auscultatory sound over an artery; produced by turbulent flow.

burn center – specialized care unit with facilities, personnel, and resources devoted to the care of patients with serious burn injuries.

burn, epidermal – first-degree burn injury that involves only the epidermal layer of the skin; does not blister; has relatively minor physiologic effects; heals without scarring.

burn, first-degree – see *burn, epidermal*.

burn, full-thickness – third-degree burn injury that involves the entire epidermis and dermis; usually requires skin grafting.

burn, partial-thickness – second-degree burn injury that involves some, but not all, of the dermis; variable in appearance, but because epidermal appendages are intact, heals if followed long enough; deep partial-thickness burns are usually treated with skin grafting.

burn, second-degree – see *burn, partial-thickness*.

burn, third-degree – see *burn, full-thickness*.

carcinoembryonic antigen – antigen produced by many gastrointestinal tumors; measured in the blood; used in surveillance for cancer recurrence.

carcinoid syndrome – carcinoid tumor that causes a syndrome of signs and symptoms that include cutaneous flushing, diarrhea, bronchospasm, skin lesions, and vasomotor instability.

cardiac output – quantity of blood pumped by the heart into the pulmonary and systemic circulation each minute.

cardiac tamponade – compression of the heart from accumulation of fluid or blood within the pericardial sac; ventricular filling is restricted; the increased pressure within the pericardial sac is transmitted to each cardiac chamber; results in equalization of the right atrial, right ventricular diastolic, pulmonary artery diastolic, pulmonary capillary wedge, left atrial, left ventricular diastolic, and intrapericardial pressures.

cardiogenic state – decreased cardiac output from inadequate function of the heart itself, rather than deficiencies in venous return.

cerebral blood flow – cerebral perfusion pressure divided by cerebrovascular resistance.

cerebrovascular accident (stroke) – region of cerebral infarction secondary to arterial atheroembolism or hypoperfusion.

Charcot's triad – triad of clinical findings that includes right upper quadrant abdominal pain, fever and chills, and jaundice; associated with cholangitis.

Child's classification – series of five parameters (serum bilirubin, serum albumin, presence of ascites, encephalopathy, and nutrition) used to grade the status of liver disease.

chin-lift maneuver – maneuver used to open the mouth so that the oral cavity can be inspected and patency assured; accomplished by placing the fingers of the left hand under the chin while the thumb is placed anteriorly below the lips; the chin is grasped and lifted forward and downward; the mouth is opened for inspection; a more secure grip on the jaw is accomplished by placing the thumb inside the mouth and behind the lower incisors.

cholangiocarcinoma – adenocarcinoma that has two types: infiltrating bile duct tumor that usually arises at the level of the bile duct bifurcation and, less commonly, solid intraparenchymal tumor within the substance of the liver.

cholangiogram – radiographic image of the bile ducts; obtained by injecting contrast material through a needle or catheter.

cholangiogram, percutaneous transhepatic – radiologic imaging of the biliary tree; obtained by inserting a needle through the abdominal wall into the liver parenchyma and injecting contrast material directly into the intrahepatic bile ducts; used to extract stones, obtain a cytology specimen, or place a catheter.

cholangitis, acute – acute infection of the bile ducts; caused by a stone, stricture, or neoplasm.

cholangitis, acute suppurative – acute infection of the bile ducts; complicated by the finding of pus; requires urgent drainage.

cholecystectomy, laparoscopic – removal of the gallbladder with a laparoscopic approach; preferred approach for most elective and many emergency situations.

cholecystitis, acute – acute infection of the gallbladder; usually caused by calculus obstructing the cystic duct.

cholecystitis, acute acalculous – acute infection of the gallbladder without underlying gallstone disease; usually occurs in patients who are being treated in intensive care units for other medical problems.

cholecystitis, acute emphysematous – acute infection of the gallbladder; caused by gas-forming bacteria; characterized by air in the wall or lumen of the gallbladder or in the bile ducts; often associated with diabetes mellitus; requires emergency cholecystectomy.

cholecystitis, acute gangrenous – acute infection of the gallbladder that progresses to gangrene; requires emergency cholecystectomy.

choledocholithiasis – presence of a stone or stones in the common bile duct; stones usually originate in the gallbladder and pass through the cystic duct into the common bile duct.

circulating nurse – usually a registered nurse; a member of the operating room team who does not directly participate in the surgical procedure, but manages activities outside the sterile field; duties include opening sterile supplies, counting sponges, making and answering calls, delivering specimens, maintaining records, and other vital tasks.

Clark system – system for microstaging malignant melanomas based on the anatomic level (I through V) of invasion of the tumor; survival is related to the depth of invasion.

claudication – reproducible pain that occurs in a major muscle group; precipitated by exercise and relieved by rest; classically, pain occurs in the posterior calves after mild to moderate exercise.

closed-gloving technique – method of donning surgical gloves in which the hands are not pushed fully through the cuffs of the surgical gown; usually practiced by surgical technicians as a self-gloving technique.

coagulation factor – substance in the blood that is necessary for clotting; numbered with Roman numerals.

coagulation pathway, common – final steps that lead to the generation of a clot; includes factors I (fibrinogen), II (prothrombin), V, and X; the end-product is fibrin.

coagulation pathway, extrinsic – part of the first stage of coagulation; requires the interaction of factor VII with tissue thromboplastin to convert factor X to factor X^a.

coagulation pathway, intrinsic – part of the first stage of coagulation; initiated by the interaction of factor XII with negatively charged surfaces; other coagulation factors in this pathway are factors VIII, IX, and XI; the eventual product converts factor X to factor X^a.

collagen – principal structural protein of the body; its production, remodeling, and maturation define the second and third stages of wound healing.

colloid – fluid for intravenous administration; consists of water, electrolytes, and protein or other molecules that are of sufficient molecular weight to exert a colloid oncotic pressure effect similar to that of endogenous albumin; packed red cells are often considered colloid, but do not meet this definition.

colonoscopy – flexible diagnostic instrument that uses light-transmitting fiberoptics; allows visualization of the entire colon and terminal ileum.

colostomy – surgical procedure in which the colon is divided and the proximal end is brought through a surgically created defect in the abdominal wall and sewn to the skin.

compartment syndrome – elevation of the pressure within a fascial compartment of the upper or lower extremity; interstitial tissue pressure becomes higher than capillary perfusion pressure, resulting in ischemia to the muscles and nerves within the fascial compartment.

competency – ability to use mental capacities to understand one's condition and the consequences of choices.

complement – system of 20 or more proteins present in the serum; when activated, these proteins stimulate lymphocytes, macrophages, and reticuloendothelial cells as part of the host defense against bacterial pathogens.

contractility – the force of cardiac muscle contraction under conditions of a predetermined preload or afterload.

contusion – soft tissue swelling and hemorrhage without violation of the skin elements.

contusion, myocardial – blunt cardiac injury associated with deceleration or crush injury to the anterior chest; associated with sternal or rib fractures; the anterior myocardium (right ventricle) is primarily involved; when severe, may lead to right-sided heart failure; difficult to diagnose by electrocardiogram because the weaker right ventricular electrical activity is overshadowed by the stronger left ventricular electrical activity.

contusion, pulmonary – injury to the lung parenchyma that causes interstitial hemorrhage, alveolar collapse, and extravasation of blood and plasma into the alveoli; causes a ventilation–perfusion mismatch that results in hypoxemia; physical examination may show blunt or penetrating injury to the chest; radiographic studies show a poorly defined infiltrate that develops over time.

Cooper's ligament – strong fibrous insertion of transversus abdominus muscle on the pectineal line of the pelvis.

Courvoisier's law – obstruction of the common bile duct by carcinoma of the pancreas or other malignancies of the distal common bile duct may lead to an enlarged palpable, nontender gallbladder; contrariwise, obstruction by stones in the common bile duct does not lead to a palpable, nontender gallbladder because scarring from chronic gallbladder inflammation prevents enlargement of the gallbladder.

Courvoisier's sign – in a small percentage of cases, obstruction of the common bile duct by carcinoma of the pancreas causes enlargement of the gallbladder; obstruction caused by stones in the common bile duct does not cause enlargement because scarring from infection prevents the gallbladder from distending.

crepitus – crackling; the sensation felt or sound heard when palpating soft tissue that contains gas or when moving fractured bones.

cricothyroidotomy – incision through the skin and cricothyroid membrane through which a small tracheostomy tube is inserted to relieve airway obstruction.

Crohn's disease – inflammatory process of the small intestine and colon; usually causes transmural involvement of the small intestinal wall; occasionally similar to acute appendicitis.

crossmatch – in vitro process of mixing donor leukocytes with recipient serum and complement; used to determine whether the recipient produces antibodies that are cytotoxic to the leukocytes, thus predicting rejection of a potential allograft.

crystalloid – fluid for intravenous administration; consists of water, electrolytes, and sometimes glucose in isotonic or hypertonic concentrations.

Cushing's disease – Cushing's syndrome (see below) caused by excess production of adrenocorticotropic hormone by an adenoma of the anterior pituitary gland; first defined in 1932.

Cushing's reflex – increase in systemic blood pressure associated with bradycardia and a slowed respiratory rate; caused by increased intracranial pressure.

Cushing's syndrome – constellation of clinical findings that result from excessive circulating glucocorticoids.

cytopenia – decreased number of cells, usually hematologic cells; anemia is decreased red cell count; leukopenia is decreased white cell count; thrombocytopenia is decreased platelet count.

dead space – potential or real cavity that remains after closure of a wound and is not obliterated by the operative technique.

debridement – technique to remove dead skin, other nonviable tissue, and debris from a wound surface; some surgeons use this term to describe excision of burns, but it usually refers only to treatment provided at the bedside, without anesthesia.

deep-space compartment – confined anatomic space; increased pressure within such a space (e.g., from edema) limits circulation and threatens tissue function and viability.

dentate line – anatomic line that delineates the conversion of squamous epithelium to cuboidal and columnar epithelium in the anal canal.

dermatofibroma – slowly growing benign skin nodule; poorly demarcated cellular fibrous tissue encloses collapsed capillaries, with scattered hemosiderin-pigmented and lipid macrophages.

dexamethasone suppression test – dexamethasone is administered to suppress cortisol secretion; in Cushing's syndrome, this suppression does not occur.

diagnostic peritoneal lavage – surgical procedure used to identify an intraperitoneal injury; under local anesthesia, a peritoneal catheter is inserted into the peritoneal cavity through a small midline incision; a syringe is attached to the catheter and aspirated; if 10 mL blood is aspirated, the test result is positive; if less than 10 mL blood is aspirated, then 1000 mL or 10 mL/kg warm lactated Ringer's or normal saline solution is infused into the peritoneal cavity; after 5 to 10 minutes, the lavage fluid is retrieved by gravity siphon technique; a 50-mL portion is sent to the laboratory for microscopic analysis, cell count, and bile and amylase analysis; the result is positive for blunt trauma if the red blood cell count is 100,000 cells/mm^3 or greater; if the white blood cell count is more than 500 cells/mm^3; if bacteria, bile, or food particles are present; or if amylase is greater than serum amylase; a negative study does not exclude retroperitoneal injury to the duodenum, pancreas, kidneys, diaphragm, aorta, or vena cava.

disseminated intravascular coagulation – hemorrhagic syndrome that occurs after the uncontrolled activation of clotting factors and fibrinolytic enzymes throughout the small blood vessels; fibrin is deposited, platelets and clotting factors are consumed, and fibrin degradation products that inhibit fibrin polymerization and clot formation are created, resulting in bleeding.

Dripps-American Surgical Association Classification – system of patient classification (I–IV); based on chronic health status; used to estimate perioperative risks.

duct of Santorini – accessory pancreatic duct.

duct of Wirsung – main pancreatic duct.

Dukes' classification – staging system that correlates the prognosis in colorectal cancer with the depth of penetration of the primary tumor.

dumping syndrome – complex myriad of symptoms; may include crampy abdominal pain and diarrhea; secondary to ablation of the pyloric sphincter mechanism.

durable power of attorney for health care – formal advance directive that names a specific person to make health care decisions for the patient if the patient becomes unable to do so.

dysphagia – difficulty in swallowing.

elemental diet – chemically defined enteral diet of high osmolarity and low viscosity; designed to meet specific nutritional and metabolic needs that cannot be achieved naturally.

embolism – occlusion or obstruction of an artery by a transported thrombus, atherosclerotic plaque, bacterial vegetation, or foreign body.

endarterectomy – surgical excision of the intima, atherosclerotic plaque, and a portion of the media of an atherosclerotic blood vessel.

endoscopic retrograde cholangiopancreatogram (ERCP) – radiologic imaging of the biliary tree and pancreatic duct by retrograde injection of contrast material through a cannula placed endoscopically in the ampulla of Vater; used to extract stones, obtain a cytology specimen, or place a catheter.

eschar – coating of dead skin, serum, and debris that forms on the surface of a burn wound.

escharotomy – incision made through burned tissue to relieve compression caused by edema formation beneath rigid eschar.

esophageal diverticulum – outpouching of all layers of the esophagus; typically located in the cervical, midthoracic, or epiphrenic region; associated with dysfunction of the cricopharyngeus muscle and lower esophageal sphincter complex; in Zenker's diverticulum, only the mucosa projects through the esophageal wall.

esophageal myotomy – incision in the muscular portion of the esophagus; performed for achalasia or another esophageal motility disorder; converts the esophagus into a larger, but passive tube.

esophageal stricture – stenosis of the esophagus; typically occurs from gastric acid reflux, from neglected reflux esophagitis, or after corrosive materials are swallowed.

excision, early – technique of burn wound treatment; burned tissue is surgically removed before spontaneous eschar separation occurs.

excision, fascial – technique of burn wound excision; the skin and subcutaneous tissue are removed to the level of the fascia.

excision, tangential – technique of burn wound excision; only burned tissue is removed with a dermatome, leaving viable dermis and subcutaneous tissue behind.

extracorporeal shock wave lithotripsy (ESWL) – fragmentation of gallstones with a shock wave; performed ultrasonographically; limitations include strict eligibility criteria, high failure rate, high recurrence rate, and the need for an expensive solvent (ursodeoxycholic acid) and expensive equipment.

false diverticulum – diverticulum characterized by mucosal outpouching through a weakened portion of the colon wall.

familial atypical mole and melanoma (FAM-M) syndrome – risk factor for hereditary melanoma; associated with mutations on chromosomes 1p and 9p.

familial medullary thyroid carcinoma – autosomal dominant condition caused by a mutation of RET; associated with medullary thyroid carcinoma, but no other endocrine abnormalities.

fasciotomy – incision through the fascia to relieve increased pressure; used to treat compartment syndrome.

feeding, postpyloric – feeding into the gastrointestinal tract distal to the pyloric valve, usually with a nasoduodenal or gastroduodenal tube.

feeding, prepyloric – feeding into the gastrointestinal tract proximal to the pylorus with a nasogastric or gastrostomy tube.

felon – infection of the pulp space of the digits in the hand.

Felty's syndrome – leg ulcers or chronic infection associated with splenomegaly and neutropenia in patients with rheumatoid arthritis.

fibrin – essential portion of a blood clot; white, fibrous protein formed from fibrinogen by the action of thrombin.

fibrinogen – factor I; globulin produced in the liver and converted to fibrin during blood clotting.

fibromuscular dysplasia – idiopathic nonatherosclerotic hyperplastic and fibrosing lesion of the intima, media, or adventitia; the most common form is medial fibroplasia.

fine-needle aspiration cytology – cytologic examination of cells aspirated from the thyroid; also the most commonly used technique to diagnose palpable breast masses; a small-gauge needle is used to extract three random samples of the breast mass; the contents of the needle are smeared on a glass slide using a technique similar to that used with a Pap smear.

fistula – abnormal connection between two epithelial-lined structures.

fistula, aortocaval – abnormal communication between the aorta and inferior vena cava.

fistula, aortoenteric – abnormal communication between the abdominal aorta and the third portion of the duodenum where it overlies the aorta; usually associated with breakdown of a previous aortic bypass graft anastomosis, although primary aortoenteric fistulae occur.

fistula-in-ano – abnormal communication between the anus at the level of the dentate line and the perirectal skin through the bed of a previous abscess.

flail chest – result of fracture of consecutive ribs in multiple places (i.e., each rib is fractured in at least two places); the free-floating, or flail, segment of the chest wall moves paradoxically with inspiration and expiration.

follicle – extracellular space within the thyroid; contains colloid; bordered by follicular cells; triiodothyronine (T3) and thyroxine (T4) are stored bound to thyroglobulin.

follicular cells – thyroid cells that process iodine into thyroid hormone.

fulminant hepatic failure – hepatic failure associated with massive hepatocyte necrosis or severe impairment; occurs within 8 to 12 weeks of the onset of symptoms; findings are not associated with chronic liver disease; unless liver transplantation is performed, may progress to coma and brain stem herniation from increased cerebral pressure.

fundoplication – operation to restore competence to the esophagogastric junction as part of the treatment of sliding hiatal hernia and reflux esophagitis; the most common is the Nissen fundoplication, in which the gastric fundus is wrapped around the lower and intraabdominal segment of the esophagus to produce an acute angle of His and other functional changes.

futility – concept that the risks of a treatment far outweigh its possible benefits.

gallstone ileus – mechanical obstruction of the intestine caused by a large gallstone that erodes through the gallbladder into the duodenum; may be associated with pneumobilia; the point of obstruction is often in the distal ileum.

gas-bloat syndrome – abdominal bloating associated with inability to vomit; may occur after gastric fundoplication.

gastric outlet obstruction – obstruction in the pyloric area of the stomach secondary to repeated bouts of acute duodenal ulcerations with subsequent scarring.

gastrin – hormone produced by the G-cells of the stomach; stimulates acid secretion by the parietal cell.

gastritis – diffuse erythema and disruption of the mucosa of the stomach; associated with the ingestion of irritating agents.

Glasgow Coma Scale – method used to classify the severity of head injuries; eye opening score 1 to 4, verbal response score 1 to 5, and motor response score 1 to 6.

globus hystericus – subjective sensation of a lump in the throat.

goiter – thyroid enlargement.

graft, heterotopic – graft placed at a site different from the normal anatomic position (e.g., renal transplant).

graft, orthotopic – graft placed in the normal anatomic position (e.g., cardiac transplant).

granulocyte colony stimulating factor – similar to erythropoietin for red cells; stimulates the maturation of white blood cells; dramatically decreases the sequelae of leukopenia after chemotherapy.

Graves' disease – autoimmune thyrotoxicosis.

H$_2$ blockade – most common modality used to treat duodenal ulcer disease; blocks the histamine receptor of the parietal cell; one-half of the total is given in the first 8 hours postburn; the rest is given over the next 16 hours.

hamartoma – benign tumor; normal tissues grow rapidly compared with surrounding normal tissues.

Harris-Benedict equations – pair of regression equations based on sex, age, height, and weight; used to estimate resting metabolic expenditure.

Hartmann's procedure – stapling or oversewing of the distal end of a sigmoid colon resection, leaving a blind rectal stump in the peritoneal cavity.

Hashimoto's thyroiditis – autoimmune thyroiditis; first described by Japanese surgeon Hakuru Hashimoto (1881–1934).

healing, primary – primary adhesion of tissue after a wound is closed by direct approximation of the edges; no granulation tissue is formed.

healing, secondary – closing of a wound by secondary adhesion; the wound is left open and allowed to heal spontaneously.

healing, tertiary – active closing of a wound after a delay of days to weeks; an open wound is closed with sutures or sterile tape before it heals; the secondary healing process is interrupted.

Heinz bodies – erythrocyte inclusions that consist of denatured hemoglobin.

Helicobacter pylori – Gram-negative bacterium associated with the pathogenesis of gastritis, gastric ulcers, and duodenal ulcers.

hemangioma – tumor composed primarily of blood vessels; can involve the small and large intestine and liver.

hemangioma, cavernous – benign, often incidentally found, tumor; consists of endothelial vascular spaces separated by fibrous septa; spontaneous rupture is rare; most patients require no specific treatment.

hemochromatosis – autosomal recessive disease; characterized by excessive absorption of iron from the intestinal tract; affects the liver, heart, pancreas, and spleen.

hemoglobinopathy – abnormality in hemoglobin structure; may lead to anemia and red cell structural abnormalities.

hemolytic anemia – anemia caused by destruction of red blood cells.

hemophilia, type A – X-linked recessive disorder of the blood; occurs almost exclusively in men; marked by a permanent tendency to hemorrhage as a result of factor VIII deficiency; characterized by prolonged clotting time, decreased formation of thromboplastin, and diminished conversion of prothrombin to thrombin.

hemothorax – blood in the pleural cavity.

hemothorax, massive – rapid loss of more than 1500 mL blood into the pleural cavity; class III or greater hemorrhage into the pleural cavity.

hepatic encephalopathy – poorly understood neuropsychiatric disorder; associated with advanced liver disease and portosystemic shunting; suspected etiologies include altered amino acid levels in the systemic circulation.

hepatocellular carcinoma (hepatoma) – tumor, usually in the setting of cirrhosis (70%–80%); accounts for 90% of all primary liver malignancies; most are advanced at presentation; fewer than 20% of patients are candidates for standard surgical resection.

her-2-neu oncogene – oncogene whose expression indicates a poor prognosis, particularly in patients with node-positive breast cancer.

hereditary spherocytosis – inherited condition that can lead to hemolytic anemia because of rigid, abnormally shaped erythrocytes that are sequestered and destroyed in the spleen.

hernia – protrusion of all or part of a structure through the tissues that normally contain it.

hernia, direct – groin hernia that results from protrusion through the attenuated posterior inguinal wall.

hernia, femoral – protrusion of intraabdominal structures through the femoral canal.

hernia, indirect – groin hernia into a patent processus vaginalis.

hernia, Richter's – hernia at any site through which only a portion of the circumference of a bowel wall, usually the jejunum, incarcerates or strangulates.

hernia, sliding – hernia in which a portion of the wall of the protruding peritoneal sac is made up of some intraabdominal organ; as the sac expands, the organ is drawn out into the hernia.

hernia, umbilical – protrusion of bowel or omentum through the abdominal wall under the skin at the umbilicus.

Hesselbach's triangle – triangular area in the lower abdominal wall bounded by the inguinal ligament below, the border of the rectus abdominis medially, and the inferior epigastric vessels laterally; site of direct inguinal hernias.

Hodgkin's disease – malignant lymphoma marked by chronic enlargement of the lymph nodes that is often local at onset and later generalized, together with enlargement of the spleen and often of the liver, no pronounced leukocytosis, and often anemia and continuous or remittent fever; associated with inflammatory infiltration of lymphocytes and eosinophilic leukocytes and fibroses.

Howell-Jolly bodies – erythrocyte inclusion of nuclear remnants; usually found on peripheral blood smears after splenectomy.

human leukocyte antigens (HLA) – antigens expressed by all nucleated cells; used to determine histocompatibility; the genetic loci that determine these antigens are located in the sixth human chromosome.

hyperparathyroidism, primary – condition caused by excess secretion of parathyroid hormone, usually from a parathyroid adenoma.

hyperparathyroidism, secondary – overactivity of the parathyroid glands in response to physiologic changes caused by chronic renal failure.

hyperparathyroidism, tertiary – autonomous overactivity of the parathyroid glands; causes hypercalcemia; usually caused by chronic renal failure.

hyperplasia, atypical – increased number of abnormal-appearing cells in the milk ducts; precedes ductal carcinoma in situ on the continuum from cells lining a normal milk duct to ductal carcinoma in situ to invasive cancer.

hyperplasia, focal nodular – benign tumor that usually contains a central scar with both ductal elements and hepatocytes; spontaneous rupture is rare; most require no specific therapy.

hyperplasia, parathyroid – diffuse enlargement and overactivity of the parathyroid glands.

hypersplenism – excess splenic function manifested by cytopenia; may be unrelated to spleen size.

hypoperfusion – inadequate blood flow to tissues.

hyposplenism – diminished splenic function; usually increases susceptibility to infection, particularly with encapsulated bacteria.

hypovolemia – decreased intravascular volume; causes decreased venous return.

ileoanal pullthrough – operative procedure of choice for ulcerative colitis; consists of total colectomy, mucosal proctectomy, creation of a storage reservoir, and anastomosis to the dentate line; obviates a permanent ileostomy.

ileocecal valve – termination of the small intestine; regulates the passage of intestinal contents into the large intestine.

immune thrombocytopenic purpura – thrombocytopenia caused by antibodies directed at platelets; leads to platelet sequestration in the spleen.

incarceration – confinement of a herniated structure to its protruded position.

indirect calorimetry – method to measure precisely the resting metabolic rate by analysis of inspired and expired gases for O_2 and CO_2; when coupled with urine urea nitrogen, can be used to compute the proportion of protein, carbohydrate, and fat substrates being oxidized.

infection – microbial phenomenon characterized by an inflammatory response to the presence of microorganisms or the invasion of normally sterile host tissue by organisms.

infection, nosocomial – infection that occurs because of or during hospitalization and treatment.

infection, overwhelming postsplenectomy – highly lethal infection (75% mortality rate) caused by encapsulated bacteria (*Streptococcus pneumoniae* is the most common); loss of the spleen increases susceptibility to these bacteria.

infection, polymicrobial – infection that is difficult to treat because it involves multiple bacterial species.

inflammation – cellular processes that are activated by a variety of cellular and tissue injuries; necessary for tissue repair and wound healing.

inflammation, severe – inflammation stimulated by cellular or tissue injury; causes total body cellular or organ malfunction.

informed consent – transfer of information between physician and patient that allows the patient to make a knowledgeable decision about a particular treatment.

inhalation injury – injury that occurs from inhaling smoke or the products of combustion; occurs as carbon monoxide poisoning, upper-airway injury, or pulmonary parenchymal injury.

inotropic drug – agent that increases the contractility of heart muscle.

internal hemorrhoids – vascular venous cushions that arise above the dentate line; often associated with swelling, bleeding, and discomfort.

iodine – element concentrated and complexed exclusively by thyroid tissue.

ischemia, reperfusion – cellular response to loss of blood flow followed by restoration of blood flow.

isograft – tissue transferred between genetically identical individuals (e.g., monozygotic twins).

jaw-thrust maneuver – maneuver used to open the mouth so that the oral cavity can be inspected and patency assured; accomplished by standing behind the patient's head, placing the fingers behind the angle of the jaw, grasping the jaw on both sides, and then lifting it forward; the thumbs are used to open the mouth by drawing the mouth and chin downward.

Kehr's sign – pain at the top of the left shoulder referred from diaphragmatic irritation (e.g., from blood from a ruptured spleen).

Kupffer cell – liver-based macrophage that accounts for 80% to 90% of the body stores of fixed macrophages; responsible for hepatic clearance of toxins, including endotoxin and specific infectious organisms; also responsible for the generation of cytokines and other inflammatory mediators.

Kussmaul's sign – increase in central venous pressure with inspiration; seen in severe cardiac tamponade.

laceration – torn or jagged wound or accidental cut wound.

leiomyoma – tumor that involves the small or large intestine or any other smooth muscle.

leiomyosarcoma – malignant tumor of smooth muscle.

lentigo maligna melanoma (Hutchinson's melanotic freckle) – malignant lesion of the elderly; arises in sun-damaged skin; occurs primarily on the face and neck.

ligament of Treitz – area of the small intestine where the duodenum meets the jejunum; located to the left of the midline in the left upper quadrant.

living will – formal advance directive that describes patient wishes regarding treatment decisions if the patient is not competent to make decisions.

lower esophageal sphincter – complex of anatomic structures that acts as a sphincter and keeps gastric acid in the stomach, yet allows swallowing, belching, or vomiting.

lymphedema – swelling caused by the obstruction of lymphatic vessels or lymph nodes and the accumulation of large amounts of lymph; lymphedema of the arm, one of the most disabling complications of axillary dissection, occurs in 2% to 3% of cases after a level I or level II axillary dissection; usually occurs 6 months to many years after the surgical procedure.

lymphoma – lymphatic malignancy that arises in the lymphoreticular components of the reticuloendothelial system.

lymphoma, non-Hodgkin's – lymphoma other than Hodgkin's disease; classified by Rappaport according to pattern (nodular or diffuse) and cell type; a working or international formulation separates lymphomas into low, intermediate, and high grades and into cytologic subtypes that reflect follicular center cell or other origin.

lyophilization – process of preserving tissue by removing its water content through freezing and rewarming in a vacuum.

magnification, compression views – special mammographic techniques used to evaluate an abnormal density seen on a routine two-view screening mammography; if a density is real, magnification and compression of the breast tissue make the lesion more discrete; if the lesion represents an area of breast parenchyma that is more dense than surrounding tissue, compression usually causes the area to appear normal and diminishes clinical concern.

mammographic microcalcifications – breast calcifications that are classified as benign, indeterminate, or pleomorphic; benign microcalcifications are isolated, smooth, round densities that need no further evaluation; pleomorphic microcalcifications are irregularly shaped and resemble broken glass; they suggest ductal carcinoma in situ and require biopsy; microcalcifications that exhibit both benign and pleomorphic characteristics are called indeterminate; they require either biopsy or mammographic reevaluation in 6 months; if not associated with ductal carcinoma in situ, these microcalcifications are seen in fibrocystic conditions.

mass contractions – contraction pattern that is unique to the colon; characterized by contraction of long segments of colon and resulting in mass movement of stool.

McBurney's point – point on the anterior abdominal wall; located between the middle and outer thirds of a line drawn between the anterior iliac spine and umbilicus; represents on the anterior abdominal wall the location of the appendix.

Meckel's diverticulum – true diverticulum of the ileum; occurs in 1% to 3% of the population; associated with bleeding, inflammation, and bowel obstruction.

medullary thyroid carcinoma – carcinoma that originates from the C-cells (calcitonin-secreting cells) of the thyroid; part of the multiple endocrine neoplasia types 2A (MEN-2A) and 2B (MEN-2B), and familial medullary thyroid carcinoma syndromes.

melanoma – malignant neoplasm of the skin; derived from the cells that form melanin.

menin – gene associated with multiple endocrine neoplasia type 1.

mitotane – adrenolytic agent used to treat adrenocortical adenocarcinoma.

multiple endocrine neoplasia (MEN) – familial endocrine tumor syndromes inherited as autosomal dominant conditions; three types: MEN-1, MEN-2A, and MEN-2B.

multiple endocrine neoplasia type 1 (MEN-1) – autosomal dominant condition associated with primary hyperparathyroidism, pituitary adenomas, pancreatic islet cell tumors, carcinoid tumors of the thymus or bronchus, and lipomas.

multiple endocrine neoplasia type 2A (MEN-2A) – autosomal dominant condition caused by a mutation of RET; associated with medullary thyroid carcinoma, pheochromocytoma, and parathyroid hyperplasia.

multiple endocrine neoplasia type 2B (MEN-2B) – autosomal dominant condition caused by a mutation of RET; associated with a characteristic phenotype, medullary thyroid carcinoma, and pheochromocytoma.

multiple organ system failure – altered organ function in an acutely ill patient; homeostasis cannot be maintained without intervention.

Murphy's sign – sharp pain on deep inspiration during palpation in the right upper quadrant; associated with acute cholecystitis.

necrotizing fasciitis – soft tissue infection that spreads along the fascia and causes necrosis; often caused by mixed aerobes and anaerobes; when the male genitalia are involved, called Fournier's disease.

Nelson's syndrome – development of an adrenocorticotropic hormone–producing pituitary tumor after bilateral adrenalectomy in Cushing's syndrome; causes aggressive growth and hyperpigmentation of the skin.

nevus, blue – dark blue or blue-black nevus covered by smooth skin; formed by melanin-pigmented spindle cells in the lower dermis.

nevus, compound – common nevus caused by nests of cells in the dermis and epidermal–dermal junction.

nevus, congenital giant hairy – large, hairy congenital pigmented nevus that often involves the entire lower trunk; high risk for melanoma.

nevus, intradermal – most common benign nevus in adults; caused by nests of melanocytes in the dermis.

nevus, junctional – slightly raised, flat, pigmented tumor; caused by nests of nevus cells in the basal layer at the epidermal–dermal junction.

nitrogen balance – nitrogen intake (g/day) minus nitrogen excretion (24-hr urine urea nitrogen plus 3 g for unmeasured nitrogen losses); crucial goal in nutritional support.

nodular melanoma – most malignant melanoma tumor; grows vertically, is blue-black, has a palpable nodular component in its earliest development, and develops quickly.

normal serum laboratory values – [in commonly used units and Système Internationale (SI) units]

serum	common units	SI units
K^+	3.5–5.0 mEq/L	3.5–5.0
Na^+	135–145 mEq/L	135–145
Ca^{++} (total)	8.9–10.3 mg/dL	2.23–2.57
Ca^{++} (ionized)	4.6–5.1 mg/dL	1.15–1.27
Mg^{++}	1.3–2.1 mEq/L	0.65–1.05
Cl^-	97–110 mEq/L	97–110
CO_2 (serum, not $Paco_2$)	22–31 mEq/L	22–31
$PO_4^=$	2.5–4.5 mg/dL	0.81–1.45
Blood urea nitrogen	8–25 mg/dL	2.9–8.9
Creatinine	0.6–1.5 mg/dL	53–133 μmol/L
Fasting glucose	65–110 mg/dL	3.58–6.05

obturator sign – clinical sign elicited during acute appendicitis by passive rotation of the flexed right thigh; an acutely inflamed appendix irritates the obturator internus.

odynophagia – pain on swallowing.

oliguria – in an adult, urine output of less than 500 mL/day.

omeprazole – potent inhibitor of hydrochloric acid production; acts by blocking the proton pump of the parietal cell.

open-gloving technique – method of donning surgical gloves when a gown is not required or when the hands have been passed fully through the cuffs of the surgical gown; usually requires an assistant because it is difficult to accomplish individually without contaminating the outside of the glove.

opsonins – proteins that bind to particulate and bacterial antigens and facilitate phagocytosis.

orthostatic (postural) hypotension – excessive decrease in blood pressure on assuming the erect position; usually marked by an increase in heart rate.

osmolality – number of osmoles per kilogram of water; total volume is 1 L plus a relatively small volume occupied by the solute.

osmolarity – number of osmoles per liter of solution; volume is less than 1 L by an amount equal to the solute volume.

pancreas divisum – congenital abnormality of the pancreas; the duct of Santorini is not fused to the duct of

Wirsung because of failure of the dorsal and ventral pancreatic buds to fuse during embryonic development.

pancreatic magna – largest branch of the splenic arteries; supplies the body of the pancreas.

pancreaticoduodenectomy (Whipple procedure) – removal of the head of the pancreas, duodenum, and distal common bile duct; performed for carcinoma of the pancreas, duodenum, or distal common bile duct, and for trauma.

pancreatitis, acute – single episode of diffuse pancreatitis in a previously normal gland.

pancreatitis, acute biliary (gallstone) – acute inflammation of the pancreas secondary to gallstones; usually caused by passage of small gallstones and sludge through the ampulla of Vater.

pancreatitis, chronic – chronic inflammatory process in the pancreas that destroys its functional capabilities; characterized by endocrine and exocrine deficiency and constant pain.

pancreatitis, gallstone – acute inflammation of the pancreas caused by gallstones occluding the ampulla of Vater.

Pappenheimer bodies – iron inclusions in erythrocytes.

paradoxical aciduria – aciduria in the late stages of hypokalemic metabolic alkalosis; the urine becomes acidic as the kidney, in an attempt to retain potassium, excretes hydrogen ions despite the overlying metabolic alkalosis (in which case hydrogen ions would be retained).

parafollicular cells – cells of neuroendocrine origin within the thyroid that secrete calcitonin.

paraganglionoma – pheochromocytoma located outside the adrenal medulla (extraadrenal pheochromocytoma).

parathyroid glands – endocrine glands in the neck that secrete parathyroid hormone.

parathyroid hormone (parathormone) – peptide hormone secreted by the parathyroid glands; primarily responsible for maintaining calcium homeostasis.

parenteral nutrition, peripheral – 3% amino acid and 10% dextrose solution with lipid emulsion; delivered into a peripheral or central vein to satisfy the nutritional needs of a nonstressed patient.

parenteral nutrition, total – high-osmolarity solution of amino acids, dextrose, and often lipid emulsion; delivered into a central vein to satisfy all of a patient's nutritional needs.

parietal cell – cell found in the fundus of the stomach; produces hydrochloric acid and intrinsic factor.

Parkland formula – widely used formula for resuscitation from burn shock: 4 mL lactated Ringer's solution × body weight (kg) × burn (percentage of total body surface area).

paronychia – local infection of the skin over the mantle of the fingernail and lateral nail folds.

PEG/PEJ – percutaneous endoscopic gastrostomy, alone or with accompanying percutaneous jejunal tube placement; feeding tube placement performed in the intensive care unit or endoscopy suite rather than with laparotomy in the operating suite, which would require a general anesthetic.

pericardiocentesis – needle puncture of the pericardium to aspirate fluid or blood to relieve cardiac tamponade.

peristaltic waves – waves of alternate circular contraction and relaxation in the gastrointestinal tract that propel food and fluids onward.

peritonitis – inflammation of the surfaces of the peritoneal cavity.

Peyer's patches – aggregates of lymphoid cells in the lymph nodes in the gastrointestinal tract; concentrated in the ileum.

phase, proliferative – second stage of wound healing; characterized by the laying down of collagen by fibroblasts.

phase, remodeling – third stage of wound healing; characterized by the maturation of collagen and flattening of the wound scar.

phase, substrate (inflammatory, lag, exudative) – first phase of wound healing; characterized by inflammation, macrophage formation, and appearance of substrates for collagen synthesis.

pheochromocytoma – neoplasm of the adrenal medulla; arises from chromaffin tissue of neural crest origin; secretes excess epinephrine, norepinephrine, dopamine, or other vasoactive amine; causes a constellation of signs and symptoms as a result of catecholaminemia;

associated with the familial endocrine syndromes multiple endocrine neoplasia types 2A (MEN-2A) and 2B (MEN-2B).

plasma – fluid (noncellular) portion of the circulating blood; distinguished from serum, which is obtained after coagulation.

plasma, fresh frozen – separated plasma, frozen within 6 hours of collection; used to replenish coagulation factor deficiencies [e.g., liver failure, excessive warfarin (Coumadin) effect].

platelet – irregularly shaped disk in the blood; has granules, but no definite nucleus; approximately one-third to one-half the size of an erythrocyte; contains no hemoglobin; known chiefly for its role in hemostasis.

platelet count – calculation of the number of platelets in 1 mm³ blood by counting the cells in an accurate volume of diluted blood; normal = 150,000 to 400,000 mL.

Plummer's disease – toxic multinodular goiter.

pneumonia – active infection within the lung parenchyma.

pneumoperitoneum – free intraperitoneal air caused by perforation of the stomach, duodenum, or other part of the intestinal tract.

pneumothorax – air or gas in the pleural cavity.

pneumothorax, open (sucking chest wound) – large chest wall defect that permits equilibration of intrapleural and atmospheric pressures; leads to lung collapse; if the defect is at least two-thirds the diameter of the trachea, resistance to flow is lower through the defect than through the trachea; air moves into and out of the pleural space instead of through the trachea, and effective ventilation is prevented.

pneumothorax, tension – air leaks out of the lung or bronchi into the pleural cavity and is trapped; intrapleural pressure rises and can exceed atmospheric pressure; the ipsilateral lung collapses; the mediastinum and trachea are pushed to the contralateral side, causing compression, distortion, and kinking of the superior and inferior vena cavae; venous return to the heart is significantly decreased; oxygen delivery is compromised; without rapid treatment, death ensues.

polycystic liver disease – autosomal dominant disorder that causes progressive formation of multiple cysts; rarely leads to hepatic failure, but can cause significant symptoms associated with the mass effect of hepatic cysts.

polyp – small mucosal excrescence that grows into the lumen of the colon and rectum.

polyp, pedunculated – polyp that is rounded at the end and attached to the mucosa by a long, thin neck.

polyp, sessile – flat polyp that is intimately attached to the mucosa.

polyvalent pneumococcal polysaccharide vaccines – vaccines that contain polysaccharide antigens from many pneumococcal types; current vaccines contain 23 common types that cause infection in humans.

portal hypertension – abnormally elevated pressure within the portal vein or its tributaries; causes gastroesophageal varices, variceal hemorrhage, and ascites.

portosystemic collateral routes – multiple sites of collateralization that arise in the setting of portal hypertension; routes include the esophageal–azygos system, splenorenal system, mesenteric–hemorrhoidal system, retroperitoneal collaterals, and caput medusae at the umbilicus.

portosystemic shunts – large-caliber connections between the portal and systemic circulatory systems; reduce portal pressure; effectively control varices and ascites, but may be associated with hepatic encephalopathy.

position, reverse Trendelenburg – positioning of a patient so that the head is elevated and the feet are lower than the heart.

position, Trendelenburg – positioning of a patient so that the head of the table is tilted at a 45° angle; the feet are elevated and the head is kept below the level of the heart.

postthrombotic syndrome – condition of the lower extremity, usually secondary to deep vein thrombosis; causes edema, pain, venous stasis, cellulitis, varicose veins, and in severe cases, ulceration.

prealbumin – plasma protein with a 4-day half-life; used to reflect visceral protein status and the effectiveness of nutritional support when measured weekly.

preload – magnitude of myocardial stretch; the stimulus to muscle contraction described by the Frank-Starling mechanism.

pressure, central venous – blood pressure measurement taken in the superior vena cava; reflects right ventricular end-diastolic pressure (preload).

pressure, cerebral perfusion – difference between mean arterial pressure and intracranial pressure.

pressure, colloid osmotic – difference in pressure between intravascular and interstitial fluid; mostly caused by albumin in the plasma, but not in the interstitium.

pressure, pulmonary artery occlusion (pulmonary capillary wedge pressure, wedge pressure) – left atrial pressure measured by advancing a balloon-tipped catheter into the pulmonary artery until it goes no further; normal pressure is 8 to 12 mm Hg.

primary aldosteronism (Conn's syndrome) – excessive, autonomous production of aldosterone by a benign adrenocortical adenoma; rarely caused by adrenocortical carcinoma; first described in 1955 by Jerome Conn at the University of Michigan.

primary biliary cirrhosis – progressive small bile duct obstruction that leads to cirrhosis, likely from cytotoxic T-cells; predominantly affects middle-aged women.

primary sclerosing cholangitis – idiopathic disease that causes a chronic fibrotic stricturing process; can involve both the intrahepatic and extrahepatic biliary tree; the only effective long-term treatment is liver transplantation.

proctocolectomy – surgical removal of the entire colon and rectum; a permanent ileostomy is left.

prophylactic antibiotics – antibiotics administered to prevent infection.

prothrombin time (PT) – time required for clotting after thromboplastin and calcium are added in optimal amounts to plasma with normal fibrinogen content; if prothrombin is diminished, the clotting time increases; PT is sensitive to levels of clotting factors V, VII, and X, prothrombin, and fibrinogen.

proximal gastric vagotomy – antiulcer operation; selectively denervates vagal stimulation to the parietal cells; maintains the function of the pyloric sphincter.

pseudoaneurysm – dilation of the artery wall that does not contain all three layers; usually forms at areas of trauma or regions of weakened arterial graft anastomosis.

pseudocyst, pancreatic – cyst (without an epithelial lining) of the pancreas or of the pancreas and adjacent structures; often the result of pancreatitis.

pseudopolyp – small island of normal mucosa surrounded by deep ulceration; creates the appearance of a polyp.

psoas sign – clinical sign used in acute appendicitis; elicited by extension of the right hip, which causes the inflamed appendix to irritate the iliopsoas muscle.

pulse oximetry – photoelectric measurement of the oxygen saturation of capillary blood.

pulsus paradoxus – decrease in systolic blood pressure, during inspiration, greater than 10 mm Hg; seen in cardiac tamponade.

pus – collection of dead phagocytic cells, fibrin, and plasma proteins; densities of both dead and viable microorganisms and bacterial products that form in a closed area at the site of bacterial invasion.

pyrosis – substernal pain or burning; usually associated with regurgitation of gastric juice into the esophagus.

radioactive iodine – isotope (^{131}I) of iodine used to evaluate or treat thyroid disease.

radionuclide biliary scan (HIDA scan) – diagnostic test in which a ^{99m}Tc-labeled derivative of iminodiacetic acid is injected intravenously; the radionuclide is excreted into the bile ducts and enters the gallbladder through the cystic duct; absence of gallbladder filling in 4 hours, along with filling of the common bile duct and passage of radionuclide into the duodenum, strongly suggests acute cholecystitis.

Ranson's criteria – in patients with pancreatitis, a group of risk factors that are present on admission or within 48 hours and aid in the prediction of major complications and death.

red pulp – anatomic portion of the spleen; contains the cords; site of removal of antibody-sensitized cells and particulate material.

reduced-size liver transplant – use of only the left lobe or the left lateral segment of a living or cadaver liver as a transplant, especially in children.

reflux esophagitis – inflammation of the lower esophagus; related to reflux of gastric acidity; contact burn related to the duration and degree of gastric acid contact.

regurgitation – flow of material in the opposite direction of normal (e.g., return of undigested food from the stomach into the mouth).

rejection, accelerated acute – destruction of a graft in the first few days after transplantation by a second set of anamnestic responses of preformed antibodies and lymphocytes.

rejection, acute – reversible attack on a transplanted organ mediated by T-lymphocytes; causes organ dysfunction.

rejection, chronic – slow, progressive immunologic destruction of a transplanted organ over years; mediated by both humoral and cellular elements.

rejection, hyperacute – destruction of a graft by the recipient through preformed antibodies (e.g., ABO, HLA, or species-specific antibodies); occurs within hours of transplantation.

resection, abdominoperineal – removal of the lower sigmoid colon, rectum, and anus, leaving a permanent proximal sigmoid colostomy.

resection, low anterior – removal of the distal sigmoid colon and upper one-half of the rectum with primary anastomosis of the proximal sigmoid to distal rectum.

respiratory quotient (RQ) – ratio of CO_2 to O_2 consumption; reflects whether the patient's energy supply is inadequate ($RQ < 1$), balanced ($RQ = 1$), or excessive ($RQ > 1$).

rest pain – pain in the distal extremities, especially the toes and metatarsal heads, when the extremity is elevated; elevation decreases the hydrostatic perfusion pressure of the lower extremities; they become ischemic, and pain occurs; symptoms are usually relieved with "dangling" of the affected extremities.

resting metabolic expenditure – energy needed by a resting, supine person after an overnight fast.

resuscitation – restoration from potential or apparent death; the airway is secured, ventilation is assured, and oxygen is administered; external blood loss is controlled with direct pressure; intravenous lines are established with a balanced electrolyte solution; Ringer's lactate is preferred in patients with traumatic injury; intravascular volume is restored; hypothermia is combated with high-flow fluid warmers; aspiration and gastric distension are reduced with the placement of a gastric tube; pulse oximetry, blood pressure, electrocardiographic readings, and urine output are monitored; in patients with traumatic injury, these measures are begun simultaneously with the primary survey.

RET – tyrosine kinase receptor oncogene; used as a gene marker for multiple endocrine neoplasia types 2A (MEN-2A) and 2B (MEN-2B) and familial medullary thyroid carcinoma.

reversible ischemic neurologic deficit – reversible changes in mentation, vision, and motor or sensory function; completely resolves within 7 days; no changes are seen on cerebral computed tomography scan.

Reynold's pentad – right upper quadrant abdominal pain, fever and chills, jaundice, hypotension, and mental confusion; associated with acute suppurative cholangitis.

ring sign (target sign) – pattern produced when a drop of bloody cerebrospinal fluid is placed on filter paper; because cerebrospinal fluid diffuses faster than blood, the blood remains in the center and one or more concentric rings of clearer (pink) fluid form around the central red spot; used to test bloody otorrhea and rhinorrhea for the presence of cerebrospinal fluid.

Rovsing's sign – clinical sign of pain seen in acute appendicitis; pressure applied to the left lower quadrant of the abdomen creates pain in the right lower quadrant.

S-phase – phase in the growth cycle of a cell; a finding of more than 6% or 7% of cells in the S-phase in a tissue sample, as measured by flow cytometry, suggests a rapidly growing tumor.

SCALP – mnemonic for remembering the five layers of the scalp; Skin, subCutaneous tissue, galea Aponeurotica, Loose areolar tissue, and Periosteum (pericranium).

scrub nurse – member of the surgical team who participates directly in the surgical procedure; manages the sterile instruments and supplies; often assists with the procedure.

Seagesser's sign – neck tenderness produced by manual compression over the phrenic nerve; caused by diaphragmatic irritation (e.g., by blood from a ruptured spleen).

seborrheic keratosis – superficial, benign, verrucous lesion; consists of proliferating epidermal cells; usually occurs in the elderly.

secretin – duodenal hormone that inhibits gastric acid secretion and gastric emptying.

selective shunts – shunts that decompress gastroesophageal varices, but maintain prograde portal profusion to the liver; best known is the distal splenorenal shunt.

Sengstaken-Blakemore tube – tube placed through the esophagus for balloon tamponade of gastric and esophageal varices; provides temporary occlusion.

sepsis – systemic response to infection as manifested by two or more of the following conditions:
1. Temperature > 37° C or < 36° C
2. Heart rate > 90 beats/min
3. Respiratory rate > 20 breaths/min or $Paco_2$ < 32 mm Hg
4. White blood cell count > 12,000 cells/mm^3, < 4000 cells/mm^3, or > 10% immature (band) forms

sepsis, burn wound – invasive infection of a burn wound; bacteria penetrate beneath the burned surface and invade viable tissue and blood vessels.

shock – inadequate organ perfusion; types include anaphylactic, cardiogenic, hemorrhagic, hypoadrenal, hypovolemic, neurogenic, and septic; total body cellular metabolism is malfunctional.

shock, burn – severe loss of intravascular volume caused by fluid sequestration in and beneath burn wounds.

shock, spinal – neurologic condition that occurs after spinal cord injury; caused by acute loss of stimulation from higher levels; this "shock" or "stun" to the injured cord makes it appear functionless; there is complete flaccidity and areflexia instead of the predicted spasticity, hyperreflexia, and positive Babinski sign that are seen in the classic upper motor neuron lesion; not a synonym for neurogenic shock, which is inadequate organ perfusion.

silver sulfadiazene (Silvadene, SSD, Thermazene) – topical antibiotic widely used in burn treatment; active against a wide range of gram-positive and gram-negative organisms and yeast; many other topical agents are also available.

singultus – hiccup.

Sister Mary Joseph's node – hard nodule at the umbilicus; associated with metastatic gastric carcinoma.

skin graft, full-thickness – graft obtained by excising an ellipse of skin and subcutaneous tissue, usually from the groin or flank; donor site is closed with sutures.

skin graft, split-thickness – graft obtained by excising tissue at the level of the dermis, leaving a base that heals spontaneously.

sodium (salt) loading – administration of more than 200 mEq sodium/day for 3 to 4 days to suppress aldosterone secretion; does not inhibit aldosteronerone secretion in patients with autonomous aldosterone production (e.g., primary aldosteronism).

somatostatin – pharmacologic agent that reduces variceal bleeding by inducing mesenteric vasoconstriction; diminishes variceal bleeding in at least 50% of patients.

splenectomy – removal of the spleen.

splenic cords (of Billroth) – reticular portion of the spleen in the red pulp that lacks endothelium; blood percolates slowly and comes in contact with numerous macrophages.

splenomegaly, congestive – enlargement of the spleen as a result of vascular engorgement (e.g., portal hypertension).

splenomegaly, infiltrative – enlargement of the spleen because of accumulation of materials within the splenic reticuloendothelial cells (e.g., Gaucher's disease with accumulation of glucocerebrosides).

spontaneous nipple discharge – discharge on clothing in the absence of breast stimulation; in contrast, elicited discharge is noted after the nipple or breast is squeezed, or after vigorous mammography; only spontaneous discharge requires evaluation.

squamous cell carcinoma – malignant neoplasm derived from stratified squamous epithelium; variable amounts of keratin are formed in relation to the degree of differentiation; if the keratin is not on the surface, a "keratin pearl" is formed.

sterile field – operative area that is covered with sterile drapes and prepared for the use of sterile supplies and equipment; classically, includes the instrument table, Mayo stand, and operative area.

sterile technique – moving, working, or functioning in a sterile environment with sterile equipment to prevent contamination of the incision site.

sterilization – physical or chemical process by which all pathogenic and nonpathogenic microorganisms are destroyed.

sterilization, dry-heat – killing of microorganisms through heat absorption.

sterilization, ethylene oxide gas – sterilization technique used for instruments or objects that are sensitive to heat or moisture; ethylene oxide is cidal to all microorganisms, but requires a longer exposure time (3–6 hours) than heat sterilization.

sterilization, moist-heat – sterilization technique that uses saturated steam under pressure (autoclave); easiest, fastest, and least expensive method of sterilization.

strangulation – vascular compromise of an incarcerated organ.

Sturge-Weber syndrome – facial hemangioma (causing a port wine stain) occupying the cutaneous distribution of the trigeminal nerve, angiomatous malformations of the brain and meninges, and occasionally pheochromocytoma.

surrogate – person empowered to make decisions for a patient who is not competent to do so.

survey, primary – rapid initial evaluation of a patient with traumatic injury; involves the diagnosis and treatment of all immediately life-threatening injuries; the essence of the "ABCDEs" of trauma management; sequentially, the physician protects the cervical spine while assessing the injured patient's Airway, Breathing, Circulation, and neurologic Disability; Exposure of the patient and prevention of hypothermia are the last steps; all immediately life-threatening injuries are treated in sequence before proceeding to the next phase.

survey, secondary – detailed, head-to-toe evaluation of a trauma patient; includes a history and physical examination to identify all injuries; begins after the primary survey is completed, resuscitation is initiated, and the airway, breathing, and circulation are reassessed; tubes or fingers are placed in every orifice; baseline laboratory studies are drawn if they were not drawn when the intravenous lines were started; portable x-rays are taken; special procedures (e.g., peritoneal lavage) are done during this phase.

syndrome of inappropriate secretion of antidiuretic hormone (SIADH) – syndrome associated with physiologically uncontrolled production of antidiuretic hormone by malignant tumors or disturbances from intracranial injury disorders.

systemic inflammatory response syndrome – syndrome that indicates systemic inflammation; caused by a variety of cellular and tissue injuries (see Chapter 6 for the criteria-based definition).

T-cell – thymus-derived cell; involved in the cellular response to foreign tissue; produces cytokines, recruits other cells, and differentiates into helper, suppressor, and cytotoxic cells.

target sign – see *ring sign*.

tenosynovitis – infection of the tendon sheath, usually of the hand.

thalassemia – deficit in the synthesis of one or more subunits of hemoglobin; leads to erythrocyte abnormalities and anemia; many types are seen, but β thalassemias are the most common.

therapy, adjuvant – systemic treatment, including chemotherapy and hormonal therapy, of cancer to prevent recurrence throughout the body; in contrast, local regional therapy (e.g., surgery, radiation treatment) prevents local recurrence.

therapy, estrogen replacement – therapy, often initiated after surgical or natural menopause, to prevent the perimenopausal and postmenopausal symptoms of estrogen withdrawal (e.g., hot flashes, vaginal atrophy, urogenital deterioration); also seems to significantly diminish osteoporosis and cardiac disease.

therapy, protein-sparing – 3% amino acid and 5% dextrose solution delivered by peripheral veins; minimizes proteolysis in a nutritionally fit, fasting patient.

thionamides – class of antithyroid drugs (e.g., propylthiouracil, methimazole); inhibit iodide organification and iodotyrosine coupling; reduce the rate of peripheral conversion of thyroxine (T4) to triiodothyronine (T3).

third-space fluid accumulation – accumulation of extracellular and intracellular fluid in response to regional or total body cellular or tissue injury; accumulation in excess of the volume of fluid that normally occupies these regions; sequestration decreases intravascular fluid volume.

third-space fluid loss – loss of intravascular or extravascular body fluid into tissue spaces or body cavities after trauma or surgery (e.g., retroperitoneal hematoma, bowel edema).

thrill – palpable turbulence within an arterial vessel as a result of disturbed flow.

thrombin time – time needed for a fibrin clot to form after thrombin is added to citrated plasma; prolonged thrombin time is seen in patients who are receiving heparin therapy, those who have factor I (fibrinogen) deficiency, and those with elevated levels of fibrin or fibrinogen split products.

thrombocytosis – platelet count greater than 400,000/mm³.

thrombosis – formation of an occlusive or nonocclusive blood clot within a blood vessel or cavity of the heart.

thrombotic thrombocytopenic purpura – disease of arteries and capillaries; characterized by thrombosis and thrombocytopenia.

thrombus – blood clot that forms within a blood vessel and remains in place, often causing an obstruction.

thyroglobulin – molecule on which iodine is complexed to form triiodothyronine (T3) and thyroxine (T4).

thyroid carcinoma (papillary, follicular, medullary, or anaplastic) – types of thyroid cancer; papillary and follicular carcinomas are well-differentiated carcinomas of follicular cells; medullary carcinomas are of parafollicular cell origin; anaplastic carcinomas dedifferentiate from follicular cells.

thyroid-stimulating hormone (TSH, thyrotropin) – hormone secreted by the pituitary to regulate thyroxine (T4) production and secretion by the thyroid.

thyroidectomy – surgical excision of the thyroid gland.

thyrotoxicosis (hyperthyroidism) – overactive thyroid.

thyroxine (T4, tetraiodothyronine) – major hormone secreted by the thyroid in response to thyroid-stimulating hormone; feeds back to regulate thyroid-stimulating hormone.

tonicity – "effective" osmolality; often used to describe intravenous fluid replacement or body fluids (e.g., hypotonic, isotonic, or hypertonic solutions or fluids mean, respectively, less effective, same, or more effective osmolality).

total body water – portion of body weight composed of water and fluids; in a typical 70-kg man, 60% of body weight is water and fluids; in women and the elderly, it is 50% to 55%.

toxic multinodular goiter – thyroid enlargement from multiple nodules that may cause compression symptoms.

transient ischemic attack – reversible changes in mentation, vision, and motor or sensory function; usually last seconds to minutes; completely resolves within 24 hours.

transjugular intrahepatic portacaval shunt (TIPS) – radiologically placed intrahepatic shunt; connects the portal vein with the hepatic vein; bypasses the increased hepatic resistance.

triangle of Calot – hepatocystic triangle bounded by the inferior margin of the liver, common hepatic duct, and cystic duct; traversed by several important normal and anomalous structures.

triiodothyronine (T3) – thyroid hormone that acts at the tissue level where it is formed by deiodinization of thyroxine (T4).

truncal vagotomy – complete transection of both vagal trunks at the gastroesophageal junction; eliminates vagal stimulation of the parietal cell.

tumor, carcinoid – most common tumor of the appendix; may cause carcinoid syndrome; often malignant.

tumor, phyllodes – breast tumor seen in younger women; usually a large, smooth, nontender mass; clinically similar to fibroadenoma, but larger; most are benign, but a small percentage are malignant; treatment involves wide excision.

ulcer, duodenal – ulcer that usually occurs in the first portion of the duodenum as a result of acid hypersecretion.

ulcer, gastric – ulcer that typically occurs on the lesser curvature of the stomach; usually secondary to mucosal breakdown of the stomach.

ulcer, Marjolin's – squamous cell cancer that arises in the inflammatory scar of a nonhealing ulcer (e.g., chronic wound, fistula-in-ano, osteomyelitis).

ulcerative colitis – mucosal disease of the colon; causes significant diarrhea and bleeding; tends to become malignant.

United Network for Organ Sharing (UNOS) – organization of transplant centers, organ procurement agencies, and professional and patient groups; regulates organ allocation and procurement in the United States.

urine urea nitrogen – 24-hour urine collection assayed for urea; used to measure nitrogen loss and calculate nitrogen balance.

vasoconstriction – reduction in the caliber of blood vessels; leads to decreased blood flow.

venous return – quantity of blood that returns to the right atrium from the systemic veins each minute.

volvulus – rotation of a segment of the intestine on the axis formed by the mesentery; causes obstruction of the bowel.

vomiting – forcible expulsion of stomach contents through the mouth.

von Hippel-Lindau disease – neuroectodermal dysplasia associated with cystic cerebellar hemangioblastoma and angiomatous malformation of the retina and pheochromocytoma.

von Recklinghausen's disease – common neuroectodermal dysplasia; multiple neurofibromas of peripheral nerves; associated with pheochromocytomas.

von Willebrand's disease – hemorrhagic diathesis characterized by a tendency to bleed, primarily from the mucous membranes; laboratory abnormalities include prolonged bleeding time, variable deficiency of factor VIII clotting activity, prolonged activated partial thromboplastin time, reduced von Willebrand's antigen and activity, and reduced ristocetin-induced platelet aggregation; inheritance is autosomal dominant, with reduced penetrance and variable expressivity.

water brash – heartburn with regurgitation of sour fluid or almost tasteless saliva into the mouth.

Wernicke-Korsakoff syndrome – syndrome caused by excessive alcohol intake; bilateral sixth cranial nerve palsy, nystagmus, diplopia, disconjugate gaze, and strabismus; ataxia is typical; mental changes include generalized apathy and lack of awareness; delirium is a late manifestation.

white pulp – anatomic portion of the spleen where lymphocytes and lymphatic follicles reside; probably site where soluble antigens are processed.

Wilson's disease – autosomal recessive disorder caused by excess copper; causes markedly diminished copper excretion into the biliary tree; correctable with liver transplantation.

wound, clean – surgical wound, made under sterile conditions, that does not enter the gastrointestinal, respiratory, or genitourinary tract; wound in which there is a break in sterile technique; wound that is not exposed to a significant bacterial population.

wound, clean-contaminated – surgical wound that enters the gastrointestinal, respiratory, or genitourinary tract without significant spillage; wound in which there is a break in sterile technique; wound that is initially clean, but is exposed to endogenous colonization during the procedure.

wound, contaminated – surgical wound in which extensive spillage from the gastrointestinal tract occurs; fresh traumatic wound; wound in which a major break in sterile technique occurs; wound in which gross contamination occurs during the procedure.

wound, dirty – wound that contains dirt, fecal material, purulence, or other foreign material; high risk of infection.

wound, infected – wound with a bacterial count of more than 10^5 organisms/g tissue.

xenograft – tissue transferred between members of different species.

xeroderma pigmentosum – eruption of exposed skin that occurs in childhood; characterized by numerous pigmented spots that resemble freckles; larger atrophic lesions eventually cause glossy, white thinning of the skin.

Zollinger-Ellison syndrome – severe variant of duodenal ulcer disease; results from the independent production of gastrin by a tumor (gastrinoma) that arises in the pancreas or paraduodenal area.

Index